The HIV Pandemic:

local and global implications

Edited By

EDUARD J BECK

NICHOLAS MAYS

ALAN W WHITESIDE

JOSÉ M ZUNIGA

Managing Editor

LYNN-MARIE HOLLAND

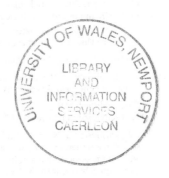

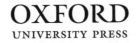

OXFORD

UNIVERSITY PRESS

OXFORD
UNIVERSITY PRESS

Great Clarendon Street, Oxford OX2 6DP

Oxford University Press is a department of the University of Oxford.
It furthers the University's objective of excellence in research, scholarship,
and education by publishing worldwide in

Oxford New York

Auckland Cape Town Dar es Salaam Hong Kong Karachi
Kuala Lumpur Madrid Melbourne Mexico City Nairobi
New Delhi Shanghai Taipei Toronto

With offices in

Argentina Austria Brazil Chile Czech Republic France Greece
Guatemala Hungary Italy Japan Poland Portugal Singapore
South Korea Switzerland Thailand Turkey Ukraine Vietnam

Oxford is a registered trade mark of Oxford University Press
in the UK and in certain other countries

Published in the United States
by Oxford University Press Inc., New York

© Oxford University Press, 2006

The moral rights of the author have been asserted
Database right Oxford University Press (maker)

First published 2006
First published in paperback 2008

British Library Cataloguing in Publication Data
Data available

Library of Congress Cataloguing in Publication Data
The HIV Pandemic: local and global implications / edited by Eduard J. Beck ... [et al.].
     p. ; cm.
Includes bibliographical references and index.
1. AIDS (Disease)–International cooperation. 2. HIV infections–International cooperation.
[DNLM: 1. Acquired Immunodeficiency Syndrome–prevention & control. 2. HIV infections–prevention
& control. 3. Cross-Cultural Comparison. WC 503.6 H67587 2006] I.Beck, Eduard J.
RA643.8.H582 2006
362.196′9792–dc22   2005036621

Typeset by Cepha Imaging Pvt Ltd, India
Printed in Great Britain
on acid-free paper by
CPI Antony Rowe, Chippenham, Wiltshire

ISBN 978-0-19-852843-2 (Hbk.)
ISBN 978-0-19-923740-1 (Pbk.)
10 9 8 7 6 5 4 3 2 1

Foreword

Almost from the time it was first described 25 years ago in the USA, AIDS has outstripped our worst fears and predictions. This disease has become one of the make-or-break issues of our times, on a par with global climate change and the persistence of mass, extreme poverty.

This timely book brings together a diversity of people who have been tackling HIV in their own country or internationally, and who possess vast—sometimes unique—experience in the field. Not a narrow academic exercise, it succeeds in being a forum for sharing and learning from their experiences.

An underlying theme that binds the essays in this book is that the response to HIV needs to be as unprecedented as the pandemic itself.

While the response must crucially involve health systems in every country, it cannot stop there—virtually every sector of society has a direct role and responsibility. This pandemic will not be overcome by health specialists acting alone.

Though many severely affected countries need assistance from international donors, it is demonstrably wrong and counterproductive to prescribe what they need to do. Domestic ownership and commitment—from the grass-roots to the highest reaches of government—are pre-conditions for success.

In every setting, success against AIDS hinges on the direct participation of community members, community-based organizations and civil society. People infected and affected by HIV are a vital part of the solution to this complex epidemic. Unless human rights such as non-discrimination, health, education and the equality of women are promoted and fulfilled, people become infected, and those living with HIV suffer even more grievous hardship.

Because of the complexity of this pandemic, the response in every country needs to be comprehensive, spanning HIV prevention, treatment and impact alleviation. Each of these elements has to be made available universally.

To maximize the collective effectiveness of all actors, countries should develop and implement a single strategic response, as encapsulated in the 'Three Ones' principles: one national HIV strategy, one national coordinating agency and one monitoring and evaluation framework.

Within countries and in global forums, spending on the response to AIDS needs to be recognized as a vital social and economic investment. The world's leaders must find ways to ensure adequate and steady financing for tackling AIDS in low- and middle-income countries.

Because this is a long-term epidemic that may last several more decades, if not several more generations, we absolutely must take a long-term perspective, anticipate longer-term challenges and plan our responses accordingly. From being largely reactive, our response must shift to being proactive. We must plan for success.

In the final analysis, countering the HIV pandemic is a political matter. We have now reached a point in the global response where we can get ahead of the epidemic. To succeed in this critical stretch, we must intensify our efforts to make HIV a key political concern in all countries, poor and rich alike.

Peter Piot
Executive Director,
UNAIDS

July 2005

Preface and Acknowledgements

Eddy Beck and Nicholas Mays commissioned and edited three series of papers collectively entitled *Healthcare Systems in Transition* and published in the UK *Journal of Public Health Medicine* (now the *Journal of Public Health*) between 1996 and 2000, which focused on 12 countries and how they responded to their respective HIV epidemics. For each country, a description of its health system was complemented by a section on its HIV epidemic; each series was accompanied by an editorial. Encouraged by the experience of commissioning these series, the two discussed a book that would expand the scope of the original series to regions and countries not covered by the initial project. The goal was to demonstrate how the response to a common, global threat is shaped by the history, culture and institutions in each country, and in particular, how the health system response to HIV reflects the arrangements that existed before the advent of each country's epidemic and continues to be influenced by the demands that the HIV epidemic and its control exact as it manifests itself in that country.

It became apparent that surprisingly little had been published in this vein. Accordingly, in March 2001, Helen Liepman, Senior Commissioning Editor at Oxford University Press, was brave enough to approve their proposal for a multi-country comparative book, which resulted in a book that comprised 28 country case studies and 22 thematic chapters on the successes, failures and lessons learned a quarter of a century into the HIV pandemic. We remain indebted to Helen for her confidence in our ability to see the book through to completion.

To further facilitate the integration of the chapters, it was considered advantageous to hold an international conference, which would allow authors to present their ideas and exchange first drafts of their country chapters. By October 2001, the International Association of Physicians in AIDS Care (IAPAC), led by its Chief Executive, José M Zuniga, had pledged its support to help organize and secure funding to make such an international gathering of country authors possible. This also brought José onto the editorial team as a co-editor. He was followed shortly thereafter by Alan Whiteside, Head of the Health Economics and HIV/AIDS Research Division of the University of KwaZulu-Natal, who joined the editorial team to broaden its expertise in light of the scale of the undertaking. With IAPAC's backing, it was possible to recruit a managing editor, Lynn-Marie Holland, who also acted as conference organizer alongside IAPAC staff. Without IAPAC's financial and in-kind support it would not have been possible to host the 6th International Conference on Healthcare Resource Allocation for HIV/AIDS, under the banner theme of *Healthcare Systems in Transition*, which took place in October 2003 in Washington, DC. The conference brought together many of the country authors who have contributed to this book, as well as global experts who addressed more macro-level issues. Also supporting the conference were the London School of Hygiene and Tropical Medicine, McGill University and the University of KwaZulu-Natal.

While IAPAC's support had made possible the crucial first phase of the project that culminated in the Washington conference, it soon became apparent that assembling a book on this scale would take far longer than originally anticipated. As a result, more support was needed and the editors set out once again to secure funds. Early in 2004, the UK Department for International Development (DFID) pledged its support, which enabled us to extend Lynn-Marie's crucial involvement. We are extremely grateful to DFID, and in particular Robin Gorna, for this support, without which it would have been impossible to assemble, edit and complete a book comprised of 50 chapters authored by some 165 authors from more than 30 countries.

As our managing editor, Lynn-Marie Holland has made an immense contribution—liaising with, cajoling, supporting and soothing authors; deftly turning editorial scribbles and annotations into revised manuscripts; helping to transform 50 idiosyncratic contributions into well presented, consistent prose; resolving abstruse linguistic niceties; and keeping the ball in play with four far-flung and often distracted editors.

In addition to Oxford University Press, IAPAC and DFID, Lynn-Marie Holland and, of course, all the many authors who contributed to this book, we are greatly indebted to a number of individuals for their invaluable contributions behind the scene. These include Mike Glass, Scott Wolfe, Harry Snyder and Mark Wagner (all formerly of IAPAC) for their role in helping to make the conference a reality; Tim Quinlan (University of KwaZulu-Natal) for serving as one of the conference co-chairs; Sundhiya Mandalia (NPMS-HHC) and Guy Harling (McGill) for their assistance at the Conference; Chris Simms for heroically stretching his participation to three chapters (two as co-author, one as sole author); Catherine Hankins (UNAIDS, Geneva) for coordinating and co-authoring two key thematic chapters with very little lead time; Richard Lessard and John Carsley (Direction de santé publique, Montreal) for facilitating Lynn-Marie's employment through the McGill MUHC Research Institute and, like Yves Souteyrand (WHO, Geneva), for supporting the completion of the book; Rebecca Fuhrer (McGill University, Joint Department of Epidemiology, Biostatistics and Occupational Health) for providing the project's home base for more than 2 years; and Jacqueline van Tongeren (IATEC, The Netherlands), Zackie Achmat and Nathan Geffen (TAC, South Africa) for all their efforts on the book's behalf. In addition, we wish to thank the many individuals who provided ongoing administrative support, including Jane Trecarten and Philip Picard (McGill MUHC Research Institute), Gisèle Dupuis and Jacques Bissonnette (DSP, Montreal), Laurie Tesseris, Marielle Olivier and Star-Ann Coleman (McGill University).

Ultimately, the value of this book must be based on its utility—we hope that each chapter proves useful to all those involved in battling the pandemic.

Thank you all.

The Editors

* The views expressed in this book are those of the authors and are not necessarily those of the organizations they work for, unless specifically stated in the text.

Illness is the night-side of life, a more onerous citizenship. Everyone who is born holds dual citizenship, in the kingdom of the well and in the kingdom of the sick. Although we all prefer to use only the good passport, sooner or later each of us is obliged, at least for a spell, to identify ourselves as citizens of the other place.

Susan Sontag
New York Review of Books
January 26, 1978

My argument is that history is made by men and women, just as it can also be unmade and rewritten, always with various silences and elisions, always with shapes imposed and disfigurations tolerated, so that 'our' East, 'our' Orient becomes 'ours' to possess and direct.

Edward W Said
Orientalism
Preface to the 25th Anniversary Edition
2003

Cover photo credits

C-2876-F1000006   : UNAIDS/W. Phillips
C-2878-F1020029   : UNAIDS/W. Phillips
C-2775-IMG00014   : UNICEF/UNAIDS
C-2743-IMG00068   : ILO/UNAIDS/L. Solmssen
C-3359-IMG0499   : UNAIDS/S. Drakborg
C-2783-IMG00012   : UNICEF/UNAIDS
C-3278-Moscow262 : UNAIDS/J. Spaull
C-1957-IMG00007   : UNAIDS/UNAIDS/Chris Sattlberger

Contents

Section V **Strengthening the Response**

The Editors

Eduard J Beck was born in Indonesia of Dutch parents. At the age of 15, having lived in The Netherlands for several years, he moved to Melbourne, Australia with his family. There he completed his secondary schooling and his undergraduate medical degree at Monash University. After moving to the UK for postgraduate work, he served as Guy's Hospital representative on a European Exchange Scheme for Junior Doctors before starting his public health training at North West Thames Region Health Authority. He completed an MSc in Community Medicine at the London School of Hygiene and Tropical Medicine and worked as a Lecturer at St Mary's Hospital Medical School, Imperial College, where he completed his PhD in Public Health and worked as a Senior Research Fellow and Senior Lecturer. In 1999, Eddy moved to Montreal, Canada to join McGill University as an Associate Professor, a joint post with Montreal's Direction de santé publique (DSP), where he is employed as a public health specialist. Though based in Montreal, he continued to work in the UK and is an Honorary Consultant at the St Stephen's Centre, Chelsea and Westminster NHS Trust, London. In 2004, he moved to Geneva to take up a post in the HIV Department of the World Health Organization, and recently joined the Monitoring and Evaluation Office at UNAIDS, Geneva.

Ever since he began his public health training in 1986, Eddy has been working in the field of HIV. While he has been involved in different aspects of HIV-related work, one of his main long-term interests has been to monitor and evaluate the use, cost and outcome of HIV service provision, which has often necessitated developing the necessary infrastructure, and which has allowed him to work in both industrialized and developing countries. *eduard.beck@mcgill.ca.*

Nicholas Mays was educated at Oxford University and the London School of Economics and Political Science. He has worked for most of his career as a health policy analyst and health services researcher at the Universities of Leicester, London and Queen's Belfast, and from 1994 to 1998 at the King's Fund, the UK's leading independent health policy and management foundation, where he served as Director of Health Services Research. After working for 20 years in the UK, he took up a post as principal adviser in the Social Policy Branch of the New Zealand Treasury in 1998. In April 2003, he was appointed Professor of Health Policy at the London School of Hygiene and Tropical Medicine in the University of London.

Professor Mays' main research interests are in primary healthcare reform and comparative health systems in high-income countries. His methodological interests include mixed-methods health services research, programme evaluation and systematic reviews of complex quantitative and qualitative evidence. *nicholas.mays@lshtm.ac.uk*

Alan Whiteside was born in Kenya and grew up in Swaziland, where he attended Waterford-Kamhlaba College. He completed a BA (Development Studies) and an MA (Development Economics) at the University of East Anglia. He holds a D Econ from the University of Natal.

From 1980 to 1983 he was an Overseas Development Institute Fellow working as a Planning Officer (Economist) in the Ministry of Finance and Development, Gaborone, Botswana. In 1983, he joined the Economic Research Unit of the University of Natal as a Research Fellow. In 1998, he established the Health Economics and HIV/AIDS Research Division at the University and he is currently the Director of this Division.

Dr Whiteside started the newsletter *AIDS Analysis Africa* in 1990 and edited it for 10 years. His major publications include *AIDS: The Challenge for South Africa*, co-authored with Clem Sunter and published by Human and Rousseau/Tafelberg in 2000; *AIDS in the 21st Century: Disease and Globalisation* (with Tony Barnett) published by Palgrave in 2002; and numerous journal articles and book chapters. He is an elected Member of Governing Council of the International AIDS Society and a member of the Governing Council of Waterford Kamhlaba College. He is also a member of the United Nations Commission on HIV/AIDS and Governance in Africa. *whitesid@ukzn.ac.za; www.heard.org.za*

José M Zuniga joined the International Association of Physicians in AIDS Care (IAPAC) in August 1997 as Deputy Director, and was appointed President and Chief Executive Officer in December 1999. Since his appointment to the IAPAC presidency, the association's membership has grown to 12,800 members in 103 countries, and its geographic reach has expanded to include offices in Chicago, Johannesburg, Amsterdam and a Technical Annex in Washington, DC.

Dr Zuniga holds a MSc degree in Public Health (MSPH) and a PhD in International Public Health Policy, and is a Visiting Professor at a number of academic institutions, including the Medical University of Southern Africa (MEDUNSA) and Northwestern University in the USA. He also serves on a number of advisory bodies, including the *JIAPAC* Editorial Advisory Board; IAPAC Board of Trustees; Humanitas Foundation Board of Directors; Center on Halsted Board of Directors; and the *Secure the Future* Technical Advisory Board. Dr Zuniga has been published in various journals and has served as a contributing editor and author for several reference books. *jzuniga@iapac.org; www.iapac.org*

List of Contributors

Endalamaw Aberra, MD, MPH
World Health Organization,
Ethiopia

Orvill Adams
Director, Orvill Adams & Associates;
Former Director of Human Resources,
Health Department, World Health
Organization
Switzerland

Michael W Adler
Professor of Genitourinary Medecine,
University College London,
UK

Victor Alfonso
BC Centre of Excellence in HIV/AIDS
Canada

Lidia Andrushchak
Social Mobilization and Partnership
Adviser,
UNAIDS,
Ukraine

Antoine Augustin
President and CEO,
March Foundation,
Haiti

Carlos Avila-Figueroa
Ministry of Health,
Mexico

Peter Barron
Health Systems Trust,
South Africa

Francisco I Bastos
Senior Researcher,
Oswaldo Cruz Foundation
Brazil

Eduard J Beck
Associate Professor of Epidemiology,
McGill University, Canada
eduard.beck@mcgill.ca

Teklu Belay, MD
HIV/AIDS Prevention and Control
Office,
National AIDS Control Secretariat
Ethiopia

Jasper Bos, PhD
Head of Product Development,
PharmAccess Foundation,
The Netherlands
j.bos@pharmaccess.org

Frédéric Bourdier
Anthropologist, Scientific Coordinator
for HIV/AIDS policies in Cambodia,
Institute for Research and Development
France

Pedro Cahn
Assistant Professor of Infectious Diseases,
University of Buenos Aires Medical
School, and Director, Fundación
Huésped
Argentina

Michel Carael
Professor of Medical Sociology,
Free University of Brussels
Belgium

Peter R Carr
PAHO/WHO Consultant (retired), and
Lecturer,
Department of Community Medicine
and Psychiatry,
University of the West Indies,
Jamaica

Robert Carr
Health Management Consultant
Jamaica
robert_carr@hotmail.com

José Carvalho de Noronha
Researcher,
Oswaldo Cruz Foundation
Brazil

Jesús Castilla
Consultant Epidemiologist,
Instituto de Salud Publica de Navarra
Spain

Venkatraman Chandra-Mouli
Coordinator, Adolescent Health
and Development
World Health Organization
Switzerland

Marie-Louise Chang
World Health Organization,
Switzerland

Fernando Antonio Compostella
Director of Regional Health
and Social Agency
(Veneto) Italy

Emma Conti, MD
Specialist, Infectious Diseases,
San Bortolo Hospital
Italy

Berhe Tesfu Costantinos
President, Centre for Human
Environment,
Ethiopia
costy@costantinos.org

Suzanne M Crowe
Professor, Macfarlane Burnet Institute for
Medical Research and Public Health
Australia

François Dabis, MD, PhD
Institut de Santé Publique,
Epidémiologie et Développement,
Université Victor Segalen,
France
francois.dabis@isped.u-bordeaux2.fr

Mario R Dal Poz
Associate Professor, Institute of Social
Medicine, University of the State of Rio
de Janeiro, Brazil; and Coordinator
of Human Resources for Health,
World Health Organization,
Switzerland
dalpozm@who.int

Ernest Darkoh MD, MPH, MBA
Chairman,
BroadReach Healthcare,
USA

Arie C de Groot
Managing Director,
Future Africa
Switzerland

Karl L Dehne, MD, PhD, MPH
UNAIDS Country Coordinator,
Zimbabwe

Paul R DeLay, MD, DTM&H (Lond)
UNAIDS,
Switzerland
delayp@unaids.org

Araya Demissie, BSc, MPH
Consultant, Health Information
and Promotion Specialist,
Ethiopia

Andrea Donatini
Economic Evaluation Unit,
LHU Parma
Italy

Sarah Dougan
Senior Scientist (Epidemiology),
Health Protection Agency,
UK
sarah.dougan@hpa.org.uk

Norbert Dreesch
Technical Officer, Human Resources
for Health Department,
World Health Organization,
Switzerland

Lilian Dudley
Managing Director/Public Health
Specialist,
Health Systems Trust
South Africa

José Esparza
Senior Adviser, HIV Vaccines,
Bill & Melinda Gates Foundation,
USA
jose.esparza@gatesfoundation.org

Dr Barry G Evans
Consultant Epidemiologist,
Health Protection Agency
UK

Timothy G Evans
Assistant Director-General,
Evidence and Information for Policy,
World Health Organization,
Switzerland

Carlos Falistocco
Medical Adviser to the National
HIV/AIDS Programme,
Ministry of Health
Argentina

Dr Bayo S Fatunmbi
Adviser on Roll Back Malaria,
World Health Organization
Nigeria

Bruce Fetter
Professor of History, University
of Wisconsin,
USA
bruf@uwm.edu

J Peter Figueroa
Ministry of Health,
Jamaica

José J Joanes Fiol
Specialist in Epidemiology,
National HIV/AIDS/STI Program,
Cuba

Daniel William Fitzgerald
Assistant Professor of Medicine,
Cornell University,
USA
dfitzgerald@gheskio.org

Julian Fleet
Senior Adviser, UNAIDS,
Switzerland
fleetj@unaids.org

Yves-Antoine Flori
Professor of Economics, Institut de Santé
Publique, d'Epidémiologie et
Développement (ISPED),
Université de Bordeaux 2 Victor
Segalen,
France

Christopher Fontaine
Communications Officer,
UNAIDS
Switzerland

Lisa Forman
Doctoral Candidate,
Faculty of Law,
University of Toronto
Canada

George France
Senior Researcher, Istituto de Studi sui
Sistemi Regionali e Federali e sulle
Autonomie,
Consiglio Nazionale delle Ricerche,
Italy
france@mclink.it

AK Ganesh
YRG Centre for AIDS Research
and Education
India

Helene D Gayle, MD, MPH
Director, HIV, TB and Reproductive
Health
Bill & Melinda Gates Foundation,
USA

Gulin Gedik
World Health Organization
Switzerland

Peter D Ghys
Manager, Epidemic and Impact
Monitoring, UNAIDS,
Switzerland

Norbert Gilmore
Professor of Medicine, McGill University
Canada
norbert.gilmore@staff.mcgill.ca

Sandra Gomez-Fraga
Ministry of Health,
Mexico

Kimberly Gray
Research Officer,
Department of Genitourinary Medicine,
King's College London
UK

Suriadi Gunawan
Senior Researcher,
National Institute of Health Research
and Development,
Indonesia
suriadig@cbn.net.id

Markus Haacker
International Monetary Fund
USA
mhaacker@imf.org

Mariana A Hacker
Junior Researcher,
Oswaldo Cruz Foundation
Brazil

Damen Haile Mariam, MD, MPH, PhD
Department of Community Health,
Faculty of Medicine,
Addis Ababa University
Ethiopia

Gabriela Hamilton
Director, National HIV/AIDS
Programme, Ministry of Health
Argentina
ghamilton@msal.gov.ar

Catherine A Hankins
Associate Director and
Chief Scientific Advisor,
UNAIDS
Switzerland
hankinsc@unaids.org

Guy Harling
Desmond Tutu HIV Center,
University of Cape Town,
South Africa
guy.harling@hiv-research.org.za

Alison Hickey
Manager, AIDS Budget Unit,
Institute for Democracy in South Africa
(Idasa)
South Africa
alison@idasact.org.za

Sheila Hillier
Professor of Medical Sociology, and Head,
Centre of Human Science and Medical
Ethics, Barts and The London School
of Medicine and Dentistry,
UK
s.m.hillier@qmul.ac.uk

Dr Robert S Hogg
BC Centre of Excellence in HIV/AIDS
Canada
bobhogg@cfenet.ubc.ca.

John Imrie
Senior Research Fellow,
University College London,
UK
jimrie@gum.ucl.ac.uk

José A. Izazola-Licea
Team Leader, Resource Tracking
and Projections Unit,
UNAIDS,
Switzerland
jizazola@aol.com

Jantine Jacobi
Senior Advisor, Country Support
for Treatment and Care,
UNAIDS
Switzerland

Jin Cheng-Gang
Associate Professor, School of Public
Health and Family Medicine,
Capital University of Medical Sciences
People's Republic of China

Anne M Johnson
Head, Department of Primary Care
and Population Sciences,
Royal Free and University College
Medical School
UK

Afework Kassa, MD, MPH
HIV/AIDS/STI Team, Disease Control
and Prevention Department,
Ministry of Health,
Ethiopia

Yayehyirad Kitaw, MD, MPH
Senior Consultant, Health Development
Ethiopia
yayehyriad@telecom.net.et

Soewarta Kosen
Chief, Health Economics & Policy
Analysis Research Group, National
Institute of Health Research
& Development
Indonesia

Yuriy Kruglov
Epidemiologist,
Ukrainian AIDS Centre
Ukraine

N Kumarasamy
Chief Medical Officer,
YRG Centre for AIDS Research and
Education
India

JMA Lange
Professor of Medicine,
AMC/University of Amsterdam,
The Netherlands
j.lange@amc.uva.nl.

Maria Isela Lantero Abreu
Specialist in Epidemiology,
and Coordinator,
National HIV/AIDS/STI Programme,
Ministry of Public Health,
Cuba
lantero@infomed.sld.cu

Valeriya Lekhan
Professor of Medicine, and Head,
Department of Social
Medicine and Health Management,
Dniepropetrovsk
State Medical Academy
Ukraine

Suszy Lessof
Project Manager, European Observatory
on Health Systems and Policies
Belgium

Jeffrey Levi
Associate Professor of Health Policy,
George Washington University,
USA
jlevi@gwu.edu

Maureen A Lewis
Senior Fellow,
Center for Global Development,
USA
mlewis@cgdev.org

Liu Min
Associate Professor,
Department of Epidemiology,
Peking University
People's Republic of China

Lu Fan
Division of Epidemiology, National
Center for HIV/AIDS Control and
Prevention, China Center
for Disease Control and Prevention,
People's Republic of China

Louisiana Lush
Senior Health and HIV/AIDS Adviser,
Department of International
Development,
UK
l-lush@dfid.gov.uk

Shao-Jun Ma, MS, PhD
Department of Epidemiology, School
of Basic Medicine, Peking Union
Medical College,
People's Republic of China

Hein Marais
Geneva, Switzerland

Nicole Massoud
Monitoring and Evaluation Adviser,
UNAIDS Secretariat
Switzerland

Nicholas Mays
Professor of Health Policy,
London School of Hygiene
and Tropical Medicine
UK
nicholas.mays@lshtm.ac.uk

David McCoy, B Med, Dr PH
Public Health Specialist,
National Health Service,
UK
dmcoy@ucl.ac.uk

Tsehaynesh Messele, BSc, MSc, PhD
Ethio-Netherlands AIDS Research
Project, Ethiopian Health
and Nutrition Research Institute
Ethiopia

Julio SG Montaner, MD
Professor of Medicine, and Chair in AIDS,
University of British Columbia
Canada

Ofelia T Monzon, MD
President Emeritus and Member
of the Board, AIDS
Society of the Philippines,
The Philippines
aidsphil@pacific.net.ph

Douglas H Morgan, MPA
Director, Division of Service Systems,
HIV/AIDS Bureau, Health Resources
and Services Administration,
US Department of Health
and Human Services,
USA

Guy Morineau
Senior Surveillance and Evaluation Officer,
Family Health International
Cambodia
morineau@fhi.org.kh

Céline Moty-Monnereau, MD
Assistant Hospitalo-Universitaire,
Université Victor Segalen, and
Centre Hospitalo-Universitaire de
Bordeaux
France

Béchir N'Daw
Programme Development Adviser,
Intellectual Property and Trade
UNAIDS
Switzerland

Marie-Louise Newell
Professor of Paediatric Epidemiology,
Institute of Child Health,
University College London
UK

Isabel Noguer
Head, HIV/AIDS Surveillance,
National Centre of Epidemiology,
Instituto de Salud Carlos III,
Spain
inoguer@isciii.es

Ellen Nolte
Senior Lecturer, London School
of Hygiene and Tropical Medicine,
UK
ellen.nolte@lshtm.ac.uk

Rosaida Ochoa Soto
Assistant Professor,
University of Havana
Cuba

Dr Adeniyi Ogundiran
Adviser on HIV/AIDS,
World Health Organization
Nigeria

Michael O'Shaughnessy, OBC, PhD
Vice President, Provincial/Tertiary
Programs and Research,
Providence Health Care
Canada

Jean William Pape
Professor of Medicine,
Division of International Medicine and
Infectious Diseases,
Weill Medical College of Cornell
University
USA

Justin O Parkhurst
Lecturer,
London School of Hygiene
and Tropical Medicine
UK
justin.parkhurst@lshtm.ac.uk

Edith Patouillard
Assistant, Institut de Santé Publique,
d'Epidémiologie et Développement
(ISPED), Université Bordeaux 2
Victor Segalen
France

David Patterson
Consultant,
Canada
david.patterson@videotron.ca

Thomas L Patterson
Professor of Psychiatry,
University of California, San Diego
USA

Jorge Perez Avila
Professor of Clinical Pharmacology and
Infectious Diseases,
Instituto de Medicina Tropical,
Cuba

Alena N Peryshkina
Director, AIDS Infoshare
Russian Federation

Dr Barry S Peters
Senior Lecturer, Guy's, Kings & St.
Thomas' School of Medicine, Kings
College London,
UK

Maya L Petersen
Doctoral Student in Epidemiology,
University of California, Berkeley,
USA
mayaliv@socrates.berkeley.edu

Wiput Phoolcharoen
Ministry of Public Health
Thailand

Peter Piot
Executive Director, UNAIDS
Switzerland

Roderick E Poblete, MD
Secretariat, Philippine National
AIDS Council
The Philippines

Ritu Priya
Associate Professor,
Centre for Social Medicine
and Community
Health, Jawaharlal Nehru University,
India
ritupriya@mail.jnu.ac.in

Imrana Qadeer
Professor,
Centre for Social Medicine
and Community Health,
Jawaharlal Nehru University,
India

Tim Quinlan
Research Director, HEARD,
University of KwaZulu-Natal
South Africa

Sergolame Lekoko Ramotlhwa
Operations Manager, National
Anti-retroviral Therapy (ART) Program,
Ministry of Health
Botswana

José Ramon Repullo
Professor and Head, Department
of Health Planning and Financing,
National School of Public Health,
Instituto de Salud Carlos III,
Spain

Timothy C Roach FRCP (Edin)
Associate Lecturer,
School of Clinical Medicine
and Research, University
of the West Indies
Barbados

Reid Austin Roberts
Treatment Literacy Researcher,
Treatment Action Campaign (TAC)
South Africa

Zachary Rosner
Pritzker School of Medicine,
University of Chicago
USA

Volodymyr Rudiy
Ukrainian Director, Health Financing
and Management EU Project
Ukraine

Deborah L Rugg, PhD
Associate Director for Monitoring
and Evaluation, Global AIDS Program,
US Centers for Disease Control,
USA

Melanie LA Rusch
Michael Smith Foundation for Health
Research, University of British Columbia,
and BC Centre for Excellence in HIV/
AIDS
Canada

R Salamon, MD, PhD
Professor of Public Health,
University of Bordeaux 2,
France

Jessica Salas Martinez, MD
Adviser to the Deputy Minister of
Health
Costa Rica

Dr Ignacio Salom Echeverria
Clinical Immunologist,
Costa Rica
nanacho@racsa.co.cr

Manuel Santin Peña
Specialist in Epidemiology,
Direccion Nacional Epidemiologica,
MINSAP
Cuba

O. Schellekens, MSc
General Director,
Centre for poverty-related communal
disease Academic Medical Centrum
PharmAccess
The Netherlands

Dr David Serwadda
Director, Institute of Public Health,
Makerere University
Uganda

Alla Shcherbinska
Professor of Medicine,
Institute of Epidemiology and Infectious
Diseases, AMS,
Ukraine

Jay J Shen
Associate Professor of Health Economics
and Policies, Governors State University,
USA

Michel Sidibe
UNAIDS
Switzerland

Chris Simms
Independent Consultant
Canada
csimms88@hotmail.com

Lee Soderstrom
Associate Professor of Economics,
McGill University
Canada

Suniti Solomon
Director, YRG Centre for AIDS Research
and Education, Voluntary Health Services
India

Papa Salif Sow, MD, MSc
Professor of Medicine, Department
of Infectious Diseases, Dakar University
Teaching Hospital
Senegal

Freddie Ssengooba
Lecturer, Health Policy Planning
& Management, Institute of Public
Health, Makerere University,
Uganda

Julie Stachowiak
Research Associate,
Johns Hopkins University
Bloomberg School of Public Health,
USA
jstachowiak@gmail.com

Karen A Stanecki, MPH
UNAIDS
Switzerland

Eileen Stillwaggon
Associate Professor of Economics,
Gettysburg College,
USA
estillwa@gettysburg.edu

Susan A Stout
Manager, Results Secretariat,
Operations Policy and Country Services
World Bank
USA

Steffanie A Strathdee, PhD
Professor and Harold Simon Chair and
Chief, Division of International Health
& Cross Cultural Medicine,
Family and Preventive Medicine,
University of California, San Diego,
USA
sstrathdee@ucsd.edu

Chutima Suraratdecha
Ministry of Public Health
Thailand

Elhadj Sy
United Nations Development
Programme
USA
elhadj.sy@undp.org

Viroj Tangcharoensathien
Ministry of Public Health,
Thailand
viroj@ihpp.thaigov.net

Francesco Taroni
Professor of Social Medicine,
University of Bologna,
Italy

Sombat Thanprasertsuk
Ministry of Public Health,
Thailand

Gonzalo Estévez Torres, MD
Deputy Minister of Public Health,
Specialist in Epidemiology,
Cuba

Rigoberto Torres Peña, Prof. MD
Specialist in Epidemiology,
Ministry of Public Health
Cuba

Andrea Tramarin MD, PhD
U O de Malattie Infettive e Tropicali,
San Bortolo Hospital (Vicenza),
Italy
tramarin@gpnet.it

Claudia Travassos
Senior Researcher,
Oswaldo Cruz Foundation,
Brazil

Maurits H van Pelt, MSc, LLM
Consultant on Health and Poverty,
Cambodia

Eric van Praag
Country Director, Tanzania
Family Health International
Tanzania
evanpraag@fhi.org

John Waller
Freelance Health Data Analyst
in the British National
Health Service
UK

ER Walrond
Professor Emeritus of Surgery,
University of the West Indies,
Barbados
ewalrond@uwichill.edu.bb

Alan Whiteside
Professor and Director of the Health
Economics and HIV/AIDS Research
Division (HEARD), University of
KwaZulu-Natal,
South Africa
whitesid@ukzc.ac.za

Dawit Wolday, MD, MSc, PhD
Senior Researcher, Ethio-Netherlands
AIDS Research Project, Ethiopian Health
and Nutrition Research Institute,
Ethiopia
dawit@enarp.com

Dr R Cameron Wolf
Senior Technical Advisor for Monitoring
and Evaluation,
USAID
USA

Robin Wood
Professor of Medicine,
University of Cape Town,
South Africa

Carlos Zala
Director, Clinical Research,
Fundación Huésped,
Argentina

Kong-Lai Zhang
Professor of Epidemiology,
Peking Union Medical College,
People's Republic of China.
konglai_zhang@163.com

José M Zuniga, MSPH, PhD
President and CEO,
International Association of Physicians
in AIDS Care,
USA
jzuniga@iapac.org

List of Figures

List of Tables

List of Boxes

Glossary of Acronyms and Abbreviations

3 by 5	WHO/UNAIDS "3 by 5 Initiative"
ABC	Abstain, Be faithful, use a Condom
AIDS	Acquired Immune Deficiency Syndrome
AMREF	African Medical and Research Foundation
AMT	AIDS management team
ANC	Antenatal clinic
ART	Antiretroviral therapy/treatment
ARV	antiretroviral drug
AusAID	Australian Government Overseas Aid Programme
AZT	Azidothymidine (=Zidovudine)
BSS	Behavioural surveillance surveys
CAREC	Caribbean Epidemiology Centre
CARICOM	Caribbean Community and Common Market
CBA	Cost-benefit analysis
CBO	Community-based organization
CCM	Country coordinating mechanism
CDC	US Centers for Disease Control and Prevention
CEA	Cost-effectiveness analysis
CFA	Communauté Financière d'Afrique (franc)
CIDA	Canadian International Development Agency
CMA	Cost-minimization analysis
C-POL	Community popular opinion leader
CSO	Civil Society organization
CUA	Cost-utility analysis
DALY	Disability-adjusted life year
DFID	Department for International Development (UK)
DHS	Demographic health surveys
DOT	Directly observed therapy
DRG	Diagnosis related group
EDS	Enquête démographique et sanitaire (demographic and health survey)
EU	European Union
FAO	Food and Agriculture Organization (UN)
FHI	Family Health International
FSU	Former Soviet Union
FSW	Female sex worker
GAVI	Global Alliance for Vaccines and Immunization
GDP	Gross domestic product
GHESKIO	Group Haïtien d'Etude du Sarcome de Kaposi et des Infections Opportunistes (Haiti)
GNP	Gross national product
GUM	Genitourinary medicine

HAART	Highly active antiretroviral therapy
HBV	HIV-B virus
HCV	HIV-C virus
HDI	Human development index
HIV	Human immunodeficiency virus
IAPAC	International Association of Physicians in AIDS Care
IAVI	International AIDS Vaccine Initiative
ICESCR	International Covenant on Economic, Social and Cultural Rights (UN)
IDA	International Development Association
IDASA	Institute for Democracy in South Africa
IDB	Inter-American Development Bank
IDC	International Donor Community
IDU	Injecting drug use/user
IEC	Information, education and communication
IFI	International Financial Institutions
IHAA	International HIV/AIDS Alliance
IMCI	Integrated management of childhood illness
IMR	Infant mortality rate
IPPPH	Initiative on Public-Private Partnerships in Health
KfW	KfW Entwicklungsbank—German Development Bank
M&E	Monitoring and evaluation
MAP	Multi-Country HIV/AIDS Program
MCH	Maternal and child health
MTCT	Mother-to-child transmission
MIM	Multilateral Initiative on Malaria
MoH	Ministry of Health
MRI	Magnetic resonance imagining
MSF	Médecins Sans Frontières
MSM	Men who have sex with men
MSW	Male sex worker
NAC	National AIDS Committee Commission
NACA	National Advisory Committee on AIDS
NACO	National AIDS Control Organization
NACP	National AIDS Control Programme
NAFTA	North American Free Trade Agreement
NASCP	National AIDS and STI control programme
NEP	Needle exchange programme
NGO	Non-governmental organization
NIH	National Institutes of Health(USA)
NNRTI	Non-nucleoside reverse transcriptase inhibitor
NRTI	Nucleoside reverse transcriptase inhibitor
NtRTI	Nucleotide reverse transcriptase inhibitor
NVP	Nevirapine
ODA	Overseas development assistance
OECD	Organisation for Economic Co-operation and Development
OI	Opportunistic infections

ORT	Oral rehydration therapy
PAHO	Pan American Health Organization
PANCAP	Pan Caribbean partnership Against HIV/AIDS
PEPFAR	US President's Emergency Plan for AIDS Relief
PHC	Primary healthcare
PI	Protease inhibitor
PIH	Partners in Health
PLHIV	People living with HIV
PMTCT	Prevention of mother-to-child transmission
PRSP	Poverty Reduction Strategy Paper
RCT	Randomized controlled trial
SAP	Structual adjustment programme
Sida	Swedish International Development Cooperation Agency
STI/STD	Sexually transmitted infection/disease
SW	Sex worker
T&C	Testing and counselling
TAC	Treatment Action Campaign (South Africa)
TASO	The AIDS Support Organization (Uganda)
TB	Tuberculosis
UN	United Nations
UNAIDS	Joint United Nations Programme on HIV/AIDS
UNDP	United Nations Development Programme
UNFPA	United Nations Population Fund
UNGASS	United Nations General Assembly Special Session
UNICEF	United Nations Children's Fund
USAID	Untied States Agency for International Development
UWI	University of the West India
VCT	Voluntary counselling and testing
WHO	World Health Organization
WIPO	World Intellectual Property Organization
WTO	World Trade Organization
ZDV	Zidovudine (= Azidothymidine)

Section I

The Pandemic

Chapter 1

The HIV pandemic and health systems: an introduction

Eduard J Beck* and Nicholas Mays

While the HIV pandemic progresses seemingly unabated, the last 5 years have seen a remarkable policy shift in terms of global containment measures. One of the most dramatic changes has been the shift from 'prevention only' as the main containment strategy, especially for middle- and lower-income countries, to a strategy that includes scaling up HIV treatment, care and prevention services in these countries, including the prescription of combination antiretroviral therapy. While providing hope for many HIV-infected people around the world, this shift in strategy has also added to the challenges that the HIV pandemic has already presented to health systems around the world, particularly in middle- and lower-income countries, since it brings into play all parts of the health system. The pandemic has forced policy-makers, healthcare professionals and users of the services to think differently about how services are financed, how resources are allocated, how systems are structured and organized, how services are delivered to patients and how the resulting activity is monitored and evaluated in order to improve the effectiveness, efficiency, equity and acceptability of the response.

There is increasingly firm evidence that this concern with the entire health system is justified. Healthcare, and the health system through which services are provided, both matter for population health, even in lower-income countries. Although physical environment, socio-economic conditions and individual lifestyles all make major contributions to health, nations with relatively better healthcare have relatively healthier populations [1]. As better data and methods have become available, studies are showing the nature of this effect more clearly. For example, Anand and Bärnighausen [2] compared maternal, infant and under-5 mortality rates in 117 mostly lower middle- and lower-income countries to assess the contribution that healthcare workers make to the health of populations. Controlling for per capita income, poverty and female literacy, they found a strong negative correlation between the density of physicians and population mortality. The contribution of nurses and midwives was smaller. Population health at the country level was most strongly related to per capita income, with physician density and female literacy ranked second and third, or vice versa, depending on which measure of mortality was being compared across countries. The results were similar if only lower middle- and lower-income countries were compared. Or [3] produced similar results for high-income countries alone, showing that real resources in the shape of physicians per capita, rather than expenditure, were associated with lower rates of premature mortality.

The significance of these findings for health systems is profound. For example, they indicate the importance of being able to achieve not only a reasonable number of staff, especially

*Corresponding author

doctors, per capita at country level, but also a reasonably equitable distribution of doctors, nurses and other trained staff geographically within countries. In addition, it is likely that the available human resources will be able to function better, the more supportive the health system infrastructure and the better the decision-making processes. Staff need equipment and facilities such as clinics, hospitals, transport and laboratories to improve health—in other words, a well-functioning health system around them.

Yet there is no perfect health system, despite recent efforts by the World Health Organization (WHO) to rank the world's 197 health systems [4]. Equally, there are few if any simple rules for an effective, high-quality system. For example, obvious features such as the amount of money spent and how it is allocated to providers, through either fee-for-service or capitation funding, do not seem to affect the quality of care in high-income countries [5] or mortality rates in all countries, though the level of funding is associated with different levels of intervention. It seems that at any level of spending, results depend on how money is spent and real resources are deployed, which, in turn, depends on how each health system enables providers to match the needs of individuals and communities with the available resources in the most appropriate and effective way. There is also the frustrating reality that systems tend to be strong in some aspects and weak in others, and that their strengths and weaknesses tend to be predictable from their basic design and orientation. Thus, traditionally, more population-focused systems such as the British National Health Service tended to do better on measures such as screening rates and management of long-term chronic conditions, whereas far more pluralistic, individually focused systems such as those found in the USA tended to do better on outcomes of treatment such as cancer survival after surgery and radiotherapy.

Changing concepts and theories of medical science and infectious disease

Even more fundamentally than its challenge to the capability and nature of health systems, the pandemic has forced people to question and revise concepts and taken-for-granted assumptions about the nature of health and disease and their causes; the nature of infection; notions of risk, vulnerability, interdependence and mutual responsibility between individuals, communities and nations; the human rights of people living with HIV; the nature and contribution of political leadership in the field of public health; the relationship between prevention and treatment; and the power, or lack of it, of health science alone to prevent and mitigate threats to public health.

The variable course and dynamics of the pandemic have highlighted the importance of the historical, social, economic and cultural context of each country and population subgroup within a country in shaping the route of transmission and a population's likelihood of being infected with HIV. The strengths and weaknesses of the pre-existing health system have proved to be an important part of that context as well as a crucial basis for any response.

The HIV pandemic has drawn stark attention to a relatively neglected insight in the health field, namely that the nature, means of implementation and consequences of the implementation of scientific health knowledge are all dependent on the historical and social context in which the knowledge is created and the response is implemented. This may be disquieting for those who believe in the modernist view of knowledge and science, with its sharp distinction between the 'objective' and 'subjective' realms, based on the idea of the existence of fixed entities independent of the observer that can be studied dispassionately. For modernists, knowledge about the world needs to be assessed independently of historical, social and other 'subjective' interpretations: knowledge is subject-based, divorced from an everyday context, super-specialized and governed by a culture of expertise [6].

Science is often described as a cumulative process; however, theory change in science is more often a non-cumulative and non-convergent process [7]. Many of the currently predominant scientific theories are considered without their historical or social context [7], but they can be subject to periodic 'paradigm shifts' [8]. The field of infectious disease and its control is no exception. As in other areas of science, the social context has shaped not only the occurrence of diseases and human responses to them, but also the way in which infectious diseases themselves have been defined, and their causes and interventions conceptualized. In turn, these changes in concepts of disease and illness have significant implications for the way in which health systems are structured and organized, and for the work that takes place within them.

Before the fifteenth century, infectious diseases in Europe were explained in terms of either humoral pathology or general theories concerning poor living conditions, such as the Greek 'miasmic' theories. While specific quarantine measures had been introduced in the Middle Ages subsequent to the outbreak of the plague in Mediterranean ports [9], it was during the fifteenth- and sixteenth-century European syphilis and typhus epidemics that a theory of contagious diseases was first formulated, pre-empting the Germ Theory of infectious diseases by three centuries [10].

The Italian Fracastorius outlined a general theory of infectious diseases in 1553 [11], and the idea of 'contagion' rapidly gained acceptance throughout Europe. During the sixteenth and seventeenth centuries, theories that considered *contagium* or *animaculae* to cause infectious diseases became widely accepted [12–14]. By the mid-eighteenth century, the predominant controversy was whether these *animaculae* could regenerate spontaneously (heterogenesis) or whether they were transmitted by fomites ('fomes'). The work of Spallanzani in 1751 [15] provided early experimental evidence of the transmission of *animaculae*, but it was not until the work of Pasteur and others in 1862 that this issue was settled [12,14] (Fig. 1.1).

By the end of the eighteenth century the anti-contagionist movement had re-emerged, questioning central tenets of the contagionist theory [12]. They specifically pointed to the inability of the orthodox contagionists to explain and devise appropriate containment strategies for three global epidemics between 1800 and 1850: yellow fever, cholera and typhus. The most popular anti-contagionist explanation for the occurrence of these epidemics was that the 'miasma' emanating from the squalor and the filthy living and working conditions operative in most European cities at the time caused disease in exposed individuals with a weak constitution, a theory dating back to ancient Greece [10]. Most of the sanitary reforms introduced in European cities during this period were the result of the work of the anti-contagionists. Ironically, despite their views concerning the above-mentioned epidemics, many anti-contagionists did not discount the infectious nature of some diseases, including syphilis and gonorrhoea [10].

Through implementation of sanitary reforms in many European cities, the impact of the anti-contagionists was enormous. However, the association between water and morbidity as demonstrated by John Snow and the isolation of *Vibrio cholera* by Pacini in 1850 and Koch in 1883 [16] were some of the factors that caused the demise of the anti-contagionist movement and the re-emergence of the Germ Theory of infectious diseases, albeit in a more specific format [12].

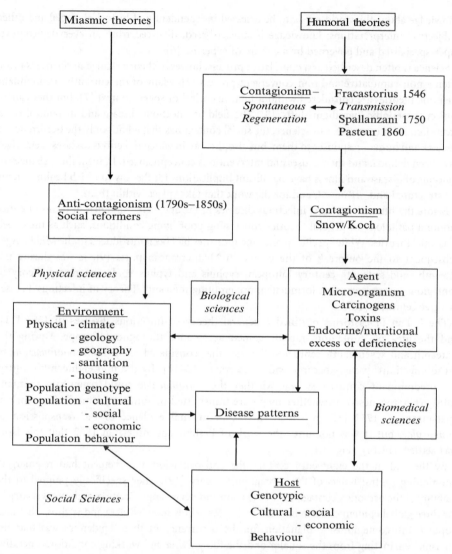

Fig. 1.1 Conceptual development of the European concepts of infectious diseases culminating in the *Ecological Model of Disease Causation*, based on the interaction of host, agent and environmental factors.

The great debate of the nineteenth century between the contagionists and anti-contagionists recently resurfaced in the debates concerning the nature and causes of AIDS. After the isolation of HIV from patients with AIDS in the early 1980s [17,18], the nature of the association between HIV and AIDS was the focus of an intense debate within the scientific community, which reverberated within the public arena. One section of the scientific community, the 'contagionists', claimed that HIV was the cause of AIDS and HIV could cause AIDS in its own right [19]; the 'anti-contagionists' claimed that HIV was a marker rather than the direct cause of AIDS [20–22]. Lifestyle characteristics of those with AIDS were considered to be the cause of immunosuppression, which, in turn, was postulated to be directly linked to drug-taking behaviour [20–22].

While this latest variant of the 'contagionist' versus 'anti-contagionist' debate has been recognized for what it is [23], often the conclusion of many medical authors merely reiterates the 'contagionist' stance and remains predominantly focused on the causative agent. What makes the comparison between the nineteenth- and late twentieth-century debates even more pertinent is that many of the 'contagionists' of the HIV debate are medical 'experts', while many of the 'anti-contagionists' are not part of the medical establishment, similar to the disposition of forces observed in the nineteenth-century debate. The latest variation of this debate involved the recent denials by some South African politicians of the causal association between HIV and AIDS, and their contention that AIDS is attributable to nutritional deficiencies [24].

Relevant to the current prospects for controlling the HIV pandemic is the fact that, though the nineteenth-century anti-contagionist miasmic theories proved to be incorrect, many of the sanitary reforms promoted by the anti-contagionists proved to be appropriate containment measures for dealing with diseases that eventually came to be related to specific agents. In effect, they had adopted the appropriate containment strategies for the wrong reasons, but, in so doing, and with the benefit of hindsight, it can be seen that their theories drew attention to important factors in community susceptibility to disease and the fact that the consequences of the same disease could be very different in different communities. Scientists such as Henle and Virchow had already pointed out during the second part of the nineteenth century that the disease agent is not synonymous with the disease process; medical scientists should therefore perhaps not only be concerned with finding 'causes' for diseases, but should also be concerned with describing the conditions in which these diseases arise and, particularly in the context of this book, the circumstances in which they may be successfully combated, including the features of the health system.

Thus, a functional framework of disease causation needs to integrate the occurrence of diseases in populations as well as in individuals, thereby also addressing the complementary role of structural versus behavioural factors that influence the occurrence of diseases while acknowledging the potential existence of tensions between a population and individualist approach. One framework that allows us to integrate the influences exerted by causal agent(s), host and environmental factors is the *Ecological Model of Disease Causation* [25,26]. This framework provides a synthesis of the 'contagionist' versus 'anti-contagionist' debate (Fig. 1.1). The interaction between agent, host and environmental factors, which includes the health system, determines the occurrence of disease patterns in individuals and populations at particular periods in time, and is embedded in the relevant biological, biomedical, social and physical sciences. This framework enables the occurrence of particular disease processes to be analysed within their broader context, and to devise, implement, monitor and evaluate the appropriateness of intervention programmes.

Over the millennia, medical practice has developed from itinerant medicine, focused primarily on the diagnosis and prognosis of disease in individuals, to the recent development of population medicine. The period after the Second World War saw the rise of the Welfare State in Europe [27]. The predominance of utilitarian risk-sharing principles, combined with technological developments during the second part of the twentieth century, resulted in a major conceptual shift of healthcare provision. Prior to the Second World War, the provision of medical care was primarily considered to be a personal responsibility; as part of the development of the Welfare State, the provision of medical care had primarily become a responsibility of the State, of which the National Health Service in the UK was a prime example [28]. The focus of responsibility for medical care had shifted from being subject-based to being inter-subjective or population-based [28], a shift that began with the sanitary reforms in the nineteenth century [12] and the introduction of compulsory insurance schemes throughout Europe in the late nineteenth and early twentieth centuries [10,29]. Furthermore, until recently, medical practitioners were primarily private practitioners paid on a fee-for-services basis, and only after the development of the Welfare State were more healthcare professionals employed as salaried practitioners in these systems.

In parallel to these developments, the prevailing concepts of disease causation have developed from broad cosmological interpretations to very narrow anthropocentric or biomolecular interpretations. Concepts of disease causation not only provide an analytic framework, but also provide the basis for intervention strategies.

While the cosmological and early anthropocentric views on disease causation integrated individuals within their social and biological context, with the development of localism in the seventeenth century, the view was promoted that individuals are individual units consisting of a collection of organs, tissues or cells, and that ill health has a single cause, namely disease. Since then, our technical understanding has undoubtedly been extended through this process, but such a reductionist framework is inadequate for addressing many contemporary challenges, including the HIV pandemic [30]. Ackerknecht summarized these developments as follows: 'What appears to have happened is that in the latter part of the nineteenth century and the first half of the twentieth century the old insights were lost in the shuffle of fascinating objective discoveries with the attendant over-mechanization and over-specialization.' [12]

The need for an integrated conceptual framework is apparent with the resurgence of the contagionist versus anti-contagionist debate within the context of the HIV pandemic. To address the HIV pandemic successfully, we need to adopt a conceptual framework that integrates the individuals within their communities, placed within their cultural and physical environment—including the health system available to them—while acknowledging the importance of their unique biological and cultural characteristics. Such a framework draws attention to the possibility that altering people's social contexts may reduce their level of ill health and, at the same time, that patients are people who can exercise choice and control over their lives—they are not inevitably passive victims of circumstance and disease processes.

Defining and classifying health systems

While also addressing some of the wider, international problems and responses to the HIV pandemic, a large part of this book focuses on relating different countries' responses to their HIV epidemic and their successes and failures to the evolution and properties of their health and healthcare systems. So, what is a 'health system'? The World Health Report 2000 [4] defines a health system as ' ... all the activities whose primary purpose is to promote, restore or maintain health.' This is a broad definition that goes beyond the healthcare system, but would tend to exclude from direct consideration, for example, the education system, whose primary purpose lies elsewhere. Most countries' health systems comprise more than one parallel subsystem either designed for different population groups, such as the military, civil servants or others, versus the general population, or based on affordability, typically the private versus public sectors, or providing for specific health needs, such as vertical programmes for specific problems like HIV, tuberculosis or malaria, connected to varying degrees to the 'mainstream' of healthcare.

It is striking how differently countries described in this book approach the structure and organization of their systems, given that each is predominantly built on a common set of assumptions about disease, medical science and other factors. It is also striking how long-standing many of these differences are. Health systems are determined by the particular historical circumstances that prevailed when they came into being in their current form. In most cases, these stem from the period when health professions were organizing and when governments, sometimes in the form of colonial administrations, became closely involved in paying for and operating health institutions. Before being able to compare the performance of different systems, it is important to have some way of classifying them to cut through the amount of detailed 'surface' difference and also increase the likelihood of comparing like with like. There are numerous approaches to classifying health systems, each highlighting different aspects to differing degrees.

Traditionally, the numerous schemes for classification tended to focus on locating a health system along a 'market–state socialist' continuum. Thus, Field [31] developed a fivefold classification of health systems based on the role of the state versus the market, the position of physicians, the role of professional associations and the ownership of facilities. The five 'ideal types', which were abstracted and generalized from more complex realities, were a fully 'private' system in which healthcare is an item of personal consumption (e.g. parts of the USA and Western European systems); a 'pluralistic' system in which healthcare is a consumer good (e.g. the USA more widely); national health insurance in which healthcare is an insured but guaranteed consumer good (e.g. France and Canada); a national health service in which healthcare is mostly a state-financed public service (e.g. the UK and Spain); and a fully socialized health service in which healthcare is a state-financed and -provided public service (e.g. the former Soviet Union, Cuba).

Roemer [32] developed a similar typology based on the level of market intervention in health policy, but added a second dimension, that of the level of economic development of a country according to its gross national product (GNP) per capita, thereby allowing a more global classification (Table 1.1).

In his matrix, four economic levels are distinguished: 'affluent industrialized', 'developing transitional', 'very poor' and 'resource-rich', meaning that the country has extensive natural resources. In addition, he identified four health system types: 'entrepreneurial and permissive', 'welfare-oriented', 'universal and comprehensive' and 'socialist and centrally planned', which are very similar to Field's categories. The country case studies in the current volume cover most of the types of national health systems in Roemer's classification.

In the body of Table 1.1 are examples of countries that Roemer regarded as broadly fitting the relevant cell in the matrix in the late 1980s and early 1990s. In many cases, countries have not altered their position, but there are notable exceptions. For example, with the fall of the Soviet Union, the Russian Federation, its constituent republics and the former Eastern Bloc countries of Europe have ceased to be 'affluent industrialized–socialist centrally planned'. Indeed, it is hard to think of a country that fits this description in the early twenty-first century. For the most part, China would now be regarded as 'developing and transitional', even 'affluent and industrialized' in some regions, rather than 'very poor', and its health system has become much

Table 1.1 Types of national health systems, early 1990s

Economic level, GNP per capita	Health system policies (types of market intervention)			
	Entrepreneurial and permissive	Welfare-oriented	Universal and comprehensive	Socialist and centrally planned
Affluent and industrialized	USA	West Germany	UK	Soviet Union
		Canada	New Zealand	Czechoslovakia
		Japan	Norway	
Developing and transitional	Thailand	Brazil	Israel	Cuba
	Philippines	Egypt	Nicaragua	North Korea
	South Africa	Malaysia		
Very poor	Ghana	India	Sri Lanka	China
	Bangladesh	Burma	Tanzania	Vietnam
	Nepal			
Resource-rich		Libya	Kuwait	
		Gabon	Saudi Arabia	

Source: [33].

more 'entrepreneurial and permissive' in parallel. Likewise, South Africa today aspires towards a more 'universal and comprehensive' approach despite a lack of resources.

Another point of note in relation to both the Field and Roemer classifications is the fact that whereas some countries fit their position in the classification fairly well—such as Cuba's health system, which is overwhelmingly 'socialist and centrally planned'—in many countries there are different types of health system side by side, often reflecting the coincidence of very different economic levels within the countries. South Africa is a good example of this since there is an 'entrepreneurial and permissive' health system for the well-off alongside much more basic health services for the poor majority that aspire to be 'universal and comprehensive' and are organized on the lines of a national health service.

More recent classifications are less exclusively organized around macro-level political differences and reflect the fact that the world is no longer so clearly divided into capitalist- and socialist-aligned countries. For example, today there might be a greater focus in attempting to distinguish health systems on the nature and extent of popular, including representative democratic, involvement in decisions affecting people's health and healthcare within each system. More recent approaches also tend to be more multidimensional and attend more closely to how health-related services are provided and controlled, and to the possibility of different forms of ownership and degrees of state control existing simultaneously within the same country, perhaps serving different population groups. Thus, Frenk and Donabedian [34] and Frenk [35] disaggregate the notion of state control into regulation, financing and delivery, allowing for the possibility, for example, of strict regulation of privately owned providers or weak regulation of state-owned providers as well as the commonly encountered phenomenon of publicly financed but private or Third Sector provision of health services (Table 1.2).

More recent approaches are still less 'Left–Right' politically oriented but focus more on the interaction between the main actors in the health system, i.e. patients, first-level providers such as primary care physicians, second-level providers such as hospitals, third-party payers and governments as regulators, and the main functions that health systems have to discharge for system maintenance, such as financing, resource allocation and payment and regulation.

Of course, in reality, there are usually many more levels of decision making constituting a health system. However, it is useful for analysis and comparison purposes to think of a health system as comprising three distinct levels with different rationales and foci: the *micro-level*, where users and professionals interact; the *meso-level*, representing the organizations that shape activity at the microlevel such as those that set budgets between different service areas; and the *macro-level*, where broad policy decisions that influence the whole system are made, such as deciding how much to spend on the public system and how to finance this spending.

A fairly complex recent example of the approach based on identifying 'functions' within the health system that take place at different levels is the framework set out in *The World Health Report 2000* [4]. This framework informed, but did not determine, the guidance given to authors of country case studies in the current book. The framework identifies three major and challenging social goals for any health system: health attainment; responsiveness to the expectations of the population; and fairness of financial contribution. In order to achieve, or help to achieve, these goals, the health system has to carry out certain key functions: *financing, provision of personal and non-personal health services*—public health programmes such as health education, vaccination and provision of a safe water supply; *resource generation*, such as forward planning to ensure that there are human and physical resources available as well as intellectual and social support for the system, such as information and programme evaluation; and *stewardship*, or the oversight function within the system to ensure its continuance. The 'financing' function in the WHO framework includes three distinct activities: *fund pooling*—spreading financial risk across the population through either taxes or insurance contributions of some sort; *revenue collection*—mobilizing and extracting money from individuals, households, corporations, governments and external donors; and *purchasing*—allocating the collected revenue to providers so that they can deliver agreed-upon services. The concept of *stewardship* is perhaps the least familiar part of this functional framework. It includes the leadership and policy direction of the system as well as setting the regulations governing behaviour and relationships, and gathering and publishing information on the performance of the system and how it can be improved. It is clear that the health system response to HIV tests

Table 1.2 Typology of healthcare modalities

Mechanism for state intervention (degree of control)	Purchasing power	Basis for population eligibility		
		Poverty/low income	Socially perceived priority	Citizenship
Regulation	Private enterprise	Private charity	Company-based services	German social insurance
Financing		US Medicaid	Incipient health insurance	National health insurance
Delivery		Public assistance	Social security (Latin American model)	Socialized (national health service)

Source: [35].

the strengths and weaknesses of all these functions in different countries. The WHO has used its framework to attempt to assess the performance of the health system of every country in the world on a comparable basis. However, there may be subtle differences between similar-seeming functions across countries that cannot so easily be captured in the WHO framework. A very different approach to thinking about the make-up of a health system is described by the acronym 'CATWOE' [36], which purports to be able to describe any human activity and its context in terms of the following: a certain *Transformation* (process) is performed for *Customers* (those who directly or indirectly benefit) by *Actors* within an *Environment* of constraints (e.g. geography, climate, wealth) and, crucially and distinctively, guided by a particular world view (*Weltanschauung*) or set of beliefs and values. CATWOE brings to the fore the norms, values and beliefs underpinning a particular system as a result of which similar-seeming functions are discharged differently with different consequences in different countries, though it says nothing about how well any system is performing.

Learning from comparative health system performance

Nolte *et al.* [37] identify three main types of comparative study at the health system level:

- *Descriptive studies* such as the European Observatory on Health Systems and Policies' series on Health Care Systems in Transition, which are structured descriptions of individual systems in Europe and other industrialized countries. Each report offers contextual information on the country followed by a description of the institutions and processes involved in financing, funding (reimbursing providers), delivering and regulating services, concluding with a review of trends in reforms in the particular system. The structure of the country case study chapters in Section III was influenced in part by the European Observatory approach as well as the WHO framework described above;

- *Quantitative studies* such as the econometric studies comparing health system performance by Anand and Bärnighausen [2] and Or [3], discussed above. These are organized around the notion of the health system as a 'production function' in which a range of inputs are used in a set of processes to explain statistically a particular health outcome measure such as mortality;

- *Focused analytical studies*, which take a single issue or aspect of health system activity or performance and try to assess the strengths and weaknesses of different countries' approaches. The approach tries to identify and learn from 'best practice' across countries while recognizing that policies, institutions and techniques of management and organization cannot simply be transported to different contexts with different histories and cultures. Instead, the research attempts to study the effects of particular policies *in situ*, identify the contextual factors that enable a policy to work in a particular country, explore whether similar factors exist elsewhere and whether the policy would need to be modified in other settings and, finally, provide some analysis of how well the policy might work in new settings before undertaking empirical evaluation of its actual impact once exported to the new settings.

What follows in this book is best seen as a largely descriptive study with some elements of focused analysis. The latter is because the subject is restricted to how health systems around the world have and are responding to the HIV pandemic, and because there is an attempt to draw lessons from this experience, albeit tentatively, given the fact that health systems are embedded in the history and governance of countries such that major changes occur relatively rarely and depend on factors in the wider political and policy environment outside the health sector [38].

Another reason for being tentative in lesson-drawing is methodological. There is relatively little experience in comparative health systems research in this area. Accurate lesson-drawing requires not only a detailed understanding of the policies being compared, but also a detailed understanding of each of the policy and system contexts in which policies are being implemented in order to discern in which circumstances a policy works well, not so well, badly or not at all, and why, before any lessons can be drawn with confidence. Doing this at a global level is a complex and daunting prospect—hence the modest pretensions of this book. Nonetheless, international comparisons offer a means for sharing experience, providing an opportunity for mutual learning, cross-fertilization or even policy transfer where appropriate [37].

The purpose of this book

While there have been thousands of articles, reports and commentaries on all aspects of the HIV pandemic since the early 1980s, there has been comparatively less description and analysis of the response as it is both shaped by, and shapes, each country's health system. While WHO/UNAIDS report annually on the pandemic and the global response, including country case studies, this book is distinctive in attempting to describe and assess a range of responses across the globe by situating them within the characteristics of each country and its health system. The breadth of this account of 28 countries provides, if nothing else, a contribution towards the historical record of an important endeavour in the history of public health. Of course, it is to be hoped that the descriptions themselves prompt further enquiry, stimulate reflection and lead to contemporary action, since the book attempts to help identify more and less effective responses at the health system level with a view to learning more about approaches that seem to be broadly positive, and in which settings, as well as something about the combination of elements and any common factors present in the more effective health system responses.

Many countries face common problems but vary in how they organize their response, which allows mutual learning to occur through the 'natural experiments' that are health systems. In addition, looking across countries should help enlarge the policy repertoire and spur improvements within countries as they discover more about the potential range of responses to common issues that have been tried in other places. Specifically, the country chapters that follow are designed to provide some raw material to begin to shed further light on the following questions:

1. Which health systems appear to have done particularly well in responding to their country's HIV epidemic, and which aspects of their health system and of their response appear to have been most influential in this?
2. Are there examples of countries that appear to be doing better or worse than their overall situation would predict, in terms of their gross domestic product (GDP) per capita, prevalence of HIV, quality of health system or other factors? If so, how are these countries managing to do this, and what lessons, if any, do such responses have for other countries?

3. Is there anything that can be generalized from the 'effective' responses either to similar countries (in terms of level of development, nature of health system, system of government, history, culture, etc.) or more widely: are there any elements of responses that appear to be universally positive or negative for HIV control?

4. Are the 'lessons' that have been drawn from the most celebrated country responses correct, and, if so, are they helpful to a wide range of countries?

The 28 countries selected for inclusion were chosen to provide the following: a geographic spread across the regions of the world; a range of high-, middle- and low-income countries; a variety of different 'types' of health system (e.g. national health service, national health insurance, social security, etc.); different stages of the epidemic—'concentrated' versus 'generalized' epidemics; different levels of incidence and prevalence; different styles of response (i.e. timing, balance between prevention and treatment, level of non-governmental organization involvement, etc.); and a range of more and less well-known country responses.

Authors were asked, as far as possible, to provide an overview of the country's health system linked to an account of the system's response to HIV. To do this, health policy or systems generalists were invited to collaborate with HIV specialists to produce an integrated description and analysis of how the country's health system had influenced the nature and effectiveness of the country's response, combining a 'top-down' health system and 'bottom-up' HIV-specific perspective. The process was similar to that used for the three *Health Care Systems in Transition* series, which were published in the *Journal of Public Health* [39–62].

Teams were asked to try, within the limits of the data available to them, to cover the topics in Boxes 1.1 and 1.2 as a minimum. They were free to include other material and themes.

Authors of most of the country chapters were brought together at a conference in Washington DC in October 2003 in order to share insights and so that health system and HIV specialist authors could discuss the implications of the health system for HIV control, and vice versa, before writing the final versions of their chapters.

The more thematic and analytical chapters in Sections I, II and IV provide an overview and some suggestions for solutions to some of the most serious outstanding issues facing health systems and the global response in the next few years. Authors of most of the thematic chapters had access to drafts of the country case studies, first drafts of which had been prepared earlier for the October 2003 Conference. The issues and institutions selected for analysis in the thematic chapters were chosen because they were well known to be critical for HIV control globally. The particular focus of each of these chapters was informed by insights from the country case studies.

Strengths and weaknesses of this book

This book is ambitious in its breadth of topics and of countries, and as such it has its limitations. It is a planned and edited series of contributions from a large and diverse group of authors that attempts to make sense as a whole, but it is not the product of original funded research or analysis by a single team. Thus, for example, while it was possible to give guidance to authors relating to their contribution, it was not possible to insist on a particular approach to the task. Authors from different backgrounds emphasized different features of their health systems, of HIV and of the response based on their interests and familiarity with specific topics.

Box 1.1 Suggested topics for country case study authors to include in their description of each country's health system

- Country context, societal organization and recent socio-economic changes;
- Key statistics on population, economy and health of the population from consistent international sources such as World Bank and OECD (e.g. population size, GDP per capita, percentage GDP on health, and a range of health measures), depending on data availability;
- Outline of the current health system in terms of finance, organization, ownership of facilities, specialization, relationships between primary, secondary and tertiary care, etc;
- Recent and current developments in terms of their positive and negative features;
- Impact of system in terms of nature of health services, accessibility, quality, etc;
- Anticipated future developments in relation to:

  1. demography, morbidity and demand for service;

  2. need for cost-containment/spending control;

  3. public and private mix of finance and delivery;

  4. use of 'market incentives';

  5. access to healthcare by the population in relation to needs;

  6. technology (cost, availability and control)

  7. accountability.

Box 1.2 Suggested topics for country case study authors to include in their description of each country's response to the HIV epidemic

- The way in which the response to HIV has been influenced by the societal and health system context, as described in the health system section;
- The current scale of the HIV problem, the populations affected and likely future trends;
- The implementation of health education, health promotion and preventive measures and their impact;
- A description of the HIV-related healthcare provided at the various stages of infection, including the involvement of the various healthcare sectors (primary, secondary and tertiary care) and the extent of population coverage;
- The extent to which antiretroviral therapy (mono, dual, triple or more therapy) or specific treatments for opportunistic illnesses have been routinely used in the management of HIV-infected individuals or in the reduction of perinatal transmission of HIV from mother to child;
- The extent to which the use of these therapies was financed through public health care provision or could only be acquired if paid for by individuals themselves;
- How the effectiveness, efficiency, equity and acceptability of the preventive and therapeutic interventions have been assessed so far and how this will be done in the future.

Although the editors attempted to highlight instances of clear disagreement between authors, there was no way that they could enforce unanimity of view. In particular, there are some tensions between the perspectives of economists and non-economists over the feasibility or desirability of taking a cost-benefit approach to the choice of interventions and balance of the response in different countries. As a result, the book does not present a single framework for analysis either within or between countries. Furthermore, no attempt was made to compare the performance of health systems' responses quantitatively by correlating indicators of disease control with system features by country, or to go from this to multivariate analyses of influences on the performance of different health systems.

Other limitations include the inevitability that parts of the book will go out of date more rapidly and substantially than others, as most of the book was written during 2004 and early 2005; the fact that not all countries of interest are represented is due to lack of space and lack of time to obtain contributions; variability between country chapters in their coverage of some of the major issues associated with health systems' responses to HIV; and the fact that the authorship varies as well as the subject matter, so that some issues are covered by clinicians in one chapter and by epidemiologists, economists or civil servants in another.

Perhaps most profoundly, the book demonstrates the challenges of undertaking comparative case studies and their interpretation in the health field. While a lot can be learned from comparative case studies and other more focused forms of analysis, there are many hurdles to be overcome even in highly circumscribed, funded research projects across countries, let alone in edited volumes such as the current one. These include:

- gaps in data, especially in relation to the quality of the actions and activities described;
- variable and potentially misleading use of common terms, such as 'nurse' or 'doctor';
- the lack of true comparability of data;
- the task of separating out the contribution of factors within the health system's control from those outside its influence over a particular period of time;
- the difficulty of generalizing the effects of policies or programmes across different contexts, because of different *Weltanschauung* and cultures, without exercising considerable care and imagination.

Yet, despite these difficulties, there are two 'fallacies' in discussions of health system and country comparisons, described by Marmor as the *World Cup* and the *Nihilist* fallacies [64], that the current venture has tried to avoid:

1. The search for a single, 'best' model—in this case for responding to HIV—is what Marmor calls the '*World Cup*' fallacy. This approach ignores the importance of context and the possibility that the best model in one setting or group of countries may not be so in another and, instead, attempts to rank countries and approaches.

2. The contrary belief that nothing can be learned from other contexts because differences in context are so crucial and the influences on health systems performance are so complex and particular as to defy generalization—Marmor describes this as the '*Nihilist*' fallacy.

This book was motivated by the belief that there is scope for comparative learning at the health system level, and that generalizations can be developed but that they require a parallel analytical process capable of identifying which settings are sufficiently similar and dissimilar for comparative generalizations to be made within groups of systems. McPake and Mills [64] refer to this as a ' "framework" for international comparisons of health systems'. They go on to argue that 'Such a framework can be constructed by developing, testing and revising models of cause and effect in health policy, and particularly by prospectively evaluating policy transfer.' For example, they describe the evolution of longitudinal, prospective research designed to identify the characteristics of country contexts, which positively and negatively affect the performance of private sector providers of care, in terms of level of economic development, population density, human resource development and the institutional legacy. The implication of this work is that the same policy to stimulate private sector involvement on the provision side of a health system will have different consequences depending on the specific features of each country context.

Since the material in this book is not the product of such a programme of prospective, comparative research on the impact of specific approaches to HIV control in different contexts, the conclusions and generalizations drawn about what works, for whom and in which context can only be tentative. The research and analysis required to develop the framework for categorizing health systems in relation to their response to HIV have yet to be undertaken—a theme picked up again in the concluding chapter of the book. Nonetheless, the thematic chapters and the concluding chapters do attempt, within the limitations of the data and analysis available, to identify some of the features of different health systems associated with more and less effective responses to HIV. Perhaps because the scope of the current volume is global, it is far harder to ignore or underplay the significance of contextual variations in the history, governance, society and health system of countries when attempting to provide useful insights at the health system level to improve the control of the HIV pandemic.

References

1. Hitiris T, Posnett J. (1992). The determinants and effects of health expenditure in developed countries. *Journal of Health Economics* 11:173–81.
2. Anand S, Bärnighausen T. (2004). Human resources and health outcomes: cross-country econometric study. *Lancet* **364**: 1603–9.
3. Or Z. (2001). *Exploring the Effects of Health Care on Mortality Across OECD Countries*. Paris: OECD.
4. World Health Organization. (2000). *The World Health Report 2000: Health Systems, Improving Performance*. Geneva: World Health Organization.
5. McGlynn EA. (2004). There is no perfect health system. *Health Affairs* 23:100–2.
6. Habermas J. (1981). Modernity versus postmodernity. *New German Critique* 22:3–14.
7. Laudan L. (1984). The aims of science and their role in scientific debate. *Science and Values* 8:103–37.
8. Kuhn TS. (1996). *The Structure of Scientific Revolutions*, 3rd edn. Chicago: Chicago University Press.
9. McNeill WH. (1979). *Plagues and Peoples*. London: Penguin Books, p160–2.
10. Temkin O. (1977). *The Double Face of Janus and Other Essays in the History of Medicine*. Baltimore, MD: The John Hopkins University Press.
11. Singer C, Singer D. (1917). The scientific position of Girolamo Fracastro with special reference to the source, character and the influence of his theory of infection. *Annals of Medical History* 1:1–34.
12. Ackerknecht EH. (1982). *A Short History of Medicine (Revised Edition)*. Baltimore/London: The Johns Hopkins University Press.

13. Selwyn S. (1974). *The Origins of Medical Microbiology in Britain and Abroad.* Proceedings of the XXIII International Congress of the History of Medicine, Wellcome Institute of the History of Medicine, London, p654–60.

14. Selwyn S and Wardlaw AC. (1983). Microbiology including virology. *Proceedings of the Royal Society of Edinburgh* **84**:267–93.

15. Singer C. (1943). *A Short History of Science to the Nineteenth Century.* Oxford: Oxford University Press, p245–7.

16. Howard-Jones N. (1972). Choleranomalies: the unhistory of medicine as exemplified by cholera. *Perspectives in Biology and Medicine* **15**:422–33.

17. Barre-Sinoussi F, Chermann JC, Rey F *et al.* (1983). Isolation of a T-lymphotropic retrovirus from a patient at risk for acquired immune deficiency syndrome (AIDS). *Science* **220**:868–70.

18. Levy JA, Hoffman AD, Kramer SM, Landis JA, Shimabukura JM, Oshiro LS. (1984). Isolation of lymphocytopathic retroviruses from San Francisco patients with AIDS. *Science* **225**:840–2.

19. Blattner W, Gallo RC. Temin HM. (1988). HIV causes AIDS. *Science* **241**:515.

20. Duesburg P. (1988). HIV is not the cause of AIDS. *Science* **241**:514.

21. Duesburg PH. (1987). Retroviruses as carcinogens and pathogens: expectations and reality. *Cancer Research* **47**:1199–1220.

22. Duesburg PH. (1989). Human immunodeficiency virus and acquired immunodeficiency syndrome: correlation but not causation. *Proceedings of the National Academy of Sciences of the USA* **86**:755–64.

23. Weiss RA, Jaffe HW. (1990). Duesburg, HIV and AIDS. *Nature* **345**:659–60.

24. Cameron E. (2005).The tragedy of AIDS denialism in South Africa. In: *Witness to AIDS.* Cape Town: Tafelberg, p103–22.

25. Beck EJ. (1985).*The Enigma of Aboriginal Health: Interaction Between Biological, Social and Economic Factors in Alice Springs Town-camps.* Canberra: Australian Institute of Aboriginal Studies, p52–3.

26. Beck EJ. (1993). Urban–rural population research: a town like Alice. In: Schell LM, Smith MT, Bilsborough A, eds. *Urban Ecology and Health in the Third World.* Cambridge: Cambridge University Press, p129–43.

27. Beveridge W. (1942). *Social Insurance and Allied Services.* London: HMSO.

28. Klein R. (1984). *The Politics of the National Health Service.* London: Longman, pp. 2–7.

29. Illich I. (1976). *Limits to Medicine.* London: Marion Boyars, p39–124.

30. Wade DT, Halligan PW. (2004). Do biomedical models of illness make for good healthcare systems? *British Medical Journal* **329**:1398–401.

31. Field MG. (1978). *Comparative Health Systems: Differentiation and Convergence.* Washington, DC: National Center for Health Services Research.

32. Roemer MI. (1977). *Comparative National Policies on Health Care.* New York: Marcel Dekker.

33. Roemer MI. (1991). *National Health Systems of the World.* New York: Oxford University Press.

34. Frenk J, Donabedian A. (1987). State intervention in medical care: types, trends and variables. *Health Policy and Planning* **2**:17–31.

35. Frenk J. (1994). Dimensions of health system reform. *Health Policy* **27**:19–34.

36. Checkland P. (1981). *Systems Thinking, Systems Practice.* Chichester, UK: Wiley.

37. Nolte E, McKee M, Wait S. (2005). Describing and evaluating health systems. In: Bowling A, Ebrahim S, eds. *Handbook of Health Research Methods: Investigation, Measurement and Analysis.* Maidenhead, UK: Open University Press, p12–43.

38. Tuohy CH. (1999). Dynamics of a changing health sphere: the United States, Britain and Canada. *Health Affairs* **18**:114–34.

39. Hillier S, Shen J. (1996). Health care systems in transition: People's Republic of China part I: an overview of China's health care system. *Journal of Public Health Medicine* 18:258–65.

40. Zhang KL, Chen W. (1996). Health care systems in transition: People's Republic of China part II: the Chinese health care system's response to HIV-AIDS. *Journal of Public Health Medicine* 18:266–8.

41. Ashton T. (1996). Health care systems in transition: New Zealand part I: an overview of New Zealand's health care system. *Journal of Public Health Medicine* 18:269–73.

42. Chetwynd J, Dickson N. (1996). Health care systems in transition: New Zealand part II: the New Zealand health care system's response to HIV-AIDS. *Journal of Public Health Medicine* 18:274–7.

43. Schut FT. (1996). Health care systems in transition: The Netherlands part I: health care reforms in The Netherlands: miracle or mirage? *Journal of Public Health Medicine* 18:278–84.

44. Danner SA. (1996). Health care systems in transition: The Netherlands part II: the response of the Dutch health care system to HIV-AIDS. *Journal of Public Health Medicine* 18:285–8.

45. Buss P, Gadelha P. (1996). Health care systems in transition: Brazil part I: an outline of Brazil's health care system reforms. *Journal of Public Health Medicine* 18:289–95.

46. Santos BR, Barcellos NT. (1996). Health care systems in transition: Brazil part II: the current status of AIDS in Brazil. *Journal of Public Health Medicine* 18:296–300.

47. Liu CT. (1998). Heath care systems in transition II. Taiwan, part I. A general overview of the health care system in Taiwan. *Journal of Public Health Medicine* 20:5–10.

48. Chang HJ. (1998). Health care systems in transition II. Taiwan, Part II. The current status of HIV-AIDS in Taiwan. *Journal of Public Health Medicine* 20:11–15.

49. Lim MK. (1998). Health care systems in transition II. Singapore, part I. An overview of health care systems in Singapore. *Journal of Public Health Medicine* 20:16–22.

50. Boudville IC, Wong SY. (1998). Health care systems in transition II. Singapore, part II. The current status of HIV-AIDS. *Journal of Public Health Medicine* 20:23–8.

51. Arai Y, Ikegami N. (1998). Health care systems in transition II. Japan, part I. An overview of the Japanese health care systems. *Journal of Public Health Medicine* 20:29–33.

52. Soda K, Mizushima S. (1998). Health care systems in transition II. Japan, part II. The current status of AIDS-HIV in Japan. *Journal of Public Health Medicine* 20:34–40.

53. Shin YS. (1998). Health care systems in transition II. Korea, part I. An overview of health care systems in Korea. *Journal of Public Health Medicine* 20:41–6.

54. Shin YO, K MY. (1998). Health care systems in transition II. Korea, part II. The current status of HIV-AIDS in Korea. *Journal of Public Health Medicine* 20:47–51.

55. Vaughan JP, Karim E, Buse K. (2000). Bangladesh part I: an overview of the health care system in Bangladesh. *Journal of Public Health Medicine* 22:5–9.

56. Hawkes S, Azim T. (2000). Bangladesh part II: Bangladesh's response to HIV-AIDS. *Journal of Public Health Medicine* 22:10–3.

57. Fernando D. (2000). Sri Lanka part I: an overview of Sri Lanka's health care system. *Journal of Public Health Medicine* 22:14–20.

58. Abeyewickreme I, de Silva K. (2000). Sri Lanka part II: the current state of HIV-AIDS in Sri Lanka. *Journal of Public Health Medicine* 22:21–4.

59. Qadeer I. (2000). India part I: the Indian experience. *Journal of Public Health Medicine* 22:25–32.

60. Maniar JK. (2000). India part II: the current status of HIV-AIDS in India. *Journal of Public Health Medicine* 22:33–7.

61. Ghaffer A, Kazi BM, Salman M. (2000). Pakistan part I: an overview of the health care system in Pakistan. *Journal of Public Health Medicine* 22:38–42.

62. Kazi BM, Ghaffer A, Salman M. (2000). Pakistan part II: Pakistan's response to HIV-AIDS. *Journal of Public Health Medicine* 22:43–7.

63. Marmor TR. (1997). Global health policy reform: misleading mythology or learning opportunity. In: Altenstetter C, Bjorkman JW, eds. *Health Policy Reform: National Variations and Globalization.* London/New York: Macmillan/St. Martin's Press, pp. 348.

64. McPake B, Mills A. (2000). What can we learn from international comparisons of health systems and system reform? *Bulletin of the World Health Organization* 78:811–20.

Chapter 2

The evolving HIV pandemic

Catherine A Hankins[*], Karen A Stanecki, Peter D
Ghys and Hein Marais

HIV is unique in recent human history in its rapid spread, its extent and the depth of its impact. Since the first AIDS case was diagnosed in 1981, the world has struggled to come to grips with its extraordinary dimensions. Early efforts to mount an effective response were fragmented, piecemeal and vastly under-resourced. Few communities recognized the dangers ahead, and even fewer were able to mount an effective response. Now, close to 25 years later, more than 20 million people are dead. At the end of 2004, 39.4 million people (range: 35.9–44.3 million) worldwide were living with HIV (Fig. 2.1) [1]. That year, an estimated 4.9 million people (range: 4.3–6.4 million) became newly infected with HIV. This is more than in any one year before. AIDS killed 3.1 million people (range: 2.8–3.5 million) in 2004 [1].

This chapter describes the global epidemic by region, highlighting the changing dynamics of HIV transmission and the diverse patterns of infection found worldwide. The epidemic remains extremely dynamic, growing and changing character as the virus exploits new opportunities for transmission. Virtually no country in the world remains unaffected. The number of people

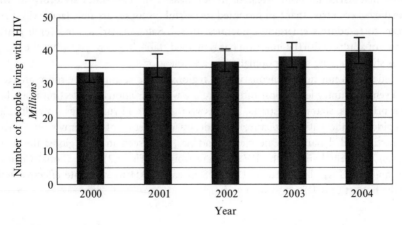

Fig. 2.1 Estimated number of people living with HIV, 2000–2004. Source: UNAIDS/WHO. AIDS Epidemic Update, 2004 [1].

* Corresponding author.

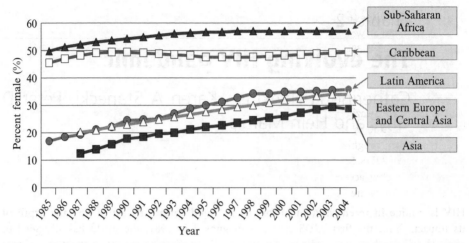

Fig. 2.2 Percentage of adults (15–49 years old) living with HIV who are female, 1985–2004. Source: UNAIDS/WHO AIDS Epidemic Update, 2004 [1].

living with HIV (PLHIV) has been rising in every region, with the steepest recent increases occurring in East Asia, Eastern Europe and Central Asia.

The number of PLHIV in East Asia rose by almost 50% between 2002 and 2004, an increase that is attributable largely to China's swiftly growing epidemic. In Eastern Europe and Central Asia, where the epidemic of injecting drug use among millions of young people is fuelling HIV transmission, there were 40% more PLHIV in 2004 than in 2002.

Some industrialized countries that have let down their guard are seeing a rise in new infections, in part due to a dangerous myth fuelled by widespread access to antiretroviral medicines that AIDS has been defeated. In Southeast Asia, epidemics are evolving, with the result that even countries that had mounted successful responses are now faced with having to shift gears to re-address emerging epidemics. In sub-Saharan Africa, the overall population percentage of adults with HIV infection has remained stable in recent years, but the number of PLHIV is still increasing as the population as a whole grows.

The epidemic is not homogeneous within regions; some countries are more affected than others. Even at country level, most often there are wide variations in infection levels between different provinces, states or districts, and between urban and rural areas. In reality, like the global epidemic, the national picture is made up of a series of epidemics with their own characteristics and dynamics. One clear trend has been seen in all regions: the increasing proportion of adults living with HIV who are women (Fig. 2.2). The Global Coalition on Women and AIDS was launched by UNAIDS in early 2004 to stimulate effective action to reduce the impact of AIDS on women and girls.

Sub-Saharan Africa

Sub-Saharan Africa, with the most advanced epidemic, remains the hardest-hit region worldwide. With just over 10% of the world's population, it is home to close to two-thirds of all PLHIV—some 25.4 million (23.4–28.4 million) people were living with HIV at the end of 2004.

Just under two-thirds (64%) of all PLHIV are in sub-Saharan Africa, as are more than three-quarters (76%) of all women living with HIV. Among young people 15–24 years of age, 6.9% of women (range: 6.3–8.3%) and 2.1% of men (range: 1.9–2.5%) were living with HIV by the end of 2003 [1].

The epidemics in sub-Saharan Africa are generally stabilizing, with HIV prevalence at around 7.4% for the entire region, although it appears to be rising in a few countries, such as Madagascar and Swaziland. However, roughly stable HIV prevalence does not necessarily mean the epidemic is slowing. On the contrary, it can disguise the worst phases of an epidemic—when roughly equally large numbers of people are being newly infected with HIV and are dying of AIDS. Southern Africa, which offers only slight hints of possible future declines in prevalence, now accounts for one-third of all AIDS deaths globally. Furthermore, the epidemics in Africa are diverse, in terms of both their scale and the pace at which they are evolving. There is no single 'African' epidemic. Some urban parts of East Africa display modest declines in HIV prevalence among pregnant women, while in West and Central Africa, prevalence levels have stayed roughly steady at lower levels than in the rest of sub-Saharan Africa. A review of national community-based studies in Africa shows that HIV prevalence in urban areas is about twice as high as in rural areas [2].

There is tremendous diversity across sub-Saharan Africa in the levels and trends of HIV infection. Southern Africa remains the worst-affected region in the world, with data from selected antenatal clinics in urban areas in 2002 showing HIV prevalence of more than 25%, following a rapid increase from just 5% in 1990. For example, in Swaziland, the average prevalence among pregnant women was 39% in 2002—up from 34% in 2000 and only 4% in 1992. In Botswana [3], weighted antenatal clinic prevalence has been sustained at 36% in 2001, 35% in 2002 and 37% in 2003. In South Africa [4], the prevalence among pregnant women was 25% in 2001, 26.5% in 2002 and 27.9% in 2003.

In Eastern Africa, the prevalence among pregnant women in urban areas has fallen to 13%, down from around 20% in the early 1990s. There are signs of a real decline in infections in some countries. This is most notable in Uganda [2], where national prevalence dropped to 4.1% (range: 2.8–6.6%) in 2003. In Kampala, prevalence was around 8% in 2002—down from 29% 10 years ago. A variety of prevention approaches were probably responsible, including community mobilization, pioneering non-governmental organization (NGO) projects and public education campaigns emphasizing delayed sexual initiation, partner reduction and condom use, combined with strong political leadership, destigmatization and open communication. Behavioural changes in the early 1990s—in particular, delayed sexual debut and reduced numbers of casual partners—reduced HIV transmission, while increased condom use played an important role in stabilizing the epidemic [5,6]. A recent study reported that increased mortality also played a role in Uganda's declining HIV prevalence [7]. No other country in the region has so dramatically reversed the epidemic as Uganda, but HIV prevalence among pregnant women has declined elsewhere at the subnational level. For example, in the Ethiopian capital, Addis Ababa, prevalence fell from a peak of 21% in 1995 to 12% in 2003 [8]. In Kenya, prevalence has also dropped in several sites and remained stable in others [9].

Prevalence in West and Central Africa has remained stable at around 5%, generally, but the epidemic remains diverse and changeable. HIV prevalence is lowest in the Sahel countries at around 1%, and highest in Côte d'Ivoire and Nigeria—the latter, with a population of more than 120 million and a national prevalence in 2003 of 5.4% (range: 3.6–8%), has the third largest number of PLHIV in the world after South Africa and India. HIV prevalence among pregnant women in Nigeria is more than 1% in all states and more than 5% in 13 states. National prevalence levels are highest in Côte d'Ivoire at 7% (range: 4.9–10%), although Abidjan recorded its lowest level (6%) in a decade in 2002. In Senegal, although the national HIV prevalence is below 1% (range: 0.4–1.7%), prevalence rose from 5% and 8% among sex workers in two cities in 1992, to 14% and 23%, respectively, in 2002 [2].

In sub-Saharan Africa, heterosexual transmission is by far the predominant mode of HIV transmission, and effective strategies addressing sexual transmission have the largest potential to turn the epidemic around in this region. Unsafe injections in healthcare settings are believed to be responsible for around 2.5% of all infections [10], and the safety of injections must be assured in all healthcare settings to prevent transmission through this route. Injecting drug use is now being reported from Nigeria, Kenya and Tanzania [11], highlighting the need to turn to demand-reduction education and harm minimization or reduction strategies to head off transmission through contaminated injecting equipment.

African women are being infected at an earlier age than men, as the gap in HIV prevalence between them continues to grow. At the beginning of the epidemic in sub-Saharan Africa, women living with HIV were vastly outnumbered by men. However, today there are, on average, 13 infected women for every 10 infected men; the difference between infection levels is more pronounced in urban areas, with 14 women for every 10 men, than in rural areas, where 12 women are infected for every 10 men [12]. Among young people 15–24 years old, the difference in infection levels is even more pronounced, with 20 young women living with HIV for every 10 men in South Africa, and 45 women for every 10 men in Kenya and Mali [13–15].

There is no single explanation for why the epidemic is so rampant in Southern Africa. A combination of factors, often working in concert, seems to be responsible. These factors include poverty and social instability that result in family disruption, high levels of other sexually transmitted infections, the low status of women, sexual violence and ineffective political and community leadership at critical points during the spread of HIV. An important factor, too, is high mobility, which is largely linked to migratory labour systems.

Migrant labour systems have aggravated women's economic dependence on their male partners to a much greater extent in Southern Africa than in other parts of the continent where women are more prominent in market trading and other forms of commercial activity. Across this subregion, income-earning opportunities for women with low educational attainment are particularly poor, and industrial sectors in which female workers predominate, such as garment manufacturing, have been hard hit by job losses related to changes in tariffs and subsidies. This has further weakened women's economic status, aggravating gender inequalities and probably heightening women's vulnerability to HIV [16].

Middle East and North Africa

With the exception of a few countries, systematic behavioural and sero-surveillance of the epidemic is not well developed in the Middle East and North Africa. Inadequate monitoring of the situation among populations at higher risk of HIV exposure, such as sex workers, injecting drug users and men who have sex with men, means that in most countries there is no early warning system for potential epidemics in these populations. Available information, based mostly on case reporting, suggests that around 480,000 people (range: 200,000–1.4 million) are living with HIV in the region, which has a prevalence of 0.2% of the adult population (range: 0.1–0.6%). Sudan is by far the worst-affected country, with an overall HIV prevalence of 2.3% (range: 0.7–7.2%). The epidemic is most severe in the southern part of the country where HIV prevalence among pregnant women is reported to be six to eight times higher than around Khartoum in the north [1].

In some countries in the region, HIV infection appears concentrated among injecting drug users. Substantial transmission through contaminated injecting equipment has been reported in Bahrain, Libya and Oman. Unsafe blood transfusion and blood collection practices still pose a risk in some countries, although efforts are being made to expand blood screening and sterile procedures in healthcare systems to full coverage. There is concern that the virus may be spreading undetected among men who have sex with men, whose sexual behaviour is illegal and widely condemned in the region.

Eastern Europe and Central Asia

Diverse HIV epidemics are under way in Eastern Europe and Central Asia, where the number of PLHIV has risen dramatically in just a few years—reaching an estimated 1.4 million people (range: 920,000–2.1 million) at the end of 2004, compared with about 160,000 in 1995. This is more than a ninefold increase in less than 10 years. Among young people aged 15–24, 0.8% of women (range: 0.4–1.6%) and 1.7% of men (range: 0.8–3.7%) were living with HIV by the end of 2004 [1].

Estonia, Latvia, the Russian Federation and Ukraine are the worst-affected countries in this region, but HIV continues to spread in Belarus, Moldova and the Central Asian Republics. The main driving force behind epidemics across the region is injecting drug use—an activity that has spread explosively in the years of turbulent change since the demise of the Soviet regime. A striking feature is the low age of those infected; more than 80% of HIV-positive people in this region are under 30 years of age. In contrast, in North America and Western Europe, only 30% of infected people are under 30.

The Russian Federation had the largest number of PLHIV in the region at the end of 2003, estimated at 860,000 (range: 420,000–1.4 million). The picture is uneven; well over half of all reported cases of HIV infection come from just 10 of the 89 administrative territories [17]. Most injecting drug users in Russia are male, but the proportion of females among new HIV cases is growing fast—up from one in four in 2001, to one in three just a year later. The trend is most obvious in the parts of Russia where the epidemic is oldest, and this suggests that sexual intercourse has been playing an increasing role in transmission. In Ukraine, although drug injecting remains the principal mode of transmission, sexual transmission is becoming increasingly common. An increasing proportion of those who become infected through unsafe sex have no direct relationship with drug users [18].

Recently, several Central Asian countries—notably Kazakhstan, Kyrgyzstan and Uzbekistan—have reported growing numbers of people diagnosed with HIV, most of them injecting drug users. Central Asia is at the crossroads of the main drug trafficking routes between East and West, and, in some places, heroin is said to be cheaper than alcohol.

Throughout the region, estimates and trends are based almost exclusively on case reporting, since there has been little investment in sentinel surveillance. This raises concerns that HIV may be spreading among people who rarely come into contact with the authorities or testing services. For example, very little is known about how the epidemic affects men who have sex with men, since sex between men is widely stigmatized and rarely acknowledged. However, in Central Europe, sex between men is clearly the predominant mode of HIV transmission in the Czech Republic, Hungary, Slovenia and the Slovak Republic [2].

Latin America

More than 1.7 million (1.3–2.2 million) people were living with HIV in Latin America at the end of 2004. Among young people 15–24 years of age, an estimated 0.5% (0.4–0.9%) of women and 0.8% (0.6–1.3%) of men were living with HIV at the end of 2004 [1]. HIV infection tends to be highly concentrated among populations at particular risk, with the majority of infections caused by contaminated drug-injecting equipment or sex between men. Two countries in this region—Guatemala and Honduras—have a national adult HIV prevalence of more than 1%. However, elsewhere, lower prevalence disguises serious, localized epidemics, not least in Brazil, which accounts for more than one-third of the PLHIV in Latin America. National prevalence is well below 1%, but infection levels above 60% have been reported among injecting drug users in some cities. In other cities, harm-reduction programmes have been associated with steep drops in HIV prevalence among injecting drug users in recent years—notably in El Salvador, where prevalence fell from 50% in 1996 to 7% in 2001 [19]. Brazil's epidemic has dispersed into all regions of the vast country and has become more varied, with women increasingly affected [20].

In Central America, HIV is spread predominantly through sex. A recent international study shows that HIV prevalence among female sex workers ranges from less than 1% in Nicaragua, 2% in Panama, 4% in El Salvador and 5% in Guatemala, to more than 10% in Honduras [21]. Among men who have sex with men, levels of HIV infection appear to be uniformly high, ranging from 9% in Nicaragua to 24% in Argentina (Fig. 2.3).

Although sex between men is the predominant mode of transmission in several countries, notably Colombia and Peru, conditions appear ripe for the virus to spread more widely, as

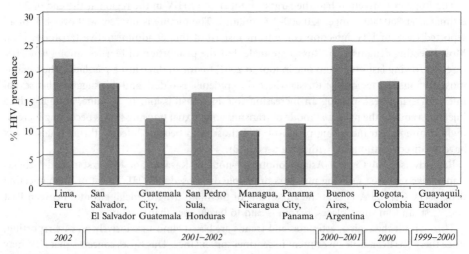

Fig. 2.3 HIV prevalence among men having sex with men, Latin America 1999–2002. Source: UNAIDS/WHO Report on the Global AIDS Epidemic, 2004 [2].

large numbers of men who have sex with men also have sex with women [22]. A study in Lima, Peru found that almost 90% of HIV-positive pregnant women had had just one or two sexual partners in their lifetimes [23]. The women's HIV risk depended almost exclusively on the sexual behaviour of their male partners, and those most at risk were young women [24]. Several urban Peruvian studies found that 87% of men who had sex with men also had sex with women; confirmed very low rates of condom use, irrespective of the partner's sex; and revealed high levels of sexually transmitted infections such as syphilis and herpes [25]. Given the consistently high HIV prevalence detected in Peru in recent years among groups of men who have sex with men—12% in Iquitos in 2002 and 22% in Lima in the same year—there is significant scope for wider HIV spread [22]. Other research suggests that similar patterns of HIV transmission could be significant factors in epidemics elsewhere in the region.

Shadowing the considerable variation in Latin America's epidemics, however, is a troubling mismatch in several countries between prevention spending priorities and the main epidemiological features of countries' epidemics. With the notable exception of Peru, most countries direct the bulk of their preventive expenditure to female sex worker programmes, despite the fact that sex between men is a driving force in the epidemic throughout the region. The disparity is most pronounced in Central America. Meanwhile, among those countries where injecting drug use features prominently in their epidemics, only Argentina and Brazil appear to have prioritized their preventive spending accordingly. Unless much better use is made of epidemiological and other pertinent data to tailor the mix of preventive programming, these countries will not slow their epidemics significantly.

The Caribbean

With average adult HIV prevalence of 2.3%, the Caribbean is the second most affected region in the world. In the Bahamas, Belize, Guyana, Haiti, and Trinidad and Tobago, national prevalence exceeds 2%, whereas in Barbados it is 1.5%. More than 440,000 (270,000–780,000) people are living with HIV in the Caribbean. Among young people 15–24 years of age, an estimated 3.1% (1.6–8.3%) of women and 1.7% (0.9–4.6%) of men were living with HIV at the end of 2004. AIDS has become the leading cause of death among adults aged 15–44 years [26]. Yet, a growing number of Caribbean countries are showing that the epidemic does yield to appropriate and resolute responses.

The Caribbean epidemic is predominantly heterosexual (almost two-thirds of all AIDS cases to date are attributed to this mode of transmission), although sex between men, which is heavily stigmatized, and in some places illegal, remains a significant—but still neglected—aspect of the epidemics. Concentrated among sex workers in many places, the virus is also spreading in the general population.

The worst-affected country is Haiti, where national prevalence is around 5.6% (range: 2.5–11.9%), with the north-west of Haiti having a prevalence as high as 13% compared with 2–3% in the south. Prevalence in the Dominican Republic, which shares the island of Hispaniola with Haiti, has declined due to effective prevention efforts that encouraged people to reduce their number of sexual partners and increase condom use. In the capital, Santo Domingo, prevalence among pregnant women declined from around 3% in 1995 to below 1% at the end of 2003.

HIV transmission through injecting drug use remains rare in the Caribbean, with the significant exception of Bermuda, where it accounts for a large share (43%) of AIDS cases, and Puerto Rico, where more than half of all infections in 2002 were associated with injecting drug use and about one-quarter were heterosexually transmitted [2,27].

The number of new HIV infections among women now outstrips those among men, with the result that roughly as many women as men are now living with HIV in this region. In Jamaica, girls are 2.5 times more likely than boys in the same age group (10–19 years) to be infected, due partly to the fact that some girls have sexual relationships with older men who are more likely to be HIV-infected, a trend that has also been documented in several other countries.

Asia

National HIV infection levels in Asia are generally low, but the populations of many Asian nations are so large that even low national HIV prevalence means large numbers of people are living with HIV. Latest estimates show some 8.2 million (5.4–11.8 million) people in Asia, of whom 2.3 million (1.5–3.3 million) were adult women, were living with HIV at the end of 2004. Among young people 15–24 years of age, 0.3% of women (0.2–0.6%) and 0.4% of men (0.3–0.8%) were living with HIV by the end of 2004 [1]. Epidemics in this region remain largely concentrated among injecting drug users, men who have sex with men, sex workers, clients of sex workers and their sexual partners.

The nature, pace and severity of HIV epidemics differ across this vast region. Some countries, such as Cambodia, Myanmar and Thailand, were hit early; others, such as Indonesia, Nepal, Vietnam and several provinces in China, have more recently begun to experience rapidly expanding epidemics and need to mount swift, effective responses. In parts of India and China, HIV has become well entrenched in some sections of society, despite modest efforts to halt the virus' spread. Other countries, such as Bangladesh, East Timor, Laos, Pakistan and the Philippines, still have extremely low HIV prevalence, even among people at high risk of exposure to HIV, and have golden opportunities to pre-empt serious outbreaks [21].

The world's most populous countries, China and India, home to some 2.4 billion people, have a low national HIV prevalence: 0.1% (range: 0.1–0.2%) in China and between 0.4 and 1.3% in India. However, both have extremely serious epidemics in a number of provinces, territories and states, and there is concern about what might be happening in the vast areas of both countries for which there are few data.

In China, the virus has spread to all 31 provinces, autonomous regions and municipalities. In Anhui, Henan and Shandong, HIV gained a foothold in the early 1990s among rural people who were selling blood plasma to supplement their meagre farm incomes. Infection levels of 10–20% have been found, rising to 60% in certain communities, and many people have already died of AIDS. Elsewhere, the virus has established a more recent but firm presence among injecting drug users and, to a lesser extent, sex workers and their clients [28]. HIV prevalence among drug injectors was between 18 and 56% in six cities in the southern provinces of Guangdong and Guangxi in 2002, while some 21% of injectors tested positive for HIV in Yunnan province in 2003 [29]. Sexual transmission of HIV from injecting drug users to their sex partners looks certain to feature more prominently in China's fast-evolving epidemic. Some 47% of surveyed female drug injectors in Sichuan province, and 21% in neighbouring Yunnan province, reported selling sex for money or drugs in the previous month, according to recent studies. In surveys of sex workers in Guangxi and Sichuan, condom use with clients was inconsistent. Little is known about the possible role of sex between men in China's epidemic. A rare survey of men who have sex with men in Beijing, conducted in 2001–2002, found that approximately 3% of the men were HIV-infected (almost all of whom had been unaware of their sero-status) [30].

There are signs that efforts to boost public knowledge about HIV are bearing fruit, but there remains much room for improvement. A 2003 survey found that two out of five Chinese men and women could not name a single way to protect themselves against infection [31]. In Sichuan province, more than one-third of sex workers (and a similar proportion of clients) did not know that condoms offer good protection against HIV. Recent moves by the government to adopt condom policies of the sort that helped Cambodia and Thailand bring their epidemics under control will be critical in shaping the course of China's epidemic.

India's epidemics are even more diverse than China's. Latest estimates show that about 5.1 million (2.5–8.5 million) people were living with HIV in India in 2003. Serious epidemics are under way in several states. In Tamil Nadu, an HIV prevalence of 50% has been found among sex workers, while in each of the states of Andhra Pradesh, Karnataka, Maharashtra, Manipur and Nagaland, HIV prevalence has crossed the 1% mark among pregnant women. In Manipur, an epidemic driven by injecting drug use has been in full swing for more than a decade and has acquired a firm presence in the wider population [32]. HIV prevalence measured at antenatal clinics in the Manipur cities of Imphal and Churachand has risen from below 1% to over 5%, with many of the women testing positive appearing to be the sex partners of male drug injectors. About 20% of female sex workers inject drugs, and many injectors are young, with 40% of male injectors surveyed in 2002 being under 25 years of age, factors which will help sustain Manipur's epidemic [21].

There are signs that injecting drug use is playing a bigger role in India's epidemics than previously thought. In the southern city of Chennai, 64% of drug injectors were found to be infected with HIV in 2003. In most cities where injecting drug users have been surveyed, at least one-quarter of them—and 46% in Chennai—said they lived with a wife or regular sex partner [21]. This has probably contributed to the fact that Chennai also has one of the highest HIV prevalence rates among pregnant women in the country.

HIV transmission through sex between men is also a major cause for concern in many areas of India. In a household-based survey in a low-income area of Chennai, 6% of men reported having sex with other men. These men were over eight times more likely to be infected with HIV than other men, and 60% more likely to be infected with other sexually transmitted infections. A high proportion of men who have sex with men also reported having sex with women [33]. For example, in a household study in India, 57% of men who reported having sex with other males were married [34].

Elsewhere in South Asia, conditions are ripe for HIV to spread. For example, in Bangladesh, where national adult prevalence is less than 0.1%, large numbers of men buy sex, and most do not use condoms in these encounters. Female sex workers report the lowest condom use in the region. Among injecting drug users, 71% of those who do not participate in needle exchange programmes use non-sterile injecting equipment, compared with 50% of attendees in central Bangladesh programmes and 25% in north-west Bangladesh programmes [35]. Surveys show that only about 65% of young people, less than 20% of married women and just 33% of married men have even heard of AIDS [2].

Pakistan has an estimated adult HIV prevalence of 0.1%, but it also has about 3 million heroin users, many of whom started injecting drugs in the 1990s. The first outbreak of HIV infection among injecting drug users was in the small town of Larkana, where 10% of 175 injecting drug users tested HIV-positive [36]. A behavioural survey in Quetta found that a high proportion of respondents used non-sterile injecting equipment, and over half of them said they visited sex workers. Few had heard of AIDS, and even fewer had ever used a condom. [37]

Injecting is the driving force behind Nepal's epidemic, with use of non-sterile injecting equipment being widespread. HIV prevalence is high (22–68% across the country in 2002) among male injectors, many of them younger than 25 [21]. Nepal's epidemic also highlights the potential links between HIV infection and mobility. Injecting drug users from cities with low prevalence, but who had injected drugs elsewhere, were found to be two to four times more likely to have acquired HIV than those who had remained in their home cities. Half of the sex workers surveyed in central Nepal who said they had worked in Mumbai (India) were HIV-infected, compared with 1.2% of those who had never been to India.

In Southeast Asia, three countries—Cambodia, Myanmar and Thailand—are experiencing particularly serious epidemics. Cambodia's national HIV prevalence is around 1.5–4.4%, the highest recorded in Asia. However, its large-scale prevention programmes addressing sexual transmission of HIV have resulted in significant reductions in risk behaviour and declining levels of new HIV and other sexually transmitted infections. Fewer men are now visiting sex workers, and there has been a significant rise in condom use in commercial sex. The combined effect has been a steep drop in sexually transmitted infections and a steady decline in HIV prevalence in Cambodia. However, little has been done to monitor the epidemic among drug users or men who have sex with men, even though HIV prevalence among male sex workers in the capital was more than 15% when last measured in 2000 [38].

HIV prevalence among military recruits can be an indication of HIV spread in the general population. Myanmar is a case in point, with 2% of new recruits testing positive at two sites in 2003 [39]. Between 45 and 80% of drug injectors tested positive for HIV infection each year between 1992 and 2003. HIV prevalence rose in sex workers from 5% to 31% over the same period. Among sexually transmitted infection clinic patients, 6% of men and 9% of women tested HIV-positive in 2003 [21,39].

Thailand has shown that a well-funded, politically supported and pragmatic response can change the course of the epidemic. National adult HIV prevalence continues to edge lower, with the latest estimates putting it at 1.5% (0.8–2.8%) at the end of 2003 [2]. This remarkable achievement came about mainly because men used condoms more, and also reduced their visits to brothels. However, there is mounting evidence that the epidemic has shifted, requiring recharged commitment and revised strategies. Half of annual, new HIV infections are occurring among co-habiting couples, as more women are infected by husbands who are, or were, clients of sex workers. One-fifth of all new HIV infections are occurring through unsafe injecting drug use, compared with about one-twentieth a decade ago [40], with little preventive activity under way. Despite the illegality of injecting drug use, a pragmatic approach such as that adopted toward sex work in the 1990s is much more likely to bring success. The same holds true for men who have sex with men, among whom HIV prevalence is as high as 17% [41].

Widespread injecting drug use by sex workers makes Vietnam's epidemic particularly explosive. In Ho Chi Minh City, 38% of almost 1000 sex workers injected drugs, and 49% of injecting sex workers were infected with HIV, compared with 8% of those who did not use any drugs. In Haiphong, nearly 40% of all sex workers said they injected drugs, as did one in six sex workers in Hanoi. Drug-using sex workers are about half as likely to use condoms as those who do not use drugs, according to another study in Ho Chi Minh City, where HIV prevalence of 8% was detected in a 2003 survey among men who have sex with men [1].

Indonesia's epidemics are unevenly distributed across this vast archipelago nation of 210 million people; six of the 31 provinces are particularly badly affected. The country's epidemic is driven largely by the use of contaminated needles and syringes for drug injection. HIV prevalence among its estimated 125,000–196,000 injecting drug users tripled from 16% to 48% between 1999 and 2003. In Jakarta, HIV prevalence ranged from 66% to 93% among injecting drug users attending testing sites in 2002 and 2003. Incarceration of drug users is frequent, and in early 2003, 25% of inmates in Jakarta's Cipinang prison were HIV-positive. A recent survey in three cities found 88% of the injectors had used non-sterile needles or syringes in the preceding week, yet less than one-third said they felt at high risk of HIV infection [42]. There is strong evidence that various sexual and injecting drug-user networks in Indonesia overlap significantly, thus creating an ideal environment for the spread of HIV. Condom use ranges from irregular to rare. HIV prevalence among sex workers in Sorong, Papua reached 17% by 2003, over five times the national average for sex workers. Household surveys of young men and women in Jayapura and Merauke suggest patterns of sexual networking that could favour dynamic HIV spread in the general population on Papua [43].

Oceania

An estimated 35,000 people (25,000–48,000) in Oceania are living with HIV. Among young people 15–24 years of age, an estimated 0.2% of women (0.1–0.4%) and 0.2% of men (0.1–0.3%) were living with HIV by the end of 2004 [1]. The annual number of new HIV diagnoses in Australia has gradually increased from 650 in 1998 to about 800 in 2002. As in New Zealand, HIV transmission continues to be mainly through sexual intercourse between men, which accounted for more than 85% of new HIV diagnoses in the 5 years up to 2002. In a survey among men who have sex with men in Sydney, 25% of respondents reported unprotected anal sex with casual partners, compared with 18% in 1998–1999. Recent gonorrhoea surveillance data, too, have pointed to a possible increase in risky sexual behaviour among men who have sex with men, underlining the need to reinvigorate prevention efforts in this population [44]. Although per capita rates of HIV diagnoses among Australian Aborigines are similar to those in non-Aboriginal Australians, Aboriginal women constitute 36% of the total HIV-infected population, compared with non-Aboriginal, who comprise 11% of the total.

Papua New Guinea, which shares an island with Irian Jaya, one of Indonesia's worst-affected provinces, has the highest prevalence of HIV infection in Oceania. An estimated 0.6% (0.3–1.0%) of adults—roughly 16,000 (7800–28,000) people of the adult population of about 2.6 million—were living with HIV at the end of 2003 [1]. In 2003, 1.4% of pregnant women at antenatal clinics in the capital, Port Moresby, tested HIV-positive, while in Lae, in the central highlands, 2.5% of pregnant women were HIV-infected [21]. More than twice as many young women (aged 15–24 years) as men have been diagnosed with HIV. Available data suggest the epidemic is centred on commercial and casual sex, most of it heterosexual. A high incidence of rape, sexual aggression and other forms of violence against women appears to be aiding the epidemic's growth. According to one study, up to 70% of women have experienced domestic violence, while other studies have put the figure even higher [45]. Action to avert a rampant epidemic that will have ramifications for years to come is now urgent.

HIV infection levels appear to be very low in other parts of Oceania, but the data are extremely limited. On remote islands, seafarers and their partners appear to be most at risk, with high rates of sexually transmitted infections detected on Vanuatu and Samoa. In such contexts, once HIV makes its way into the tiny populations of island nations in Oceania, diffuse epidemics are likely to follow. Prevention strategies that reduce and treat sexually transmitted infections, and that quickly bolster AIDS knowledge among the population at large, are urgently needed.

High-income countries

An estimated 1.6 million people (range: 1.1–2.2 million) are living with HIV in North America and in Western and Central Europe. Among young people 15–24 years of age, 0.1% of women (range: 0.1–0.2%) and 0.2% of men (range: 0.1–0.5%) were living with HIV by the end of 2004 [1].

In high-income countries, where the great majority of people who need antiretroviral treatment do have access to it, PLHIV are staying healthy and surviving longer than infected people elsewhere. Widespread access to life-extending antiretroviral treatment kept the number of AIDS deaths at between 15,000 and 32,000 in 2004. However, prevention efforts are not keeping pace with the changing epidemics in several countries. Sex between men is the most common route of infection in Australia, Canada, Denmark, Germany, Greece and the USA. Patterns of HIV transmission are changing, with an increasing proportion of people becoming infected through unprotected heterosexual intercourse. In Belgium, Norway and the UK, the increase in heterosexually transmitted infections is dominated by people from countries with generalized epidemics, predominantly sub-Saharan Africa. In the USA, about half of all newly reported infections are among African Americans, who make up 12% of the population. Their HIV prevalence is 11 times higher than among whites. In New York City, over 1% of the adult population, and almost 2% of Manhattan's, was HIV-positive in 2001.

Drug injecting accounted for more than 10% of all reported HIV infections in Western Europe in 2002, and in Portugal it was responsible for over 50% of cases. In Canada and the USA, about 25% of HIV infections are attributed to drug injecting. Infections transmitted through contaminated injecting equipment are particularly frequent among indigenous people, who are often among the poorest and most marginalized inhabitants of the industrialized world.

Conclusion

Worldwide, HIV continues to spread. A massive effort is needed to increase coverage of proven interventions to achieve a response on a scale that matches that of the global AIDS epidemic. Virtually every region, including sub-Saharan Africa, has several countries where the epidemic is still at a low level or at an early enough stage to be held in check by effective preventive action. This calls for programmes that can thwart the spread of HIV among the most vulnerable population groups. However, in many countries, inadequate resources and a failure of political will and leadership still bar the way—especially where HIV has established footholds among marginalized and stigmatized population groups such as women who sell sex, drug injectors and men who have sex with men. Unless reticence is rapidly replaced with pragmatic and forward-looking approaches, HIV will spread more extensively in many countries that, until now, had escaped with only minor epidemics.

In the coming years, as access to life-prolonging antiretroviral treatment increases, more people will be living with HIV. Providing treatment is both a humanitarian and a rights issue. Without effective prevention to avert new HIV infections today, the goal of scaling up access to antiretroviral medications for all those living with HIV in need of treatment will be impossible to reach as long as the numbers of those falling ill with HIV-related disease continue to climb.

Acknowledgement

The authors would like to thank Valerie Manda for her assistance with references in the final manuscript.

References

1. UNAIDS. (2004). *AIDS Epidemic Update.* Geneva: UNAIDS.
2. UNAIDS. (2004). *Report on the Global AIDS Epidemic. 4th Global Report.* Geneva: UNAIDS.
3. The National AIDS Coordinating Agency, Botswana. (2003). *Second Generation HIV/AIDS Surveillance, A Technical Report.* Gaborone: The National AIDS Coordinating Agency.
4. The South African Department of Health Study. (2003). Available at: http://www.avert.org/safricastats.htm. Accessed March 2, 2005.
5. Shelton JD *et al.* Partner reduction is crucial for balanced 'ABC' approach to HIV prevention. *British Medical Journal* **328**: (10).
6. Singh S, Darroch JE, Bankole A. (2003). *A, B and C in Uganda: The Roles of Abstinence, Monogamy and Condom Use in HIV Decline.* Washington: The Alan Guttmacher Institute. Available at http://www.synergyaids.com/documents/UgandaABC.pdf.
7. Wawer MJ, Gray R, Serwadda D *et al.* (2005). *Declines in HIV Prevalence in Uganda: Not as Simple as ABC.* In: Book of Abstracts, 12th Conference on Retroviruses and Opportunistic Infections, February 22–25, 2005. Boston, MA.
8. Ministry of Health of Ethiopia. (2004). *AIDS in Ethiopia.* Fifth Report. Addis Ababa: 9. Ministry of Health, Disease Prevention and Control Department.
9. National AIDS and STDs Control Programme. (2005). *National HIV Prevalence in Kenya.* Nairobi, Kenya.
10. Schmid GP, Buve A, Mugyenyi P, Garnett GP, Hayes RJ, Williams BG *et al.* (2004). Transmission of HIV-1 infection in sub-Saharan Africa and effect of elimination of unsafe injections. *Lancet* **363**:482–8.
11. McCurdy SA, Williams ML, Timpson SC, *et al.* (2005). Perceived homelessness and STIs among injecting female heroin injectors, Dar es Salaam, Tanzania. In: *Abstract Book, AIDSIMPACT 2005.* Cape Town, South Africa.
12. Stover J. (2004). Projecting the demographic consequences of adult HIV prevalence trends: the Spectrum Projection Package. *Sexually Transmitted Infections* **80**: i14–18.
13. Kenya Demographic and Health Survey. (2003). Available at http://www.cbs.go.ke/kdhs2003.html. Accessed March 2, 2005.
14. Mali Enquète Démographique et de Santé. (2001). Available at http://www.measuredhs.com/hivdata/surveys/survey_detail.cfm?survey_id=159. Accessed March 2, 2005.

15. Pettifor AE, Rees HV, Steffenson A *et al.* (2004). *HIV and Sexual Health Behaviour Among Young South Africans: A National Survey of 15 to 24 Year Olds.* Johannesburg: Reproductive Health Research Unit, University of Witwatersrand.

16. Hunter M. (2002).The materiality of everyday sex: thinking beyond 'prostitution'. *African Studies* 61:99–120.

17. AIDS Foundation East-West. Officially registered HIV cases by region of the Russian Federation, 1 January 1987 through 22 March 2004. Available at http://hivinsite.ucsf.edu/global?page=cr03-rs-00. Accessed on March 2, 2005.

18. EuroHIV. (2003). *HIV/AIDS Durveillance in Europe.* Saint-Maurice: Institut de Veille Sanitaire (Mid-year Report 2003, No. 69). Available at http://www.eurohiv.org. Accessed March 2, 2005.

19. Ministerio da Saude do Brasil. (2001). *A Contribuicao dos Estudos Multicentricos Frente e Epidemia de HIV/AIDS entre UDIs no Brasil: 10 Anos de Pesquisa e Reducao de Danos.* Brasilia: Ministerio da Saude do Brasil. Available at www.aids.gov.br/final/biblioteca/avalia8/rio/parte % 2011/introducao.htm.

20. Marins JR, Barros MB, Jamal LF *et al.* (2003). Dramatic improvement in survival among adult Brazilian AIDS patients. *AIDS* 17:1675–82.

21. Monitoring the AIDS Pandemic (MAP) Network. (2004). Available at http://www.mapnetwork.org/docs/MAP_AIDSinAsia2004.pdf. Accessed March 3, 2005.

22. HIV infection and AIDS in the Americas: lessons and challenges for the future. MAP report 2003. Available at http://www.mapnetwork.org/MAPLACDraftApril9.2003%20to%20print.doc. Accessed March 4, 2005.

23. Alarcon JO, Johnson KM, Courtois B, Rodriguez C, Sanchez J, Watts DM, Holmes KK. (2003). Determinants and prevalence of HIV infection in pregnant Peruvian women. *AIDS* 17:613–8.

24. Johnson KM, Alarcon J, Watts D, Rodriguez C, Velasquez C, Sanchez J. (2003). Sexual networks of pregnant women with and without HIV infection. *AIDS* 17:605–12.

25. Guanira JV, Pun M, Manrique H. (2004). Second generation of HIV surveillance among men who have sex with men in Peru during 2002. In: Abstract WePe. Proceedings of the XV International AIDS Conference, July 11–16 2004, Bangkok, Thailand.

26. Caribbean Epidemiology Centre (CAREC)/PAHO/WHO. (2004). *Status and Trends, Analysis of the Caribbean HIV/AIDS Epidemic 1982–2002.* Caribbean Epidemiology Centre, Trinidad and Tobago. 2004; Available at http://www.carec.org/. Accessed March 3, 2005.

27. Caribbean Epidemiology Centre. The Caribbean HIV/AIDS epidemiological status—success stories: a summary. CAREC Surveillance Report. Available at http://www.carec.org/documents/csr_supplement.pdf. Accessed March 3, 2005.

28. Zhang KL, Ma SJ and Xia DY, (2004). Epidemiology of HIV and sexually transmitted infections in China. *Sexual Health* 1: 39–46.

29. China National Centre for HIV/STD Control and Prevention. (2003). *Questionnaire Survey of Injecting Drug Users in a Compulsory Detoxification Centre and Non-treatment Locations in Beijing.* Beijing: World Health Organization.

30. Choi K, Hui Liu, Guo Y, Han L, Mandel JS, Rutherford GW. (2003). Emerging HIV-1 epidemic in China in men who have sex with men. *Lancet* 361:2125.

31. Shengli C, Shikun Z, Westley SB. (2004). HIV/AIDS awareness is improving in China. *Asia Pacific Population and Policy* 69:1–5.

32. UNAIDS/WHO. (2003). AIDS Epidemic Update 2003. Geneva:UNAIDS/WHO.

33. Go VF, Srikrishnan AK, Sivaram S *et al.* (2004). High HIV prevalence and risk behaviors in men who have sex with men in Chennai, India. *Journal of Acquired Immune Deficiency Syndrome* 35:314–9.

34. National AIDS Control Organisation (NACO). National baseline high risk and bridge population behavioural surveillance survey part II: men who have sex with men and injecting drug users.2002; Available at http://www.nacoonline.org/publication/51.pdf. Accessed March 3, 2005.

35. Dhaka (2003). *HIV in Bangladesh: Is Time Running Out?* National AIDS/STD Programme of the Directorate General of Health Services, Ministry of Health and Family Welfare, Government of the People's Republic of Bangladesh.

36. Shah SA, Altaf A, Mujeeb SA, Memon A. (2004). An outbreak of HIV infection among injection drug users in a small town in Pakistan: potential for national implications. *International Journal of STD and AIDS* 15:209–10.

37. Zafar T, Brahmbhatt H, Imam G, Hassan S, Strathdee S. (2003). HIV knowledge and risk behaviors among Pakistani and Afghani drug users in Quetta, Pakistan. *Journal of Acquired Immune Deficiency Syndrome* 32:394–8.

38. Girault P, Saidel T, Song N *et al.* (2004). HIV, STIs, and sexual behaviors among men who have sex with men in Phnom Penh, Cambodia. *AIDS Education and Prevention* 16:31–44.

39. Department of Health. (2003). *Myanmar Sentinel Surveillance Data for March–April 2003.* AIDS Prevention and Control Project. Myanmar Ministry of Health.

40. Brown T, Peerapatanapokin W (Thai Working Group on HIV Estimation and Projection). (2001). *Projections for HIV and AIDS in Thailand: 2000–2020.* Bangkok: AIDS Division, Ministry of Public Health.

41. UNDP. (2004). Thailand's response to HIV/AIDS: progress and challenges. Bangkok, UNDP. Available at http://www.undp.or.th/documents/HIV_AIDS_FullReport_ENG.pdf. Accessed March 3, 2005.

42. Pisani E, Dadun, Sucahya PK, Purwa K, Kamil O, Jazan S. (2003). Sexual behavior among injection drug users in 3 Indonesian Cities carries a high potential for HIV spread to noninjectors. *Journal of Acquired Immune Deficiency Syndrome* 34:403–6.

43. Indonesia Central Bureau of Statistics and MACRO International. Indonesia young adult's reproductive health survey 2002–2003. Available at http://www.measuredhs.com/pubs/pdf/FR157/00FrontMatter.pdf. Accessed March 4, 2005.

44. HIV/AIDS, viral hepatitis and sexually transmitted infections in Australia: annual surveillance report 2003. Available at http://www.med.unsw.edu.au/nchecr/Downloads/03ansurvrpt.pdf. Accessed March 3, 2005.

45. Brouwer EC; Harris BM; Tanaka S, eds. (1998). *Gender Analysis in Papua New Guinea.* Washington, DC: The World Bank.

Chapter 3

Social and economic impact of the HIV pandemic

Tim Quinlan and Alan Whiteside[*]

Introduction

In early 2003, an outbreak of a new disease, severe acute respiratory syndrome (SARS), caused panic around the world. In Asia, there was huge disruption to international travel. For example, Cathay Pacific, the major airline flying from Hong Kong, saw passenger numbers fall from 35,000 per day in June 2002 to 8000 per day in June 2003 [1]. A localized outbreak in Toronto led to a rapid mobilization of the public health system and imposition of quarantines. The resulting restrictions included the cancellation of a number of sporting and cultural events and hit the local economy. When the disease was finally brought under control and the costs were totalled, SARS had claimed 321 lives in 26 countries [2]. The estimated cost to the global economy was between US$40 billion and US$140 billion [3].

In contrast, HIV has been recognized for over 20 years. The first cases were seen in 1981 and the test to identify antibodies was available as of 1983. The early extensive press coverage and concern that the disease represented a threat to the developed world has been replaced by the realization that the disease mainly affects those in resource-poor settings and does not represent a threat to the global economy. It is estimated that there were between 34 and 46 million people infected as of December 2003 [4]. Since the epidemic began, there have been perhaps 60 million infections and 20 million deaths. The HIV epidemic has not been brought under control, and the toll continues to mount. Yet, this disease has not had the level of global, social and economic response that SARS had. Nor, we argue, is it likely to. This chapter explains why this is the case, but first we need to look at the impacts of the pandemic.

What is the economic and social impact?

Measuring the economic impact—the effect on nations' economic development, the production of firms, and household economies—of AIDS should, in theory, be reasonably easy. For instance, the cost of treating people who have fallen ill is measurable in monetary terms. There are also techniques to assess the cost of lost production because a person is ill or because they have died. The reality is rather different; we lack data and are not always sure how to interpret the limited information we do have available. How to use data is an issue which we cannot explore in detail here, but it is an issue that needs to be highlighted. Much research still uses restrictive concepts such as 'household', orphans as children under the age of 15 years, and

* Corresponding author.

'affected' versus 'non-affected' individuals/families/households. This is problematic because they fail to explain, or indeed even capture, the profound multiple effects of HIV across society.

When we discuss economic impact, we can look at various levels. These range from households, through community and firm, to the macro or national economy.

Microeconomic impact

Scientists' ability to measure the impacts of death or illness of a breadwinner stems from the fact that the root causes of many diseases are known, often effectively treatable and, importantly, medical science generally has long experience in working out how to manage their effects on individuals and society at large. AIDS is somewhat different [5–7]. Its origins and pathology are hidden for several years. It is a relatively new 'disease', and there is as yet no cure.

The first papers to postulate micro-level impact appeared in the early 1990s. Over the past few years, a second phase of household studies, particularly in Africa, has produced new data [8–12]. These studies show that there is a close relationship between a household being affected by HIV and its subsequent impoverishment. Children in such households are particularly vulnerable. In a phrase, AIDS is bad news for affected households.

Nonetheless, there are problems with household economic impact assessments. They tend to concentrate on rural households and ignore the urban and peri-urban areas; are mainly *economic* studies concentrating on monetary measures; look at *households* and thus exclude information about relationships between households; and methods do not capture the most seriously affected households, for example those that have already disintegrated due to the impact of the disease. However, most seriously, they do not capture the dynamics of a deteriorating situation—locally, regionally and globally—described in other chapters. Only in Uganda, Brazil and Thailand has mortality from national epidemics peaked and begun to fall. Relatively small epidemics are controlled in North America and Western Europe, but the threat of extended outbreaks remains. In Eastern Europe and Asia, national and regional epidemics are spreading. There is a pandemic throughout Southern and Central Africa, some indications that HIV is currently under control in a few West African countries, and epidemics in North Africa that are perceived to be slowly spreading, but limited—though there is little information to substantiate this.

A survey of households affected by HIV in South Africa, released in 2002, gives a clear indication of the impoverishing nature of the epidemic in developing countries [13]. The study surveyed more than 700 households with at least one person already sick with AIDS. Significantly, the sample was drawn from households already in contact with non-governmental organizations (NGOs). It was a snapshot of HIV-affected families and, if anything, underestimated impacts. Key findings are shown in Box 3.1.

South Africa is fortunate in that there is a formal social safety net, however imperfect, in the form of child grants and pensions. Despite this, millions of South Africans face growing misery. The situation is replicated across the rest of the continent and becoming evident in Eastern Europe, Asia and Central America. The negative economic and social consequences of this disease are not well understood, and many of them are still evolving, but there is some evidence accumulating. In Malawi, for instance, there is a small but growing body of empirical work that highlights the inexorable impoverishment of much of the population [11]. In turn, this economic strain has far-reaching social impacts. Recent studies in Mexico, Thailand, Botswana and South Africa highlight the psychosocial stress on individuals and families [14–18]. More generally, the World Food Programme has shown that the poor are

---

Box 3.1 **Key findings-Survey of households affected by HIV in South Africa, 2002**

1. Two-thirds of the households in the survey reported loss of income as a consequence of HIV.

2. Almost half reported not having enough food and that their children were going hungry.

3. Almost a quarter of all children under age 15 in the sample had already lost at least one parent.

4. In 12% of the households, children were sent away to live elsewhere; in 8%, children under 18 were the primary caregivers; and in 25% of households, caregivers were over 60.

5. More than two-thirds of the people with AIDS in the survey were women and girls, with an average age of 33.

6. Only about 50% of the respondents had acknowledged publicly that the sick person they were caring for had HIV; one in 10 reported hostility and rejection.

7. Less than 16% of households in the survey were receiving government grants of any kind, even though all qualified for some form of assistance.

8. Some 55% of AIDS-affected households had paid for a funeral in the last year, spending, on average, four times their total monthly income on the funeral [13].

---

getting poorer in Southern Africa, to the point that food aid is essential because, even if the effects of HIV on people's existing vulnerability to drought and war are not well understood, starvation is a reality [19].

In sum, the household economic impact assessments undertaken to date have been flawed and incomplete. Furthermore, such studies seldom provide a clear indication of how the impact of HIV on households can be mitigated. Greener summarizes this neatly:

> It is clear, however, that the most serious impacts of HIV/AIDS are felt at the level of households, who are more likely to fall into poverty, or firms, who face higher employment costs, and of governments, who are likely to face falling revenue and rising expenditure demands. The extent of these effects will form important research areas in the coming years, and are probably more important than further studies of impact on aggregate GDP [20].

Between the macro and the micro

When national accounts are reviewed, production is divided by sectors, typically manufacturing, services, agriculture, government, and so on. The measured wealth of the country is produced by individuals, companies and the government, who respectively grow the crops, make the goods and provide the services. The small-scale subsistence farmer, diamond mine and government hospital all contribute to the national economy. Not included in national accounts are informal care and domestic labour carried out mainly by women outside the formal labour market. In short, conventionally productive activities take place between the macro- and micro-levels of a national economy. The impact of AIDS at this level needs to be considered, yet there is surprisingly little information.

At the firm level, we know that AIDS can add substantially to payroll costs, thereby increasing the cost of doing business [21]. While there have been studies on the impact of AIDS on large companies, there is little information on small companies, the informal sector and subsistence agriculture because of the difficulties of designing research for these sectors. With regard to subsistence agriculture, there are a few studies. The findings are similar; for example, a study for the Zimbabwe Farmers' Union in one small and communal farm area found that any adult death had an adverse effect on output, but that, in the case of AIDS, this effect was worse. An adult death resulted in a 45% decline in marketed output of maize but, where the cause of death was identified as AIDS, there was a 61% loss [22]. We assume that this greater impact was due to the nature of AIDS. People die at younger ages, the period of illness is protracted, and there is evidence that productive assets are more likely to be sold to provide for the household and the patient.

With regard to the impact of AIDS on productivity, we are aware of only one study, on a tea plantation in Kericho district in Kenya [23]. The researchers reviewed records of workers' health and output over a 5-year period. The principal finding was that during the last years of life, tea pluckers who died due to AIDS were absent from work almost twice as often as other tea pluckers. Most (58%) of this difference comprised unpaid and unauthorized leave. Output began to fall as early as 3 years before death for those who were HIV-infected.

The impact on productivity among other workers has not been addressed. Of great concern is the public sector, where job security is often seen as a substitute for salary. People accept lower pay and expect other benefits, including substantial sick leave. In normal times, this can be and is factored into planning production in the government and parastatal sector. However, AIDS means times are not normal, and it is probable that governments will operate increasingly inefficiently, with all the attendant consequences for the business environment, competitiveness and output. For example, there may be delays in clearing goods through customs at borders or posts. The issuing of permits to do business and for tax clearance may become tardier.

A South African study on the impact of HIV on the education system in one province, KwaZulu-Natal, has highlighted the diverse costs of teacher illness and death on teaching activities, schools and, notably, the capacity of the education department to deliver on its mandate [24]. Also, the demand for healthcare is rising at a time when capacity to provide care, particularly in resource-poor countries, is under threat. Health workers are falling ill and dying from AIDS in a period of marked international mobility of doctors and nurses. There is discernible evidence of many other health workers leaving state services and emigrating in response to public and private sector incentives, particularly to North America and Western Europe [25–27]. The increase in adult mortality is creating large numbers of orphans, and they, in turn, need government support. The elderly are facing ever-larger demands on their pensions as they take in grandchildren.

Macroeconomic impact

Will AIDS cause national economies as a whole to grow more slowly? AIDS advocates and activists have suggested that evidence of macroeconomic impact will persuade people to respond to the epidemic. To governments they say, 'AIDS means that economic growth will be slower than expected, you will have less money to spend and your people will be poorer than they would have been in the absence of AIDS'. To company chief executive officers, the suggestion is that they need to respond to the disease because 'AIDS will put up the cost of labour, decrease productivity and affect markets'. To mobilize the international community they say, 'Africa's per capita growth is 0.7% per annum lower than it would have been in the absence of AIDS'.

As early as 1992, economists predicted that AIDS would slow economic growth, although the extent would depend on who was infected and the degree to which the response to the illness was funded from savings, thereby limiting investment [28,29]. One World Bank economist suggested that AIDS had reduced Africa's economic growth by 0.8% per annum in the 1990s and that HIV and malaria combined had resulted in an annual 1.2% decrease in gross domestic product (GDP) growth between 1990 and 1995 [30].

Most empirical work on the macroeconomic impact of the disease comes from South Africa. The headline finding is that AIDS will cause an economy to grow more slowly than it would otherwise, but not by very much—the current estimates point to a decline in the growth of GDP of around 0.5% per annum [30]. Of course, over time, this compounds to produce a significant impact. The analytical problem is that there are so many other things going on in an economy that it is hard to disentangle the AIDS impact even with hindsight, let alone predict it into the future. The South African Bureau for Economic Research has recently concluded:

> While the economic impact of HIV is negative, we are far from witnessing a doomsday scenario. The negative impact on real GDP growth is gradual and the economy could continue to register 3 per cent average real GDP growth (or better) over the next 10 to 15 years; inflation could still average around 7 per cent (in line with the past 5–6 years); real interest rates may only be marginally higher; the current account deficit could average below 2 per cent of GDP and the budget deficit below 3 per cent of GDP [31].

Despite the inevitable uncertainties of macroeconomic studies, there is growing interest in them. The reasons are simple:

1. The scale and growth of the epidemic is worse than expected. The number of people infected with HIV in 2004 was considerably above that predicted in 1990.

2. Known demographic effects are now such that recognition of economic consequences is unavoidable. For example, in South Africa, mortality has doubled due to AIDS and most deaths are of people in their 30s and 40s. Population growth is slowing and structures are changing.

3. There is similar evidence of impact at micro-levels, making calculations of macro-impacts credible. If sufficient numbers of households are impoverished or dissolving, then it must have an effect on local markets. As the cost of business rises—because workers fall sick, are less productive or their benefits rise—this must be factored into investment decisions.

The complexity of the disease and the scope of its consequences are better understood. For example, loss of key government workers means work is not done efficiently, investment is reduced and economic growth slows [32–36]. The example of customs delays given above is an immediate impact. In the longer term, if the education sector operates less efficiently due to teacher illness and death, then this will have effects on the next generation of workers.

Others have bleaker predictions, arguing, for example, that conventional economics misses the complexity and full significance of the epidemic [37]. When the epidemic was in its early stages, projections based on scenarios computed 'with AIDS' and 'without AIDS' were reasonable, but such comparisons are no longer valid. The disease cannot be treated as an exogenous influence that can be tacked on to models derived on the presumption that the workforce is not infected with HIV. HIV is now an endogenous influence on most African countries. Macpherson *et al.* [37] point out that rising prevalence of HIV lowers worker efficiency, raises costs and reduces individual savings and firms' profits. The problem with an economic downturn is that once it begins, it is not easy to halt. AIDS has the potential to push economies into decline and then keep them there.

A recent paper from the World Bank suggests that the long-term economic costs of AIDS are almost certain to be very much higher than predicted to date, and may be devastating [38]. The paper presents a model that is then applied to South Africa. It emphasizes the importance of human capital, i.e. the skills and aptitudes of people, and how it is transmitted across generations. AIDS, the authors say, will severely retard economic growth because:

+ it destroys existing human capital, particularly of young adults;
+ it wrecks the mechanisms that generate human investment in children and young people through the death of parents and loss of income;
+ as children become adults with little education and little knowledge, they are less able to raise their own children and invest in their education.

This long report proposes three instruments to avoid economic collapse. These are:

+ spending on measures to contain the disease and treat infected people, a point particularly significant for this book;
+ aiding orphans in the form of income support or subsidies;
+ taxes to finance the programme.

However, these proposals raise policy and political questions to which, as other chapters intimate, many governments have given inadequate answers. Importantly, the questions and answers highlight why the world does not, and will not, respond to HIV as it did to the SARS outbreak, as described at the outset of the chapter.

For instance, the proposals challenge governments to consider the revival of 'welfare state' policies and the reorientation of national budget allocations towards more social spending in a world driven by market forces [39–41]. South Africa is a notable example of these challenges in view of the contentious political statements of its President and the vociferous public debate on, and legal challenges to, government policies in the context of the HIV epidemic [42,43]. More broadly, the funding, development and elaboration of national programmes that include provision of antiretroviral treatment (ART) is a challenge that has yet to be well understood. We can predict that if ART is made available widely, then some of the increase in morbidity, mortality and its sequelae will be postponed. However, this will have a very significant cost. Resources spent on ART, be they financial, staff or infrastructural, cannot be used for other things, although they may represent a saving on other expenditure.

The 2001 report of the Commission on Macroeconomics and Health made the compelling argument that investing in health could result in macroeconomic growth [44]. It provided evidence to suggest that good health is necessary but not sufficient for economic growth. Historical evidence from Europe, the USA and other Organization for Economic Cooperation and Development (OECD) countries suggests that economic take-off was supported by breakthroughs in public health, disease control and better nutrition. The Commission argued that poor societies with a heavy burden of disease face many severe impediments to economic progress. Most striking was the statement that: 'A typical statistical estimate suggests that each 10% improvement in life expectancy at birth (LEB) is associated with a rise in economic growth of at least 0.3 to 0.4 percentage points per year, holding other growth factors constant' [44, p. 24]. In the high-income countries, life expectancy at birth is 75 years for men and 81 for women and rising; in sub-Saharan Africa, it is 49 years for men and 52 for women and falling [45]. 'Thus the difference in growth will be about 11.6 percentage points per year, and this will cumulate rapidly. In short, health status seems to explain an important part of the difference in economic growth rates, even after controlling for standard macroeconomic variables' [44].

Table 3.1 HIV expenditure and prevalence in selected countries

Country	Adult HIV prevalence (%) 2001	GDP per capita (US$) 2001	Health expenditure per capita (US$) 2000	% of GDP 2000
Canada	0.31	27,130	2534	6.5
USA	0.61	34,320	4499	5.8
France	0.33	23,990	2380	7.2
UK	0.10	24,160	1804	5.9
Italy	0.37	24,670	2028	5.9
Spain	0.50	20,150	1547	5.4
Barbados	1.20	15,560	909	4.2
Argentina	0.69	11,320	1091	4.7
Chile	0.30	9190	697	3.1
Costa Rica	0.55	9460	474	4.7
Mexico	0.28	8430	477	2.5
Cuba	<0.10	5259	193	6.1
Russia	0.90	7100	405	3.7
Thailand	1.79	6400	237	2.1
Brazil	0.65	7360	631	3.4
Philippines	<0.10	3840	167	1.5
Ukraine	0.99	4350	152	2.9
Jamaica	1.22	3720	208	2.6
China	0.11	4020	205	2.0
Guyana	2.70	4690	198	4.2
South Africa	20.10	11,290	663	3.7
Indonesia	0.10	2940	84	0.6
India	0.79	2840	71	0.9
Botswana	38.80	7820	358	3.7
Cambodia	2.70	1860	97	1.0
Haiti	6.10	1860	56	2.4
Nigeria	5.80	850	15	0.5
Uganda	5.00	1490	38	1.6
Senegal	0.50	1500	56	2.6
Ethiopia	6.41	810	14	1.1

Source: United Nations Development Programme (UNDP) *Human Development Report*, 2003 [46].

It is clear, though, that the impacts will evolve. It will take a generation or so before we will be able to assess what the epidemic has meant. It is also clear that the impact is not going to be uniform. The contrast in countries is considerable, as is illustrated in Table 3.1.

The impact of the disease will depend on two primary factors: the size of the epidemic and the ability of the country to mobilize resources to deal with it. For example, Zambia has an HIV prevalence of 22%, which is more than 20 times that of Brazil at 0.7%. Furthermore, the GDP per capita of Zambia is US$780, which is many times smaller than that of Brazil at US$7360.

The conclusion is simple: the economic impact of AIDS has to be looked at in the context of each country. Some countries have very small epidemics that will probably remain small, for example Senegal and the Philippines. Some countries either have resources to deal with the disease or have been able to mobilize resources from the international community—Thailand, Brazil, Botswana and South Africa provide examples, although the political will has been lacking in South Africa.

This chapter has not covered the development consequences of HIV. Measurement of a country's progress in development terms is more than an economic issue. 'Economic growth is the promise that governments offer to people. Continued delivery of growth affords legitimacy to government. Economic growth is the means; "development", improved living standards, better quality of life—all these are the ends' [47]. This was recognized by the United Nations Development Programme (UNDP), which began publishing a Human Development Report in 1990. The first report opened with the statement: 'The real wealth of a nation is its people. And the purpose of development is to create an enabling environment for people to enjoy long, healthy and creative lives. This simple but powerful truth is too often forgotten in the pursuit of material and financial wealth' [48]. The Human Development Index (HDI) introduced in 1990 is designed to capture as many aspects of human development as possible in one simple composite index combining:

- life expectancy, which is a proxy indicator for longevity;
- educational attainment, which is proxied by literacy and enrolment rates;
- standard of living, which is proxied by real GDP per capita.

The measure that will be affected first is life expectancy, consequent to increased infant and child mortality and premature deaths among adults. The UNDP's Human Development Reports track how life expectancy has fallen with the resulting decline in HDI and changes in the ranking of countries. This is shown in Table 3.2 for selected African countries.

At the UN Millennium Summit in 2000, 189 countries adopted eight Millennium Development Goals. HIV means that it will be very difficult for many African countries to achieve these goals, and some may now be beyond the reach of some countries on the continent. Thus, although the economic consequences of the disease are severe, they are more than economic.

AIDS, security and sustainability

Recently, HIV has been proclaimed a global security issue in addition to being a major development challenge. Again, the proclamations belie a global, comprehensive effort to contain the pandemic, as was the case with SARS. However, just as arguing that AIDS is the most important development challenge amidst a plethora of other challenges of varying significance to different countries, so too it is problematic to argue that AIDS is a security

Table 3.2 Life expectancy and place in the Human Development Index (HDI)

	1996 Report (1993 data)		1999 Report (1997 data)		2001 Report (1999 data)		2003 Report (2001 data)	
	Life expectancy	HDI (rank)	Life expectancy	HDI (rank)	Life expectancy	HDI (rank)	Life expectancy	HDI (rank)
Botswana	65	0.741 (71)	47.4	0.678 (97)	41.9	0.577 (114)	44.7	0.614 (125)
Nigeria	50.6	0.400(137)	50.1	0.391 (142)	51.5	0.455 (136)	51.8	0.463 (152)
South Africa	63.2	0.649(100)	54.7	0.717 (89)	53.9	0.701 (94)	50.9	0.684 (111)
Swaziland	57.8	0.586 (110)	60.2	0.597 (115)	47	0.583 (113)	38.2	0.547 (133)
Zimbabwe	53.4	0.534 (124)	44.1	0.507(130)	42.9	0.554 (117)	35.4	0.496 (145)

Source: UNDP reports [48,49].

issue. In an insightful discussion, Professor Gwyn Prins of the London School of Economics and Columbia University noted:

> During the last twenty years, there has often been an uneasy relationship between the claim that an issue is important and that it is a security issue. That is because the political stakes of so doing are high, but so too are the costs. If an issue can be 'securitised', it is the equivalent of playing a trump at cards, for at once it leap-frogs other issues in priority. But the unavoidable cost of this is, first, that to obtain that priority, people must be persuaded to be afraid of the threat, and to see it as a 'real and present danger', secondly, it throws the solution into the hands of state—or state-derived and mediated—structures, for they alone command the resources to satisfy the scale and urgency of the 'securitised' threat once accepted as such [50].

AIDS has been made a security issue in the theoretical sense and at a political level. In 2000, it was discussed at a special session of the United Nations Security Council. Subsequently, AIDS has been the subject of two reports issued by the US National Intelligence Council [51,52]. It is, however, difficult to understand exactly what calling AIDS a security threat will mean in practical terms. For instance, the Health Economics and HIV/AIDS Research Division (HEARD) of the University of KwaZulu-Natal has convened a number of meetings to discuss this topic. There was a great deal of concern, but no evidence of whether such a threat exists [53].

Of equal importance is the issue of sustainability, or ensuring that support can be maintained for as long as necessary. The rush to provide ART is the one area where this is not being addressed. The moral argument is that as much treatment as possible for as many people as possible should be provided. While this is laudable, it has to be understood that commitment to treatment means committing resources for as long as people can tolerate the drugs and continue to thrive. The economic costs of sustaining such treatment alongside associated treatment and support, such as nutrition, have not been calculated anywhere. Indeed, work has only just begun on the broader questions of how to devise appropriate strategies and programmes that integrate the multiple factors, such as institutional restructuring, coordination of different activities or 'mainstreaming', that need to be addressed.

Conclusion

In summary, the reasons for the different response to SARS compared with HIV can be discerned from assessing the efforts to understand the consequences of the HIV pandemic. There is a relative lack of data compared with SARS. There are limitations to research methods. These limitations are known, and there are continual efforts to refine and improve them. However, this is a process that takes time in view of the difficulties of designing research and, in turn, practical interventions that take into account the diverse consequences of the pandemic. Equally, despite warnings from scientists, and from populations that are experiencing the devastation caused by AIDS, the sorts of effects that make policy-makers and governments take notice take time to reveal themselves. Furthermore, piling up the evidence does not necessarily invoke a concerted response. The challenge of what ought to be done includes a demand for more social welfare-oriented policies and programmes. For example, there is a need to consider providing financial grants for at-risk families. Even food packages may be necessary. However, this runs counter to global market economic forces. At root, the effects vary greatly from country to country and take time to accumulate, unlike those of SARS and other global influenza-type threats, where deaths and illness occur in a matter days or weeks.

The limitations of economic impact assessments have been described, and the social impacts are even less understood or measured. One of the key problems in looking at these impacts is that the epidemic is still evolving. The long incubation period between infection and illness means that some 7–8 years will elapse before people begin to fall ill and show up in the health system. This means that the epidemic's impacts will take many more years to emerge.

The risk is that discussion over the next decade will centre on various forms of treatment and what these mean for healthcare systems. This may be problematic if, as a result, it ignores the many wider impacts of the disease outlined in this chapter, and how they may be reduced by other means.

References

1. *Pacific Business News*, 5 June 2003.
2. World Health Organization. (2003). *Report by the Secretariat to the 113th Session of the Executive Board of the WHO, 27 November.* Geneva: WHO.
3. *Straits Times*, 2 October 2003. Singapore.
4. UNAIDS. (2003). *Epidemic Update December 2003.* Geneva: UNAIDS.
5. World Bank (1997). Coping with the impact of AIDS. In: *Confronting AIDS: Public Priorities in a Global Epidemic.* World Bank: Washington, DC.
6. UNAIDS. (2000). Consultation on STD interventions for preventing HIV: what is the evidence? *UNAIDS Best Practice Collection.* Geneva: UNAIDS, p26–7.
7. Morrison SJ. (2002). *Expanding Antiretroviral Treatment in Developing Countries Creates Critical New Challenges.* Washington, DC: Center for Strategic and International Studies (CSIS), CSIS HIV/AIDS Task Force.
8. Booysen F le R, Van Rensburg D, Bechmann M, Engelbrecht M, Steyn F. (2002). The Socio-Economic Impact of HIV/AIDS on Households in South Africa: Pilot Study in Welkom and Qwaqwa, Free State Province. University of the Free State, South Africa, May 2002. *MRC AIDS Bulletin* 11(1).
9. Yamano T, Jayne TS. (2003) Measuring the Impacts of Prime-Age Adult Death on Rural Households in Kenya. Paper presented at the scientific meeting on Empirical Evidence for the Demographic and Socio-Economic Impacts of AIDS, Durban, March 2003.
10. Mushati P, Gregson S, Mlilo M, Lewis J, Zvidzai C. (2003). Adult mortality and erosion of households viability in towns, estates and villages in eastern Zimbabwe. Paper presented at the scientific meeting on Empirical Evidence for the Demographic and Socio-Economic Impacts of AIDS, Durban, March 2003.
11. Floyd S, Crampin A, Glynn J *et al.* (2003). The Impact of HIV on Households Structure in Rural Malawi. Paper presented at the scientific meeting on Empirical Evidence for the Demographic and Socio-Economic Impacts of AIDS, Durban, March 2003.
12. Hosegood V, Herbst K, Timaeus I. (2003). The Impact of Adult AIDS Deaths on Household Structure and Living Arrangements in Rural South Africa. Paper presented at the scientific meeting on Empirical Evidence for the Demographic and Socio-Economic Impacts of AIDS, Durban, March 2003.

13. Steinberg M, Johnson S, Schierhout G *et al.* (2002). *Hitting Home: How Households Cope with the Impact of the HIV/AIDS Epidemic: A Survey of Households Affected by HIV/AIDS inSouth Africa.* Durban: Health Systems Trust, and Washington, DC: The Kaiser Family Foundation.

14. Akintola G. (2004). Home-based care: a gendered analysis of informal caregiving for people living with HIV/AIDS in a semi-rural South African setting. PhD thesis, University of KwaZulu-Natal. Paper presented at the Empirical Evidence for the Demographic and Socio-Economic Impacts of AIDS, Durban, March 2003.

15. Gertler P, Levine D, Martinez S, Bertozzi S. (2003). The Presence and Presents of Parents: Do Parents Matter More than Their Money? Paper presented at the scientific meeting on Empirical Evidence for the Demographic and Socio-Economic Impacts of AIDS, Durban, March 2003.

16. Daniel M. (2003). Children Without Parents in Botswana: The Safety Net and Beyond. Paper presented at the scientific meeting on Empirical Evidence for the Demographic and Socio-Economic Impacts of AIDS, Durban, March 2003.

17. Knodel J, Im-Em W. (2003). The Economic Consequences for Parents of Losing an Adult Child to AIDS: Evidence from Thailand. Paper presented at the scientific meeting on Empirical Evidence for the Demographic and Socio-Economic Impacts of AIDS, Durban, March 2003.

18. Nyamukapa C, Gregson S, Wambe M. (2003). Extended Family Child Care and Orphan Education in Eastern Zimbabwe. Paper presented at the scientific meeting on Empirical Evidence for the Demographic and Socio-Economic Impacts of AIDS, Durban, March 2003.

19. De Waal A, Whiteside A. (2003). New variant famine: AIDS and food crisis in southern Africa. *Lancet* 362(11):1234–7.

20. Greener R. (2002). AIDS and macroeconomic impact. In: Forsythe S, ed. *State of The Art: AIDS and Economics, The Policy Project.* Washington, DC: IAEN.

21. Rosen SB, MacLeod W, Vincent J, Fox M, Thea D, Simon J. (2002*).* Investing in the Epidemic: The Impact of AIDS on Businesses in Southern Africa. Paper presented at the XIV International AIDS Conference, Barcelona, July 2002.

22. Kwaramba P. (1998). *The Socio-economic Impact of HIV/AIDS on Communal Agricultural Production Systems in Zimbabwe.* Harare: Friedrich Ebert Stiftung. Economic Advisory Project, Working Paper 19.

23. Fox M, Simon J, Bii M *et al.* (2003). The Impact of Labour Productivity in Kenya. Paper presented at the scientific meeting on Empirical Evidence for the Demographic and Socio-Economic Impact of AIDS, Durban, March 2003.

24. Badcock-Walters P, Desmond C, Wilson D, Heard W. (2003). Educator Mortality In-service in KwaZulu-Natal: A Consolidated Study of HIV/AIDS Impact and Trends. Paper presented at the scientific meeting on Empirical Evidence for the Demographic and Socio-Economic Impact of AIDS, Durban, March, 2003.

25. Brown R, Connell J. (2003). The migration of doctors and nurses from South Pacific Island nations. School of Economics, University of Queensland. Unpublished.

26. Mowatt R, Quinlan T. (2003). *A Rapid Appraisal of the Cost of HIV/AIDS Treatment to the KwaZulu-Natal Public Health Services.* Durban: HEARD.

27. Jinabhai C, Whittaker S, Sasha Y, Govender M, Green-Thompson R, Bourne D. (2002). *The Impact of the HIV/AIDS Epidemic on Hospital Services in South Africa: Responses, Coping Strategies and Behaviour of Management and Health Professionals.* Durban: School of Family and Public Health, Nelson Mandela School of Medicine, University of KwaZulu-Natal. (Report for the World Health Organization).

28. Over M. (1992). *Macroeconomic Impact of AIDS in Sub-Saharan Africa.* Washington, DC, World Bank, Africa Technical Department, Population, Health and Nutrition Division, (Technical Working paper, 3).

29. Bonnell R. (2000). HIV/AIDS and economic growth: a global perspective. *Journal of South African Economics* **68**:820–55.

30. ING Barings. (2000). *Economic Impact of AIDS in South Africa: A Dark Cloud on the Horizon.* Johannesburg: ING Barings.

31. Bureau for Economic Research. (2001). *The Macro-economic Impact of HIV/AIDS in South Africa.* University of Stellenbosch.

32. Cohen D. (2002). *Human Capital and HIV Epidemic in Sub-Saharan Africa, ILO Programme on HIV/ AIDS and the World of Work.* Geneva: ILO.

33. Government of Swaziland. (2002). *Assessment of the Impact of HIV/AIDS on the Central Agencies of the Government of the Kingdom of Swaziland: Executive Summary.* Mbabane: Government of Swaziland.

34. Husain I, Badcock-Walters P. (2002). Economics of HIV/AIDS Impact Mitigation: Responding to Problems of Systemic Dysfunction and Sectoral Capacity. Paper presented at the XIV International HIV/AIDS Conference, Barcelona, July 7–12, 2002 Available on HEARD website: http//www.heard.org.za/papers.

35. Malawi Institute of Management and UNDP. (2001). *The Impact of HIV/AIDS on Human Resources in the Public Sector in Malawi.* Lilongwe: Malawi Institute of Management.

36. Stover J, Johnston A. (1999). *The Art of Policy Formulation: Experiences from Africa in Developing National HIV/AIDS Policies.* Washington, DC: The Futures Group.

37. MacPherson MF, Hoover DA, Snodgrass DR. (2000). *The Impact on Economic Growth in Africa of Rising Costs and Labor Productivity Losses Associated with HIV/AIDS.* Boston, MA: Harvard Institute of International Development.

38. Bell C, Devarajan S, Gersbach H. (2003). *The Long-run Economic Costs of AIDS: Theory and an Application to South Africa.* Washington, DC: The World Bank.

39. International Centre for Trade and Sustainable Development and the International Institute for Sustainable Development. (2003). *Intellectual Property Rights, Doha Round Briefing Series.* Available at: www.wto.org.

40. OXFAM. (2002). *Generic Competition, Price and Access to Medicines: The Case of Antiretrovirals in Uganda.* Oxfam Briefing Paper 26. Available at www.oxfam.org.

41. Perez-Casas C, Macé C, Berman D, Double J. (2001). *Accessing ARVs: Untangling the Web of Price Reductions for Developing Countries.* Geneva: Médecins Sans Frontières.

42. Willan S. (2003). Briefing: recent changes in the South African government's HIV/AIDS policy and its implementation. *African Affairs* **104**:109–17.

43. Quinlan T, Willan S. (2005). Finding ways to manage HIV/AIDS: South Africa 2004–5. In: Daniel J, Southall R, Lutchman JM, eds. *The State of the Nation 2004–2005.* Pretoria: Human Sciences Research Council.

44. World Health Organization. (2001). *Macroeconomics and Health: Investing in Health for Economic Development.* Report of the Commission on Macroeconomics and Health. Geneva: WHO.

45. World Bank. (2000). *World Development Report.* New York: Oxford University Press.

46. United Nations Development Programme. (2003). *Human Development Report.* New York: Oxford University Press.

47. Barnett T, Whiteside A. (2002). *AIDS in the Twenty-first Century: Disease and Globalization.* Basingstoke: Palgrave Macmillan.

48. United Nations Development Programme. (1999). *Human Development Report.* New York: Oxford University Press, p1.

49. United Nations Development Programme. (1996, 2001, 2003). *Human Development Report.* New York: Oxford University Press.

50. Prins, G. (2004). AIDS and global security. *International Affairs (London)* **80**:931–52.
51. National Intelligence Council. (2002). *Global Trends 2015: A Dialogue About the Future with Non-government Experts*. National Intelligence Council. NIC 2000–02, December.
52. The next wave of HIV/AIDS: Nigeria, Ethiopia, Russia, India and China. ICA 2000–04 D, September.
53. Health Economics and HIV/AIDS Research Division, University of KwaZulu-Natal. (2003). *Report of the Workshop on HIV/AIDS, Democracy and Development in South Africa*. Durban: University of KwaZulu-Natal. URL: www.heard.org.za.

Chapter 4

Determinants of the HIV pandemic in developing countries

Eileen Stillwaggon

It is no coincidence that the highest prevalence of HIV and the highest rates of increase in HIV infection are in countries with myriad other problems. The majority of people living with HIV and AIDS and most of those newly infected with HIV live in countries beset by economic and social crises. This chapter demonstrates how the economic and social environment of low- and middle-income developing and transitional countries makes them more vulnerable to epidemic diseases, including HIV. After a discussion of the status of economic and health systems in developing and transitional countries, it shows some of the ways in which poverty not only influences risk-taking behaviour but also creates a riskier environment for poor people. A few solutions that illustrate how to address the causes of risky behaviours and the risky environment conclude this chapter.

Protecting the health of a population is not primarily a medical problem. The solutions to the vast majority of health problems are already known. Whether a population can share in those solutions is determined chiefly by income and the access that income gives to adequate food, clean water, safe housing and communities, sanitary infrastructure, health information and medical services. The allocation of national resources to the health needs of the population is an economic and political decision. Laws and institutions also play a major role in population health because they influence the success of the economy and the access of all members of society to the protections afforded by state and non-state institutions. The HIV epidemics are fuelled by the same economic and social conditions that impede other facets of national and individual development.

Despite variation in geography and economic levels among the countries of the developing world, there is much in common in the living conditions of the poorer half of their populations. Poor people live in overcrowded, insanitary apartments, cardboard or plastic shanties or mud-and-stick huts in nearly 100 countries. They drink contaminated water, have food insufficient in quality or quantity and lack affordable or accessible health services. Much of the developing world also shares a history of failed economic policies, chronic stagnation, high unemployment and underemployment, vulnerability to world markets, dependence on few exports, lack of capital and poorly equipped labour forces.

Policies of fiscal austerity and privatization introduced in the 1980s worsened conditions for poor people in many countries, in particular in sub-Saharan Africa and Latin America. The reform of those economies was necessary, but it was often carried out in a corrupt, mean-spirited and short-sighted way [1]. The burden of economic policy was borne by poor and middle-income people. To satisfy, or to appear to satisfy, demands for fiscal restraint, governments slashed health and education spending, even though those expenditures had never been important contributors to the soaring fiscal deficits.

The 1980s were a lost decade for Africa and Latin America, and many countries fared no better in the 1990s. In numerous countries, gross domestic product (GDP) and GDP per capita fell during those decades [2]. Economic growth dissolved into crisis in South-East Asia in the late 1990s. The collapse of the Soviet Union precipitated a period of economic transition with calamitous decreases in output in the 1990s in the former Soviet Union (FSU) and Eastern Europe. In these settings of economic decay and personal hardship we find the highest levels of HIV prevalence or the fastest rates of increase in HIV infection.

Economic and health status of developing and transitional countries

Africa

Most of the poorest countries in the world are in sub-Saharan Africa; in 2001, 31 countries had a per capita GDP below US$500. In 15 African countries, more than half the population lives on less than US$1 a day, and in 25 countries more than two-thirds of the people live on less than US$2 a day [2]. Those African countries with relatively higher GDP per capita—South Africa, Botswana and Zimbabwe among them—have very unequal distributions of income [3,4]. A quarter of Botswana's population and more than one-third of the populations of Zimbabwe and Namibia live on less than US$1 a day [2]. Both individually and nationally, low income is a good predictor of poor health outcomes [5]. In the case of HIV, however, inequality in the distribution of income is more highly correlated with HIV prevalence than is the level of income [6,7].

In the 1970s and 1980s, when the AIDS pandemic had its origins, sub-Saharan Africa suffered worsening poverty, drought and malnutrition. Between 1970 and 1997, per capita calorie intake fell by 1.5% and per capita protein consumption by 4% in sub-Saharan Africa, the only world region to experience a decline in either calorie or protein consumption in that period [8]. Thirty per cent of the population of sub-Saharan Africa was malnourished in the 1990s.

Civil and cross-border wars produced 18 famines in Africa in the last quarter of the twentieth century, with massive flows of refugees, food shortages and crowding in insanitary camps [9] that precipitated epidemics of communicable diseases such as measles, cholera and other gastrointestinal diseases, malaria and respiratory infections [10]. The economies of sub-Saharan Africa continued to decline in the 1990s. In 24 countries in the region, per capita income in 2001 was lower than in the 1970s or 1980s [2].

Latin America and the Caribbean

Most Latin American and Caribbean countries are ranked as middle-income and of medium human development, but that ranking results from simply averaging the affluence of a small wealthy class and the extreme poverty of the majority or significant minority. The average income obscures the extent of poverty in the hemisphere because Latin America has the most unequal distribution of income in the world. In most of the region, income is concentrated in the top decile, there is no significant middle class, and the bottom 20–40% of the population lives in extreme poverty. In Brazil, for example, the bottom decile of the population receives only 0.8% of the country's income, and the bottom quintile receives only 1.7%, while the top decile receives 47% of national income [11]. Brazil has one-third of the population in Latin America and the Caribbean, and one in 10 Brazilians lives on less than US$1 a day. Latin America exhibits a veneer of affluence, but 10 countries in the region report more than 14% of the population living on less than US$1 a day [2].

In the region as a whole, 12% of the total population was undernourished in 2000 [2]. In shanty towns throughout Latin America, rates of stunting, wasting and psychomotor problems are not only much higher than official data indicate for young children, but the problems are even more severe in children between 5 and 12 years old, an age group often overlooked [1].

A quarter of children under 5 years of age in Latin America and the Caribbean are deficient in vitamin A [12]. Iron-deficiency anaemia affects more than 50% of the population in some countries, reducing work capacity, resistance to disease, and maternal and fetal survival rates [13]. More than 77 million children and women in Latin America and the Caribbean are anaemic, and the proportion of infants and young children who are iron deficient ranges from 9% in Chile to 33% in Mexico and Argentina. Hookworm and other parasites contribute to the prevalence of anaemia in the population [12]. In Latin America as a whole, 46% of the population is poor and over half of the poor are indigent, which means that the entire family income is insufficient to buy 80% of the minimum food requirement [14].

Safe drinking water is not available for rural and suburban areas throughout the region, and almost 90% of sewage is dumped untreated directly into streams and rivers. Intestinal worms infect 20–30% of the population of all the countries in the region and 60–80% of people in highly endemic regions. Virtually 100% of children in poor neighborhoods without clean water and sanitary services have intestinal worms. Malaria is endemic in 21 American countries, and 20% of people in the region live in areas of moderate or high malarial risk [13].

Eastern Europe and the former Soviet Union

The world region experiencing the most rapid increase in HIV infection comprises the former Soviet republics and the formerly socialist countries of Eastern Europe, which are undergoing a transition from centrally planned economies to market systems. The HIV epidemics in Eastern Europe and the FSU differ from those in sub-Saharan Africa and other developing areas in that, until recently, they were driven primarily by injecting drug use (IDU) and sex work [15].

A focus on drug and sex behaviours in the transitional countries has the effect of emphasizing individual choices. Overlooked are the causes of those behaviours or the context of poverty that not only motivates the behaviour, but also makes it more dangerous. The HIV epidemics in the FSU and Eastern Europe, just as in the developing world, are spreading in the context of weak economies with collapsing income and provision of social services.

Before the transition, the former socialist countries were industrialized, but they were not affluent [16]. The abrupt change from party-run, planned economies to open, market economies precipitated a sharp decline in output and a substantial increase in inequality. By 2001, only seven countries had regained their pre-transition levels of output, while 11 of the countries were still at less than 70% of their 1989 output [17].

Failing economies and a dismal record in civil and human rights had made economic and political transition necessary, but the process of economic reform also imposed unnecessary costs on the economy and the population, as it did in most of Africa and Latin America. In most transitional countries, government officials and well-positioned managers stripped state enterprises of assets and secured the gains of privatization for themselves, leaving few resources for much-needed social services or maintaining the infrastructure of the public sector.

The privatization and closure of state enterprises and cutbacks in state spending increased unemployment. In half the transitional countries, official unemployment rates were in excess of 10% in 2000 [17]. In Central and Eastern Europe, by 1999, there were 18 million people between 15 and 24 years of age who were neither in school nor employed [18]. In all 23 countries for which data were available for 1989–2000, real wages fell, and in 10 countries real wages in 2000 were less than half of what they had been in 1989 [17].

During the socialist era, the state provided most, if not all, of the physical and organizational infrastructure—educational, cultural, sports, leisure and transportation facilities—by which people were integrated into society. When the state collapsed or withdrew, it left a vacuum for the provision of services, and people faced an economic and social crisis in which there were no institutions for support, recreation or community involvement.

Nutrition was inadequate even before transition, and iodine, calcium and iron deficiencies continue to affect 30–40% of the populations in several of these countries [19–21]. Sexually transmitted infections (STIs) have increased dramatically. In Russia, the incidence of syphilis increased over 30-fold in the 1990s [22]. In all of the rest of the FSU, the incidence of syphilis and gonorrhoea in 2000 was higher than in 1989 and, in some countries, two or three times as high [17].

Since 1992, the prevalence of tuberculosis (TB) has increased 10–15% per year in Russia [22]. Not only is TB prevalence very high in most of the countries, but TB incidence is increasing rapidly. In 14 countries, TB incidence has increased more than 40% since 1989, and TB incidence has more than doubled in the Baltic States, the Caucasus and Russia [17]. In the transition era, there has been a widening of socio-economic differences in mortality, for the most part driven by a large increase in deaths due to alcohol, injuries, violence, and parasitic and infectious diseases [21].

The epidemic of IDU in the FSU follows decades during which alcoholism was a serious problem in the Soviet Union. Organized crime groups have increased the supply of drugs, but the social crisis has produced the demand. The transitional countries are facing parallel epidemics of youth suicide and drug and alcohol abuse. It is essential to ask what is causing suicidal levels of drinking and drug-using behaviour, a question that is obscured by a focus on individual lifestyle choices. The increases in AIDS, accidents, homicide and suicide, together with morbidity and mortality related to the abuse of alcohol, tobacco and drugs, are occurring in countries in the throes of a social crisis of enormous proportions. A chief casualty of that crisis has been the healthcare system [23]. As in the developing world, the success of economic and political reform itself is threatened by inequities in the process.

Asia

In contrast to the FSU, the prevalence of HIV in Asia is still relatively low. In East Asia, prevalence among adults is less than 0.2%, and in South and South-East Asia, it is 0.6%. Only Cambodia and Thailand report adult prevalence in excess of 2% [24]. The vast numbers of people in Asia and the widespread conditions of extreme poverty, however, make it essential to address the epidemics there.

Most of the world's poor people live in Asia. The economies of the region are very diverse, but most have achieved substantial economic growth over the past 30 years. In 2002, GDP per capita for East Asia and the Pacific was US$4768, and for South Asia, US$2658. Regional averages are useful in indicating the contributions made by successful agricultural revolutions and industrialization. In East Asia, substantial investment in primary education also contributed to higher national incomes. However, the averages, as elsewhere in the world, hide the vast numbers of people living in extreme poverty. In India, GDP per capita is US$2670, but 80% of the population live on less than US$2 a day, and 35% live on less than US$1 per day. In Cambodia, Bangladesh and Nepal, the proportions of people in extreme poverty are about the same as in India. Even in some of the fastest-growing economies, China, the Philippines and Indonesia, about half of the population lives on less than US$2 per day [25].

The region's poverty is reflected in the large proportion of malnourished children; almost half of the children in India, Bangladesh, Nepal and Cambodia are underweight for their age. In much of the region, the majority of the population lacks access to a reliable source of clean water or sanitation. Infectious and parasitic diseases continue to be the major source of morbidity and mortality in all Asian countries, including the more advanced economies [25]. All of the conditions that made the other regions fertile ground for epidemics of HIV are present in Asia. The burden of multiple parasites weakens children and adults. Malaria is endemic in much of the region. STIs, including ulcerative diseases such as chancroid, go untreated for lack of access to healthcare. TB is widespread and undertreated. In addition, IDU continues to be a grave problem in Southeast Asia and China.

Urban–rural inequalities continue to produce large streams of migrants. There are approximately 130 million internal migrants in China. Ongoing reforms include the restructuring of state-owned enterprises, leading to an increase in urban unemployment [26]. In some countries, such as the Philippines, violence in the countryside motivates people to migrate to the city for safety. International migration within Asia has been a major factor in the development boom, but migrants do not generally become permanent residents. They cannot bring their families with them, and their migrant status limits their access to healthcare services. Thailand has an estimated 1 million migrant workers from surrounding countries. The Philippines has exported labour for decades, and about 8 million Filipinos work abroad [26]. The low social and economic status of women, as elsewhere in the world, is also an important contributor to the epidemic of HIV in Asia [2,24].

The state of health systems

A characteristic of underdevelopment and economic crisis common to most, if not all, of the countries with serious HIV epidemics is an inadequate healthcare delivery system. Most of the developing and transitional countries already had weak healthcare systems before the economic crises of the 1980s and 1990s, but in others, good health infrastructure deteriorated as health spending was cut during economic austerity programmes. In half the sub-Saharan African countries for which data are available, real per capita expenditure on health fell between 1980 and 1985. Most of the decline occurred in non-wage recurrent expenditure, such as for drugs [27]. In Zambia in 1986, government spending on drugs was only 10% of what it had been in 1983 [28]. In Zimbabwe, the Ministry of Health budget fell 35% in real terms from 1991 to 1993 [29].

Cutbacks in public health spending in the Americas were even greater than in Africa. In Argentina, decades of economic decline, the policies of the military government (1976–1983) and the Menem administration (1989–1999) left public health centres and hospitals without medicines, sterilizing equipment, sinks for washing hands, reagents for testing blood, gloves and disposable syringes, and some even without running water [1].

Most of the formerly socialist countries maintained public health spending as a proportion of GDP over the first decade of transition. The calamitous decreases in GDP, however, meant commensurate decreases in absolute levels of public spending on health, in total and per capita. Some of the countries did not even maintain public health spending as a share of their shrinking GDPs [17].

The developing and transitional countries share many problems of healthcare delivery, as the country chapters will demonstrate. Worsening shortages of doctors and other medical personnel are reported in Russia, South Africa, Botswana and China. Inadequate funding and poor organization plague health systems as diverse as those of Brazil, India, South Africa and Russia. Economic reform in Ukraine included the removal of subsidies for essential inputs, including electricity, raising the cost of providing healthcare. In addition, health spending has fallen in Ukraine and, as in sub-Saharan Africa, infrastructure and payroll take up most of the budget, leaving little funding for medicines. A number of countries, including Brazil, South Africa and China, have very unequal access to healthcare between income levels, between regions and between rural and urban areas. Serving remote areas requires a well-devised system and political will.

Another weakness common to the healthcare systems of the developing world and transitional countries is the low priority placed on preventing or treating communicable disease. South Africa has a very low TB cure rate; in India, only half the people identified with TB infections are treated; and in China's rural areas, TB continues to be the leading killer. Failure to deliver TB therapy could be seen as a prime indicator of failure of a healthcare system.

Constrained choices

There are two routes through which social and economic conditions promote the spread of HIV. The first is through the constraints that poverty and underdevelopment impose on people's choices. Prevention policies limited to information, education and provision of condoms can succeed only if people have the power to make decisions about their lives, including about their sexual behaviour. The second route is the direct effect that poverty has on health and vulnerability to disease. People who eat poorly and are burdened with infections and parasites are more susceptible to HIV just as they are to other infectious diseases. Moreover, poor people have less access to preventive and curative healthcare services. This section addresses some of the ways that economic and social factors influence risk-taking behaviours. The following section describes the environment of biomedical risks in which those behaviours occur.

We have seen that economic conditions in developing countries produce dire social consequences. Poor people have inadequate private goods, such as food, clothing and shelter, and they also have poorer access to the protections of society at large, such as personal safety, legal protection, education and healthcare, even when those goods are publicly provided. To be poor in a developing or transitional country presents multiple risks because the institutions of civil and social protection may be less developed, and they may exclude or discriminate against people on the basis of gender, ethnicity or sexual identity. This lack of protection further marginalizes poor people and makes their environment riskier.

Legal systems in many countries perpetuate the inferior economic and social status of women. While gender inequality is a worldwide problem, it is aggravated in those countries in which women have no rights to property. Women are the primary agriculturalists and the main source of support for their children in many parts of the world, but women in many countries do not have rights to land apart from their fathers or husbands. Although they may know the risk of having unprotected sex with their husbands, refusing them risks personal injury and abandonment, leaving them without land to farm or other means of support.

After 20 years of AIDS prevention programmes based on information and education, there have been few signs of success in halting the epidemic. While in Botswana condoms are widely available, HIV infection continues to spread. Although in most countries people are now aware of the causes of HIV infection, their behaviour has not changed because the chief determinants of that behaviour are economic and social, not informational.

Key institutions that could protect people from HIV are lacking or inadequately accessible. Education protects young people from risks in numerous ways. Children are generally safer in school than out, especially if they live in shanty towns where there are gangs or widespread drug use. Young people in school are more likely to postpone initiation of sex, and schooling provides the opportunity for instruction about sexuality and safe sex. Literacy and learning empower people—girls in particular—to have control over their health and that of their children. Yet, some countries have instituted school fees, which have the perverse effect of motivating some girls who want to stay in school to accept the sexual advances of school administrators or of affluent men who pay their fees in return for sex.

There are other legal or regulatory impediments common to less-developed and transitional countries that might seem unrelated to health conditions but, in fact, have serious repercussions for health. In many countries, trade regulations, corrupt officials or outdated methods of clearing goods across national or provincial borders also promote the spread of HIV. Trucking routes have been an important path of HIV spread, in part because delays that can last for days keep truckers away from home, and they can often save money by staying with sex workers at border crossings instead of in hotels.

Another factor contributing to the spread of HIV and other diseases has been population movement due to economic and political causes. Government spending has tended to favour urban areas and populations. Many governments have kept producer prices low for agricultural products through commodity marketing boards, overvalued exchange rates and other means, making farming non-remunerative and encouraging people to leave the land for the cities. Concentrated land ownership and the failure of governments to reform land holding leave little opportunity for young people, who migrate to cities in search of work. Some of the causes of rural poverty are international. Volatile world markets, external pressure to open markets too quickly, and trade barriers erected by the USA, Japan and the European Union to the agricultural exports of poor countries have all contributed to the collapse of sustainable rural systems. Individual poverty and national underdevelopment are exacerbated by those external forces.

Migration creates conditions that encourage the spread of many different diseases, including HIV. Poor people crowd into refugee camps, urban slums and suburban shanty towns. Water supply, sanitation and other infrastructure do not keep up with population increase. Infectious and parasitic diseases spread under such conditions, worsening malnutrition.

In some regions, migration is circular. Workers from all over Southern Africa were recruited to work in the mines and factories of South Africa. The apartheid regime made no provision for the workers' families, so men lived in single-sex barracks and returned to their wives perhaps 1 month a year. After apartheid ended, the labour system of Southern Africa did not change rapidly enough to prevent the spread of HIV in the region. Throughout Africa, mines, factories and plantations rely on circular migrant streams, and similar labour systems fuel Asia's economic boom and the spread of infectious diseases.

In the Americas, circular migration also contributes to the spread of HIV. The Dominican Republic and Haiti send many thousands of workers to the USA, especially to New York and Miami. Dominicans and Haitians return to their homes and bring HIV with them. Ecuador also has thousands of workers who return after a few years of work in the USA with enough money to build a house or start a small business. Until recently, most of the people with HIV in Ecuador were returnees from the USA or their family members.

In all of the developing regions and some of the transitional countries, wars, civil conflicts and natural disasters have led to the dislocation of populations, with attendant effects on health status and social cohesion. Colombia alone has more than 1 million people internally displaced by the civil war, the fourth largest internally displaced population in the world [30].

Another form of labour migration that promotes HIV is the forced trafficking of women and children. The International Office for Migration estimates that 35,000 women have been trafficked from Colombia, 50,000 from the Dominican Republic and 75,000 from Brazil, primarily for work in Europe [31]. With the breakdown of the economic and social fabric, an epidemic of sex work and trafficking in women and children has engulfed the transitional countries of Eastern Europe and the FSU. Poverty, increasing stress, alcoholism and drug use in these countries are also producing more dysfunctional families that permit, and even promote, the trafficking of their daughters for sex work to Western Europe, Great Britain and Japan [32].

In the cities, there is not enough work, there are few opportunities for women, and there are few remunerative positions for the many migrants with little education. Consequently, many people—men, women and children—see no option for survival other than to engage in commercial sex with local clients and tourists. Poverty compels people to prioritize risk. Survival today for themselves or their children through selling sex may win out over the risk of illness and death in the future from AIDS. For women and children, and for racial and ethnic minorities, low social status compounds the powerlessness of poverty.

The economic and legal vulnerability of the sex worker makes negotiating safe sex extremely difficult. Foreign exchange earnings make governments less interested in taking action against predatory sex tourism, which continues to be an important industry in Thailand and is on the increase in South America, Central America, the Caribbean and Eastern Europe. In the Dominican Republic, with a population of 8.5 million people, the Health Ministry estimates that more than 200,000 women and men work as prostitutes, especially in the tourist trade [33].

There are an estimated 40 million children in Latin America who work and live on the street and engage in 'survival sex' with adults to secure food, clothing and shelter. The prevalence of HIV and other STIs is very high among street children in Honduras, Guatemala, Costa Rica and the Dominican Republic [31,34,35]. In Brazil, over 500,000 prostitutes under the age of 17 work on the streets. In Mexico City, as a result of child prostitution and sexual abuse, 5% of street children are infected with HIV, and none of the children has access to state health services [35].

Dangerous environments

Not only do poverty and underdevelopment create an environment conducive to unhealthy behaviours, they also directly contribute to poor health. An overemphasis on individual behaviour has plagued the discourse on the sources of the AIDS epidemic. Behaviour is an important part of the AIDS epidemics, and the social and economic determinants of behaviour are important, but HIV infection is also a biomedical problem. Susceptibility to infection, no matter how the disease is transmitted, is influenced by a person's overall health, nutrition and access to healthcare, all of which are determined chiefly by income and wealth in the absence of effective public services and welfare supports.

Increased susceptibility to infection results from deficiencies of macronutrients, protein and energy malnutrition, and deficiencies of vitamins and minerals. There is a synergy between infection and malnutrition; minor illnesses can induce anorexia (lack of appetite) or diarrhoea, and poor nutrition weakens the immune response. Even mild protein-energy malnutrition and micronutrient deficiency weaken the immune system [36–38]. Iron is essential in promoting resistance to infection. The lack of iron is the most widespread nutritional deficiency in the world and is especially common in women and children [39]. Even a mild zinc deficiency can cause a decrease in the cellular immune response [36,40]. Zinc deficiency also impedes wound healing and weakens resistance to parasite infection, both of which aggravate malnutrition [37]. Vitamin A deficiency reduces the number of natural killer cells and T lymphocytes, and the integrity of the skin and mucosa, which makes people more susceptible to STIs, including HIV [41].

Overall malnutrition and micronutrient deficiency are widespread in developing and transitional countries. Malnourished people are more vulnerable to transmission of infectious bacterial and viral diseases because their immune systems are weakened by malnutrition and by the synergistic effects of other infectious and parasitic diseases.

Parasitic diseases are common in developing countries, and they aggravate the nutritional and immune status of poor people, especially in tropical areas. Malnourished people are more susceptible to parasites, and parasites worsen the afflicted person's nutritional status [42]. Of the 300–500 million cases of malaria occurring annually worldwide, more than 90% are in tropical Africa. Of the more than 200 million people with schistosomiasis (bilharzia), more than 80% live in sub-Saharan Africa [43]. Intestinal parasites of many kinds are extremely widespread among poor populations in tropical areas, with an estimated 3.5 billion people infected worldwide. People often carry several different parasites, resulting in aggravated malnutrition and retarded development [44–46]. Besides undermining nutrition, parasites also depress the immune response by reducing epithelial integrity and the production of natural killer cells, B cells and T cells.

Poverty and underdevelopment promote not just infectious disease in general, but transmission of HIV in particular, through deficiencies of the health sector and through the health environment of poor people. Inadequate health systems and individual poverty promote HIV infection through direct iatrogenic transmission, through the recourse of poor people to informal health providers and through deficiencies in access to diagnosis and treatment.

In many countries, government hospitals and health posts use non-sterile medical equipment and contaminated blood products that have caused a significant number of infections over the past two decades. The lack of access to affordable healthcare has also had a direct impact on the spread of HIV. Poor people sometimes seek medical attention from untrained injectionists who inject vitamins, antibiotics and sometimes just dirty water and also contribute to iatrogenic transmission of HIV and other infections [47–51]. In China, 30% of injections in some health facilities are reportedly administered without precautions for infection control. The combination of poverty and poor state oversight led to the infection of perhaps 1 million people in Henan and surrounding provinces through unsafe blood collection methods.

The deficiencies of the health sector in providing diagnosis and treatment of STIs also directly affect HIV transmission. In Africa and South and South-East Asia, genital ulcer diseases such as chancroid constitute a much larger proportion of STIs than in affluent countries [5]. Health services are inadequate, drugs are not available, and people do not get treatment for STIs, increasing the likelihood of transmission of an ulcerative STI and HIV.

For an HIV-negative person, STIs provide easy entry for HIV [52], and they enhance HIV transmission [53] because they have an inflammatory effect on genital tissue, attracting T cells to the site where they can be most easily infected. Co-infection with other STIs in an HIV-infected person also increases the likelihood of transmission of HIV because STIs promote more viral shedding in the genital tract of HIV-positive people [53,54].

While nutrition is important for resistance to disease in general, it has also been demonstrated to affect HIV transmission directly. Malnutrition increases viral load and viral shedding, increasing the likelihood of mother-to-child transmission [55,56].

Parasitic infections not only weaken overall immune response, but also directly enhance HIV transmission. Malaria stimulates HIV replication, and HIV viral loads are significantly higher in malarial patients, even after treatment [57]. Those with malaria are consequently more likely to transmit HIV to unprotected partners. People with worm infections—the majority in most poor communities—are more susceptible to HIV infection and more vulnerable to progression to AIDS once infected [58,59].

Schistosomiasis promotes HIV transmission in the same way that STIs do, by producing genital lesions and by the inflammatory effect of attracting CD4 cells to the genital area. Schistosomiasis is highly endemic in many poor, tropical regions, especially in sub-Saharan Africa: 60–75% of women with urinary schistosomiasis also have reproductive tract infections of schistosomiasis, with infestation of worms and ova in the vagina, uterus, vulva or cervix [60–64], constituting a very large population with increased susceptibility to HIV.

One-third of the world's population is infected with TB, and 5–10% of those infected will develop active cases of the disease. Sub-Saharan Africa is the region with the highest prevalence of TB, but prevalence is also extremely high in parts of Latin America, Asia and the former Soviet republics. HIV promotes the activation of latent TB, and TB infection accelerates the progression of HIV to AIDS and death, which has serious implications for the spread of the HIV epidemic.

Poor countries and poor people also have less access to antiretroviral treatment for HIV, which can reduce viral load and viral shedding, thereby reducing the risk of sexual and vertical transmission [65]. Treatment is complementary to other forms of prevention and improves the cost-effectiveness of other prevention programmes.

Solutions

Because the HIV epidemics in the developing and transitional countries arise from, and are sustained by, economic and social conditions, i.e. from 'upstream' causes, stopping them requires 'upstream' solutions. There has been considerable bewilderment in AIDS policy circles that interventions to change behaviour through information and education, with few exceptions, do not seem to be working. Without changing the context in which behaviours occur, however, we should not expect changes in behaviour. To the extent that the risk of transmission is increased by biological factors, including nutrition, endemic diseases and the lack of access to healthcare, there is a need for upstream interventions that change the biomedical risk environment as well.

There are numerous actors who can change the environment in which the HIV epidemics are spreading. Agents outside the developing and transitional countries include the international organizations and the affluent countries. Poor and transitional countries are saddled with a crushing burden of external debt, the result of bad decisions and corruption or manipulation on the part of their own past governments or lenders. There is reasonable reluctance on the part of lenders to provide a lesson that sovereign states need not take responsibility for their actions. Repayment, however, inflicts suffering on the poor and powerless, not on the rich and powerful who were responsible for acquiring the debt. It is not beyond the talents of economists and lawyers to devise and monitor a system of debt-for-health and debt-for-education swaps. Heavily indebted and HIV-affected countries can be enabled and required to redirect resources from debt repayment to the broad array of needed investments. Sanitation, institutional reforms, including legal protections for women and children, and modernization of the communication and commercial infrastructure would all contribute to poverty eradication and improve the environment for health and education.

Another clear example of a change that can be made outside the affected countries is the reform of trade restrictions and subsidies that make it impossible for developing countries to compete in world markets. Protecting farmers in rich countries is costly, inefficient and harmful to developing countries.

Rich countries currently contribute a very small percentage of their national budgets and an even smaller proportion of their GDPs to foreign aid. Stopping HIV will require a serious commitment to more and better-designed foreign aid programmes from governments and philanthropic organizations for poverty eradication, social reform and government modernization. The European Union is well prepared to provide technical assistance for trade facilitation. An excellent use of the resources of the Bill & Melinda Gates Foundation would be to assist countries with the computerization of trade logistics to speed regional truck transport and reduce unnecessary border delays.

Rich nations in search of ways to help developing and transitional countries battle HIV and other health problems should, first, do no harm. Rich countries actively recruit nursing graduates and, even worse, nursing instructors trained at public expense in developing countries. The freedom to migrate should not be denied to health workers, but rich nations should not raid poor nations' skilled labour resources. As in the case of agricultural subsidies and tariffs, rich countries are solving structural imbalances of their own labour and capital markets at the expense of poor countries.

There are many structural changes that need to be made within developing and transitional countries. The ways to advance human development and economic growth are well established in the development literature and will only be outlined briefly here. Countries need to control waste and corruption in order to yield resources for investment in education and health. Those investments will be repaid many times over in the form of capable workers. Transparency must extend to modernizing the regulatory apparatus that strangles regional trade and local initiative. Outmoded regulations serve only special interests and are part of the morass of underdevelopment that keeps people poor in spite of how hard they work every day. Legal systems must be reformed to give women and other marginalized people equal rights. It will be argued that cultural barriers make that impossible, but culture is a reflection of the economic power that men hold over women. It should not be romanticized and used as a justification for oppression. Institutional and economic reform can lead and culture will follow.

Even the nature of the required investments in education and health is already known. The most important investment in education is at the primary level, and the same is true for health [1,5]. The most cost-effective way to provide the broad array of services needed by poor people and populations as a whole is through horizontally integrated health services. In the long term, stand-alone programmes such as separate STI or reproductive health clinics waste valuable resources and address only a narrow category of needs. Of what use is a clinic that houses only a population-control programme to a woman who is losing her only child to diarrhoea? The biggest constraint on eradication of schistosomiasis and other parasites has been the lack of an adequate institutional framework for implementing control programmes [66]. However, that is the same constraint that discourages investment in myriad complementary programmes. Building healthcare systems that address the broad spectrum of health needs of poor people maximizes the return from health investment [67].

The venues, personnel and equipment needed to deliver medications for opportunistic infections and antiretroviral treatment for HIV are part of the same set of resources that are needed to provide cheap deworming medications, nutritional supplements, routine gynaecological attention, treatment for injuries, substance abuse and depression, and education for maintaining clean water supplies or practising safe sex. Antiretroviral treatment requires staff and laboratory facilities that are more sophisticated than most other healthcare services, but without a system of primary care, delivery of antiretroviral medication is almost impossible. There are numerous synergies to exploit in an integrated healthcare system. Treatment for TB, for example, addresses a pressing need in most of the developing and transitional countries and has been shown to be effective in reducing viral load and improving survival in HIV-positive individuals.

There will continue to be a need for special programmes to eradicate parasitic diseases, especially those that are highly endemic and act as cofactors for HIV, including malaria, schistosomiasis and worm infection. Investment in safe water and sanitation is necessary to reduce malnutrition, morbidity and mortality from infectious and parasitic diseases, and improve overall well-being. However, a system of preventive and curative healthcare delivery that integrates vertical programmes into a part of the integrated healthcare system is essential.

The proximate cause of HIV transmission clearly is behaviour such as unprotected sex or the use of contaminated blood, medical equipment or drug paraphernalia. Those behaviours occur in a social and economic setting that influences both the behaviour and the risk that behaviour entails. Ultimately, the HIV epidemics derive from economic, political and social as well as biological causes. The solutions, therefore, must address those issues. Poor and powerless people face a hierarchy of risk. What we now offer many of them is the opportunity to make a rational decision on time to death: to choose surviving through risky behaviours in a risky environment until they succumb to HIV. We offer information, but not alternatives. It will be much easier to change behaviours if the economic and social pressures that produce them are alleviated. Even behaviours that do not change can present less risk if the biological environment is altered through changing the economic and social conditions.

References

1. Stillwaggon E. (1998). *Stunted Lives, Stagnant Economies: Poverty, Disease, and Underdevelopment.* New Brunswick, NJ: Rutgers University Press.
2. United Nations Development Programme. (2003). *Human Development Report.* New York: Oxford University Press. URL: http://www.undp.org/hdro/ indicators.html.

3. World Bank. (1997). *Confronting AIDS: Public Priorities in a Global Epidemic.* Oxford: Oxford University Press.

4. World Bank. (1999). *World Development Report 1998–1999.* New York: Oxford University Press.

5. World Bank. (1993). *Investing in Health: World Development Report 1993.* Washington, DC: World Bank.

6. Stillwaggon E. (2000). HIV transmission in Latin America: comparison with Africa and Policy Implications. *South African Journal of Economics,* Special Edition on the Economics of HIV/AIDS, 68:985–1011.

7. Stillwaggon E. (2002). HIV/AIDS in Africa: fertile terrain. *Journal of Development Studies* 38(6):1–22.

8. United Nations Development Programme. (2000). *Human Development Report.* New York: Oxford University Press.

9. von Braun J, Teklu T, Webb P. (1999). *Famine in Africa: Causes, Responses, and Prevention.* Baltimore: Johns Hopkins University Press.

10. Centers for Disease Control and Prevention. (1992). Famine-affected, refugee, and displaced populations: recommendations for public health issues. *Morbidity and Mortality Weekly* **41** (RR-13).

11. Inter-American Development Bank. (1998). *Facing up to Inequality in Latin America.* Economic and Social Progress in Latin America, 1998–1999 Report. Washington, DC: Johns Hopkins Press.

12. Pan American Health Organization. (2002). *Health in the Americas: Volume I.* Scientific Publication No. 569. Washington, DC: Pan American Health Organization.

13. Pan American Health Organization. (1998). *Health in the Americas: Volume I.* Scientific Publication No. 569. Washington, DC: Pan American Health Organization.

14. Barraclough S. (1997). Food and poverty in the Americas: institutional and policy obstacles to efficiency in food aid. *Development in Practice* 7:117–29.

15. UNAIDS (Joint United Nations Programme on HIV/ AIDS). (2002). *Report on the Global HIV/AIDS Epidemic.* Geneva: United Nations. URL: http:// www.unaids.org.

16. World Bank. (1991). *World Development Report: The Challenge of Development.* Oxford: Oxford University Press.

17. TRANSMONEE Data Base. UNICEF/IRC. URL: http://www.unicef.org.

18. Central and Eastern European Harm Reduction Network. (2002). *Injecting Drug Users, HIV/AIDS Treatment and Primary Care.* Vilnius, Lithuania: CEEHRN.

19. Eidukiene V. (2002). Poverty and welfare trends over the 1990s in Lithuania. Background Paper for *Social Monitor (2002).* UNICEF.

20. Sekula W, Babinska K, Petrova S. (1997). Nutrition policies in central and Eastern Europe. *Nutrition Reviews* 55(11):S58–73.

21. Shkolnikov V, Leon D, Adamets S, Andreev E, Deev A. (1998). Educational level and adult mortality in Russia: an analysis of routine data 1979 to 1994. *Social Science and Medicine* 47:357–69.

22. Zbarskaya I. (2002). Poverty and welfare trends in the Russian Federation over the 1990s. Background paper for the *Social Monitor (2002).* UNICEF.

23. Shaw M, Dorling D, Smith GD. (1999). Poverty, social exclusion, and minorities. In: Marmot M, Wilkinson RG, eds. *Social Determinants of Health.* Oxford: Oxford University Press, p211–39.

24. Joint United Nations Programme on HIV/AIDS. (2004). *Report on the Global HIV/AIDS Epidemic.* URL: http://www.unaids.org.

25. United Nations Development Programme. (2004). *Human Development Report.* New York: Oxford University Press.

26. International Organization for Migration. (2000). *World Migration Report.* Geneva: IOM.

27. Jespersen E. (1992). External shocks, adjustment policies and economic and social performance. In: Cornia GA, Van der Hoeven R, Mkandawire T, eds. *Africa's Recovery in the 1990s: From Stagnation and Adjustment to Human Development.* New York: St. Martin's Press, p9–50.

28. Sanders D, Sambo A. (1991). AIDS in Africa: the implications of economic recession and structural adjustment. *Health Policy and Planning* 6:157–65.

29. World Bank. (1993). *Sexually Transmitted Infections: Prevention and Care Project, Zimbabwe.* Staff Appraisal Report No. 11730-ZIM.

30. Deng F. (1999). Don't overlook Colombia's humanitarian crisis. *Christian Science Monitor* 6 October.

31. Pan American Health Organization. (2003). Trafficking of Women and Children for Sexual Exploitation in the Americas. URL: http://www.paho.org/English/ HDP/HDW/TraffickingPaper.pdf.

32. International Organization for Migration. (2002). *Public Perception and Awareness of Trafficking in Women in the Baltic States.* Vilnius: IOM.

33. Abel D. (1999). Aids linked to infidelity in Dominican Republic. *Boston Globe,* 28 December, pA2, A4.

34. Scanlon T, Tomkins A, Lynch M, Scanlon F. (1998). Street children in Latin America. *British Medical Journal* 316:1596–600.

35. Seitles MD. (1997/1998). Effect of the Convention on the Rights of the Child upon street children in Latin America: a study of Brazil, Colombia, and Guatemala. *In the Public Interest* 16:159–93.

36. Beisel W. (1996). Nutrition and immune function: overview. *Journal of Nutrition* 126:2611S–5S.

37. Chandra RK. (1997). Nutrition and the immune system: an introduction. *American Journal of Clinical Nutrition* 66:460S–3S.

38. Woodward B. (1998). Protein, calories, and immune defenses. *Nutrition Reviews* 56(1, Part 2): S84–92.

39. Scrimshaw N, SanGiovanni JP. (1997). Synergism of nutrition, infection, and immunity: an overview. *American Journal of Clinical Nutrition* 66:464S–77S.

40. Cunningham-Rundles S. (1998). Analytical methods for evaluation of immune response in nutrient intervention. *Nutrition Reviews* 56(1, Part 2):S27–37.

41. Semba R. (1998). The role of vitamin A and related retinoids in immune function. *Nutrition Reviews* 56(1, Part 2):S38–48.

42. Storey DM. (1993). Filariasis: nutritional interactions in human and animal hosts. *Parasitology* 107(Supplement):S147–58.

43. World Health Organization. (1998). *Schistosomiasis Control.* URL: http:// www.who.int/ctd/html/ schisto.html.

44. Hlaing T. (1993). Ascariasis and childhood malnutrition. *Parasitology* 107(Supplement):S125–36.

45. Oberhelman RA, Guerrero ES, Fernandez ML *et al.* (1998). Correlations between intestinal parasitosis, physical growth, and psychomotor development among infants and children from rural Nicaragua. *American Journal of Tropical Medicine and Hygiene* 58:470–5.

46. World Health Organization. (1998). *Intestinal Parasites Control.* URL: http://www.who.int/ctd/html/ intest.html.

47. Brewer D, Brody S, Drucker E *et al.* (2003). Mounting anomalies in the epidemiology of HIV in Africa: cry the beloved paradigm. *International Journal of STD and AIDS* 14:144–7.

48. Drucker E, Alcabes P, Marx P. (2001). The injection century: massive unsterile injections and the emergence of human pathogens. *Lancet* 358:1989–92.

49. Gisselquist D, Potterat J, Brody S, Vachon F. (2003). Let it be sexual: how health care transmission of AIDS in Africa was ignored. *International Journal of STD and AIDS* 14:148–61.

50. Luby S. (2001). Injection safety. *Emerging Infectious Diseases* 7(3, Supplement), URL: http:// www.cdc.gov/ncidod/eid/vo17no3_supp/luby.htm.

51. Moore A, Herrera G, Nyamongo J *et al.* (2001). Estimated risk of HIV transmission by blood transfusion in Kenya. *Lancet* **358**:657–60.

52. Hitchcock P, Fransen L. (1998). *Preventing HIV Infection—What are the Lessons from Mwanza and Rakai?* URL: http://www.iaen.org/partmat/ mwanza.htm.

53. Fleming D, Wasserheit J. (1999). From epidemiological synergy to public health policy and practice: the contribution of other sexually transmitted diseases to sexual transmission of HIV infection. *Sexually Transmitted Infections* **75**:3–17.

54. Corbett E, Steketee R, ter Kuile F, Latif A, Kamali A, Hayes R. (2002). HIV-1/AIDS and the control of other infectious diseases in Africa. *Lancet* **359**:2177–87.

55. Nimmagadda A, O'Brien W, Goetz M. (1998). The significance of vitamin A and carotenoid status in persons infected by the human immunodeficiency virus. *Clinical Infectious Diseases* **26**:711–8.

56. Semba R, Miotti P, Chiphangwi J *et al.* (1994). Maternal vitamin A deficiency and mother-to-child transmission of HIV-1. *Lancet* **343**:1593–7.

57. Whitworth J, Morgan D, Quigley M *et al.* (2000). Effect of HIV-1 and increasing immunosuppression on malaria parasitaemia and clinical episodes in adults in rural Uganda: a cohort study. *Lancet* **356**:1051–6.

58. Bentwich Z, Kalinkovich A, Weisman Z, Borkow G, Beyers N, Beyers A. (1999). Can eradication of helminthic infections change the face of AIDS and tuberculosis? *Immunology Today* **20**(11):485–7.

59. Borkow G, Leng Q, Weisman Z *et al.* (2000). Chronic immune activation associated with intestinal helminth infections results in impaired signal transduction and anergy. *Journal of Clinical Investigation* **106**:1053–60.

60. Feldmeier H, Poggensee G, Krantz I, Helling-Giese G. (1995). Female genital schistosomiasis. *Tropical and Geographical Medicine* **47**(2, Supplement):2–15.

61. Feldmeier H, Leutscher P, Poggensee G, Harms G. (1999). Male genital schistosomiasis and haemospermia. *Tropical Medicine and International Health* **4**:791–3.

62. Feldmeier H, Helling-Giese G, Poggensee G. (2001). Unreliability of PAP smears to diagnose female genital schistosomiasis. *Tropical Medicine and International Health* **6**:31–3.

63. Harms G, Feldmeier H. (2002). Review: HIV infection and tropical parasitic diseases—deleterious interactions in both directions? *Tropical Medicine and International Health* **7**:479–88.

64. Mosunjac M, Tadros T, Beach R, Majmudar M. (2003). Cervical schistosomiasis, human papilloma virus (HPV), and human immunodeficiency virus (HIV): a dangerous coexistence or coincidence? *Gynecologic Oncology* **90**:211–4.

65. Fiore J, Suligoi B, Monno L, Angarano G, Pastore G (2002). HIV-1 shedding in genital tract of infected women, *Lancet* **359**:1525–6.

66. World Health Organization. (1996 last updated/ 2003 accessed). *Schistosomiasis*. Fact Sheet No. 115, URL: http://www.who.int/inf-fs/en/ fact115.html.

67. World Health Organization. (2001). *Macroeconomics and Health: Investing in Health for Human Development*. Geneva: Commission on Macroeconomics and Health, WHO.

Section II

Prevention, Treatment and Care: Advances in Knowledge

Chapter 5

HIV prevention programmes: an overview

Steffanie A Strathdee*, Marie-Louise Newell, Francisco Inacio Bastos and Thomas L Patterson

Background

Since the beginning of the HIV epidemic, interventions to reduce high-risk behaviours have focused mainly on individuals, although, in some cases, prevention programmes have been developed for the general population, with examples including mass media- and school-based education campaigns and voluntary HIV testing and counselling. Preventive interventions have also been developed or tailored for particular populations based on the route of exposure, such as the development of needle exchange programmes for injecting drug users (IDUs), or the provision of prophylactic antiretroviral therapy (ART) to HIV-infected pregnant women.

With growing understanding of attitudes, social norms and behaviours, approaches to HIV interventions have become more sophisticated and complex. Behavioural interventions based on various theoretical models have been developed to promote HIV awareness, the use of condoms, avoidance of contaminated injecting equipment and entry into drug abuse treatment, or to delay the onset of sexual behaviour. Combinations of interventions have also been tested in both developed and developing countries, such as the integration of voluntary HIV testing and counselling with cognitive–behavioural interventions or interventions to reduce mother-to-child transmission (MTCT).

Increasingly, structural interventions targeting conditions that increase vulnerability to HIV transmission, or the 'risk environment', have gained attention [1]. These interventions include changes in policies or laws that directly or indirectly influence risk behaviours, such as 100% condom campaigns introduced in brothels, and laws permitting access to sterile injection equipment for IDUs.

In this chapter, we provide a brief overview of interventions aimed at the general population and populations at high risk of HIV infection. Our focus is primarily in prevention of MTCT (PMTCT), and specific groups such as IDUs, men who have sex with men (MSM) and sex workers. The majority of infections globally are caused by heterosexual transmission, and this issue is not specifically addressed here. Our review is by no means exhaustive, but is meant to provide a context for more detailed examples outlined in subsequent chapters. When appropriate, we discuss the implications of these findings for healthcare systems, and make suggestions for future research.

---

* Corresponding author

Media campaigns

Messages diffused by mass media and social marketing have the potential to reach a large and diverse audience through television, radio, print or commercial advertising and, more recently, the Internet. For this reason, mass media represent a critical component of a concerted effort to disseminate accurate and culturally appropriate information, foster behaviour change and modify social norms.

Media campaigns have been used in different societies and cultures as a key component of national strategies to prevent HIV, prejudice and discrimination. Media campaigns have aimed to dispel myths about ways in which HIV is transmitted and to encourage condom use and HIV testing [2].

By highlighting prominent public figures who have HIV, television and print campaigns have helped 'put a face' on the epidemic. Increases in health-seeking behaviour have been documented following targeted campaigns using peer images [3]. In Côte d'Ivoire, television soap operas on AIDS, such as *SIDA dans la Cité*, have been found to be an important tool for promoting condom use, since the programme was most appealing to viewers who engaged in risky behaviours [4].

Yet, mass media campaigns can also have unintended consequences. In France, respondents to a survey who reported being influenced by media campaigns on HIV were less likely to believe in HIV transmission through casual contact and to express discriminatory attitudes towards people living with HIV (PLHIV), but were more likely to support mandatory HIV screening for the general population [5]. Promotion of the female condom by the STOP AIDS Project in San Francisco led to its uptake among MSM, despite the fact that efficacy of the product had not been established for anal sex [6].

Unfortunately, in many societies, preventive messages still face opposition from conservative forces. The complexity of contemporary societies, where many different perspectives and mores co-exist, poses a challenge to health professionals, policy-makers and media experts in disseminating sound and culturally sensitive HIV education messages. In 2002, the popular children's television programme *Sesame Street* introduced the first HIV-positive Muppet, 'Kami', to promote education about HIV in Africa and elsewhere. Although UNICEF recognized the Muppet as a 'champion for children', members of the US Congress and other viewers expressed concern. Ironically, the controversy seemed to extend the reach of the Muppet's educational messages, but, nevertheless, this example illustrates how controversial HIV education can be.

Perhaps due to the aforementioned difficulties, truly integrated campaigns such as those implemented in Switzerland [2] have been the exception rather than the rule. Even well-planned campaigns have seldom been evaluated. The Swiss STOP AIDS campaign can be viewed as a paradigm of both planning and evaluation. This campaign was one of the first to include messages directed both towards the general public as well as each of the major populations at risk, such as MSM or IDUs, was disseminated simultaneously in several languages and included an awareness campaign to minimize stigma directed toward PLHIV. While this campaign appeared to have no real effect on the rate of sexual activity of adolescents over a 5-year period, it nevertheless had a positive effect on the use of contraception and condoms [7].

Well-designed mass media initiatives have reached hard-to-reach populations such as IDUs, usually viewed as a population refractory to mainstream preventive messages [8].

In the USA, 40% of IDUs reported that their most common source of HIV information was the television. In the same study, exposure to mass media sources and small media materials was related to HIV knowledge and HIV testing, especially among males [9]. The 'No Piques' ('Don't shoot') campaign implemented in Spain in the late 1980s [10] can be considered an example to be emulated by other campaigns targeting marginalized and impoverished populations.

In recent years, the Internet has become a powerful media tool for disseminating HIV prevention messages. HIV education can be found on websites, list-servs and chat rooms in a multitude of languages that are targeted to both broad and specific audiences. In Los Angeles, California, public health officials have even used the Internet to notify sex partners of people with sexually transmitted infections (STIs) who were otherwise anonymous [11]. Other researchers are using the Internet to recruit subjects at high risk for HIV infection and to promote and reinforce changes in behaviour. Although one challenge of Internet-based activities is the potential for the spread of misinformation, it is becoming one of the most important ways to educate people.

Voluntary counselling and testing

Voluntary HIV counselling and testing (VCT) lays the foundation for increasing access to appropriate HIV care among infected people, preventing MTCT and fostering behaviour change among both HIV-positive and HIV-negative people. According to the World Health Organization (WHO), 180 million people should be tested and counselled annually by 2005 to reach targets for enhanced prevention and increased access to ART [12].

Abundant literature has shown that VCT is an essential component of any concerted effort to foster behaviour change. A randomized trial carried out in African resource-limited communities demonstrated that VCT is an effective means of changing behaviour toward safer sex [13]. However, sustaining protective behaviours usually requires enhanced prevention strategies, addressing both couples [14] and the community at large [12].

Ongoing efforts carried out by the WHO and its partners to increase access to ART substantially in resource-poor settings require the continuous development and evaluation of innovative, ethically sound and cost-effective VCT alternatives. Several countries have developed guidelines for VCT—such as Brazil, Russia and South Africa—that include both pre- and post-test counselling. The recent introduction of several types of rapid HIV tests has increased uptake of VCT in both developed and developing countries [15,16]. Another strategy is to provide pre-test information in a standardized format, including the provision of information or videos for groups of clients [12].

Implications for health systems

Steps to offer potent ART to large numbers of HIV-infected individuals in developing countries have contributed to reducing discrimination and stigma among PLHIV, attracting new individuals to VCT and shortening the time lag between VCT and effective entry into treatment. Successful initiatives have been shown to be cost-effective in very poor settings such as Haiti, Trinidad, Tanzania and Kenya [17–19]. In this context, VCT can be expanded and incorporated into venues such as primary healthcare, antenatal and STI clinics, and needle exchange and drug treatment programmes [12]. In particular, VCT should accompany

STI testing among high-risk individuals. Syndromic treatment of STIs has also been evaluated as an HIV prevention strategy in Uganda and Tanzania [20]; however, the impact of this approach on HIV incidence may depend on the prevalence of curable STIs in the population [21].

Increased access to treatment does not necessarily translate into increased uptake of VCT and less discrimination. An integrated attempt to mobilize communities and educate people about HIV prevention is pivotal in any strategy for VCT scale-up, early diagnosis and improved treatment [22]. As documented in Haiti, dissemination of concrete benefits of ART in terms of longer and healthier lives of PLHIV receiving ARVs may increase the demand for VCT and further enrolment of clients into treatment [17].

VCT should be translated into concrete benefits for those being tested, linking testing to treatment, care and support. However, scarcity of funds and lack of infrastructure have compromised this goal in many countries. Optimal VCT delivery also faces challenges such as a persisting high rate of non-return [23], the need to better integrate counselling and screening of HIV and tuberculosis [24], and improving capacity to attract vulnerable and stigmatized populations. Recent efforts to provide VCT in African rural settings [25] and on-site VCT for drug users from residential programmes [26] should be replicated and further evaluated.

As in any other field of public health, all initiatives must be carefully monitored to prevent unintended consequences of VCT, such as misperceptions about oral HIV transmission after saliva testing [27]. Experience has shown that previously insurmountable challenges, such as optimal VCT for inmates [28], can be successfully addressed. Health systems must be prepared to overcome these barriers if the WHO goals for VCT are to be realized.

Mother-to-child transmission

In the absence of specific interventions, rates of MTCT range from 15 to 40% [29]. HIV substantially contributes to infant and child mortality in many African countries and has reversed recent trends towards improved survival, highlighting the importance of PMTCT. With the identification of risk factors associated with MTCT, including breastfeeding practices [30], maternal plasma viral load [31], high titre of cell-associated HIV in the genital tract [32], low CD4 count [31] and maternal malaria [33], a number of interventions have been developed that aim to reduce the risk. These include recommendations about breastfeeding practices, elective Caesarean section delivery and the administration of antiretroviral prophylaxis antenatally to the mother and neonatally to the infant. Below, we briefly review these interventions and their applications.

Prophylactic antiretroviral therapy

Results of three randomized, open-label trials in Africa evaluated the use of intrapartum and postnatal prophylactic ART to reduce MTCT. Preliminary results from West Africa and Thailand have indicated the short-term effectiveness of boosting short-course zidovudine (AZT) or AZT + 3TC with peripartum nevirapine (NVP) [34,35], with MTCT rates at 6–8 weeks of 4.6% where short-course AZT + 3TC was boosted by NVP. An evaluation of post-exposure prophylaxis of either NVP or NVP and AZT given to newborns whose mothers did not receive antenatal care or peripartum ART prophylaxis showed NVP + AZT to be more effective than NVP alone [36].

Elective Caesarean delivery

There is evidence of a substantial effect of elective Caesarean section delivery before labour and before membrane rupture on the risk of MTCT [37,38]. The number of elective Caesarean section deliveries in the USA increased significantly, from 20% in 1996 to 48% in 2000 [39]. Elective Caesarean rates in Europe among HIV-infected women have been considerably higher at around 70–80%, although there may have been a recent decline in women who already receive highly active antiretroviral therapy (HAART) [40].

Variations in elective Caesarean rates reflect the debate around its potential side effects, which some argue no longer outweigh the benefits in terms of reduced MTCT for infected women successfully treated with HAART who have undetectable viral loads. However, in a European setting, two case–control studies comparing HIV-infected with uninfected women delivering by elective Caesarean and vaginally showed that, although infected women have an increased risk of complications following elective Caesarean delivery compared with uninfected women, they also had an increased risk of post-partum morbidity, and especially fever, compared with controls after vaginal delivery [41].

Breastfeeding interventions

In developed country settings where formula-feeding is safe, affordable and feasible, HIV-infected women are advised to avoid breastfeeding. However, in much of the developing world, infants born to HIV-infected mothers would be at greater risk of illness and death if they were not breastfed, as compared with the risks posed by HIV infection. In settings with high breastfeeding prevalence, postnatal HIV transmission may reduce overall long-term efficacy of prophylactic perinatal ART [32], and new approaches involving prophylaxis for HIV-exposed breastfeeding infants are being investigated [42]. In a phase I/II open-label randomized trial that evaluated three different 6-month regimens of NVP prophylaxis (once weekly, twice weekly and once daily) for breastfeeding, NVP was found to be safe and well tolerated [43]. Preliminary results from a trial in Kampala and Kigali, Uganda, where breastfeeding HIV-negative infants born to HIV-infected women who had received double ART prophylaxis in late pregnancy were given NVP or 3TC for 6 months, showed a 1% rate of postnatal HIV transmission between birth and 6 months [44], which was substantially lower than the 3–4% rate between 4 weeks and 6 months without ART in an earlier meta-analysis [45].

VCT in antenatal care

With the effectiveness of short-term antiretroviral prophylaxis to prevent MTCT now established, there is a need to scale up preventive MTCT programmes to include improved access to antenatal care and VCT. With the exception of mass single-dose NVP intrapartum and neonatal treatment that has been piloted in Lusaka, Zambia [46], all preventive MTCT interventions require identification of infected women, preferably during pregnancy, but also around the time of delivery. Recent trends favour the adoption of the 'opt-out' approach by making VCT a standard procedure of regular antenatal care, except for patients who explicitly refuse testing.

However, high VCT uptake rates do not necessarily translate into successful MTCT programmes, as pregnant women need to return for their test results, accept the intervention offered and then actually use it, if self-administered, such as single-dose NVP in many settings, for the programme to be effective. Rapid HIV tests with same-day results may significantly increase the proportion of women actually receiving their results compared with conventional testing [47].

One year after the introduction of single-dose NVP into clinical practice in a tertiary hospital in Kenya, although 97% of pregnant women had undergone HIV testing, only 30% of infected women and their infants eventually received NVP. Reasons included non-return for test results, non-return for receipt of NVP and non-adherence [47]. Similarly, evaluation of the first year of an MTCT prevention programme in Lusaka, Zambia showed that, despite successful integration within existing antenatal services and a 72% testing uptake rate, a significant minority of infected women did not collect their NVP [46]. Such findings underscore the need to reduce patient attrition and non-compliance. In a study in Kenya, partner involvement and the provision of support and education regarding MTCT were identified as potentially improving compliance with perinatal interventions

In resource-rich settings, problems remain with respect to late identification of HIV-infected pregnant women and suboptimal use of MTCT interventions. Assessment of the use of interventions in nearly 5000 infants born to HIV-infected mothers in the USA identified a missed opportunity for prevention in 20% of deliveries, which was associated with increased MTCT risk [48]. In a French study, 4% of HIV-infected pregnant women enrolled since 1996 received no antenatal antiretroviral prophylaxis, accounting for 20% of all infected infants born; key reasons identified were refusal and unmonitored pregnancy, including cases where the woman was aware of her infection status prior to pregnancy [49]. Canadian researchers estimated that less than half (46%) of preventable vertical transmissions were actually prevented in Ontario in 2001, primarily due to low uptake of antenatal screening [50].

Point-of-care HIV testing in the labour room using a rapid HIV test requiring 20 minutes to develop was found to be both feasible and accurate in a US study involving 380 women. This approach allows undiagnosed infected women to have their test results and receive intrapartum prophylaxis [39]. Such approaches are now even more pertinent following studies that indicate the feasibility and efficacy of post-exposure prophylaxis in the infant [36].

Implications for health systems

The extent to which current VCT programmes in antenatal care can and will contribute to a decline in the rate of global MTCT is unknown. The UN special assembly has targeted a 20% reduction in new infections in children by 2005, and 50% by 2010. Although virtual elimination of MTCT of HIV infection is theoretically possible in developed country settings, early identification of HIV-infected pregnant women is essential for the optimal application of interventions. Even in these settings, there are substantial numbers of women with inadequate antenatal care or access to antenatal HIV testing who are identified late in pregnancy, during labour or in the postnatal period [12].

In less-developed countries, many women are not tested for HIV and other STIs, or are unaware of their serostatus [51]. There is also a problem where women tend to deliver at home. It is challenging to ensure that the mother receives her single-dose NVP according to instructions, and there is no easy single-dose NVP preparation for the infant. Thus, contact with the healthcare system is still needed within a few days of delivery.

Consensus is emerging that even women presenting a few hours before delivery should benefit from VCT through the use of rapid tests, prompt initiation of prophylaxis and further counselling, if applicable, about the proper management and care of newborns at risk for HIV infection [12]. To obtain informed consent and to counsel pregnant women in the very moment of labour and delivery represent enormous challenges, but such challenges must be faced given the high percentage of women presenting very late in obstetric facilities world-wide. For example, many successful attempts have been made in Brazil to integrate rapid testing, brief counselling, prompt intervention and psychosocial support to such women [15]. Recent findings from India [16] corroborate the idea that such initiatives are not only desirable but well accepted in different cultures and settings and should be integrated into maternity units as routine procedures. Recent advances in rapid HIV testing and post-exposure prophylaxis may result in at least some vertical infections being prevented in such women, but should not be seen as an alternative to improving antenatal HIV screening programmes.

Men who have sex with men

MSM have been disproportionately affected by the HIV pandemic [51,52]. Approximately 65% of those living with AIDS in the USA are MSM, and 67% of new HIV diagnoses among individuals living in states with name-based HIV reporting are MSM [53]. Apparent reductions in high-risk behaviours have been offset by increases in STIs due to unprotected sex and increased numbers of new HIV infections among MSM [51,54]. Despite these patterns, relatively few interventions designed to reduce the number of new infections have been tested. Three general intervention approaches have been tested: individual, group and structural interventions. Interventions targeting MSM have tended to focus on primary prevention, or preventing new infections, although recently, secondary prevention interventions have been developed that seek to reduce transmission behaviours among HIV-positive MSM in an effort to interrupt the chain of HIV transmission. Since a large number of interventions have been developed and evaluated for MSM populations, we provide illustrative examples of various approaches to changing risky behaviour.

Individual-level interventions

Interventions that target individuals have the advantage of being able to target problems unique to each individual. Ideally, interventions are based on behavioural theories that guide their development, implementation and evaluation. For example, the EXPLORE study, a random-ized trial conducted among MSM in the USA, was designed to test the efficacy of a 10-session behavioural intervention in preventing HIV infection [55]. This intervention was based on the information–motivation–behaviour model and social learning theory, and promoted safer sex by addressing behaviour change in areas in which individuals might be ambivalent through the use of motivational interviewing and training individual skills, including communication to partners about condoms. The first three sessions were used to establish rapport between the counsellor and the individual while identifying those factors most salient to unsafe sex and effective self-protective behaviour.

Using factors relevant to the individual, counsellors selected pertinent modules for subsequent sessions from six domains: (i) individual perception of risk behaviour in their previous sexual behaviour; (ii) work to modify attitudes and skills that facilitate or impair communication of risk limits; (iii) beliefs about sero-status and its role in sex practices; (iv) the role of substance use in risk behaviour; (v) contextual aspects of risk behaviour, such as partner types, events and places; and (vi) planning for adherence to safer sex.

Thus, in this approach, the precise delivery of the intervention was guided by the individual's needs. For example, MSM engaging in the use of 'club drugs'—e.g. Ecstasy (methylenedioxy-methamphetamine) and GHB (gamma-hydroxybutyrate)—that are frequently used in high-risk situations such as circuit parties [56] may require focused interventions that take into account the extent to which these drugs are related to unsafe sex [57].

However, a disadvantage to individual-level interventions is that they often require highly skilled interventionists, the delivery and standardization of the intervention is complex, and they tend to be expensive. As a result, the utility and sustainability of such interventions in resource-poor settings may be limited.

Group-based interventions

Interventions that utilize a group format have a number of advantages, including the ability to intervene with more than one person at a time and the opportunity for participants to problem solve and role play with others. In a review of MSM intervention studies, Johnson *et al.* [58] reported that interventions targeting small groups produced significant improvements in sexual risk behaviour. Kalichman and colleagues [59] tested the effectiveness of an intervention based on Social Cognitive Theory to reduce sexual risks among HIV-infected individuals. Individuals were randomly assigned to either a five-session, group-based, safer sex intervention condition or a time- and contact-equivalent social support group condition, each including 6–10 participants. Participants in the risk-reduction intervention condition had significantly lower rates of unprotected sex, fewer total sex acts, fewer HIV-uninfected partners and a larger percentage of sex acts involving condom use at 6-month follow-up, compared with the control condition.

As this example illustrates, group-based interventions have the potential to reach a larger number of people with HIV risk-reduction interventions in a standardized format. However, these interventions are not always lower in cost compared with interventions involving individuals, since both time and expense are required to screen and locate eligible participants, especially if a minimum number is required for an appropriate group size.

Community-level interventions

Community-level interventions seek to reduce the prevalence of high-risk behaviours by reaching large numbers of vulnerable individuals with HIV risk-reduction messages. Such interventions have the potential to change the behaviour of whole groups by providing education, increasing motivation and creating new social norms. Based on the ideas of Rogers [60], who suggested that behavioural innovations often originate among a subgroup of individuals who are the communities' popular opinion leaders, Kelly and colleagues [61,62] developed and tested such an intervention for MSM they termed the Community Popular Opinion Leader (C-POL) model.

In the C-POL model, key gatekeepers and informants observed bar patrons and identified individuals who were seen most frequently and positively to interact with others in the same setting. These opinion leaders were then approached and invited to attend a four-session group programme that taught skills for communicating HIV prevention messages to friends and acquaintances during regular interactions. The effectiveness of the intervention was determined by pre- and post-intervention surveys of MSM and suggested reductions in high-risk sex of about 35% [61], and 2-year follow-up data suggested that these changes were maintained [63].

An alternative approach is that of structural interventions, which aim to modify the environment in ways that promote safer behaviours. For example, the Mpowerment Project was a community-level HIV prevention intervention for young gay/bisexual men that was implemented in four US communities [64]. The theoretical framework was based on diffusion of innovation theory, community organizing, peer influence and personal empowerment. The project promoted the norm for safer sex through a variety of social, outreach and small group activities run by a 'core group' of 12–15 young gay and bisexual men who, along with volunteers, designed and carried out all project activities. Following the intervention, the proportion of men engaging in any unprotected anal intercourse decreased from 41% to 30%. In contrast, significant increases in unsafe sex occurred in the comparison communities during the same period [65].

This study highlights the potential importance of structural interventions and suggests that HIV prevention messages should be embedded in the social activities of the targeted community. Further research is needed on structural interventions and methods for determining the mechanisms underpinning behavioural change at the population level.

Implications for health systems

A meta-analysis of behavioural interventions designed to reduce high-risk sexual behaviour among MSM concluded that interventions that promoted interpersonal skills, were delivered in community-level formats or focused on younger individuals or those at higher risk were most effective [58]. Yet, none of these approaches or those described above has been widely implemented. This is true despite the fact that the US Centers for Disease Control (CDC) has endorsed a number of interventions, including C-POL. Furthermore, few studies have been conducted to assess the efficacy of these interventions in settings outside the US. Cultural taboos against homosexuality may drive MSM underground, making this population more difficult to reach.

High rates of HIV/STI among MSM suggest that medical care settings may provide a valuable target for prevention efforts. The CDC, the Health Resources and Services Administration, the National Institutes of Health (NIH) and the HIV Medicine Association of the Infectious Diseases Society of America have recommended that HIV prevention be incorporated into the medical care of all HIV-infected individuals. To this end, they have made a number of recommendations that are relevant to MSM of all ages, ethnicities and nationalities: (i) screening for HIV transmission risk behaviours and STIs; (ii) providing brief behavioural risk-reduction interventions in the office setting; and (iii) referring selected patients for additional prevention interventions and other related services, and facilitating notification and counselling of sex and needle-sharing partners of infected persons [52].

The social landscape within which prevention messages are delivered is constantly changing in the MSM community, suggesting the need for re-evaluation. The increased prevalence of 'barebacking', or intentional unprotected anal sex, is evidenced among gay men, particularly those who are HIV-positive, by the number of Internet sites devoted to this practice and the growing number of men seeking sexual partners through the Internet [66]. As previously mentioned, future interventions using the Internet as a virtual venue for delivering HIV prevention messages may be particularly well suited for MSM populations.

Injecting drug users

The major types of interventions aimed to reduce drug-related harm include drug abuse treatment programmes, needle exchange programmes (NEPs), outreach and network-oriented interventions. Below, we review the effectiveness of drug abuse treatment and NEPs in reducing HIV risk behaviours. Readers interested in more detailed reviews of these and the remaining interventions are referred to a number of excellent sources [67–71].

Drug abuse treatment

Since cessation of injecting drug use is the only sure way to reduce the probability of HIV transmission through contaminated injection equipment to zero, drug abuse treatment is the most widely endorsed intervention to reduce HIV-associated risk behaviours among IDUs [70]. Over the past two decades, research has consistently shown associations between enrolment in substance abuse treatment and reductions in HIV transmission risk behaviours, which can be attributed to reductions in injecting drug use [72–75]. Moreover, the longer the duration of substance abuse treatment, the greater the protective effects [70,75]. Detoxification alone appears to be insufficient to provide protection from HIV infection unless it is followed by a longer course of treatment [70].

Worldwide, the most consistent reductions in HIV-related risk behaviours have been observed for medication-assisted therapies that block opiate receptors, particularly maintenance programmes offering methadone [73–76] or buprenorphine [77,78]. More recently, buprenorphine maintenance has been shown to be just as effective as methadone in reducing ongoing use of opiates [77,78].

While drug abuse treatment is considered to be an effective HIV prevention strategy, its impact has varied dramatically between and even within countries. In Amsterdam, a decline in HIV incidence among IDUs was associated with a combination of widespread access to low-threshold methadone maintenance, needle exchange and voluntary HIV testing and counselling [79]. Likewise, in New York City, the reversal of a major HIV epidemic that began in the early 1980s has been attributed to a combination of expanded methadone maintenance and increased access to sterile syringes and outreach [80]. Unfortunately, as little as 15–20% of active drug users in the USA are enrolled in drug abuse treatment at any given time [81].

Needle exchange programmes

NEPs allow IDUs to exchange potentially contaminated syringes for sterile ones. An important aim of NEPs is to decrease the circulation of contaminated injection equipment, thereby reducing the spread of blood-borne pathogens in the community. Since the first NEP was introduced in Amsterdam in 1984, at least 46 regions, countries and territories reported having at least one NEP by the end of 2000 [69]. By 2002, there were 178 exchanges in 36 US states, Washington, DC and Puerto Rico, according to the North American Syringe Exchange Network [Dave Purchase, personal communication, 2004].

The overwhelming majority of studies provide strong evidence of the effectiveness of NEPs in reducing high-risk injection behaviours among HIV-seronegative and HIV-seropositive IDUs. In 1988, Buning and colleagues from Amsterdam reported declines in needle sharing and injection frequency associated with NEP participation [82]. Other studies subsequently reported reductions in incidence of HIV, hepatitis B virus (HBV) and hepatitis C virus (HCV) infections [67,83–88], decreased needle sharing among HIV-negative and HIV-positive people [87–90], decreases in syringe re-use [91] and increased rates of entry into drug treatment programmes [81,91]. Despite variations among programmes, a recent international comparison showed that in 29 cities with established NEPs, HIV prevalence decreased on average by 5.8% per year, but increased on average by 5.9% per year in 51 cities without NEPs [92]. There appears to be no published evidence that NEPs can cause negative societal effects such as increases in drug use, discarded needles, crime or more permissive attitudes towards drugs among youth [87,93–95]. A national policy of funding NEPs, pharmacy sales and syringe disposal in the USA was estimated to cost US$34,278 per HIV infection averted, which is well below the lifetime costs of treating an individual's HIV infection [96].

Implications for health systems

International experience with both drug abuse treatment and NEPs offers important insights for healthcare systems. The public health impact of substance abuse treatment has been severely hampered because access to these programmes is severely limited. At least in the USA, most communities have no adequately funded treatment services, and, in some cases, funding for substance abuse treatment programmes has actually diminished during the course of the HIV epidemic. Additionally, the lack of third-party reimbursement for substance abuse treatment limits access for some HIV-positive drug users [81].

In some parts of the world, public policy restricts certain modalities of drug abuse treatment. For example, in Russia, agonist treatments for drug abuse such as methadone and buprenorphine are prohibited [70]. In many countries in Asia that have reported explosive HIV epidemics among IDUs, such as Thailand or China, there is almost no access to opiate agonist therapies. It is not surprising that each of these countries is experiencing ongoing explosive HIV epidemics among IDUs. Therefore, expansion of medication-assisted drug abuse treatment services is needed, perhaps through innovative approaches such as mobile vans [97].

More recently, medically supervised prescription of heroin to IDUs who have failed in the use of traditional opiate agonist therapies has been evaluated and has shown remarkable success in reducing injecting drug use and its associated ill effects in Switzerland [98], where it has been adopted as part of the country's overall public health response to treating heroin addiction. Heroin maintenance trials are also under way in The Netherlands, Germany and Canada [99]. Heroin maintenance may be an appropriate treatment modality for 'hard core' drug users whose behaviour is hardest to change.

In many settings, NEPs tend to attract higher-risk IDUs who engage in riskier behaviours compared with IDUs who tend to obtain syringes from other sources [100–102], which is considered an advantage because these individuals are precisely those who need to be linked to HIV prevention and care. Apart from increasing access to sterile syringes, NEPs can provide crucial ancillary services such as condoms, on-site HIV testing and counselling, screening for medical conditions such as STIs and tuberculosis, provision of HBV and HAV vaccines, abscess care, overdose prevention and multivitamins. NEPs have served as a pivotal entry point for drug treatment and rehabilitation, provided that adequate numbers of treatment slots are available [81,91,103]. Altice *et al.* recently reported that provision of HAART to IDUs attending mobile NEPs in New Haven, Connecticut was feasible; a similar project is under way in Baltimore, Maryland [104].

Yet, in both developed and developing countries, there exist intentional and unintentional barriers to the provision of sterile syringes to IDUs. Although global expansion of NEPs has occurred since the first NEP was introduced two decades ago, NEPs exist in less than half the countries reporting HIV among IDUs, and coverage of these programmes is typically very low [105]. In the USA, a federal ban on funding for NEPs was enacted in 1988, which has been upheld despite the fact that several US government-commissioned reports have specifically called for the ban to be lifted [65,106–109].

The ban on US federal funding for NEPs has affected HIV prevention and treatment for IDUs. In a survey of 81 NEPs across the USA, Paone and colleagues [110] reported that NEPs that operated illegally were significantly less likely to offer ancillary services such as on-site HIV testing and counselling and formal arrangements for referrals to drug abuse treatment. Therefore, even in settings where access to sterile syringes is legally offered through pharmacies, physician prescription or syringe vending machines, NEPs are worthwhile interventions since they can offer both HIV prevention and treatment when supported as part of a comprehensive health programme.

Sex workers

Commercial sex work has changed little since biblical times. Sex workers are ubiquitous in many cultures, and high rates of STIs and HIV infection have been documented in this population. Interventions designed to slow the spread of HIV in this high-risk population have, for the most part, been promising.

Some environmental interventions have been designed to expand the economic power of female sex workers as a way to extend their employment opportunities beyond sex work and increase their ability to negotiate safer sex. For example, in Zambia, women fish traders were often forced into sex in exchange for fish from fishermen. In order to combat this, economic cooperatives were set up to bargain collectively for fish and provide credit to women, which led to reductions in sexual exploitation [111]. In Bangladesh, a bank provided access to credit for rural women which resulted in increased use of contraception [112].

National-level responses have shown great promise in Thailand, where the HIV epidemic in the heterosexual population spread exponentially in the 1980s. A high proportion of HIV cases were linked to sex work, a problem that was compounded by the fact that clients offered sex workers more money for unprotected sex. In response, the Thai government established the '100% Condom Policy', which mandates and enforces condom use in all commercial sex establishments. This programme, which is an example of an environmental–structural intervention, began with a nationwide condom advertising campaign that was soon followed by the 100% condom use policy. In addition, STI services and over-the-counter antibiotics were made widely available. Use of condoms in brothels rose from 14% before the programme to 91% in 1993, and was accompanied by an 85% decrease in the number of male STI cases presenting at government clinics [113]. Successes were subsequently reported from a similar programme in the Dominican Republic [114], which is now being widely implemented in several countries in Africa and Asia.

Conclusions

In the third decade of the HIV pandemic, health systems in both developed and developing countries face several challenges to prevention, which include the difficulty in implementing HIV preventive interventions that have already been proven effective. For example, although there are ample studies in a variety of settings that demonstrate the cost-effectiveness of VCT and programmes to reduce MTCT, NEPs and drug abuse treatment, these interventions have not been implemented as widely as they need to be to reduce the global burden of HIV infection significantly. As we have described in this chapter, a combination of problems contributes to the lack of coverage, including lack of resources, poor health infrastructures and lack of political will. Clearly, scaling-up of these and other programmes is urgently needed.

Further research is also needed in a number of key areas. For example, interventions for HIV-positive individuals have only received attention in recent years and are especially relevant in communities where HIV prevalence is already high. Structural interventions that mediate on multiple levels may prove it possible to reduce the incidence of HIV and other conditions such as STIs, or the behaviours and conditions that increase vulnerability to HIV infection, such as unprotected sex, drug abuse or homelessness.

Finally, it should be recognized that an integrated approach is needed to HIV prevention; no single intervention operating in isolation is likely to have a significant impact on HIV incidence in a population. What works today may not work tomorrow. The constantly changing dynamic of the HIV pandemic reflects the need to revisit and revise existing interventions so that they are culturally appropriate and sensitive to the needs of local communities. For these reasons, ongoing evaluations including HIV and behavioural surveillance are needed to help inform both programmes and policies.

Acknowledgements

SA Strathdee acknowledges support from the Foundation for the Harold Simon Chair and the National Institute on Drug Abuse (DA12568 and DA09225); FI Bastos is partially supported by a National Research Council (CNPq) salary grant and a FIOCRUZ grant PAPES III 250.250.122; TL Patterson acknowledges grant support from the National Institute on Drug Abuse (DA012116) and the National Institute on Mental Health (MH061146); M-L Newell acknowledges support from the European Commission (QLK2-CT-2000-00002) and the Medical Research Council (UK).

References

1. Rhodes T, Stimson GV, Crofts N, Ball A, Dehne K, Khodakevich L. (1999). Drug injecting, rapid HIV spread and the 'risk environment'. *AIDS* **13**(Supplement A):S259–69.

2. Kocher KW. (1993). *STOP AIDS. The STOP AIDS story 1987–1992*. Zurich: Swiss AIDS Foundation and Federal Office for Public Health.

3. McOwan A, Gilleece Y, Chislett L, Mandalia S. (2002). Can targeted HIV testing campaigns alter health-seeking behaviour? *AIDS Care* **14**:385–90.

4. Shapiro D, Meekers D, Tambashe B. (2003). Exposure to the 'SIDA dans la Cite' AIDS prevention television series in Côte d'Ivoire, sexual risk behaviour and condom use. *AIDS Care* **15**:303–14.

5. Moatti JP, Dab W, Loundou H, Quenel P, Beltzer N, Anes A, Pollak M. (1992). Impact on the general public of media campaigns against AIDS: a French evaluation. *Health Policy* 21:233–47.

6. Gibson S, McFarland W, Wohlfeiler D, Scheer K, Katz MH. (1999). Experiences of 100 men who have sex with men using the Reality condom for anal sex. *AIDS Education and Prevention* 11:65–71.

7. Hausser D, Michaud PA. (1994). Does a condom-promoting strategy (the Swiss STOP-AIDS campaign) modify sexual behavior among adolescents? *Pediatrics* 93:580–5.

8. Montoya ID, Trevino RA, Ataabadi AN. (1997). The impact of public health media campaigns on drug users. *Mark Health Services* 17(4):20–7.

9. Wolitski RJ, Fishbein M, Johnson WD, Schnell DJ, Esacove A. (1996). Sources of HIV information among injecting drug users: association with gender, ethnicity, and risk behaviour. AIDS Community Demonstration Projects. *AIDS Care* 8:541–55.

10. Conde F. (1989). *Investigacion sobre la Campaña de Publicidad 'No Piques'.* Madrid: Ministerio de Sanidad y Consumo España.

11. US Centers for Disease Control and Prevention (CDC). (2004). Using the Internet for partner notification of sexually transmitted diseases in Los Angeles County, California, 2003. *Morbidity and Mortality Weekly Reports* 53(6):129–31.

12. World Health Organization. (2003). *Treating 3 Million by 2005. Making it Happen: The WHO Strategy.* Geneva: WHO.

13. The Voluntary HIV-1 Counselling and Testing Efficacy Study Group. (2000). Efficacy of voluntary HIV-1 counselling and testing in individuals and couples in Kenya, Tanzania, and Trinidad: a randomised trial. *Lancet* 356:103–12.

14. Allen S, Meinzen-Derr J, Kautzman M et al. (2003). Sexual behaviour of HIV discordant couples after HIV counseling and testing. *AIDS* 17:733–40.

15. Nogueira SA, Lambert JS, Albuquerque AL et al. (2001). Assessment of a rapid HIV test strategy during labour: a pilot study from Rio de Janeiro, Brazil. *Journal of Human Virology* 4:278–82.

16. Shankar AV, Pisal H, Patil O et al. (2003). Women's acceptability and husband's support of rapid HIV testing of pregnant women in India. *AIDS Care* 15:871–4.

17. Mukherjee J, Colas M, Farmer P et al. (2003). *Access to Antiretroviral Treatment and Care: The Experience of the HIV Equity Initiative, Cange, Haiti—Case Study.* Geneva: WHO.

18. Farmer P. (2003). *Pathologies of Power: Health, Human Rights, and the New War on the Poor.* Berkeley: University of California Press.

19. Sweat M, Gregorich S, Sangiwa G et al. (2000). Cost-effectiveness of voluntary HIV-1 counselling and testing in reducing sexual transmission of HIV-1 in Kenya and Tanzania. *Lancet* 356:113–21.

20. Grosskurth H, Gray R, Hayes R, Mabey D, Wawer M. (2000). Control of sexually transmitted diseases for HIV-1 prevention: understanding the implications of the Mwanza and Rakai trials. *Lancet* 355:1981–7.

21. Orroth KK, Korenromp EL, White RG et al. (2003). Higher risk behaviour and rates of sexually transmitted diseases in Mwanza compared to Uganda may help explain HIV prevention trial outcomes. *AIDS* 17:2653–60.

22. Kalichman SC, Simbayi LC. (2003). HIV testing attitudes, AIDS stigma, and voluntary HIV counselling and testing in a black township in Cape Town, South Africa. *Sexually Transmitted Infections* 79:442–7.

23. Hightow LB, Miller WC, Leone PA, Wohl D, Smurzynski M, Kaplan AH. (2003). Failure to return for HIV post-test counseling in an STD clinic population. *AIDS Education and Prevention* 15:282–90.

24. Suggaravetsiri P, Yanai H, Chongsuvivatwong V, Naimpasan O, Akarasewi P. (2003). Integrated counseling and screening for tuberculosis and HIV among household contacts of tuberculosis

patients in an endemic area of HIV infection: Chiang Rai, Thailand. *International Journal of Tubercular Lung Disease* 7(12 Supplement 3):S424–31.

25. Matovu JK, Kigozi G, Nalugoda F, Wabwire-Mangen F, Gray RH. (2002). The Rakai Project counselling programme experience. *Tropical Medicine and International Health* 7:1064–7.

26. Strauss SM, Des Jarlais DC, Astone J, Vassilev ZP. (2003). On-site HIV testing in residential drug treatment units: results of a nationwide survey. *Public Health Reports* 118:37–43.

27. Clair S, Singer M, Huertas E, Weeks M. (2003). Unintended consequences of using an oral HIV test on HIV knowledge. *AIDS Care* 15:575–80.

28. Burchell AN, Calzavara LM, Myers T *et al.* (2003). Voluntary HIV testing among inmates: socio-demographic, behavioural risk, and attitudinal correlates. *Journal of Acquired Immune Deficiency Syndrome* 32:534–41.

29. Newell ML, Dabis F, Tolley K, Whynes D. (1998). Cost-effectiveness and cost-benefit in the prevention of mother-to-child transmission of HIV in developing countries. Ghent International Working Group on Mother-to-Child Transmission of HIV. *AIDS* 12:1571–80.

30. Nduati R, John G, Mbori-Ngacha D *et al.* (2000). Effect of breastfeeding and formula feeding on transmission of HIV-1: a randomized clinical trial. *Journal of the American Medical Association* 283:1167–74.

31. Fiore J, Soligoi B, Saracino A *et al.* (2003). Correlates of HIV-1 shedding in cervicovaginal secretions and effects of antiretroviral therapies. *AIDS* 17:2169–76.

32. Tuomala R, O' Driscoll P, Bremer J *et al.* (2003). Cell-associated genital tract virus and vertical transmission of human immunodeficiency virus type 1 in antiretroviral-experienced women. *Journal of Infectious Diseases* 187:375–84.

33. Brahmbhatt H, Kigozi G, Wabwire-Mangen F *et al.* (2003). The effects of placental malaria on mother-to-child HIV transmission in Rakai, Uganda. *AIDS* 17:2539–41.

34. The Petra study team. (2002). Efficacy of the three short-course regimens of zidovudine and lamivudine in preventing early and late transmission of HIV-1 from mother to child in Tanzania, South Africa and Uganda (Petra Study): a randomized, double-blind, placebo-controlled trial. *Lancet* 359:1178–86.

35. Moodley D, Moodley J, Coovadia H *et al.* (2003). A multicenter randomized controlled trial of nevirapine versus a combination of zidovudine and lamivudine to reduce intrapartum and early postpartum mother-to-child transmission of human immunodeficiency virus type 1. *Journal of Infectious Diseases* 187:725–735.

36. Taha TE, Kumwenda NI, Gibbons A *et al.* (2003). Short postexposure prophylaxis in newborn babies to reduce mother-to-child transmission of HIV-1: NVAZ randomized clinical trial. *Lancet* 362:1171–7.

37. The European Mode of Delivery Collaboration. (1999). Elective Caesarean section versus vaginal delivery in preventing vertical HIV-1 transmission: a randomised clinical trial. *Lancet* 353:1035–9.

38. The International Perinatal HIV group. (1999) Mode of delivery and vertical transmission of HIV-1: a meta-analysis from fifteen prospective cohort studies. *New England Journal of Medicine* 340:977–87.

39. Cohen MH, Olszewski Y, Branson B *et al.* (2003). Using point-of-care testing to make rapid HIV-1 tests in labour really rapid. *AIDS* 17:2121–4.

40. European Collaborative Study. (2001). HIV-infected pregnant women and vertical transmission in Europe since 1986. *AIDS* 15:761–70.

41. European HIV in Obstetrics Group (Fiore S, Newell ML, Thorne C and other collaborators). (2004). Higher rates of post-partum complications in HIV-infected than in uninfected women irrespective of mode of delivery. *AIDS* 18:933–8.

42. Gaillard P, Fowler MG, Dabis F *et al.* for the Ghent IAS working group on HIV in women and children. (2004). *Journal of Acquired Immune Deficiency Syndrome* 35:178–187.

43. Shetty AK. (2003). Safety and trough concentrations of nevirapine prophylaxis given daily, twice weekly or weekly in breast-feeding infants from birth to 6 months. *Journal of Acquired Immune Deficiency Syndrome* 34:482–90.

44. Vyankandondera J, Luchters S, Hassink E *et al.* (2003). Reducing Risk of HIV-1 Transmission from Mother to Infant Through Breastfeeding Using Antiretroviral Prophylaxis in Infants (SIMBA). Presented at the 2nd IAS Conference on HIV Pathogenesis and Treatment, Paris, 13–16 July 2003 [Abstract LB7].

45. Coutsoudis A, Dabis F, Fawzi W *et al.* (2004). Late postnatal transmission of HIV-1 in breast-fed children: an individual patient data meta-analysis. *J infect Dis* 189(12): 2154-66.

46. Stringer EM, Sinkala M, Stringer JS *et al.* (2003). Prevention of mother-to-child transmission of HIV in Africa: successes and challenges in scaling-up a nevirapine-based programme in Lusaka, Zambia. *AIDS* 17:1377–82.

47. Malonza IM, Richardson BA, Kreiss JK, Bwayo JJ, John-Stewart GC. (2003). The effect of rapid HIV-1 testing on uptake of perinatal HIV-1 interventions: a randomized clinical trial. *AIDS* 17:113–8.

48. Peters V, Liu KL, Dominguez K, Frederick T *et al.* (2003). Missed opportunities for perinatal HIV prevention among HIV-exposed infants born 1996–2000, pediatric spectrum of HIV disease cohort. *Pediatrics* 111:1186–91.

49. Mayaux M J, Teglas JP, Blanche S. (2003). Characteristics of HIV-infected women who do not receive preventive antiretroviral therapy in the French perinatal cohort. *Journal of Acquired Immune Deficiency Syndrome* 34:338–343.

50. Remis RS, King S, Vernich L *et al.* (2003). Epidemiologic modelling to evaluate prevention of mother-infant HIV transmission in Ontaria. *Journal of Acquired Immunodeficiency Syndrome* 34:221–30.

51. Stoto MA, Almario DA, McCormick MC (eds). (1999). *Reducing the Odds. Preventing Perinatal Transmission of HIV in the United States*. Washington, DC: National Academy Press.

52. US Centers for Disease Control and Prevention (CDC); Health Resources and Services Administration; National Institutes of Health; HIV Medicine Association of the Infectious Diseases Society of America. (2003). Incorporating HIV prevention into the medical care of persons living with HIV. Recommendations of CDC, the Health Resources and Services Administration, the National Institutes of Health, and the HIV Medicine Association of the Infectious Diseases Society of America. *Morbidity and Mortality Weekly Reports* 52(RR-12):1–24.

53. Kippax S, Race K. (2003). Sustaining safe practice: twenty years on. *Social Science and Medicine* 57: 1–12.

54. Ciesielski CA. (2003). Sexually transmitted diseases in men who have sex with men: an epidemiologic review. *Current Infectious Diseases Report* 5:145–152.

55. Chesney MA, Koblin BA, Barresi PJ *et al.* (2003). EXPLORE Study Team. An individually tailored intervention for HIV prevention: baseline data from the EXPLORE Study. *American Journal of Public Health* 93:933–8.

56. Mansergh G, Marks G, Colfax GN, Guzman R, Rader M, Buchbinder S. (2002). 'Barebacking' in a diverse sample of men who have sex with men. *AIDS* 16:653–9.

57. Ross MW, Mattison AM, Franklin DR Jr. (2003). Club drugs and sex on drugs are associated with different motivations for gay circuit party attendance in men. *Substance Use and Misuse* 38: 1173–83.

58. Johnson WD, Hedges LV, Ramirez G *et al.* (2002). HIV prevention research for men who have sex with men: a systematic review and meta-analysis. *Journal of Acquired Immune Deficiency Syndrome* 30:S118–29.

59. Kalichman SC, Rompa D, Cage M *et al.* (2001). Effectiveness of an intervention to reduce HIV transmission risks in HIV-positive people. *American Journal of Preventive Medicine* 21(2):84–92.

60. Rogers EM. (1985). *Diffusion of Innovation.* New York: Free Press.

61. Kelly JA, St Lawrence JS, Stevenson LY *et al.* (1992). Community AIDS/HIV risk reduction: the effects of endorsements by popular people in three cities. *American Journal of Public Health* 82:1483–9.

62. Kelly JA, Murphy DA, Sikkema KJ *et al.* (1997). Randomised, controlled, community-level HIV-prevention intervention for sexual-risk behaviour among homosexual men in US cities. Community HIV Prevention Research Collaborative. *Lancet* 350:1500–5.

63. St. Lawrence JS, Brasfield TL, Diaz YE *et al.* (1994). Three-year follow-up of an HIV risk reduction intervention that used popular peers. *American Journal of Public Health* 84:2027–8.

64. Hays RB, Rebchook GM, Kegeles SM. (2003). The Mpowerment Project: community-building with young gay and bisexual men to prevent HIV1. *American Journal of Community Psychology* 31:301–12.

65. Kegeles SM, Hays RB, Coates TJ. (1996). The Mpowerment Project: a community-level HIV prevention intervention for young gay men. *American Journal of Public Health* 86:1129–36.

66. Halkitis PN, Parsons JT. (2003). Intentional unsafe sex (barebacking) among HIV-positive gay men who seek sexual partners on the Internet. *AIDS Care* 15:367–78.

67. Normand J, Vlahov D, Moses LE (eds). (1995). *Preventing HIV Transmission: The Role of Sterile Needles and Bleach.* Washington, DC: National Academy Press.

68. Latkin CA. (1998). Outreach in natural settings: the use of peer leaders for HIV prevention among injecting drug users' networks. *Public Health Reports* 113(Supplement 1):151–9.

69. Bastos FI, Strathdee SA. (2000). Evaluating effectiveness of syringe exchange programs: current issues and future prospects. *Social Science and Medicine* 51:1771–82.

70. Metzger DS, Navaline H. (2003). Human immunodeficiency virus prevention and the potential of drug abuse treatment. *Clin Infect Dis* 37(Suppl 5):S451–6.

71. Semaan S, Des Jarlais DC, Sogolow E *et al.* (2002). A meta-analysis of the effect of HIV prevention interventions on the sex behaviors of drug users in the United States. *Journal of Acquired Immune Deficiency Syndrome* 30(Supplement 1):S73–93.

72. Booth RE, Crowley T, Zhang Y. (1996). Substance abuse treatment entry, retention, and effectiveness: out-of-treatment opiate injection drug users. *Drug and Alcohol Dependence* 42:11–20.

73. Metzger DS, Woody GE, McLellan AT *et al.* (1993). Human immunodeficiency virus seroconversion among in- and out-of-treatment intravenous drug users: an 18-month prospective follow-up. *Journal of Acquired Immune Deficiency Syndrome* 6:1049–56.

74. Ball JC, Lange WR, Myers CP *et al.* (1988). Reducing the risk of AIDS through methadone maintenance treatment. *Journal of Health and Social Behavior* 29:214–26.

75. National Consensus Development Panel on Effective Medical Treatment of Opiate Addiction. (1998). Effective medical treatment of opiate addiction. *Journal of the American Medical Association* 280:1936–43.

76. Langendam MW, van Brussel GH, Coutinho RA, van Ameijden EJ. (1999). Methadone maintenance treatment modalities in relation to incidence of HIV: results of the Amsterdam cohort study. *AIDS* 13:1711–6.

77. Carrieri MP, Rey D, Loundou A, Lepeu G, Sobel A, Obadia Y. (2003). The MANIF-2000 Study Group. Evaluation of buprenorphine maintenance treatment in a French cohort of HIV-infected injecting drug users. *Drug and Alcohol Dependence* 72: 13–21.

78. Johnson RE, Chutuape MA, Strain EC, Walsh SL, Stitzer ML, Bigelow GE. (2000). A comparison of levomethadyl acetate, buprenorphine, and methadone for opioid dependence. *New England Journal of Medicine* 343:1290–7.

79. van Ameijden EJC, Watters JK, van den Hoek JAR, Coutinho RA. (1995). Interventions among injecting drug users: do they work? *AIDS* 9(Supplement A):S75–84.

80. Des Jarlais DC, Marmor M, Friedmann P, *et al.* (2000). HIV incidence among injection drug users in New York City, 1992–1997: evidence for a declining epidemic. *American Journal of Public Health* 90:352–9.

81. Shah N, Celentano DD, Vlahov D *et al.* (2000). Correlates of enrollment in methadone maintenance programmes differ by HIV-serostatus. *AIDS* 14:2035–43.

82. Buning EC, Coutinho RA, van Brussel GH, van Santen GW, van Zadelhoff. (1986). Preventing AIDS in drug addicts in Amsterdam. *Lancet* 1:1435.

83. Van Ameijden EJC.and Coutinho RA. (1998). Maximum impact of HIV prevention measures targeted at injecting drug users. *AIDS* 12:625–33.

84. Lurie P, Reingold AL, Bowser B *et al.* (1993). *The Public Health Impact of Needle Exchange Programmes in the United States and Abroad. Summary, Conclusions and Recommendations.* Berkeley CA: School of Public Health, University of California.

85. Des Jarlais DC, Hagan H, Friedman SR, Friedmann P *et al.* (1995). Maintaining low HIV seroprevalence in populations of injecting drug users. *Journal of the American Medical Association* 15:1226–31.

86. Hagan H, DesJarlais DC, Friedman SR *et al.* (1995). Reduced risk of hepatitis B and hepatitis C among injection drug users in the Tacoma Syringe Exchange programme. *American Journal of Public Health* 85:1531–37.

87. Vlahov D, Junge B, Brookmeyer R *et al.* (1997). Reductions in high-risk drug use behaviors among participants in the Baltimore needle exchange programme. *Journal of Acquired Immune Deficiency Syndrome and Human Retrovirology* 16:400–406.

88. Drucker E, Lurie P, Wodak A, Alcabes P. (1997). Measuring harm reduction: the effects of needle and syringe exchange programmes and methadone maintenance on the ecology of HIV. *AIDS* 12(Supplement A):S217–30.

89. Bluthenthal RN, Kral AH, Gee L, Erringer EA, Edlin BR. (2000). The effect of syringe exchange use on high-risk injection drug users: a cohort study. *AIDS* 14:605–11.

90. Vertefeuille J, Marx MA, Tun W, Huettner S, Strathdee SA, Vlahov D. (2000). Decline in self-reported high risk injection-related behaviors among HIV seropositive participants in the Baltimore needle exchange programme. *AIDS and Behavior* 4:381–8.

91. Heimer R. (1998). Can syringe exchange serve as a conduit to substance abuse treatment? *Journal of Substance Abuse Treatment* 15:183–91.

92. Hurley S, Jolley D, Kaldor J. (1997) Effectiveness of needle-exchange programmes for prevention of HIV infection. *Lancet* 349:1797.

93. Marx MA, Crape B, Brookmeyer RS *et al.* (2000). Trends in crime and the introduction of a needle exchange programme. *American Journal of Public Health* 90:1933–36.

94. Doherty MC, Junge B, Rathouz P, Garfein RS, Riley E, Vlahov D. (2000). The effect of a needle exchange programme on numbers of discarded needles: a 2-year follow-up. *American Journal of Public Health* 90:936–9.

95. Marx MA, Brahmbhatt H, Beilenson P *et al.* (2001). Impact of needle exchange programmes on adolescent perceptions about illicit drug use. *AIDS and Behavior* 5:379–386.

96. Lurie P, Gorsky R, Jones TS, Shomphe L. (1998). An economic analysis of needle exchange and pharmacy-based programmes to increase sterile syringe availability for injection drug users. *Journal of Acquired Immune Deficiency Syndrome* 18(Supplement 1):S126–32.

97. Kuo I, Brady J, Butler C *et al.* (2003). Feasibility of referring drug users from a needle exchange programme into an addiction treatment programme: experience with a mobile treatment van and LAAM maintenance. *Journal of Substance Abuse Treatment* 24:67–74.

98. Guttinger F, Gschwend P, Schulte B, Rehm J, Uchtenhagen A. (2003). Evaluating long-term effects of heroin-assisted treatment: the results of a 6-year follow-up. *European Addiction Research* 9(2):73–9.

99. Fischer B, Rehm J, Kirst M *et al.* (2002). Heroin-assisted treatment as a response to the public health problem of opiate dependence. *European Journal of Public Health* 12:228–34.

100. Bruneau J, Lamothe F, Franco E *et al.* (1997). High rates of HIV infection among injection drug users participating in needle exchange programmes in Montreal: results of a cohort study. *American Journal of Epidemiology* 146:994–1002.

101. Schechter MT, Strathdee SA, Cornelisse PG *et al.* (1999). Do needle exchange programmes increase the spread of HIV among injection drug users? An investigation of the Vancouver outbreak. *AIDS* 13(6):F45–51.

102. Hahn JA, Vranizan KM, Moss AR. (1997). Who uses needle exchange? A study of injection drug users in treatment in San Francisco, 1989–1990. *Journal of Acquired Immune Deficiency Syndrome and Human Retrovirology* 15:157–64.

103. Brooner R, Kidorf M, King V, Beilenson P, Svikis D, Vlahov D. (1998). Drug abuse treatment success among needle exchange participants. *Public Health Reports* 113(Supplement 1):129–39.

104. Altice FL, Springer S, Buitrago M, Hunt DP, Friedland GH. (2003). Pilot study to enhance HIV care using needle exchange-based health services for out-of-treatment injecting drug users. *Journal of Urban Health* 80:416–27.

105. Strathdee SA, Vlahov D. (2001). The effectiveness of needle exchange programmes: a review of the science and policy. *AIDScience* 1(16):1–33.

106. National Commission on AIDS. (1991). *The Twin Epidemics of Substance Sbuse and HIV*. Washington, DC: National Commission on AIDS.

107. US General Accounting Office. (1993). *Needle Exchange Programmes: Research Suggests Promise as an AIDS Prevention Strategy*. Washington, DC: US Government Printing Office (Publication no. GAO/HRD 93–60).

108. Office of the Surgeon General. (2000). Evidence-based findings on the efficacy of syringe exchange programmes: an analysis from the Assistant Secretary for Health and Surgeon General of the scientific research completed since April 1998. Washington DC. Available at: http://www.harmreduction.org/surgreview.html.

109. NIH Consensus Development Program. (1997). Interventions to prevent HIV risk behaviours. *NIH Consensus Statement* 15:1–41.

110. Paone D, Clark J, Shi Q, Purchase D, Des Jarlais DC. (1999). Syringe exchange in the United States, 1996: a national profile. *American Journal of Public Health* 89:43–6.

111. Msiska R. (1994). *An Intervention Study to Develop and Test the Benefits of an Enabling Approach in Reducing HIV Transmission in a Fish Trading Community in Zambia*. Lusaka: National AIDS programme.

112. Schuler SR, Hashemi SM. (1994). Credit programmes, women's empowerment and contraceptive use in rural Bangladesh. *Studies in Family Planning* 25:65–76.

113. Hanenberg R, Rojanapithayakorn W, Kunasol P, Sokal D. (1994). Impact of Thailand's HIV-control programme as indicated by the decline in sexually transmitted diseases. *Lancet* 344:243–245.

114. Kerrigan D, Ellen JM, Moreno L *et al.* (2003). Environmental–structural factors significantly associated with consistent condom use among female sex workers in the Dominican Republic. *AIDS* 17:415–23.

Chapter 6

Antiretroviral treatment and care of HIV

Joep MA Lange

Introduction

The success of highly active antiretroviral therapy (HAART) is an illustration of the fact that quantitative factors can make a dramatic qualitative difference. Effective antiretroviral agents have been available since 1987 [1]. First-generation antiretrovirals—nucleoside analogue reverse transcriptase inhibitors (NRTIs) such as zidovudine (ZDV) and didanosine (ddI)—are still components of many antiretroviral drug regimens today. The antiviral efficacy of HAART is not only due to the appearance of drugs with new mechanisms of action, such as HIV protease inhibitors (PIs) or non-nucleoside reverse trascriptase inhibitors (NNRTIs), but primarily to using combinations of at least three anti-HIV drugs that inhibit viral replication to such an extent that development of viral drug resistance is smothered [2]. This already implies that the ability to measure the amount of virus in blood and other body compartments has been of crucial importance in the development of effective antiretroviral therapy. Use of NNRTIs in a regimen that does not suppress viral replication to minimal levels leads to the appearance of majority populations of NNRTI-resistant mutants in just a few weeks, whereas this may be prevented if they are used in more suppressive regimens [3].

The introduction of HAART is one of the great success stories of modern medicine. Its impact on HIV-related morbidity and mortality can almost be compared with that of the introduction of penicillin on pneumococcal pneumonia half a century earlier. However, in contrast to pneumococcal infections, HIV infections are chronic, therapy is not curative, and antiretroviral therapy, unlike a penicillin course, is a lifelong affair.

The introduction of HAART in the developed world has led to striking reductions in HIV-related morbidity and mortality [4]. Consequently, prophylaxis and treatment of opportunistic infections associated with HIV infection are less of an issue in the HAART era than they were before. However, this is not true for developing countries, where the introduction of HAART is still limited to a minority of the population in need and which also have to deal with a dual epidemic of HIV and tuberculosis (TB) [5]. Thus, we will also briefly discuss prophylaxis and treatment of opportunistic infections in resource-poor settings and specifically deal with HIV/TB dual infections.

Antiretroviral drugs and drug regimens

Currently licensed antiretroviral drugs belong to four classes: (i) nucleoside or nucleotide analogue reverse transcriptase inhibitors (NRTIs and NtRTIs, respectively); (ii) NNRTIs;

(iii) PIs; and (iv) fusion inhibitors (FIs) [6]. The point of action of the respective classes of antiretrovirals is shown in Fig. 6.1; individual drugs are listed in the legend.

NRTIs and NtRTIs act by terminating viral DNA chain elongation and as competitive inhibitors of reverse transcriptase. NRTIs and NtRTIs are administered to patients as precursor compounds that are phosphorylated to their active triphosphate form by cellular enzymes [7]. They are the oldest class of antiretrovirals.

NRTIs comprise the following drugs: zidovudine (ZDV), didanosine (ddI), zalcitabine (ddC), lamivudine (3TC), stavudine (d4T), abacavir (ABC) and emtricitabine (FTC). There is currently only one NtRTI on the market: tenofovir disoproxil fumarate (TDF). There are variable levels of cross-resistance among NRTIs/NtRTIs [8].

NNRTIs bind to the catalytic site of reverse transcriptase and act as non-competitive antagonists of enzyme activity. The two most commonly used NNRTIs are efavirenz (EFZ) and nevirapine (NVP). The third NNRTI, delavirdine, is only licensed in North America. Available NNRTIs are all highly specific inhibitors of HIV-1 and have no activity against other lentiviruses, including HIV-2 [9]. There is virtually complete cross-resistance among NNRTIs [8].

PIs interfere with the process of cleavage of the viral gag–pol polyprotein precursor by the viral aspartic acid protease enzyme, which occurs late in the virus life cycle. Protease-mediated cleavages are essential for viral maturation, as viral mutants devoid of protease activity generate

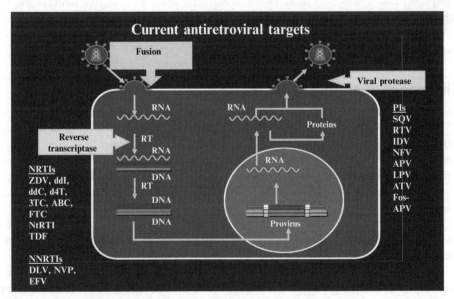

Fig. 6.1 Targets of currently licensed antiretrovirals. NRTIs = nucleoside analogue reverse transcriptase inhibitors, ZDV = zidovudine, ddI = didanosine, ddC = zalcitabine, d4T = stavudine, 3TC = lamivudine, ABC = abacavir, FTC = emtricitabine. NtRTI = nucleoside RT inhibitor, TDF = tenofovir. NNRTIs = non-nucleoside RT inhibitors, DLV = delavirdine, NVP = nevirapine, EFZ = efavirenz. PIs = protease inhibitors, SQV = saquinavir, RTV = ritonavir, IDV = indinavir, NFV = nelfinavir, APV = amprenavir, LPV = lopinavir, ATV = atazanavir, Fos-APV = fos-amprenavir. There is currently one fusion inhibitor on the market: the polypeptide T-20 or enfuvirtide.

virions containing the normal complement of viral RNA and protein, but are non-infectious [10]. Licensed PIs comprise the following drugs: saquinavir (SQV), indinavir (IDV), ritonavir (RTV), nelfinavir (NFV), amprenavir (APV), lopinavir (LPV) in a fixed-dose combination with low dose RTV (Kaletra®), fosamprenavir (fos-APV) and atazanavir (ATV). RTV is a potent inhibitor of hepatic cytochrome P450 3A4 and 2D5 enzymes, which mediate PI metabolism [11]. The drug is now almost exclusively used in low doses to boost levels of other PIs; conversely, PIs other than NFV are now mainly or almost exclusively used in RTV-boosted regimens [6]. Boosting provides a pharmacological barrier against development of viral drug resistance and may also be used to overcome certain levels of PI resistance. There are variable levels of cross-resistance among PIs [8].

The fusion inhibitor enfuvirtide (ENF, T-20) is the first active agent in a new class of antiretrovirals. Despite potent antiviral activity, it is mainly reserved for patients with advanced HIV disease because it has to be administered subcutaneously twice a day [12,13].

Currently recommended first-line regimens consist of two NRTI/NtRTIs plus either an NNRTI or a PI (usually RTV-boosted) [6]. Such regimens have been shown to be superior to triple NRTI-based regimens [14,15]. With the most successful initial HAART regimens, virological response rates in intent-to-treat analyses may be over 70%, even with prolonged follow-up [16–18]. Choice of second-line and subsequent regimens is often guided by the history of prior therapy, as well as by resistance assays [8]

NRTIs are relatively metabolically inert, although the NtRTI TDF has exhibited some unexpected interactions with other antiretrovirals (ddI and ATV) [19,20]. NNRTIs and PIs exhibit multiple interactions, both with antiretrovirals and with drugs from other classes [6,21]. Physicians and patients need to be continuously aware of potential interactions and seek expert guidance when changing regimens or introducing new drugs.

Challenges of antiretroviral therapy

The fact that antiretroviral therapy needs to be taken lifelong, together with the particularities of HIV infection, poses formidable challenges. First of all, there is the problem of patient adherence: taking drugs according to prescription every day proves difficult for many. Yet there are few diseases where strict adherence is as important as in HIV infection [22]. Lapses may lead to rapid development of drug resistance, which not only undermines the efficacy of the current regimen but, because of cross-resistance among drugs, is also likely to compromise that of future regimens.

Secondly, in 1998, after a few years of carefree prescribing, it became apparent that chronic use of antiretrovirals was often associated with development of chronic toxicity, such as the disfiguring lipodystrophy syndrome [23]. Use of particular antiretroviral agents could also lead to a rise of blood lipid levels and increased risk for cardio- and cerebrovascular morbidity and mortality [24]. Mitochondrial toxicity of NRTIs can be associated with several bothersome manifestations, such as peripheral neuropathy and myopathy and, in the worst case, development of hepatic steathosis with lactic acidosis, which is often lethal [25]. In other words, the success of HAART comes at a price. This should not make us lose sight of the fact that the benefits of HAART still far outweigh the disadvantages, but it has undoubtedly led to a certain reluctance to be very aggressive in starting antiretroviral therapy. Therapy is now generally initiated later in the course of infection than it was a few years ago, and therapy guidelines have been modified accordingly [6].

The success of a particular antiretroviral regimen is directly dependent on the number of active drugs in that regimen. Unfortunately, there is a growing population of HIV-infected patients who harbour virus with resistance to one or more currently available antiretroviral agents [26]. Usually the drug resistance mutations are acquired during periods of suboptimally suppressive therapy, but patients may also be infected with drug-resistant strains [27]. For a substantial proportion of patients, it has become difficult or impossible to constitute antiretroviral drug regimens that will give sufficient and durable suppression of viral replication. Somewhat surprisingly, these people are often still doing better on 'failing' drug regimens than they would have without antiretrovirals. Viral resistance mutations may be associated with loss of viral fitness—in other words, they may make the virus less virulent. In such cases, despite the virological failure, CD4 cell decline may be relatively slow. As long as drug pressure is available, drug-resistant viruses will form the majority virus population in such patients. If therapy is taken away, the more virulent wild-type virus may quickly take over again, leading to a rapid decline of CD4 cells and associated clinical progression [28]. Apart from the chronic toxicity, finding ways to treat patients with drug-resistant viruses is the major challenge of antiretroviral therapy today. Over the past few years, patient adherence has been made easier by the development and appearance of greatly simplified regimens involving only a few pills a day. Single-pill, once-a-day, fixed-dose combinations (FDCs) of first-line HAART regimens are being developed.

Dealing with hepatitis virus co-infections becomes an increasing challenge in the HIV-infected population. Hepatitis C virus (HCV) co-infections occur in 25–30% of the HIV-infected population in Europe and the USA, and in 50–90% of individuals who acquired their HIV infection from injecting drug use [29].

In the developed world, the relative contribution of liver-related mortality to mortality of HIV-infected subjects has risen greatly since the advent of HAART [30,31]. This may be explained in part by a decline in traditional opportunistic disease manifestations, but it is also due to the fact that the prolonged survival of HAART recipients allows the natural history of the hepatitis virus infections to take its course. The HIV-related immunodeficiency accelerates progression to cirrhosis and end-stage liver disease in HCV co-infected patients, whereas HAART may reverse this acceleration [32,33]. The net result, however, remains a relative increase in the contribution of liver disease to morbidity and mortality in the HAART era in the developed world. In addition, about 5–10% of HIV-infected homosexual men in the USA and Europe are chronic carriers of the hepatitis B virus (HBV), and the prevalence rates of HBV infections are also high in Asia and sub-Saharan Africa [34]. Effective strategies to treat people with dual HCV/HIV and dual HBV/HIV infections are thus of the utmost importance. Both HCV and HBV co-infections increase the 'hepatotoxicity' of HAART regimens [35], but this may often be a manifestation of immune reconstitution disease rather than pure drug toxicity [36]. Unfortunately, response rates to standard HCV therapy with peginterferon-α plus ribavirin are considerably lower than in the non-HIV-infected population, particularly in HCV genotype 1 infections [37–39]. Moreover, treatment of HCV infections complicates treatment with HAART, and vice versa, because of additive and overlapping toxicities. Treatment options for HBV/HIV co-infections are improving because TDF, 3TC and FTC all have antiviral activity against both HIV and HBV [40–42], allowing for TDF/3TC- or TDF/FTC-containing HAART regimens with dual drug activity against HBV. One should take the anti-HBV effect of these particular drugs into account when initiating or changing HAART regimens in HBV-co-infected patients; withdrawal may lead to serious hepatitis flare-ups [43].

Lastly, there is controversy regarding the effect of HCV co-infections on the natural history of HIV disease and on HAART treatment responses [44–46].

New antiretrovirals

Both chronic drug toxicity and the widespread circulation of multidrug-resistant viral strains are strong incentives for the development of new antiretroviral agents. These may either be agents belonging to classes already on the market (NRTIs, NtRTIs, PIs, NNRTIs and FIs) or drugs with new mechanisms of action (Fig. 6.2). In the long run, expectations are highest for the latter category, although some of the new drugs from established classes that are in clinical development appear to exhibit substantial activity against drug-resistant viruses [47–49]. Examples of drugs with new mechanisms of action that are in pre-clinical or clinical development are: (i) attachment inhibitors, agents that interfere with the first step of viral entry, binding of the viral envelope glycoprotein gp120 to the cellular CD4 receptor [50]; (ii) CCR5 or CXCR4 inhibitors that interfere with the subsequent step of viral entry, binding of gp120 to the cellular co-receptor [51–55]; (iii) integrase inhibitors that interfere with the viral integrase enzyme and inhibit integration of viral DNA in the host cell genome [56]; and (iv) maturation inhibitors that block the conversion of the HIV-1 capsid precursor (CA-SP1, p25) to mature capsid protein (p24) late in the replicative cycle, like the PIs leading to release of non-infectious virus particles [57]. Fortunately, a number of pharmaceutical companies are still committed to developing new anti-HIV agents. As is the case for bacterial infections and antimicrobials, stagnation in drug development would mean that gains made in the treatment of HIV infections would be lost over time.

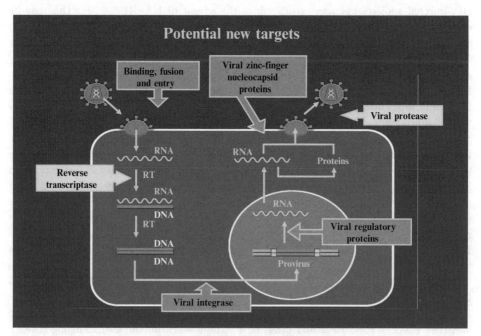

Fig. 6.2 Promising new antiretroviral targets in addition to established targets.

Alternative approaches

Because of the shortcomings of HAART, a lot of research on immunomodulatory approaches to supplement HAART is currently being carried out. An example is the use of cycles of the T-cell growth factor interleukin-2 (IL-2). IL-2 use may lead to considerable rises in $CD4^+$ cell numbers [58,59]; whether this confers clinical benefit is being investigated in several large clinical trials.

Because of growing concerns about the chronic toxicity of HAART, clinical research on HAART-sparing approaches has become popular. Here, IL-2 also figures. Another immuno-logical approach that is being explored is the use of therapeutic HIV vaccines that purportedly boost and broaden HIV-specific immunity [60,61]. A completely different approach is the use of immunosuppressive agents such as cyclosporin or mycophenolate mofetil (MMF) [62–64]. The aim here is to inhibit activation of target cells. MMF might also potentiate the activity of the NRTIs abacavir and ddI, but could antagonize that of ZDV and stavudine (d4T). The role of the various immunomodulatory approaches in the treatment of HIV infection is far from established.

A separate category is the so-called 'structured treatment interruptions'. These were studied for different purposes in different stages of HIV infection:

- in acute HIV infection, to boost and broaden HIV-specific immunity [65];
- in chronic infection with HAART suppression of viral replication to minimal levels, to boost and broaden HIV-specific immunity [66] and as a HAART-sparing approach [67,68];
- in chronic HIV infection where HAART has not succeeded in suppressing viral replication to minimal levels (i.e. in drug-resistant cases), to achieve a better virological response to renewed HAART exposure [69].

The usefulness of structured treatment interruptions for all of these indications is now highly doubtful, and in some patients they may in fact be dangerous [66,68,70–74].

When to start antiretroviral therapy?

This has been a contentious issue from the very beginning. Even during the ZDV monotherapy period, some promoted early treatment, while others were more conservative. In the years following the introduction of HAART, the pendulum swung towards early and aggressive treatment ('hit hard, hit early') [75] but, due to concerns about long-term toxicity of antire-trovirals as well as a realization of the fact that eradication of HIV infection with a few years of HAART was not feasible [76], guidelines have gradually become more conservative again [6]. It is clear, however, that waiting too long is not a good idea. Several studies have shown that disease progression and mortality are lessened when HAART is initiated when the CD4 cell count is above $200/mm^3$ [77,78]. Moreover, baseline plasma HIV-1 RNA levels higher than 100,000 have been independently associated with death [79]. Even when guidelines for the treatment of chronic HIV infection became more conservative, an exception was made for the treatment of acute HIV infections.

Based on a small uncontrolled study, it was believed that only with immediate treatment during acute infection could HIV-specific CD4 cell responses, and consequently HIV-specific CD8 cell responses, be maintained [65]. In a recent study, it was found that such responses do not protect against eventual viral escape [70]. Moreover, it has become clear that by the time acute HIV infection manifests itself clinically, the greatest damage, i.e. destruction of gut-associated lymphoid tissue, has already been done [80]. Thus, the validity of initiating anti-retroviral therapy during acute HIV infection is far from established and, fortunately, is now being studied in randomized controlled clinical trials.

Bringing HAART to resource-poor settings

In light of the devastation HIV is causing in developing countries, which is not only a humani-tarian but also an economic and developmental disaster on an unprecedented scale, pressure has grown to make HAART available in resource-limited settings as well. Since the year 2000, this has culminated in a number of important developments: (i) increased political commitment to the fight against HIV/AIDS on an international and national level; (ii) the establishment of new and substantial funding mechanisms, such as the World Bank's Multi-country AIDS Program (MAP), the Global Fund to Fight AIDS, Tuberculosis and Malaria (Global Fund) and US President Bush's Emergency Plan for AIDS Relief (PEPFAR); (iii) considerable reductions in prices of antiretro-virals for the poorest countries; and (iv) the uptake of antiretrovirals in the Essential Medicines list and the development of a public health approach to treatment of HIV infections by the World Health Organization (WHO) [81–83].

Despite these important and essential developments, the antiretroviral scale-up is fraught with difficulties. WHO's public health approach simplifies antiretroviral treatment and the monitoring thereof, and does not require a sophisticated healthcare infrastructure. However, in quite a few sub-Saharan countries, essential supportive functions such as reliable drug supply lines are lacking. Hopefully, the current momentum to increase access to HIV treatment will eventually lead to the building of sustainable health systems, including sustainable financing mechanisms for healthcare, in the countries concerned.

From a purely medical perspective, treating HIV infection in resource-poor settings also poses specific challenges. Most people only present when severely ill. There are several reasons for this: (i) they often do not know their HIV status; (ii) CD4 cell numeration is not widely available, so it is impossible to let the CD4 cell count, rather than clinical symptoms, drive the decision to initiate antiretroviral treatment; (iii) where co-payment is required, people postpone the initiation of treatment until the very last moment; and (iv) from a mistaken cost-effectiveness perspective, withholding treatment until symptoms appear is often official policy [83].

The enormous burden of concomitant HIV and TB infection adds to the problem. The result of the late initiation of antiretroviral treatment in developing countries, together with a high TB burden, is a high rate of immune reconstitution disease [36]. The lack of adequate laboratory facilities to diagnose specific infections is another complicating factor. Consequently, mortality rates during the first months of HAART are high [84]. The development of cheap and simple laboratory tests that could serve to identify those eligible for HAART before they develop symptoms, and to monitor treatment, is thus of utmost importance.

Another issue is the choice of drug regimen. The cheapest FDC available is d4T/3TC/NVP. Ease of use and good short-term tolerance add to its attraction. Furthermore, d4T does not lead to anaemia, unlike ZDV, and NVP only leads to fulminant hepatitis in those with higher CD4 cell counts. As a result, this combination is currently the 'market leader' in sub-Saharan Africa.

However, d4T is a major cause of lipoatrophy and mitochondrial toxicity [17,25,85], so choosing the cheapest option at the outset may in fact be paid for dearly by the patients later. There is an urgent need to develop effective FDCs of well-tolerated, safe and effective antiretrovirals, even if they have to be a little more expensive. There is also an urgent need to develop effective and affordable second-line regimens, which are now often missing.

A special problem is posed by paediatric treatment. The number of antiretroviral drugs with paediatric formulations is limited, and generic drug makers often do not develop them at all. In practice, paediatric treatment often involves the breaking of FDC adult tablets, which is a highly unsatisfactory and outright dangerous form of dosing. Here, too, urgent global action is required.

Use of antiretrovirals to prevent HIV infections

The use of antiretrovirals for the prevention of mother-to-child transmission (PMTCT) has been highly successful. It all started in 1994 with the US/French ACTG 076 study, which showed that a complex regimen of ZDV monotherapy given during the later part of pregnancy and intrapartum to mothers, and 6 weeks postpartum to infants, reduced the transmission of HIV-1 from non-breastfeeding mothers to infants by two-thirds [86]. The ZDV regimen was felt to be too complex and expensive for developing countries, which led to several studies that demonstrated the relative efficacy of simple short-course regimens in reducing HIV-1 transmission [87–95]. The simplest of these is maternal intrapartum and neonatal single-dose NVP, which reduces peripartum trans-mission from mother to child by almost 50% [90]. Because of its simplicity, it has become the regimen of choice in most developing countries.

A problem with single-dose NVP is that one of the characteristics which makes this regimen effective—the long terminal half-life of the drug—also leads to development of viral NVP resistance in a significant proportion of mothers and infants exposed in this manner [96,97]. The fact that in the absence of selective pressure, resistance mutations tend to disappear as a majority viral species over time led many to doubt the significance of NVP resistance develop-ment in this context [97]. A recent study, however, confirmed that intrapartum NVP has a negative impact on success rates of subsequent maternal treatment with NVP-containing HAART [98]. Since first-line HAART regimens in developing countries are virtually all NNRTI-based, this poses a serious problem. Strategies to maximize the benefits of both antiretroviral prophylaxis against MTCT of HIV-1 and chronic antiretroviral therapy for mothers and HIV-infected children are urgently needed [99].

Another issue that was initially downplayed in the exultation over the success of short-course peripartum antiretroviral regimens in reducing MTCT of HIV-1 is subsequent transmission via breastfeeding in populations where this practice is the norm and where formula feeding is not an alternative. In the Petra study, it was shown that a significant amount of the peripartum efficacy is indeed lost during subsequent breastfeeding. As might be expected, this applies particularly to the more effective peripartum interventions [92]. The Simba study has shown that daily single-agent antiretroviral prophylaxis—for example, NVP or 3TC— given to HIV-1-negative infants born to HIV-1-infected mothers during the period of breastfeeding may minimize this risk [100].

Similarly, oral antiretroviral pre-exposure prophylaxis (PREP) may also be effective in preventing sexual transmission of HIV. This approach is currently being investigated with

TDF in several high-risk populations across the globe. Although earlier animal studies with TDF suggested the utility of this drug for PREP [101], results from a recent macaque study with repeated rectal simian/human immunodeficiency virus (SHIV) challenges showed that TDF delayed, but did not prevent, the occurrence or manifestation of infection [102].

The outcome of ongoing PREP studies is eagerly awaited, as there is a great need for female-controlled prevention technologies. Condoms have been shown to be highly effective in preventing HIV-1 transmission [103], but their use is highly dependent on consent of the male partner. Vaginal microbicides are another potential female-controlled prevention technology [104–106]. Unfortunately, first-generation microbicides were all based on non-specific spermicides such as nonoxynol-9, which, in studies in high-risk populations, at worst led to increased HIV-1 transmission [107], or at best were ineffective [108]. The newest generation of vaginal microbicides under investigation utilize classes of HIV-specific inhibitors that are also used in, or developed for, therapeutic purposes [109,110].

Prophylaxis and treatment of opportunistic disease manifestations

As previously stated, the prophylaxis and treatment of opportunistic infections has become less relevant in the developed world since the advent of HAART, as their incidence has gone down dramatically. In addition, the incidence of Kaposi's sarcoma has also decreased dramatically [4,111,112]. Nevertheless, even in the developed world, significant proportions of HIV-infected people only present themselves at the clinic once they have developed symptomatic disease [113]. A thorough knowledge of options to prevent and treat these diseases in HIV-infected individuals is therefore essential for those practising HIV medicine. For detailed recommendations, the reader is referred to authoritative and comprehensive guidelines that are regularly updated [114–116].

In resource-poor settings, the treatment of opportunistic infections is hampered not only by a relative lack of medicines, but also by the fact that diagnostic facilities are also limited. One often has to take a 'syndromic' empirical approach. It is obviously far better to prevent than to treat infections, and studies of co-trimoxazole prophylaxis in HIV-positive patients with smear-positive TB conducted in the late 1990s in the Côte d'Ivoire and South Africa showed significant reductions in morbidity and mortality [117,118]. A study conducted in Malawi, however, showed reductions in mortality with a 'package' consisting of voluntary counselling, HIV testing and adjunctive co-trimoxazole for HIV-positives in TB patients, but failed to do so for smear-positive cases [119]. Moreover, as a consequence of the co-trimoxazole prophylaxis, *Escherichia coli* resistance to that drug increased significantly in the study population [120]. Overall, however, the original UNAIDS/WHO recommendation to use co-trimoxazole prophylaxis in those in Africa with symptomatic HIV-related disease or CD4 cell counts of less than 500/mm^3 still seems sensible [121]. Of note, a recent study from rural South Africa looking at the effectiveness of co-trimoxazole prophylaxis in reducing mortality in adults with TB irrespective of HIV status had a positive outcome [122].

Dual HIV/TB infections present an exceptional challenge. Worldwide, 14 million people are co-infected with these pathogens, and TB is a leading cause of death among people living with HIV [5]. HIV infection increases the risk of reactivating latent *Mycobacterium tuberculosis* infection, placing HIV-positive people at increased risk for developing TB [123]. HIV infection also increases the risk of rapid TB progression after primary *M.tuberculosis* acquisition or re-infection [124]. TB may accelerate the progression of HIV disease via immune activation, and is associated with higher mortality and shorter survival in HIV-positive people [125]. The risk of TB increases as CD4 cell counts decrease; similarly, the highest mortality rates associated with TB occur in those with the lowest CD4 cell counts [126]. However, there is already a rapid increase in TB incidence soon after infection with HIV [127,128]. The presentation of TB in those with advanced HIV disease is often atypical, and a documented bacteriological diagnosis may be more difficult to make [129].

Concomitant treatment of HIV and TB also poses difficulties. As mentioned above, in those with dual infections who initiate antiretroviral treatment in advanced stages of HIV infection, there is a high rate of immune reconstitution disease [36]. There are also overlapping drug toxicities [130]. Rifampin, through cytochrome P450 enzyme pathway induction, reduces blood levels of PIs and NNRTIs [21], considerably narrowing antiretroviral treatment choices in those who need concomitant treatment. In patients whose CD4 cell counts allow for a delay in HAART initiation, it is obviously very tempting to treat the TB first. However, delaying HAART initiation in patients with low CD4 lymphocyte counts in a developed country setting appeared to be associated with higher morbidity and mortality [131]. Moreover, the optimal duration of treatment for HIV-related TB remains controversial. Such patients appear to respond well to standard 6-month treatment regimens [132], but it is unclear whether this also applies to patients with advanced HIV disease and TB [115]. Several studies on the optimal timing of HIV/TB treatment in developing countries are ongoing.

TB case loads may be brought down with treatment of latent infections. There is convincing evidence that standard 6-month prophylactic treatment with isoniazid (INH) reduces the risk of TB in tuberculin skin test (TST)-positive people with HIV infection, whereas no such benefit has been clearly demonstrated in TST-negatives [123]. However, in high TB prevalence and incidence areas, the effectiveness of this intervention appears to wane over time [133,134]. The duration of effect may be prolonged through use of rifampin-containing combinations as prophylactic regimens [134]. In a number of developing countries, INH preventive therapy of latent TB infections in HIV-positive individuals is official policy; in others, it is not. An argument for the latter is that exclusion of active TB may be too difficult, and the risk of developing drug resistance thus too high. A case has been made for post-treatment preventive INH therapy for HIV-positives, since recurrent TB after curative treatment of active TB is more common in these subjects, especially when they already have HIV-related symptoms [135,136]. Benefits of various forms of TB preventive therapy notwithstanding, a far more effective and straightforward way to bring down the TB case load would be the widespread introduction of HAART in the settings concerned; it has been shown that the introduction of HAART may reduce the incidence of HIV-1-associated TB by more than 80% in areas where TB and HIV are endemic [137].

Concluding remarks

Despite the enormous benefits of HAART, drug regimens have suffered from poor tolerability, severe short-term and long-term toxicities, and from development of viral drug resistance. The latter was an inevitable consequence of using suboptimally suppressive drug regimens in the pre-HAART era, or from poor adherence to therapy. Fortunately, it is now certainly possible to devise simple, well-tolerated, first-line drug regimens that do not appear to carry a high risk of developing severe metabolic and mitochondrial toxicity [17]. We have an obligation not only to scale up access to antiretroviral therapy in resource-poor countries, but also to close the gap between first-rate regimens for those who live in affluent societies and second-rate regimens for those who are less fortunate. Furthermore, since poor adherence is one of the main causes of drug resistance in the HAART era, and since this leads to rapidly diminishing treatment options, we should intensify our efforts to help patients adhere. In this respect, community-based approaches that have been explored successfully in resource-poor settings [138] deserve a place in other settings as well. These types of approaches will reduce the demand for second- and third-line HAART regimens, which, unfortunately, are hardly available in many resource-poor settings at present. We also need to reconsider the moment of antiretroviral therapy initiation: from a medical perspective, with current drug options, a clear case can be made for starting antiretroviral therapy earlier than is currently recommended in both the developed and the developing world [139].

One of the great dramas of our time is the extent to which HIV prevention efforts are falling short. In 2004, more new HIV infections occurred than in any previous year. It is thus essential that the HAART scale-up go hand in hand with an increase in prevention services and measures. Ultimately, however, only an effective preventive vaccine will be able to 'break' the HIV epidemic. The major challenge here is to develop immunogens that are capable of neutralizing primary HIV isolates from all genetic subtypes and regions of the world. Fortunately, there is increasing global commitment to, and coordination of, HIV vaccine development [140].

References

1. Fischl MA, Richman DD, Grieco MH *et al.* (1997). The efficacy of azidothymidine (AZT) in the treatment of patients with AIDS and AIDS-related complex: a double-blind placebo-controlled trial. *New England Journal of Medicine* 317:185–91.

2. Lange JMA. (1997). Current problems and the future of antiretroviral drug trials. *Science* 276: 548–50.

3. Montaner JSG, Reiss P, Cooper D *et al.* (1998). A randomized, double-blinded trial comparing combinations of nevirapine, didanosine and zidovudine for HIV infected patients—the Incas trial. *Journal of the American Medical Association* 279:930–7.

4. Palella FJ, Delaney KM, Moorman AC *et al.* (1988). Declining morbidity and mortality among patients with advanced human immunodeficiency virus infection. *New England Journal of Medicine* 338:853–60.

5. The Stop TB Partnership. TB/HIV: facts at a glance. Available at: http://www.stoptb.org/events/internationalaidscon InfoPack/1GB.pdf.

6. Yeni PG, Hammer SM, Hirsch MS *et al.* (2004). Treatment for adult HIV infection: 2004 recommendations of the International AIDS Society USA Panel. *Journal of the American Medical Association* 292:251–65.

7. Göte M, Spira S, Wainberg MA. (2002). Nucleoside inhibitors of reverse transcriptase and the problem of drug resistance. In: Emini EA, ed. *The Human Immunodeficiency Virus: Biology, Immunology and Therapy*. Princeton: Princeton University Press, p100–31.

8. Hirsch MS, Brun-Vézinet F, Clotet B *et al.* (2003). Antiretroviral drug resistance testing in adults infected with human immunodeficiency virus type 1: 2003 recommendations of the International AIDS Society USA Panel. *Clinical Infectious Diseases* 37:113–28.

9. Balzarini J. (2002). Non-nucleoside reverse transcriptase inhibitors of HIV-1. In: Emini EA, ed. *The Human Immunodeficiency Virus: Biology, Immunology and Therapy*. Princeton: Princeton University Press, p132–71.

10. Condra JH, Vacca JP. HIV-1 protease inhibitors. In: Emini EA, ed. (2002). *The Human Immunodeficiency Virus: Biology, Immunology and Therapy.* Princeton: Princeton University Press, p172–222.

11. Hsu A, Granneman GR, Bertz RJ. (1998). Ritonavir: clinical pharmacokinetics and interactions with other anti-HIV agents. *Clinical Pharmacokinetics* 35:275–91.

12. Lalezari J, Henry K, O'Hearn M *et al.* (2003). Enfuvirtide, an HIV-1 fusion inhibitor, for drug-resistant HIV infection in North and South America. *New England Journal of Medicine* 348:2175–85.

13. Lazzarin A, Clotet B, Cooper D *et al.* (2003). Efficacy of enfuvirtide in patients infected with drug-resistant HIV-1 in Europe and Australia. *New England Journal of Medicine* 348:2186–95.

14. Van Leeuwen R, Katlama C, Murphy RL *et al.* (2003). A randomized trial to study first-line combination therapy with or without a protease inhibitor in HIV-1 infected patients. *AIDS* 17:987–99.

15. Gulick RM, Ribaudo HJ, Shikuma CM *et al.* (2004). Triple-nucleoside regimens versus efavirenz-containing regimens for the initial treatment of HIV-1 infection. *New England Journal of Medicine* 350:1850–61.

16. Hicks C, King MS, Gulick RM *et al.* (2004). Long-term safety and durable antiretroviral activity of lopinavir/ritonavir in treatment-naïve patients: 4 year follow-up study. *AIDS* 18:775–9.

17. Gallant JE, Staszewski S, Pozniak AL *et al.* (2004). Efficacy and safety of tenofovir DF vs stavudine in combination therapy in antiretroviral naïve patients: a 3-year randomized trial. *Journal of the American Medical Association* 292:191–201.

18. Ananworanich J, Ruxrungtham K, Siangphoe U *et al.* (2004). A Prospective Cohort Study of Efficacy and Safety of 2 NRTIs Plus Once-daily Ritonavir-boosted Saquinavir Hard Gel Capsule (SQV-HGC-r) at 24 weeks. Presented at the XV International AIDS Conference. July 11–16, 2004, Bangkok, Thailand. Abstract TuPeB4469.

19. Kearney B, Flaherty J, Sayre J *et al.* (2001) A Multiple-dose, Randomized, Crossover, Drug Interaction Study Between Tenofovir DF and Lamivudine or Didanosine. Presented at the 1st International AIDS Society Conference on HIV Pathogenesis and Treatment, July 8–11, 2001, Buenos Aires, Argentina. Abstract 337.

20. Taburet AM, Piketty C, Chazallon C *et al.* (2004). Interactions between atazanavir–ritonavir and tenofovir in heavily pretreated human immunodeficiency virus-infected patients. *Antimicrobial Agents and Chemotherapy* 48:2091–6.

21. De Maat MM, Ekhart GC, Huitema AD, Koks CH, Mulder JW, Beijnen JH. (2003). Drug interactions between antiretroviral drugs and co-medicated agents. *Clinical Pharmacokinetics* 42:223–82.

22. Paterson DL, Swindells S, Mohr J *et al.* (2000). Adherence to protease inhibitor therapy and outcomes in patients with HIV infection. *Annals of Internal Medicine* 133:21–30.

23. Carr A, Samaras K, Burton S *et al.* (1998). A syndrome of peripheral lipodystrophy, hyperlipidemia and insulin resistance in patients receiving HIV protease inhibitors. *AIDS* 12:F51–8.

24. The Writing Committee of the Data Collection on Adverse Events of Anti-HIV Drugs (D:A:D) Study Group. (2004). Cardio- and cerebrovascular events in HIV-infected persons. *AIDS* 18:1811–7.

25. Brinkman K, Smeitink JA, Romijn JA, Reiss P. (1999). Mitochondrial toxicity induced by nucleoside-analogue reverse-transcriptase inhibitors is a key factor in the pathogenesis of antiretroviral therapy-related lipodystrophy. *Lancet* 354:1112–5.

26. Richman DD, Morton SC, Wrin T *et al.* (2004). The prevalence of antiretroviral drug resistance in the United States. *AIDS* 18:1393–401.

27. Little SJ, Holte S, Routy JP *et al.* (2002). Antiretroviral drug susceptibility and response to initial therapy among recently HIV infected subjects in North America: a study from the Acute Infection and Early Disease Research Program (AIEDRP). *New England Journal of Medicine* 347:385–94.

28. Deeks SG, Wrin T, Liegler T *et al.* (2001). Virologic and immunologic consequences of discontinuing combination antiretroviral drug therapy in HIV-infected patients with detectable viremia. *New England Journal of Medicine* 344:472–80.

29. Sulkowski MS, Thomas DL. (2003). Hepatitis C in the HIV-infected person. *Annals of Internal Medicine* 138:197–207

30. Bica I, McGovern B, Dhar R *et al.* (2001). Increasing mortality due to end-stage liver disease in patients with human immunodeficiency virus infection. *Clinical Infectious Diseases* 32:492–7.

31. Macias J, Melguizo I, Fernandez-Rivera FJ *et al.* (2002). Mortality due to liver failure and impact on survival of hepatitis virus infections in HIV-infected patients receiving potent antiretroviral therapy. *European Journal of Clinical Microbiology and Infectious Diseases* 21:775–81.

32. Graham CS, Baden LR, Yu E *et al.* (2001). Influence of human immunodeficiency virus infection on the course of hepatitis C virus infection: a meta-analysis. *Clinical Infectious Diseases* 33:562–9

33. Qurishi N, Kreuzberg C, Lüchters G *et al.* (2003). Effect of antiretroviral therapy on liver-related mortality in patients with HIV and hepatitis C virus coinfection. *Lancet* 362:1708–13.

34. Maynard JE, Kane MA, Alter MJ *et al.* (1988). Control of hepatitis B by immunization: global perspectives. In: Zuckerman AJ, ed. *Viral Hepatitis and Liver Disease*. New York: Alan R Liss, p967–9.

35. Den Brinker M, Wit FW, Wertheim-van Dillen PM *et al.* (2000) Hepatitis B and C virus coinfection and the risk for hepatotoxicity of highly active antiretroviral therapy in HIV-1 infection. *AIDS* 14:2895–902.

36. French MA, Price P, Stone SF. (2004). Immune restoration disease after antiretroviral therapy. *AIDS* 18:1615–27.

37. Torriani FJ, Rodriguez-Torres M, Rockstroh J *et al.* (2004). Peginterferon alfa-2a plus ribavirin for chronic hepatitis C virus infection in HIV-infected patients. *New England Journal of Medicine* 351:438–50.

38. Chung RT, Andersen J, Volberding P *et al.* (2004). Peginterferon alfa-2a plus ribavirin versus interferon alfa-2a plus ribavirin for chronic hepatitis C in HIV-coinfected persons. *New England Journal of Medicine* 351:451–9.

39. Laguno M, Murillas J, Blanco JL *et al.* (2004). Peginterferon alfa-2b plus ribavirin for treatment of HIV/HCV co-infected patients. *AIDS* 18:F27–36.

40. Dore G, Cooper D, Barrett C, Goh L, Thakar B, Atkins M. (1999) Dual efficacy of lamivudine treatment in HIV/hepatitis B virus-coinfected persons in a randomized, controlled study (CAESAR). *Journal of Infectious Diseases* 180:607–13.

41. Dore G, Cooper D, Pozniak A *et al.* (2004). Efficacy of tenofovir disoproxil fumarate in antiretroviral therapy-naïve and -experienced patients coinfected with HIV-1 and hepatitis B virus. *Journal of Infectious Diseases* 189:1185–92.

42. Gish R, Leung N, Wright T *et al.* (2002). Dose range study of pharmacokinetics, safety and preliminary antiviral activity of emtricitabine in adults with hepatitis B virus infection. *Antimicrobial Agents and Chemotherapy* 46:1734–40.

43. Bessesen M, Yves D, Condreay L, Lawrence S, Sherman K. (1999). Chronic active hepatitis B exacerbations in HIV-infected patients following development of resistance to or withdrawal of lamivudine. *Clinical Infectious Diseases* 28:1032–5.

44. Grueb G, Ledergerber B, Battegay M *et al.* (2000). Clinical progression, survival, and immune recovery during antiretroviral therapy in patients with HIV-1 and hepatitis C virus coinfection. *Lancet* 356:1800–5.

45. Sulkowski M, Moore R, Mehta SH, Chaisson RE, Thomas DL. (2002). Hepatitis C and progression of HIV disease. *Journal of the American Medical Association* 288:199–206.

46. Yoo TW, Donfield S, Lail A, Lynn HS, Daar ES. (2005). The Hemophilia Growth and Development Study. Effect of hepatitis C virus (HCV) genotype on HCV and HIV-1 disease. *Journal of Infectious Diseases* **191**:4–10.

47. Gazzard BG, Pozniak AL, Rosenbaum W *et al.* (2003). An open-label assessment of TMC 125—a new, next generation NNRTI, for 7 days in HIV-1 infected individuals with NNRTI resistance. *AIDS* **17**:49–54.

48. Cooper D, Hicks C, Cahn P *et al.* (2005). 24 Week RESIST Study Analyses: The Efficacy of Tipranavir/ Ritonavir is Superior to Lopinavir/Ritonavir, and the TPV/r Treatment Response is Enhanced by Inclusion of Genotypically Active Antiretrovirals in the Optimized Background Regimen. Presented at the 12th Conference on Retroviruses and Opportunistic Infections. February 22–25, 2005, Boston, USA. Abstract 560.

49. Katlama C, Berger D, Bellos N *et al.* (2005). Efficacy of TMC114/r in 3-class Experienced Patients with Limited Treatment Options: 24-week Planned Interim Analysis of 2 96-week Multinational Dose-finding Trials. Presented at the 12th Conference on Retroviruses and Opportunistic Infections. February 22–25, 2005, Boston, USA. Abstract 164LB.

50. Hanna G, Lalezari J, Hellinger J *et al.* (2004). Antiviral Activity, Safety and Tolerability of a Novel, Oral Small Molecule HIV-1 Attachment Inhibitor BMS-488043, in HIV-1 Infected Subjects. Presented at the 11th Conference on Retroviruses and Opportunistic Infections. February 8–11, 2004, San Francisco, USA. Abstract 141.

51. Westby M, Whitcomb J, Huang W *et al.* (2004). Reversible Predominance of CXCR4 Utilizing Variants in a Non-responsive Dual Tropic Patient Receiving the CCR5 Antagonist UK-427,857. Presented at the 11th Conference on Retroviruses and Opportunistic Infections. February 8–11, 2004, San Francisco, USA. Abstract 538.

52. Schurmann D, Rouzier R, Nougarde R *et al.* (2004). SCH D: Antiviral Activity of a CCR5 Receptor Antagonist. Presented at the 11th Conference on Retroviruses and Opportunistic Infections. February 8–11, 2004, San Francisco, USA. Abstract 140LB.

53. Demarest J, Adkinson K, Sparks S *et al.* (2004). Single and Multiple Dose Escalation Study to Investigate the Safety, Pharmacokinetics and Receptor Binding of GW873140, a Novel CCR5 Receptor Antagonist, in Healthy Subjects. Presented at the 11th Conference on Retroviruses and Opportunistic Infections. February 8–11, 2004, San Francisco, USA. Abstract 139.

54. Schols D, Vermeire K, Fransen S *et al.* (2005). Multi-drug Resistant HIV is Sensitive to Inhibition by Chemokine Receptor Antagonists. Presented at the 12th Conference on Retroviruses and Opportunistic Infections. February 22–25, 2005, Boston, USA. Abstract 545.

55. Moore JP, Doms RW. (2003). The entry of entry inhibitors: a fusion of science and medicine. *Proceeedings of the National Academy of Sciences of the USA* **100**:10598–602.

56. Little S, Drusano G, Schooley R *et al.* (2005). Antiviral Effect of L-000870810, a Novel HIV-1 Integrase Inhibitor, in HIV-1-infected Patients. Presented at the 12th Conference on Retroviruses and Opportunistic Infections. February 22–25, 2005, Boston, USA. Abstract 161.

57. Martin D, Jacobson J, Schurman D, *et al.* (2005). PA-457, the First-in-class Maturation Inhibitor, Exhibits Antiviral Activity Following a Single Oral Dose in HIV-1 Infected Patients. Presented at the 12th Conference on Retroviruses and Opportunistic Infections. February 22–25, 2005, Boston, USA. Abstract 159.

58. Kovacs JA, Vogel S, Albert JM *et al.* (1996). Controlled trial of interleukin-2 infusions in patients infected with the human immunodeficiency virus. *New England Journal of Medicine* **335**:1350–8.

59. Chun TW, Engel D, Mizell SB *et al.* (1999). Effect of interleukin-2 on the pool of latently infected, resting CD4+ T cells in HIV-1-infected patients receiving highly active anti-retroviral therapy. *Nature Medicine* **5**:651–5.

60. Jin X, Gao X, Ramanathan M Jr, Deschenes GR, Nelson GW, O'Brien SJ. (2002). Safety and immunogenicity of ALVAC vCP1452 and recombinant gp160 in newly human immunodeficiency virus type 1-infected patients treated with prolonged highly active antiretroviral therapy. *Journal of Virology* 76:2206–16.

61. Lévy Y, Gahéry-Ségard H, Durier C *et al.* (2005). Immunological and virological efficacy of a therapeutic immunization combined with interleukin-2 in chronically HIV-1 infected patients. *AIDS* 19:279–86.

62. Rizzardi GP, Harai A, Capiluppi B *et al.* (2002). Treatment of primary HIV-1 infection with cyclosporin A coupled with highly active antiretroviral therapy. *Journal of Clinical Investigation* 109:681–8.

63. Chapuis AG, Paolo RG, D'Agostino C *et al.* (2000). Effects of mycophenolic acid on human immunodeficiency virus infection *in vitro* and *in vivo*. *Nature Medicine* 6:762–768.

64. Sankatsing SUC, Jurriaans S, van Swieten P *et al.* (2004). Highly active antiretroviral therapy with or without mycophenolate mofetil in treatment naïve HIV-1 patients. *AIDS* 18:1925–31.

65. Rosenberg ES, Altfeld M, Poon SH *et al.* (2000). Immune control of HIV-1 after early treatment of acute infection. *Nature* 407:523–6.

66. Oxenius A, Price DA, Gunthard H *et al.* (2002). Stimulation of HIV-specific cellular immunity by structured treatment interruptions fails to enhance viral control in chronic HIV infection. *Proceedings of the National Academy of Sciences of the USA* 99:13747–52.

67. Dybul M, Nies-Kraske E, Daucher M *et al.* (2003). A Randomized, Controlled Trial of Long Cycle Structured Intermittent Versus Continuous ARV Therapy for Chronic HIV Infection. Presented at the 10th Conference on Retroviruses and Opportunistic Infections. February, 2003, Boston, USA. Abstract 681b.

68. Ananworanich J, Nuesch R, Le-Braz M *et al.* (2003). Failures of 1 week on 1 week off antiretroviral therapies in a randomized trial. *AIDS* 17:F33–37.

69. Miller V, Sabin C, Hertogs K *et al.* (2001). Virological and immunological effects of treatment interruptions in HIV-1-infected patients with treatment failure. *AIDS* 14:2857–67.

70. Kaufmann DE, Lichterfeld M, Altfeld M *et al.* (2004) Limited durability of viral control following treated acute HIV infection. *PloS Medicine* 1:137–48 (e36).

71. Koup RA. (2004). Reconsidering early HIV treatment and supervised treatment interruptions. *PloS Medicine* 1:109–10 (e41).

72. Nuesch R, Ananworanich J, Sirivichayakul S *et al.* (2005). Development of HIV with drug resistance after CD4 cell count-guided structured treatment interruptions in patients treated with highly active antiretroviral therapy after dual nucleoside analogue treatment. *Clinical Infectious Diseases* 40:728–34.

73. Worthington MG, Ross JJ. (2003). Aseptic meningitis and acute HIV syndrome after interruption of antiretroviral therapy: implications for structured treatment interruptions. *AIDS* 17:2145–6.

74. Kilby JM, Goepfert PA, Miller AP *et al.* (2000). Recurrence of the acute HIV syndrome after interruption of antiretroviral therapy in a patient with chronic HIV infection. *Annals of Internal Medicine* 133:435–8.

75. Ho DD. (1995). Time to hit HIV, early and hard. *New England Journal of Medicine* 333:450–1.

76. Finzi D, Blankson J, Siliciano *et al.* (1997). Latent infection of CD4$^+$ T cells provides a mechanism for lifelong persistence of HIV-1,even in patients on effective combination therapy. *Nature Medicine* 5:512–7.

77. Palella FJ, Deloria-Knoll M, Cmiel JS *et al.* (2003). Survival benefit of initiating antiretroviral therapy in HIV-infected persons in different CD4+ cell strata. *Annals of Internal Medicine* 138:620–6.

78. Sterling TR, Chaisson RE, Keruly J, Moore RD. (2003). Improved outcomes with earlier initiation of highly active antiretroviral therapy among human immunodeficiency virus-infected patients who

achieve durable virologic suppression: longer follow-up of an observational cohort study. *Journal of Infectious Diseases* **188**:1659–65.

79. Wood E, Hogg RS, Yip B *et al.* (2003). Higher baseline levels of plasma human immunodeficiency virus type 1 RNA are associated with increased mortality after initiation of triple-drug antiretroviral therapy. *Journal of Infectious Diseases* **188**:1421–5.

80. Mehandru S, Poles MA, Tenner-Racz K *et al.* (2004). Primary HIV-1 infection is associated with preferential depletion of CD4+ lymphocytes from effector sites in the gastrointestinal tract. *Journal of Experimental Medicine* **200**:761–70.

81. United Nations General Assembly on HIV/AIDS. (2001). *Declaration of Commitment on HIV/AIDS, no. 55,* 25–27 June, 2001.

82. World Health Organization. (2003). *Treating 3 Million by 2005: Making it Happen.* Geneva: WHO.

83. World Health Organization. (2002). *Scaling up Antiretroviral Therapy in Resource-limited Settings: Guidelines for a Public Health Approach.* Geneva: WHO.

84. Arnaud J, Loretxu P, Calmy A *et al.* (2005). Clinical and Virological Outcomes of Patients on HAART in a Large-scale Simplified Treatment Program in a Rural District of Malawi. Presented at the 12th Conference on Retroviruses and Opportunistic Infections. February 22–25, 2005, Boston, USA. Abstract 625b.

85. Van der Valk M, Casula M, Weverling GJ *et al.* (2004). Prevalence of lipoatrophy and mitochondrial DNA content of blood and subcutaneous fat in HIV-1-infected patients randomly allocated to zidovudine- or stavudine-based therapy. *Antiviral Therapy* **9**:385–93.

86. Connor EM, Sterling RS, Gelber R *et al.* (1994) Reduction of maternal–infant transmission of human immunodeficiency virus type 1 with zidovudine treatment. *New England Journal of Medicine* **331**:1173–80.

87. Shaffer N, Chuachoowong R, Mock P *et al.* (1999). Short-course zidovudine for perinatal HIV-1 transmission in Bangkok, Thailand: a randomized controlled trial. *Lancet* **353**:773–80.

88. Dabis F, Msellati P, Meda N *et al.* (1999). 6-Month efficacy, tolerance and acceptability of a short regimen of oral zidovudine to reduce vertical transmission of HIV in breastfed children in Côte d'Ivoire and Burkina Faso: a double-blind placebo-controlled multicentre trial. *Lancet* **353**: 786–92.

89. Wiktor S, Ekpini E, Karon J *et al.* (1999). Short-course oral zidovudine for prevention of mother-to-child transmission of HIV-1 in Abidjan, Côte d'Ivoire: a randomized trial. *Lancet* **153**:781–5.

90. Guay LA, Musoke P, Fleming T *et al.* (1999). Intrapartum and neonatal single-dose nevirapine compared with zidovudine for prevention of mother-to-child transmission of HIV-1 in Kampala, Uganda: HIVNET 012 randomised trial. *Lancet* **354**:795–802.

91. Lallement M, Jourdain G, Le Coeur S *et al.* (2000). A trial of shortened zidovudine regimens to prevent mother-to-child transmission of human immunodeficiency virus type 1. *New England Journal of Medicine* **343**:982–91.

92. Petra Study Team. (2002). Efficacy of three short-course regimens of zidovudine and lamivudine in preventing early and late transmission of HIV-1 from mother-to-child in Tanzania, South Africa, and Uganda (Petra study). *Lancet* **359**:1178–86.

93. Moodley D, Moodley J, Coovadia H *et al.* (2003). A multicenter randomized controlled trial of nevirapine versus a combination of zidovudine and lamivudine to reduce intrapartum and early postpartum mother-to-child transmission of human immunodeficiency virus type 1. *Journal of Infectious Diseases* **187**:725–35.

94. Lallement M, Jourdain G, Le Coeur S *et al.* (2004). Single-dose perinatal nevirapine plus standard zidovudine to prevent mother-to-child transmission of HIV-1 in Thailand. *New England Journal of Medicine* **351**:217–28.

95. Mofenson LM, McIntyre JA. (2000). Advances and research directions in the prevention of mother-to-child HIV-1 transmission. *Lancet* 355: 2237–44.

96. Jackson JB, Becker-Pergola G, Guay LA *et al.* (2001). Identification of K103N resistance mutation in Ugandan women receiving nevirapine to prevent HIV-1 vertical transmission (HIVNET 012). *AIDS* 14:F111–5.

97. Eshleman SH, Mracna M, Guay LA *et al.* (2001). Selection and fading of resistance mutations in women and infants receiving nevirapine to prevent HIV-1 vertical transmission (HIVNET 012). *AIDS* 15:1951–7.

98. Jourdain G, Ngo-Giang-Huong N, Le Coeur S *et al.* (2004). Intrapartum exposure to nevirapine and subsequent maternal responses to nevirapine-based antiretroviral therapy. *New England Journal of Medicine* 351:229–40.

99. McIntyre J. (2005). Controversies in the Use of Nevirapine for the Prevention of Mother-to-child Transmission. Presented at the 12th Conference on Retroviruses and Opportunistic Infections. February 22–25, 2005, Boston, USA. Abstract 8.

100. Vyankadondera J, Luchters S, Hassink E *et al.* (2003). Reducing Risk of HIV-1 Transmission Through Breastfeeding Using Antiretroviral Prophylaxis in Infants (SIMBA Study). Presented at the 2nd IAS Conference on HIV Pathogenesis and Treatment. July 13–16, 2003, Paris, France. Abstract LB7.

101. Tsai C-C, Follis KE, Sabo A *et al.* (1995). Prevention of SIV infection in macaques by (R)-9-(2-phosphonylmethoxypropyl)adenine. *Science* 270:1197–9.

102. Subbarao S, Otten R, Ramos A *et al.* (2005). Chemoprophylaxis with Oral Tenofovir Disoproxil Fumarate Delays But Does Not Prevent Infection in Rhesus Macaques Given Repeated Sexual Challenges of SHIV. Presented at the 12th Conference on Retroviruses and Opportunistic Infections. February 22–25, 2005, Boston, USA. Abstract 136LB.

103. Weller SC. (1993). A meta-analysis of condom effectiveness in reducing sexually transmitted HIV. *Social Science and Medicine* 36:1644–53.

104. Shattuck RA, Moore JP. (2003). Inhibiting sexual transmission of HIV-1 infection. *Nature Reviews in Microbiology* 1:25–34.

105. Moore JP. (2005). Topical microbicides become topical. *New England Journal of Medicine* 352:298–300.

106. Smith RJ, Bodine EN, Wilson DP, Blower SM. (2005). Evaluating the potential impact of vaginal microbicides to reduce the risk of acquiring HIV in female sex workers. *AIDS* 19:413–21.

107. Kreiss J, Ngugi E, Holmes K *et al.* (1992). Efficacy of nonoxynol 9 contraceptive sponge use in preventing heterosexual acquisition of HIV in Nairobi prostitutes. *Journal of the American Medical Association* 268:477–82.

108. Van Damme L, Ramjee G, Alary M *et al.* (2002). Effectiveness of COL-1492, a nonoxynol-9 vaginal gel, on HIV-1 transmission in female sex workers: a randomized controlled trial. *Lancet* 360: 971–7.

109. Di Fabio S, Van Roey J, Giannini G *et al.* (2003). Inhibition of vaginal transmission of HIV-1 in hu-SCID mice by the non-nucleoside reverse transcriptase inhibitor TMC120 in a gel formulation. *AIDS* 17:1597–1604.

110. Lederman MM, Veazey RS, Offord R *et al.* (2004). Prevention of vaginal SHIV transmission in rhesus macaques through inhibition of CCR5. *Science* 306:485–7.

111. Mocroft A, Vella S, Benfield TL *et al.* (1998). Changing patterns of mortality across Europe in patients infected with HIV-1. *Lancet* 352:1725–30.

112. Dore GJ, Li Y, McDonald A *et al.* (2002). Impact of highly active antiretroviral therapy on individual AIDS-defining illness incidence and survival in Australia. *Journal of Acquired Immune Deficiency Syndrome* 29:388–95.

113. Egger M, May M, Chene *et al.* (2002). Prognosis of HIV-1-infected patients starting highly active antiretroviral therapy: a collaborative analysis of prospective studies. *Lancet* **360**:119–29.

114. Masur H, Kaplan JE, Holmes KK. (2002). Guidelines for preventing opportunistic infections among HIV-infected persons—2002. Recommendations of the US Public Health Service and the Infectious Diseases Society of America. US Public Health Service, Infectious Diseases Society of America. *Annals of Internal Medicine* **137**:435–77.

115. Benson CA, Kaplan JE, Masur H, Pau A, Holmes KK. (2004). Treating opportunistic infections among HIV-infected adults and adolescents. Recommendations from CDC, the National Institutes of Health, and the HIV Medicine Association/Infectious Diseases Society of America. *Morbidity and Mortality Weekly Reports* **53**(RR-15):1–112.

116. Mofenson L, Oleske J, Serchuck L, Van Dyke R, Wilfert C. (2004). Treating opportunistic infections among HIV-exposed and infected children. Recommendations from CDC, the National Institutes of Health, and the Infectious Diseases Society of America. *Morbidity and Mortality Weekly Reports* **53**(RR-14):1–92.

117. Wiktor SZ, Sassan-Morokro M, Grant AD *et al.* (1999). Efficacy of trimethoprim–sulfamethoxazole prophylaxis to decrease morbidity and mortality in HIV-1-infected patients with tuberculosis in Abidjan, Cote d'Ivoire: a randomized controlled trial. *Lancet* **353**:1469–75.

118. Badri M, Maartens G, Wood R, Ehrlich R. (1999). Co-trimoxazole in HIV-1 infection. *Lancet* **354**:334.

119. Zachariah R, Spielmann M-P L, Chinji C *et al.* (2003). Voluntary counseling, HIV testing and adjunctive cotrimoxazole reduces mortality in tuberculosis patients in Thyolo, Malawi. *AIDS* **17**:1053–61.

120. Zachariah R, Harries AD, Spielmann MP *et al.* (2002). Changes in *Escherichia coli* resistance to co-trimoxazole in tuberculosis patients and in relation to co-trimoxazole prophylaxis in Thyolo, Malawi. *Transactions of the Royal Society of Tropical Medicine and Hygiene* **96**:202–4.

121. UNAIDS. (2000). *Provisional WHO/UNAIDS Secretariat Recommendations on the Use of Cotrimoxazole Prophylaxis in Adults and Children Living with HIV/AIDS in Africa.* Geneva: UNAIDS.

122. Grimwade K, Sturm AW, Nunn AJ, Mbatha D, Zungu D, Gilks CF. (2005). Effectiveness of cotrimoxazole prophylaxis on mortality in adults with tuberculosis in rural South Africa. *AIDS* **19**:163–8.

123. Bucher HC, Griffith LE, Guyatt GH *et al.* (1999). Isoniazid prophylaxis for tuberculosis in HIV infection: a meta-analysis of randomized controlled trials. *AIDS* **13**:501–7.

124. Daley CL, Small PM, Schecter GF *et al.* (1992). An outbreak of tuberculosis with accelerated progression among persons infected with the human immunodeficiency virus: an analysis using restriction-fragment length polymorphisms. *New England Journal of Medicine* **326**:231–5.

125. Whalen CC, Nsubuga P, Okwera A *et al.* (2000). Impact of pulmonary tuberculosis on survival of HIV-infected adults: a prospective epidemiologic study in Uganda. *AIDS* **14**:1219–28.

126. Shafer RW, Bloch AB, Larkin C *et al.* (1996). Predictors of survival in HIV-infected tuberculosis. *AIDS* **10**:269–72.

127. Srikantiah P, Charlebois E, Havlir DV. (2005). Rapid increase in tuberculosis incidence soon after infection with HIV—a new twist in the twin epidemics. *Journal of Infectious Diseases* **191**:147–9.

128. Sonnenberg P, Glynn JR, Fielding K, Murray J, Godfrey-Faussett P, Shearer S. (2005). How soon after infection with HIV does the risk of tuberculosis start to increase? A retrospective cohort study in South African gold miners. *Journal of Infectious Diseases* **191**:150–8.

129. Jones BE, Young SM, Antoniskis D, Davidson PT, Kramer F, Barnes PF. (1993). Relationship of the manifestations of tuberculosis to CD4 cell counts in patients with human immunodeficiency virus infection. *American Review of Respiratory Diseases* **148**:1292–7.

130. Lee WM. (2003). Drug-induced hepatotoxicity. *New England Journal of Medicine* **349**:474–85.

131. Dheda K, Lampe FC, Johnson MA, Lipman MC. (2004). Outcome of HIV-associated tuberculosis in the era of highly active antiretroviral therapy. *Journal of Infectious Diseases* **190**:1670–6.

132. Perriens JH, St. Louis ME, Mukadi YB *et al.* (1995). Pulmonary tuberculosis in HIV infected patients in Zaire: a controlled trial of treatment for either 6 or 12 months. *New England Journal of Medicine* **332**:779–84.

133. Quigley M, Mwinga A, Hosp M *et al.* (2001). Long term effect of preventive therapy for tuberculosis in a cohort of HIV infected Zambian adults. *AIDS* **15**:215–22.

134. Johnson JL, Okwera A, Hom DL *et al.* (2001). Duration of efficacy of latent tuberculosis infection in HIV-infected individuals. *AIDS* **15**:2137–47.

135. Fitzgerald DW, Desvarieux M, Severe P, Joseph P, Johnson WD Jr, Pape JW. (2000). Effect of post-treatment isoniazid on prevention of recurrent tuberculosis in HIV-1-infected individuals. *Lancet* **356**:1470–4.

136. Churchyard GJ, Fielding K, Charalambous S *et al.* (2003). Efficacy of secondary isoniazid preventive therapy among HIV-infected Southern Africans: time to change policy? *AIDS* **17**:2063–70.

137. Badri M, Wilson D, Wood R. (2002). Effect of highly active antiretroviral therapy on incidence of tuberculosis in South Africa: a cohort study. *Lancet* **359**:2059–64.

138. Farmer PE, Leandre F, Mukherjee JS *et al.* (2001). Community-based approaches to HIV treatment in resource-poor settings. *Lancet* **358**:404–9.

139. Holmberg SD, PalellaF, Lichtenstein KA, Havlir DV. (2004) The case for earlier treatment of HIV infection. *Clinical Infectious Diseases* **39**:1699–704.

140. Coordinating Committee of the Global HIV/AIDS Vaccine Enterprise. (2005). The Global HIV/AIDS Vaccine Enterprise: Scientific Strategic Plan. *PloS Medicine* **2**:111–21.

Chapter 7

HIV vaccines: development and future use

José Esparza[*], Marie-Louise Chang and Helene D Gayle

Introduction

Soon after HIV was identified as the cause of AIDS, there was an expectation that an effective vaccine would be easily developed and rapidly deployed. Such optimism was expressed by the US Secretary of Health and Human Services, Margaret Heckler, when she indicated in 1984 that 'such a vaccine will be ready for testing in approximately two years' [1]. Secretary Heckler was right in that the first small-scale phase I trial of an HIV vaccine was initiated in 1987, but she could not have predicted that the actual development of an effective HIV vaccine would take much longer. In fact, no one knew at that time that HIV was much more complex than any other viral disease for which vaccines had been successfully developed. Some of these scientific complexities are related to the apparent inability of natural immune responses to control HIV infection or progression to disease, and to the enormous adaptability of the HIV genome, which allows the virus to escape normal mechanisms of immune protection.

Nevertheless, numerous clinical trials of experimental vaccines continued to be conducted, and a large amount of information on the virology, immunology and pathogenesis of HIV was obtained in subsequent years. That wealth of information provided renewed optimism that led US President Clinton to proclaim, in 1997, the national goal of finding a vaccine for AIDS within the next 10 years. President Clinton acknowledged, however, that this was going to be a difficult task, and compared it with President Kennedy's call to put a man on the moon before the end of the 1960s. Despite important progress made since 1997, it has now become evident that the development of an HIV vaccine remains one of the most difficult scientific challenges confronting biomedical science, and that the deadline of 2007 will not be met.

To tackle the enormous HIV vaccine development challenge, an international group of scientists proposed, in 2003, the creation of the Global HIV Vaccine Enterprise [2,3]. This proposal was motivated by the recognition that scientific progress is creating new opportunities that can be harnessed through better coordination of global efforts. However, these efforts need to be of a magnitude and intensity without precedent in biomedical research, with the Human Genome Project as a useful model. Critical to success will be a more collaborative effort that shares information, systematically builds on research results, links

* Corresponding author.

clinical trials with standardized laboratory evaluation in an iterative fashion and prioritizes the most promising approaches for clinical trials.

An increased vaccine development effort should be considered an integral part of the global response to the HIV pandemic [4]. Together with the urgent need to expand access to existing preventive and therapeutic interventions, it is also important to recognize that most of the existing interventions are far from ideal and that we still need to support research to develop novel and more effective strategies, including better treatments and expanded prevention tools such as microbicides and vaccines. Ultimately, a safe, effective and accessible vaccine will be critical to the successful containment of the HIV pandemic.

Scientific challenges in the development of an HIV vaccine

The major stumbling block for the rational development of an HIV vaccine has been the lack of information on the immune responses that could be responsible for protection against HIV, the so-called immunological correlates of protection. With most vaccine-preventable diseases, naturally occurring or vaccine-induced immune responses correlate with protection against infection or disease. In contrast, even though most people infected with HIV develop a broad range of immune responses against the virus, in most cases these immune responses neither control the infection nor prevent progression to disease. Natural history studies and animal protection experiments have failed to produce conclusive results about immune correlates of protection, although most scientists believe that a combination of the two main types of immune responses—humoral and cell-mediated—may be needed for effective protection. This, in turn, could be improved if a mucosal immune component were added. Ongoing HIV vaccine development strategies are targeting these two major types of immune responses [5].

The other major scientific challenge to HIV vaccine development is related to the genetic variability exhibited by HIV, especially in the gene coding for the envelope glycoproteins gp120 and gp41 (the *env* gene). This genetic variability complicates vaccine development in two different ways. First, the variability of the *env* gene has resulted in the emergence and circulation of different genetic groups and subtypes of HIV-1. Most HIV-1 infections in the world are caused by viruses belonging to HIV-1 group M (or 'major'), which, in turn, is divided into at least nine pure genetic subtypes or clades (A–D, F–H, J and K) and a number of inter- and intra-subtype recombinants with mosaic genomes. These pure subtypes and recombinant forms have unequal geographical distribution, with subtype B being prevalent in the Americas and Europe, subtype C in Southern Africa and India, the recombinant subtype E in Thailand and neighboring countries, and subtypes A and D in East Africa [6] (see Fig. 7.1). What is unclear at the present time is how the genetic variability of HIV could relate to potential vaccine-induced protection. For example, it is not known whether the HIV genetic subtypes define immunological subtypes, or whether specific vaccines will need to be designed for each subtype.

The second aspect in which the genetic variability of HIV complicates vaccine development is related to the high rate of mutations that results in the emergence of HIV strains that eventually escape an otherwise successful immune response. Those 'escape mutants' can be a major problem in vaccines that fail to prevent infection completely but induce a reduction in virus load, as could be the case with most current candidate vaccines designed to induce cell-mediated immunity. The scientific challenge is to develop vaccines that induce potent, broad, persistent antibodies, as well as long-term memory T cells that suppress viral replication and escape.

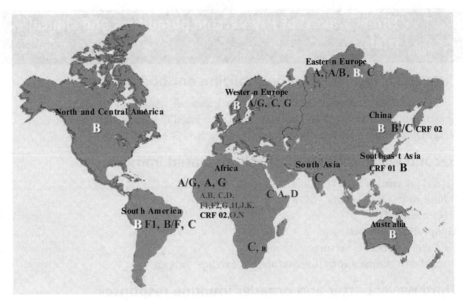

Fig. 7.1 HIV-1 diversity: non-B viruses are predominant. Source: C Rouzioux, 2005.

Evolution of vaccine paradigms and clinical trials

Despite the difficulties discussed above, a number of candidate vaccines have been developed in the laboratory and are being tested in animal models. The most promising products have also moved to clinical trials in humans. Since the first HIV vaccine trial was conducted in the USA in 1987, approximately 20,000 healthy human volunteers in different parts of the world have participated in more than 80 phase I/II trials to evaluate the safety of over 30 different candidate vaccines and their ability to reduce anti-HIV-specific immune responses (immunogenicity), and, in two phase III trials, to assess the ability of the candidate vaccines to protect against HIV infection (protective efficacy). Phase I/II trials have shown that the candidate vaccines are safe, but, unfortunately, only a few induce sufficiently high levels of HIV-specific immune responses to warrant further evaluation of their protective efficacy against HIV.

The current HIV vaccines originate from more than 16 years of clinical trials experience, with many lessons learned over the years. A variety of HIV vaccine concepts have been tested in three successive overlapping 'waves' of clinical trials that have been dominated by different vaccine development paradigms (Box 7.1) [5,7].

First wave: induction of neutralizing antibodies

The first wave of HIV candidate vaccines and clinical trials was based on the concept that antibodies that neutralize the infectivity of the virus (neutralizing antibodies) would be sufficient to confer protection against HIV infection or development of AIDS. This paradigm resulted in the design of candidate vaccines based on the envelope glycoproteins of HIV, especially gp120, or on synthetic peptides representing highly immunogenic

---

Box 7.1   Three 'waves' of HIV vaccine paradigms and clinical trials

First wave: induction of neutralizing antibodies

Recombinant gp160 produced in a baculovirus/insect cell system;
Several recombinant gp120 and gp160 proteins produced in mammalian cell systems;
V3/gp120 peptides (synthetic or produced in bacterial systems).

Second wave: induction of cell-mediated immunity

Several poxvirus vectors (vaccinia, canarypox, fowlpox);
'Modified vaccinia Ankara' (MVA) vectors;
DNA constructs;
Lipopeptide constructs;
First generation BCG vectors;
Prime-boost combinations (live vectors and envelope antigens).

Third wave: better and broader immune responses

Replication-incompetent adenovirus vectors;
Other viral vectors (VEE, SFV, AAV, VSV);
Candidate vaccines based on regulatory proteins (TAT);
Novel DNA constructs;
Novel envelope-based immunogens;
Multiple prime-boost combinations.

Sources: [5,6].

---

regions of gp120, such as its third hypervariable (V3) loop. The first generation of envelope vaccines included mainly monomeric gp120 molecules based on laboratory-adapted strains of HIV-1, or X4 strains, which, in addition to the CD4 molecule, use the CXCR4 molecule as co-receptor for entry into the target cells and are produced by genetic engineering in insect or mammalian cells. With the elucidation of the co-receptor use by different strains of HIV-1, novel envelope candidate vaccines also included in their design envelopes from clinical or primary isolates of HIV-1 R5 strains, which use CD4 and the CCR5 co-receptor.

Envelope-based candidate vaccines were found to induce neutralizing antibodies in 100% of volunteers, but not cytotoxic T lymphocytes (CTLs), whose function is to search for and destroy virus-infected cells. However, the antibodies induced by the first generation of envelope-based vaccines were mostly directed to laboratory-adapted strains of HIV, with weak or no ability to neutralize clinical isolates, which are thought to be the most relevant for vaccine development.

In fact, the only two phase III efficacy trials of an HIV vaccine conducted to date were implemented in the USA and Thailand using monomeric gp120 molecules developed by VaxGen. Results from these two trials became available in 2003, providing conclusive clinical evidence that these candidate vaccines were not significantly protective [8].

Second wave: induction of cell-mediated immunity

The second wave of HIV vaccine research started in the mid-1990s, with the recognition of the importance of cell-mediated immune responses (CTLs) in the control of HIV infection. This paradigm led to the development or refinement of live recombinant viral vectors, especially poxvirus vectors, capable of inducing CTLs. The antigens expressed by these candidate vaccines include products of the *env* gene, but more often from *gag*, which codes for the more conserved internal core protein, and from other regulatory and functional genes of HIV-1 (*pol, tat* and *nef*). Prime examples of this approach have been the different constructs of replication-deficient canarypox–HIV recombinant vectors, collectively known as ALVAC-HIV from Aventis-Pasteur. Other, more recent candidate vaccines being developed under the cell-mediated immunity paradigm include different types of DNA constructs, vectors based on the attenuated modified vaccinia Ankara (MVA), and lipopeptide vaccines.

Different ALVAC-HIV vectors have been tested extensively in clinical trials, often in prime-boost regimes together with gp120 products. These trials have shown that the ALVAC vectors are capable of inducing CTL responses to different HIV-1 proteins, but generally only in less than 50% of the immunized volunteers. MVA vectors have generally, but not always, shown better ability than the ALVAC vectors to induce CTLs, as measured by the γ-interferon ELISPOT assay. However, recent data suggest that this assay, which is the one that has been extensively used in these trials, may not adequately assess cell-mediated immune responses [9].

We may need to develop and validate new multiparametric assays to test multiple mechanisms of the cell-mediated immune response, including interleukin-2 and other cytokines. In any case, the third phase III efficacy trial of an HIV vaccine was initiated in Thailand late in 2003 to test the protective efficacy of a prime-boost regime consisting of a subtype-E ALVAC vector in combination with gp120 envelope proteins based on subtype B and E viruses. This trial will enrol up to 16,000 volunteers, and the results should be available around 2008–2009.

Third wave: better and broader immune responses

The third wave of HIV vaccines is now starting, and it should see much work aimed at optimizing immune responses by existing or yet to be developed candidate vaccines. The goals of this new wave are to develop candidate vaccines that can induce antibodies capable of neutralizing clinical (R5) strains from all HIV-1 subtypes or high levels of long-lasting, cross-reactive CTLs against different structural and regulatory proteins of HIV.

A range of novel candidate vaccines are being developed to meet that challenge, and some are already moving to human trials. One of these novel candidate vaccines is represented by a replication-incompetent adenovirus type 5 vector expressing different HIV-1 proteins, mostly designed to induce cell-mediated immunity. The major challenge, however, would be the development of envelope-based candidate vaccines capable of inducing the appropriate type of neutralizing antibodies, a problem that is being approached by a highly sophisticated interaction of structural biology, peptide chemistry, basic immunology and genetic engineering.

Logistical and financial challenges in the development and evaluation of HIV vaccines

Although the major challenges encountered in the development of an HIV vaccine are the scientific issues discussed above, other challenges that need to be addressed are of a logistical and financial nature.

Logistical challenges

The logistical challenges are mainly related to the complexities of conducting multiple trials in healthy human volunteers, especially large-scale phase III efficacy trials in developing countries. Trials in developing countries are necessary because: (i) the vast majority of HIV infections are occurring in these countries, where an effective vaccine is most needed; (ii) efficacy trials need to be conducted in populations with high HIV incidence, many of which are in developing countries, because sufficient new infections are needed to be able to conclude that the candidate vaccine has a real impact in preventing these infections; (iii) the genetic variability of HIV may impose the need to test different candidate vaccines in different areas of the world where different HIV subtypes and strains circulate; and (iv) it may be necessary to evaluate how different routes or cofactors of transmission and host genetic background could influence vaccine-induced protection [10].

A renewed global effort on HIV vaccines will require the expansion of existing vaccine evaluation sites in industrialized and developing countries, and the identification of new sites with the necessary epidemiological characteristics, such as high HIV incidence, well characterized HIV subtypes and the ability to recruit and retain a sufficient number of volunteers. These sites, especially in developing countries, need to be prepared with the long-term aim of building site capacity in general, rather than just preparing for specific trials. They should include additional activities in major areas of public health in order to address the needs of individual communities and countries. Sites need to be developed with full involvement of the local authorities and community, including training of scientific staff.

It is also essential to address the regulatory and ethical challenges associated with the conduct of highly complex trials in developing countries, many of which lack the necessary expertise, processes and other systems needed to make regulatory decisions expeditiously.

Financial challenges

The global investment in HIV vaccine research and development was tentatively estimated to be of the order of US$550 million in 2002, with the public sector accounting for more than 67% of these funds, the pharmaceutical industry for approximately 15% and the remainder from the philanthropic sector [11]. Although this amount is certainly important, especially when compared with investments in other vaccines, it still is not commensurate with the magnitude and socio-economic consequences of the AIDS pandemic or with the estimated financial requirements to mount an enhanced research and development effort that would have a real possibility of developing an effective vaccine in the foreseeable future.

Initial estimates indicate that such an enhanced HIV vaccine research and development effort would require an annual investment of the order of US$1.3 billion over the next 10 years, or more [12]. It is appreciated, however, that although additional funding is needed, use of existing resources could be optimized with better planning and more coordinated implementation. Since an effective overall global response to the epidemic may require US$12–20 billion per year [4], an HIV vaccine research and development programme with real chances of success would only represent approximately 5–10% of the total investment.

If history is of any relevance to this case, it would be important to remember that from 1938 to 1962, the successful National Foundation for Infantile Paralysis, better known as 'The March of Dimes', invested 59% of its funds to treat the children affected by poliomyelitis, including orthopaedic surgery and the purchase of 'iron lungs'. However, they were wise enough to invest 11% of their resources to support research on new interventions, which, in 1955, resulted in the successful development of the Salk polio vaccine. An additional 8% of their funds was dedicated to professional training and 13% to fund-raising [13].

Society will have to decide what proportion of existing resources should be used now to expand access to existing interventions to prevent and treat HIV, and what proportion of resources are needed to support research to develop new interventions. Based on previous programmatic experiences, we believe that a 90%/10% proportion could be in the appropriate range, but we also recognize that rigorous economic analysis will be needed to define the ideal proportion so that we do not deny access to existing interventions to people who need them today but, at the same time, we do not deny future generations the more effective interventions that research would undoubtedly develop, including a vaccine.

Planning for future access to an HIV vaccine

From our previous discussion, it should be evident that it will take several years before a highly effective HIV vaccine is finally developed. It is believed, however, that even a preventive vaccine with low or moderate efficacy of the order of 30–50% could be a valuable prevention tool, especially if targeted at populations at higher risk of HIV infection [14].

Early planning is essential to ensure that, when such a vaccine is developed, it is made available to all populations in need without unnecessary delays, and that the vaccine is made available simultaneously both in the 'North' and in the 'South'. However, the strategies to make vaccines available worldwide would have to differ from those that have been generally used for most drugs, which are first made available in the 'North', where higher prices can be charged and research and development expenditures recouped, and only after a number of years do they become available in the 'South', in regions of the world that often need them the most. This 'trickle-down' effect will be unacceptable once an HIV vaccine is developed.

To ensure global availability of future HIV vaccines, a number of actions must take place now, including the identification of policies and strategies for vaccine introduction and use in different communities, countries and regions, as well as the development of estimates of needs and probable vaccine uptake according to different levels of vaccine efficacy. Of special importance would be to ensure that the introduction of a future vaccine is coordinated with, and complementary to, the overall response to the HIV pandemic. In particular, the use of any vaccine would be complementary to the use of antiretroviral therapy.

Estimates of need and potential uptake

A first approximation to how an HIV vaccine could be used in developing countries, and how many doses would be required to initiate a global vaccination campaign, was obtained from a study conducted during 2001–2002 by the WHO/UNAIDS HIV Vaccine Initiative, in collaboration with the International AIDS Vaccine Initiative (IAVI) [15].

In this study, key informants were consulted through workshops conducted in four different regions of the world, with participants spanning a broad range of areas of expertise. Participants were presented with two hypothetical scenarios of vaccine efficacy, partial efficacy and high efficacy, and were asked which population groups should be considered for vaccination. The ensuing discussions were used to estimate needs for future HIV vaccines based on anticipated policies regarding target populations. The estimated needs were then adjusted for accessibility and acceptability in the target populations, to arrive at an estimate of probable uptake, i.e. courses of vaccine likely to be delivered.

Participants in the study suggested that a future HIV preventive vaccine with partial efficacy could be used in specific vulnerable populations such as men who have sex with men, sex workers and injecting drug users. In Latin America and Africa, patients with sexually transmitted infections were also identified as potential target populations. Additional groups in Africa identified as potential target groups for a partially effective vaccine were truck drivers, postnatal women and, in some cases, adolescents when other preventive interventions were not widely available. Depending on the HIV epidemiology in different regions, a highly effective vaccine could be used in larger segments of the population, such as adolescents and young adults, military recruits, discordant couples, prisoners and healthcare workers.

Based on the identified target populations, initial estimates suggest that with a high-efficacy HIV vaccine, global needs would be of the order of 690 million full immunization courses in the first 5 years of an immunization campaign, targeting 22% and 69%, respectively, of adults worldwide and in sub-Saharan Africa. On the other hand, with a low/moderate-efficacy vaccine targeting populations at higher risk of HIV infection, the global needs were estimated to be 260 million full immunization courses, targeting 8% of adults worldwide and 41% of adults in sub-Saharan Africa [15].

The current estimate of probable uptake for hypothetical HIV vaccines using existing health services and delivery systems is 38% of the estimated need for a high-efficacy vaccine, and only 19% for a low/moderate-efficacy vaccine. Bridging the gap between the estimated need and the probable uptake for HIV vaccines will represent a major public health challenge for the future. These early estimates should also help in calculating future financial needs related to vaccine procurement and delivery.

Cost-effectiveness and delivery issues

The WHO/UNAIDS HIV Vaccine Initiative is currently engaged in a pilot study in five countries—Brazil, China, Kenya, Peru and Thailand—to assess their potential capacity to deliver future HIV vaccines. These studies are supported by a mathematical model (VaccSim), which is a simulation model used to investigate optimal distribution patterns for limited quantities of HIV vaccines under various HIV epidemic scenarios [16]. The model can be used to compare the effect on the epidemic when delivering a vaccine of variable efficacy to different target groups.

As part of these pilot studies, cost-effectiveness features will be integrated into the VaccSim model. Cost-effectiveness analyses could then be used to guide policy processes. Rather than supporting a policy decision merely because it appears to be effective, or because it enjoys broad political support, systematic analysis pushes another—and perhaps more useful—question to the fore: what is the best use of available resources?

An economic evaluation will assist policy-makers in making evidence-based decisions on immunization strategies and in assessing the cost implications. When an HIV vaccine initially becomes available on the market, it is predicted that supply will fall short of demand. An important outcome of this analysis will be to guide policy-makers on the most cost-effective use of limited vaccine supply. For example, shortly after a vaccine is licensed for use, it is expected that it will be available only in limited quantities. In this period, and until the manufacturing facilities are scaled up, phase IV trials could be conducted to address the effectiveness of the vaccine in non-experimental conditions, including the uncertainties about the practical generalizability of vaccine performance, community effects and potential behavioural disinhibition.

Another possibility is to initiate a vaccination campaign targeting populations at high risk of HIV infection, where vaccination would result in immediate individual benefit to the vaccine recipients, but also in potentially important public health benefits by interrupting the chain of transmission of the virus, preventing the infection of many others. At a later stage, routine vaccination of lower-risk populations could be initiated. The potential advantages and disadvantages of targeted versus universal vaccination will have to be considered in the future, including the potential risk of stigmatizing groups identified for targeted immunization.

In exploring the cost-effectiveness of different delivery strategies, it is also necessary to assess the country's capacity to deliver future HIV vaccines. Delivery might prove to be a significant challenge to public health authorities and communities. The logistical and practical barriers to delivering an HIV vaccine are enormous and raise a number of questions about immunization services in the future.

Pre- and early adolescents will be one of the main target groups for future HIV vaccines, i.e. before the age of exposure to the virus [17]. Historically, however, immunization has mainly focused on infants. Indeed, vaccines have only occasionally targeted adolescents systematically, even in industrialized countries. Delivering vaccines to pre-adolescents and adolescents in developing countries would be, to a great extent, a new challenge.

A number of possibilities exist for delivery of a future HIV vaccine. Relying on traditional health clinics is not likely to result in the high uptake of an HIV vaccine in most developing countries. In addition, many of the countries that need an HIV vaccine the most might lack the necessary infrastructure and require significant resources to build the necessary capacity. Both vaccines and antiretroviral therapy will need good healthcare infrastructure for successful delivery. The choice of vaccination delivery setting and vaccination provider will obviously vary depending on the situation. The current options for the delivery of a future HIV vaccine appear to be: (i) existing HIV prevention and care facilities; (ii) reproductive health clinics; and (iii) national immunization programmes. There are advantages and disadvantages—and complications—for all three of these options, and, depending on the type of vaccine and vaccination strategies, the possible delivery channels will have to be assessed and strengthened.

Issues to consider in accelerating future introduction

The previous discussion serves to emphasize that to accelerate the development and future availability of safe, effective and affordable HIV vaccines, it is essential to address not only the associated biomedical obstacles, but also the many logistical aspects concerning the introduction and use of those vaccines in the future, as discussed during a consultation organized by the WHO/UNAIDS HIV Vaccine Initiative and the US CDC in November 2002 [18].

> Box 7.2 **Logistical issues that need to be addressed to accelerate the development and future availability of HIV vaccines: recommendations from a WHO/UNAIDS–CDC consultation**
>
> ### Manufacturing and licensing
>
> Strengthen regulatory framework in selected countries;
> Facilitate validation of potential end-points for vaccine trials;
> Expand assessments of HIV vaccine demand by regions and over time;
> Catalyse discussion aimed at increasing global vaccine manufacturing capacity;
> Develop a position on HIV vaccine-related intellectual property and patents.
>
> ### Acceptability and social marketing
>
> Develop broad-based global platform for planning future vaccine introduction;
> Adapt global platform to needs of individual countries;
> Establish international partnership to implement future programmes.
>
> ### Immunization strategies and delivery
>
> Develop national policies supporting HIV vaccination programmes;
> Ensure that future vaccines are delivered along with other prevention programmes;
> Develop strategies for initial introduction of vaccines with limited availability;
> Develop pilot methods for evaluation of future HIV immunization programmes;
> Encourage programmes to bundle HIV vaccines with other appropriate vaccines.
>
> ### Access and economic issues
>
> Ensure the goals of global availability and maximum public health benefit;
> Conduct research on cost-benefit, demand and resource implications;
> Explore different financial options;
> Collaborate with the vaccine industry and identify appropriate incentives;
> Facilitate evaluation of infrastructures for future vaccine delivery;
> Ensure community involvement in the whole process.
>
> Source: [18].

Participants identified a number of logistical issues that need to be addressed in four different areas: (i) vaccine manufacturing and licensing; (ii) vaccination acceptability and social marketing; (iii) immunization strategies and delivery; and (iv) access and economic issues (Box 7.2).

It is important to appreciate, for instance, that in order for a safe and efficacious vaccine to be adopted for public health use, it must be licensed by the national regulatory authorities in the countries where it will be used. Obtaining the data required to support licensing should be planned before conducting phase III efficacy trials if there is to be a rapid deployment of an efficacious vaccine. This assessment should also include risk-benefit evaluations in the context of differing epidemic dynamics, and country needs and resources.

In addition, whether or not a future HIV vaccine will be accepted by the target population will depend on a number of variables such as efficacy, side effects, price per full course of vaccination to the consumer, duration of protection, and other considerations. Communication materials will need to convey all known facts in a transparent and concise way, managing information to avoid creating unreasonable expectations.

Addressing the set of complex issues that will arise once an effective vaccine is developed will require the participation of multiple stakeholders in the public and private sectors, and in industrialized and developing countries. These actions, however, would be essential to ensure widespread and rapid access to HIV vaccines globally, soon after their efficacy is demonstrated in clinical trials.

Conclusions

Emerging during the last quarter of the twentieth century, the HIV pandemic has now extended into the twenty-first century and is still progressing. As has been the case with many other infectious diseases, a safe, effective and accessible preventive vaccine represents the best long-term hope for the control of the HIV pandemic. The development of an HIV vaccine, however, has faced a number of difficult scientific challenges that have been compounded by additional logistical and financial difficulties. To address the scientific challenges, there is a need to coordinate the current research effort better so that the scientific creativity of individual investigators is complemented by a more global, collaborative strategy aimed at developing and testing novel candidate vaccines faster and more efficiently.

This HIV vaccine development effort needs to be positioned in the context of the overall global response to the HIV pandemic alongside expanded access to existing preventive and treatment interventions and other research efforts, including developing better drugs and preventive tools, microbicides and behavioural interventions. A defined proportion of the global resources invested in HIV prevention and control, perhaps of the order of 10% of the total, needs to be used to develop novel and more effective interventions, including vaccines, which will be needed for successful control of the pandemic.

However, the development of more effective tools will not be enough to control the pandemic unless those tools are made available to all people in need, anywhere in the world. If the development of an HIV vaccine has been a difficult challenge, making it available worldwide could be just as onerous. We believe that it is not too early to begin planning how to use a future vaccine and that sufficient foresight could make it possible to reduce the gap between the discovery of the vaccine and its widespread use. Failure to do so could have serious public health consequences.

References

1. Cohen J. (2001). *Shots in the Dark, the Wayward Search for an AIDS Vaccine.* New York: Norton, p7–13.
2. Klausner RD, Fauci AS, Corey L *et al.* (2003). The need for a global HIV vaccine enterprise. *Science* 300:2036–9.
3. Coordinating Committee of the Global HIV/AIDS Vaccine Enterprise. (2005). The Global HIV/AIDS Vaccine Enterprise: scientific strategic plan. *Public Library of Science Medicine* 2:e25. URL: http://www.plosmedicine.org.

4. Piot P, Feachem RGA, Jong-wook L, Wolfensohn JD. (2004). A global response to AIDS: lessons learned, next steps. *Science* **304**:1909–10.

5. Esparza J. (2004). The quest for a preventive vaccine against HIV/AIDS. In: de Quadros C, ed. *Vaccines: Preventing Disease, Protecting Health.* Washington: Pan American Health Organization, p189–99.

6. Osmanov S, Patou C, Walker N, Schwardlander B, Esparza J. (2002). Estimated global distribution and regional spread of HIV-1 genetic subtypes in the year 2000. *Journal of Acquired Immunodeficiency Syndrome* **29**:184–90.

7. Esparza J, Osmanov S. (2003). HIV vaccines: a global perspective. *Current Molecular Medicine* **3**:183–93.

8. The rgp120 HIV Vaccine Study Group. (2005). Placebo-controlled phase 3 trial of a recombinant glycoprotein 120 vaccine to prevent HIV-1 infection. *Journal of Infectious Diseases* **191**:654–65.

9. Van Rompay KK, Abel K, Lawson JR *et al.* (2005). Attenuated poxvirus-based simian immunodeficiency virus (SIV) vaccines given in infancy partially protect infant and juvenile macaques against repeated oral challenge with virulent SIV. *Journal of Acquired Immunodeficiency Syndrome* **38**:124–34.

10. Esparza J, Osmanov S, Pattou-Markovic C, Toure C, Chang ML, Nixon S. (2002). Past, present and future of HIV vaccine trials in developing countries. *Vaccine* **20**:1897–8.

11. Bing A, Gold D, Lamourelle G, Rowley J, Sadoff S. (2004). Quantifying global expenditures on AIDS vaccines R&D. Poster presented at the XV International AIDS Conference, Bangkok. Abstract no. TuPeE5325.

12. International AIDS Vaccine Initiative. (2004). *Scientific Blueprint 2004.* New York: IAVI, p28.

13. Wilson JR. (1963). *Margin of Safety: The Fight Against Polio.* London: Collins, p66.

14. Vermund SH. (1998). Rationale for the testing and use of a partially effective HIUV vaccine. *AIDS Research and Human Retroviruses* **14**(Supplement 3):S321–3.

15. Esparza J, Chang ML, Widdus R, Madrid Y, Walker N, Ghys PD. (2003). Estimation of 'needs' and 'probable uptake' for HIV/AIDS preventive vaccines based on possible policies and likely acceptance (a WHO/UNAIDS/IAVI study). *Vaccine* **21**:2032–41.

16. Barth-Jones DC, Longini IM. (2002). Determining optimal vaccination policy for HIV vaccines. In: *Proceedings of the International Conference on Health Sciences Simulation,* San Antonio, Texas, p63–79.

17. Clements CJ, Abdool-Karim Q, Chang ML, Nkowane B, Esparza J. (2004). Breaking new grounds: are changes in immunization services needed for the introduction of future HIV/AIDS vaccines and other new vaccines targeted at adolescents? *Vaccine* **22**:2822–6.

18. Chang ML, Vitek C, Esparza J *et al.* (2003). Public health considerations for the use of a first generation HIV vaccine: report from a WHO–UNAIDS/CDC consultation, Geneva, 20–21 November 2002. *AIDS* **17**:W1–10.

Chapter 8

Ethical issues and HAART

Norbert Gilmore

Introduction

The availability of treatment can strongly influence the ethical issues raised by a disease. This can be seen with the discovery of, and improvements in, HIV treatment. Those treatment changes have defined three phases in the evolution of the HIV pandemic. The earliest or pre-treatment phase, before 1987, pre-dated the discovery and availability of HIV antiviral drugs [1,2]. The second phase, ending in 1996, was characterized by the availability of single or double drug treatments that mostly produced unsustainable or partially effective outcomes. The third and most recent phase began in 1996 with the availability of effective multi-drug therapy, highly active antiretroviral therapy (HAART). HIV infection outcomes changed with these treatment changes, progressing from an untreatable, relentlessly fatal infection to a likely, but variably, fatal one and, most recently, to a chronic illness.

HAART has helped restore many immunodeficient individuals to seemingly normal health [3]. It has prevented HIV transmission to a substantial proportion of newborn children from HIV-infected mothers [4], prevented infection in healthcare workers accidentally exposed to HIV [5–7] and in partners following unprotected sexual exposure to HIV [8,9]. These successes have not been without financial and biological costs, particularly in the forms of medication intolerance, toxicity and financial burden. There also appear to be unexpected returns from making HAART available. For example, free, universal access to HAART in Brazil has, to date, helped reduce HIV transmission, resulting in a lower than expected HIV prevalence [10–12]. Brazil also shows that HAART can help reduce treatment costs by reducing morbidity, premature mortality, need for hospitalization and other healthcare needs, though it extends the duration of treatment, which is lifelong.

Ethical concerns have been a prominent feature of the debate about the HIV pandemic [13]. Articles examining some of those concerns were being published within 2 years of the discovery of AIDS [14–18]. Publications increased rapidly thereafter. Index Medicus, for example, lists 4957 citations published between 1981 and 2004 for MESH headings 'HIV' and 'AIDS' that are restricted to 'bioethics'. After 1982, the citations increased each year until 1988 (564 citations), then decreased steadily, with only 57 citations listed for 2004. Most ethical issues had already been analysed by 1996, when HAART became available [19], but few of those issues have been re-analysed since then. Also, few of the newer issues raised by HAART itself have been analysed exhaustively [20,21]. These issues include concerns about the generation and communication of personal information, rights to, and in, care of people infected with HIV, as well as rights in relation to prevention and vaccine research. The capacity of HAART to prevent infection following a variety of HIV exposures raises concerns about HIV testing and disclosure of personal information. Some issues arise from the availability of HAART, whereas others arise from its unavailability, especially in developing countries. Many healthcare and research concerns involve standards of care, namely the conflict between local standards where HAART may be inaccessible and developed country standards where HAART, and the monitoring of its safety and effectiveness, is widely accessible. This chapter briefly examines the principal issues that HAART highlights as a basis for encouraging future investigations and discussion. Ethical issues related to basic research, classical prevention campaigns and conflicts of interest are not discussed, since HAART appears to have little direct impact on them.

Generation of information

The generation of personal information related to HIV infection, whether voluntary, mandatory, compulsory or research-based, has raised—and continues to raise—ethical concerns. This often occurs when someone has been exposed to HIV unexpectedly and information is needed to help answer the crucial question: will the immediate use of HAART be lifesaving for the exposed person by stopping infection from happening, or is HAART unnecessary, thereby avoiding risks and harms from HAART while conserving scarce resources?

Individuals who have been sources of exposure will often consent to answer questions about their HIV status and treatment, or be tested for HIV infection. Sometimes the voluntary generation of information will not be feasible. The source person may be unavailable, unable, or refuse to consent due to being demented, comatose or, having refused testing earlier, may now be incapable of changing that decision. There are times when information could be generated from earlier blood samples or from medical records but, again, there may be no consent to generate this information. Involuntary generation of personal information has been considered unjustifiable, in general and for HIV-related information in particular, because of its intrusiveness, its disrespect for the subject of the information, and because risks and harms generally outweigh benefits for that person [22].

This situation may be changing. There are at least three legislated exceptions to this earlier prohibition: compulsory testing of babies born to mothers in New York and Connecticut who have refused antenatal or perinatal HIV testing [23,24]; compulsory testing of individuals who are the sources of occupational exposure of healthcare workers in Virginia and Florida [25]; and compulsory testing of arrested individuals in Georgia when their victims or peacekeepers have suffered a potentially 'significant' HIV exposure [26]. A British court has also ordered an infant to be tested who was born to an HIV-infected mother who refused HIV prophylaxis and planned to breastfeed her infant [27]. More and more demands for involuntary testing are likely, as negative HIV test results are increasingly being used to justify avoiding or stopping post-exposure prophylaxis [7,8,28,29].

Preventing mother-to-child HIV transmission

Antiretroviral treatment of HIV-infected pregnant women can save the majority of their infants from infection during pregnancy and childbirth, but it is less clear what should be done to ensure all exposed fetuses and infants can benefit from prophylaxis. One possibility is to treat all pregnant women without testing them or knowing who is infected. Another possibility is to test all pregnant women, but treat only those who are infected. A 'test no one–treat all' approach exposes uninfected women and their babies to risks and harms from prophylaxis without benefits, and increases costs. A 'test first, then treat' approach spares uninfected women risks and harms while benefiting exposed babies, but it adds risks and harms that can include false-positive or false-negative results, being forced to learn one is infected, having to notify partners and having results disclosed accidentally or maliciously. Testing newborns instead of mothers occurs too late for intrauterine prophylaxis, but postnatal prophylaxis, while unproven, is possible, and testing could help minimize further exposure to HIV by helping to identify mothers who need to avoid breastfeeding.

Mothers can still be treated if they refuse to be tested or to be informed of their test results, whereas refusing prophylaxis is much more problematic. Compulsory treatment of uninfected women is unjustifiable, so that testing becomes a prerequisite for involuntary treatment. Compulsory testing without compulsory prophylaxis is ethically dubious in most situations because of the risks and harms from testing for the mother and the absence of preventive benefits for the fetus when prophylaxis is refused. Testing has sometimes been made compulsory, but, so far, prophylaxis has not. Implementing involuntary prophylaxis would be a major change to the almost universally accepted voluntary response approach to the HIV pandemic [30,31]. It would also threaten maternal autonomy.

The choice of antenatal–perinatal prophylaxis is also a problem. Beginning HAART during pregnancy and continuing it through childbirth is the standard intervention in developed countries. This is not a feasible intervention in developing countries, whereas single-dose nevirapine has been both effective and feasible. Unfortunately, nevirapine does not prevent intrauterine transmission. Also, resistance to nevirapine has developed in more than one-third of infected mothers, threatening its future prophylactic and therapeutic usefulness [32], and some women treated with nevirapine have developed progressive, sometimes fatal, hepatitis [33]. Hopefully, these concerns will be short-lived if increasing availability of, and access to, HAART allows safer and more effective prophylactic interventions to be implemented.

Preventing HIV infection following occupational exposure of a health worker

Preventing post-exposure HIV infection of providers of healthcare, emergency, safety or security services can be cost-effective by avoiding infection and conserving scarce service resources. Beginning HAART requires knowing that the source of exposure is HIV-infected, presumed to be infected, or the absence of infection cannot be proven. Successful prophylaxis can require knowing, or presuming, the infecting HIV is sensitive, or likely to be sensitive, to the prophylactic medications that will be used. That, in turn, requires knowing what HIV treatment, if any, the source of exposure has received, the efficacy of that treatment to control HIV replication, and any laboratory data such as genotyping [34,35]. Prophylaxis can begin and continue in the absence of such information, but a successful outcome may depend on knowing this information [36]. Stopping or avoiding prophylaxis also depends on knowing that the source of exposure is uninfected. Risks and harms from generating this information are greater than when there has not been an exposure. The exposed person, for instance, may have no obligation to keep source information confidential, may not keep it confidential or may disclose it inadvertently by using HAART. There can be an additional benefit, however, in the altruism of helping to prevent HIV infection. Often this information will be generated voluntarily, but sometimes the source person will refuse or cannot consent to its generation. In many situations, it is likely that generating information involuntarily may be justifiable, and may become the norm. Virginia and Florida, for example, already authorize compulsory post-exposure testing [25].

Preventing HIV infection following accidental exposure of a patient

Preventing exposure to the blood of HIV-infected providers of healthcare, emergency, safety or security services during the provision of their service has been analysed repeatedly, in particular by professional medical associations and licensing bodies. A consensus emerged that whenever there is a risk of exposure, i.e. by an 'exposure-prone' invasive procedure, HIV-infected professionals must 'disclose or withdraw' [37,38], i.e. they must refuse to perform those procedures, other than in a genuine emergency situation, or perform them only after patients have been informed and given consent to the infected professional performing the procedure. Infected professionals are expected to consult experts to determine what procedures require disclosure–withdrawal. This policy is the norm today, but it needs to be reviewed now that HAART can reduce the risk of HIV transmission by suppressing HIV production to undetectable levels and post-exposure prophylaxis can prevent infection.

Professionals have to inform their patients whenever they injure or expose them to avoidable risks and harms such as being exposed to the provider's HIV. This can include being offered effective HAART and being told that prompt treatment can be lifesaving [39–41]. Determining if prophylaxis is needed, and what type is needed, requires information about the service provider's infection. The provider has an obligation to disclose information if it is known, or to generate it when it is feasible to do so. Conflicts of interest also require disclosure, or the intervention of other professionals, when the source of exposure is the provider responsible for services to the exposed person.

Testing service providers prospectively as a condition of professional practice has generally been rejected, although some universities in Thailand require HIV testing of their medical students [42]. While testing would identify HIV-infected service providers, it is not known how much it would reduce the incidence of HIV transmission, or at what cost. The risk is already tiny and will be even smaller where HAART is routinely available such that service providers' HIV replication is undetectable, and when HAART prophylaxis can prevent infection.

Preventing HIV infection following sexual or parenteral exposure

Anyone with a sexually or parenterally transmissible disease has an obligation to avoid exposing others, unless exposed individuals knowingly consent to the risks involved. Starting and completing prophylaxis promptly whenever exposure is likely and cannot be excluded would seem prudent [8]. Sometimes, generating information may be necessary to establish that an exposing partner is infected or which medications may be required for prophylaxis. This carries the additional risk of further, unwanted disclosure along with an additional benefit of knowing the information can help prevent infection or spare the exposed person weeks of prophylaxis.

Involuntary generation of information for prophylaxis may have been questionable before HAART became available, but a persuasive argument can be made now for mandatory or compulsory generation of information. The success of prophylaxis depends on using effective medications, which, in turn, requires knowing the treatment history of the exposing person, including data on medication resistance. Recent studies emphasize the seriousness of this situation. Nearly half of the adults in a recent study who had detectable HIV viral loads while being treated with HAART were infected with HIV resistant to two classes of HAART drugs, while 13% were infected with HIV resistant to three drug classes [43].

Individuals can also be exposed to HIV non-consensually by rape, sexual aggression or violence that results in exposure to an aggressor's blood or sexual fluids. Generating information in this situation appears similar to that following accidental or consensual exposure, although it is complicated by the intent implicit in the exposure, by its non-consensual nature and by the aggressor's egregious disrespect of the victim. The situation is likely to be dominated by legal issues such as accusations, criminal charges and collection of evidence, but the central issues here are whether the victim (or aggressor) needs HAART, what regimen is likely to be effective and how quickly it can be started, or avoided if not needed [44].

Communication of information

Voluntary disclosure of personal information rarely poses ethical concerns, unlike involuntary disclosure. The effectiveness of HAART can make the need for disclosure a compelling and pressing issue, and a difficult ethical conundrum.

Disclosure to benefit a partner at risk

The need to inform a sexual or injection equipment-sharing partner that she/he has been exposed to a serious risk or harm—in this case, HIV infection—is a classic public health dilemma. Disclosure gives the exposed partner an opportunity to make appropriate healthcare and other personal decisions. Those decisions can include avoiding further exposure and seeking healthcare, including HIV testing and starting post-exposure prophylaxis. There may be urgency to disclose information because starting HAART promptly is necessary, otherwise prophylaxis is likely to fail [8]. The exposing partner should inform the exposed partner or consent to allowing someone else to do it, such as a healthcare provider, since refusal to do so is likely to result in involuntary disclosure by the exposing partner's physician or by a public health official.

Disclosure to benefit a patient at risk

While much less likely today, patients may still be exposed to blood or tissue from an HIV-infected patient, such as when receiving a rare blood component or transplant, or by exposure to inadequately cleaned medical or surgical equipment previously used on an infectious patient. Exposed patients have to be informed about the error and provided with the information necessary to prevent or limit further harm. This can include information necessary for successful prophylaxis, such as data on prior HAART use and drug resistance. Some situations may raise conflicts of interest that need to be disclosed or avoided.

Disclosure to benefit service providers at risk

Providers of healthcare, emergency, safety or security services may find themselves exposed to infections such as HIV. Promptly starting HAART can be lifesaving. Knowing that the source of exposure is uninfected can bring great relief and make HAART unnecessary. When the source of exposure cannot, or refuses to, consent, someone else will have to disclose the information so that the exposed provider has an opportunity to begin, continue or stop prophylaxis. That information may be unknown, but can be generated in a timely manner from the source of exposure, such as through questioning or HIV testing; known in confidence by a healthcare professional, such as the source's physician; or present in hospital or other medical records. Since the risks and harms from disclosure are likely to be far less than the resulting benefits, namely preventing infection or avoiding the need for prophylaxis, then justification of disclosure is likely.

Disclosure to benefit an HIV-infected patient

HIV-infected patients can sometimes benefit from disclosure of confidential information when, for example, successful HAART would be stopped or medications would be prescribed unknowingly that could interfere with HAART metabolism, thereby predisposing to HIV resistance or jeopardizing the efficacy of HAART. The patient may be reluctant to disclose this information due to fear of being discriminated against—in particular, being refused care or receiving an inferior standard of care. Alteratively, the patient might be unresponsive, demented or otherwise unable to communicate information. A similar situation could arise when a patient develops side effects from HAART that might not be treated appropriately without knowing the patient is using HAART.

A very different issue can arise when patients would be placed at risk or harmed were information to be disclosed that they are HIV-infected or using HAART. For example, an employer, family or friend might want to know if a patient is infected, receiving HAART or has HAART-related side effects. Some patients are reluctant to use HAART because of lipodystrophy [45]. Choosing or changing treatments to those less likely to produce this side effect, when it is feasible to do so, can be an example of protecting patients' best medical interests and privacy.

Rights to care

HAART is amplifying many ethical issues relating to the availability of, and access to, care and treatment of HIV-infected people. Many of these issues are articulated as financial ones, namely who can or should pay for HAART—where treatment and monitoring can cost as much as US$20,000 a year [46–48]—since HAART is rarely affordable without assistance from governments, private insurance plans or charitable programmes. Nowhere is this more obvious than in the developing world. For example, less than 4% of HIV-infected Africans were estimated to be receiving HAART in 2004 [49,50].

Determining who should receive care and treatment when resources are extremely limited is a very difficult ethical dilemma that is not specific to HIV. One or more of the following approaches could conceivably be used:

+ random allocation, i.e. using a lottery to select individuals to be treated first;

+ queuing, i.e. treating those first in line;

+ treating, first, those most in need, i.e. those who are sickest or in greatest danger of dying;

+ treating, first, those likely to benefit the most, i.e. those likely to show the greatest improvement;

- treating, first, those likely to benefit others the most, e.g. mothers, midwives or service providers, a Prime Minister or a Nobel laureate, ahead of others.

Qualifiers may also be used, such as blanket eligibility and exclusion criteria, which relate to these more general approaches. In the case of HIV, these might include having clinical immunodeficiency, CD4 lymphocytes below a particular threshold or a very high HIV viral load. Treatment might be modified or withheld when an individual is hypersensitive to one or more medications such as abacavir or nevirapine, has advanced liver disease or severe non-HIV dementia, has a treatment-resistant disease such as cancer or emphysema, or is unlikely to comply with the treatment regimen and, so, waste medication. Other approaches might include using HAART as post-exposure prophylaxis before using it to treat established infection, or treating younger patients before older ones. Most countries would exclude from general health services coverage people who are not recognized as permanent citizens. Refugees and asylum seekers should be considered as special populations eligible for treatment like nationals, since they did not choose to migrate.

Even with robust criteria to identify who would be treated, there is still the issue of how much to spend on each patient. Is it ever justifiable to treat patients with a lower standard of care in order to maximize treatment rates rather than offering fewer patients the maximum benefit possible? There is no 'right' answer to this dilemma, but good data on the costs and effectiveness over time of different approaches to HAART would assist decisions. Additional concerns include trying to decide what resources will be allocated to diagnosing HIV infection, monitoring the safety and efficacy of HAART, and investigating and treating side effects of HAART. Despite careful allocation, treatment can remain wasteful if people are treated without adequate education and support to encourage and maintain treatment adherence, or by continuing unsuccessful treatment regimens that fail because of HIV resistance.

Are developed countries obliged to assist developing ones?

HAART has quickly come to be regarded as an essential tool to help control the HIV pandemic because of its capacity to help prevent HIV transmission, morbidity, premature death, new healthcare needs and many of the pandemic's costly socio-economic consequences. Yet, many countries lack the infrastructure to identify who needs HAART and the resources needed to deliver and monitor its safety and effectiveness [51]. They urgently need assistance from better-off countries to help them slow the pandemic, and states are justified in assisting other states or individuals in need, providing them with foreign aid or international assistance. Reasons for doing so can include self-imposed multilateral or bilateral obligations, charity, altruism or national self-interest. The United Nations, individual states and some charities are funding developing countries to help increase access to, and monitoring of, HAART [51]. However, are developed countries obliged in any way to help developing countries make HAART available? This is probably an unanswerable question due mostly to a lack of universally accepted ethical values and principles on which to base such an obligation [52]. Differences in national or regional values, principles and beliefs make ethical analyses jurisdictional, with analysis in one country not necessarily applying elsewhere. Analyses need not differ in their conclusions, but can differ when dominant values differ, such as, say, those of a strictly Islamic country and those of a staunchly Catholic one, or those of developing and developed countries. One example of this discrepancy has been the differences in informed consent requirements in Africa and in industrialized countries [53]. Fundamental human rights, while considered to be universally binding [54], do not help solve this conundrum. They do not oblige states explicitly to assist others outside their borders [55]. Nor do they inform states about what particular responses to the HIV pandemic, or other health problems, might be necessary and justified. One exception to this situation may be the evolving, but controversial and disputed, right to intervene when human rights are being abused [56]. The movement to globalize ethics [57] may, some day, help solve this conundrum.

> Unfortunately, the HIV pandemic has come too soon for globalization to persuade the world that national borders cannot be barriers to helping people in developing countries, just as we help each other within our own national borders. Can we, today, claim an ethical responsibility to help others that is based upon a future world arrangement? International policing and peacekeeping, humanitarian aid and a right to intervene across borders, international trade agreements and economic unions could be affirmative arguments, but most might say that it is still too early to claim borders do not limit ethical justifications. Making healthcare, in general, and drug treatment, in particular, available and accessible globally would be another important step in this journey [58].

Is profiting from the sale of HAART justifiable?

The unaffordability of HAART in developing countries has become an international cause, spearheaded, in part, by Médecins Sans Frontières [59], along with a consortium of community groups and activists, particularly in South Africa [60]. At the heart of this issue has been the demand that pharmaceutical companies reduce medication prices; that medications be manufactured without respecting pharmaceutical company patent or proprietary rights; and that international assistance help make HAART universally accessible.

Brazil, India and South Africa have been some of the major battlegrounds for these initiatives. The Brazilian government funded the manufacture and distribution of HAART medications, while disregarding patent protection. Cipla Ltd, an Indian manufacturer of generic drugs, pioneered production and inexpensive marketing of HAART medications, regardless of pharmaceutical company property rights [61]. In South Africa, pharmaceutical companies went to court to secure their proprietary rights but, in the end, dropped their suit [62,63]. Meanwhile, the pharmaceutical industry has responded with differential pricing, where medication prices appear to be linked to levels of national income. The World Trade Organization passed a resolution in 2003 recognizing public health emergencies as a valid exception to respecting pharmaceutical patent rights [64]. Also, the United Nations is soliciting funds to fight HIV infection, tuberculosis and malaria, especially trying to make HAART universally accessible [51,65]. Nonetheless, a huge gap remains between the need for, availability of and access to HAART [66].

Prevention campaigns have failed to fully control the spread of HIV infection [67], so that without an effective preventive vaccine, HAART is the only other tool available to help control this infection. Yet, its lifesaving benefits are unaffordable to almost everyone in developing countries. What, then, should be the limits of proprietary rights—in this case the patent monopoly on HAART medications—in the face of such a relentless, ravaging pandemic? Clearly, the pharmaceutical industry cannot squander its resources, nor can it be expected to market its products at a loss, except for, say, its own altruistic reasons. It is already showing its generosity by offering many of its medications at prices that not only preclude profits, but also may incur losses [68]. Boerhinger Ingelheim has gone further, offering free nevirapine to

Southern African governments to help prevent mother-to-child transmission of HIV [69]. Here, the question is not about how the world arranges itself with regard to profits in general [70], but whether profiting from a product or service is justifiable when it is the only lifesaving one available. Profits from luxury goods that are unnecessary for survival, such as, say, cosmetic BOTOX® injections and erectile dysfunction drugs, would seem easily justifiable, with profits determined by what the marketplace will tolerate. The question, then, that needs ethical analysis is: can a necessary public good ever be a profitable one?

Is the exclusive funding of HIV interventions justifiable?

More and more resources in both developing and developed countries are being directed to control HIV transmission and its devastating consequences. This includes resources for HAART. This allocation may be justifiable, despite so many other life-threatening diseases, because:

- the HIV pandemic is an expanding one, unlike the stable prevalence of many other diseases;
- many of the pandemic's burdens are new and increasing, unlike the more stable burdens from many other diseases;
- entire family units are at great risk of being infected and destroyed by HIV, a situation that rarely occurs with other diseases;
- suppressing HIV infection can reduce further HIV transmission, morbidity and premature mortality;
- escalating economic losses attributable to HIV infection are threatening to erode other development and security resources [71,72].

Responses to the HIV pandemic that deprive or destabilize other health and social assistance or development situations would be ethically questionable were the consequences to be more harmful than the consequences avoided by responding to the HIV pandemic. Not responding to the pandemic, however, can worsen those other needs, such as controlling tuberculosis, or jeopardize responses to them. HAART is showing benefits that would have been unexpected a decade ago; growing costs are being controlled, and sometimes reduced, while complementing prevention efforts. It is becoming clearer that treatment is not an alternative to prevention efforts; instead, it complements these efforts. How, then, should scarce resources be allocated between these needs? There is probably no overarching resolution to this dilemma, since it is inherently an operational one, subject to research and evaluation in the context of each country's epidemic and health system. Some situations may favour greater preventive efforts, whereas others may favour a greater emphasis on treatment, but neither, alone, can be considered sufficient to control the spread of HIV infection.

Rights in care

Unlike rights *to* care that concern the availability of, and access to, health services, rights *in* care concern the quality of those services. Justice prohibits wrongful discrimination in the provision of services, just as it does for access to services. This means that services in general, or a particular service, may sometimes be withheld, restricted or modified, but only when it is clearly justifiable to do so. For example, providing unnecessary or futile treatment is unethical, such as prescribing HAART when HIV is fully resistant to the medications prescribed, or providing prophylaxis weeks after an HIV exposure. Refusing, delaying or reducing treatment without a valid justification, such as using dual therapy, or refusing to treat someone who is considered undesirable, such as an HIV-infected, convicted paedophile or rapist, is also unethical. Falsely economizing treatment costs by using treatment intermittently or by refusing to monitor its safety and efficacy is just as unacceptable.

Standards of care can vary widely, from those used to treat local health problems to national or international standards, with particular standards often reflecting local resources. Which standard should apply in a given locale, and under what circumstances, is an ethical dilemma that has been intensified by the unavailability of HAART in many developing countries. Like the universality of science, treatment standards should be universal [73], but HAART is rarely so. At times it may be geographically inaccessible; natural disasters, wars and other calamities may make it unavailable; or the infrastructure to deliver it may be inadequate. Most often, however, HAART is wholly or partially unaffordable, so that lesser standards, if any, are used. In the end, the dramatic efficacy of HAART brings us face to face with an age-old ethical dilemma, namely, should fewer people be treated with the best standard available, and, if so, who should be treated, or is treating more people with a lesser standard ever justifiable?

HIV rarely becomes resistant to HAART when medications are prescribed and taken meticulously and at adequate doses. Resistance may develop when HIV replication is not suppressed completely due to inadequate dosing, drug interactions that lower drug concentrations to ineffective levels, or intermittent treatment. So, patients and research subjects can expect to be prescribed appropriate medications at adequate doses and to be monitored appropriately for treatment safety and efficacy [74–76]. Deviations from this standard would be ethically unacceptable unless the deviation can be clearly justified.

When respecting such a standard is not feasible, what, then, should be done? Until additional resources are secured, rationing of treatment may be the only necessary option available. Treating fewer people would allow those treated to receive appropriate medications and monitoring while avoiding inadequate therapy, thereby minimizing the risks of treatment failure, resistance and wasted resources. This, in turn, poses an all too familiar and anguishing dilemma, namely, who should be treated, and when?

Research

Clinical research can make HAART available to some people, but not to everyone needing it. So who should be eligible to participate in a clinical trial, and how should that be decided? And what standard of care should apply to research subjects in a developing country when the research is designed, organized or funded elsewhere? Should the standard be that of developing countries, where HAART is practically unavailable, or that of developed countries, where it is abundant [77]?

Ethical concerns have increased along with clinical HIV research in developing countries. Some concerns are straightforward, such as when research is designed, organized and carried out in a single country or region and its results are mostly generalizable to that locale. More complex concerns often arise when research is carried out in different jurisdictions or in a developing country, but the research is designed, organized or sponsored elsewhere. Then, conflicts between developed and developing country standards are likely to arise. This 'double standard' dilemma has been studied extensively, but it remains unresolved [51,78–80]. The guidelines from the Council for International Organizations of Medical Sciences (CIOMS), for example, were revised in 2002 after protracted debate about research in developing countries. The United States National Bioethics Advisory Committee issued a report in 2001 on US-sponsored, developing country research [53]. The World Medical Association revised its *Helsinki Declaration* in 2000 in order to address some of these concerns [20,81]. UNAIDS also produced guidelines in 2000 for HIV-related vaccine research in developing countries [82]. The guidelines did not resolve the dilemma. For instance, UNAIDS' guidance point 16 states: 'Care and treatment for HIV/AIDS and its associated complications should be provided to participants in HIV preventive vaccine trials, with the ideal being to provide the best proven therapy, and the minimum to provide the highest level of care attainable in the host country....' [82].

Access to HAART is bringing a new momentum to this debate, as a recent joint World Health Organization–UNAIDS Consultation reported:

[w]hile there is now broad, though not unanimous agreement among sponsors of HIV vaccine trials that antiretroviral therapy (ART) and a clinical care package should be provided to those who become infected during conduct of a trial, certain issues remain unresolved:

◆ Who should pay for ART?

◆ How long should ART be provided for?

◆ Does treatment extend outside of ART?

◆ What else should be included in the standard of care package and who should pay for it?

◆ Who should provide treatment and care? [51, at pW2].

The Consultation clarified many of these issues and, in doing so, it moved the 'double standards' debate forward, concluding: '[t]he consensus that emerged from the presentations and discussions was that volunteers who participate in HIV preventions trials and become HIV-infected during the conduct of such trials should have access to good quality treatment and care, including antiretroviral therapy, within the framework of the WHO guidelines' [51, pW11].

Risks and harms are common to research and to healthcare interventions, while benefits for research subjects may often be absent, uncertain or unlikely. Consequently, great effort is made to protect research subjects [83]. This includes stringent ethics committee review, oversight of research protocols, meticulous attention to informed consent procedures, full disclosure of conflicts of interest and of commitment, participation by research subjects or their communities in the design and execution of research protocols, and ensuring that there are opportunities to share fairly in whatever benefits might result from their participation in the research.

Research is generally unacceptable whenever research subjects or their communities are excluded from the benefits and potential benefits arising from their participation in the research, or whenever benefits are not shared fairly [84]. It would be unacceptable for research to help save or rescue people in the developed world while exploiting research subjects or their communities in developing countries by depriving them of the same benefits. Those benefits may involve access to HAART during and following a clinical trial. For subjects already being treated successfully with a study medication, this would mean being able to continue treatment as long as it is medically necessary and remains effective, and until it can be obtained elsewhere [84].

Since HIV treatment is considered lifelong, it would be unethical to stop successful treatment simply because a trial ends or HAART becomes commercially available but unaffordable. Subjects randomized to less effective or less safe treatments can also claim access to the study's better treatment after the trial. For all subjects, appropriate follow-up is indicated or else benefits may be lost through toxicity, side effects, resistance or inefficacy. Subjects failing treatment during a study should expect effective treatment when it becomes available to developed country research subjects. Vaccine research has also faced a 'double standard' concern. The concern here is whether lifelong HAART will be available to research subjects who are infected because of vaccine failure or being in a control or placebo arm of a trial. HAART would undoubtedly be available to vaccine research subjects living in developed countries, but not necessarily to subjects living in developing countries [85].

The communities to which research subjects belong, or their countries, may sometimes benefit from research, but not at the expense of research subjects who expose themselves to risks and harms. These benefits could include an improved infrastructure with which to deliver and monitor the safety and efficacy of HAART, greater expertise in the use of HAART, less morbidity and premature mortality, and fewer healthcare burdens from HAART that is available to research subjects and possibly others.

How, then, can scarce resources such as HAART be allocated fairly as a research benefit or, more generally, as a public good? This is a classic ethical conundrum that rarely has a static solution. It will change as circumstances change, such as wider availability of medication, changes in the number of people who need treatment, changes in resources to secure and deliver treatment, and the discovery and availability of newer, more effective treatments.

The use of placebos has also been a controversial research concern. It erupted again when clinical trials were being designed to establish the best intervention to prevent mother-to-child HIV transmission in developing countries. The standard intervention in developed countries was too complex, expensive and unmanageable for developing country use, even as a standard to compare with simpler interventions [86–88]. Yet, using a placebo rather than the developed country standard was considered unethical. This impasse ended when research showed that simpler interventions could be used that were feasible and effective in resource-poor locales. Single-dose nevirapine treatment of mother and newborn was found to be as efficacious in preventing perinatal, but not antenatal, transmission as the very complex developed country standard involving weeks of oral HAART, intravenous treatment at the time of childbirth and weeks of neonatal treatment thereafter [89]. This research shows that the placebo issue is a contentious one, but sometimes it is possible to avoid it.

Conclusion

HAART has brought dramatic benefits to HIV-infected children and adults. Those benefits are accompanied by an array of ethical dilemmas. Some are new and need to be studied, but most are older, had already been analysed before HAART was discovered, and now need to be revisited. The dramatic impact of HAART to help reduce or stop the seemingly inescapable morbidity, premature mortality, suffering and devastating social and economic consequences of this pandemic pleads for more definitive study of these ethical dilemmas. HAART can also influence public responses to the pandemic along with ethical concerns that arise from the design, management and delivery of health services, and the development of public policy and public health interventions. Those ethical issues also need much more study.

References

1. Anonymous. (2005). *The History of AIDS*. 1981–1986. Available at www.avert.org/his81_86.htm.

2. Anonymous. (2005). *The History of AIDS*. 1987–1992. Available at www.avert.org/his87_92.htm.

3. Enanoria WTA, Ng C, Saha SR, Colford JM Jr. (2004). Treatment outcomes after highly active antiretroviral therapy: a meta-analysis of randomized controlled trials. *Lancet Infectious Diseases* 4:14–25.

4. Thorne C, Newell ML. (2004). Prevention of mother-to-child transmission of HIV infection. Current opinion. *Infectious Diseases* 17:247–52.

5. Bassett IV, Freedberg KA, Walensky RP. (2004). Two drugs or three? Balancing efficacy, toxicity, and resistance in postexposure prophylaxis for occupational exposure to HIV. *Clinical Infectious Diseases* 39:395–401.

6. Gerberding JL. (2003). Clinical practice. Occupational exposure to HIV in health care settings. *New England Journal of Medicine* 348:826–33.

7. Centers for Disease Control. (2001) Updated US Public Health Service guidelines for the management of occupational exposures to HBV, HCV, and HIV and recommendations for postexposure prophylaxis. *Morbidity and Mortality Weekly Report* 50(RR11):1–42.

8. Centers for Disease Control. (2005). Antiretroviral postexposure prophylaxis after sexual, injection-drug use, or other nonoccupational exposure to HIV in the United States. *Morbidity and Mortality Weekly Report* 54(RR-2):1–20.

9. Katz MH, Gerberding JL. (1998). The care of persons with recent sexual exposure to HIV. *Annals of Internal Medicine* 128:306–12.

10. Teixeira PR, Vitoria MA, Barcarolo J. (2004). Antiretroviral treatment in resource-poor settings: the Brazilian experience. *AIDS* 18(Supplement 3):S5–7.

11. The World Bank. (2003). *Provision of ARV Therapy in Resource-limited Settings: The Challenges of Drug Resistance and Adherence*. Meeting Report. Geneva: Global HIV/AIDS Program of the World Bank, 17–18 June 2003.

12. Ortells P. (2003). *Brazil: A Model Response to AIDS*. New York: Global Policy Forum. URL: www.globalpolicy.org/socecon/develop/aids/ 2003/04aidsbrazil.htm.

13. Reamer FG (ed.). (1991). *AIDS & Ethics*. New York: Columbia University Press.

14. Purtillo R, Sonnabend J, Purtillo DT. (1983). Confidentiality, informed consent and untoward social consequences in research on a 'New Killer Disease' (AIDS). *Clinical Research* 31:462–72.

15. Bayer R. (1983). Gays and the stigma of bad blood. *Hastings Center Reports* 13(2):5–7.

16. Bayer R, Levine C, Murray TH. (1984). Guidelines for confidentiality in research on AIDS. *IRB: A Review of Human Subjects Research* 6(6):1–7.

17. Novick A. (1984). At risk for AIDS: confidentiality in research and surveillance. *IRB: A Review of Human Subjects Research* 6(6): 10–11.

18. Plumeri PA. (1984). The refusal to treat: abandonment and AIDS. *Journal of Clinical Gastroenterology* 6:281–4.

19. US Food and Drug Administration, Center for Drug Evaluation and Research. FDA Drug and Device Product Approvals. Available at URL: www.fda.gov/cder/da/ ddpa.htm.

20. Wolfe LE, Lo B. (2001). HIV Policy: Ethical dimensions of HIV/AIDS. In: Peiperl L, Volberding P, eds. *HIV InSite Knowledge Base*. San Francisco: University of California. Available at URL: www.hivinsite.ucsf.edu/ InSite?page=kb-08.

21. Selwyn PA, Meyer HS, Morse DH. (2004). Book review: *The AIDS Pandemic: Complacency, Injustice, and Unfulfilled Expectations* by LO Gostin. Chapel Hill, NC: University of North Carolina Press. *Journal of the Americn Medical Association* 292:276–278.

22. Susman E. (2002). AMA unit says 'no' to mandatory HIV testing. News. *AIDS* **16**:N–N6.

23. Abramson D. (1999). Passing the test. New York's newborn HIV testing policy, 1987–1997. In: Stoto MA, Almario DA, McCormick MC, eds. *Reducing the Odds: Preventing Perinatal Transmission of HIV in the United States*, Appendix L. Washington, DC: Committee on Perinatal Transmission of HIV, Commission on Behavioral and Social Sciences and Education, National Research Council, Institute of Medicine, p313–40.

24. Cameron T. (2002). Mandatory HIV testing of newborns in New York state: what are the implications? *Journal of Health Social Policy* **14**:59–78.

25. Moloughney BW. (2001). Transmission and postexposure management of bloodborne virus infections in the healthcare setting: where are we now? *Canadian Medical Association Journal* **165**:445–51.

26. Anonymous. (1998). Georgia statute compelling submission to an HIV test upheld. *Hospital Law Newsletter* **16**:4–6.

27. Brahams D. (1999). Court order for HIV-1 test for baby. *Lancet* **354**:884.

28. Greub G, Gallant S, Zurn P *et al.* (2002). Spare non-occupational HIV post-exposure prophylaxis by active contacting and testing of the source person. *AIDS* **16**:1171–6.

29. Greub G, Maziero A, Burgisser P, Telenti A, Francioli P. (2001). Spare post-exposure prophylaxis with round-the-clock HIV testing of the source patient. *AIDS* **15**:2451–2.

30. Walensky RP, Freedberg KA, Losina E *et al.* (2004). Voluntary HIV testing as part of routine medical care—Massachusetts, 2002. *Morbidity and Mortality Weekly Report* **53**:523–526.

31. Bayer R. (1999). Clinical progress and the future of HIV exceptionalism. *Archives of Internal Medicine* **159**:1042–8.

32. Eshleman SH, Jackson JB. (2002). Nevirapine resistance after single dose prophylaxis. *AIDS Rev* **4**:59–63.

33. Boxwell D, Haverkos H, Kukich S, Struble K, Jolson H. (2001). Serious adverse events attributed to nevaripine regimens for postexposure prophylaxis after HIV exposures—worldwide, 1997–2000. *Morbidity and Mortality Weekly Report* **49**:1153–6.

34. Anonymous. *Transmission of Resistant HIV.* URL: http://www.aidsmap.com/en/docs/27A9FF69-3C3D-4F68-ACA1-CC7AA10A260E.asp.

35. Little SJ, Koelsch KK, Ignacio CC *et al.* (2004). Persistence of Transmitted Drug-resistant Virus Among Subjects with Primary HIV Infection Deferring Antiretroviral Therapy. Presented at the Eleventh Conference on Retroviruses and Opportunistic Infections, San Francisco, 2004, abstract 36LB.

36. Little SJ, Holte S, Routy JP *et al.* (1999). Reduced antiretroviral drug susceptibility among patients with primary HIV infection. *Journal of the American Medical Association* **282**:1142–9.

37. American Medical Association Council on Scientific Affairs. (2004). *Report 10 of the Council on Scientific Affairs (I-98): Bloodborne Pathogen Transmission to and from Health Care Workers.* Chicago, IL: American Medical Association.

38. American Medical Association Council on Scientific Affairs. (2004). American Medical Association Policy H-20.912: *Guidance for HIV-infected Physicians and other Health Care Work.* Chicago IL: American Medical Association.

39. National Academy of Sciences Institute of Medicine. (2000). *To Err is Human: Building a Safer Health System.* Washington, DC: Institute of Medicine.

40. Hébert PC, Levin AV, Robertson G. (2001). Bioethics for clinicians: 23. Disclosure of medical error. *Canadian Medical Association Journal* **164**:509–3.

41. Pietro DA, Shyavitz LJ, Smith RA, Auerbach BS. (2000). Detecting and reporting medical errors: why the dilemma? *British Medical Journal* **320**:794–6.

42. Daoruen P. (1977). Thailand: HIV Tests for Medical Students Stirs Rights Debate. InterPress News Service, Tuesday, December 30, 1997, as quoted by Aegis.com at URL: www.aegis.com/news/ips/ 1997/ IP971206.html.

43. Richman DD, Morton SC, Wrin T *et al.* (2004). The prevalence of antiretroviral drug resistance in the United States. *AIDS* **18**:1393–401.

44. *Gender News* (Nov 2002) 6(2), from the Community Law Centre of the University of the Cape, SA). Available at URL: www.communitylawcentre.org.za/gender/ gendernews2002/2002_2_testing.php.

45. Carr A, Samaras K, Thorisdottir A *et al.* (1999). Diagnosis, prediction, and natural course of HIV-1 protease-inhibitor-associated lipodystrophy, hyperlipidaemia, and diabetes mellitus: a cohort study. *Lancet* **353**:2093–9.

46. Bozzette SA, Berry SH, Duan N *et al.* (1998).The care of HIV-infected adults in the United States. HIV Cost and Services Utilization Study Consortium. *New England Journal of Medicine* **339**:1897–904.

47. Gebo KA, Chaisson RE, Folkemer JG, *et al.* (1999). Costs of HIV medical care in the era of highly active antiretroviral therapy. *AIDS* **13**:963–9.

48. Paltiel AD, Weinstein MC, Kimmel AD *et al.* (2005). Expanded screening for HIV in the United States—an analysis of cost-effectiveness. *New England Journal of Medicine* **352**:586–95.

49. World Health Organization. (2004). *The 3 by 5 Initiative.* Available at URL: http://www.who.int/3by5/en/.

50. World Health Organization Regional Office for Europe. (2004). *Treatment and Care: Access to Care.* Available at URL: http://www.euro.who.int/eprise/main/WHO/Progs/SHA/treatment/20040116_2?PrintView=1&.

51. Anonymous. (2004). Treating people with intercurrent infection in HIV prevention trials. Report from a WHO/UNAIDS consultation, Geneva 17–18 July 2003. *AIDS* **18**:W1–12.

52. Baker R. (1998). A theory of international bioethics: multiculturalism, postmodernism, and the bankruptcy of fundamentalism. *Kennedy Institute of Ethics Journal* **8**:201–31.

53. US National Commission on Bioethics. (2001). *Ethical and Policy Issues in International Research: Clinical Trials in Developing Countries.* Washington, DC: National Commission on Bioethics.

54. Stork J. (1999). Human Rights and U.S. Policy. *Foreign Policy in Focus* **4**(8):1–3. Available at URL: www.fpif.org/pdf/vo14/ 08ifhr-a.pdf.

55. World Health Organization. *Constitution of the World Health Organization in Basic Texts.* Forty-Fourth Edition. Geneva: World Health Organization. Available at URL: policy.who.int/cgibin/ om_i-sapi.dll?hitsperheading=on&infobase=basicdoc&record={21}&softpage=Document42.

56. Kouchner B. (1999). The right to intervention: codified in Kosovo. *New Perspective Quarterly* **16**(4), as reprinted in Anonymous: Establish a Right to Intervene Against War, Oppression. *Los Angeles Times*, 18 October 1999.

57. Baker R. (1998). A theory of international bioethics: the negotiable and non-negotiable. *Kennedy Institute of Ethics Journal* **8**:233–73.

58. Gilmore N. (2001). *Analysis of Ethical Issues Raised by the Impending Availability of Drug Treatment of HIV Infection and its Consequences in Resource Poor Settings.* Background paper for a World Health Organization International Consultative Meeting on HIV/AIDS Antiretroviral Therapy. Geneva: World Health Organization, 22–23 May 2001, p28.

59. Médecins Sans Frontières. (2004). *Campaign for Access to Essential Medicines.* London: Médecins Sans Frontières. Available at URL: www.accessmed-msf.org.

60. Achmat Z. (2002). Commentary: most South Africans cannot afford anti-HIV drugs. *British Medical Journal* **324**:217–8.

61. Specter M. (2001). India's plague. *The New Yorker*, 17 December, 2001, p74–85.

62. Brown PJ. (2002). Access to medicines is not the business of the pharma industry. *Journal of the International Association of Physicians in AIDS Care* **1**(1):9–11.

63. Singhal N. (2002). Access to medicines is not a business. *Journal of the International Association of Physicians in AIDS Care* 1(1):12–4.

64. World Trade Organization. (2003). Intellectual Property Decision removes final patent obstacle to cheap drug imports. Press Release. *World Trade Organization News*, 30 August 2003 (Press/350/Rev.1). Geneva: WTO.

65. Global Fund to Fight AIDS, Tuberculosis and Malaria. (2005). URL: www.theglobalfund.org.

66. Joint United Nations Programme on HIV/AIDS (UNAIDS). (2004). *Financing the Expanded Response to AIDS.* Geneva: UNAIDS.

67. Valdiserri RO, Ogden LL, McCray E. (2003). Accomplishments in HIV prevention science: implications for stemming the epidemic. *Nature Medicine* 9:881–6.

68. Fleshman M. (2001). Drug price plunge energizes AIDS fight. *Africa Recovery* 15(1–2):1.

69. Joint United Nations Programme on HIV/AIDS (UNAIDS). (2000). *UNAIDS Welcomes Boehringer Ingelheim's Commitment to Offer Nevirapine Free of Charge to Developing Countries for Prevention of Mother-to-child Transmission of HIV.* Press Release, 28 November. Geneva: UNAIDS.

70. Angell M. (2000). The pharmaceutical industry—to whom is it accountable? *New England Journal of Medicine* 342:1902–1904.

71. International Crisis Group. (2001). *HIV/ AIDS as a Security Issue.* Brussels: International Crisis Group.

72. Food and Agriculture Organization, United Nations Development Programme. (2004). *African-Asian Agriculture against AIDS.* Bangkok: United Nations Development Programme.

73. Brewer TF, Heymann SJ. (2004). Editorial: the long journey to health equity. *Journal of the American Medical Association* 292:269–71.

74. Panel on Clinical Practices for Treatment of HIV Infection. (2004). *Guidelines for the Use of Antiretroviral Agents in HIV-1-Infected Adults and Adolescents.* Washington, DC: US Department of Health and Human Services. URL: www.aidsinfo.nih.gov/guidelines/ default_db2.asp?id=50.

75. Yeni PG, Hammer SM, Hirsch MS *et al.* (2004). Treatment for adult HIV infection: 2004 recommendations of the International AIDS Society-USA panel. *Journal of the American Medical Association* 292:251–65.

76. British HIV Association Writing Committee. (2003). *BHIVA guidelines for the treatment of HIV-infected adults with antiretroviral therapy.* London: British HIV Association (BHIVA). URL: www.bhiva.org/guidelines/ 2003/hiv/index.html.

77. Wendler D, Emanuel EJ, Lie RK. (2004). The standard of care debate: can research in developing countries be both ethical and responsive to those countries' health needs? *American Journal of Public Health* 94:923–8.

78. Bhutta ZA. (2002). Ethics in international health research: a perspective from the developing world. *Bulletin of the World Health Organization* 80:114–20.

79. Macklin R, McCall-Smith A. (2004). *Double Standards in Medical Research in Developing Countries.* New York: Cambridge University Press.

80. Schüklenk U. (2004). The standard of care debate: against the myth of an 'international consensus opinion'. *Journal of Medial Ethics* 30:194–7.

81. Levine RJ, Carpenter WT, Appelbaum PJ. (2003). Clarifying standards for using placebos. *Science* 300:1659–1661.

82. Joint United Nations Programme on HIV/AIDS (UNAIDS). (2000). *Ethical Considerations in HIV Preventive Vaccine Research.* Geneva: UNAIDS.

83. Institute of Medicine. (2002). *Responsible Research.* Washington, DC: Institute of Medicine.

84. Council for International Organizations of Medical Sciences. (2002). *International Ethical Guidelines for Biomedical Research Involving Human Subjects.* Geneva, CIOMS. URL: www.cioms.ch/frame_guidelines_nov_2002.htm.

85. Bloom BR. (1998). The highest attainable standard: ethical issues in AIDS vaccines *Science* 279:186–9.

86. Angell M. (1997). The ethics of clinical research in the Third World. *New England Journal of Medicine* 337:847–9.

87. Lurie P, Wolfe SM. (1997). Unethical trials of interventions to reduce perinatal transmission of the human immuno-deficiency virus in developing countries. *New England Journal of Medicine* 337:853–56.

88. Varmus H, Satcher D. (1997). Ethical complexities of conducting research in developing countries. *New England Journal of Medicine* 337:1003–5.

89. Department of Reproductive Health and Research. (2004). Monthly Survey of PMTCT Publications and Abstracts. Geneva: World Health Organization. URL: www.who.int/reproductive-health/rtis/ MTCT/ monthly_publications /listing_mtct_reports.htm. Accessed 18 May 2005.

Chapter 9

Legal and human rights implications

David Patterson* and Lisa Forman

Introduction

Any contemporary discussion of the relationship of law to HIV and health systems must situate the national legal framework that regulates the provision of healthcare and services within the international legal and human rights framework by which all countries are, to a greater or lesser extent, bound. Domestic law is directly and indirectly influenced by international treaty and customary law, and indeed there is no polity in the world that operates outside the parameters of international law. The international system is overseen by specialized treaty committees, which have given guidance on national obligations relating to HIV in both their general comments and when reviewing periodic country reports.

The international community has consistently affirmed that all human rights are universal, indivisible, interdependent and interrelated, and it follows that HIV cannot be addressed independently of other health, social, economic or development challenges. The founding Charter of the United Nations itself makes clear that national sovereignty is subject to over-riding considerations of global peace, security and human rights, and HIV no less than terrorism should be seen in this way. In July 2000, the Security Council stressed that 'the HIV pandemic, if unchecked, may pose a risk to stability and security' [1].

Similarly, in June 2001, at a United Nations Special Session on HIV, 189 states recognized that 'the global HIV/AIDS epidemic, through its devastating scale and impact, constitutes ... one of the most formidable challenges to human life and dignity, as well as to the effective enjoyment of human rights, which undermines social and economic development throughout the world...' [2].

For many in the front lines of HIV prevention, education and healthcare provision, the statements of international bodies may seem remote, even irrelevant, to their daily work. Yet, as this chapter will illustrate, international human rights law often has direct application to domestic laws and policies affecting the provision of HIV services, as well as to the international response to HIV. This is now a pandemic, requiring international solidarity and a concerted global response [2]. Moreover, countries most affected by HIV are often dependent upon international development assistance to support their national response, and development assistance is increasingly linked to internationally recognized good practice and approaches that support human rights.

International human rights also play a background role in shaping policies on development and HIV. For example, in 1998, the United Nations Secretary-General launched a broad, rights-based approach to development, intended to help governments and development agencies redirect their development thinking [3]. Many international donors require that the rights of

*Corresponding author.

women and girls be integrated into their development programmes, although not all use the language of human rights to express this. The UK Department for International Development (DFID), the Swedish International Development Agency (Sida) and the Canadian International Development Agency (CIDA) are but some of the donors that have either considered or have adopted human rights-based approaches to their development assistance programmes.

A commitment to human rights-based approaches to development assistance has practical implications for the formulation of national and international policies. For example, in accordance with the fundamental human rights principle of community participation in decisions that affect them, civil society representatives have been included in the country and regional coordinating mechanisms, and governance structures, of the Global Fund to Fight AIDS, Tuberculosis and Malaria.

Finally, national health systems are situated in a domestic legal and constitutional context that potentially regulates every aspect of planning and delivery, including budgets and spending, taxation, procurement, approval of drugs and diagnostic equipment, licensing of facilities and practitioners, transparency, accountability, and civil and criminal liability. All of these areas are subject to the increasing influence of international law and practice [4]. Many countries are directly bound by treaty obligations on health, and, in many other countries, international law is applied and enforced by domestic courts [5].

This chapter discusses both the content and implications of international law for the provision of national HIV services. It considers the linkages between health and human rights; limitations on rights to protect public health; law and human rights on HIV-related health services in resource-poor countries; and international and domestic accountability mechanisms.

Health, human rights and ethics

Perhaps the appropriate starting point for any discussion on law and rights relating to HIV is with the growing understanding of the mutually reinforcing connections between health and human rights, particularly in the protection of human dignity and privacy [6,7]. Human rights and laws on health are often directly relevant to the content and scope of the HIV health services that front line health professionals deliver, and in many cases overlap and reinforce interpersonal bioethical considerations such as doctor–patient confidentiality.

Indeed, there are increasing synergies between health ethics and international human rights law, particularly in the nascent development of global public health ethics, which promote equity not only through social and economic rights, but through a greater attention to international justice, duties and interdependence [8–10].

This overlap has particular relevance for national and international policy-makers who determine the content and scope of HIV health services, requiring them to consider their actions not simply as health providers bound by interpersonal and global ethical considerations, but also as duty bearers under international human rights law. International law has long recognized individual responsibility for violations of international legal standards during war-time and in performing acts of terrorism [11,12]. Indeed, international human rights standards can apply to health professionals, irrespective of the domestic legal order. For example, in the 1990s, the South African Truth and Reconciliation Commission (TRC) held hearings on the role of the health sector during apartheid, looking at both institutions and individual health professionals. The TRC found that the health sector, through apathy, acceptance of the status quo and acts of omission, allowed the creation of an environment in which the health of millions of South Africans was neglected, even at times actively compromised, and in which violation of moral and ethical codes of practice was frequent, facilitating violations of human rights [13]. In this context, the breach of ethical obligations by health professionals was seen to be intimately connected to breaches of human rights standards. A contemporary South African example of this link is the Mbeki government's refusal to provide antiretroviral therapy (ART) in the public health sector and its active opposition to health workers who did so. This was a serious violation of the government's right-to-health obligations and led to a considerable outcry from the medical profession, which argued that this forced health workers to breach their ethical duties to act in the best interests of their patients [14,15].

HIV and human rights in international law

International law cannot, of course, guarantee good health. Instead, it places obligations on governments to assure the conditions under which the highest possible standard of physical and mental health can be attained [16]. This includes providing an adequate standard of healthcare as well as addressing the socio-economic and environmental factors that promote conditions in which people can lead healthy lives [17].

The obligation to ensure universally accessible and affordable public health and healthcare facilities may be implemented progressively, depending upon available resources. Nonetheless, the UN Committee on Economic, Social and Cultural Rights has noted that governments have core obligations to ensure that health facilities, goods and services are provided equitably and without discrimination, and that national plans developed through participatory and transparent processes are in place to address the health concerns of the whole population as resources become available [16]. The Committee also identified the provision of essential medicines, defined by the World Health Organization (WHO) as a core obligation, with the duty to prevent, treat and control epidemic disease held to be of comparable importance [16]. A tragic example of the inadequacy of national planning is the failure of many countries to prepare for the recent precipitous drop in the price of ARTs by, for example, expanding voluntary counselling and testing facilities, integrating HIV and tuberculosis (TB) services, and strengthening health systems generally to deliver these medications to those who can benefit from them.

The right to health is not, however, dependent upon the recognition of international health rights *per se*, and is also noted explicitly in other international treaties that address a range of civil, political, economic, social and cultural rights [18,19]. Similarly, while the national constitutions of approximately 100 countries protect health and health-related rights [20], the right to health is also implied in every constitution and legal system that prohibits discrimination and protects equality, dignity, freedom, life and bodily security.

This inherent protection of health reflects the interdependent nature of all human rights— civil, political, economic and social. HIV in particular illustrates this interdependence by the broad range of civil and economic rights violations commonly experienced by people who have, or are perceived to have, HIV, including unfair dismissals, the denial of healthcare and gender-related violence.

The right to HIV-related health services thus involves other rights, such as freedom of speech and the right to accurate information about HIV infection, or non-discrimination and the right to equal treatment irrespective of race, colour, sex, language, religion, political or other opinion, national or social origin, property, birth or other status. The United Nations Commission on Human Rights has affirmed repeatedly that 'other status' in this context includes HIV status.

Overcoming HIV-related stigma and discrimination is now recognized as a key challenge in the national responses to HIV, and discrimination in the provision of health services must be prohibited by law and reinforced by policies, training and effective mechanisms for redress. Legislation and policies prohibiting discrimination can be put in place relatively quickly, and this obligation is of immediate application.

Other legal aspects affecting national HIV-related health systems include the provision of an enabling legal and regulatory environment for comprehensive HIV prevention, care and treatment, as well as research. Workplace policies should be developed that protect healthcare workers from occupational exposure while protecting patient confidentiality and patient rights to physical integrity. Policies should anticipate and provide for occupational exposure and subsequent care, treatment and support [21]. Institutional policies should provide HIV-infected healthcare workers with clear guidance on measures to protect their own health and to avoid HIV transmission in the healthcare setting. Needless to say, the failure to institute and observe adequate institutional policies can lead to civil or even criminal action against staff, management and the healthcare institution itself.

HIV poses particular challenges for health systems because the groups most vulnerable to HIV infection, e.g. men who have sex with men, injecting drug users, sex workers, street children and other groups, often also have difficulty accessing appropriate health services. Confusion also persists in some countries around the legality of harm minimization initiatives for injecting drug users, such as needle and syringe programmes and safe injecting sites. Laws should be reformed or clarified to remove real or perceived impediments to effective HIV prevention interventions [22–26].

While international law obliges governments to assure the best possible HIV healthcare and services, there is no assumption that these services will be provided through either a predominantly public or private model. Nonetheless, approaches to development based in human rights stress the need for government transparency and accountability, and empowerment and participation of civil society, in determining healthcare priorities and programmes. Specifically, people living with HIV and groups most vulnerable to HIV infection and the impact of AIDS should be involved in the design and delivery of HIV health services. Governments are thus increasingly accountable for both the *processes* and the *results* of their efforts to improve HIV health systems.

The right to HIV-related health services, therefore, not only depends on the protection of individual rights, but also relies more generally on open and democratic governance in which people can freely protest government failures to provide HIV services, and in which HIV and AIDS-related information is freely accessible. Democratic institutions such as free media and civil society can and do play critical roles in monitoring the appropriateness and influencing the content of a government's provision of HIV services.

Limitations on rights under international law to protect public health

International law provides that certain rights, such as the right to freedom of movement, can be limited to protect public health, but only after strict tests have been satisfied. The Siracusa Principles require that the limitation be:

• provided for and carried out in accordance with the law;

• based on a legitimate interest;

• proportional to that interest and constituting the least intrusive and least restrictive measure available, and actually achieving that interest in a democratic society [27].

Some rights, such as the right to freedom from torture, cannot be restricted under any circumstances. The focus is, therefore, on the nature of the right to be limited and the legal justification for the proposed limitation, rather than a purported conflict between the rights of individuals and society. For example, international guidelines provide that public health legislation ensures that people are not subjected to coercive measures such as isolation, detention or quarantine based on their HIV status. Where freedom of movement is to be restricted, in exceptional cases, on public health grounds, due process protections such as notice, rights of review and appeal, fixed rather than indeterminate periods of orders, and rights of representation should be guaranteed by law [28,29].

HIV-related health services, law and human rights in resource-poor countries and settings

Concerned that 'HIV exceptionalism' might result in the imposition of inappropriate approaches in resource-poor countries, some commentators have rejected the application of human rights approaches to the provision of HIV-related health services in these settings [30]. However, as noted above, human rights are universal. The recognition that the protection of women's human rights requires gender-specific approaches would support measures that enable women to make informed decisions whether to have an HIV test during an antenatal examination. These principles are all the more important today, now that the advent of cheaper therapies makes treatment access for millions of people possible [31].

The importance of adopting human rights approaches to the provision of HIV services is suggested, in particular, by the prevalent stigma that continues to attach to HIV, affecting both the quality of healthcare provided and the willingness of people to be tested for HIV and, where infected, to engage with the healthcare system. The reciprocal relationship between the protection of human rights and effective prevention and treatment of HIV has long been recognized [32]. It is also illustrated in practical terms by the extent to which the effective provision of HIV services depends upon adequate and appropriate counselling and testing services in a non-discriminatory and non-coercive environment.

Criminal, public health and other relevant legislation should be introduced or amended to reflect international guidance and best practice. Government policies, often easier to introduce and amend than laws, should also respect and protect HIV-related rights. Tools have been developed to measure the appropriateness of legal and policy frameworks, including effective legal protection against discrimination [33,34]. Governments must not only recognize health rights, but must also provide effective judicial and administrative remedies for alleged violations of these rights.

Specific obligations exist to prevent, treat and control epidemic and endemic diseases. These include the obligation to undertake or facilitate HIV-related research to improve treatments, as well as research on preventive interventions such as HIV vaccines and microbicides. The rights of patients and research subjects must at all times be preserved.

HIV has accelerated and focused attention on the right to health, including a focus on its social and economic determinants. This is illustrated generally by the disproportionate preponderance of HIV infection in developing countries, and amongst poor and marginalized communities in developed countries. More specifically, the lack of access to antiretroviral medicines in developing countries has focused attention on the inequalities in access to healthcare between rich and poor countries. In 2002, the growing focus on the right to health at the international level resulted in the appointment of the United Nations Special Rapporteur on the Right to Health, who has since chosen to include a focus on HIV in his reports on the right to health. The Special Rapporteur's work promises to clarify the scope of the right and the related nature of obligations it places on national health policy-makers, as well as to indicate practical mechanisms for integrating right-to-health considerations into, for example, domestic trade policies [35].

There has also been a growing emphasis in international law on the obligations of developed nations to assist poorer countries in fulfilling their human rights obligations. This is not, however, a novel recognition, and the Charter of the United Nations itself, as well as subsequent international treaties, recognizes the obligations on richer countries to cooperate and assist poorer countries in realizing the right to health, through both financial aid and the transfer of technology. These obligations have been confirmed repeatedly in international forums addressing HIV, human rights and related issues such as intellectual property [36–38]. The Canadian government's initiative to enable generic production and export of antiretroviral medicines to sub-Saharan African countries should be seen in this light, as illustrating a developed country's fulfilment of its international obligations of cooperation and assistance.

International and domestic accountability frameworks for human rights

There are a number of mechanisms and processes at the international level that provide for increased national accountability for HIV service provision. Every country has obligations under one or more international treaties that directly or indirectly address aspects of national health systems and is, therefore, required to prepare periodic reports on measures taken to respect, protect and fulfil the relevant aspects of the right to health. UN committees that review these reports are paying increasing attention to HIV and publish public comments on both achievements and areas for greater attention. The reporting process requires states to account for their policies publicly, and the treaty bodies' observations contribute cumulatively to the normative development of specific rights, including health. Likewise, in developing and reviewing funding proposals, both donors and recipient governments should consider relevant observations of international human rights committees on country situations.

Within the treaty system, national health systems are coming under increasing international scrutiny as to their ability to respond to the needs of groups particularly vulnerable to HIV. Both the UN Committee on the Elimination of Discrimination against Women and the UN Committee on the Rights of the Child have stressed the importance of recognizing and responding to the differential impact of HIV on women and girls, which should be reflected in the provision of gender-sensitive and child-friendly HIV and related health services, including sexual and reproductive health services. When reporting on HIV health services, gender-disaggregated data should be provided to enable an evaluation of the degree to which these services meet the specific needs of women and girls [39].

The Committee on the Rights of the Child has noted that children are more likely to use services that are friendly and supportive, provide a wide range of services and information, are geared to their needs, give them the opportunity to participate in decisions affecting their health, are accessible, affordable, confidential and non-judgemental, do not require parental consent and are not discriminatory. Taking into account the evolving capacities of the child, the Committee has urged that health services employ trained personnel who fully respect the rights of the child to privacy and non-discrimination in access to HIV-related information, voluntary counselling and testing, knowledge of their HIV status, confidential sexual and reproductive health services, and free or low-cost contraceptive methods and services [40].

The UN Human Rights Committee (HRC) has also addressed HIV in its observations on country reports. In 2004, the HRC signalled to both Namibia and Uganda that their response to HIV was not adequate for the magnitude of the problem, and that this infringed on the right to life of its citizens [41,42]. In particular, the HRC recommended that national governments in these countries adopt comprehensive measures to enable greater numbers of people with AIDS to obtain adequate antiretroviral treatment.

The HRC, like the Committee to Eliminate Discrimination against Women and the Committee to Eliminate Racial Discrimination, can accept individual complaints in countries that have accepted its jurisdiction in this regard. This offers the potential for international enforcement of HIV health-related claims, both in relation to discrimination—for instance, concerning access to health services—and on other substantive grounds. The HRC's expressions of concern in concluding observations 'tend to support a conclusion of a treaty violation' [43], and the HRC's observation that access to ART is a right-to-life issue indicates the potential for its complaints mechanism to be used to make claims for access to treatment. While there is as yet no prompt and effective mechanism at the international level for redress regarding a lack of health services under the International Covenant on Economic, Social and Cultural rights (ICESCR) [44], there are alternative international mechanisms that can enforce HIV- and health-related claims.

Similarly, international political commitments that contain global health goals should be seen as not simply assisting in the achievement of developing country health goals, but also as providing accountability mechanisms by which state responses to HIV can be transparently monitored. For example, the Millennium Development Goals contain a global commitment to have halted and begun to reverse the spread of HIV by 2015, which was confirmed and expanded in the 2001 United Nations General Assembly Special Session on HIV 'Declaration of Commitment on HIV/AIDS' (Declaration of Commitment). Under the latter, states are invited to report to the General Assembly annually on their progress in implementing the Declaration of Commitment, and national indicators have been developed to measure national funds expended on sexually transmitted infection (STI) control activities, HIV prevention, HIV clinical care and treatment, and HIV impact mitigation. To promote transparency and accountability in reporting, in 2003 UNAIDS posted over 100 such national reports on its website. Further research is now possible on national health systems using standardized indicators. Disparities in countries with comparable per capita incomes must reflect, in part, the role of political commitment in the national response.

Outside the international human rights system, other forums also offer the possibility for enforcing human rights norms. The Inter-American human rights system has been successfully invoked to require the provision of HIV treatment, including antiretroviral therapy, through national health systems in a number of countries [45,46]. Both the African and European human rights systems offer similar regional forums.

In states with a firm commitment to the rule of law and to democratic institutions, domestic courts may offer the best option for enforcing HIV-related human rights. At the national level, constitutional protections of rights in many countries may require health systems to address HIV prevention and treatment for certain groups, such as indigenous populations. This may occur either through the direct protection of health rights, as in South Africa and several Latin American countries, or through the indirect protection of health through civil and political rights, as in India [47,48].

These human rights protections have the capacity to alter domestic policies on HIV services significantly, both through guiding policy and through judicial enforcement. For example, in South Africa's Treatment Action Campaign case, the Constitutional Court found that the state's failure to make the drugs and counselling necessary to prevent mother-to-child transmission (MTCT) of HIV available nationally violated constitutional healthcare rights [49]. This case successfully challenged the South African government's failure to provide comprehensive measures to prevent MTCT where extensive political advocacy and protest had failed, illustrating the potential for health rights litigation to secure HIV health services even in the face of considerable governmental opposition.

Similarly, in the Cruz Bermudez case, the Venezuelan Supreme Court held that the government's failure to provide people with HIV with access to ART violated their right to health protected in international and constitutional law, and the government was ordered to provide medicines, develop treatment policies and programmes, and reallocate budget sufficient to carry out the court's decision [50]. Other domestic courts have similarly ordered governments to provide ART under human rights claims. Indeed, court action has often been critical in challenging discriminatory practices and in generating the national political will necessary to provide appropriate HIV-related healthcare.

Implications for health systems

Upper-income countries should ensure that the full range of HIV services are available through national health systems, whether these are predominantly public, private or a combination of both, and that these services are affordable for all, including socially disadvantaged groups. Middle- and lower-income countries must take all possible steps to introduce prevention, treatment and care services progressively, including ART and other HIV-related medical treatments where possible. Brazil has demonstrated the feasibility of comprehensive national prevention, care and treatment programmes, including universal access to ART, in resource-limited settings with great social, economic and geographical disparities. While scarce resources may constrain the realization even of core obligations in less-developed countries, countries are nonetheless bound to take immediate steps to fulfil these obligations, including the provision of essential medicines, and to ensure non-discriminatory access to whatever healthcare services are provided.

Reflecting the Declaration of Commitment, by 2003 all countries were to have developed comprehensive multisectoral national strategies and financing plans to strengthen health, education and legal system capacity, and were to have adopted legislation, regulations and other measures to prohibit HIV-related discrimination. Regrettably, many countries, particularly those in the regions most affected, have yet to introduce much-needed legislative reforms.

Conclusion: evolving responses and obligations

Clearly, HIV cannot be addressed independently of other health challenges, and a sustainable and equitable response consistent with international legal obligations requires investment in health services that address the continuum of HIV prevention, care, treatment and support within the context of a prioritized health agenda based on local needs and determined through inclusive and consultative processes.

While the right to health in the ICESCR continues to suffer from a lack of enforceability in the international arena, rights related to health are increasingly enforceable at the international level, and enforcement is also possible within domestic and regional forums. The right to health also offers a powerful normative framework by which to assess the conduct of states playing critical roles in relation to the provision of HIV services. This normative framework has had an impact both on the formulation of rights in domestic and regional jurisdictions, and in the interpretation of domestic rights to create state obligations to provide HIV services. The cross-pollination between international and national legal systems has also resulted in domestic judicial interpretations of health rights in relation to HIV informing the interpretations adopted by the UN human rights bodies.

Less-developed countries seeking international assistance for health systems development will be better placed to make these claims if they can demonstrate progress in implementing their immediate and progressive obligations to respect, protect and fulfil the right to health of their citizens. There is an increasing focus on the means by which health systems responding to HIV are designed, implemented and evaluated. This includes an increasing expectation, consistent with international law, that the groups most affected by, and vulnerable to, HIV infection and AIDS will be meaningfully involved in the aspects of health system design, delivery and evaluation that affect them. It is crucial that in reforming health systems to respond to HIV, the legal and human rights environment in which health systems are situated, and which also significantly determines HIV vulnerability and impact, is also reviewed and reformed consistent with international law and evolving best practices.

References

1. United Nations Security Council Resolution 1308. (2000).
2. UN General Assembly. (2001). *Declaration of Commitment on HIV/AIDS*. (UNGASS Declaration). New York: United Nations, A/RES/S-26/2.

3. United Nations. (1998). *Report of the Secretary-General on the Work of the Organization.* New York: United Nations, A/53/1.

4. Commonwealth Secretariat. (1988). *Bangalore Principles. Developing Human Rights Jurisprudence: Conclusions of Judicial Colloquia and other meetings on the Domestic Application of International Human Rights Norms and on Government under the Law 1988–1992.* London: Commonwealth Secretariat. URL: http://www.thecommonwealth.org.

5. Knop K, Moran M. (2004). *Influential Authority and the Estoppel-like Effect of International Law.* Presented at the University of Toronto Faculty of Law Conference, The Migration of Constitutional Ideas, 15–16 October 2004. Unpublished manuscript.

6. Tarantola D. (2000). *Building on the Synergy Between Health and Human Rights: A Global Perspective.* Working Paper No. 8. Boston: François Xavier Bagnoud Center for Health and Human Rights. URL: http://www.hsph.harvard.edu/fxbcenter/working_papers.htm.

7. Mann JM, Gruskin J, Grodin MA, Annas GJ, eds. (1999). *Health and Human Rights: A Reader.* New York: Routledge.

8. Benatar SR, Daar AS, Singer PA. (2003). Global health ethics: the rational for mutual caring. *International Affairs* 79:1(107–138):108,132.

9. Wikler D. (1997). *Bioethics, Human Rights and the Renewal of Health for All: An Overview.* In: *Council for International Organizations of Medical Sciences, Ethics, Equity and Health for All, Proceedings of the XXIXth CIOMS Conference.* Geneva: CIOMS, p21–30.

10. Nixon S, Forman L. (2005). Exploring the Synergies between Human Rights and Public Health Ethics: A Whole Greater than the Sum of its Parts? Unpublished manuscript.

11. *Trials of War Criminals before the Nuremberg Military Tribunals under Control Council Law No. 10, 1946–1949,* Vol. III. (1951).

12. Convention to Prevent and Punish the Acts of Terrorism Taking the Form of Crimes Against Persons and Related Extortion that are of International Significance 27 U.S.T. 3949, T.I.A.S. No. 841313. (1971).

13. Truth and Reconciliation Commission of South Africa Report Volume 5. (1998). Cape Town: TRC. Quoted in: Baldwin-Ragaven L, de Gruchy J, London L. (1999). *An Ambulance of the Wrong Colour: Health Professionals, Human Rights and Ethics in South Africa.* Cape Town:University of Cape Town Press, p6.

14. Stoppard A. (2002). *Doctors Defy Ban on Anti-retroviral Drugs.* Inter Press Service.

15. Physicians for Human Rights. (2002). *South African Doctors' Rights to Care for Patients.* URL: http://www.phrusa.org/campaigns/aids/action040202.html.

16. Leary J. (1994). The right to health in international human rights law. *Health and Human Rights* 1(1). URL: http://www.hsph.harvard.edu/fxbcenter/V1N1.htm.

17. Committee on Economic, Social and Cultural Rights. (2000). General Comment 14, *The Right to the Highest Attainable Standard of Health.* UN Doc. E/C.12/2000/4. New York: United Nations.

18. *Convention on the Elimination of All Forms of Discrimination Against Women.* (1979). U.K.T.S. 1989 No. 2, 19 I.L.M. 33 1980 (entered into force 3 September 1981).

19. *Convention on the Rights of the Child.* (1989) U.K.T.S. 1992 No. 44, 28 I.L.M. 1448 1989 (entered into force 2 September 1990).

20. Commission on Human Rights. (2003). *The Right of Everyone to the Enjoyment of the Highest Attainable Standard of Physical and Mental Health.* Report of the Special Rapporteur, Paul Hunt, submitted in accordance with Commission resolution 2002/31. UN Doc. E/CN.4/2003/58, para.20.

21. International Labour Office. (2001). *Code of Practice on HIV/AIDS and the World of Work.* Geneva: International Labour Office.

22. Canadian HIV/AIDS Legal Network. (1999). *Injection Drug Use and HIV/AIDS: Legal and Ethical Issues.* Montreal: Canadian HIV/AIDS Legal Network.

23. Butler WE. (2003). *HIV/AIDS and Drug Misuse in Russia: Harm Reduction Programmes and the Russian Legal System.* London: International Family Health.

24. Marks SP. (2003).*The Human Rights Framework for Development: Seven Approaches.* Working Paper Series. Boston MA: François-Xavier Bagnoud Center for Health and Human Rights.

25. Office of the UN High Commissioner for Human Rights, UNAIDS. (1996). *International Guidelines on HIV/AIDS and Human Rights: Second International Consultation on HIV/AIDS and Human Rights.* HR/PUB/98/1, Geneva: OHCHR and UNAIDS. (International Guidelines).

26. Office of the UN High Commissioner for Human Rights, UNAIDS. (2002). *HIV/AIDS and Human Rights International Guidelines: Revised Guideline 6–Access to Prevention, Treatment, Care and Support.* UNAIDS/02.49E, Geneva: OHCHR and UNAIDS.

27. United Nations Economic and Social Council. (1985). *Siracusa Principles on the Limitation and Derogation Provisions in the International Covenant on Civil and Political Rights.* UN Doc. E/CN.4/1985/4, Annex.

28. International Guidelines, para 27(d).

29. UNAIDS. (1999). *Handbook for Legislators on HIV/AIDS, Law and Human Rights.* Geneva: UNAIDS, p45–7.

30. De Cock KM, Mbori-Ngacha D, Marum E. (2002). Shadow on the continent: public health and HIV/AIDS in Africa in the 21st century. *Lancet* **360**:67–72.

31. Csete J, Schleifer R, Cohen J. (2004). 'Opt-out' testing for HIV in Africa: a caution. *Lancet* **363**:493–4.

32. Kirby M. (1996). Human rights and the AIDS paradox. *Lancet* **348**:1217.

33. UNAIDS. (2000). *Protocol for the Identification of Discrimination Against People Living with HIV.* Geneva: UNAIDS.

34. Watchirs H. (1999). *A Rights Analysis Instrument to Measure Compliance with the International Guidelines on HIV/AIDS and Human Rights.* Canberra, Australia: Australian National Council on AIDS, Hepatitis C and Related Diseases.

35. Commission on Human Rights. (2004). *The Right of Everyone to the Enjoyment of the Highest Attainable Standard of Physical and Mental Health*: Report of the Special Rapporteur, Paul Hunt— Addendum Mission to the World Trade Organization. E/CN.4/2004/49/Add.1.

36. United Nations. (1945). *The Charter of the United Nations.* Can. T.S. 1945 No. 7 (entered into force on 24 October 1945).

37. Commission on Human Rights. (2001). *Access to Medication in the Context of Pandemics Such as HIV/AIDS.* E/CN.4/RES/2001/33.

38. World Trade Organization. (2001). Ministerial Declaration. Geneva: World Trade Organization. WT/MIN(01)/DEC/1. (Doha Declaration), para. 7.

39. UN Committee on the Elimination of Discrimination against Women (CEDAW). General Recommendation No. 15 (1990) and General Recommendation No. 24 (1999).

40. Committee on the Rights of the Child. (2003). *HIV/AIDS and the Rights of the Child.* General Comment No. 3. CRC/GC/2003/3.

41. Committee on the Rights of the Child. (2004). *Concluding Observations on Namibia.* 30/07/2004. UN Doc. CCPR/CO/81/NAM.

42. Committee on the Rights of the Child. (2004). *Concluding Observations on Uganda.* 04/05/2004, UN Doc. CCPR/CO/80/UGA.

43. Bayesfsky AF. (2002). *How to Complain to the UN Human Rights Treaty System.* Ardsley Park: Transnational Publishers, Inc, p156.

44. Commission on Human Rights. (2004). Report of the open-ended working group to consider options regarding the elaboration of an optional protocol to the International Covenant on Economic, Social and Cultural Rights on its first session. UN Doc. E/CN.4/2004/44.

45. Jorge Odir Miranda Cortez *et al.* v. El Salvador, Case 12.249, Report No. 29/01, Inter-Am. C.H.R., Annual Report 2000, OEA/Ser./L/V/II.111, Doc. 20 Rev. 2001.

46. Torres, MA. (2004). Access to Treatment in Latin America: Using the Legal System to Access Antiretroviral Treatment. Presentation at University of Toronto, Faculty of Law, World AIDS Day Conference. Unpublished.

47. Paschim Banga Khet Mazdoor Samity and others. v. State of West Bengal and another. 1996 AIR SC 2426.

48. Shah SS. (1999). Illuminating the possible in the developing world: guaranteeing the human right to health in India. *Vanderbilt Journal of Transnational Law* 32: 435, p462.

49. Minister of Health and other v. Treatment Action Campaign and others [2002] 5 S.Afr.L.R. 721 (S.Afr.Const.Ct).

50. Cruz Bermudez *et al.* v. Ministerio de Sanidad y Asistencia Social. (1999). Supreme Court of Justice of Venezuela, Case No. 15.789, Decision No. 916.

Chapter 10

Strategic information for HIV programmes

Paul R De Lay[*], Nicole Massoud, Deborah L Rugg,
Karen A Stanecki and Michel Carael

Introduction

Over the past decade, pressure for rapid and visible action against local HIV epidemics has led many national AIDS programmes to consider evaluation as a low priority. It was assumed that what is effective was known, and that the only challenge was to make interventions widely available to populations. There was ongoing pressure to spend external funds on much-needed prevention and treatment activities, and investments in monitoring and evaluation were perceived as an unnecessary research activity or an attempt to control the use of external donor funds.

HIV monitoring and evaluation (M&E) activities were often limited to the production of episodic reports on HIV prevalence and of clinical records of AIDS cases detected, and could be grossly underestimated. These disease prevalence surveys were generally treated as data used to support requests by donors and often not widely disseminated. It often took years for the communities being tested to have access to information on local HIV prevalence. National reviews of HIV Strategic Plans were the only programme monitoring activities conducted to assess progress towards goals and objectives, looking at management capacities, processes and planned activities. Monitoring is usually defined as the routine tracking and reporting of a programme's priority information and its intended inputs, outputs, outcomes and impacts. As most national AIDS programmes were still under the ministry of health, monitoring efforts were focused on the improvements of the health information system. By 2002, the proportion of countries with a fully implemented HIV sero-surveillance system was 58%, 34% and 10% in countries with a generalized, concentrated and low-level epidemic, respectively [1].

Improvements to extend HIV surveillance to the monitoring of risk behaviours largely came from international efforts to standardize data collection and tools. In the early 1990s, the Global Programme on AIDS, based at the World Health Organization (WHO), developed a set of priority prevention indicators covering knowledge of preventive practices, sexual behaviour, case management of sexually transmitted infections (STIs), condom availability and use, and STI/HIV prevalence. These indicators required, in addition to health facility

* Corresponding author.

surveys, repeated surveys of the general population or of specific subpopulations. These indicators were further developed and incorporated in most of the Demographic and Health Surveys (DHS). In countries with low or concentrated HIV epidemics, behavioural surveillance surveys (BSS) among selected groups at higher risk of HIV became a standard practice. However, at the country level, these population data were often not linked with the results of HIV surveillance activities, nor used as part of a coherent monitoring and evaluation system. The integration of the results of sentinel sero-surveys with behavioural data has been promoted in recent years as part of what is called 'second-generation surveillance systems', but it is still only in early development in many countries.

Concerns about establishing more coherent national M&E systems for HIV have accelerated in recent years, due to at least three interlinked factors:

1. The continuous increase and heterogeneity of the HIV epidemics around the world despite the efforts of national AIDS programmes against HIV created doubts about the effectiveness and relevance of the implemented strategies. This perceived lack of impact on the reduction of new HIV infections called for more attention to the national policy environment of HIV activities and to intermediate outcomes such as increased knowledge, awareness and behavioural change. It also required more focus on input and output indicators, reflecting the extent to which activities were effectively implemented at a scale that would allow the measurement of an effect at population level.

2. There was a change of paradigm in the way HIV was perceived and acted upon: it moved from solely an infectious disease to a global threat to security and socio-economic development. This shift in thinking created an expansion of the sectors involved in the response to HIV far beyond the health sector. Ministries such as education, tourism, planning and finance became actively involved. This expansion also created an increased demand for data as diverse as the impact of HIV on poverty, of poverty on HIV, and the costs and the effectiveness of programmes.

3. The recent international mobilization around HIV has created concern at country level that multiple, parallel M&E systems would be implemented in diverse sectors by numerous organizations. The HIV community has recently attempted to address this lack of coordination by using the 'Three Ones Principle': one action framework for all HIV programmes, one national authority and one M&E system.

The emerging concept of a strategic information system for HIV at country level described in this chapter will encompass a much broader scope than the monitoring of behavioural and epidemiological trends. The notion of strategic information is derived from the military and the private sectors, where information plays a crucial role in formulating, implementing and evaluating strategies. In HIV, strategic information is now being seen as the cornerstone of an evidence-based approach to the decision making required for designing and implementing effective prevention and care programmes. The data sources and methods used in collecting strategic information vary, but typically rely on data from surveillance systems and special surveys, health management information systems, programme monitoring and operational research. It can be defined as acquiring, analysing and making use of relevant, consistent, accurate, timely and affordable information from multiple sources in support of HIV strategies for the purpose of programme improvement.

Biological surveillance

Use of sentinel and population biological data to track the epidemic and the response

The most common measure of the HIV epidemic is the prevalence of HIV infection among a country's adult population—the percentage of the adult population living with HIV. Prevalence of HIV provides a good picture of the overall state of the epidemic. Obtaining an estimate of the number of people infected with HIV in a country or region is important for the purpose of evaluation, programme planning and advocacy. Because epidemics develop differently in different countries, the surveillance systems can also differ [2]. Currently, epidemics are categorized into three types: *low-level*, where no identifiable group has an HIV prevalence greater than 5%; *concentrated*, where prevalence among pregnant women is below 1% in urban areas, but some groups at high risk have a prevalence greater than 5%; and *generalized*, where transmission is sustained outside of 'at-risk' groups with prevalence among pregnant women consistently over 1%.

In countries where HIV is uncommon, biomedical surveillance and behavioural data can provide an early warning of a possibly impending epidemic. Where HIV is concentrated in subgroups with high-risk behaviour, surveillance can provide valuable information for designing focused interventions. In generalized epidemics, sentinel HIV surveillance among the general population can provide essential information for planning care and support, and to indicate the success of the current response [3].

In the mid-1980s, facility-based sentinel surveillance of HIV was recommended by the WHO for monitoring the HIV epidemic, mainly because of easy access to people attending public health facilities and the possibility of measuring trends over time. In most countries with generalized epidemics, annual HIV surveillance among pregnant women attending public sector antenatal clinics has since become the primary source of data on the spread of HIV [4]. At various times and in various countries, sentinel surveillance has also included blood donors, military recruits and personnel, patients attending STI clinics, sex workers, tuberculosis patients and hospitalized patients.

However, the use of some of these subpopulations could be misleading. For example, sentinel surveillance among blood donors is generally not recommended due to inherent biases in this subpopulation. The distribution by age and sex of blood donors is generally not representative of the general population. Also, over time, countries have instituted blood screening programmes that actively eliminate the most vulnerable populations, resulting in HIV prevalence rates among blood donors much lower than among the general population. For example, in Bujumbura, Burundi, HIV prevalence among blood donors declined from 9.2% in 1988 to 0.2% in 2001, whereas among pregnant women in Bujumbura, HIV prevalence remained around the same level, just over 15% between 1988 and 2001 [5]. In addition, the type of blood donor will also bias the results. Blood donors can be volunteer, paid or replacement donors. More and more, countries are eliminating paying for blood donations because of higher risk behaviours among those selling blood. Replacement donors are family members who donate blood at the time of hospitalization. In high-prevalence countries, a substantial proportion of patients are hospitalized due to HIV complications. HIV prevalence among family members can be higher than in the general population due to the increased potential for sexual transmission. For example, in Eritrea, in 2000, HIV prevalence among replacement blood donors was 5%, compared with 1.6% among volunteer donors. Changes in the blood donor profiles over time have made it difficult to monitor changes in the HIV epidemic in these countries.

Prevalence among pregnant women can be measured easily and cheaply and has been shown to be a good approximation to prevalence among sexually active men and women aged 15–49 years [6]. Because the collection of data among antenatal clinic attendees is relatively simple and inexpensive, it has often been the primary means of assessing the state of a national epidemic. As the epidemic has spread and more resources have become available, countries have expanded the surveillance system by increasing the number of sites in urban as well as rural areas.

Concerns about the representativeness and accuracy of national HIV estimates derived from antenatal clinic surveillance have led to an increased demand for more surveys and more data on the prevalence and distribution of HIV in the whole population. The demand by decision makers for better data on the burden of HIV in countries and the limitations of antenatal surveillance systems with respect to geographical coverage, under-representation of rural areas and the absence of data for men have led to an interest in including HIV testing in national population-based surveys. Technological developments such as the use of dried blood spots for HIV sample collection, oral fluids and urine tests, and rapid HIV testing have greatly facilitated HIV testing in population-based surveys.

In recent years, the number of population-based surveys that included collection of biological specimens for HIV testing has increased. Many of these surveys covered women aged 15–49 years and men aged 15–59, and used dried blood spots for specimen collection (Table 10.1).

Because large-scale population-based surveys and sentinel surveillance both have weaknesses, combining the two sources of data will yield the most accurate estimates of HIV prevalence [7]. Population-based surveys can provide reasonable estimates of HIV prevalence for generalized epidemics, where HIV has spread throughout the general population in a country. However, for low-level and concentrated epidemics, these surveys will underestimate HIV prevalence because HIV is concentrated in high-risk groups and these groups are usually not adequately sampled in household-based surveys. For example, HIV prevalence obtained from a national household population-based survey in the USA conducted between 1999 and 2001 is thought to have underestimated HIV prevalence by about 30% because of the exclusion of certain high-risk groups such as the military and prison populations. The survey

Table 10.1. Population-based surveys incorporating HIV testing

Zambia	2001/2002
Burkina Faso	2003
Cameroon	2004
Dominican Republic	2002
Ghana	2003
Mali	2001
Rwanda	2005
Tanzania	2003/2004
Uganda	2005

Source: USAID Measure DHS, ORC Macro 2005.

estimate of HIV prevalence was 0.43% among people aged 18–49 years [8], as compared with the UNAIDS estimate of 0.6% based on the US Centers for Disease Control (CDC) HIV case surveillance.

Linking biological surveillance with M&E

HIV sero-surveillance provides the overall picture of the magnitude of the HIV epidemic and its geographical spread. Serial seroprevalence data in young pregnant women can give some insight on HIV incidence, providing that sample sizes are large enough, and recognizing that this sexually active group may be atypical of other youth in some countries. New laboratory methods to measure incident infection can be used on cross-sectional samples to assess which persons are newly infected and to estimate HIV incidence. These data are critical to monitor the impact of interventions over time.

With the rapid expansion of voluntary counselling and testing (VCT) services and increased access to prevention of mother-to-child transmission (PMTCT) treatment and antiretroviral therapy (ART), possible new data sources such as improved AIDS case reporting and service-related data can be incorporated into sero-surveillance systems. To measure the progress in access to treatment, health systems will need to monitor: coverage, as measured by the number of HIV-infected persons receiving ART divided by the number of HIV-infected people who are symptomatic; morbidity, as measured by a decrease in persons developing symptomatic HIV infection; AIDS mortality, as measured by increased survival and a decrease in the number of persons dying of HIV; and HIV drug resistance.

Overview of coherent M&E systems

Over the past 20 years, an increased range of partners have played an instrumental role in the struggle against HIV, from communities and people living with HIV, to governments, the United Nations and the private sector. A sense of common purpose has emerged, culminating in the adoption by 189 States of a Declaration of Commitment (DoC) on HIV/AIDS at the June 2001 United Nations General Assembly Special Session (UNGASS) [9]. By setting hard and time-bound targets, the DoC has put pressure on countries to implement and scale up interventions and report on achievements on a regular basis [10]. Similar targets related to HIV have been included in the Millennium Development Goals declaration (MDG) [11].

Scaling up national HIV programmes to achieve an expanded and comprehensive response may now be feasible, with the increased funding through the Global Fund to Fight AIDS, Tuberculosis and Malaria (Global Fund), the World Bank Multi-Country AIDS Program (MAP), the US President's Emergency Plan for AIDS Relief (PEPFAR) and other major funding mechanisms. Yet, such rapid expansion of new resources requires effective M&E anchored within strong information systems, which are currently lacking in most countries affected by the epidemic.

Indeed, the current national monitoring and evaluation systems are not ready for this challenge, as revealed by the UNAIDS *Progress Report on the Global Response to the HIV/AIDS Epidemic, 2003* [12]. The establishment of a coherent monitoring and evaluation system was among the top four challenges for reaching the targets set by the 2001 UN DoC on HIV. A number of barriers to the roll-out of a common, unified and coherent M&E system to support National AIDS Programmes with reliable information were reported.

However, recent negotiations among representatives of major donor organizations and many developing countries led to the adoption, on 25 April 2004, of three principles as the overarching framework for improved coordination (Box 10.1) [13]. The principles agreed upon—in particular, the underlying commitment made by all stakeholders—will help countries develop robust M&E systems, urgently needed for scaling up based on evidence.

This chapter focuses on the advantages and features of coherent M&E systems, the status of current national M&E systems in terms of infrastructure and practices, and suggests some concrete actions to fill the gaps.

Box 10.1 The Three Ones

- One agreed HIV/AIDS action framework that provides the basis for coordinating the work of all partners;

- One national AIDS coordinating authority, with a broad-based, multisectoral mandate; and

- One agreed country-level monitoring and evaluation system.

Source: [13].

Advantages of coherent, unified systems

The importance of creating, implementing and strengthening a single and coherent M&E system at the country level cannot be overemphasized. A unified system could enhance:

- collection of data based on national needs rather than those of individual donors, thus avoiding vertical and isolated initiatives;

- production of higher quality, relevant, accurate and timely data;

- submission of reports to international bodies as part of a unified global effort;

- efficient and effective use of data and resources;

- greater coordination, transparency and communication among different groups involved in the national response to AIDS.

Setting up a robust M&E system may be costly initially; yet, this will help governments in ensuring continued funding—especially with the recent introduction by the Global Fund and others of performance-based disbursement—but also, and most importantly, in planning and programming through continued learning and identification of best practices.

It is, however, essential to use existing systems if they can provide timely and credible information. If new systems must be established, planners must ensure that they complement and reinforce those that already exist. This applies to existing management information systems in health, education and other sectors containing information on HIV and related areas.

Features of coherent monitoring and evaluation systems

For a national M&E system to be coherent, all stakeholders should agree on the required infrastructure [14–16], briefly described below.

1. *One monitoring and evaluation unit:* M&E activities implemented by various partners; the unit should be responsible for planning, coordinating overall data collection and analysis,

and disseminating strategic information to different target audiences. Expertise in epidemiology, behavioural or social science, data processing and statistics, data dissemination or communication should exist in or be affiliated with the unit. This unit should also establish a working group composed of representatives from appropriate ministries, statistics bureaus, research institutions, universities, non-governmental organizations (NGOs), donors and the private sector to ensure coordination of M&E efforts among all partners and to complement other health information systems that may exist. If the establishment of such a unit proves to be difficult, other means for effective coordination and integration of M&E efforts should be identified.

2. *One national multisectoral M&E plan* built into the national strategic plan at the design stage, with clear goals and targets and for which funding is secured. The recommended M&E budget is 5–10% of the national HIV/STI budget; the M&E plan should include data collection, dissemination and use strategies.

3. *One national set of standardized indicators* endorsed by all stakeholders and reflecting the country's needs; there is no point in collecting data on areas that are not relevant to the local context in view of the costs involved. The selection of those indicators should also take into account the existing data collection and analysis capacities. The use of such indicators permits triangulation of findings and allows local inconsistencies and differences to be noted and addressed. Standard indicators and data collection tools are also critical for comparability over time and across countries.

4. *One national-level information system* that can link key data and databases, which contain information on serological surveillance, behavioural surveillance, coverage of essential services, financial tracking, socio-economic impact of the epidemic and its impact on a number of sectors including health and education. This network of information sources will allow the appropriate synthesis of various types of data and ensure adequate linkage with existing health and management information systems. An effective information system provides a solid basis for evaluations of large-scale programmes, ultimately leading to improved planning and decision making.

5. *Effective information flow* between subnational and national levels and among different national-level actors feeding into the national information system, based on operational guidance issued to national and subnational partners (Fig. 10.1). Quality subnational-level data provide a valuable indication of trends and can be useful for programme planning and implementation.

6. *Coordinated M&E capacity-building* strategy among all the training providers at global, regional and national levels to avoid duplication of efforts. The strategy should include agreement on the agency that needs to take the lead in skill development at national level, support mechanisms for cascading training at lower levels, and follow-up plan, including mentoring, to ensure the utilization of skills provided at a specific training activity.

Key categories of strategic information

Eight key categories of strategic information are essential to determine the current state of the epidemic and to monitor the progress and impact of our collective response (Box 10.2). It is not expected that each M&E system in each country will collect all this information in the

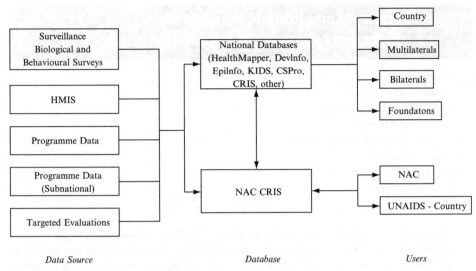

Fig. 10.1 Strategic information flow. Source: Country Response Information System (CRIS)/ UNAIDS.

short term. Key strategic questions may take a longer time to answer and may require more rigorous evaluation methods, but planning for the most important to be collected while launching the less complex information activities should be a strategic decision taken at country level.

1. *Epidemiology.* What is happening with the epidemic? The most basic information requirements include estimating the number of people who are currently infected, determining the number of new infections and whether transmission is decreasing, increasing or levelling off. Age and sex disaggregated data are also critically needed to target programmes.

2. *Prevention effectiveness.* Do people have the knowledge, skills and tools to protect themselves from getting or transmitting HIV infection? Are prevention interventions having an effect on risk behaviours? The effectiveness of prevention interventions must be assessed on an ongoing basis. There is a wide range of tools now available to measure the levels of risk behaviour included in the M&E guidelines that assess such factors as age of sexual debut, number of sexual partners or use of condoms in risky encounters.

3. *Service delivery and coverage.* Are pregnant women getting services to reduce transmission to their newborns? Data are needed to estimate how many women should receive these services; how many actually get tested; and, most importantly, how many mothers and newborns receive the essential antiretroviral drugs needed to prevent transmission. Data are also needed to estimate the number of people who have access to testing for HIV infection, to basic information on AIDS and ways to protect themselves, and the number of infected persons who have access to ART.

4. *Treatment effectiveness.* Are people who are infected receiving quality care and treatment? Not only must we measure the number of people who started and remain on treatment, but key processes must also be monitored, such as the equitable provision of treatment while

Box 10.2 **National monitoring and evaluation: Eight key categories of information**

Epidemiology
Prevention effectiveness
Service delivery and coverage
Treatment effectiveness
Support to those affected by AIDS
Resource allocation
General health sector performance
Policy environment

demand exceeds supply. Adherence to the prescribed drug regimens is important, both to improve the quality of care and to avoid drug resistance. This information can provide an early warning system to signal possible drug 'stock-outs' before they occur, and to determine whether treatment failures are rising. The impact of treatment must be tracked. Are people able to return to work? Is their quality of life improving? It is important that data on the scale-up of treatment actually contribute to improving patient management, and that the issue of confidentiality of health information is being adequately addressed.

5. *Support to those affected by AIDS.* Are those family members who are most affected receiving services, especially vulnerable children whose parents are sick, dying or deceased? We must assess the number of children who are receiving basic support services and the number of children who would be eligible to receive such services. At the same time, we need to know whether the services being delivered are having an impact. For example, are children orphaned by AIDS receiving adequate nutrition? Are they staying in school?

6. *Resource allocation.* Are resources being spent in the right places and for the most effective activities to reach the targets that have been set? International financial resources need to be tracked from their sources—bilateral donors, the Global Fund, foundations, the World Bank—to the country and project level. Determining domestic resources, be they from the public sector or out-of-pocket, is important in assessing the changing ratios of funding and assuring efficiencies and equities.

7. *General health sector performance.* What is happening to the health sector in general as a result of the epidemic and the response? The advent of dramatically increased resources for the country response can lead to both negative and positive impacts on health sectors. Donors and countries will need to track key information, such as the changing of staffing patterns, distribution of medical supplies and the cost of services and commodities over time. Are other key health services such as childhood immunizations and treatment of malaria improving or suffering? Are drugs and the delivery of services getting cheaper due to economies of scale, or are prices actually rising over time? We need to know if the scaling-up of AIDS programmes is improving health delivery and, if not, how to correct it.

8. *Policy environment.* Have countries developed multisectoral strategies to combat HIV? Have they integrated HIV into their general development plans? Is there a functional

national multisectoral HIV body for a coordinated response among all partners? Are there policies or strategies covering prevention, treatment, care and support, and cross-cutting issues such as gender and human rights? Without a favourable policy environment, countries will not be able to implement their HIV programmes effectively.

Ideally, a mixed quantitative and qualitative monitoring and evaluation approach should be applied when collecting these categories of information. Qualitative information should complement, validate, provide a richer understanding of quantitative findings and allow us to listen to the voice of those most affected by the epidemic [17].

Current monitoring and evaluation infrastructure and practices

Status of monitoring and evaluation at global level

During the 1990s, except for HIV surveillance, many bilaterals and UN organizations developed their own M&E frameworks and tools in relative isolation from each other. Monitoring tools, programme reviews, studies and surveys were commissioned at national level by a range of different partners at different times to meet different needs. This lack of cohesion led to differences in M&E concepts and definitions, designs, fieldwork and practices, and outputs. This was a source of confusion and frustration for many users at national and international level.

Since the establishment of the Joint United Nations Programme on HIV/AIDS (UNAIDS) in 1996, harmonization of M&E strategies at global level has been seen as a priority task, mainly through the guidance of the Monitoring and Evaluation Reference Group (MERG) composed of the UNAIDS Secretariat, M&E focal points of UNAIDS co-sponsors, the Global Fund, key bilateral agencies, research institutes and individual experts. With its broad membership, the MERG guided the assessment of monitoring and evaluation data needs at country and international level, current data collection strategies, and the potential for integration and further development.

As a result, a standardized set of M&E general and thematic guidelines was jointly developed and endorsed by most agencies and organizations within the four broad categories of prevention, care and treatment, HIV transmission, and health and survival. Additional guides and tools address M&E systems and data collection methods. These guidelines were widely disseminated and are used with varying degrees of success at country level. The MERG has also ensured the cohesion of existing standard tools with other internationally agreed-upon frameworks such as the Millennium Development Goals, and the reporting on progress towards the UN General Assembly Special Assembly Declaration of Commitment.

There are a number of other global reference groups whose primary mandate is to improve the coordination of activities, the harmonization of tools—common definitions and standards—and the collaborative synthesis of data. The UNAIDS/WHO Working Group on Global HIV/AIDS and STI Surveillance focuses on strengthening national, regional and global structures and networks for improved monitoring and surveillance of HIV and STIs in order to avoid duplication of activities and foster the involvement of other partners and bodies. The UNAIDS Reference Group on Estimates, Modelling and Projections advises UNAIDS, WHO and other international organizations on the most appropriate methods and assumptions for their global estimates on HIV prevalence and projections. They represent the consensus reached among representatives from the UN Population Division, the US Census Bureau, UNICEF, WHO and UNAIDS, among others.

Monitoring and evaluation of HIV has been dominated by the production—at global level—of general and thematic guidelines within the four broad categories mentioned above. To date, there are over 15 UNAIDS M&E guidelines focusing on specific thematic areas such as services for children orphaned or made vulnerable by AIDS, care and treatment, young people and preventive MTCT. These guidelines constitute valuable tools for country partners in need of field-tested standard indicators to monitor and evaluate their HIV programmes. Also, guidelines on sampling methodologies that address problems in determining denominators when working with hidden populations such as men who have sex with men, or with low and concentrated epidemics, have been published.

One widely accepted conceptual framework constitutes the basis for all of these guidelines: the input–process–output–outcome–impact framework, where results at one level are expected to lead to results at the next level, leading to the achievement of the overall programme or project goal. For each stage of the framework, a list of standard indicators and related methods of data collection are proposed. Those indicators have been developed with the specific purpose of minimizing information demands on countries, while also assuring that indicators address specific international needs. Figure 10.2 depicts the array

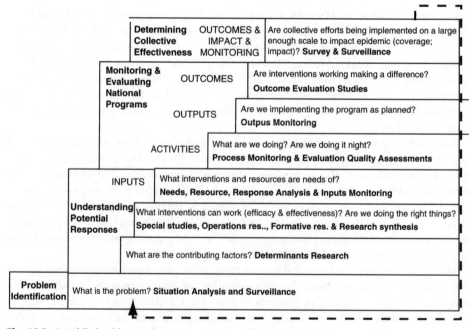

Fig. 10.2. A public health questions approach to unifying AIDS M&E. Source: [18]

of essential information needed for the planning of data collection over time, serving as a 'roadmap' with which the answers to questions at one step provide the basis for the questions and strategic information required at the next step. It also allows all involved to identify their respective roles and contributions to the development and implementation of a unified national M&E system.

A general agreement has also been reached on the issue of attributing results directly to a project or to resources from a specific donor. Only input and output results can be associated with funding sources, as these activities are often directly funded by a donor and are relatively easy to track. However, a culture of collective responsibility for actions and measurement of collective achievements has been promoted for outcome and impact indicators in view of the difficulty in attributing those outcomes to one single donor (Fig. 10.2).

Status of monitoring and evaluation at country level

In the 2003 UNGASS [12], most countries (85%) reported having a dedicated M&E unit and M&E focal points, with Central and South America lagging slightly behind. However, experience has shown that government M&E staff lack the required skills to coordinate and implement M&E activities effectively.

Some 43% of countries reported having an M&E plan, while only 24% indicated that they had an M&E budget to carry out these activities, according to the same survey. Although a significant improvement in the development of national M&E plans has been noted over the last 2–3 years, partly because of intensive regional M&E workshops and increased funding for M&E programmes, additional work is needed to make those plans more feasible, to secure additional funding for M&E activities and, most importantly, to accelerate implementation of those plans.

Most countries (88%) indicated they have a formal health information system (HIS). However, almost half of them do not have an HIS operational at the subnational level, making it difficult to obtain standardized national-level programme monitoring data.

While coordination at the global level has substantially improved, national-level collaboration between the same partners remains weak. In some countries, however, national M&E reference or working groups have emerged and have proved useful. Most of them have a broad composition, with representatives from the National AIDS Council, ministry of health, other key ministries and implementing partners, UN Theme Group members, bilateral or multilateral donors, NGOs, academic or research institutions and people living with HIV (PLHIV) groups. The main role of the national M&E reference groups is to advise the government on the development and implementation of national M&E plans and to advocate for more M&E resources.

Currently, the dissemination of monitoring data primarily consists of producing a set of national and global reports covering the status of the HIV epidemic and presenting new data during key events such as the International Conferences on AIDS or the UNGASS on HIV at global level, and through workshops at national level. An efficient dissemination strategy requires a framework for regular sharing of information with different target audiences through various means. It also calls for harmonized donor reporting requirements using common definitions and common outcomes. While such efforts have been relatively successful for the development of indicators, this remains a significant challenge for the reporting phase. Ideally, all donors should support not only a coherent data-to-action planning process, but also a concerted and coordinated effort to develop a single national HIV report that includes data contributed by all parts of the M&E system. This will ultimately be beneficial to them as well, since data feeding international databases may reach recipients in a more timely manner.

Another serious challenge is the translation of data into action. To date, not enough effort has been put into ensuring the appropriate use of collected information for strategic planning and programme improvement. Data have primarily been used more for advocacy and generating resources than for attributing changes to specific interventions for programme improvement. Among the factors that have contributed to this situation are the lack of government ownership throughout the data collection process, insufficient time allocated to this topic in most training activities, and inadequate resources allocated for the data-use plan. [19]

Also, countries have not given enough attention to the evaluation and operations research agenda. Most of them have not been able to conduct an evaluation of their national HIV programmes for a number of reasons, including lack of funding, status of implementation and lack of a culture of performance. Extensive project evaluations are sometimes carried out at the request of a specific donor using external funding and without the results ever being shared in the field or linked to an overall system.

Evaluation and operations research: setting an agenda for a multilevel participatory approach

Global and national AIDS partners must give more attention to the evaluation of interventions and programmes. A comprehensive evaluation agenda needs to be developed based on an assessment of existing data and needs, and then endorsed by the major stakeholders and donors. Operations research that systematically applies this information to improve service delivery is a critical component for ensuring optimal programme operations. This is especially critical now for scaling up small but effective programmes to a national scale.

In addition to a lack of funding, some of the delays in establishing strong programme evaluations stem from confusion about the differences between monitoring and evaluation and operations research, as well as lack of an organizing framework to develop a systematic agenda for evaluation [20].

One of the important roles that can be played at the global level is to review and synthesize existing international literature producing recommendations regarding the effectiveness of interventions, and to be explicit with the public and with policy-makers about HIV prevention successes and failures. There is increased recognition that evaluating the effectiveness of prevention interventions will necessarily entail the use of designs other than randomized controlled trials (RCTs) and various types of evidence, often used in combination [21]. Most interventions in HIV prevention are multifaceted, and the pathways to impact are complex, reflecting the intricacy of the relationship between HIV and risk behaviours [22]. Plausibility evaluation, which documents impact and tries to rule out alternative explanations by including a comparison group, historical or geographic, and by addressing confounding variables, is often more appropriate than RCTs. Evaluations that document time trends in the expected direction, following introduction of a programme or retrospectively, are often the only possibility.

Observational data provide evidence of behavioural change at the population level that is plausibly related to interventions such as information and education provided by NGOs, social institutions, peers and the media. Observational data at national level, from the few countries that have documented behavioural change and declines in HIV infection, are often difficult to interpret and can therefore be misconstrued. For example, documented declines in HIV prevalence in Uganda, Thailand and Cambodia have been attributed to a variety of interventions, from communications strategies to condom promotion, but the type and magnitude of behavioural changes are still not clear, nor is it clear which interventions produced these changes. In addition, it is likely that it was a specific combination of intervention strategies, including involvement by high-level political and other community leaders, behavioural change communication and condom promotion, which produced significant changes [22].

One of the critical weaknesses in measuring the effectiveness of behavioural interventions is that nearly all behavioural outcomes are self-reported, which raises questions about their validity. This was recently demonstrated by the results of a community randomized trial of an adolescent sexual health programme in Mwanza, Tanzania, where both behavioural and biological outcomes were assessed and compared. This comprehensive intervention included in-school sexual and reproductive health education, youth-friendly reproductive health services, community-based condom promotion and distribution, and other community activities to create a supportive environment for youth. Evaluation results showed that the intervention had a significant impact on knowledge, reported attitudes and reported behaviours, but when HIV or other STI outcomes were measured in the intervention and control communities, there were no significant differences between the two arms [23].

The complexity of interventions and the inadequacy of their evaluation mean that policy decisions are often taken with partial or imperfect evidence. The more controversial the intervention, the stronger the evidence that would be required to support it.

Efforts to review, assess and conduct research on effectiveness are just now beginning to increase. The Talloires Evaluation Group, a group of 40 experts, reviewed the international prevention literature, producing a list of 23 interventions for young people in low-income countries that were rated accordingly [24]. This translated into practical application. The group developed four categories: *Go, Ready, Steady* and *Don't Go*. 'Go' means there is sufficient evidence to recommend widespread implementation now. 'Ready' means that the evidence suggests the interventions are effective, but large-scale implementation must be accompanied by further evaluation to clarify their effect and mechanisms. 'Steady' means the interventions are promising, but further intervention development, pilot testing and evaluation are needed before they can move into the 'Ready' category. 'Don't Go' means there is evidence of ineffectiveness of these interventions.

There will be a continuous need for collecting, analysing, and disseminating evidence of intervention effectiveness.

Conclusions and recommendations

The politics of monitoring and evaluation

It is important to note that there are additional challenges that must be confronted when establishing a credible and effective M&E framework, including the various political influences exerted upon M&E. These can have both negative and positive effects. Political leaders can endorse and support more accurate and timely collection of data. The effect of these political influences may also suppress, limit, delay, manipulate or selectively use M&E outputs [18].

Although relatively simple and inexpensive methods of HIV testing have been available over the past decade, some national governments have been hesitant to release the identified levels of HIV infection, or have even denied the presence of HIV. Prevalence numbers have been lowered or suppressed, reports delayed, or it is implied that the infected individuals are primarily 'foreign'. These problems are, however, not unique to HIV [25]. There are many reasons for such denial: to protect the reputation of the country and culture; embarrassment about discussing the modes of transmission; the perceived negative impact on tourism and economic investment; and being forced to acknowledge the presence of marginalized or 'illegal' subpopulations, such as men who have sex with men and injecting drug users. These dynamics have occurred in every region of the world, among both developing and developed countries. However, over time, this situation has improved, and the most recent prevalence data reflect a more accurate assessment of the state of the epidemic.

There are other pressures on how data are collected and used. The data needs that are most useful to programme implementers for decision making are not necessarily the most useful for accountability to international donors. Undoubtedly, donor countries need to demonstrate the value of their contributions in order to justify these expenditures and be able to seek increased funding. There is now an active effort to reconcile these different data needs and ensure that both donors and programme managers have access to the most appropriate information available. Many of these recent changes can be attributed to increased involvement of national and subnational programmes in the design and implementation of surveys that are funded by an interested international donor.

The tracking of financial resources is becoming a key component of basic monitoring and evaluation activities. Linking the expenditure of resources with delivery of services allows critical analyses of allocative efficacy and allocative equity, and can support the study of specific concerns such as economies of scale. However, the increased inclusion of financial data within routine M&E must be planned and tracked with sensitivity. Early in the implementation of such data collection efforts there may be a misperception that the focus is on unmasking possible corruption, the channelling of funding into other activities and being able to analyse the equity of resource allocation among different populations, geographical locations and for specific interventions. These concerns can lead to difficulties in credibly analysing resource flows within an M&E programme [26].

As major new funding initiatives are launched, such as the Global Fund and PEPFAR, we are witnessing a shift in how funds are disbursed. There is more reliance on performance- or results-based disbursements, and the release of funding will be carefully linked to specific, time-defined indicators and targets. The pressure to perform and to report on specified targets can be overwhelming, particularly in low-resource settings where healthcare and community services are already fragile [27].

While it is easy to criticize some of the negative influences on accurate monitoring that are presented in this section, it must always be remembered that epidemics, and our monitoring of them, occur in a very real world. Protecting the economic stability of a country is not a minor issue, and, with the continued lack of critical evaluation research on the efficacy of various interventions, it is also understandable that politicians and programme planners will seize upon the limited available data that best support their personal views.

Increased involvement of stakeholders at all levels, especially civil society, can improve the accuracy and use of such data. As monitors of the implications of selected data, and by providing qualitative information on the quality and equity of access to services, community members and NGOs can play a powerful role in furthering the collection and dissemination of essential information about the epidemic and the services that are currently provided.

As the need for clinical service delivery and coverage data increases, it will be important that programme staff be part of the process of developing these monitoring systems.

Timely, accurate and relevant data should be seen to serve rather than harm programmes. As monitoring and evaluation programmes are strengthened at national and subnational level, political bodies must be brought into the dialogue. HIV is politically charged in most countries. Important religious and political lobbies, along with the general population, may initially oppose specific interventions. Their views must be taken into consideration and mutually satisfactory solutions found. It is in this context that M&E is perhaps most useful of all. Only careful measurement and recording of the success of existing initiatives will persuade policy-makers to expand programme efforts using the most effective interventions available.

Recommendations for future action

While significant progress has been made in monitoring and evaluation, most achievements have not been linked to other relevant sources at country level, such as HIV sero-surveillance, behavioural surveys, clinical records, programme monitoring, operations research and evaluations. This isolated and vertical approach will hopefully be addressed with the recent commitment to the 'Three Ones'. The fact that major donors have recognized the importance and benefits of coherent monitoring and evaluation systems and, as a result, have allocated additional resources for such a purpose constitutes a move in the right direction. The following agenda is proposed in order to fill the gap between the current and needed monitoring and evaluation strategy for HIV programmes.

1. *Move from planning to implementation as soon as possible.* The days of lengthy processes to develop conceptual frameworks are gone. It is time rapidly to operationalize and implement these frameworks.

2. *Strengthen existing management information systems at both national and subnational levels.* This calls for increased focus on both national and subnational capacity building in monitoring to ensure quality aggregated data. Dedicated M&E staff must be recruited and trained at all levels.

3. *Develop key simple and standardized monitoring tools* to ensure the production of sound data on coverage, quality of service delivery, distribution of infection, disease and death for programme planning and policy-making, including the equity dimension, i.e. ensuring that women benefit from fair and equitable representation and access to services and treatment.

4. *Give more attention to evaluation and operations research.* A comprehensive evaluation agenda needs to be developed based on an analysis of current gaps in M&E, and harmonized among major stakeholders. Also, operations research should be used more often for scaling-up purposes.

5. *Invest more time and resources on data-use strategies.* More efforts should be made in data presentation and packaging for different target audiences, ultimately leading to their use for planning and programming.

References

1. Garcia-Calleja JM, Zaniewski E, Ghys PD, Stanecki K, Walker N. (2004). A global analysis of trends in the quality of HIV sero-surveillance. *Sexually Transmitted Infections* **80**(Supplement 1):25–30.

2. UNAIDS/WHO. (2000). *Second Generation Surveillance for HIV: The Next Decade.* Geneva: UNAIDS.

3. Chin J, Mann J. (1989). Global surveillance and forecasting of AIDS. *Bulletin of the World Health Organization* **67**:1–7.

4. WHO/UNAIDS. (2003). *Guidelines for Conducting HIV Sentinel Serosurveys Among Pregnant Women and Other Groups.* Geneva: UNAIDS.

5. US Census Bureau. (2005). HIV/AIDS Surveillance Data Base, 2005.

6. Grassly NC, Morgan M, Walker N *et al.* (2004). Uncertainty in estimates of HIV/AIDS: the estimation and application of plausibility bounds. *Sexually Transmitted Infectections* **80**(Supplement 1): 31–38.

7. UNAIDS/WHO Working Group on Global HIV/ AIDS/STI Surveillance. (2005). *Guidelines for Measuring National HIV Prevalence in Population Based Surveys.* Geneva: UNAIDS.

8. McQuillan G, Kottiri B, Kruszon-Moran D. (2005). The Prevalence of HIV in the United States Household Population: The National Health and Nutrition Examination Surveys, 1988 to 2002. Presented at the 12th Conference on Retroviruses and Opportunistic Infections, February 2005, Boston, MA.

9. UNAIDS. (2001). *UNGASS Declaration of Commitment on HIV/AIDS.* Geneva: UNAIDS.

10. UNAIDS. (2002). *Monitoring the Declaration of Commitment on HIV/AIDS. Guidelines on Construction of Core Indicators.* Geneva: UNAIDS.

11. United Nations Development Programme (UNDP). (2004). *The Millennium Development Goals.* Available at http://www.undp.org/millenniumgoals/.

12. UNAIDS. (2003). *Progress Report on the Global Response to the HIV/AIDS Epidemic, 2003. Follow Up to the 2001 UNGASS on HIV/AIDS.* Geneva: UNAIDS.

13. UNAIDS. (2004). *The Three Ones Principle.* Available at http://www.unaids.org/en/ about+unaids/ what+is+unaids/ unaids+at+country+level/ the+three+ones.asp.

14. UNAIDS. (2000). *National AIDS Programmes: A Guide to Monitoring and Evaluation.* Geneva: UNAIDS.

15. Global Fund to Fight AIDS, Malaria and Tuberculosis. (2004) *Monitoring and Evaluation Toolkit for HIV/AIDS, Tuberculosis and Malaria.* Geneva: Global Fund.

16. UNAIDS/WHO. (2004). *Guidelines for Effective Use of Data from HIV Surveillance systems.* Geneva: UNAIDS/WHO Working Group on Global HIV/AIDS/STI Surveillance. Geneva: UNAIDS.

17. Needle RH, Trotter RT, Singer M *et al.* (2003). Rapid assessment of the HIV/AIDS crisis in racial and ethnic minority communities: an approach for timely community interventions. *American Journal of Public Health* **93**:970–79.

18. Rugg D, Peersman G, Carael M, eds. (2004). Global advances in HIV/AIDS monitoring and evaluation. *New Directions for Evaluation* **103**:13–31.

19. UNAIDS/World Bank. (2002) *National AIDS Councils (NACs) Monitoring and Evaluation Operations Manual.* Geneva: UNAIDS/World Bank.

20. Rehle T, Lazzari S, Dallabetta G, Asamoah-Odei E. (2004). Second-generation surveillance: better data for decision-making. *Bulletin of the World Health Organization* **82**(2):1–7.

21. Victora CG, Habicht JP, Brice J. (2004). Evidence-based public health: moving beyond randomized trials. *Public Health Matters* **94**:400–405.

22. Carael M and Holmes K, eds. (2001). The multicentre study of factors determining the different prevalences of HIV in sub-Saharan Africa. *AIDS* **15** (Supplement 4).

23. Plummer ML, Ross DA, Wight D *et al.* (2004). A bit more truthful: the validity of adolescent sexual behaviour data collected in rural northern Tanzania using five methods. *Sexually Transmitted Infections* **80** (Supplement 2):49–56.

24. *Using Evidence for Policies and Programmes for Achieving Global Goals on HIV/AIDS: The Evidence of Intervention Effectiveness Among Young People.* Results of an Expert Consultation Report, May 2004, Talloires.

25. Sabatier R. (1988). *Blaming Others.* London: Panos.

26. Marais H, Wilson A, for Joint United National Programme on HIV/AIDS. (2002). 'Meeting the Need'. In: *Report on the Global HIV/AIDS Epidemic.* Geneva: UNAIDS.

27. Kapriri L, Norheim OF, Heggenhougen K. (2003) Public participation in health planning and priority setting at the district level in Uganda. *Health Policy and Planning* **18**:205–213.

Chapter 11

The contribution of cost-effectiveness analysis

Guy Harling* and Lee Soderstrom

Introduction

Organizations worldwide are struggling to cope with the HIV pandemic. They are confronted by a scarcity of resources that is particularly acute in Africa and in other developing countries. This chapter focuses on the extent to which economic evaluations can help these organizations deal with this fundamental economic constraint.

This discussion is timely because, despite the steady growth of economic evaluation, its usefulness in relation to the HIV response has recently been questioned. When cost-effectiveness analyses (CEAs) were used to argue that Africa should focus primarily on prevention rather than treatment [1,2], it was roundly attacked [3–5]. Subsequently, WHO/UNAIDS launched the treatment-centred '3 by 5' programme [6].

We assess the relevance of CEA by considering the extent to which it can help domestic and international decision makers deal with two important problems. The first is determining the overall funding available for all HIV programmes in a developing country, which will be the result of the decisions of both domestic and foreign organizations. Much has been written about the funding 'needed' for HIV programmes and about how much donor countries 'ought' to make available, but little has been said about what determines the funding that countries actually provide. This is surprising: there is no country today where available resources are as great as HIV advocacy groups believe they should be. We explore the extent to which CEAs can help decision makers determine total HIV funding made available to a country.

The decision makers' second problem is determining the allocation of the total HIV funds available to the country among the various prevention and treatment programmes, i.e. deciding upon the mix of programmes funded. At present, notwithstanding the WHO's recent focus on treatment, most planners agree that both treatment and prevention spending should be increased [7]. Even if more total funding becomes available in the coming years, each country's decision makers must still decide how much should be spent on each possible programme. The role of highly active antiretroviral therapy (HAART) is a central issue in this field. To illustrate some ideas about the extent to which CEAs can facilitate good decisions about programme mix, we therefore show its implications for decisions regarding HAART and a generic prevention programme. These ideas are, however, equally applicable to decisions about any prevention and treatment programmes.

*Corresponding author.

Decisions shaping total funding are linked to decisions about programme mix because donor countries are often willing to fund some types of programmes, but not others. Although we make allowance for this, we also discuss each of the two problems separately, as each has unique features that contribute to a fuller understanding of the usefulness of CEAs. We first discuss decisions about programme mix, and then those regarding total funding.

Our discussions draw heavily on experiences in sub-Saharan Africa, as it is the region where the prevalence and impact of HIV have been greatest [8], and it is where almost all cost-effectiveness research in the less-developed world has been conducted [9]. Nevertheless, the ideas advanced here are relevant for decision makers everywhere concerned about HIV, particularly those in lower-income settings.

Resource scarcity

Decision makers are constrained by a basic economic fact: resources are scarce. The funds—and more fundamentally, the resources such as infrastructure, staff and others required as part of an HIV programme—have an 'opportunity cost', in that their use in that programme means that their use to provide some other health or non-health programmes must be forgone. This scarcity generates the two problems we are discussing. In the case of the first problem, if a country devotes more of its own resources to HIV programmes, it must cut back spending on other activities. Similarly, if a donor nation provides more funding for HIV programmes abroad, it must reduce spending on domestic programmes or on other programmes abroad. In the case of the second problem, since the total level of funds available for HIV programmes is fixed at any given moment in time, decision makers must choose among programmes irrespective of the level of resources. For example, spending more on prevention of mother-to-child transmission (PMTCT) means spending less on condom distribution, treating opportunistic infections (OIs), or other HIV containment programmes.

Resource scarcity does not dictate what decisions makers must do with respect to either problem, but it does constrain their options. Economic growth does not eliminate this scarcity; even the richest countries today limit their domestic spending on HIV because they want to use available resources for other socially desirable goods and services as well [10], as demonstrated in the chapters from industrialized countries in this book.

These resource constraints are often neglected in HIV policy discussions. Having determined the funding believed to be needed on clinical grounds, planners concerned about HIV in the developing world often argue that social equity demands that donor countries should provide the requisite funds [11]. Moreover, they add, the funds needed are only a tiny fraction of the donor nations' total incomes, so providing them should not impose a major burden on these countries [12]. This view, however, neglects the fact that in all countries there are other attractive, competing uses for the same resources—uses that may also be justifiable on equity grounds, such as domestic HIV programmes.

Economic evaluation

The four different methods of economic evaluation are often loosely referred to as CEA, although in fact only one is strictly a cost-effectiveness method. Each method is outlined in Box 11.1, and further information can be found in Drummond *et al.* [13]. While this chapter refers only to CEA in the strict sense, the ideas developed here apply to all four methods.

Box 11.1 An overview of economic evaluations

Health services researchers evaluating a health programme seek to determine whether its benefits are sufficient to justify its costs. Evaluations are performed by calculating the ratio of the change in costs resulting from the introduction of the programme to the change in benefits arising from it. Costs are evaluated in the same manner in all four approaches, but benefits are treated differently in each one.

♦ **Cost-minimization analysis** (CMA) makes no allowance for any differences in the health benefits of these programmes. It compares the cost of the programme in question with those for alternative programmes, in order to discover which one is least costly. CMA is therefore most appropriate when evaluating programmes that yield the same type and quantity of benefits.

♦ **Cost-effectiveness analysis** (CEA) calculates the benefits of each programme in terms of a particular health benefit. The cost-effectiveness ratio calculated is the added cost per unit of health benefit gained by using the programme. In HIV research, the benefit is usually either infections averted or life years gained (LYG). The ratios for two programmes can be compared only if both involve the same type of health benefit. Thus, CEA is most appropriate when only one type of benefit is important or feasible to measure.

♦ **Cost-utility analysis** (CUA) involves the calculation of programme benefits in terms of a gain in life expectancy, adjusted for the value placed on the added LYG for individuals. The most common such measures used are quality-adjusted life years (QALYs) and disability-adjusted life years (DALYs). This approach facilitates the evaluation of programmes which have multiple, important health outcomes. It also allows for the comparison of programmes which involve diverse health benefits.

♦ **Cost-benefit analysis** (CBA) places monetary value on a programme's benefits. Researchers then compare the value of the programme's benefits and its costs. This approach allows comparisons to be made between health and non-health programmes with widely differing outcome measures.

The frequent use of CEA in HIV research can be explained by the fact that for many HIV programmes, a single health benefit, such as LYG or infections avoided, is of major importance. Its popularity is also due to the fact that it is simpler to conduct than CUA or CBA, which require sophisticated, sometimes controversial, techniques to value benefits using QALYs, DALYs, or in cash.

It is often said that programmes subjected to a CEA can be ranked according to their cost-effectiveness ratios, the programmes with the lowest ratio being the most cost-effective. However, as we explain in this chapter, the preferred programmes sometimes are not the ones with the lowest CE ratios.

The many economic evaluations of HIV programmes have recently been reviewed in detail elsewhere [9]. This literature is summarized in Box 11.2. Most of these evaluations are CEAs, and the results obtained using the other methods are consistent with those for CEAs.

Box 11.2   **A summary of HIV cost-effectiveness studies[†]**

Prevention strategies

Prevention interventions are very cost-effective when focused on those at highest risk of infection.

◆ **Community-based behaviour change** interventions to prevent HIV infection among high-risk, vulnerable adults are frequently cost-effective in both high-income and sub-Saharan African countries; this result is less robust for interventions in more general populations.

◆ **Voluntary counselling and testing** (VCT) at clinics to avert subsequent transmission of HIV and other sexually transmitted infections (STIs) or of other health problems is generally cost-effective in both high- and low-income countries.

◆ **Testing healthcare workers** routinely for HIV does not have low cost-effectiveness ratios in either high- or low-income countries.

◆ **Blood screening** programmes are generally cost-effective in high-income nations, as are measures to screen donors and test blood locally in sub-Saharan Africa.

◆ **Prevention of mother-to-child transmission** is cost-effective, if not cost-saving, across a broad range of settings. The use of elective Caesarean section deliveries in high-income settings, and of short-course ART in Africa, is particularly worthwhile.

Treatment strategies

Treatment strategies tend to have higher cost-effectiveness ratios than the most effective prevention interventions, although cost-effectiveness ratios vary widely.

◆ **Highly active antiretroviral therapy** (HAART) has low cost-effectiveness ratios in high-income countries, relative both to no treatment and to other ART regimes. In sub-Saharan Africa, HAART falls within commonly used criteria for being considered cost-effective in such settings.

◆ **Post-exposure prophylaxis** (PEP) with antiretrovirals is cost-effective for people at occasional high risk, such as healthcare workers, but not for those at high risk on a regular basis.

◆ **Prophylaxis for opportunistic infections** (OIs) such as *Pneumocystis carinii* pneumonia, toxoplasmosis and *Mycobacterium avium* complex is generally cost-effective in developed countries. Fluconazole for fungal infections is of questionable cost-effectiveness, and ganciclovir for cytomegalovirus has a very high cost-effectiveness ratio. In the only study to evaluate prophylaxis for tuberculosis in Africa, providing isoniazid for 6 months was cost-effective.

Source: [9].

[†]A programme is termed 'cost-effective' if the available cost-effectiveness ratios for it are either low relative to those for other programmes in the same setting, or within the guidelines generally used for identifying cost-effectiveness programmes. These guidelines are discussed later in this chapter.

HAART and 'spill-over' effects

A particularly important issue today is the role of HAART in developing countries' HIV programmes. Its benefits are impressive in increasing the quality of life and longevity of people living with HIV (PLHIV), but treatment with HAART is expensive, particularly in developed countries. Although outpatient monitoring replaces more costly inpatient stays, the savings are generally not sufficient to offset the high price of the drugs [14–16]. Moreover, because HAART increases life expectancy, the lifetime cost of treatment rises. However, recent reductions in drug prices have improved the cost-effectiveness of HAART in developing countries [16].

HAART and prevention programmes can have 'spill-over' effects. Treatment programmes may encourage prevention activities; for example, the expanded availability of HAART may increase the willingness of individuals to be tested, and reduced viral load may lower the risk of transmission during sexual acts or birth [7]. On the other hand, if people live longer with fewer symptoms, they may engage in additional risky behaviours [17,18]. Similarly, prevention programmes may make people more aware of HIV and its consequences, thereby reducing stigma and increasing people's willingness to be tested and to seek treatment when necessary. However, no allowance will be made for these effects in this discussion, as evidence regarding their extent is limited and doing so would not change our underlying arguments.

Problem: determination of HIV programme mix

Suppose decision makers in a high HIV prevalence country know the level of domestic and foreign funding available, i.e. total HIV funding available is pre determined. They must decide how much to spend on each possible HIV intervention. If more is spent on programme A, less can be spent on programme B. Thus, decision makers face a trade-off: to obtain more of the benefits of A, they must sacrifice some of the benefits of B. The greater the cost of programme A relative to that of B, the greater the benefits of B that must be sacrificed. Decision makers must choose between A and B because resources are limited, not because of CEA.

Though this trade-off does not dictate programme mix, it means that decision makers must decide whether putting more resources into A would yield sufficient additional benefits to compensate for those forgone due to fewer resources being available for B. Given the decision makers' perceptions of the trade-off in benefits, their decisions about programme mix depend on the relative values they attach to the benefits of A gained and the benefits of B sacrificed. The greater the value attached to the benefits of A relative to those of B, the more of A decision makers prefer. A variety of factors determine those values, including decision makers' perceptions of social values in their country, political considerations and their own personal preferences.

CEAs can aid decision makers in choosing among programmes because it provides them with explicit information about the extent of the trade-off confronting them. Without this information, decision makers' perceptions of the trade-off may be erroneous. Suppose that the primary health benefit of programmes A and B is life years gained (LYG). The trade-off between them then depends on the cost per LYG of each programme. If CEA indicates that the cost per LYG using A is US$10 and using B is US$1, then to obtain one more LYG by expanding A will require sacrificing 10 LYs because of the necessary reduction in spending on B. If decision makers valued equally an LYG provided by A and an LYG provided by B, they would prefer programme B. In the absence of such a CEA, decision makers might act on the basis of erroneous beliefs they held about each programme. If they thought the cost per LYG using B were US$15, then they might incorrectly elect to spend more on programme A.

If competing HIV programmes had the same measure of outcome, say LYG, then the above analysis would suggest that: first, all competing programmes should be ranked according to their cost-effectiveness ratios; and, secondly, funds should be allocated to each in turn, progressing from the programme with the lowest ratio towards the one with the highest, until all available funds are exhausted. This would maximize the LYG with the available funds. However, as we explain below, there are problems with this procedure; some of the most desirable programmes may not be the ones with the lowest cost-effectiveness ratios.

To illustrate the use of CEAs, consider their role in decision making relating to HIV prevention and HAART programmes. Taking at face value existing evidence that cost-effectiveness ratios for HAART are higher than those for many prevention programmes, the implication is that treating one more existing case will lead to several new cases because less can be spent on prevention. For example, a recent South African study of the benefit of HAART compared with no treatment in a community setting found the cost per LYG to be US$1113 (2002 US$), and the cost per additional case treated to be US$6745 [16]. CEAs of various prevention programmes in Africa report incremental costs of less than US$100 per LYG, and less than US$1000 per case avoided [1]. These results suggest that as long as the settings are comparable, more than 11 LYG could be lost through prevention interventions forgone for each LYG via treatment, and that more than six new cases could occur for each additional case treated. However, not all prevention programmes are found to be more cost-effective than HAART. Söderlund *et al.* estimated that in South Africa, VCT and formula feeding at 6 months post-partum for preventive MTCT would cost over US$1100 per LYG [19].

Despite these results, decision makers clearly do not—and should not—deny funding to all HAART programmes. To understand why, consider the special case in which four conditions are satisfied: (i) the outcomes and the costs of the programmes being considered are correctly measured in the CEAs; (ii) these outcomes fully reflect all important social benefits of each programme; (iii) decision makers are indifferent to which social group, such as newborns or PLHIV, reaps the benefits; and (iv) donor countries have no preferences regarding the type of HIV programmes that recipient countries adopt. In this case, decision making is straightforward: choose the programme with the lowest cost-effectiveness ratio. In reality, we argue below, all four conditions are generally violated. Consequently, decision making is not straightforward; programmes should not be ranked merely by their cost-effectiveness ratios.

Limitation 1: methodological problems in existing analyses

Four examples indicate that decision makers reviewing CEA results must make allowance for various methodological problems, some of which are discussed in more detail elsewhere [13].

1. The data regarding the effects of the programme evaluated on clinical outcomes and health service utilization are often of mixed quality [9]. Only a minority of CEAs use effectiveness data drawn from a single study—most mix data from several studies involving different populations. Few researchers consider the quality of the studies from which their effectiveness data are drawn; estimates may reflect not only the impacts of the programme, but also biases arising from the study design used. In addition, researchers must sometimes make assumptions about important programme effects. In clinical studies of HAART, the follow-up periods have often been insufficient to determine its effect on longevity, so researchers doing CEAs of HAART must make assumptions about those effects [16,20,21]. Prevention programmes frequently

measure cases averted using changes in questionnaire responses, not changes in confirmed HIV infections [22].

2. Evaluations of programmes are often made in experimental settings, where the motivations of patients and staff may differ from those in an implemented programme. Consequently, compliance may be a greater problem in practice than experimental studies suggest. Similarly, these evaluations have focused on the effects of initial interventions in various populations, but such 'naïve' populations are becoming rare. The benefits of the first HIV education programme in an area are likely to differ from those of the second or third such programme.

3. Studies in Africa frequently combine North American evidence of programme effectiveness with African cost data. If effectiveness differs between continents—because of differences in patient compliance or in the training and availability of health personnel—programme benefits in Africa will differ from those in North America.

4. Costs and benefits measured in studies are often incomplete. Costs are sometimes measured from the perspective of the programme, sometimes from that of the health system, but seldom from a societal perspective. For example, allowance is seldom made for costs borne by patients' families. Likewise, measures of benefits rarely make allowance for productivity gains. In reality, when PLHIV receive HAART, they can work more intensively and for longer.

At minimum, the first three problems create uncertainty about the reliability of reported cost-effectiveness ratios. This uncertainty will never be eliminated, because avoiding all significant methodological problems would be too difficult, costly and time consuming. It is, however, lessened by two results from the literature. First, multiple evaluations of the same type of programme often yield similar results, though this may partly stem from the studies using some of the same clinical and financial data. Secondly, results from sensitivity analyses often show that results remain unaffected when alternative, plausible assumptions are made about key parameters. For example, the differential between prevention and HAART cost-effectiveness ratios would apparently remain even if drug costs were substantially lower: Cleary *et al.* reported that if drug costs were 45% lower, the additional cost per LYG would be US$778—still well above many prevention programmes' cost-effectiveness ratios [16].

The fourth problem is more worrisome, suggesting that reported results are probably biased upwards. CEAs generally ignore any effect of prevention and treatment programmes on people's ability to work. Thus, if a programme does increase hours worked more than the alternative programme being considered, thereby reducing net social costs, CEAs for that programme overstate its real cost. In an early CEA of HAART using Swiss data, Sendi and colleagues found that the treatment increased HIV patients' ability to do paid work and that when allowance was made for this, the intervention was cost-saving [23]. Similarly, prevention interventions could raise productivity. Clearly, more attention should be given to such productivity gains.

Limitation 2: limited scope of available CEAs

It is sometimes difficult to compare alternative programmes because there are no CEAs for them. Worldwide, only a small number of studies have been completed, with over 60% of them focusing on North America [9]. Very few involve programmes in Africa, and even fewer Asia. Encouragingly, evaluations of the same type of programme in different continents often yield similar results, though this may again be an artefact of different researchers using some of the same data sources.

The literature has several other, similar shortcomings. Most existing studies reflect experiences in large institutional settings, whereas most high-prevalence countries require evidence from community-based interventions [16,20]. Children and adolescents, a key demographic group for heterosexually transmitted HIV, have been largely ignored. Little evidence exists on the prophylaxis or treatment of opportunistic infections outside North America; attention particularly needs to be given to the interactions between HIV and OIs in low-income, high disease burden settings [9]. Furthermore, the rapidly declining cost of HAART in developing countries may quickly render existing studies obsolete, requiring frequent updating. Finally, when establishing a programme, planners would like to set eligibility criteria in order to target people who would benefit most from it. For many programmes, the available CEAs do not provide results for pertinent subpopulations.

Limitation 3: no consideration of equity

Although decision makers are frequently not indifferent as to which social group benefits from HIV programmes, CEA makes no allowance for concerns about equity. The same weight is attached to each individual: an LYG by people targeted by programme A is assumed to be as important as one gained by people targeted by programme B. CEA only indicates which programme would be less costly per LYG. There are, however, various ethical reasons why decision makers may favour one group over another. One is that they do not want to discriminate against people with low incomes or older people. Another is the 'rule of rescue', which implies that current, identifiable patients should receive more attention than possible future patients who are currently only abstractions. Thus, in the case of HIV, even though HAART has higher cost-effectiveness ratios than prevention, some spending on it may be desirable.

However, when decision makers are tempted to ignore the CEAs on ethical grounds, they should consider two issues. First, providing HAART on ethical grounds implies that PLHIV are viewed differently from people living with other health problems. The ethical argument for HAART is often based on the proposition that, because HAART prolongs life, it is unethical to deny treatment to PLHIV. There are, however, many people worldwide with other life-threatening health problems for which effective treatment exists, but for which access to those treatments is not widely available. Examples in Africa include chemotherapy for tuberculosis, oral rehydration for diarrhoea and angioplasty for cardiac disease. A complete ethical argument for prioritizing HAART should justify differential treatment for PLHIV.

Secondly, ethical concerns do not eliminate the trade-off caused by scarcity of funding, so the weight attached to those concerns should take into account the magnitude of the trade-off. When considering prioritizing HAART over prevention, decision makers should consider whether the ethical concerns are sufficient to justify the additional HIV cases that would result from spending less on prevention. Favouring HAART on ethical grounds seems easily justifiable if treating an additional existing patient would result in only one more new infection occurring. However, given current evidence indicating that the figure is rather higher, that case may be harder to make.

Similar issues arise if there are ethical concerns within a country about certain types of HIV interventions, for example, if promoting the provision and use of condoms is seen as promoting liberal sexual mores. When deciding about programme mix, decision makers must take any such concerns into account just as they do concerns about equity.

Limitation 4: no allowance for donor countries' preferences

Similarly, some donor countries have preferences regardimg programme mix for various reasons. As a result, the level of funding which they offer a recipient country may be influenced by the willingness of that country to adopt their preferred mix. Decision makers in the recipient country should take these preferences into account when setting domestic spending priorities, recognizing that the benefits of implementing the donors' preferred mix would include those resulting from the donor's willingness to provide additional dollars. CEAs make no allowance for such benefits.

Relevance of CEA

Given these limitations, a strict ranking of HIV programmes according to their cost-effectiveness ratios—where they are available—seems undesirable. The use of cost-utility analysis (CUA) or cost-benefit analysis (CBA) would not remove these limitations, which are the result of funding constraints, not the method of economic evaluation. In the final analysis, the quality of decisions about programme mix will always depend on the judgement of decision makers, who must make allowance for these limitations when choosing among programmes.

Nevertheless, CEA is still important. Without it, decision makers would not have explicit evidence concerning the extent of the trade-off confronting them when they consider funding a particular programme. Certainly, the assumptions and methods of each study should be critically appraised. However, judging by the reported sensitivity analyses and the similarity of results among evaluations of the same programmes, the technical limitations of most available CEAs are not so serious that their results should be ignored. A caveat to this is the lack of CEAs that make allowance for the productivity effects of HIV programmes.

Problem: determination of total HIV funding

The other major problem facing decision makers is the determination of total HIV funding for a particular country. This problem is particularly acute for those countries with a widespread or fast-growing epidemic, where domestic funding, whether from government or private sources, is often limited by low per capita incomes. As a result, such countries depend heavily on public and private support from more developed nations [8,24,25]. While funding from all sources for these countries has increased in recent years, funds available remain less than those perceived to be needed [8].

In brief, two factors determine public and private funding decisions of a donor country. First, because resources are scarce domestically, the donor faces a trade-off between the benefits achieved from expenditures on HIV programmes abroad and those gained from alternative spending options, including other foreign aid, domestic HIV programmes and private domestic consumption. The higher the cost of HIV programmes relative to the costs of other programmes, the greater the cut-backs in benefits from other programmes required to expand the HIV programmes.

Secondly, given their perceptions about this trade-off, decision makers in the donor country then determine funding by comparing the perceived value of the benefits of the HIV programmes abroad to the donor country with those of other forms of spending. Similarly, funding decisions in a recipient country are determined by its income constraint and by its decision makers' preferences. Although a more sophisticated view of decision making is possible, it would yield the same fundamental conclusion: funding for HIV programmes must compete for support with donor and recipient countries' other priorities.

Cost-effectiveness analysis

CEA can help decision makers determine total funding to the extent that it provides them with useful information about the trade-off between the benefits of funding HIV programmes and the benefits of funding other options. However, the usefulness of CEA here is limited by the technical limitations already described and by equity concerns related to spending on HIV compared with other priorities. It is further reduced by two additional limitations.

Limitation 1: difficulties in comparing different types of programmes

To characterize explicitly the trade-offs facing decision makers, CEAs would have to exist for both HIV and alternative programmes. Planners could then compare the benefits of spending US$10 million on HIV with spending US$10 million on education, infrastructure or private consumption. Unfortunately, few CEAs exist for competing non-HIV programmes, and most of those that do are for alternative health programmes in developed countries.

To overcome the paucity of CEAs for competing programmes, health planners in developed countries often compare the cost-effectiveness ratio of a proposed new HIV intervention with those of existing health services currently funded in their country. These planners argue that some decision makers have already decided that it was better to use some available resources for those existing programmes than for alternatives. They further argue that if the new HIV programme has a lower cost-effectiveness ratio than some existing health programmes, it is at least as attractive as those programmes are. Thus, the planners conclude, decision makers should fund the new HIV programme, in part by cutting back less cost-effective heath programmes, and in part by shifting resources from the provision of other goods and services. Guidelines have been developed to facilitate such comparisons [13]. In developed countries, many HIV prevention and treatment programmes have cost-effectiveness ratios within these guidelines [26]. It is therefore not surprising that such programmes are widely used in North America and Western Europe.

The available cost-effectiveness ratios for the same programmes when provided in Africa are also generally within the industrialized countries' guidelines. Consequently, as long as there are unfunded HIV programmes with such cost-effectiveness ratios in developing countries, some HIV planners argue that donor countries and international donor organizations should provide developing countries with more funding for HIV. This is sometimes justified on equity grounds: what is available in donor countries should be available elsewhere.

There is, however, no precedent in Africa for health programmes being funded at the same level as that in donor countries simply because they have cost-effectiveness ratios within the donor countries' guidelines. To understand funding decisions, it is more relevant to compare the cost-effectiveness ratios of HIV programmes in Africa with those for other health services that are actually provided there and are extensively donor-funded. Suppose most health services receiving substantial funding from abroad have cost-effectiveness ratios of US$10 or less per LYG, i.e. special equity concerns aside, suppose donor countries showed little willingness to pay more than US$10 per LYG. In this case, there is no reason to expect donors to provide massive funding for a programme with a cost-effectiveness ratio of US$2000, even though that ratio is less than US $50,000, a cut-off commonly used in North America.

Limitation 2: difficulties in accounting for 'macro' effects of HIV

The pandemic in Africa today is so widespread that it has caused significant social and economic disruption at the 'macro' level. Consequently, implementing HIV programmes that affect a significant fraction of the population of an African country may reduce this disruption, as well as increase life expectancy. When considering funding for such programmes, decision makers should consider both benefits. CEAs, however, make no allowance for the benefits resulting from reduced 'macro' disruptions, thus understating the attractiveness of funding these programmes in countries where such disruptions are considerable.

These 'macro' benefits come from a number of sources. For example, HIV programmes may directly or indirectly reduce the number of HIV-related orphans, thereby reducing the social and economic burden they represent. In addition, by reducing the prevalence of HIV and increasing the capacity of PLHIV to work, HIV programmes may increase the incentive for people to invest in their own education and formal training, thereby facilitating greater economic growth. Moreover, maintaining a larger, healthier population may facilitate the transfer of skills and knowledge to others via informal training [27]. However, due to limited research to date, the extent of these 'macro' effects is uncertain.

It is possible to make allowances for some non-healthcare benefits when conducting a CEA. For example, most evaluations of preventive MTCT programmes focus only on cases averted or LYG, but South African researchers found that such an intervention also yielded substantial savings to the government through reduced welfare payments for HIV-positive children [28].

We are unaware of any CEA in which full allowance is made for the impact of the programme evaluated on 'macro' economic and social problems. Such effects are technically difficult to measure, and the nature of CEA itself has not encouraged analysts to try to measure them. Analysts have used the same approach to evaluate HIV programmes as they have used for other health programmes. In these latter evaluations, analysts are generally concerned about the consequences of implementing only a single programme, which benefits only the small group of people directly involved in the programme. The 'macro' benefits of such programmes are negligible. Current policy discussions, on the other hand, relate to the funding of a set of HIV programmes affecting, directly or indirectly, a significant fraction of the population. In this case, the 'macro' benefits may be considerable. As a result, it may be unwise to base funding decisions solely on CEAs, which make no allowance for these potentially major benefits.

Relevance of CEA

As a result of these two limitations, CEA is probably less useful for decisions about the overall level of HIV funding than for choices regarding programme mix. Nevertheless, it does provide a starting point for decision makers concerned about funding. Using the cost-effectiveness ratios for the programmes a donor country is considering funding, planners can calculate the dollars needed to achieve any particular level of benefits. Then, to determine what funding that country will provide, its decision makers will also need to consider two issues for which CEA can be of little help. One is the perceived effect of its HIV spending on the 'macro' problems of the pandemic in the recipient country. The other is the benefit that the donor country would have to forgo because of the reduction in resources available for other desirable things.

In principle, using CBA avoids the first limitation of CEA for funding decisions [13], but it does not overcome the second. Health service researchers conducting economic evaluations have traditionally assumed that the programmes being evaluated affect only a small group of people—that their 'macro' effects are negligible.

Conclusion

Financial constraints confront decision makers concerned with scaling up HIV programmes in countries with the greatest need. These constraints are not caused by CEA, but by the scarcity of resources. CEA can help decision makers deal with these constraints—although more so when making decisions about programme mix than those about overall funding—because it can provide decision makers with useful information about the trade-offs confronting them. The usefulness of CEA is, however, circumscribed by two classes of difficulties. The first, the current state of the cost-effectiveness evidence base, can be mitigated by tackling some methodological difficulties and by expanding the range of CEAs. The second is the inability of CEA to account for ethical concerns, for the effects of programme mix on funding and for the impact of large-scale programmes on the 'macro' social and economic disruptions caused by HIV. These difficulties cannot be averted using CEA or other economic evaluation methods.

These shortcomings of CEA do not mean decision makers can ignore the scarcity of resources. They do, however, mean that the quality of HIV-related decision making depends heavily on the judgement of the decision makers. This illustrates a central theme of this volume: without building and maintaining staff expertise, the HIV pandemic will not be brought under control. The task here is great because choices about programme mix and funding involve a wide range of decision makers in the heavily affected countries, in the donor nations and in major international agencies and non-governmental organizations (NGOs).

Acknowledgements

When preparing this text, the authors benefited greatly from discussions with Mira Johri and Eddy Beck concerning the ideas developed here. However, the authors retain full responsibility for the final text, including all opinions expressed herein.

References

1. Creese A, Floyd K, Alban A, Guiness L. (2002). Cost-effectiveness of HIV/AIDS interventions in Africa: a systematic review of the evidence. *Lancet* **359**:1635–1642.
2. Marseille E, Hofmann PB, Kahn JG. (2002). HIV prevention before HAART in sub-Saharan Africa. *Lancet* **359**:1851–1856.
3. Piot P, Zewkie D, Türmen T. (2002). HIV/AIDS prevention and treatment (Letter). *Lancet* **360**:86.

4. Goemaere E, Ford N, Benatar SR. (2002). HIV/AIDS prevention and treatment (Letter). *Lancet* 360:86–87.

5. Gonsalves G. (2002). HIV/AIDS prevention and treatment (Letter). *Lancet* 360:87.

6. World Health Organization/UNAIDS. (2003). *Treating 3 Million by 2005: Making It Happen: the WHO Strategy.* Geneva: WHO, p55.

7. Moatti JP, N'Dove I, Hale P, Kazatchkine MD. (2003). Antiretroviral treatment for HIV-infected adults and children in developing countries: some evidence in favor of expanded diffusion. In: Forsythe S, ed. *State of the Art: AIDS and Economics.* The Policy Project/International AIDS-Economics Network, p96–117. Available from: www.policyproject.com/pubs/other/ SOTAecon.pdf (Accessed 5 Apr 2005).

8. UNAIDS. (2004). *2004 Report on the Global AIDS Epidemic.* Geneva: UNAIDS, p231.

9. Harling G, Wood R, Beck EJ. (2005). A review of the efficiency of interventions in HIV infection, 1994–2004. *Disease Management & Health Outcomes* 13(6): 371–394.

10. Johri M, Paltiel DA, Goldie SJ, Freedberg KA. (2002). State AIDS Drug Assistance Programs: equity and efficiency in an era of rapidly changing treatment standards. *Medical Care* 40:429–41.

11. France T, Ooms G, Rivers B. (2002). The Global Fund: which countries owe how much? *Aidspan Global Fund Document 15.* Available from: http://www.aidspan.org/ gfo/docs/gfo15.htm (Accessed 5 April 2005).

12. Boelaert M, Van Damme W, Meessen B, Van der Stuyft P. (2002). Editorial: the AIDS crisis, cost-effectiveness and academic activism. *Tropical Medicine and International Health* 7:1001–2.

13. Drummond MF, O'Brien B, Stoddart GL, Torrance GW. (1997). *Methods for the Economic Evaluation of Health Care Programmes,* 2nd edn. Oxford: Oxford University Press, p305.

14. Beck EJ, Mandalia S. (2003). The cost of HIV treatment and care in England since HAART. *British Journal of Sexual Medicine* 27:19–23.

15. Bozzette SA, Joyce G, McCaffrey DF, *et al.* (2001). Expenditures for the care of HIV-infected patients in the era of highly active antiretroviral therapy. *New England Journal of Medicine* 344:817–823.

16. Cleary S, Boulle A, McIntyre D, Coetzee D. (2004). Cost-effectiveness of antiretroviral treatment for HIV-positive adults in a South African Township. Health Economics Unit, School of Public Health and Family Medicine, University of Cape Town. Available from: http://www.hst.org.za/ upload/files/ arv_cost.pdf (Accessed 5 April 2005).

17. Do AN, Hanson DL, Dworkin MS *et al.* (2001). Risk factors and trends in gonorrhea incidence among persons infected with HIV in the United States. *AIDS* 15:1149–1155.

18. Dodds JP, Nardone A, Mercey DE, Johnson AM. (2000). Increase in high risk sexual behaviour among homosexual men, London 1996–8: cross-sectional, questionnaire study. *British Medical Journal* 320:1511–1512.

19. Söderlund N, Zwi K, Kinghorn A *et al.* (1999). Prevention of vertical transmission of HIV: analysis of cost effectiveness of options available in South Africa. *British Medical Journal* 318:1650–6.

20. Wood E, Braitstein P, Montaner JSG *et al.* (2000). Extent to which low-level use of antiretroviral treatment could curb the AIDS epidemic in sub-Saharan Africa. *Lancet* 355:2095–2100.

21. Boulle A, Kenyon C, Skordis J *et al.* (2002). Exploring the costs of a limited public sector antiretroviral treatment programme in South Africa. *South African Medical Journal* 92:811–7.

22. Pinkerton SD, Holtgrave DR, Bloom FR. (1998). Cost-effectiveness of post-exposure prophylaxis following sexual exposure to HIV. *AIDS* 12:1067–78.

23. Sendi PP, Bucher HC, Harr T *et al.* (1999). Cost-effectiveness of highly active antiretroviral therapy in HIV-infected patients. *AIDS* 13:1115–22.

24. Schwartlander B, Stover J, Walker N *et al.* (2002). Resource needs for HIV/AIDS. *Science* 292:2434–2436.

25. Gutiérrez JP, Johns B, Adam T *et al.* (2004). Achieving the WHO/UNAIDS antiretroviral treatment 3 by 5 goal: what will it cost? *Lancet* **364**:63–4.

26. Pinkerton SD, Holtgrave DR, DiFranceisco W *et al.* (2000). Cost–threshold analyses of the National AIDS Demonstration Research HIV Prevention Interventions. *AIDS* **14**:1257–1268.

27. Bell C, Devarajan S, Gerbach H. (2003). The long-run economic costs of AIDS: theory and an application to South Africa. *World Bank Working Paper 3152.* Washington, DC: World Bank, p118.

28. Skordis J, Nattrass N. (2002). Paying to waste lives: the affordability of reducing mother-to-child transmission of HIV in South Africa. *Journal of Health Economics* **21**:405–422.

Section III

Country Responses

Chapter 12

Botswana

Louisiana Lush[*], Ernest Darkoh and Segolame L Ramotlhwa

Background

Botswana has the unfortunate distinction of having one of the highest rates of HIV in the world. Antenatal sero-surveillance put prevalence among pregnant women aged 15–49 at 39% in 2000, 36% in 2001, 35% in 2002 and 37% in 2003 [1–3]. In 2001, the UN estimated that 300,000 adults and 28,000 children were living with HIV. Life expectancy at birth is 39 years, which would have been 72 in the absence of HIV [4]. In the face of this crisis, the Botswana government in 2002 became the first in Africa to offer comprehensive HIV care and treatment to all its population.

Botswana, formerly a British protectorate, gained its full independence in 1966. Since then, it has been a stable democratic country governed under a parliamentary system, led by President Festus Mogae at the time of writing. At independence, the landlocked country in Southern Africa was one of the poorest in the world, but during the last 30–40 years, it has enjoyed one of the world's highest growth rates, thereby transforming itself into a middle-income country. In 2002, per capita gross domestic product (GDP) was US$9500 (at purchasing power parity) and growing at 6% each year. This economic success is fuelled by diamonds, which, along with other minerals, currently account for more than a third of the GDP and 90% of export earnings. Other economic sectors are tourism, cattle and subsistence farming. Like other countries heavily dependent on mineral resources, there are significant problems of unemployment and poverty: unemployment is officially 21%, but unofficial estimates place it at closer to 40%.

In 2001, the population was 1.6 million, of which just under half was living in urban areas. Life expectancy at birth rose to over 60 years before the impact of HIV reduced it to 39 in 2001, with infant mortality at 58 per 1000 live births [5]. The population is, nonetheless, well educated and has widespread access to water, indicating the high level of infrastructural development across the country. The main ethnic group is the Tswana, who make up nearly four-fifths of the population, with Kalanga, Basarwa and others making up the remainder. The capital, Gaborone, is one of 10 administrative districts, of which four are town councils (see Table 12.1).

The health system

The Botswana public health system is under the authority of the Ministry of Health (MoH) and the Ministry of Local Government, Lands and Housing (MLGLH), both guided by the

* Corresponding author.

The views expressed in this chapter are those of the authors and are not necessarily those of the organizations they work for, unless specifically stated in the text.

Table 12.1 Demographic indicators for Botswana

	2001
Population mid-year (millions)	1.6
Average annual growth rate	1.7
Life expectancy at birth (years)	39
Infant mortality (per 1000 live births)	58
Child malnutrition (% of children under five)	17
Illiteracy (% of adults)	22
Gross primary enrolment (% of school-age population)	108

Source: [6].

National Health Policy [7]. The MoH is responsible for determining the National Health Policy and has direct authority over referral, district and primary hospital services. In addition, it supports a number of specialist programmes, of which the AIDS/sexually transmitted infection (STI) unit, epidemiology [including tuberculosis (TB)], health planning, national health research, maternal and child/family planning and manpower units are all key for HIV policy.

The MLGLH runs basic health services, including primary healthcare clinics, health posts and other community services within a district health system. It is also responsible for social welfare services, and councils have specific responsibility for health promotion, basic curative services, referrals to higher healthcare levels, counselling, family health and social welfare. They also manage a district health team that includes a communicable diseases officer focusing on HIV and TB.

District, city and town councils plan, provide and evaluate basic health services in consultation with the MoH and in accordance with the National Health Policy and guidelines. The system is expected to function coherently and to link to social services, but problems remain. The main forum for consultation between the various authorities is the Primary Health Care Coordinating Committee, which meets quarterly and is chaired by the Deputy Permanent Secretary for Health. The health system is oriented towards primary healthcare to deliver maximum social benefit from resources. Difficulties of defining roles and responsibilities are acknowledged in the Policy [8].

While the MoH remains the lead policy agency in policy and programme development for HIV, the National AIDS Council (NAC) is responsible for coordinating a multisectoral response to the HIV epidemic. Co-chaired by the Minister of Health, the NAC also has representation from the MLGLH, Office of the President, Ministry of Finance and Development Planning, as well as senior representation from all other ministries, business and civil society. At district level, District Health Services Coordinating Committees (DHSCCs), which include representation from hospitals and clinics, meet quarterly and are the main forums responsible for coordinating district health services. District Multisectoral AIDS Committees have also been established and are responsible for coordinating all HIV-related activities at the district and subdistrict level.

Health expenditure has risen markedly in recent years, rising to 6% of GDP in 2000, of which nearly two-thirds was from the public sector [9]. Health expenditure per person in 2000 was US$191. The country currently has two referral hospitals, one specialist psychiatric hospital, one private hospital, 12 district hospitals—four of which are non-government, there being two mine and two mission hospitals—and 16 primary hospitals. All hospitals are staffed by doctors, nurses and other relevant health workers. In addition, in 2000, Botswana had 222 clinics, 330 health posts and 740 mobile stops countrywide staffed primarily by nurses [7]. Around 90% of the population has access to healthcare, defined as living within 15 km of a facility. However, access remains a problem, particularly for referred services, since a large sector of the population lives in remote districts.

In 1998, 14,200 people were employed in the health sector [7], absorbing 53% of the health budget, although in all areas of the health system, personnel accounted for a shrinking proportion of recurrent spending through the 1990s. Scarcity of trained health workers is recognized as the main constraint on improving equity and levels of healthcare in Botswana. Despite improvements in the doctor–patient or nurse–patient ratios since the 1980s (Table 12.2), skills scarcity persists in a number of crucial areas, especially at primary healthcare level [7]. Although Botswana's primary healthcare system is relatively well developed, its main focus has been preventive care, with varying supplies of drugs and expertise in facilities. Partly in compensation, family welfare educators have been recruited within communities and receive basic preventive care training to work in the community. Frequently, despite very little capacity for curative care, they have moved to clinics to cover for absent professional nurses. In 1998, a study found that 14% of clinics did not have posts for staff with professional qualifications and 17% had not had a nurse in post for 3 months [7]. Nurse practitioners and community nurses with post-basic training tended not to be adequately deployed at primary healthcare levels and may not have the capacity needed to coordinate HIV/STI and TB services as required.

In sum, in Botswana, compared with elsewhere in sub-Saharan Africa, a relatively large proportion of the population has quite good access to healthcare. Although the population has been growing rapidly, relative economic security has meant that healthcare has expanded in line with increases in numbers needing treatment. Nevertheless, as in many countries, HIV has a heavy impact on health services and poses particular challenges.

Table 12.2 Numbers of health workers, 1987–1997

	1987	1992	1997	% increase 1987–1997
Doctors	166	316	424	155%
Nurses	1946	3057	4130	112%
Family Welfare Educators	670	692	749	12%

Source: [8].

The HIV epidemic

Current scale of the problem, populations affected and likely future trends

The first case of AIDS in Botswana was reported in 1985, when it was still seen as a disease affecting male homosexuals in the West or other African countries. Subsequently, the astonishingly high rates of HIV in Botswana rose from around 5% in 1990, when sentinel surveillance data started to be collected nationally [4]. In 2001, contrary to initial projections of a plateau at around 25% prevalence, urban antenatal surveillance sites reported a median prevalence of 45%, with minimum 39% and maximum 56% [4] (Fig. 12.1). In rural areas, figures were slightly lower. In all districts, more than a fifth of pregnant women were infected, and in some more than half. In 2002, the government estimated that about 258,000 Batswana were living with HIV and declared it a national emergency [10]. While preliminary evidence from younger age groups suggests a slight decline in incidence and prevalence from 2001 to 2002, incidence continues to be high among all age groups. Data on other population groups are limited, and estimates of national prevalence rely on antenatal surveillance systems.

The determinants of this extraordinary epidemic are linked to fundamental elements of the Batswana culture and social structure. The National Strategic Framework cites four categories of determinant: stigma and denial; socio-cultural determinants; socio-economic determinants; and demographic mobility [10]. The majority of those infected in Botswana continue to be ignorant of their status and continue to infect their sexual partners. Those with the disease suffer severe stigma, and few talk openly about their experiences. Women are particularly vulnerable in a culture which subordinates their needs to those of men and in which they have little economic independence. Society at large accepts men having multiple partners and places women under great pressure when they try to protect themselves by changing their own and their partners' sexual practices. Alcohol consumption, especially among the young, is high and has been shown to increase levels of casual, unprotected sex [10].

Socio-economic factors involved in the spread of HIV in Botswana can be represented by a cycle of real or perceived needs and exploitation. People with high levels of disposable income are at risk, since they can exploit situations of relative inequality and exert advantage in the pursuit of sex. Poorer people, however, are also vulnerable, since they may adopt high-risk survival strategies in order to meet their daily needs. This infection cycle also has a gender element, since it is often richer, older men providing support to poorer, younger women in return for sexual favours [10]. In addition, the rapid economic growth over the last 20 years in Botswana has taken place in a highly mobile population. Traditionally, the Batswana often migrated in search of fertile agricultural land. This mobility grew during the colonial era when men migrated to South Africa in search of jobs. More recently, government policy of transfer-

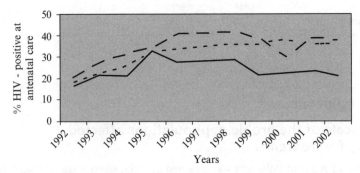

Fig. 12.1 Trend in HIV prevalence among pregnant women, 1992–2002. Solid line, 15–19 years old; dashed line, 20–24 years old; dotted line, 15–49 years old. Source: [4]

ring workers around the country, either on promotion or to ensure equitable availability of services in remote areas, has further contributed to the high mobility. Botswana is also a landlocked country at the centre of the Southern African region, which has been particularly hard hit by the epidemic. Good quality transport networks between countries such as Zimbabwe, South Africa, Namibia and Zambia have contributed to the spread of the epidemic along routes and among transport workers and their sexual partners.

Demographic, economic and health system impact of HIV

The demographic impact of HIV can be seen in the changing structure of the population and its growth rate. Mortality has risen in all age groups. If nothing is done, a third of the current population will die within 10 years and there will be increasing proportions of young and old relative to working-age adults. Life expectancy at birth is a mere 39 years, and it has been estimated that by 2010, life expectancy could be as low as 29 years [5]. By 2015, AIDS deaths will also more than double the national death rate. In 2001, the World Bank projected that by 2015, the population of Botswana would be 1.7 million—some 67% lower than it would have been in the absence of AIDS [5].

The macroeconomic and social impact of HIV acts through its effect on the labour force and is greater than other diseases, since the sexually active population it so disproportionately affects is also the working-age population. The return on government investments to promote foreign direct investment, diversify the economy and create employment will decline during the next 5–10 years as the adult population shrinks, taking with it crucial skills and experience [10]. Apart from directly reducing the number of working people, AIDS will also change the dynamics of skills accumulation in the labour market, making the labour force younger and less skilled or experienced. However, because the Botswana labour force is largely unskilled at the moment, this impact appears lower than might be expected, although it will hinder efforts to raise productivity [5]. AIDS will also affect savings and investment relations, as expenditure by households and governments will reduce the amount of capital. Botswana has succeeded, historically, in building up revenues from diamonds to act as a buffer in periods of lower savings; between 1987 and 1997, gross fixed capital formation averaged 28% of the gross domestic product (GDP). AIDS-related expenditure will erode this safety net [5].

The epidemic will also increase poverty and human suffering within households and communities. Nearly all households in Botswana have now experienced the illness and death of a family member. The number of AIDS orphans was 78,000 in 2002 and is predicted to rise to over a fifth of all children by 2010 [10]. An analysis by the Botswana Institute for Development Policy Analysis showed that HIV will cause a decrease of 8–10% in household per capita income between 2000 and 2010 [11]. HIV forces households to spend more on health and to lose income, with many being pushed over the poverty line as a result. Poor households will be disproportionately affected by the costs of AIDS care and funerals as well as the loss of productive family members [11].

The largest economic impact has been and will be felt in public expenditure, particularly in the health and education sectors. AIDS has weakened the government's capacity to deliver essential services to sustain human development, and, by 2003, Botswana had slipped down the United Nations Development Programme (UNDP) Human Development Index rankings to 125th (from 71st in 1996) out of a total of 171 countries [10]. While Botswana is lucky in having a cushion of high levels of foreign exchange reserves, erosion of these could further hinder local economic investment.

High levels of morbidity and mortality among teachers threaten to reduce the number of staffed classrooms and the quality of teaching, as well as requiring the government to train over 20% more teachers than they would have in the absence of AIDS [5]. As more children are either infected or caring for sick relatives, or supporting their families, school enrolments are expected to decline. Those at school may be traumatized and less able to learn.

The national health system is creaking, and an increasing proportion of public and private health resources are devoted to the care and treatment of HIV patients, who have longer than average hospital stays—9 days as opposed to 5 days for non-HIV patients—and can displace other patients [7]. Identifying the impact of HIV on hospitals is complicated by under-reporting of HIV-positive patients, but in 2000, UNDP published a report showing dramatic rises in hospital death rates among neonates and the 15–44 age group. Confirmed AIDS deaths rose 300% between 1992 and 1997, and by 1996, AIDS was the second most common cause of neonatal hospital deaths [7]. Most hospitals reported rising occupancy rates and overcrowding as well as long hospital stays. Over two-thirds of hospitals reported inadequate staff for increased patient loads and staff burn-out.

A projection of acute hospital bed-day requirements was made in 1999, showing a rise from 323,400 bed days in 1999 to 616,800 in 2010 under a low estimate, or 1,703,000 in 2010 under a high estimate [7]. Such rises have the potential to increase hospital costs massively—with and without antiretrovirals. Hospital costs include simple bed-day management as well as drugs, blood and diagnostic tests. In 2000, real budgets for HIV-related hospital care were expected to double by 2010 [7].

The impact of HIV on primary healthcare services was also assessed in 2000, in terms of both increased volume of patients and a different range of complaints. In Botswana, anecdotal evidence suggests that HIV patient load has increased substantially and that the majority of patients seen are in an advanced stage of disease—in fact often bypassing primary care and going directly to hospitals [7].

The system's response

Overall policy framework and political leadership

Before 1990, when little was known about the spread of the epidemic, the focus of HIV activities was on screening blood to eliminate blood transfusion risks. From 1989 to 1997, under the first Medium Term Plan, other preventive activities, including information campaigns, were initiated, but the response was still fairly narrowly focused. In 1993, the government adopted the Botswana National Policy on AIDS and revised it in 1998 [10]. Subsequently, the health response expanded to include comprehensive education and prevention programmes as well as the initiation of care and treatment, including the provision of antiretroviral therapy (ART). In addition, the second Medium Term Plan (MTP II), which covered the period 1997–2002, established a multisectoral response that aimed to reduce HIV transmission and mitigate the impact of AIDS at all levels of society.

The highest policy-making body regarding HIV is the NAC. Leadership from all sectors in the country is represented in the NAC, which is chaired by the President and co-chaired by the Minister of Health. In 2000, the National AIDS Coordinating Agency (NACA—formerly the National AIDS Control Programme, NACP) was given responsibility for mobilizing and coordinating the multisectoral national response to the epidemic. NACA falls under the Office of the President and is the secretariat for the NAC. High-level political support for the AIDS effort is a new feature of the Botswana response. President Festus Mogae, convinced of the severity of the emergency by a number of economic and demographic studies, personally committed himself to increasing the level of financing and services provided by the AIDS Programme. The President personally chairs the NAC and administers a work plan against which each sector reports progress. At a minimum, meetings are held quarterly, with *ad hoc* meetings arranged for discussion and resolution of special high-priority issues. The personal intervention of the President ensures alignment and maintains performance pressure and a sense of priority across a broad range of stakeholders.

In addition to mandating the introduction of ART, the President has managed to accomplish an about-turn in the national psyche by elevating the level and sophistication of dialogue regarding HIV nationally. However, despite the exemplary political leadership, the country still faces some formidable challenges. The most significant challenge is that most people in Botswana still do not know their sero-status, and prevention programmes to date do not seem to have attained the desired impact. Low testing rates, linked with failure to change behaviour, in the context of such a large burden of disease continue to drive unprecedentedly high incidence rates. The main factors hindering effective implementation and execution of prevention programmes are the lack of skills or expertise in the public sector, lack of non-governmental organization (NGO) and civil society capacity to offer large-scale services, and an overall lack of performance-based incentives for ensuring results.

In 2002, the NAC commissioned a review of the MTP II before publishing its new National Strategic Framework to cover the period 2003–2009. The review recognized the MTP II as a document that provided a conceptual framework for Botswana's national response to HIV but criticized its lack of any formal objectives, implementation structures and processes, and monitoring indicators. Its emphasis on multisectoral involvement in the battle against the epidemic has had a lasting impact, but, beyond that, it has failed to allocate clear responsibilities among the many agencies for specific interventions. Criticisms also included:

- institutional capacity and structures that did not allow for an emergency response;
- a lack of realistic human resource planning;
- inadequate legal and administrative support for stakeholders to deliver their mandates;
- lack of clear target groups for the communication strategy;
- slow scale-up of ART due to inadequate human capacity and systems;
- limited support groups for people living with HIV to break down stigma and denial;
- a weak legal, ethical and human rights framework;
- ongoing gender inequalities and failure to empower women culturally, socially and economically.

In 2003, the National Strategic Framework was published in response to these criticisms [10]. The Framework was developed through a highly consultative strategic planning process, which brought together stakeholders at all levels and in all sectors of society. Key innovations include:

- a greater management focus;
- clear identification and allocation of implementation responsibility;
- mainstreaming of HIV in district and urban development plans;

- provision of indicative resource requirements;
- clear, measurable impact indicators across objectives in all intervention areas.

Its purpose is to inform both the public and implementing agencies with a clear vision of how it intends to reduce HIV incidence in Botswana and its harm by 2016. It includes basic minimum packages for each level of the health system and a monitoring plan, including the establishment of the Botswana HIV Information Management System (BHRIMS) to guide implementation of the national response [12].

While each ministry has a role to play in the HIV response, the new framework puts the health system at the centre (Table 12.3). There are five goals:

- prevention of HIV infection;
- provision of care and support;
- strengthened management of the national response;
- psycho-social and economic impact mitigation;
- provision of a strengthened legal and ethical environment.

All of these goals contain some element for which the health system is responsible. The MoH is charged with a wide range of interventions to prevent, manage and treat HIV (Table 12.3). It is also responsible for surveillance and epidemiological research and provides technical support to the HIV programmes of other organizations.

The Ministry of Local Government is the other key ministry for implementing the Framework through providing care and support to families and orphans affected by HIV and ensuring that HIV is mainstreamed throughout District Development Plans. As a consequence, it is responsible for coordinating all HIV activities at district level. District multisectoral AIDS committees (DMSACs) have been established to coordinate the district-level response, and the village-level response is organized through the village development committee (VDC) and the village AIDS committee (VAC). However, it is not currently clear how specific officials, such as district health officers, will balance the expectations of both DMSAC and MoH plans in their work. This lack of clarity presents a threat to the effective achievement of the Framework's ambitious goals (Table 12.4).

Health education, health promotion and preventive measures and their impact

Prevention programmes in Botswana include public education and awareness, education for young people, condom distribution and education, and prevention of mother-to-child transmission (PMTCT). General public awareness has been based on the 'ABC' (Abstain, Be faithful, use Condoms) model of prevention, promoted through advertising billboards and posters throughout the country. To date, however, little impact has been seen and many people still engage in unsafe sex. Efforts are being made to target public health messages more effectively, including a radio drama, *Makgabaneng*, and workplace peer counselling [13].

The Youth Health Organization (YOHO) is a youth-run NGO that has provided information and sex education to young people at school throughout the country. With their collaboration, the Botswana Ministry of Education has developed HIV education materials. The Ministry of Education has also developed a teacher capacity-building programme with the UNDP and

Table 12.3 Organizations involved in the national multisectoral HIV response

Organization	Role
National AIDS Council (NAC)	Established 1995. Membership includes government, NGO, private sector and PLHIV. Chaired by the President. Overall oversight of implementation of national HIV response. Goal to achieve AIDS-free generation by 2016.
Parliamentary Select Committee on HIV/AIDS (PSC)	Established 1998. Goal to ensure that HIV remains on the economic and political agenda of the government. Meets twice a year, undertakes publicity campaigns and fund raising.
National AIDS Coordinating Agency (NACA)	Established 1999 initially under the MoH. In 2002 shifted to the Office of the President under the Ministry of the State President. Acts as secretariat to the NAC. Specific responsibilities: policy development; coordination and facilitation of implementation; monitoring and evaluation of expanded response; mobilization of resources.
Sector Committees	Several ministries have established HIV committees to guide and develop sectoral responses. Challenges include limited high-level support and participation, lack of clear mandate, funding constraints and lack of HIV coordinators.
AIDS/STI Unit (ASU), Ministry of Health	Established 1992 with the merging of AIDS and STI units. Located in the Department of Primary Health Care Services. Seven technical subunits: clinical management, STIs, home-based care, counselling, IEC, surveillance and research, and NGO coordination. Currently too low ranking—likely to be elevated to department reporting directly to Director of Health Services.
AIDS Coordination Unit (ACU), Ministry of Local Government	Established 2001. Acts as the interface between the districts and the central level. Provides technical assistance to the districts.
District Multisectoral AIDS Committees (DMSACs)	Established 2002/03 in all districts and most subdistricts. Membership includes Heads of Departments, District Councils, NGOs, traditional authorities, the Land Board and Members of Parliament. Participation is not mandatory and there are weak implementation mechanisms. No legal responsibility or accountability for performance.

Sources: [10,12].

supported by the African Comprehensive HIV/AIDS Partnership (ACHAP), the Bill & Melinda Gates Foundation, Merck & Co. and the Botswana government programme that aims to improve teachers' knowledge and de-stigmatize HIV as well as to break down cultural beliefs about sex and sexuality [13].

A social marketing campaign has successfully marketed both male and female condoms in Botswana, and they are widely available. Peer education was conducted through schools, at fairs and festivals, and in shopping malls, workplaces and bars. ACHAP, Population Services International (PSI) and the University of Botswana recently undertook a market research campaign to investigate national attitudes towards sex and condom use that indicated

Table 12.4 Goals of the National Strategic Framework

Goals and impact indicators	Baseline (%) 2001/02	Target (%) 2006	Target (%) 2009
Goal 1: prevention of HIV infection			
% adoption of HIV prevention behaviours of people aged 15–49	34	50	50
% reduction of infants born to HIV-infected mothers who are infected at 18 months	38	50	100
% decrease of the average HIV prevalence in transfused blood and blood products	1	100	100
% decrease in HIV incidence among sexually active population	6	50	80
% decrease in STI incidence among sexually active population	2	50	100
Goal 2: provision of care and support			
% of PLHIV on HAART returning to productive life	n/a	100	100
% reduction in the national bed occupancy rates	50–70	25–50	13–30
% reduction in the national crude mortality rate	12.4/1000	12	11
Goal 3: management of the national response to HIV			
% increase in the number of sectors, ministries, districts and parastatals implementing the NSF minimum HIV response packages	n/a	100	100
% increase in the number of sectors, ministries, districts and parastatals implementing annual planned HIV activities at all levels	n/a	100	100
Goal 4: HIV psycho-social and economic impact mitigation			
% of households with registered orphans receiving care and support for orphans	n/a	100	100
% absenteeism and sickness in government ministries, parastatals and the private sector	n/a	10	5
% reduction of the impact of the epidemic on the economy	n/a	n/a	n/a
Goal 5: provide a strengthened legal and ethical environment			
Composite policy index on number of policies on ethical, legal and human rights issues relating to HIV in circulation to support the implementation of the NSF	0.25	1.0	1.0
National composite index	0.25	1.0	1.0

Sources: [10,12].

considerable unmet need. In response, the government, with assistance from ACHAP, will install 10,500 condom dispensers to provide free condoms to the public [13].

A collaboration between USAID, the African Youth Alliance, the Botswana National AIDS Service Organization (BONASO) and NACA, seven ministries, the defence force, the police force, the University of Botswana, the US Centers for Disease Control (CDC) and ACHAP will initiate a programme targeting mobile populations. Known as the Corridors of Hope, interventions will concentrate on treating STIs, condom promotion and education on safe sex throughout Southern Africa [13].

PMTCT has become a huge priority, with high rates of infection among pregnant women. In 2000, GlaxoSmithKline began providing the antiretroviral drug zidovudine (AZT) free of charge to Botswana for PMTCT, and, although Boehringer Ingelheim donated nevirapine (Viramune®) free of charge from 2001 onward, AZT remains the principal drug used. In the last two quarters of the fiscal year 2003/04, rates of enrolment in the PMTCT programme have varied between 3% and 42% [14,15]. Reasons for non-enrolment include issues associated with fear, type and quality of counselling, socio-cultural norms around breastfeeding, and stigma [8]. A further explanation for poor attendance may be found in cultural attitudes and gender power imbalances. Many women lack the power within relationships to negotiate decisions about sexuality or even their own health. Attitudes toward preventing transmission are complicated further by the need to formula-feed babies, which is highly stigmatized in Botswana society. It is likely that, as treatment becomes more widely available for mothers, their babies and extended families, these attitudes toward prevention may shift. These issues are being addressed through a combination of training, awareness, behaviour change interventions and policy changes.

HIV-related healthcare, including effectiveness, efficiency and acceptability

Comprehensive HIV care and treatment is a central element of the Botswana National AIDS Policy. The programme is made up of voluntary counselling and testing (VCT), preventing, managing and treating opportunistic infections, and ART. VCT is one of the main entry points for accessing other HIV care and, since 2000, the Botswana government, with CDC support, has established a network of *Tebelopele* centres providing immediate, high-quality, confidential services for sexually active Batswana aged 18–49. By January 2004, over 100,000 tests had been conducted across 16 VCT centres. The *Tebelopele* centres are supported by a 'Know Your Status' campaign to encourage people to be tested, marketed throughout the country and on the radio by PSI. Other testing centres are being set up by the Botswana Christian AIDS Intervention Programme, and 250 staff have been trained through ACHAP support since July 2001.

Management of opportunistic infections is also provided free of charge at health centres throughout the country. Tuberculosis (TB) is the leading cause of death among AIDS patients: it is estimated that 75% of TB patients are co-infected with HIV, and about 36% of AIDS patients die of TB [7]. HIV has reversed the gains made by what was previously a very successful TB programme. The annual notification rose from 444 cases per 100,000 population in 1996 to 595 per 100,000 in 2000, an average increase of 8% per year over 4 years, which, if unabated, was expected to result in 11,000 cases per year by 2003. In response, the MoH implemented a National TB Register and piloted an Isoniazid Preventive Therapy programme, which is currently being rolled out to the whole country.

In health facilities, fluconazole (Diflucan®), donated by Pfizer, and co-trimoxazole are available at no cost. However, the impact of these preventive therapy programmes is hampered by low uptake of HIV testing and weak referral linkages between VCT centres and health facilities. Furthermore, most individuals who present to hospitals already have advanced disease and have, therefore, missed the benefits of preventive therapy. The introduction of ART has provided an impetus for testing and may serve as an entry point to promote and increase uptake of preventive therapy services.

Provision of antiretroviral therapy

In March 2001, President Mogae announced that the Botswana government would provide antiretroviral medicine to all those who needed it. The government conducted a needs assessment and committed to paying the bulk of the programme's costs. Ambitious targets were set for programme implementation, and the programme became known as *Masa*, Setswana for 'New Dawn'. The aim in the first year was to build capacity, in terms of human resources, infrastructure, equipment and systems, to serve 19,000 patients at four sites. It was unclear what the actual uptake would be when the programme began. High-priority groups were identified in advance so that health providers would know which patients to prioritize in cases where excess demand required the tightening of eligibility criteria. Adult inpatients with CD4 counts under 200 or AIDS-defining illnesses were prioritized along with those suffering from TB, mothers, children and partners. Otherwise, the programme was launched on a first-come, first-served basis.

In January 2002, the first antiretrovirals were dispensed in Gaborone at the Princess Marina Hospital, and by September 2002, 2200 people had been enrolled and 1500 were on triple therapy. A year later, in September 2003, 12,000 people had been enrolled and over 8000 were receiving treatment across six sites. As of September 2004, over 32,000 people were on ART, plus another 6000 patients on ART in the private sector.

Despite these considerable successes, the Botswana experience also sheds light on the challenges of providing ART, beyond ensuring the availability and affordability of drugs, particularly the recruitment of sufficient trained staff, the maintenance of adequate infrastructure and health system support for service delivery. For example, the initial cohort of patients entering the *Masa* programme was very sick, with an average CD4 count of 50–60 cells/mm^3, requiring 5–10 times more resources than would be required for patients who present with higher CD4 counts. This is driven by low levels of knowledge of HIV status within the population, with most individuals only becoming aware of their status when they fall critically ill. This, in turn, sets up a scenario of perpetually insatiable demand in the absence of significant improvements in testing rates and enhanced links between preventive and treatment programmes. In response to this, Botswana was the first country to implement a national policy of routine opt-out testing, starting at all health facilities in January 2004. Through this policy, HIV is treated like any other disease whereby patients are evaluated, informed of the investigations that are felt to be necessary to determine what is wrong with them—which may include an HIV test—then, barring any objections, are given the necessary diagnostic tests and informed of the results. HIV-negative patients are encouraged to stay negative, and seropositive patients are enrolled in the national antiretroviral programme either for follow-up for those not treatment eligible yet, or for immediate ART for those eligible. The enrolment process involves intensive counselling and preparation of the patient to ensure they understand all the implications of their HIV-positive status, the need to adhere strictly to their treatment protocol, and the need to practise safe sex to prevent infecting partners or possibly transmitting or acquiring resistant strains of virus. All patients are strongly encouraged to identify a treatment 'buddy' who goes through all the initial sessions with the patient and acts as their adherence supporter in the community.

Compared with elsewhere in sub-Saharan Africa, Botswana currently has relatively good capacity in terms of numbers of health workers and facilities. Although achieving the full complement of staff to run the programme will require additional recruitment and infra-structure, there are enough staff to launch the programme and run it for some time, especially if utilization of existing capacity is improved through introduction of efficiency measures. On the other hand, the lack of ART-specific training for staff is a key limitation to scaling the programme up, and the current model of care is concentrated in specialist centres and medically-led. A community-based model that used supervised mid-level providers could dramatically increase capacity, but bureaucracy, labour legislation and health professionals' attitudes toward changing job descriptions have hindered movement in this direction.

The infrastructure for delivering ART is based around hospitals and clinics, which are run through two different ministries. Most hospitals continue to insist on managing routine follow-ups, which would be much better carried out at clinic level to reduce hospital workload and release capacity for new patients. While the cost of drugs is less of an issue for Botswana than elsewhere in the region, upgrading hospitals and clinics to have adequate secure storage and drug management systems remains a major constraint.

In terms of health system support for ART services, lack of in-service ART training and the large number of fragmented and vertical programmes, each with associated non-integrated training programmes, seriously reduce the numbers of functional staff available for individual programmes, even in situations where aggregate staffing appears sufficient. Vertical pro-grammes are partly the result of development partners' concerns with control over resources and implementation as well as programme monitoring. Nonetheless, monitoring and evalu-ation of ART delivery currently needs much more attention and is also a limiting factor in the roll-out of the programme.

Financing HIV services

The cost of paying for HIV varies according to types of treatment, length of incubation period and type of opportunistic infections, and treatment costs have been found to vary between one and four times the Botswana per capita GDP, which is around US$10,000 at purchasing power parity [5]. Public expenditure is also dependent on drug costs and choices, the degree to which AIDS care is in hospital or at home, the degree to which costs are met by private sources—insurance or out-of-pocket—and the ability of the public health service to manage its functions and spend the budgets provided. Before the *Masa* programme, the only ART available in Botswana was through the private sector, largely funded through workplace-related medical insurance schemes. For example, the Debswana Diamond Company covered 90% of costs and employees paid 10%. Healthcare was provided through private practitioners who often had to procure the drugs themselves from South Africa. With the introduction of the National ART Programme, overall availability of anti-retrovirals has improved dramatically. There are currently over 6000 patients receiving

ART in the private sector, and there is a movement to integrate private practitioners into the national programme.

The government anticipates that human resource costs will rise due to the larger number of staff needing training and increased wages among skilled health workers as the labour force declines. The World Bank estimated that 22% more people would need to be trained than would be the case without HIV [5]. Tables 12.5–12.7 provide details of laboratory, drug and other costs according to the most recent data available.

Table 12.5 Costs of laboratory tests

Test	Cost per assay (US$)	Frequency in 1 year	Total (US$)
Screening ELISA	$8.00	1	$8.00
Viral load	$40.00	4	$160.00
CD4	$5.00	4	$20.00
Chemistry	$8.00	4	$32.00
Haematology	$2.50	4	$10.00
Hepatitis	$8.00	1	$8.00
Syphilis	$3.00	1	$3.00
Resistance	$300.00	0	$0.00
Total cost per patient per year			$241.00

ELISA = enzyme-linked immunosorbent assay.
Source: [15].

Table 12.6 Drug costs per patient

Therapy	Components	Cost in US$/year (in 2003)[a]
First line male and post-menopausal[b]	Combivir + EFV	$861
First line pre-menopausal women and children	Combivir + NVP	$329
Second line	DDI + D4T + Nelfinavir	$1335
Third line	Ritonavir + Saquinavir	$1054

Source: [16].
[a]Prices have dropped significantly over the last 2 years.
[b]Male patients on first-line therapy are currently on efavirenz which is donated by Merck & Co.

Table 12.7 Estimated costs of selected policy interventions

Category	Cost per year (million Pula in 1999/2000 prices)	(In millions of US$)	% GDP
Selected prevention			
Preventive MTCT	10	2.1	0.03
Sex education	233	50.3	0.6
Condoms	43	9.3	0.1
VCT	228	49.2	0.7
Selected mitigation			
Orphan care	605	130.7	1.8
Hospital care for PLHIV	1473	318.3	4.3
Old age pension for PLHIV	47	0.1	0.1

Source: [5].

Current data are inadequate, but health expenditure was estimated by the World Bank in 2001 [5] to increase by 80–300% as a result of HIV. Assuming the government would meet 85% of costs, the recurrent health budget would increase 70–270% by 2010. This estimate was made before ART became available and excluded the capital costs of the necessary expansion in health service facilities; for example, in 2001, 60% of hospital beds were occupied by AIDS cases [5].

The financial sustainability of the ART programme was in question from the start. The World Bank suggested [5], before ART was introduced, that healthcare would need to be rationed based on projections of the number of hospital bed-days rising from around 500,000 to 900,000. These estimates will be lower as a result of ART, which, while expensive in itself, saves the health system the cost of managing opportunistic infections.

The government of Botswana currently finances over 95% of the *Masa* ART programme, which is free to all citizens. In addition, ACHAP provided about US$12 million or, 50% of required budget, to support the first year of the roll-out. Building capacity to deliver ART was estimated to cost US$24.5 million in 2002 to cover 19,000 people, with plans for additional capacity for at least 20,000 to be added each year subsequently. It is clear that unless the number of new infections starts to fall, the government will be unable to sustain the necessary expansion to cover all those who need treatment.

A number of donors traditionally supported the Botswana effort to develop HIV communication, health service and mitigation initiatives. These included multilateral agencies such as the World Health Organization (WHO), United Nations Children's Fund (UNICEF), United Nations Population Fund (UNFPA), UNDP and the World Bank. Bilateral agencies, including the US CDC, the Swedish International Development Agency (Sida), the UK Department for International Development (DFID), and the Japanese and German governments, are also present but are not giving substantial sums as Botswana is a middle-income country.

In 2001, a unique programme was established between the Botswana government, the Bill & Melinda Gates Foundation and Merck & Co. to help the country comprehensively combat HIV. The programme is called the ACHAP and provided US$100 million over 5 years to support prevention, ART, care and support programmes in Botswana. Merck & Co. also offered to donate two of its antiretroviral drugs at no cost. In addition to driving many prevention and support programmes, ACHAP provided the necessary technical expertise to the MoH to develop the ART strategy, launch the programme and drive the nationwide roll-out. In December 2004, Botswana rolled out ART to all hospitals in the country.

Conclusion

The government of Botswana is faced with a crisis of emergency proportions. The burden of HIV is one of the highest in the world, and the epidemic is fully generalized throughout the population. There is scant evidence to show that behaviour is changing, although estimates of incidence based on antenatal sero-surveillance among younger age groups suggest it may be beginning to decline, as elsewhere in Southern Africa. This context presents huge challenges for both prevention and treatment programmes, which must develop and scale up in parallel for sustainability and for any impact to be seen.

In Botswana, as elsewhere, an initially weak response rooted in a medical view of public health disease control and centred on the national health system gradually gave way to a multisectoral approach, coordinated by the Office of the President, but lacking adequate resources or a concerted drive for programme implementation. During this time, the role of the health system was largely to spread awareness and engage in a range of apparently ineffective preventive activities among its traditional clients. A number of NGOs and the private sector supported this work, but the multisectoral emphasis of the late 1990s undermined the central role of the national health system. Since 2002, under the new National Strategic Framework, the health system has once again been placed at the centre of the battle against the disease.

The public sector health system of Botswana enjoys the advantage of being relatively adequately resourced in terms of financial and human capacity. A middle-income country as a result of its mineral wealth, Botswana has been prudent with its finances and, as a result, has substantial public savings on which it can draw. The current President, Festus Mogae, has appraised the enormity of the problem and put his full political weight behind the HIV programme.

Nonetheless, this brief review has demonstrated that even in this relatively favourable context, the challenges of managing a multisectoral, comprehensive and effective HIV programme are large. The overall management and structure of the health system is less than optimal and run by clinical staff with little to no management, policy, financial, administrative or planning training. Hospitals and ministries have not appreciably updated management paradigms and systems despite the large change in population size in the last 40 years. As a result, despite having respectable levels of staff and infrastructure on paper, the system has difficulty managing non-epidemic routine health issues and has been extremely stretched in trying to manage the large-scale emergency posed by HIV. International assistance partners, while providing welcome financial resources, inadvertently contribute to health system fragmentation through their requirements for vertical management structures and monitoring and evaluation systems. The need to improve the overall health system is highlighted by the numerous challenges faced in scaling up the ART programme and the ongoing difficulties with developing an effective prevention response.

In conclusion, to date, considering the limitations of its health system's capacity, Botswana has performed very well. In a 2-year period, it has managed to create one of the fastest growing ART programmes in the world and has enrolled a large proportion of its HIV-positive population in therapy, compared with all other similar initiatives in Africa. The country will have to continue to face the challenges dictated by a complex disease affecting 35% of adults and still spreading. Based on the early and strong start that has been made, Botswana should continue to be a source of lessons and inspiration for many other initiatives across the continent.

References

1. Masupu K, Seiphone K, Roels T et al., eds. (2001). *Botswana 2001: HIV/AIDS Surveillance Reports.* Gabarone: National AIDS Coordinating Agency.
2. Masupu K, Seiphone K, Roels T et al., eds. (2002). *Botswana 2002: HIV/AIDS Surveillance Reports.* Gabarone: National AIDS Coordinating Agency.
3. Masupu K, Seiphone K, Roels T et al., eds. (2003). *Botswana 2003: HIV/AIDS Surveillance Reports.* Gabarone: National AIDS Coordinating Agency.
4. UNAIDS. (2002). *Epidemiological Fact Sheet on HIV/AIDS and STIs: Botswana.* Geneva: UNAIDS.
5. Sackey J, Raparla T. (2001). *Botswana: Selected Development Impact of HIV/AIDS.* Washington, DC, World Bank: Macroeconomic and Technical Group, Africa Region.

6. World Bank. (2002). *Botswana at a Glance*. Washington, DC: World Bank.

7. United Nations Development Programme. (2000). *The Impact of HIV/AIDS on the Health Sector in Botswana*. Gaborone: UNDP.

8. United Nations Development Programme. (2000). *Botswana Human Development Report 2000: Towards an AIDS-free Generation*. Gaborone: UNDP.

9. World Bank. (2003). *Health, Nutrition and Population Statistics at a Glance: Botswana*. Washington, DC: World Bank.

10. National AIDS Coordinating Agency. (2003). *Botswana National Strategic Framework for HIV/AIDS 2003–2009*. Gaborone: NACA.

11. Botswana Institute for Development Policy Analysis. (2000). *Macroeconomic Impacts of the HIV/AIDS Epidemic in Botswana: Final Report*. Gabarone: Botswana Institute for Development Policy Analysis.

12. Masupu K, Gboun M, Boadi E, Segotso M. (2002). *Botswana HIV Response Information Management System (BHRIMS): National Plan (2003–2009)*. Gaborone: National AIDS Coordinating Agency.

13. AVERT. (2003). HIV & AIDS in Botswana. URL: www. AVERT.org.

14. Botswana Ministry of Health. (2003). *Primary Health Care Quarterly Report: October–December 2003*. Gaborone: Ministry of Health.

15. Botswana Ministry of Health. (2004). *Primary Health Care Quarterly Report: January–March 2004*. Gaborone: Ministry of Health.

16. Ryan M, Merry C, Coakley P and Barry M. (2003). *Evaluation of Public Private Partnership Models for the Provision of Antiretroviral Therapy in Botswana*. Dublin: National Centre for Pharmacoeconomics.

Chapter 13

Ethiopia

Yayehyirad Kitaw[*], Damen Haile Mariam, Araya Demissie, Dawit Wolday[*], Tsehaynesh Messele, Endalamaw Aberra, Teklu Belay and Afework Kassa

Background

Socio-economic context

With an area of 1.1 million km^2 and situated very close to the equator, Ethiopia shares similar health problems with many tropical countries (Table 13.1). However, since more than 50% of the land, which comprises the water reservoir of the region, is above 1500 m [1], it also shares the health problems of more temperate climates [2].

Ethiopia is home to one of the most ancient settlements of the human race [3,4] and has 3000 years of state history, most of which is characterized by wars of external aggression and internal regional or civil conflicts. In the last 50 years alone, there have been quite a number of civil wars, repeated wars with Somalia and, more recently, with Eritrea, all with clear impact on health development [5–9].

Ethiopia presents a complex picture of ethnic cultures due to influences and exchanges that have taken place among its over 70 ethnic groups and early contacts with various civilizations [8] at different historical periods [7]. In 2002, the population of Ethiopia was estimated to be 67.2 million, of whom 14% live in urban areas. The population is young, with only 5% being over 50 years of age. Fertility, at 6.1 children per woman, is very high, and the current population growth is 2.9% per year. Over 80% of the population resides on the highlands, which comprise only 40% of the land mass; 60% is Christian and 34% Muslim [10,11].

Since 1991, Ethiopia has been engaged in a process of political reform fostering pluralism in politics and decentralization and democracy in governance. The new Constitution (1995) guarantees extensive human and political rights. The Federal State is composed of nine Regional states—structured, essentially, along ethno-linguistic lines—and two autonomous administrations. The government structure is highly decentralized, with extensive powers given to regional states and *woreda*, or district, governments that exist in some 68 zones. The democratization and decentralization process is expected to facilitate a focus on grass-roots problems and ensure more responsive and responsible governance [12–14].

Ethiopia is one of the poorest countries in the world, with real gross domestic product (GDP) per capita of US$810 in 2001 purchasing power parity terms. With a human

---

[*] Corresponding authors.

Table 13.1 Selected health system indicators

Indicators	1996–1997	2001–2002	2015 (estimated)
Estimated population (millions)	58.3	67.2	90
Rural population (as % of total)	—	84.5	—
Population growth rate (%)	2.9	2.6*	2.0
Land area (1000 km²)	1101.0	1101.0	1101.0
Infant mortality (per 1000 live births)	110–128	116*	50
Maternal mortality ratio (per 100,000 live births)	500–700	871	300
Life expectancy at birth	52	45.5*	64
Daily calorie supply per capita	—	1610.0*	—
Underweight children for age, under age 5 (%)	—	47	—
Malaria, no. of cases per 100,000 people	—	556*	—
TB, no. of cases per 100,000 people	—	179*	—
Physicians per 100,000 people	2.6	1.7/2.8	6.8
Population with access to health services, %	45/53	62	90
Population with access to improved water sources, %	—	24*	—
Population with access to adequate sanitation facilities, %	—	15*	—
Contraceptive coverage, %	8	14.6	40
Immunization coverage, %	67	55	90
No. of hospitals (beds)	89	115 (11,710)	—
No. of HCs	246	412	3161
No. of HPs/HSs	2291	3763	15,805
No. of physicians	1470	1888	4405
No. of surgeons and obstetricians/gynaecologists	68	119	—
No. of Health Officers	30	484	3161
No. of nurses	3114	12,823	38,940 + 16,117(J)
Health expenditure (government): total (US$ million)	60.36	69.57	—
Health expenditure (government): per capita (US$)	1.04	1.04	—
Health expenditure: as % of GDP	2.7	—	—
GDP per capita PPP (US$) 2001	—	810*	—
Literacy rate (%)	27.3	29.4	—
Elementary school (7–14 years) gross enrolment ratio (%)	30.1	61.6	—

Source: various Ethiopian government publications and reference [15].
PPP = purchasing power parity.
* UNDP 2003.
(J)=Junior nurses

development index of 0.359, it is ranked 169th out of 174 countries by the United Nations Development Programme (UNDP) [15]. Malnutrition is rampant, with a daily per capita calorie supply of 1610, or less than 75% of daily requirement, and high rates of stunting, wasting and worsening malnutrition in children [16]. Devastating drought and famine strike periodically. Life expectancy is only 54 years and is probably declining because of HIV [10]; the UNDP places life expectancy as low as 45 years [15]. The infant mortality rate of 113 per 1000 is one of the highest in the world. Less than 40% of the population is literate, and the gross enrolment ratio is about 60%.

Smallholder agriculture is the backbone of the economy, contributing to about 48% of GDP, 85% of employment and 90% of export earnings in the mid-1990s. Almost all Ethiopians are poor. The government puts the absolute poverty level at less than US$100 per annum and, by this standard, 45% of Ethiopians—about 30 million people—are below the poverty line. A recent assessment shows that poverty is on the increase as a result of rising unemployment, increased insecurity and rising food prices in urban areas, rainfall variability, declining land fertility, and distance from roads and markets in rural areas.

It is against this background of dire poverty and rural hopelessness that healthcare in Ethiopia must be viewed. The government has formulated an agriculture-led, market-driven economic policy and strategy to alter the situation. The strategy emphasizes the role of the private sector, reducing and redirecting the role of the state, which was dominant in the previous regime, to a regulatory one, to create an enabling environment aimed at reducing market distortions and rigidities and providing incentives to economic growth [10,15–19].

Health system

The health status of the Ethiopian population is very bad. While infant and child mortality, though still high, has decreased sharply over recent decades, adult mortality, on the other hand, has risen sharply, mostly because of HIV and civil conflicts [19]. The maternal mortality rate is one of the highest in the world (Table 13.1) and has shown no significant reduction in the last three decades. Most of the burden of disease is due to infections and malnutrition. The leading causes of disease and death are malaria (556/100,000), tuberculosis (TB) (179/100,000), acute respiratory infections and diarrhoea. Malnutrition is a major underlying factor. Since the first report on the population's health published in 1984, HIV has grown into one of the most important public health problems in the country, affecting a large segment of the urban population and expanding into rural areas [20]. Few have access to safe water, sanitation and health services. Only about 60% of the population live within 10 km of primary healthcare services.

History

The great majority of Ethiopian people still use traditional medicine, self- or lay care. While traditional medicine has time-tested procedures that could usefully be integrated into primary healthcare, there are also some harmful practices such as female genital mutilation, uvula cutting, tonsil scraping and milk teeth extraction [21]. The Ethiopian health authorities formally recognized traditional medicine as early as 1942, but it is still little known and unintegrated.

'Modern' healthcare services, which have had to adapt to various and repeated shocks, including wars and civil strife, were introduced at the end of the nineteenth century, particularly after the Battle of Adwa (1896) in which Italy was defeated, marking a break in colonial aspirations in Ethiopia. From mostly urban, curative and hospital-centred services after the Italian Occupation of the Second World War (1936–1941), attempts were made to move towards more rural and prevention-oriented services with the adoption of the basic health services principle in the early 1950s. The idea was to reach the population through health stations (HS)—one per 10,000 people, or at least one per *woreda* (district)—and health centres (HCs)—one for every 10 health stations, or one per *awraja* (province)—supported by rural and referral hospitals.

Some vertical programmes were initiated. Of these, the Smallpox Eradication Programme was a success. The Malaria Eradication Programme, on the other hand, was an unmitigated failure leading to the serious outbreaks the country is facing today. While the Leprosy Control Programme could claim some qualified success, the TB and sexually transmitted infection (STI) control programmes never really took off. All have been, or are in the process of being, integrated into the general health services.

Twenty years after the adoption of the basic health services principle, at the time of the 1974 revolution, less than 15% of the population had access to health services. The Socialist government (1974–90) adopted the Primary Health Care approach, expanded HSs and HCs, started health posts (HPs) staffed by community health agents (CHAs) and trained traditional birth attendants.

When the current government came to power in 1991, only 43% of the population had physical access to health services. HPs and the CHA system had almost totally collapsed, and health services were still highly hospital- and urban-oriented. The government adopted a sector-wide approach to strategy and has completed its first Health Sector Development Plan (HSDP I, 1998–2002). It is slowly trying to consolidate services in a four-tier system consisting of:

+ Primary Health Care Units, consisting of an HC with five satellite HPs, with comprehensive primary healthcare for 25,000 people;

+ district hospitals with comprehensive out patient and in patient general practitioner care for 250,000 people;

+ zonal hospitals with major specialty care for 1,000,000 people;

+ central specialized hospitals.

Organization and quality of healthcare services

The main healthcare provider is the government, which owns most of the 3563 health stations or HPs, 412 HCs and 115 hospitals. There are also some 1235 private clinics and a relatively large number of drug outlets, of which the rural drug shops, managed by health assistants, constitute an important source of treatment for a large proportion of the population [22].

Modern health services only cover about 60% of the population, with low access in most of the rural, nomadic pastoralist and fringe areas. Coverage is calculated as the estimated number of people living within a 10 km radius of an HC or HS, or normatively with each HC supposedly serving 25,000 people, and each HS 10,000. In fact, because of the very rugged nature of the terrain, the lack of roads—75% of farms are half a day's walk from any road—and lack of transportation, a much lower proportion of the population has real access to these services. In addition, there are financial and cultural barriers, including cost of transport, user-fees, an alien environment, male decision makers and male providers, even for obstetrics.

Currently, most of the facilities, except for the major hospitals, are underutilized, despite the enormous and increasing needs. Whatever is available is often of poor quality and concentrated in urban areas, leading to the paradox of underutilization of scarce resources. The average outpatient consultation rate is only 0.25 visits per person per year and admissions less than one per 100 persons per year. Outpatient care is provided at all facilities, while only hospitals have

24-hour services. Some HCs have beds, mostly for maternity cases. Only the major hospitals and a few of the district hospitals provide emergency surgical or obstetric services because of lack of essential inputs. Only a limited number have, for example, blood transfusion facilities [23]. Even though the new design provides for emergency surgery at the HC level, none has yet started because of lack of trained medical staff. The referral system is weak to non-existent because of distance and poor transport.

Child health services are limited and underutilized. Polio is on the verge of eradication, but the Expanded Programme of Immunization (EPI), which started in 1980 with the aim of full coverage by 1990, has stagnated, with DPT3 coverage (diphtheria, pertussis and tetanus vaccines, three doses) of less than 10% in some regions. It is hoped that it will be reinvigorated by the recent review and support from the Global Alliance for Vaccines and Immunization (GAVI). Integrated management of childhood infections (IMCI) is slowly being implemented.

Antenatal care coverage is low at 34%; less than 25% of pregnant women receive tetanus toxoid (TT2) vaccination, and the number of supervised deliveries remains extremely low at about 10%. None of the HSs and only 40% of HCs provide essential emergency obstetrics or post-abortion care. Family planning services are provided in almost all health facilities, even though choices tend to be limited at lower levels. Community-based distribution is being expanded in most regions, and social marketing of condoms and contraceptive pills has developed quite extensively.

The World Health Organization's (WHO) Roll Back Malaria strategy has been adopted. Treatment is given in all facilities, but most strains are becoming resistant to chloroquine. The Tigray region uses CHAs to give symptomatic treatment. Insecticide-treated nets are being introduced. DDT, in spite of growing resistance, and malathion are sprayed in high-prevalence areas, but these are often discontinued due to logistical problems.

TB and leprosy programmes were integrated into the general health system in 1994. The directly observed treatment, short course strategy for TB (DOTS) and multiple drugs therapy (MDT) for leprosy are being implemented in all regions and have reached 92% of zones and over 90% of woredas, but only in health facilities. All public hospitals and 86% of HCs implemented DOTS, while only 42% of HSs provided treatment due to a lack of acid-fast bacilli (AFB) microscopy. Almost all facilities in prevalent areas provided MDT.

The government promotes the syndromic approach for treating sexually transmitted infections (STIs), and a national STI management guideline was prepared in 2001. A validation study of the approach is under way with support from the US Centers for Disease Control and Prevention (CDC). Overall, STI service provision is limited, particularly in preventive and educational activities, with only about 80% of health facilities, 76% of HSs, 85% of HCs and 80% of hospitals providing treatment.

Quality of care has been a constant concern. To date, no comprehensive quality assessment study has been initiated, even though some have been carried out in specific areas, such as family planning and EPI, or in specific localities. However, given the chronic shortage of essential drugs, the reported inadequacy and poor quality of curative care offered at the lowest levels of the system, the lack of safe water supply at many facilities, the shortage or inappropriate mix of staff in HSs and HPs, the high attrition rates and turnover of staff and the lack, or low quality, of supervision, it is reasonable to assume that the quality of service provided is low [24,25]. The focus in the second Health Sector Development Programme (HSDP II) will be on quality, and the Ministry of Health has recently launched a project on quality of services.

Human resources

There are about 30,000 health workers, excluding those at the lowest level, in the country, or about 45 per 100,000 population, which is very low even by East African standards. The urban centres receive the lion's share. Thus, while the national average of population per doctor is 1 per 59,000, it is about 1 per 110,000 for Afar, an emerging region, as compared with Addis Ababa with 1 per 11,000, Dire Dawa with 1 per 9000, and Harari with 1 per 4000.

Most health facilities are grossly under- or inappropriately staffed, according to Ministry standards. Staffing norms are not based on workload and often lead to false expectations and frustrations among health staff and the population. The adequacy and quality of training of lower cadres have been questioned and are being reviewed. The need to train or re-train general practitioners and health officers in emergency surgery or obstetrics is well recognized, as is correcting the gender imbalance in the workforce.

The public sector has a problem retaining trained staff. In 2002–2003, for example, there were fewer doctors and pharmacists in government employment than there had been 5 years previously at the launching of HSDP I. Certain improvements have been observed with reforms made by government, but continuous monitoring and adjustment will be required. The 'brain drain' of higher-category staff is also a problem.

There is no specific human resource development policy even though there are major unresolved policy issues, including managing the impact of decentralization, intersectoral collaboration, e.g. with the Ministry of Education, which produces a large proportion of health staff, and the implication of the newly introduced cost-sharing scheme for higher education students. Until 2003, higher education had been free, with graduates expected to serve the government for a number of years. As of 2003–2004, students are expected to finance their own studies.

HIV brings additional challenges in terms of requiring more health workers, upgrading training and, more importantly, creating an enabling and supportive environment to motivate workers to apply new knowledge and skills to meet HIV-related needs

Pharmaceuticals

The main priorities of the National Drug Policy (1993) include provision of essential drugs, control of drug distribution and use, capacity building, promoting rational drug use, institutional and technical support for strengthening the drug sector through research and development, improvement of local production, operational research, and review of pharmacy legislation and regulations. All procurement, storage and distribution of drugs for the public health sector is done by the Pharmaceutical Administration and Supply Services, a unit within the Ministry of Health. The Drug Administration and Control Authority, a recently established autonomous institution responsible to a Board chaired by the Minister of Health, is the leading institution for drug policy, regulatory affairs, information, development activities, training and supervision, as well as traditional medicines and veterinary drugs.

The total drug spending per capita amounts to US$1.70 at 2003 prices, of which $0.17 is from the public sector (US$1 = Birr 8.50). Drug expenditure is about 23% of total public expenditure on health. Recently, pharmaceutical funding has increased, from US$7.1 million in 1996–1997 to US$28.8 million in 2001–2002. A substantial part of that increase came from the government's own revenues, which grew from US$7.1 million in 1996–1997 to US$12.2 million in 2001–2002. In the same year, the remaining US$16.6 million came from International Development Agency (IDA) funds and other loans and grants. The objectives of the National Master Plan for Drugs (2002), which is the pharmaceutical component of the HSDP, include regular and adequate supply of effective, safe and affordable essential drugs of high quality in both the public and private sectors, with emphasis on policy, effective drug management and quality assurance. Its main target is to raise the annual public per capita expenditure on drugs from the current level to US$1.25 by 2017 by generating additional and new sources of revenue.

Shortage of drugs and supplies due to inadequate resources and problems in management is the main feature of the pharmaceutical sector in Ethiopia. In addition, lack of adequate and motivated human resources in the public sector makes implementation very difficult. There are also delays in port clearance and inadequate drug storage facilities. Nevertheless, availability of essential drugs has improved over the last few years. Local production is not adequate and currently covers less than 30% of the demand with the production of some 62 items. Quality control is difficult to implement because of lack of personnel and information about drug use. In 2002, there were about 49 private importers of drugs, 311 pharmacies, 314 drug shops and 1876 rural drug shops. Public capacity for supervising the private sector is not adequate, and the quality of the private providers is questionable.

Information, education and communication and environmental health

The importance of health communication as a tool for increasing knowledge and changing attitudes and behaviour towards better health has been recognized in Ethiopia since the adoption of the basic health service concept in the 1950s. Health education and environmental sanitation were the major components of HC activities in those early days. Health education was also given due emphasis, at least on paper, when the primary healthcare approach was adopted in the late 1970s and early 1980s. In the HSDP, the objective of the information, education and communication (IEC) component is to support the development and implementation of a national plan that would improve health knowledge, attitudes and practices regarding hygiene and environmental health and basic knowledge of common illnesses and their causes. Promoting political and community support for health services through advocacy at various levels is also emphasized. A Health Education Centre, a semi-autonomous institution established by the Ministry of Health to develop a national 'strategic vision' for IEC, coordinates all organizations involved in IEC. It is also responsible for producing and disseminating print and electronic materials and providing leadership in monitoring and evaluation, and technical assistance in IEC.

Despite the seemingly high recognition given to IEC, its implementation has faced a number of challenges and constraints. There is no strategically designed health communication intervention programme at national or regional level. In the first phase (1998–2002) of HSDP, it was envisaged that broad national and region-specific IEC strategies would be developed. However, due mainly to lack of local expertise and appropriate leadership, the plan has not been realized. There is an acute shortage of trained and qualified IEC professionals at all levels. To alleviate the problem, the government, with the support of the United Nations Population Fund (UNFPA), started training health education specialists at the Jimma University Health Science Institute in the 2003/04 academic year.

Efforts so far at the national and regional levels have not moved beyond the production of materials whose relevance to the vast majority of the rural, illiterate population with diverse cultures and languages is highly questionable. In most cases, these materials are not based on market research and, therefore, fail to address the health communication needs of the various segments of the population. There is little or no use of folk and traditional media for disseminating health messages. There is also little coordination among the different players in IEC, resulting in duplication of efforts and conflicting messages.

Provision of a safe and adequate supply of water, development of safe solid and liquid waste disposal mechanisms, promotion of the health and safety of workers through sanitary education, and proper inspection of imported foodstuffs and establishments where food is prepared have been identified as the ways of promoting environmental health in the HSDP. Although nationally the number of trained sanitation workers has shown a modest increase, 75% of their time is spent on inspection of catering establishments, leaving very little time for other important environmental health activities. There is very little involvement of donors, non-governmental organizations (NGOs) and other stakeholders in this work.

Management: monitoring and evaluation

The HSDP is governed by a Central Joint Steering Committee (CJSC) consisting of representatives of the Ministry of Health and the Ministry of Finance and Economic Development (MOFED), plus donors. These includes the World Bank, WHO, USAID and the government of Norway, and one NGO representative. Joint Steering Committees (JSCs) were established at regional level but had difficulties remaining functional. There is a plan to establish *woreda*-level JSCs. Previously, the CJSC used to oversee both health and education, but separate CJSCs were established with the recent reform of government structure.

With the decentralization and structural adjustment programme of the early 1990s, the Ministry of Health was slimmed down and most of its administrative responsibilities devolved to the regions. However, it retained responsibility for formulation of policies and supervision of their implementation, determination of standards, issuing of licences and qualification of professionals, and establishing standards for research and training, even though most of its technical departments were downsized or amalgamated with others. Thus, for example, HIV had a dedicated department with a relatively large technical staff. With restructuring, HIV came under the AIDS and Other STI Prevention and Control Team in the Department of Disease Prevention and Control.

Under the federal system, Regional Health Bureaus (RHBs) responsible to their Regional Councils are in charge of health systems in their respective regions. Regions are organized on similar lines to the Ministry of Health. Decentralization below regions to *woreda* levels was launched in 2002–2003, and *woreda* health offices are expected to become the main actors in the health system. The *woreda* health management system is evolving, with variation in structure and staffing patterns between regions. The most important challenge in the next few years will be capacity building to improve the skills of, and give support to, health managers, and empowerment of *woreda* health offices, especially in human resources and finance. However, regional training centres have been weakened as staff are transferred to *woreda* health offices, making it more difficult to provide training to *woreda*-level staff.

Financing and expenditure

In 2000–2001, public expenditure in Ethiopia as a percentage of the GDP was 1.8% on health, 4.8% on education and 6.8% on the military [15]. The Ethiopian health sector is financed through government revenues, aid from donors, external loans and user-fees. Health insurance payments and other local contributions are not significant sources of financing. The total health expenditure in 2002–2003 was US$171 million, representing approximately US$2.64 per capita per annum. Of this, about 52% was private out-of-pocket spending. On average, about 61% of the recurrent health budget was allocated to salaries and 26% to medical supplies and drugs. A large part of the recurrent expenditure, about US$21 million (34%), was spent on the country's 82 public hospitals, while only US$17 million was spent on primary healthcare services. Capital expenditures also appeared skewed, with about US$7.2 million spent on hospitals in 2001–2002 compared with US$3.1 million for primary care facilities.

A Health Care Financing Secretariat within the Ministry of Health is working to identify and obtain additional resources for the health sector. Innovative ways of complementing and increasing efficiency in the use of public resources, such as revolving drug funds and community insurance schemes, are being explored. There may also be scope to increase user-charges at public facilities that have proper strategies for assuring quality of services and provide a waiver mechanism for the poor. In addition, the new Health Extension Programme is expected to result in a major shift of public sector resources from high-cost curative services to preventive services, as well as rectify the highly pro-urban bias in the current resource allocation pattern.

Future development

The Ethiopian population is expected to reach 90 million by 2015, but no major demographic transition is expected, even though the contraceptive prevalence rate will reach 40%. In the HSDP II period, the trend is toward expansion of services focusing on HCs and modified HPs. Improvement in quality of services by improving the technical competence of health workers and ensuring regular supplies of drugs and medical supplies is stressed. By the end of HSDP II, an additional 1460 HPs, 140 HCs and six district hospitals are planned, increasing coverage from the current 52% to 65%.

To improve the health status of the majority of the population, the government is giving greater priority to the prevention and control of communicable disease through active community participation. To achieve these objectives, the government has introduced a Health Extension Package (HEP) as a component of the Primary Health Care Unit policy. Through the HEP, it is hoped to provide communities with equitable access to essential preventive health services. The active involvement of communities will ensure sustained preventive health actions and increased health awareness. The extension services are provided as a package, focusing on preventive health measures such as health education, sanitary education, immunization, family planning, and prevention of HIV, malaria and TB, and targeting households, in particular women/mothers at the *kebele* (neighbourhood) level. A new category of exclusively female health workers, called Health Extension Agents, will be trained and deployed. There will be two Health Extension Agents in each *kebele*, and they will be accountable to the nearest HC.

The significance of the HEP is that the government has recognized the importance of community-based health services and has committed resources to them. Previous initiatives to train and deploy community health agents were on a voluntary basis and supported mostly by NGOs or donor agencies. It was not possible to ensure their sustainability as there was no government financial commitment.

The HSDP goal is to achieve total coverage by 2015, with 3161 Primary Health Care Units. This was projected to require a minimum of US$1.5 billion, but will have to be revised as HSDP II alone is estimated to cost US$0.8 billion.

The government's ability to reach these spending levels for HSDP II is based on expectations that external loans and grants will finance about 21% of the 3-year programme and that facility revenues will bring in another 11%. This calls for, among other things, cost containment and efficient utilization of resources. Budgeting, resource management and financial accounting procedures need to be strengthened at health facility levels.

In Ethiopia, the government has been the major provider, as well as funder, of the health sector. However, with the recognition of the existing under-financing and the inability of the government to meet the growing need for modern care, the government is encouraging the participation of the private sector in the delivery and financing of the sector. The number of private institutions in the country is expected to increase rapidly. In 2001, there were 12 (10%) private and eight (7%) NGO hospitals, and 1235 (23%) private clinics in the country.

It is unlikely that there will be any significant increase in government allocations to the health sector. Instead, methods to increase efficiency in the use of existing resources, such as the use of market incentives in public health facilities, including subcontracting of facilities, creating conditions for hospital autonomy and privatizing some components of the public healthcare delivery system, are expected to multiply. Other measures include revisions to the user-fee exemption system and raising the level of, or instituting new, user-fees in addition to updating the level of financial accounting, budgeting and resource management at all levels. The heads of RHBs are accountable to their respective Councils, and there has been a rapid turnover in RHB leadership because of the political nature of appointments. In some regions, transparency in funding and human resources management has been questionable. The most glaring deficiency has been in financial and activities reporting due to lack of trained staff and high turnover. This has put the fund absorption capacity of the system under strain. It is hoped that recent civil service reform will correct major deficiencies.

The HIV epidemic

The current scale of the HIV problem and populations affected

HIV infection in Ethiopia is acquired predominantly through heterosexual contact and perinatal transmission from infected mother to child. As in several other developing countries, surveillance results conducted among pregnant women attending antenatal clinics are the main indicators of the scale of the HIV problem in Ethiopia [26,27]. According to the Ministry of Health, based on results of sero-surveys from 66 sites, the national adult HIV prevalence rate for the year 2003 among pregnant women aged 15–49 was estimated at 4.4% [28]. The average prevalence rate for urban areas was 12.6%. In Addis Ababa, the capital of Ethiopia, the prevalence of HIV among ANC attendees was 12.3% in 2003, while in the rural areas the average prevalence was 2.6%.

Age-specific HIV prevalence rates show that the highest burden is among the age group 15–24 years and, to a slightly lesser extent, among the age group 25–34 years, indicating that the population in the most productive age group is the most affected by the HIV epidemic. Females are generally infected at a younger age than males.

The results from most recent surveillance data indicate that the HIV epidemic has affected a large segment of the urban population aged 15–49 years. Current estimates from UNAIDS using a range of data sources put the national prevalence at between 3 and 7% in this age group.

Of 72,000 army recruits, 10,000 of whom lived in urban and 62,000 in rural areas prior to recruitment, the HIV prevalence was 7.2% in urban recruits, ranging from 4.3% to 10.5% depending on the region. Among rural recruits, HIV prevalence was 3.8%, but the majority were farmers (57%) and students (18%) with an HIV prevalence of 2.7% and 2.6%, respectively [29]. Regional rural HIV prevalence ranged from 3.2 to 4.3%, with marked differences at zonal levels.

It is known that over 90% of HIV in children is acquired through mother-to-child transmission (MTCT). It has, however, been estimated that the rate of vertical transmission is between 29 and 47%, although further data are absent [30]. The prevalence of HIV infection among adolescents and young adults is also not well known.

Trends

The HIV epidemic in Ethiopia started during the early 1980s. The first two HIV cases were identified in 1984 from sera collected from patients presenting with Bell's palsy [31]. The first two AIDS cases were reported in 1986 [32]. Although the prevalence of HIV was low in the 1980s, thereafter the epidemic increased steadily in various population groups in the major urban areas throughout the country. For instance, in Addis Ababa, the HIV prevalence rate increased from 4.6% in 1989 to 12.3% in 2003 (Fig. 13.1) [28,33–35]. However, the prevalence of HIV infection declined in young women aged 15–24 years in Addis Ababa between 1995 and 2003 (Fig. 13.2). The findings indicate reductions in newly acquired infections in Addis Ababa, most probably attributable to changes in sexual behaviour, since similar trends were observed with respect to syphilis seroprevalence in this population [36]. However, prevalence in rural areas is increasing.

Data on reported AIDS cases from hospitals around the country are available for the years 1986–2003 [28]. More than 90% of the affected patients are aged between 15 and 49 years, with the male to female ratio being almost equal. The peak ages for AIDS cases are 25–29 years for both males and females. In addition, there have been a significant number of AIDS cases reported among young children. At the end of 2001, 15,202 new AIDS cases were reported and a cumulative total of 107,575 AIDS cases had been officially reported to the Disease Prevention and Control Department of the Ministry of Health [28]. However, these reported cases represent only the tip of the iceberg. There is no doubt that the number of reported cases is substantially lower than the actual number of cases due to problems in recognition, diagnosis and reporting of AIDS. Thus, the Ministry of Health estimated that by the end of 2003, the number of AIDS cases was approximately 219,400. The number of people infected with HIV is even more uncertain and is officially estimated to be 1.5 million, of whom 170,000 are thought to be children [28]. Current WHO/UNAIDS estimates ranged between 950,000 and 2.3 million.

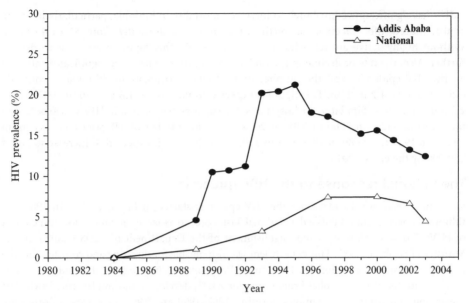

Fig. 13.1 Trends in HIV prevalence, 1984–2003.

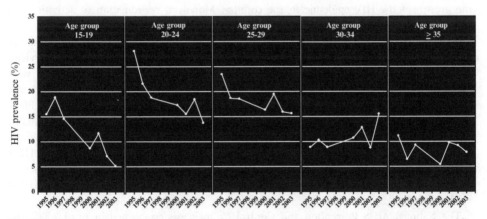

Fig. 13.2 Temporal trends in age-specific HIV prevalence rates in antenatal clinic attendees in Addis Ababa, 1995–2003.

Projections

The epidemic in Ethiopia was characterized by a steep rise in the HIV infection rate between 1984 and 1994. This was followed by a moderate increase between 1994 and 2003. It has been projected that the epidemic will level off at a prevalence rate of around 7%. In addition, it is estimated by WHO/UNAIDS that the number of AIDS cases will increase to about 300,000 in 2010 and the number of people living with HIV (PLHIV) will increase from around 2.0 million to 2.6 million in 2006 and to 2.9 million by the end of 2010.

HIV has significantly contributed to increased mortality in Ethiopia, particularly in young adults. Indeed, life expectancy at birth has decreased significantly, from 53 to 45 years. Without highly active antiretroviral therapy (HAART), this figure is expected to decline further. Also, the rate of decline in the under-5 mortality rate has been significantly affected by the HIV epidemic, and the number of HIV-related orphans in Ethiopia is currently estimated to be 1.2 million. This figure is expected to increase to 1.8 million in 2007 and to 2.5 million in 2014. Similarly, the hospital bed occupancy rate related to HIV was expected to increase from 42% in 2000 to 54% in 2004 [37]. The number of TB cases increased from 50,000 in 1984 to 82,680 in 1989 and to 150,000 in 2001. It is expected to increase to about 250,000 by the end of 2014.

The national response to the HIV epidemic

It has now been two decades since the HIV epidemic started in Ethiopia [31]. In 1985, the Ethiopian government established a National Task Force to assist in the prevention and control of HIV. This was followed by the establishment of the Department of AIDS Control in the Ministry of Health in 1987. This department was responsible for directing and coordinating the implementation of the National AIDS Control Programme. The Ministry of Health, in collaboration with the WHO's Global Programme for AIDS, developed and implemented two HIV prevention and control programmes covering 1987–1990 and 1992–1996 [38]. Efforts were made in the areas of IEC, condom promotion, surveillance, patient care and expansion of HIV testing laboratories. Despite the above efforts, however, the interventions had little impact on the growth of the HIV epidemic in the country. Moreover, coordination of activities and programme integration between stakeholders were not adequately addressed.

With the HIV epidemic situation worsening and the Ethiopian government realizing the enormous implications in terms of human suffering, social effects and costs of health services, the Ministry of Health drafted a National HIV/AIDS Policy, through consultation with stakeholders, accompanied by an implementation strategy. During the first half of 1998, the Ministry of Health and the Regional Health Bureaus formulated HIV/AIDS Strategic Plans for the period 2000–2004 for all nine regions and two city administrations [39–41]. Finally, National AIDS Priority Strategies for the period 2001–2005 were identified. This provided a national strategic framework for implementation of the Ethiopian Multi-Sectoral HIV/AIDS Project (EMSAP) [42]. The government approved a comprehensive HIV policy in August 1998 to provide an enabling environment for a multisectoral approach to the epidemic [43].

The National AIDS Prevention and Control Council was established in April 2000. The Council is headed by the President and consists of members from sector ministries, regional states, NGOs, religious bodies and representatives of civil societies and associations of people living with HIV. The council oversees the implementation of the federal and regional HIV plans, examines and approves annual plans and budgets, and monitors plan performance and impact. The Council has also appointed a National HIV/AIDS Board of Advisors to oversee the plan. A National HIV/AIDS Prevention and Control Secretariat (NACS) was also established under the Prime Minister's Office to coordinate and facilitate the EMSAP, supported by the World Bank [44]. In 2002, NACS was restructured and renamed the HIV/AIDS Prevention and Control Office (HAPCO). The EMSAP is one of the first two multicountry HIV programmes financed by the World Bank in sub-Saharan Africa. The EMSAP approach has been used as a model for many other HIV projects in Africa [44].

Priority intervention areas to prevent the spread of the epidemic include:

- IEC and behavioural change;
- condom promotion and distribution;
- voluntary counselling and testing;
- management of STIs;
- blood safety and universal precautions;
- prevention of MTCT (PMTCT) of HIV infection;
- care and support of PLHIV;
- human rights legislation;
- surveillance and research.

HIV care and treatment

HIV prevention and control activities in the country are financed by various partners that include the government, external agencies, donors, and civil and religious organizations. The total budget was set at US$37 million for 2001–2002 and US$43 million for 2002–2003. In addition, about US$20 million was directly channelled through NGOs and donors in 2001–2002. Even though substantial funding seems to be available for these activities, utilization usually lags behind, mainly due to low implementation capacity. According to projections, the country needs approximately US$140 million per year for preventive programmes and an additional US$30 million per year for antiretroviral treatment (ART) in order to reduce the current level of HIV prevalence of 6–7% to 5% in 2010 and to 3% in 2020.

Several guidelines for HIV care and treatment have been developed. These include guidelines on voluntary counselling and testing (VCT), PMTCT, home-based care, prevention and treatment of opportunistic infections and ART. In 2002, the Ministry of Health issued a policy on supply and provision of antiretroviral drugs in Ethiopia [45]. This policy emphasizes the government's key role not only in ART supply, but also in the coordination and facilitation of international research collaborations to develop an ART programme that is feasible and clinically appropriate for Ethiopia. Specifically, the policy on supply of antiretroviral drugs in Ethiopia states that:

- government shall supply ART for PMTCT to the appropriate healthcare institutions;
- antiretroviral drugs shall be exempted from taxation, shall be supplied at a reduced price through government negotiation with manufacturers, importers and distributors, and shall be purchased through a system of bulk and generic substitutions;
- government shall encourage the establishment of international antiretroviral initiatives and programmes in Ethiopia;
- government shall create an enabling environment for international research in Ethiopia so that citizens can access antiretroviral drugs by willingly participating in research projects.

The policy also specifies that ART should be started in a few centres of excellence to allow for adequate analysis of basic clinical, epidemiological and socio-behavioural aspects of ART in Ethiopia.

In February 2003, the Ministry of Health prepared a guideline for use of antiretroviral drugs in Ethiopia [46]. Since then, training on ART has been given to more than 800 healthcare workers, comprising clinicians, nurses, counsellors, laboratory technicians and pharmacists. A total of 31 public and private hospitals have started prescribing ART. Moreover, as an initial step toward a national ART programme, the Ministry of Health established a series of regional HIV laboratories to monitor ART treatment countrywide. These 13 sites are equipped with facilities for CD4 count and HIV viral load determination and will serve as referral centres. After evaluating the initial ART programme, it was extended to district hospitals and HCs.

Currently, generic antiretroviral drugs are available at a cost of around US$30–40 per month from private institutions only. The low price was achieved through government negotiations with drug companies. A total of 9500 people are now being treated with ART. The Ministry of Health is planning to increase access to drugs for non-paying patients through several mechanisms, such as involving NGOs, the Global Fund to Fight AIDS, Tuberculosis, and Malaria, and the US President's Emergency Plan for AIDS Relief. In 2005, a total of 45,000 patients will benefit from the programme and, by the end of 2008, it is anticipated that a total of 250,000 patients will be receiving ART [47].

The Tikur-Anbessa Teaching Hospital, affiliated to the Faculty of Medicine of Addis Ababa University, has been very active in preventive MTCT over the last 2 years. The NIGAT project, in collaboration with The Johns Hopkins University, is conducting the biggest nevirapine clinical trial in the country, involving the Tikur-Anbessa Hospital and several HCs within the vicinity of Addis Ababa. In addition, four hospitals and 18 satellite HCs near Addis Ababa, in collaboration with UNICEF, have recently initiated PMTCT programmes that include nevirapine. The Ministry of Health, in collaboration with CDC-Ethiopia, has initiated a project called HAREG involving an additional 23 health facilities throughout the country [48].

Conclusion

Overall, the government of Ethiopia has shown great commitment in tackling the problems posed by the HIV pandemic in the country. The magnitude of the epidemic in the major urban settings appears to be stabilizing or even lessening, but in rural settings it is on the increase. Although much effort has gone into overcoming the problems described above, much still needs to be done to strengthen these efforts, particularly to reduce the effects of HIV in rural areas. This will call for more national, international and bilateral organizations to work together.

References

1. Mesfin Wolde Mariam. (1972). *An Introductory Geography of Ethiopia.* Addis Ababa: Haile Selassie I University.
2. Kloos H, Zein ZA, eds. (1993). *The Ecology of Health and Disease in Ethiopia.* Boulder, CO: Westview Press.
3. Greenfield R. (1965). *Ethiopia: A New Political History.* London: Pall Mall Press.
4. Johansson D, Edey M. (1981). *Lucy: The Beginnings of Mankind.* New York: Warner Book Edition.
5. Rubenson S. (1976). *The Survival of Ethiopian Independence.* Addis Ababa: Kuraz Publishing Agency.
6. Tadesse Tamirat. (1972). *Church and State in Ethiopia, 1270–1527.* Oxford: Clarendon Press.
7. Levine DN. (1974). *Greater Ethiopia.* Chicago: The University of Chicago Press.
8. Pankhurst R. (1990). *A Social History of Ethiopia.* Addis Ababa: Institute of Ethiopian Studies.

9. Bahru Zewede. (1991). *History of Modern Ethiopia, 1855–1974*. Addis Ababa: Addis Ababa University Press.

10. Ministry of Health. (2002). *Health and Health Related Indicators*. Addis Ababa: Ministry of Health.

11. Central Statistical Authority (CSA). (1998). *The 1994 Census*. Addis Ababa: CSA.

12. Transitional Government of Ethiopia (TGE). (1994). *The System of Regional Administration in Ethiopia*. Addis Ababa: TGE.

13. Federal Democratic Republic of Ethiopia. (1995). Proclamation to Pronounce the Coming into Effect of the Constitution of the Federal Democratic Republic of Ethiopia (FDRE), Proclamation No. 1/1995. Addis Ababa.

14. Tafesse Olinka *et al.* (2003). *Topics in Contemporary Political Development in Ethiopia*. Addis Ababa: Addis Ababa University Press.

15. United Nations Development Programme. (2003). *Human Development Report 2003*. New York: Oxford University Press.

16. Central Statistical Authority and OCR Macro. (2001). *Ethiopia Health and Demographic Survey 2000*. Addis Ababa: CSA/OCR Macro.

17. Ministry of Finance and Economic Development. (2002). *Sustainable Development and Poverty Reduction Programme*. Addis Ababa: MOFED.

18. Ministry of Finance and Economic Development. (2002). *Development and Poverty Profile of Ethiopia*. Addis Ababa: MOFED.

19. United Nations Economic Commission for Africa. (2002). *Economic Report on Africa, 2002*. Addis Ababa: ECA.

20. Ministry of Health. (2002). *HIV/AIDS in Ethiopia*. Addis Ababa: Ministry of Health.

21. Buschkens WFL, Slikkerveer LJ. (1982). *Health Care in East Africa: Illness Behaviour of the Eastern Oromo in Harraghe (Ethiopia)*. London: Van Gorcum Assen Publishers.

22. Kloos H, Etea A, Degefa A. (1987). Illness and health behaviour in Addis Ababa and rural central Ethiopia. *Social Science Medicine* 25(9):103–9.

23. Ministry of Health/World Health Organization. (1999). *An Assessment of Reproductive Health Needs in Ethiopia*. Geneva: WHO.

24. Health Sector Development Plan. (2001). *Report of the Mid-term Review Mission*. Addis Ababa: Ministry of Health.

25. Health Sector Development Plan. (2003). *Report of the Final Evaluation of HSDP I*, Vol. 1. Addis Ababa: Ministry of Health.

26. Ministry of Health. (1999). *National Sentinel Surveillance Guideline for Ethiopia*. Addis Ababa: Ministry of Health.

27. Kebede D, Aklilu M, Sanders E. (2000). The HIV epidemic and the state of its surveillance in Ethiopia. *Ethiopian Medical Journal* 38:283–302.

28. Ministry of Health. (2004). *AIDS in Ethiopia*, 5th edn. Addis Ababa: Ministry of Health.

29. Abebe Y, Schaap A, Mamo G *et al.* (2003). HIV prevalence in 72,000 urban and rural male army recruits, Ethiopia. *AIDS* 17:1835–40.

30. Muhe L. (1997). A four-year study of HIV seropositive Ethiopian infants and children: clinical course and disease patterns. *Ethiopian Medical Journal* 35:103–15.

31. Tsega E, Mengesha B, Nordenfelt E *et al.* (1988). Serological survey of human immunodeficiency virus infection in Ethiopia. *Ethiopian Medical Journal* 26:179–84.

32. Lester FT, Ayehunie S, Zewdie D. (1988). Acquired immunodeficiency syndrome: seven cases in an Addis Ababa Hospital. *Ethiopian Medical Journal* 26:139–45.

33. Ministry of Health. (1998). *AIDS in Ethiopia: Background, Projections, Impacts, Intervention*, 2nd edn. Addis Ababa: Ministry of Health.

34. Ministry of Health. (1996). *AIDS in Ethiopia: Background, Projections, Impacts, Intervention.* Addis Ababa: Ministry of Health.

35. Wolday D, Messele T, Melesse H *et al.* (2003). Temporal trends in HIV seroprevalence in women attending prenatal clinics 1995–2003, Addis Ababa, Ethiopia. Unpublished ENARP data.

36. Tsegaye A, Rinke de Wit TFR, Mekonnen Y *et al.* (2002). Decline in prevalence of HIV-1 infection and syphilis among young women attending antenatal care clinics in Addis Ababa, Ethiopia: results from sentinel surveillance, 1995–2001. *Journal of Acquired Immune Deficiency Syndrome* **30**:359–62.

37. Ministry of Health. (2000). *AIDS in Ethiopia: Background, Projections, Impacts, Intervention,* 3rd edn. Addis Ababa: Ministry of Health.

38. Ministry of Health. (1991). *The National AIDS Control Programme of Ethiopia, Second Medium Term Plan 1992–1996.* Addis Ababa: Ministry of Health.

39. Ministry of Health. (1999). *Summary. Federal Level Multi-Sectoral HIV/AIDS Strategic Plan 2000–2004.* Addis Ababa: Ministry of Health.

40. Ministry of Health. (1999). *Summary. Regional Multi-Sectoral HIV/AIDS Strategic Plan 2000–2004.* Addis Ababa: Ministry of Health.

41. Ministry of Health. (1999). *Strategic Framework for the National Response to HIV/AIDS in Ethiopia for 2000–2004.* Addis Ababa: Ministry of Health.

42. National AIDS Council. (2001). *Strategic Framework for the National Response to HIV/AIDS in Ethiopia (2001–2005).* Addis Ababa: NACS.

43. Government of the Federal Republic of Ethiopia. (1998). *Policy on HIV/AIDS of the Federal Republic of Ethiopia.* Addis Ababa.

44. Okubagzhi G, Singh S. (2002). Establishing an HIV/AIDS programme in developing countries: the Ethiopia experience. *AIDS* **16**:1575–86.

45. Ministry of Health. (2002). *Policy on Antiretroviral Use in Ethiopia.* Addis Ababa: Ministry of Health.

46. Ministry of Health. (2003). *Guidelines for Use of Antiretroviral Drugs in Ethiopia.* Addis Ababa: Ministry of Health.

47. Ministry of Health. (2004). *Antiretroviral Therapy Implementation Plan for Ethiopia.* Addis Ababa: Ministry of Health.

48. Centers for Disease Control-Ethiopia. (2004). *President's Emergency Plan for AIDS Relief (PEPFAR)— Country Operational Plan for Ethiopia.* Addis Ababa: CDC-Ethiopia.

Chapter 14

Nigeria

Adeniyi Ogundiran, Bayo Fatunmbi and Berhe
T Costantinos[*]

Background

The Federal Republic of Nigeria is the most populous black nation in Africa, with a population of 120 million in 2002 [1]. It occupies an area of approximately 924,000 km^2 just north of the equator, between the Republic of Benin, Niger Republic, Chad and the Cameroon, and is bordered on the south by the Atlantic Ocean. Its tropical climate supports agricultural activities all year round.

There are an estimated 30 million children under 5 years of age living in Nigeria. The annual population growth rate is 3%, and adult literacy averages 56%. Two-thirds of the population (66 million) lived below the poverty line in 1996, as compared with one-third (18.3 million) in 1980. Over 60% of the population, including 54% of Nigeria's poor and 85% of the very poor, live in rural areas.

Agriculture was the main source of revenue in Nigeria until the 1970s. Since then, oil has become the main source of income and accounts for over 90% of national government revenue. Other sources of income are industry, solid minerals and small-scale enterprises.

System of government

Nigeria was defined as a nation following the amalgamation of the southern and northern protectorates of the British West African colony in 1914 and became independent in 1960. It is made up of 36 states and one federal capital territory, Abuja, and is divided into six geopolitical zones for administrative purposes (Fig. 14.1). Lagos remains the major commercial capital.

The country has been governed under both parliamentary and military systems in recent times. In 1999, the country moved to a democratic, presidential system of government after 13 years of military rule. The President and Head of State, who is also the Commander-in-Chief of the Armed Forces, heads the Federal Executive Council consisting of the ministers and heads of the army, police and national parastatals. There are two federal legislative houses—the Senate and the House of Representatives—which are responsible for enacting laws in line with the constitution. The President also chairs the meetings of the Council of States, comprising Governors of the 36 states and the Minister of the Federal Capital Territory.

The states constitute the second tier of government. Each state has its executive, the State Executive Council headed by the Governor; legislature, State House of Assembly headed by the

* Corresponding author.

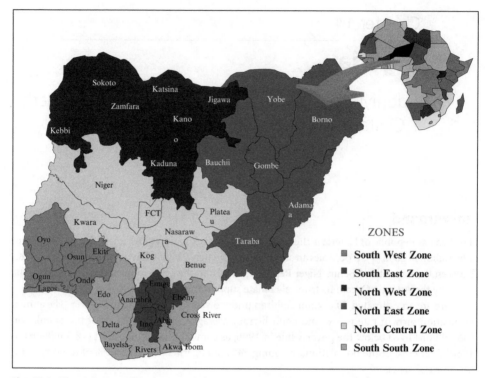

Fig. 14.1. Nigeria's geopolitical zones and states. Source: [2].

Speaker; and judiciary, headed by the State Chief Judge. The states are semi-autonomous, in line with the federal constitution. Local councils constitute the third tier of government, under the supervision of the State government. There are 774 Local Government Areas (LGAs).

The health system

History

The colonial era (1900–1960)

British colonial rule began around 1900, and with it came health services provided by the British Army Medical Services, mainly for colonial officials, local civil servants and, later, their relatives. These services were subsequently extended to the indigenous population who lived in neighbouring areas. This arrangement, complemented by the efforts of missionaries, formed the foundation of Nigeria's healthcare delivery system.

In 1946 came the first attempt at formulating a 10-year welfare development plan, managed by colonial officers with no involvement of the general populace. Although the plan was a failure, largely due to lack of coordination and broad involvement, it served as the basis for subsequent plans. By 1960, missionary organizations accounted for about 75% of health facilities, although these Western-style services were considered culturally unacceptable and, therefore, were grossly underutilized.

Post-independence (1960–1999)

During the immediate post-independence period of the early 1960s, effective community participation gradually increased, and health-related matters were given more attention in a series of National Development Plans, culminating in the adoption in 1988 of the National Health Policy and Strategy to Achieve Health for All by the Year 2000. The adoption of this historic document under the leadership of Professor Olikoye Ransome-Kuti, then Minister of Health, was influenced by the population's overall poor state of health and the resulting negative impact on all sectors of Nigeria's economy. The situation was characterized by high mortality rates from common preventable diseases, a high crude birth rate and low life expectancy of 50 years.

The period from 1988 to 1993 saw significant improvements in the health sector. However, a sudden downturn in the Nigerian economy, which had hitherto relied heavily on oil, had negative effects, compounded by an unstable political environment and the withdrawal of external assistance from some bilateral donor agencies. The situation worsened with the imposition of sanctions on the Nigerian government. All of these actions dealt a severe blow to the physical, mental and socio-economic well-being of average Nigerians [3]. The brain drain from vital professions, especially in the health sector, accelerated in the early 1990s, affecting the economy as a whole, and health workforce development and healthcare provision in particular.

By the mid-1990s, the population's poor state of health was exacerbated by a rapidly decreasing rate of immunization coverage, from over 80% in the early 1990s to less than 50% a few years later, an indicator that the healthcare system was working poorly. The increasing scourge of fatal diseases, including HIV, prompted a National Health Summit in September 1995, which resulted in the Abuja Health Declaration. According to Ekpo, the objectives of the Summit were to appraise the national health system, examine the factors militating against its improvement and plan strategies for an effective, efficient and equitable system [4]. The result was a revised National Health Policy and the Developed Health Plan of Action.

Emerging democracy (1999 to the present)

Nigeria's emerging democracy has brought about increased involvement of diverse stakeholders, including civil society groups and communities, in all levels of governance. The decision-making process, particularly in matters relating to health, is no longer restricted to military juntas and their civilian cohorts. Elected representatives of the people in the executive and legislative arms of government are fast adjusting to the democratic culture of consultation and negotiation under the watchful eyes of the judiciary.

In coalition with other democratic governments, regional and global initiatives have been established or strengthened to promote democracy and development. An environment favourable to foreign investment is being promoted, and political stability is attracting technical and financial support from development partners. Legislation to promote healthy living and prevent harmful practices has been drafted, a good example of which is the New Partnership for African Development (NEPAD). Despite recent democratic developments, the health system remains weak. In 2000, the WHO ranked Nigeria's health system 187th out of 191 countries in the world [5]. Box 14.1 summarizes the current health of the population.

Box 14.1 **Health indicators, 2003**

Infant mortality rate	100/1000 live births
Under-5 mortality rate	201/1000 live births
Maternal mortality rate	800/100,000 live births
Life expectancy at birth	53 years
Crude birth rate	40/1000 population
Total fertility rate	5.7
Full immunization coverage of children aged 12–23 months	13%

Source: [6].

The current system

Philosophy

The guiding principle behind the organizational structure and the strategy to achieve 'Health for All' is that the health sector is vital to the development of other socio-economic sectors. The principle states that: 'Federal, State and Local Government shall support in a coordinated manner a three-tier system of health care. Essential features of the system shall be its comprehensive nature, multisectoral inputs, community involvement and collaboration with non-governmental providers of health care' [7]. This principle was fully upheld in the revised Nigerian National Health Policy and Health Plan, in which the roles of other sectors were given prominence.

Financing and expenditure

Health has always been viewed as a social service, to be paid for from recurrent government tax revenues in a Beveridge-style system. Previous administrations, especially civilian ones, tended to declare free universal healthcare to be a citizen's right, without always being clear how this commitment was to be paid for. As a result, households still face substantial user-charges to access services.

Public expenditure

A vital indicator of a government's commitment to health is the amount it allocates to health services and health-related activities, in both absolute and relative terms (see Tables 14.1 and 14.2). The relatively weak financial commitment to the health system is illustrated by the low health budget over the years, much lower than the World Health Organization's (WHO) recommended minimum of 5% of the gross domestic product (GDP). Public spending on health is less than US$5 per capita per year compared with the US$14 recommended internationally. Compared with the other sectors such as defence, communications, transport and industry, health is poorly financed. There is great disparity between the allocations approved and the actual amount released, and a tendency for more to be spent on health than budgeted

Table 14.1 Actual expenditure as a percentage of approved budget allocations to the Federal Ministry of Health

Year	Health budget as % of total national expenditure	Actual amount released as % of approved budget (%)	
		Recurrent	Capital
1980	1.9	94	71
1981	2.6	99	78
1982	2.0	127	65
1983	2.3	107	69
1984	1.8	121	83
1985	1.1	106	92
1986	2.4	103	162
1987	1.4	137	181
1988	2.0	146	64
1989	1.8	106	95
1990	2.4	121	163
1991	1.4	109	264
1992	1.1	187	100
1993	2.3	100	100
1994	2.8	150	101

Source: [8].

Table 14.2 Trend in relative sectoral allocation of Federal Government capital expenditure (%)

Sector	Capital expenditure (%)						
	1988	1989	1990	1991	1992	1993	1994
Health	1.9	1.5	1.3	0.5	0.6	0.6	1.5
Agriculture	7.9	11.5	6.7	4.3	2.4	4.4	4.3
Transport and communication	5.6	3.7	1.8	1.6	0.9	2.2	2.1
Education	3.9	2.6	1.7	1.1	1.3	2.4	4.0
Housing	9.3	8.0	5.4	3.2	2.9	4.8	3.6

Source: Central Bank of Nigeria (CBN), 1994; and UNDP 1997.

for. Also, health recurrent and capital spending appears to be rising as a percentage of the federal budget.

Public–private mix in expenditure

In 1990, according to the World Bank, the private sector paid for 60% of total health expenses, the public sector paid for 34%, while international aid accounted for 6% [9]. Per capita expenditure on health at that time was as low as US$10 per year. The pattern of private healthcare financing has not been well documented. A study in Oyo State, for example, showed that the main sources of funding were revenue generation from user-charges, drug revolving fund schemes, loan systems such as the Health System Fund Project, which was World Bank-assisted, community financing and charitable donations from local and international development partners.

Despite the abundance of resources in the Nigerian private health sector, a coordinated mechanism for harnessing these resources to serve the wider population, especially the poor, is yet to be established. The National Health Insurance Scheme (NHIS), a pre-paid healthcare financing and cost-sharing mechanism that aims to ensure that the vast majority of the poor who are in serious need of health services are covered by the contributions of the few healthy rich, tries to address this. This is currently limited to pilot projects organized by the Federal Ministry of Health (FMoH). The success of this cost-sharing strategy will depend on the commitment of all concerned in the NHIS.

Organization of provision

Public sector healthcare is provided at three levels, corresponding to the three tiers of government described above. Each tier of government provides technical support to the tier below it. There is a parallel private healthcare system as well as traditional medicine. At the tertiary level, highly specialized services for specific diseases are provided at the teaching hospitals and specially designated centres such as the National Orthopedic Hospital, Lagos. They offer specialized medical services and workforce training in all fields to health personnel from within and outside the country. They sometimes have community outreach affiliates. Regular research activities are undertaken at this level. Secondary healthcare services include general medical, surgical, paediatric and community health services, and are available at the district and zonal levels within the 36 states and the Federal Capital Territory. The activities are supported by specialized services such as laboratory, diagnostic, blood bank, mortuary and physiotherapy, among others. They also serve as administrative and referral centres for the peripheral primary healthcare centres, the majority of which, due to lack of resources, are not able to cope with these responsibilities.

The cornerstone of provision is primary healthcare. At the primary healthcare level, preventive, curative, health promotion and rehabilitative services are carried out and backed up by referral support services. Under an integrated health services approach, the following services are delivered: general health education to promote health; immunization; food supply and balanced nutrition; adequate supply of potable water and maintenance of sanitation; provision of essential drugs; maternal and child health, and family planning; treatment of minor ailments and injuries; and control of communicable diseases. Mental and oral health provision have recently been added.

Inter-sectoral collaboration is encouraged between health and other sectors such as agriculture, finance, science and technology, public works and housing, education, communication and information. Public health policies, rather than healthcare policies, are developed to promote health, prevent diseases and enhance the quality of healthcare services.

Public–private mix of provision

Ownership of healthcare facilities varies with the level of care. According to Olumide [10], in some urban centres as much as 96% of secondary (acute) healthcare is in the hands of private providers. These providers include allopathic healthcare providers such as hospitals, medical clinics, maternal and child welfare centres, pharmacies and physiotherapy clinics, among others, owned by voluntary, not-for-profit non-governmental organizations (NGOs) and private for-profit individuals and groups. The 'non-orthodox' healthcare providers include the traditional healing homes, maternity homes and spiritual healing centres.

In terms of the number of hospitals and clinics, the private for-profit sector has 56 units, followed by the 42 local government, 17 state and seven mission hospitals and clinics. However, the number of patients served in each sector is inversely related to the number of units. This may be explained by the size of the hospitals and the case mix type in terms of patients treated, among other factors.

In 1991, there were 203,184 allopathic, Western-style healthcare workers practising in Nigeria, of whom 9% were physicians and dentists, 31% registered nurses, 26% registered midwives and 16% other primary care workers [11]. A fifth of these health workers were in private practice [12]. This contrasts markedly with the high numbers of 'non-orthodox' healers, estimated by Ademuwagun [13] to constitute about 4% of urban and 10% of rural populations. In 1996, the Management Development and Policy Advisory Agency (MAPAA) reported that in Oyo State, missions (NGOs) served 58% of all the patients sampled, state government hospitals and clinics treated 20%, private for-profit 13% and local government hospitals 10% of patients sampled [14].

The HIV epidemic

Prevalence

The first AIDS case in Nigeria was reported to the FMoH and was made public by the Minister of Health in April 1986. It was reported in a 13-year-old female hawker. Neither the route of transmission nor other determinants could be established prior to death. Subsequently, isolated studies on various aspects of HIV supported by donors and bilateral government agencies were undertaken. Notable among these was the series of government-driven nationwide sentinel studies defining the point prevalence and trend of the epidemic in the country. National sentinel surveys were conducted according to WHO guidelines and with the participation of personnel from the WHO, the US Centers for Disease Control (CDC), universities and various other technical partners. The estimates and projections were based on the following:

- current population figures for the states obtained from the national census;
- annual demographic health survey for the calculation of growth rate;
- data from the National Populations Commission for the calculation of urban and rural populations and distribution;
- the assumption that infection rates for males and females were equal.

The national prevalence rates were obtained by determining the median rates from all 86 sentinel sites in the country in 2001. Averages of the values from 2–5 sites in each state were used to estimate the prevalence rate for each of the states.

The first survey conducted in limited sites across the country in 1991 showed a national prevalence rate of 1.8% among women attending antenatal clinics (ANCs). The values increased to 3.8% (1993), 4.8% (1995), 5.4% (1999) and 5.8% (2001; Fig. 14.2). New sites have been recruited over time, providing wider coverage and, consequently, greater credibility to the results.

During the early stages of the epidemic, the rates were generally below 2% in all states. However, the sites surveyed were limited, with a slight bias towards urban centres. By 1993, figures as high as 10% were emerging in some states. In 1999 and 2001, the survey detected

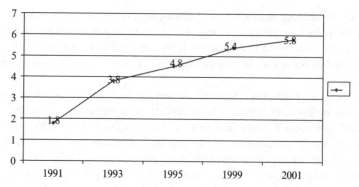

Fig. 14.2 Trend of HIV prevalence among antenatal care attendees, 1991–2001.

more sites with prevalence above 10%, while there were still sites with prevalences below 1%. In general, the North West (below 5%) and South West (below 10%) zones of the country had low prevalences. However, it appears that there were high and low prevalences at both urban and rural sites. Indeed, one of the conclusions of the 2001 survey was that there was no significant difference between the urban and rural prevalence rates in Nigeria. There is need, therefore, for future assessment to address issues relating to urban–rural spread.

There appear to have been different but simultaneous epidemics in different parts of the country. While the epidemic reached high levels in the centre of the country in 1995 (7.5–10%), these levels remained stable until 2001. In other parts of the country, prevalence remained below 5%, even by 2001. However, the prevalence rates continued to increase in many areas. It is estimated that the national prevalence ranged between 4 and 8% in 2003.

The differences between the sites with low and high prevalence rates are not readily explicable, although varying socio-cultural factors could plausibly account for them. Some of these factors include: access to information; access to facilities; access to preventive interventions, such as condoms; literacy rates; socio-cultural practices; separation from families; and prevalence of other sexually transmitted infections (STIs).

In Nigeria, as in all other parts of the globe, there is no age limit to HIV infection. Both HIV and AIDS have been reported among a range of age groups in the country. However, the modal group for HIV infection still remains young adults. The groups most affected are between the ages of 15 and 29, with the highest preponderance in pregnant women aged 25–29 years attending ANCs (Fig. 14.3). This is so across the country. In comparisons within the country, the HIV prevalence rates among youth aged 15–19 were highest in the South South zone of the country in 2001.

HIV prevalence rates seem to be the same for both sexes. However, since there are not many studies, this area needs more attention, especially when women seem disproportionately affected by the impact of widowhood and make up 52% of people living with HIV (PLHIV). The estimated number of PLHIV aged between 15 and 49 years and alive in 2003 was between 2.4 million and 5.4 million out of a total population of 120 million.

National studies are not yet available on the prevalence of HIV among children and infants. An estimated 100,000 HIV-positive children are born annually, and thus it is estimated that one HIV-positive child is born every 5 minutes. According to UNICEF, at the end of 2001, 270,000 children under 15 years of age were HIV-infected and a million were orphaned. A WHO

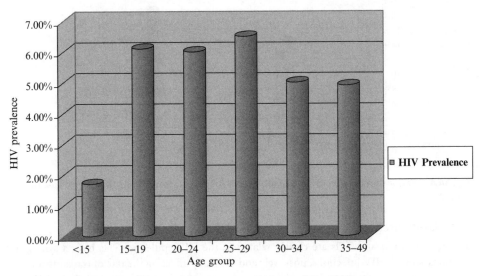

Fig. 14.3 Age distribution of HIV prevalence among ANC attendees, 2000.

Monitoring Mission, which reviewed the Antiretroviral Drug Access Programme in September 2002, recognized the lack of programmes for Nigerian children affected by HIV and recommended development and implementation of a paediatric antiretroviral drug programme.

The HIV virus

Both types of HIV are present in the country, and they are found in all zones. However, the more predominant of the two is HIV-1. National prevalence of HIV-1 in 2001 was 97.5%, while HIV-2 was 0.4% and mixed HIV1/2 was 0.1%. The distribution by zones is shown in Table 14.3.

Table 14.3 Zonal HIV prevalence by type in Nigeria

Zones	HIV-1	HIV-2	Co-infection
South East	92.90%	7.10%	0.00%
South West	98.00%	2.00%	0.00%
South South	98.10%	0.97%	0.00%
North East	99.00%	0.70%	0.00%
North West	96.40%	3.60%	0.00%
North Central	97.80%	1.50%	0.70%

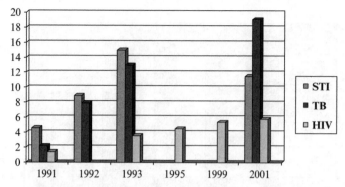

Fig. 14.4 Relationship between HIV, STI and TB in Nigeria. Source: Federal Ministry of Health (2003).

Associated diseases

Tuberculosis (TB) and STIs are closely related to the HIV epidemic. STIs have a synergistic relationship with HIV infections, positively and mutually affecting the rate of transmission and disease progression. Studies were carried out to describe trends in TB between 1991 and 2001 by the TB unit of the Ministry of Health. Figure 14.4 shows increasing prevalence rates of TB and HIV during the period. Although the prevalence rates are higher for TB than for HIV in all years, both infections increased during the period of comparison.

For STIs, different organisms show different rates across the country. The most common ones, however, are gonorrhoea and chlamydia. Attempts were also made to capture the rates of syphilis during the ANC seroprevalence surveys. The rates are similar to those of HIV over the years. However, it should be noted that they are only indicative of cumulative infections, as the tests used are antibody-based. As shown in Fig. 14.4 the prevalence rate of STIs generally rose, in line with TB and HIV, between 1991 and 1999. There was a decline in the rate in 2001.

Impact of the epidemic

The effect of the HIV epidemic in Nigeria is multifaceted, involving social, economic and medical dimensions. Although not many studies have been carried out on its impacts, evidence has accrued to indicate that the epidemic has generated orphans, increased medical expenditure, affected many officers and men of the Nigerian Army and is possibly affecting national productivity.

Response to the epidemic

In 1986, the military government set up a Technical Advisory Committee to advise the government on HIV. Later, the National AIDS Programme was established in the FMoH, subsuming an existing STI unit. A national coordinator was appointed. Correspondingly, State AIDS Programme Coordinators and Local Government and Action Managers were approved by state health ministries and local government health departments. However, the level of response in this period was very low. Emphasis was on health education and prevention of infection. Most programmes and interventions were driven by the WHO, the UK Department for International Development (DFID), the European Union (EU) and Family Health International's AIDS

Control and Prevention (AIDSCAP) project. The federal government drew up plans and made pronouncements, but without serious financial backing.

Upon the re-establishment of democratic government in 2000, a Presidential Committee on AIDS was established, chaired by the President and composed of key ministers. A technical arm of this committee, the National Action Committee on AIDS (NACA), was also established to advise the presidency. NACA is a multisectoral body involving representatives from all relevant line ministries, including Health. Its role is to implement a multisectoral response to the epidemic alongside the National AIDS and STI Control Programme (NASCP), which is responsible for the health sector's part in the response.

In collaboration with partners, NACA developed the interim HIV Emergency Action Plan (HEAP) that identified over 200 activities for implementation between 2001 and 2004. Most of the activities were conceived as short-term, high-impact interventions to form the basis for a medium-term strategic plan for HIV.

The health sector response under NASCAP involved the establishment of the following programmes:

- Antiretroviral Access Programme coordinated by the ARV Committee;
- Prevention of mother-to-child transmission (PMTCT) of HIV, coordinated by the PMTCT Task Force;
- Voluntary counselling and confidential testing (VCT) coordinated by the VCT Task Team;
- Surveillance, coordinated by the Central Management Committee;
- Other sectoral supports in the Education, Labour, Youth and Sports ministries.

In 2002, the Nigerian government started its antiretroval therapy (ART) programme. In early 2005, 25 public centres provided ART to an estimated 13,500 people. Other centres that provide ART include the private sector. While the annual cost per person for prescribing ART is around US$750 in the public sector, the cost is around US$2500 per annum in the private sector. In December 2004, the National ART Scale-up Plan was launched, with a national consensus meeting in February 2005 on the Health Sector HIV Strategic Plan. The government is dealing with generic companies for the procurement of generic ART drugs, while plans have also been drawn up for the local manufacturing of ART drugs.

The current national targets for putting people on ART are 200,000 by the end of 2005 and 1 million by 2010. The government has been able to mobilize both local and international partners for scaling up HIV therapeutic and preventive services, including the US President's Emergency Plan for AIDS Relief (PEPFAR), the World Bank, DFID and other multilateral, bilateral and local organizations.

The recent strengths of the Nigerian response have are a strong national level of political commitment, a network of health facilities, a pool of human resources, high demand for treatment and the potential for local production of antiretroviral drugs. However, on the whole, the pace of scale-up of ART has been slow, with a limited monitoring and evaluation system unable to track ART status adequately in the private and public sectors. Procurement processes, including supply chain management, are weak, though this is currently being addressed, while the cost of treatment remains high for most people. Implementation of grants from the Global Fund to Fight AIDS, Tuberculosis and Malaria has been problematic, and to date the private for-profit and not-for-profit sectors have not really been involved in the response.

Conclusion

The health system in Nigeria is widely regarded as ineffective and inefficient. To stand any chance of developing a more effective response to HIV, the system needs extensive reform. This needs to be built on strategic partnerships within and between the local, state and national levels of all actors involved in health and development. The capacities of ministries to support the overall national HIV response need to be improved. Also, despite recent attempts to galvanize the private sector to support the ongoing national response, its involvement is still very low and needs to increase.

Some of the components of any effort to develop a more effective response include:

+ active social mobilization, communication, consultation and involvement of national and local stakeholders in decision making;

+ better, more effective management systems to ensure policy implementation and improved use of resources;

+ development and transfer of appropriate health technology to enhance community development;

+ developing a financing system based on private and public sector collaboration, and with increased public spending on the health system;

+ defining a 'minimum package of services' with particular emphasis on HIV and other priority diseases.

It appears that if these directions are diligently pursued, the health system in Nigeria will be able to respond appropriately not only to the HIV epidemic, but also to other diseases.

References

1. The Federal Government of Nigeria/National Population Commission. (2002). *National Population Data by States.*

2. The Federal Government of Nigeria/National Malaria Control Programme. (2001). *Strategic Plan to Control Malaria in Nigeria 2001–2005.*

3. Odebiyi AI, Ojofeitimi EO, Ragun. (1996). Effect of political crises on health in Nigeria. *Nigerian Journal of Health Planning and Management* 1(2).

4. Ekpo M. (1996). The National Health Summit: a strategy for the development of a national health plan. *Nigerian Journal of Health Planning and Management* 1 (2).

5. World Health Organization. (2000). *Health Systems: Improving Performance.* Geneva: WHO.

6. National Population Commission. (2002). *Nigeria–2003 Demographic and Health Survey, Key Findings.* Abuja: NPC.

7. WHO/UNICEF. (1978). *Alma Ata 1978. Primary Health Care.* Geneva:WHO.

8. Federal Ministry of Health. (1995). *National Health Plan, 1996–2005.* Abuja: Ministry of Health.

9. World Bank. (1994). *Statistical Indices. Development in Practice. Better Health in Africa—Experience and Lessons Learned.* Washington, DC: World Bank.

10. Olumide E, Aderonke A. (1996). Improving the Nigerian health care system. Discussion paper. In: Dare OO, Kale OO, Fatunmbi BS, eds. *Better Health in Africa: Nigerian Perspective.* Ibadan: CHESTRAD.

11. Federal Ministry of Health. (1991). *Nigerian Health Profile.* Abuja: Ministry of Health.

12. Erinosho L. (1996). Managing human resources, infrastructures and equipment in Nigeria. In: Dare OO, Kale OO, Fatunmbi BS, eds. *Better Health in Africa: Nigerian Perspective.* Ibadan: CHESTRAD.

13. Ademuwagun ZA. (1969). The relevance of Yoruba medicine men and public health practice in Nigeria. *Public Health Reports* **84**(12).

14. Management Development and Policy Advisory Agency (MAPAA), Oyo State HSF, World Bank. (1996). *Detailed Cost Analysis of Selected Health Facilities in Oyo State, Nigeria.* Technical Report (Survey).

Chapter 15

Senegal

Chris Simms, Papa Salif Sow and Elhadj Sy*

Background

Sex, blood and procreation are important elements of every African culture. They constitute milestones in the life cycle, and shape people's personal relationships and social bonds. They express values and beliefs about life and death, friendship, love, care and support, and call for self-esteem and respect for others. They are, however, surrounded by mystical and metaphysical considerations that make it difficult for most societies to talk about them openly. HIV strikes at the very heart of this complex system, and thus leaves nobody unmoved. Individuals, families and nations react in the face of the epidemic. Reactions range from fear, denial, stigma and discrimination, to the best responses for prevention and care.

Senegal is one of a handful of countries that have adequately responded to the epidemic and have so far successfully contained the spread of HIV. Over the last two decades, it has maintained prevalence rates in the total population at about 1%, one of the lowest rates in sub-Saharan Africa. The social cohesion and stability of the country provided fertile ground for a timely, robust and effective response to the crisis, which constitutes a model of best practice.

Senegal's response to the epidemic was influenced by the country's history, culture and institutions, and reflects the arrangements for healthcare that existed before the pandemic. Political leadership and conservative sexual mores were both important in the fight against HIV, together with Senegal's long tradition of taking a pragmatic and participatory approach to primary prevention. At the same time, there are a number of challenges that the government and people of Senegal will need to confront in order to contain the threat of HIV fully, and avoid the risk of rising prevalence rates particularly generated by periods of economic crisis.

Government and society

Senegal is located on the tip of West Africa, bordering the North Atlantic Ocean, between Guinea-Bissau and Mauritania. It has a population of 10.8 million that is growing by 2.5% annually, and a fertility rate of 4.84 births per woman. With independence from France in 1960, Senegal inherited the French administrative structure: 10 regional administrative units, each with three department administrative districts that are, in turn, divided into *arrondissements*. It

* Corresponding author.

also inherited a legal system based on French civil law whereby the head of state is the President, who selects the head of government, the Prime Minister.

Senegal's strong democratic tradition and vocal free press since independence have made it attractive to the international community; consequently, it has received large amounts of aid, about twice the average for Africa. From a civil society point of view, Senegal has a tradition of participation by people and their different organizations in socio-economic life. This has resulted in a peaceful co-existence between the market and civil society in every aspect of life, including trade and health. Organizations such as trade unions, non-governmental organizations (NGOs), professional societies, microfinance organizations, farmers' groups, private schools and private medical practices are strong. Senegal has a modern, well-educated and broadly informed elite in addition to, by regional standards, a sizeable middle class. The political system, in addition to being democratic, is broadly participatory.

Economy

Senegal is a poor country, with a gross national product (GNP) per capita of US$600. Fifty-seven per cent of the population lives below the poverty line. More than 60% of the adult population is illiterate, and there is low primary school enrolment, especially for girls. It ranks 154th on the United Nations Development Programme (UNDP) Human Development Index, mainly due to its literacy deficits. The first two decades of development post-independence were loosely based on a policy of a 'state-controlled and regulated economy, national economic planning, and "African Socialism", a system based on nationalization of the peanut trade and rural cooperative development, while still leaving room for foreign capital and the private sector' [1]. During the period 1967–1993, the long-term rate of real per capita income growth was a dismal –0.35%. Senegal is seen by the World Bank as having tremendous potential, much of which, however, has been squandered by poor economic policies. The economic situation has only improved since the 50% devaluation of the Communauté Financière d'Afrique (CFA) franc in 1994, which has led to a significant fall in inflation.

Senegal's economic record is typical of many countries in sub-Saharan Africa during the first decades after independence. In the late 1970s and early 1980s, confronted with a huge debt burden, world recession, an oil crisis and falling commodity prices, the government adopted the World Bank's and International Monetary Fund's stabilization and structural adjustment programmes (SAPs). While the contribution of these policies to economic growth is questionable, there is a widely held view that they had a negative impact on the livelihoods of already vulnerable populations by reducing incomes and increasing unemployment, increasing prices for essential goods and contributing to a decline in government social services. The World Bank [2] and International Monetary Fund [3] now acknowledge serious errors in SAPs by failing to take proactive steps to protect services that benefit the poor, such as primary healthcare (PHC), to deal explicitly with the social dimensions of adjustment, and to take into account the distributional effects of their policies on the lives of ordinary people. The World Bank now concludes that by the late 1990s, 'after a decade and a half of structural adjustment, there seem to be too few positive and sustainable results, particularly in sub-Saharan Africa' [4].

As a case in point, the 1994 devaluation of the CFA franc by 50% in francophone countries impoverished urban households that could no longer afford imported produce, and forced them to switch to local, less nutritious produce. Research shows that this loss of nutritional quality led to significant increases in malnutrition [5]. Poor Senegalese households were hit hard by the fact that cheaper local rice was less nutritious [6]. UNDP reports that in urban areas between 1992 and 1996, there was a 27% and 21% rise in the proportion of children who were stunted and underweight, respectively; there was, in addition, a rise in urban infant mortality. Risk analysis of the social and economic factors that influence levels of vulnerability to HIV indicates that, as a result of the economic upheaval caused by the CFA devaluation, some of the poor and newly impoverished were forced into prostitution. This analysis also showed that the devaluation made Senegal more affordable to tourists and business visitors, which in turn led to a rise in the number of local women becoming sex workers (SWs), on either a professional or a casual basis [7].

In addition to poor economic growth and high levels of poverty, Senegal is a country of significant inequalities. It is repeatedly described as a country of two nations: 'One is approaching middle-income levels. It has access to a middle-class level of education, public services, health care, housing, financial services, social protection and urban amenities. The other, larger nation exists near or below the poverty line. It is rural or lives in urban slums and is ill-fed, ill-clothed, ill-housed, insecure and uneducated' [8]. The Gini index of income inequality is 41.3 (range 0–100). National survey data from 2001 showed that the lowest income quintile was responsible for 5.2% of consumption, while the highest bought 50% of consumer goods; in rural areas, where 59% of the population lived, 42% of private consumption was observed; Dakar had 23% of the population and 38% of private consumption. In Dakar, the daily expenditure was 7285 CFAF compared with 3779 CFAF in rural areas [8].

Gender inequalities are also evident in Senegal: women's income level is 55% that of men; economic participation is 62% that of men; and women's literacy rate is 58%. Senegal ranks 128th on UNDP's Gender-related Development Index. Table 15.1 presents data showing the percentage of women receiving delivery assistance at birth by area of residence and level of education for the 5 years preceding district health system surveys carried out in 1986, 1991 and 1997. Insofar as 'rural' and 'uneducated' can act as proxies for 'poor', these data are consistent with the notion that urban and educated women have substantially better access to healthcare than women living in rural sectors and those with no education.

Health

Despite poor economic growth, Senegal had made enormous improvements in some human welfare indicators. During the period 1960–1995, infant mortality fell from 174 to 70 deaths per 1000 live births, and under-5 mortality from 303 to 110 deaths per 1000 live births, while life expectancy at birth increased from 38 to 50 years. Key to explaining these improvements were large increases in health expenditure devoted to primary prevention activities, including maternal and child healthcare and simple curative interventions. In fact, Senegal is frequently cited by demographers as a classic example of a country able to achieve huge mortality reductions by providing essential healthcare rather than better standards of living. For example, a study of a rural area of Senegal shows that under-5 mortality rates fell from 350 to 81 per 1000 live births between 1960 and 1990 [10]. It concluded that the 'drop in mortality mainly results from improved access to new and efficient health services—a dispensary and a maternity clinic—and from growth of surveillance, health education, vaccination and malaria programmes initiated in the 1960s and 1970s. Although socio-economic conditions have changed in the area, the

Table 15.1 Percentage of women receiving delivery assistance at birth, by area of residence and level of education for the 5 years preceding surveys in 1986, 1991 and 1997

	Total	Area of residence		Level of education	
		Urban	Rural	No education	Secondary or higher
EDS-I 1986	21.8	47.5	8.1	17.2	54.9
EDS-II 1991	45.4	80.6	26.8	38.2	82.4
EDS-III 1997	43.8	74.1	29.0	36.2	70.8

Source: Enquête démographique et sanitaire (EDS) 1986, 1991, 1997 [9].

influence of classical factors such as women's educational level and improvement in transportation has probably been limited' [10].

These impressive gains notwithstanding, cross-country data show that compared with other countries in the region, and taking into account levels of per capita income, human development indicators are generally weak. For example, maternal mortality rates remain high at 690 per 100,000 births, and only about one-third of rural women receive trained delivery service at births. Some human development indicators worsened in the 1990s: UNICEF reports that the infant mortality rate had increased from 74 to 79 deaths per 1000 live births, and under-5 mortality from 127 to 138 deaths per 1000 live births, respectively, between 1996 and 2002. The percentage of underweight children increased from 22% to 23%; stunting, from 23% to 25%; and wasting, from 7% to 8% during the same period [11]. The World Health Organization (WHO) reported that childhood immunization rates also worsened: Bacillus Calmette–Guerin (BCG) coverage that had averaged 90% in the 1980s and mid-1990s was 77% in 2003; measles coverage rates were 60% in 2003, lower than the reported 70% and 80% levels of the mid-1980s and mid-1990s; DPT3 and Polio3 coverage rates were 73%, lower than the 80% achieved in the mid-1990s, but had improved from the 49–52% level of 2000–2001 [12]. However, the percentage of women receiving trained assistance at births increased from 46% (1990–96) to 58% (1995–2002), and access to safe water and sanitation also improved over the last decade.

The health system

Structure and organization

Senegal's health system is pyramidal. At the top are the agencies of central government, such as the Office of the Minister of Health and other government departments; a second, strategic level is made up of 10 medical regions covering the 10 administrative units; and third is the operational level, made up of 52 districts. [13] There is also a three-tiered system of facilities. At the first level are 750 health posts that provide basic curative care, care for the chronically ill, antenatal care and family planning. Also at the first level are 55 district health centres that receive first-level referrals from the health posts and provide limited hospitalization services. At the second level, seven regional hospitals, with a capacity of 100–150 beds, are located mainly in provincial cities and provide some specialized care. At the third level are one teaching hospital and six general hospitals in the capital city, Dakar [14]. In addition, a number of Christian church-based facilities provide healthcare, especially to low-income households. [15]

Expenditure and financing

Large investments in the health sector in the first decades after independence, which contributed to a remarkable improvement in life expectancy and child survival, came under pressure in the second half of the 1980s. Economic crisis and fiscal austerity measures led to reductions in per capita health spending: health's share of the total government budget decreased from about 4.7% to 3.3% and, as a percentage of gross domestic product (GDP), it fell from 0.9% to 0.6%. Capital spending was 27% higher during the period 1981–1985 than in 1986–1990 [16]. In the 1990s, assisted by a 152% increase in external aid to the health sector, these trends reversed, as they did in many other countries in sub-Saharan Africa: health's share of the total government budget increased from less than 4% in 1988 to 8.4% in 1997; furthermore, improvements were made in the allocation of resources away from large hospitals and the wages of their staff. Tertiary care decreased from 60% to 40% of expenditure, while basic services increased from 22% to 32%.

These allocation improvements had only minimal impact on improving access to effective healthcare due to the system's inability to organize and integrate, and the fact that services were poorly equipped and managed. As a result, they were underutilized, with 0.4 visits per person and low bed-occupancy rates [17]. However, the deterioration in childhood survival and immunization rates in the 1990s was probably more the result of reduced incomes than reduced access to effective healthcare. In its Poverty Reduction Strategy Paper (PRSP) of 2002, the government stated that:

> Even though Senegal has been cited as a reference country in Africa as regards the campaign against HIV, the health system is faced with serious constraints. Fresh outbreaks of local endemic diseases are being observed and malnutrition is becoming increasingly common, especially among those who are most vulnerable. Poor individual and collective hygiene and environmental sanitation conditions together with food shortages are responsible for the deterioration of the population's health [18].

Overall, Senegal's health sector is underfinanced. Out-of-pocket expenditures by households and government subsidies are the main sources of finance in the system. Formal user-fees, which have existed since 1972, have been based on the Bamako Initiative since 1991. They have made a modest contribution to revenues—less than 5% of recurrent revenue. In light of the fact that there are no official exemptions available for the poor, who often cannot afford to pay for healthcare, the World Bank has repeatedly cited the need to lower user-fees and introduce exemptions to protect low-income households [17,19].

Other key resource constraints that are preventing progress towards the Millenium Development Goals (MDGs) are: poor management of human and financial resources that cut absorptive capacity and prevent improvement in service quality; a failure to delegate budgetary authority away from the centre; and limited organizational capacity at district level. [19]

It is noteworthy that 80% of the Senegalese population consult traditional healers and use traditional medicine, either exclusively or in combination with modern Western medicine. Beliefs about the mystical origins of diseases are still present, and medicinal herbs have proved effective for certain pathologies. Traditional medicine is tolerated, though it is not fully recognized in law. The lack of an HIV cure has put traditional medicine in the limelight, and the Ministry of Health is increasingly collaborating with traditional healers to promote behaviour change for prevention, counselling for mutual care and support, treatment of opportunistic infections, and experiments involving herbal and traditional treatments for AIDS.

Rapid urbanization has, however, led to greater anonymity, eroded some traditional community norms and facilitated the emergence of false traditional healers who take advantage of desperate families affected by HIV. Genuine traditional healers have organized themselves into associations to fight this phenomenon and exercise peer control to encourage the ethical practice of traditional medicine.

The HIV epidemic

Epidemiology

According to WHO/UNAIDS [20], there were an estimated 44,000 (22,000–89,000) adults and children living with HIV in Senegal in 2003, of whom approximately half were women. This gives an adult (15–49 years) prevalence of 0.8% (0.4–1.7%), little changed from 2001 estimates. Prevalence among SWs in the capital city, Dakar, was estimated to be much higher at 14% in 2002. Again according to WHO/UNAIDS, there had been 3500 (range 1900–6500) AIDS deaths, up from approximately 2800 (range 1500–5300) in 2001, and 17,000 AIDS orphans aged between 0 and 17 years of age.

Social context

Senegal is a socially cohesive society, about 94% Muslim and 5% mainly Catholic, most of whom practise their religion. Many observers claim that the adherence of Senegalese Muslims and Christians to their religious traditions has had a direct bearing on the epidemic, in that male circumcision is widespread, alcohol consumption is low and sexual matters are guided by conservative mores [21]. Women in Senegal traditionally do not have sex before marriage, and the more educated they are, the longer they wait. A behavioural study in Dakar showed that 68% of women and 10% of men were virgins at marriage. On average, men tend to marry 10 years later than women. Once married, women in Senegal tend to have no sexual partners other than their husbands. In a study undertaken in Dakar in 1997, 99% of married women reported that they had had sex only with their husband during the preceding year, while 12% of married men reported having had an additional sexual partner [22].

Senegal's religious leadership and structure is enormously influential, and a substantial portion of social activity in the country is organized around religious associations. Traditionally, these associations are involved in many aspects of development, including health and education, often targeting youth and women. Literally hundreds of NGOs, religious and otherwise, are involved in social development with the ability to reach deep into their communities. UNAIDS takes the view that Senegal was able to mount a swift and comprehensive response to the HIV crisis because the political leadership worked with the pre-existing social leadership and organizations. It 'laid the foundation for productive dialogue with religious and community leaders' [21]. As a result, a long and active tradition of community participation in health and development was able to be mobilized around AIDS prevention activities.

Maximum use was made of existing structures to provide information and services to communities at high risk, especially SWs. Most civil society organizations and community-based groups generously mobilized and engaged in the fight against AIDS as early as 1985, even before the first AIDS case was officially reported. In 1989, the government had already begun to collaborate with religious organizations and discuss its AIDS prevention strategy. There is now an inter-faith coalition against AIDS composed of both Islamic and Christian religious leaders. The coalition is very active and runs some of the most effective prevention, counselling, care and support programmes. Religious leaders have contributed substantially to creating a supportive and enabling environment in Senegal, leading the fight against stigma and discrimination, and involving people living with HIV in the response.

Strong participation by community, political and religious leaders in development, and in the health sector in particular, has long been a hallmark of the Senegalese infrastructure, involving many experienced associations, movements and community organizations. NGOs—of which there are about 400 women's groups and thousands of youth and sports associations—represent an important part of the health delivery system. From the outset of the epidemic, they were well positioned to provide information, education and communication programmes and reach vulnerable groups such as SWs, youth, female domestic workers and vendors, truck drivers and others. Traditional NGOs integrated HIV very early on into their work, and many HIV NGOs and networks were formed in the course of the last 20 years. Today, they constitute a major force for change, working closely with the National AIDS Programme, but maintaining their independence and quite often challenging the government response. Recently, major AIDS NGOs and networks built a common platform called the 'national AIDS Observatory', which aims to assure the quality of the national response to HIV.

Health system context

Several other features of Senegal's government and healthcare system provided, both structurally and process-wise, a framework that facilitated the design and implementation of a timely and comprehensive response to the HIV crisis in the late 1980s:

- the fact that the health sector had been reforming itself since independence and had demonstrated a capacity to anticipate health developments, as exemplified by its early embrace of prevention and primary healthcare and, later, its community financing and local health management committees that pre-dated World Bank reform initiatives by a decade;
- adherence to democratic principles and good governance in the polity as a whole;
- strong public participation and consultation in social sectors;
- a pragmatic, no-nonsense approach to public health issues;
- openness to Western influences.

This pragmatic approach to public health, emphasizing prevention and provision of essential services, formed the foundation to strengthen efforts at sexually transmitted infection (STI) control and widespread promotion of condoms [22].

The government of Senegal had made investments in primary prevention activities beginning in the 1960s and 1970s. In addition to addressing key elements of PHC, as later elaborated at Alma-Ata in 1978, the government seems to have captured the development spirit of the PHC movement by encouraging participation, working at the grass-roots level, identifying high-risk or vulnerable groups and stressing comprehensive and integrated services. For example, achievements in its childhood immunization programme and malaria campaigns are partially explained by the emphasis given to health education [10]. Some have observed an 'anticipatory attitude' towards new health developments [21]. For instance in 1984, Senegal was able to integrate the pyramidal health service delivery system of PHC with the training of District Medical Officers (DMOs) in public health and the reorganization of district system [23]. Similarly, it was able to act immediately on the WHO recommendations for the decentralization of services in 1991, which entailed the adoption of a more autonomous district system and the transfer of management powers from the centre to the peripheral level. This is the basic integrated unit for providing PHC. Because districts were designed to be fairly autonomous in terms of planning, implementing and managing resources and service delivery, they were well suited to deal with the HIV crisis. The district system provides an effective framework for the decentralization of HIV activities because it facilitates implementation at the periphery while at the same time including HIV activities in the district's integrated activities package. The distribution of resources for HIV in 2000 showed that the peripheral level was allocated nearly three times more resources than the regional level—a good indicator of the genuine decentralization of resources. [13]

In addition, key elements for the prevention and control of HIV were already part of the health service infrastructure well before the first cases were confirmed in 1985. For instance, since the 1970s, Senegal's national blood supply system had been routinely tested for syphilis and hepatitis, and, in 1987, it started to be tested for HIV. Blood banks throughout the country have the equipment and trained personnel for HIV testing in order to prevent the transmission of HIV through blood transfusions.

Sex work, which is an important source of HIV infection in many African countries, has been legal in Senegal since 1969. As a result, registered SWs are required to undertake quarterly medical examinations; if they are diagnosed with curable STIs, they are treated. This registration system has meant that SWs as a group are enormously easier to educate and target with health promotion materials than if they were earning a living illegally and were not registered. This is exemplified by the ability to promote condom use among SWs. Before the onset of HIV in 1985, the use of condoms was virtually non-existent. Officials seeking to take immediate measures to promote the use of condoms, especially within vulnerable groups, were able to build on the regular contact between SWs and the health system and found SW groups receptive to new information and amenable to change. A behavioural study in 2001 found that 99% of registered SWs had used a condom with their last client [22].

Treatment and care

The Senegalese Antiretroviral Drug Access Initiative (ISAARV) was launched in August 1998. The pilot phase of this project was made possible because of several factors: the government's willingness to allocate an annual budget for the purchase of antiretrovirals and reagents, CD4 and plasma viral load kits; reduction in the price of antiretroviral therapy (ART); and the development of an effective collaboration between technical experts required to execute the programme and partners from the North. After an 18-month trial with a cohort of 180 patients, the results showed good clinical, immunological and virological effectiveness. Moreover, adherence was good, comparable with that in developed countries [24].

In 2001, Senegal went on to adopt a holistic, decentralized approach to treatment and care. Testing at hospitals, health centres and larger health posts was established, with syndromic management without formal testing at smaller health posts. This dual approach has improved service quality and increased awareness about HIV and STIs among the general population. Programmes to prevent mother-to-child transmission (MTCT) were also set up, along with alternative strategies for the determination of CD4 counts. In addition, protocols for the treatment and care of people living with HIV (PLHIV) were defined for use throughout the country, in both the public and private sectors. From 1998 to 2001, all patients identified for treatment were referred to the National Hospital (CHU) in Dakar on a pilot basis. Following evaluation of the pilot phase, treatment was decentralized to include regional hospitals in the referral system. Since then, antiretrovirals have become available on referral to district hospitals.

In December 2003, the government demonstrated its high level of commitment to the improvement of treatment and care by providing testing, access to ART and follow-up monitoring with CD4 counts and viral load, all free of charge. In December 2004, 2800 patients were receiving ART. The objective of the programme is to have 7000 of the 44,000 HIV-infected people currently estimated to live in Senegal on ART by 2006,

In order to increase the scale of treatment, more staff need to be trained. To date, many activities have been implemented to strengthen the decentralized system of HIV treatment and care, including:

- theoretical and practical training of regional teams in charge of treatment and care;
- standardizing techniques for measuring CD4 counts;
- harmonizing drug protocols and antiretroviral prescription schemes;
- review of treatment guidelines with a clear definition of treatment and care activities;
- setting a system of regional networks of national experts;
- appointing a technical coordinator for treatment at the regional level;
- continuous supervision and training by experts supporting each region.

The training of teams in charge of treatment and care at the regional level is multidisciplinary and involves doctors, biologists, pharmacists, social workers, nurses and midwives, and includes both theoretical and practical sessions.

The quality of theoretical training is assured by experts who are based in the capital of the selected region. The modules of theoretical training cover:

- pathophysiology of HIV infection;
- history of HIV infection;
- diagnosis and treatment of opportunistic infections;
- psycho-social support for PLHIV;
- antiretroviral drugs: type and pharmacokinetic studies;
- modalities and indications for antiretrovirals;
- side effects of antiretrovirals and treatment monitoring;
- accidents with blood exposure: risk assessment, administrative procedures, proposal for antiretroviral treatment;
- support system for adherence;
- role of laboratories in monitoring ART;
- resistance to antiretrovirals;

- treatment and care of children living with HIV;
- prevention of MTCT;
- palliative care;
- role of communities in prevention, treatment and care of patients living with HIV;
- set up of a treatment and care system for PLHIV

    at the health post level;

    at the health centre level;

    at the regional hospital level;

    at the national hospital level;

- role of the pharmacist in the antiretroviral prescription system.

This 7-day training uses formal presentations, clinical case studies and group discussion. The practical training follows the theoretical training and takes place in the centres in charge of treatment, care and support in Dakar. It includes participating in medical examinations of PLHIV, supervision of antiretroviral prescription and visits to treatment and care facilities.

A 'sponsorship' scheme for personnel newly trained in the prescription of antiretrovirals has been established and consists of selecting an expert in treatment and care at the national level who is responsible for ensuring continuous supervision of the quality of care of new staff in a particular region. This expert should also identify, along with his or her colleagues, the regional needs in terms of treatment and care to assure the continuum of care, i.e. testing, diagnosis and treatment of opportunistic infections, availability of drugs for these infections, and ART. The expert aims to be in regular contact with colleagues in the region by telephone or the Internet in order to offer advice and guidance in response to possible problems occurring in treatment in general, and in the prescription of antiretrovirals in particular. The expert visits the region to supervise every 3 months. This mission is an opportunity to review antiretroviral therapeutics protocols and the quality of medical records, and to discuss procedures to adopt regarding non-optimal clinical and immunological reactions as well as ways to deal with side effects.

Conclusion

Senegal's experience is especially important for the lessons that can be learned, particularly as regards why has it been successful and what aspects of this success can be 'duplicated' elsewhere. Social and cultural factors, low alcohol consumption, circumcision, conservative attitudes toward sexuality and, consequently, low levels of STIs are some of the key features, but presumably have limited transferability.

Responses that included condom distribution, STI control programmes and antiretrovirals have been effective, especially because they were immediate and comprehensive. Political leadership and very strong participation by social and religious groups seem key to explaining the quality of the response: the leadership made good use of existing advantages by bringing on board and entering into dialogue with stakeholders and building on health system infrastructure.

It is also noted that the government has always taken a pragmatic, no-nonsense approach to public issues. The sector is constantly reforming itself, and it seems to anticipate reforms in terms of PHC, healthcare financing, decentralization and other aspects not confined to the health sector. Issues of equity and inequalities remain challenges.

In terms of civil society, an open and free press, strong democratic traditions and high levels of public participation and openness to reform are evidence to support the notion that Senegal, while fully retaining its social and cultural integrity, has managed to extract from the West those 'import items' that would enhance its development and make them Senegalese, while ignoring the rest that are on offer. This indigenization process, which is the essence of good development, helps explain Senegal's smart leadership. It is in this context that Senegal has become a reference point in the fight against AIDS.

Senegal has also demonstrated that it is possible to implement large-scale ART programmes in resource-constrained settings The declaration of free and universal access to ART by the President in December 2003 has boosted the national response to the epidemic. Voluntary counselling and testing (VCT) centres have started receiving more clients and their decentralization in the provinces has accelerated. ART provides a real incentive for people to want to know about their sero-status, and gives hope to people with HIV. In a continent where some 80% of people living with HIV do not know their status, ART will help drive the epidemic out of the underground and strengthen both prevention and care programmes. The Senegalese experience has been well documented and constitutes an interesting source of knowledge for countries with similar socio-economic conditions.

References

1. Hemenway D. (1997). *Senegal and Structural Adjustment: For Better or For Worse?* Department of Urban Region Planning: Planning for Developing Areas. Tallahassee, FL: Florida State University. http://garnet.acns.fsu.edu/~dhh4266/Senegal.htm.

2. World Bank. (1996). *Social Dimensions of Adjustment: World Bank Experience.* Washington, DC: World Bank, Operations Evaluation Department.

3. Collier P, Gunning JW. (1999). The IMF's role in structural adjustment. *Economic Journal* 109(459):F634–51.

4. World Bank. (2003). *Toward Country-led Development: A Multi-partner Evaluation of CDF.* Synthesis Report. Washington, DC: World Bank.

5. Martin-Prevel Y, Delpeuch F, Traissac P et al. (2000). Deterioration in the nutrition for young children and their mothers in Brazzaville, Congo following the devaluation of the CFA franc. *Bulletin of the World Health Organization* 78:108–18.

6. Delpeuch F, Martin-Prevel Y, Fouere T et al. (1996). Complementary nutrition for the young child following the devaluation of the CFA franc (African Financial Community): 2 case studies in the Congo and Senegal urban environment. *Bulletin of the World Health Organization* 74:67–75.

7. Risk Analysis HIV/AIDS country profile: Senegal. (1996). *AIDS Analysis Africa* 6(6):4–7.

8. World Bank. (2003). *Memoranda of the President of IDA to Executive Directors on Country Assistance Strategy for Republic of Senegal.* Report 25498-SE. Washington, DC: World Bank.

9. EDS website: http://www.measuredhs.com/.

10. Pison G, Trape JF, Lefebvre M, Enel C. (1993). Rapid decline in child mortality in a rural area of Senegal. *International Journal of Epidemiology* 22(1):72–80.

11. UNICEF. (1998, 2004) *State of the World's Children. Statistical Tables.* New York: UNICEF.

12. WHO/UNICEF. (2004). *Review of National Immunization Coverage 1980–2003 Senegal.* Geneva: WHO.

13. Mbengue C, Gamble Kelley A. (2001). *Funding and Implementing HIV/AIDS Activities in the Context of Decentralization: Ethiopia and Senegal.* Bethesda, MD: Abt Associates Inc., Partnerships for Health Reform.

14. World Bank. (1997). *Staff Appraisal Report, Republic of Senegal Integrated Health Sector Development Program.* Report No. 16756-SE, Human Development 2, Africa Region. Washington, DC: World Bank.

15. Bitran R. (1995). Efficiency and quality in the public and private sectors in Senegal. *Health Policy and Planning* 10:271–283.

16. World Bank. (1993). *Public Expenditure Review.* Document No.11559. Washington, DC: World Bank.

17. World Bank. (1997). *Staff Appraisal Report, Republic of Senegal Integrated Health Sector Development Program.* Report No. 16756-SE, Human Development 2, Africa Region. Washington, DC: World Bank.

18. Republic of Senegal, Poverty Reduction Strategy Paper, 2002. Available at: http://www.worldbank.org/ afr/SenegalCG2003/PRSP-English.pdf

19. World Bank. (2003). *Memoranda of the President of IDA to Executive Directors on Country Assistance Strategy for Republic of Senegal.* Report 25498-SE. Washington, DC: World Bank.

20. WHO/UNAIDS. (2004). Report on the Global AIDS Epidemic. Geneva: WHO.

21. Niang CI, van Ufford PQ. (2002). The socio-economic impact of HIV/AIDS in a low prevalence context: the case of Senegal. In: *AIDS Public Policy and Well-being,* Chapter 4. New York: UNICEF. pp. 1–27. Available online at www.unicef-icdc.org/research/ESP/aids/chapter4.pdf.

22. UNAIDS. (1999). *Acting Early to Prevent AIDS; the Case of Senegal.* Geneva: UNAIDS.

23. Unger JP, Daveloose P, Ba A, Toure-Sene NN, Mercenier P. (1989). Senegal moves nearer the goals of Alma-Ata. *World Health Forum* 10:456–63.

24. Laurent C, Diakhate N, Ndeye Fatou Ngom Gueye *et al.* (2002). The Senegalese government's highly active antiretroviral therapy initiative: an 18-month follow-up study. *AIDS* 16:1363–70.

Chapter 16

South Africa

David McCoy[*], Robin Wood, Lilian Dudley and Peter Barron

David McCoy*, Robin Wood, Lilian Dudley and Peter Barron

Background

South Africa is a young constitutional democracy, having recently emerged from its apartheid past in 1994. It has three levels of government, national, provincial and local, each accountable to its own legislature or council. There are nine provinces, six metropolitan and 47 district municipalities. The roles, responsibilities and powers shared across the three levels of government are constitutionally determined. South Africa has an independent judiciary and a free press.

South Africa has a population of 45.5 million. With a per capita gross domestic product (GDP) of over US$3000 per annum, South Africa is regarded as a middle-income country [1]. However, deep socio-economic inequalities continue to exist, with large segments of the population living in poverty. The poorest 40% of households, covering 50% of the population, receive only 11% of the country's total income, while the richest 10% of households, covering 7% of the population, receive over 40% of the total income [1,2]. Approximately 65% of South Africans (29.5 million people) live below the poverty line, almost all of whom are black. These 19 million people, or 46% of the total population, appear to be 'trapped in poverty', living on less than US$55 per adult per month [1]. Racial socio-economic disparities are illustrated by the variation in unemployment rates as shown in Fig. 16.1. The racial categories of African, coloured, Indian and white, still used in South Africa, are used throughout this chapter.

There are also geographical socio-economic disparities, with 72% of the poor living in rural areas. This is reflected in inter-provincial disparities, with the provinces of Limpopo, KwaZulu-Natal and Eastern Cape, which include large sections of the rural black homelands of the apartheid era, remaining relatively disadvantaged and underdeveloped. A process of rapid urbanization has meant that poverty is increasingly concentrated in peri-urban informal settlements. Finally, poverty also has gender dimensions, with female-headed households having a 50% higher poverty rate than male-headed households.

Although the new government has made significant progress towards extending access of households to basic public utilities and services, gaps in provision remain. For example, in 2001, only 32% of households had access to piped water in the dwelling, and 54% to a flush or chemical toilet [4]. Furthermore, a sixfold difference exists between the richest and poorest income quintiles in terms of access to basic services.

*Corresponding author.

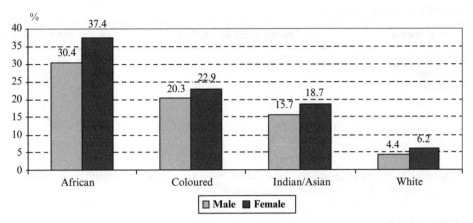

Fig. 16.1 Unemployment rate (official definition) by population group and gender: September 2003. Source: [3].

Inequities in socio-economic development are reflected in poor aggregate health indicators, as well as disparities in health status. For example, the infant mortality rate (IMR) of 59 per 1000 live births is high for a middle-income country [5]. The variation in IMR among provinces, ranging from 30 in the Western Cape to 72 per 1000 live births in the Eastern Cape, roughly correlates with the variation in socio-economic development between provinces.

The health system

Financing

South Africa spent approximately 8% of its GDP on healthcare in 2002 [6]. Its per capita health expenditure in the public sector was approximately R830 in 2001/2002, in excess of US$100, which is high by African standards. Health financing is shared among government, households, employers, donors and non-governmental organizations (NGOs), in the proportions shown in Table 16.1.

Most public health financing comes from national government revenue and taxation. Provincial governments do not raise taxation for the purpose of healthcare, and local government taxes contribute to less than 3% of total public health financing. Government financing is almost exclusively spent in the public sector.

Households are the second biggest source of financing. Lower-income groups tend to make direct out-of-pocket payments for user-charges, whilst middle-income and upper-income groups mainly make contributions through private health insurance. Most of the out-of-pocket payments made by households are to private providers, as public sector primary care is free [7]. Because the government contribution to health financing has stagnated in the past few years, resulting in a decline in public per capita expenditure between 1999 and 2001 [7,8], an increasing burden has been placed on households and employers at a time when the burden of disease is increasing as a consequence of the HIV epidemic.

Employers contribute mainly through the subsidization of private health insurance for employees, although some also directly finance clinical services for employees. However, the costs of providing healthcare benefits to employees have been increasing rapidly, with inflation

Table 16.1 Sources of financing

Source of finance	1999/00 prices (US$ billion)	% of total sources
Government	4.82	44.3
Households	4.25	39.0
Employers	1.87	16.6
Donors/NGOs	.01	0.1
Total	10.90	100.0

Source: [7].

in the health sector outstripping general inflation, threatening to shift an even greater burden of care onto the already overstretched public services.

Expenditure

Healthcare expenditure in South Africa remains inequitable. There are large differences in per capita health expenditure between socio-economic groups as a result of different levels of health expenditure in the public and private sectors. For example, in 1998/1999, 59% of total healthcare expenditure was in the private health sector [7], benefiting approximately 20% of the population, most of whom use private health insurance (Fig. 16.2). The public–private divide is sharply reflected in the distribution of health personnel, as shown in Fig. 16.3. In 1998, the ratio of medical practitioners to the population served was 1:389 in the private sector and 1:4452 in the public sector [9].

Within the public sector, the bulk of expenditure is on hospitals, with non-hospital primary care accounting for only 11% of public sector health expenditure. There are also considerable geographic inequities in resource allocation. Historically well-resourced provinces, particularly

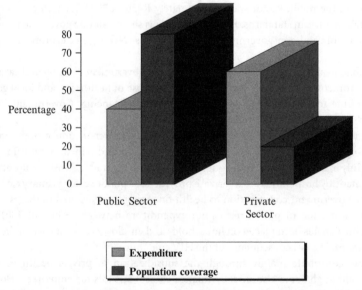

Fig. 16.2 Health expenditure and coverage between the private and public health sectors.
Source: [7].

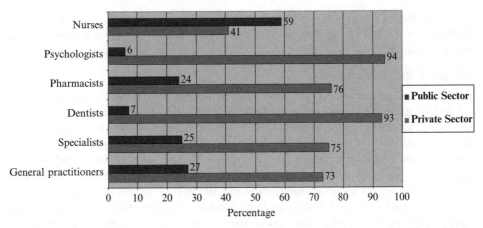

Fig. 16.3 Healthcare personnel expenditure and coverage between the private and public health sectors, 1999. Source: [9].

Gauteng and Western Cape, have higher spending levels than the previously disadvantaged and predominantly rural provinces of Limpopo and Eastern Cape.

These provincial inequities are starkly illustrated when comparing dedicated primary health-care (PHC) funding. In Gauteng and Western Cape, largely urbanized provinces, per capita average expenditure on PHC is more than R200 (US$31), whilst in the largely rural provinces of Limpopo and Eastern Cape, per capita expenditure is estimated to be R70 (US$11) and R91 (US$14), respectively. There are also large variations within provinces, mainly reflecting urban–rural differences. For example, the difference between the PHC per capita spending of the richest and poorest health districts ranges from R190 (US$29) to R75 (US$12) in the Northern Cape, and fromk R118 (US$18) to R40 (US$6) in the Eastern Cape [10].

Performance

Although many health indicators are indicative of broader socio-economic development as well as standards of healthcare, two indicators considered to be reasonably specific measures of the performance of the health system are immunization coverage rates and maternal mortality. On both counts, South Africa compares poorly with other countries (Table 16.2).

Table 16.2 Country comparison of health sector expenditure and performance

	Per capita health expenditure (2001)* (US$)	Measles immunization coverage (2002)+	Maternal mortality (2000)†
South Africa	222	84%	230
Thailand	69	97%	44
Sri Lanka	30	99%	92
Egypt	46	97%	84
Malaysia	143	92%	41

Source:* [12]; +[13]; †[14].

Low tuberculosis (TB) cure rates (64%) are another indicator of a relatively poorly functioning health system [11]. The following sections describe the key reasons for this from a health systems perspective.

The public health sector

One of the challenges of the South African health system has been to build an appropriate and efficiently organized and managed public health sector on the foundation of an inefficient and inequitable apartheid health system [15,16]. Following the democratic elections in 1994, 10 homeland and four provincial health administrations had to be integrated and reorganized into a single public system. A national Department of Health (DoH) was established primarily to develop policy and provide strategic oversight, while responsibility for the bulk of public sector healthcare delivery was to lie with nine new provincial DoHs. A number of municipalities that provided selected PHC services also had to be integrated into the new post-apartheid health system. Furthermore, in many parts of the country, there had also been a fragmentation of preventive and curative primary level services, each with separate management structures, which required integration after 1994.

A district health system (DHS) was promoted as the key health system policy to provide a decentralized and geographically based framework for public health services. However, a protracted process of local government reform and a lack of clarity about the scope of healthcare responsibilities to be devolved to local government delayed the implementation of the DHS. In 2004, the National Health Act finally defined local governments' responsibility for health as limited to environmental health services, with provincial governments responsible for the bulk of healthcare delivery.

In addition to administrative fragmentation, the health system inherited a bias towards the hospital-dominated, curative services favoured by the privileged white minority population. Meanwhile, PHC services in the rural and predominantly black areas were under-resourced, which is one reason for the poor healthcare indicators described earlier.

The cost of providing a basic basket of PHC services, excluding HIV-related services, has been estimated to be approximately R125 (US$19) per person per year [10]. Financially, the public provision of even an extended package of PHC services should be well within South Africa's grasp. However, current levels of PHC financing mean that the poorest and most disadvantaged districts cannot fund the basic PHC package. According to the national PHC facility survey of 2000, while 73% of urban clinics had functioning telephones, this was true for only 54% of rural clinics, and 73% of urban clinics experienced an uninterrupted supply of electricity as opposed to 60% of rural clinics [17]. The lack of a good PHC infrastructure is compounded by the low rate of utilization of PHC facilities, which stands at 1.8 visits per capita per year, well below the nationally established PHC norm of 3.5 [17].

Another constraint to improving access and quality of care is the limited human resource capacity in the health sector. The numbers of health personnel employed in the public sector declined in the late 1990s along with declining public sector health budgets [6]. In 2002, 43% of public sector health posts were vacant [18]. In addition to the absolute shortage of human resources, there is also an inequitable distribution. The difficulties in shifting resources to the under-resourced parts of the health system, key to any improvement in overall health system performance, have been largely due to the difficulty in shifting personnel from urban areas to rural areas, as well as a relative reluctance amongst policy makers and the medical establishment to shift resources out of large hospitals towards the primary level [19].

However, the variability in the quality of care is not simply a function of resource levels. This was illustrated clearly by the country's experience in implementing the national prevention of mother-to-child transmission of HIV (PMTCT) pilot programme, where equivalent financial resources were allocated to each province to implement PMTCT in two sites. An evaluation of the programme shows how the differences in management capacity, leadership and organization were also at the root of provincial variations in the effectiveness and efficiency of PMTCT programme implementation, pointing to the fundamental importance of human resources [20]. Other important reasons for poor quality of care are inadequate levels of clinical skills; low levels of morale and motivation, especially amongst those working in under-resourced settings and high HIV prevalence areas; inadequate systems of support and supervision to front line PHC providers; and a lack of coordination of training and policy interventions between different PHC programme areas [21].

Some of the strategies implemented by the DoH to address the shortfall in health professionals include compulsory community service for new medical, pharmacy and nursing graduates, the deployment of foreign doctors in rural underserved areas and provision of financial incentives to attract scarce skills and health professionals to underserved areas. However, the design and effective implementation of a comprehensive human resources strategy that incorporates improvements to technical capacity, morale and motivation as well as an appropriate distribution and skill mix of health workers remains key to South Africa meeting its health needs.

The private sector

A major challenge for South Africa has been to improve the efficiency of the private sector and extend the health resources available in the private sector to a wider section of the population. The barriers to this are primarily financial, with private sector costs and insurance premiums rising above the rate of inflation as a result of increasing medical costs, especially in the hospital sector, as well as overservicing due to an inadequately regulated fee-for-service reimbursement system [9].

In January 2000, the government began to implement reforms designed to increase the level of risk-pooling amongst medical scheme beneficiaries and prevent the industry from 'cherry-picking' segments of the population that were most likely to be profitable. It is now compulsory for schemes to accept all eligible applicants ('open enrolment') and only to charge differentiated premiums on the basis of income and number of dependants, not on age or the risk of ill health. In addition, it is now compulsory for every scheme to cover a comprehensive package of hospital and outpatient services, known as the Prescribed Minimum Benefits (PMBs), and monetary limits to benefits have been outlawed for certain essential services. It is hoped that this will lead to schemes competing with each other on the basis of efficiency and bring down the high costs. However, in spite of these progressive reforms, the high cost of insurance premiums has continued to lock private sector resources into a health system that services a minority of the population.

The HIV epidemic

Against this background of a fragmented and inequitable health system that failed to adequately provide for the health needs of the majority of the population, the HIV epidemic began to have a measurable impact in the early 1990s. The epidemic spread rapidly throughout the country, aided by a highly mobile population, a large migrant labour workforce and an efficient national transport network. South Africa has more people living with HIV (PLHIV) than any other country, with an estimated 5.2 million individuals living with the virus in 2002, or 12% of the total population [22]. This includes 2.95 million women and 2.3 million men between 15 and 49 years of age, as well as approximately 100,000 babies infected through MTCT.

National HIV prevalence estimates based on annual surveys of antenatal attendees in the public sector have increased from 0.7% in 1990 to 27% in 2002 (Fig. 16.4). Of the nine provinces, KwaZulu-Natal has consistently had the highest prevalence and the Western Cape the lowest, at 36% and 12.4%, respectively, in 2002.

A population-based national household survey in 2002 found an HIV prevalence of 16% in adults, with a rate of 16% in women compared with 14% in men [23]. HIV prevalence was found to be 13% in black Africans, 6% in whites, 6% in 'coloureds' and 2% in Indians. Geographically, urban informal settlements were most affected, with an adult HIV prevalence of 28%. Current estimates of prevalence range between 10 and 24%.

AIDS accounts for 25% of all adult deaths in South Africa and 40% of deaths between 15 and 49 years of age [24]. As a result, there has been a significant shift in the pattern of mortality from the old to the young, which is more pronounced in females. The death rate of women aged 25–29 years increased 3.5-fold from 1985 to 2000. The high adult mortality resulted in close to 1 million children under the age of 15 who had lost one or more parents to AIDS by 2005 [25].

Impact of HIV

The impact on the public sector is largely felt through increased numbers of people seeking healthcare and increased social spending in the form of grants and care for orphans. Actuarial extrapolations estimate that by 2010 over 8 million South Africans will be HIV-infected and the health services will need to care for 1.3 million people with AIDS [26]. In 2002, 46% of patients in public hospitals were HIV-infected [27]. The increased patient load due to HIV has tended to 'crowd out' non-HIV patients in the public sector and increase the costs of care associated with increased length of stay in hospitals.

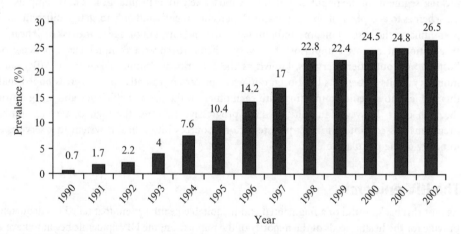

Fig. 16.4 HIV prevalence trends among antenatal clinic attendees, 1990–2002. Source: [22].

In addition, 16.3% of health workers in public facilities were HIV-infected in 2002 [27]. Increased absenteeism, low staff morale and increased mortality in health workers will increasingly undermine the sector's attempts to respond effectively to the demands for healthcare. This disproportionately affects provinces that are already financially under-resourced and have fewer health workers. Inequities in health and healthcare are therefore further exacerbated by the HIV epidemic.

The impact of HIV at the household level has been devastating. Household surveys suggest that 64% of people with AIDS are women, many of whom are also the head of the household [28]. Large numbers of caregivers also take time off work or school to care for the sick, with a consequent impact on family income and schooling of children. In one survey of households affected by HIV, it was found that more than a third had no regular income or no income except for state grants [29], and an average of 34% of household income was spent on healthcare, with rural households spending proportionally 54% compared with 29% in urban households [28]. The incapacity or loss of a breadwinner to HIV, coupled with the need for caregivers to take time off work and the increased expenditure on health, can push many households into a downward poverty spiral. Although the state provides some social security in the form of old-age pensions and children's grants, social security nets in South Africa are generally inadequate.

The full effect of the AIDS epidemic on the broader economy is only just beginning to be felt as increasing numbers of workers and professionals succumb to the disease. Direct costs to companies include increases in contributions to pension, life, disability and medical benefits. Indirect costs include higher recruitment and training costs, labour turnover, lost skills, increased absenteeism and lower productivity, amongst others. A large proportion (39%) of South African businesses report that HIV has resulted in lower labour productivity and increased absenteeism, and about a third feel that employee benefit costs have increased [30].

The response to the HIV epidemic

The government and DoH response

Overall, South Africa's response to the HIV epidemic has been a failure. A country with South Africa's wealth and level of infrastructure should have done better to curb the rise in prevalence. Although South Africa's violent and troubled history of apartheid is a significant mitigating factor, the actions of the government and DoH have often been inadequate.

The first specific response to HIV was in 1991, in the form of a national network of 18 AIDS Training, Information and Counselling Centres (ATICCs). In 1992, a National AIDS Co-ordinating Committee (NACOSA) was convened, consisting of representatives of government, NGOs, AIDS service organizations and other interest groups, with a mandate to develop a National AIDS Strategy. This eventually resulted in a comprehensive National AIDS Plan, adopted by the government in 1994.

However, the period between 1994 and 2000 was marked by a failure to implement the plan fully, for several reasons. For a start, the political transition from apartheid to democracy consumed most of the political attention during the early stages of the epidemic. Even after the 1994 elections, the new and inexperienced government was preoccupied with the massive challenge of restructuring the government and addressing the socio-economic needs of the population. The desire to attract foreign direct investment and enjoy the post-apartheid euphoria of democracy may have also resulted in a subconscious downplaying of the threat of HIV.

In the DoH, although there was a huge challenge to reorganize and restructure the public health system, there was also inadequate HIV leadership. In addition, the public health sector responses were implemented within the financial constraints of the Growth, Employment and Redistribution Strategy (GEAR), which sought to maintain the tax-to-GDP ratio and limit growth in public health expenditure, and within the context of having to transform the health system as a whole. As a result, the epidemic received a lower priority than it warranted during the years of the Nelson Mandela government. Prevention efforts were largely unsuccessful, under-resourced or inadequately implemented.

By the time the HIV epidemic had become an undeniable public health emergency, government expenditure on HIV had increased significantly. For example, real spending on provincial HIV conditional grants has increased more than 10-fold between 2000 and 2002, from R18 million (US$2.8 million) to R342 million (US$53.1 million). However, the government's response became hampered by a strange denial of the epidemic by President Mbeki. The relationship between government and an extensive network of 600 civil society organizations that had informed the policy response in the early 1990s grew increasingly strained [31]. This came to a head in 2000, when the President openly questioned the link between HIV and the AIDS epidemic. In the same year, several thousand local and international scientists signed the Durban Declaration at the 2000 International AIDS Conference in Durban, stating that the evidence that HIV causes AIDS was incontrovertible. However, the Durban Declaration was subsequently publicly dismissed by the Minister of Health. Since then, the AIDS epidemic has continued to be dogged by obfuscation, controversy and tension between the political leadership and the medical, scientific and NGO sectors in South Africa [32].

Furthermore, the challenges of transforming and restructuring the public sector health bureaucracy continued to undermine efforts to deliver a coordinated health sector response to the HIV epidemic. Provincial DoHs experienced frequent structural and personnel changes; the DHS continued to flounder because of the division of responsibilities between the provincial and local levels of government; and the lack of a coordinated human resource development plan contributed to an ongoing lack of human capacity within the public health system.

The second 5-year HIV/AIDS/STI Strategic Plan for South Africa was released by the Minister of Health in May 2000 [33]. The plan outlined four main priority areas: prevention; treatment and support; monitoring and research; and human and legal rights. Prevention priorities included a multimedia information, education and communication (IEC) campaign in collaboration with NGOs, a school-based 'life skills' programme, increased access to syndromic management of sexually transmitted infections (STIs), the distribution of condoms via non-traditional outlets and development of clinical guidelines for PMTCT.

In more recent years, there has been some evidence of success in implementing some of these strategies through the public health sector. In particular, STI management and condom distribution were strengthened during this period, and voluntary counselling and testing (VCT) was introduced in the public sector. However, the quality of STI treatment and HIV counselling remains suboptimal [34]. The 2000 National Primary Health Care Facilities Survey found wide provincial variations in the availability of VCT services (Fig. 16.5).

Perhaps the most convincing evidence of behaviour change is the dramatic increase in the distribution and use of condoms. The allocation of condoms by the DoH rose from 198 million in 2000 to an estimated 275 million by 2002, and the Nelson Mandela/Human Sciences

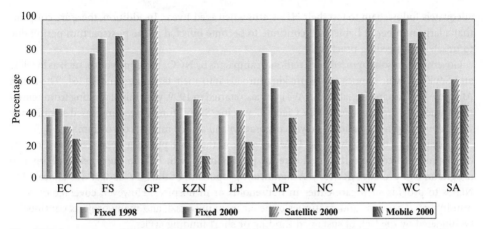

Fig. 16.5 Percentage of fixed, satellite and mobile clinics providing HIV testing, by province. Source: [17].

Research Council (NM/HSRC) study found that 97.9% of respondents aged 15–24 and 96.1% of those aged 25–49 knew where to obtain condoms should they need them [23]. Comparisons between the South Africa Demographic and Health Survey (SADHS) conducted in 1998 and the 2002 NM/HSRC survey (Table 16.3) show significant increases in condom use in all age groups over the 5 years between surveys, particularly among women [35].

A controversial aspect of the government response was the national PMTCT strategy, which initially did not include the use of antiretroviral therapy (ART). A PMTCT programme using ART was, however, initiated in the Western Cape Province in 2000, despite central government opposition. In 2000, the government finally agreed to establish a pilot PMTCT programme consisting of two sites in each province. The pilot phase of the programme has now ended and a national roll-out begun. Unfortunately, an evaluation of the PMTCT programme showed significant deficiencies in the delivery of PMTCT services as well as inequities in the quality of services between provinces. At present, the effectiveness of the PMTCT programme remains unknown due to the lack of data. Many of the babies who received nevirapine at birth are not

Table 16.3 Percentage of females who have ever used a condom and percentage who used a condom at last intercourse among females who have had sex in the past 12 months, 1998 and 2002

	2002 (NM/HSRC survey)	1998 (SADHS)
Ever condom use		
15–19 years	68.3	28.4
20–24 years	63.3	32.4
25–29 years	60.3	28.4
Condom use at last intercourse		
15–19 years	47.9	19.5
20–24 years	47.4	14.4
25–29 years	33.7	7.6

Source: [35].

adequately followed up to test their HIV status when aged 1 year. In addition, there are concerns that a large number of babies will continue to become infected in the post-partum period due to unsafe breastfeeding practices.

Government also supported large national campaigns by NGOs targeting youth, such as loveLife and SoulCity, which appear to be making inroads into their target audiences [36]. The South African AIDS Vaccine Initiative (SAAVI) was also started in 1999, with initial funding from central government, to produce a local HIV Clade 'C' vaccine. SAAVI funding was increased significantly with support from the national power corporation and a large mining consortium.

In addition to the emphasis on HIV prevention, the DoH placed a heavy emphasis on the development of community-based care for people living with HIV in the absence of any real programme to provide ART [37]. A significant proportion of the HIV budget was allocated to NGOs to provide such care either in households or in hospices. However, coverage of community-based care was and continues to be far from universal, and many projects continue to be hindered by the lack of sustained funding or short funding cycles.

Civil society response

Partly as a result of the inadequate government response to the epidemic and the political controversies, an active, vibrant and powerful civil society movement around HIV and treatment access has developed. The Treatment Action Campaign (TAC) and the AIDS Law Project have been spearheading a successful activist alliance fighting for the rights of people living with HIV and AIDS. Notable successes of its campaigns have been the provision of free Diflucan® within public sector health facilities by Pfizer, a Constitutional Court instruction in 2000 that the Minister of Health initiate an ART-based PMTCT programme throughout the public sector, and its support to the government as a 'friend of the court' in a successful court defence against the South African Pharmaceutical Manufacturers' Association. TAC continues to campaign for access to ART through the public sector, and for access to affordable drugs. In addition, TAC and its allies have also taken the government to court for failing to roll out the PMTCT pilot programme.

Beyond the treatment activist groups, the role of civil society in meeting the challenges of the HIV epidemic is mixed. On the one hand, civil society is meeting the brunt of the epidemic through the care that is provided to sick and dying people in countless numbers of homes. A variety of NGOs and community-based organizations (CBOs) play active roles in behavioural change strategies. The government recognizes the need to work in partnership with NGOs and has dedicated budgets for supporting such partnerships, although more could be done to improve the reliability and sustainability of such funding.

However, in terms of civil society leaders, there are a number of high-profile leaders speaking out and providing education about HIV, including Archbishop Desmond Tutu, Nelson Mandela, local community leaders, tribal leaders, clergymen and traditional healers. Local government leaders are perhaps still not speaking out strongly and frequently enough. This reflects the stigma still associated with HIV, as well as the lack of clear political leadership from the most senior levels of government.

With a few notable exceptions, the response of the business sector has been slow. Only a quarter of South African companies have an HIV policy, 18% provide a VCT programme, 13% provide an HIV care, support and treatment programme, and 6% provide ART in the workplace [30]. Access to ART in the private sector increased in 1998, when a large managed-care organization began to reimburse for ART. Initially, because of high ART costs, treatment was limited to dual nucleoside therapy. This strategy was demonstrated to be cost-saving, with the costs of ART being discounted by a decrease in private hospitalization costs. Reduction in ART costs within the South African market has allowed triple therapy to be substituted for dual therapy, and currently 12,000 people living with HIV are receiving triple therapy within the private sector [38].

Expanding access to ART

From 1996 to 2000, access to ART was limited to the private health sector. Several externally funded ART public sector pilot sites were started in 2001 in the Western Cape, where programmes supported by Médicins Sans Frontières and other groups in Khayelitsha, a peri-urban informal settlement, successfully demonstrated the feasibility of integrating ART into public sector HIV management. By July 2003, 24 sites in the not-for-profit sector were providing ART for approximately 1454 patients and claimed to have a capacity to treat a further 2720 [40]. The sites reflect current inequities, with 21 being urban-based and in the better-resourced provinces of Western Cape (13 sites), Gauteng (four sites) and KwaZulu-Natal (five sites).

The government's plans to provide ART has been mired in controversy and conflict, mainly centred around the President's and Minister of Health's refusal to acknowledge the effectiveness of antiretroviral drugs. However, after a prolonged struggle spearheaded by the TAC, the government's position changed in the second half of 2003 following the Minister of Finance's announcement of a budget provision of R3 billion (US$465 million)per annum for 3 years for the DoH to develop a nationwide ART programme [40]. In November 2003, a national Operational Plan for Comprehensive Care, Management and Treatment, which for the first time included provision of ART in the public sector, was approved by Cabinet [41]. The ART plan envisaged establishing at least one ART service point in each of the 53 health districts in the country during 2004, to be expanded to 207 service points by 2008. Service points are to provide a continuum of treatment and prevention based on six pillar strategies: education and community mobilization; expanding programmes aimed at boosting the immune system, including use of traditional health treatments; improved opportunistic infection management; intensified support of families affected by HIV; and provision of antiretrovirals to those who need them.

Substantial resources have been allocated to the 2003 Plan, but health messages continue to be inconsistent at the highest levels of government, and initial milestones have not been met [42]. The reported number of people receiving ART in September 2003 was 15,000 out of an estimated 837,000 who need it. The magnitude of the epidemic, the numbers of people with AIDS needing urgent access to healthcare, together with the current inequities and backlogs in health infrastructure, will require a concerted national and international effort on an unprecedented scale if the plan is to succeed.

Conclusion: challenges and priorities

Within the current macroeconomic context, the public sector will find itself increasingly constrained in its ability to meet existing needs, let alone new demands generated by the HIV epidemic. There is a need to increase the portion of GDP spent on health and social support, as South Africa is still short of the target set by the Abuja Declaration. Critically, the profound link between AIDS and poverty must be recognized and broken, and there is an urgent need for a national multisectoral response that goes well beyond the current public health response and engages the private sector and employers.

While prevention efforts have been strengthened in recent years, there is still much more improvement required to promote healthy and safe sexual behaviour. The national antenatal HIV surveillance system has been showing a decline in the prevalence of HIV amongst the younger age groups, which suggests that the incidence of HIV infection might be decreasing. However, the prevalence rates still suggest that tens of thousands of people are being infected with the virus every year.

It will be important that the attention paid to expanding access to ART not result in a diversion of resources and attention away from prevention strategies. Similarly, an ongoing challenge for the health sector will be to ensure that the broader goal of comprehensive healthcare, including ensuring safe deliveries and effective child healthcare, is not undermined by a narrow, vertical focus on HIV and access to ART. It will also be important that information systems to monitor the systems-wide effects of expanding access to ART be rapidly established.

Within the health sector as a whole, there remain several challenges to strengthen and improve the capacity of the public health system to deliver essential core health services, as well as ART. The inequitable and inappropriate distribution of health resources still requires urgent attention. The primary level of the health system, particularly in the under-resourced provinces and rural areas, is inadequately funded.

Another important dimension of the healthcare infrastructure that needs greater attention and strengthening is the DHS. Strong, capable and effective district health management structures are required in every health district to provide local leadership for the translation of policy into implementation, as well as to help ensure that the multiple demands being made upon hospital and clinic staff are adequately integrated and prioritized to meet the local and specific needs of each health district.

The government needs to continue to work towards the reform of the private health sector so that the resources that are currently locked into the coverage of a small proportion of the population can be released to cover a larger number of people. In addition, there is a need to introduce a reimbursement system that promotes efficiency and evidence-based clinical practice; reduce the high level of administrative and transactional costs; and popularize the use of disease management programmes for chronic conditions such as HIV.

Because of the lack of capacity in the public sector and the degree of urgency required to respond to the epidemic, the government should encourage active partnerships with the not-for-profit NGO sector. However, it will be important that such partnerships be constructed in a way that does not detract from capacity development of the public sector, nor displace state responsibility onto the NGO sector. The commercial and business sectors should also be increasingly harnessed to complement the initiatives of the public sector by making bigger financial commitments to prevention and treatment activities. A sense of corporate social responsibility should be enhanced in this regard. Lastly, leadership uniting all sectors behind a national response to the HIV epidemic in South Africa is desperately needed.

References

1. United Nations Development Programme. (2004). *Human Development Report, 2004*. New York: Oxford University Press. Available online at www.undp.org.
2. Department of Health. (1999). *South Africa Demographic and Health Survey. Preliminary Report*. Pretoria: Department of Health, Medical Research Council, Macro International.
3. *Labour Force Survey*. (2003). Pretoria: Statistics South Africa.

4. Census 2001. (2003). *Census in Brief.* Pretoria: Statistics South Africa.

5. Dorrington RE, Bradshaw D, Budlender D. (2002). *HIV/AIDS Profile of the Provinces of South Africa—Indicators for 2002.* Cape Town: Centre for Actuarial Research, University of Cape Town.

6. *Intergovernmental Fiscal Review.* (2003). Pretoria: National Treasury, Republic of South Africa.

7. Doherty J, Thomas S, Muirhead D, McIntyre D. (2002). Health care financing and expenditure. In: Ijumba P, Ntuli A and Barron P, eds. *South African Health Review.* Durban: Health Systems Trust pp 13–40. Available online at http://www.hst.org.za/upload/files/chapter2.PDF.

8. Thomas S, Muirhead D. (2000). *National Health Accounts Project: The Public Sector* Report. Pretoria: Department of Health.

9. Cornell J, Goudge J, McIntyre D *et al.* (2001). *National Health Accounts: The Private Sector Report.* Pretoria: Department of Health.

10. Thomas S, Mbatsha S, Muirhead D *et al.* (2004). *Primary Health Care Financing and Need Across Health Districts in South Africa.* An output of the local government and Health Consortium. Health Systems Trust, Centre for Health Policy and Health Economics Unit, University of Cape Town.

11. Kironde S, Bamford L. (2002). Tuberculosis. In: Ijumba P, Ntuli A, Barron P, eds. *South African Health Review 2002.* Durban: Health Systems Trust, pp 279–304.

12. World Health Organization. (2003). *World Health Report.* Geneva: WHO. Available online at www.who.int/whr/en/.

13. UNICEF. (2003). *State of the World's Children.* New York: UNICEF.

14. World Health Organization, UNICEF, United Nations Population Fund. (2000). *Maternal Mortality in 2000.* Geneva: WHO.

15. McCoy D. (1999). Restructuring the health services of South Africa: the district health system. In: Khosa M, ed. *Infrastructure Mandate for Change, 1994–1999.* Pretoria: Human Sciences Research Council, pp 141–59.

16. Van Rensburg HC, Harrison D. (1995). The history of health policy. In: Harrison D, ed. *South African Health Review,* 1995. Durban: Health Systems Trust, pp 95–118.

17. Viljoen R, Heunis C, van Rensburg EJ *et al.* (2000). *The National Primary Health Care Facilities Survey.* Durban: Health Systems Trust.

18. Day C, Gray A. (2002). Health and related indicators. In: Ijumba P, Ntuli A, Barron P, eds. *South African Health Review, 2002.* Durban: Health Systems Trust, pp 411–532.

19. van Rensburg D, van Rensburg N. (1999). Distribution of human resources. In: Crisp N, Ntuli A, eds. *South African Health Review,* 1999. Durban: Health Systems Trust, pp 201–232.

20. McCoy D, Besser M, Doherty T, Visser R. (2002). *Interim Findings on the National PMTCT Pilot Sites. Summary of Lessons and Recommendations.* Durban: Health Systems Trust.

21. Lehman U, Sanders D. (2002). Human resource development. In: Ijumba P, Ntuli A and Barron, eds. *South African Health Review,* 2002. Durban: Health Systems Trust, pp 119–134.

22. Department of Health. (2003). *National HIV and Syphilis Sero-prevalence Survey of Women Attending Public Antenatal Clinics in South Africa.* Pretoria: Department of Health.

23. Shisana O, Simbayi L. (2002). *Nelson Mandela/HSRC Study of HIV/AIDS—South African National HIV Prevalence: Behavioural Risks and Mass Media.* Household Survey. Cape Town: Nelson Mandela Foundation and Human Sciences Research Council. Available online at http:www.hsrcpublishers.co.za/hiv.html.

24. Dorrington R, Bourne D, Bradshaw D *et al.* (2001). *The Impact of HIV/AIDS on Adult Mortality in South Africa.* Technical Report of the Burden of Disease Research Unit. Medical Research Unit, South Africa. Available online at www.mrc.ac.za/bod.

25. Bradshaw D, Johnson L, Schneider H *et al.* (2002). *Orphans of the HIV/AIDS Epidemic.* MRC Policy Brief. Available online at http://www.mrc.ac.za.

26. Dorrington RE. (1990). ASSA600: an AIDS model of the third kind? *Transactions of the Actuarial Society of South Africa* 13:99–153.

27. Shisana O, Hall EJ, Maluleke KR *et al.* (2002). *Report on the Impact of HIV/AIDS on the Health Sector: National Survey of Health Personnel, Ambulatory and Hospitalised Patients and Health Facilities.* Report prepared for the South African Department of Health, Human Science Research Council. Available online at www.hsrcpublishers.ac.za.

28. Steinberg M, Johnson S, Schierhout S *et al.* (2002). *Hitting Home. How Households Cope with the Impact of the HIV/AIDS Epidemic: A Survey of Households Affected by HIV/AIDS in South Africa.* Washington, DC: The Henry Kaiser Family Foundation.

29. Giese S, Meintjies H *et al.* (2003). *Report on Health and Social Services to Address the Needs of Orphans and Other Vulnerable Children in the Context of HIV/AIDS.* Cape Town: Child Health Institute, University of Cape Town.

30. *The Economic Impact of HIV/AIDS on Business in South Africa.* (2003). Stellenbosch: Bureau for Economic Research.

31. Trengove Jones T. (2001). *Who Cares? AIDS Review.* Pretoria: Centre for Study of AIDS, University of Pretoria.

32. Ntuli A, Ijumba P, McCoy D *et al.* (2003). *HIV/AIDS and Health Sector Responses in South Africa. Treatment Access and Equity: Balancing the Action.* Durban: Health Systems Trust.

33. *HIV/AIDS/STD Strategic Plan for South Africa 2000–2005.* (2000). Pretoria, Department of Health.

34. Sonko R, McCoy D, Gosa E *et al.* (2003). Sexually transmitted infections. In: Ijumba P, Ntuli A, Barron P, eds. *South African Health Review, 2002.* Durban: Health Systems Trust, pp 257–278.

35. Doherty T, Colvin M. (2004). HIV/AIDS. In: Ijumba P, Day C, Ntuli A, eds. *South African Health Review, 2003.* Durban: Health Systems Trust, pp 191–211.

36. Africa Strategic Research Corporation and Kaiser Family Foundation. (2001). *The 2001 LoveLife National Awareness and Impact Survey Among Youth 12–17 Years.* Johannesburg: Africa Strategic Research Corporation and Kaiser Family Foundation.

37. Russell M, Schneider H. (2001). Models of community-based HIV/AIDS care and support. In: Ntuli A Crisp N, Clarke E and Barron P, eds. *South African Health Review, 2000.* Durban: Health Systems Trust, pp 327–349.

38. Cowlin RG, Regensberg LD, Hislop MS. (2003). Counting the cost of care: do HIV/AIDS disease management programmes deliver. *AIDS Management Report* 1(3):20–23.

39. Poole C, Abdool Karim Q, Darder M *et al.* (2003). Anti-retroviral Therapy Provision in the Public Sector and the Generic Antiretroviral Procurement Project (GARPP). Presented at the South African Aids Conference, Durban, South Africa.

40. National Department of Health. (2003). Statement of cabinet on a plan for comprehensive treatment and care for HIV and AIDS in South Africa. Government communications. URL: http//www.gov.za.

41. Operational Plan for Comprehensive HIV and AIDS care, management and treatment for South Africa. (2003). Pretoria: Department of Health. URL: http://www.gov.za.

42. Stewart R, Padarath A, Bamford L. (2004). *Antiretroviral Treatment, Southern Africa.* Presentated at the SAHARA Conference, Cape Town, South Africa.

Chapter 17

Uganda

Justin O. Parkhurst[*], Freddie Ssengooba and David Serwadda

Background

Uganda is a land-locked East African nation lying on the equator and bordering Lake Victoria along with two other East African states, Kenya and Tanzania. With its neighbouring countries—Sudan to the north, Democratic Republic of Congo to the west, and Rwanda to the south-west—Uganda is part of a region characterized as a crisis zone due to past or ongoing conflicts. It has a multi-ethnic population of 24 million with over 20 different indigenous languages.

Uganda gained its independence in 1962 but soon faced a series of civil conflicts that would devastate much of the country. It was not until 1986, when President Yoweri Museveni and the National Resistance Movement came to power, that stability returned to the majority of the country. However, the health system had been destroyed by the years of civil war and conflict. There were few remaining health services, despite the country at one time having had one of the best health infrastructures in sub-Saharan Africa [1,2]. As a result of this breakdown of the sector, donors and international actors rushed into the newly liberated Uganda in 1986, establishing numerous health projects, often in disregard of existing state structures or planning [2].

The 1980s and 1990s also saw Uganda facing heavy debt burdens, as was the case in many African nations. The government implemented a wide-scale structural adjustment programme at the instigation of the World Bank and International Monetary Fund (IMF). Part of their structural adjustment plans stipulated the so-called 'rolling back of the state', whereby state involvement in provision of services was reduced in an attempt to reduce inefficiency [3]. Just as the country was attempting to rebuild, there was pressure to reduce state involvement and spending in many social services.

Uganda's political, economic and social turmoil of the 1970s and early 1980s had far-reaching consequences for the health system and health status of the country. Poorly functioning health systems, combined with the resurgence of previously controlled infectious diseases such as malaria, emergence of new diseases such as HIV and the increase in non-infectious chronic diseases have all contributed to the falling outputs of the health system and the worsening health status in the country [4,5]. For example, by the early 1980s, immunization rates had fallen to below 20%, and, in 1991, the infant mortality rate was 122 per 1000 live births. Maternal mortality was above 500 per 100,000 live births when

* Corresponding author.

estimated in 1995 and 2000–2001 [6]. Malaria accounted for more than 56% of the total disease burden, with an incidence of 164 per 1000 persons in the year 2000. Acute respiratory infection, intestinal infection and diarrhoea comprised 12%, 6% and 5%, respectively, of the total disease burden [7,8].

Another prominent factor contributing to low health system outputs and the poor health status has been persistent poverty. Despite economic recovery, with an average growth of 6.5% per annum in the 1990s, household incomes and health expenditures are still low. Household surveys show that the proportion of households living below the 'dollar per day' poverty line was 35% in 2000, from a high of 56% in 1992/1993 and 44% in 1997/1998. The distribution of household expenditure is characterized by very pronounced inequalities, with the bottom 50% of the population generating 20% of total household expenditure, and the highest 10% generating 40% of total expenditure [9]. Uganda's social indicators (Table 17.1) reflect the picture of poverty and poor health.

The health system

Health system capacity and ownership

Uganda has a mixed healthcare system made up of public and private service provision. The Ministry of Health (MoH) oversees the healthcare system, which is made up of referral and district public hospitals, private not-for-profit (PNFP) hospitals and primary healthcare facilities (Table 17.2). Although the private for-profit sector is rapidly growing, its scope and capacity are not fully understood by the government. The private sector operates nearly as many facilities as the public sector, with the role of private actors particularly noteworthy at

Table 17.1 Selected social indicators

Indicator	Performance
Total population (2002)*	24,748,977
Life expectancy (years)[†]	47
Infant mortality rate (death per 1000 live births)[+]	88
Under-5 mortality rate (out of 1000)[+]	150
Fully immunized at first birthday (%)[+]	44
Maternal mortality ratio (per 100,000 live births)[+]	504
Total fertility rate[+]	6.9
Contraceptive prevalence (%)[+]	15
Teenage pregnancy (%)[†]	43
HIV male-to-female ratio[+]	1:1.5
Population per nurse/midwife[+]	2900
Population per physician[+]	18,700
Population per hospital bed[‡]	965
Birth attended by professional providers (%)[+]	39
Households within 5 km of health facility (%)[†]	49
Out-patient Department per capita visits (in year 2000)[‡]	0.45
Per capita health expenditure (including households)[‡]	US$ 12

Sources: *[10]; [+][6]; [†][11]; [‡][8].

Table 17.2 Number and ownership of different types of health facilities by population levels

Facility level	Population served	Public	Private not-for-profit	Private for-profit
National teaching hospital	24,300,000	2	0	0
Regional referral hospital	2,000,000	11	0	0
District hospital	500,000	42	49	5
Health centre IV	100,000	143	13	3
Health centre III	20,000	614	147	26
Health centre II	5000	781	365	879
Total		1593	574	913

Source: [12].

lower levels of care (Health Centre IIs), which provide much of the primary healthcare and preventive services.

The hospital sector includes two university teaching hospitals, district and regional referral hospitals, and PNFP and private for-profit hospitals. Most of the hospitals are in urban settings. Government provides a subsidy to the PNFP hospitals to provide care for poor population groups as a measure to expand service coverage and reduce the burden of user-fees charged by PNFP hospitals.

Financing

Funding is divided between public budget, contribution from development partners (DPs), statutory and private insurance and out-of-pocket payments (Fig. 17.1). The major source of funding is government revenue raised through taxation and DP contributions. Insurance funds account for nearly 5% of the healthcare budget [13]. Out-of-pocket expenditure funds about 60% of the non-development (recurrent) expenditures on health services, with an average household health expenditure of Sh. 5320 (US$4) per capita per year [9]. Population and epidemiological weightings such as infant mortality rates and district poverty indices are used to allocate public funds between districts [14].

The MoH, as the major financier and provider of primary care and curative services, targets rural and low-income groups. Private health insurance makes a very small contribution to health financing and essentially covers curative services for the 5% of the population that is formally employed and receiving regular wages [13]. There is little information regarding the private for-profit sector, but it represents a very mixed group of actors, from a handful of hospitals to several formal and informal providers such as unregistered clinics, drug shops and illicit drug pedlars. The formal private for-profit sector is paid by fee-for-service, is concentrated in the urban areas and serves the rich. Informal health provision includes drug shops and traditional healers who depend on fees-for-service and who are largely unregulated [15,16]. As much as two-thirds of the total number of outpatient department (OPD) contacts are in the private for-profit sector [9]. There is scanty information on the size and extent of service utilization of so-called 'traditional', non-allopathic medicine, but it is claimed that there is one traditional healer for every 300 Ugandans [17]. Before 2001, when government attention was drawn to this sector, most traditional healing was largely informal and unregulated. There are very recent attempts to integrate traditional and allopathic medicine, particularly in the fields of maternal and HIV care, counselling and referral.

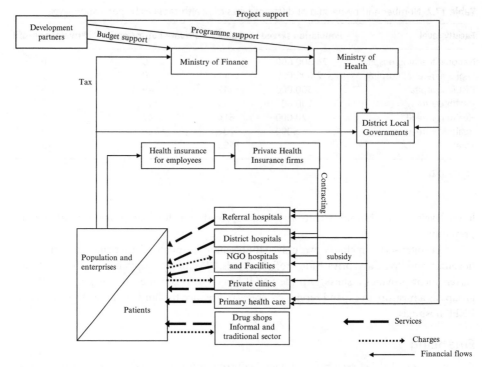

Fig. 17.1 Financial flows in the Ugandan health system.

The financing of the health sector is constrained by the overall amount of revenue raised through taxation and the competing claims on the relatively small national budget. Overall, absolute recurrent and investment health expenditures increased at an annual average of 9% between 2000/2001 and 2004/2005 [4]. Given the resources needed for the provision of the minimum healthcare package that the government has committed itself to providing to all its population, a 15% budget share over the next 20 years is required to close the resource gap.

Primary healthcare financing is among the government priority programmes for poverty reduction. Other programmes under the Poverty Action Fund (PAF) umbrella are universal primary education, access to water and sanitation, agricultural services for poor farmers and rural feeder roads [18]. The PAF has been created by the government as a strategy to guarantee that priority sectors' allocations increase over the medium term and are also protected from budget cuts prompted by revenue shortfalls. Since its inception in 1997/1998, funds from the Highly Indebted Poor Country (HIPC) debt relief initiative, as well as funds contributed by development partners and government's own tax revenues, have contributed to the 50% increase in funds allocated to the PAF, from 17% in 1997/1998 to 32% in 2001/2002 [19]. As a result of the PAF, the health sector allocation for primary healthcare has radically increased (Fig. 17.2), but at the expense of allocation to hospitals. Their budgets have been capped at the 1993/1994 level to improve allocative efficiency [20]. Concerns about poor emergency obstetric care and overall poor performance of public hospitals in the context of improvements in primary healthcare have shifted attention back to the insufficient funding of hospitals and a

Billion Shillings (US$1 = 1730 Shillings average)

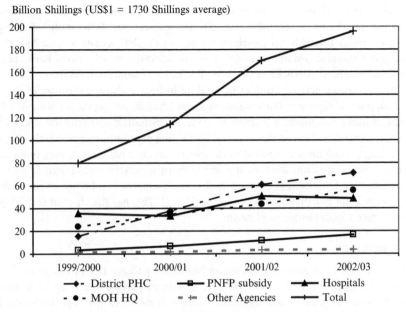

Fig. 17.2 Allocation of government budget 1999/2000 to 2002/2003. Source: [4].

need to develop an integrated healthcare system where hospitals are capable of playing their part in the continuum of care [4,21].

In the context of a highly decentralized Ugandan system of governance, about 80% of the funding to local district and municipal governments is conditional grants tied to poverty reduction priority programmes. Since 2001, the practice of charging user-fees in public health facilities has been outlawed to improve access for the poor. User-fees had been implemented by district governments in the early 1990s as a means of generating additional revenue to sustain health services during a time of very low public budget outlays to the sector. The current policy is to allow client charges and cost recovery only in the private wings of public hospitals [14].

The general picture of health financing in the 1990s can be summarized as low per capita expenditure on health as a result of a constrained government budget, with a fairly high contribution from donors and households (Table 17.3).

Table 17.3 Health system resources in the 1990s

Funding source	Per capita expenditure on health (US$)			
	1990	1995/1996	1997/1998	1999/2000
Government of Uganda	0.88	2.43	2.20	2.88
Donors	2.12	3.52	4.73	3.53
Households	3.18		4.07	4.00
Total	6.18		11.00	10.41

Source: [14].

The main donors to the health sector are bilateral organizations such as the US Agency for International Development (USAID), the UK Department for International Development (DFID), the Danish International Development Agency (DANIDA) and Iceland Aid, although some support is also obtained from multilateral organizations such as the World Bank, the United Nations Children's fund (UNICEF) and the World Health Organization (WHO).

The major consequences of insufficient funding include a chronic shortage of drugs and essential supplies. Drug expenditure stands at about US$0.80 per capita per year, which is far below the required minimum estimated at US$3.50, excluding antiretroviral drugs [14]. A barrage of reforms aimed at coordinating and liberalizing drug imports and establishing a pull-system of drug procurement controlled by the user institutions has recently been implemented. Another consequence of low levels of funding is that patients are encouraged to pay fees to avoid long queues. For example, primary healthcare is supposed to be free of charge, but, in practice, formal and informal fees are common [22,23]. This has the effect of excluding poor people who face a high burden of ill health.

Health services

Government policy is to provide a minimum healthcare package free of charge to the whole population, i.e. universal free medical care. A minimum package made up of services that address the major morbidity and mortality burdens is delivered through the public health system under the control and stewardship of the district and municipal authorities. The package of essential healthcare services was drawn from an analysis of the most cost-effective interventions to address the major disease burdens [24]. The essential health services typically include preventive services such as childhood immunization, health promotion and education, as well as treatment and control of common and infectious diseases such as malaria, HIV and tuberculosis (TB). Universal coverage is the goal, although financing and infrastructure limitations mean that urban populations have better access. On average, 49% of Ugandans live within 5 km of a health facility, but the quality and range of services vary widely, so that access remains variable. For example, the National Household Survey results presented in Table 17.4 indicate both geographical and income-related inequity in coverage.

Overall, public health facilities contribute 25% of medical services provided to households, while private facilities—hospitals, clinics, drug shops—contribute 44% of medical consultations. The remainder is made up of those not seeking care (8%) or those who are self-medicating (23%). The households in the richest 10% of the population are more than 50% less likely to self-medicate or take no action when sick compared with those in the poorest 10% (Table 17.4). This utilization pattern is consistent with a mixed system of service provision and a failure to implement universal access to free medical services in practice. It also implies the presence of significant access costs, particularly among poor households.

Human resources

Local authorities have the responsibility for service provision under the decentralized system of government. However, due to resource constraints facing local governments, paying salaries and the control of human resources is still a function of the central ministries of Health, Public Service and Finance [20]. Current established positions for professional staff are only 46% filled, illustrating the vast need to expand human resources, especially in the rural areas [4]. Civil service employment standards, i.e. permanent and pensionable employment terms, are

Table 17.4 Type of medical attention sought by the poorest and richest deciles, 1999/2000

Total	Poorest 10% of population			Richest 10% of population		
	Rural	**Urban**	**Total**	**Rural**	**Urban**	**Total**
None	28.7%	13.1%	28.5%	2.9%	1.9%	2.6%
Home treatment	26.2%	15.9%	26.1%	16.3%	14.6%	15.7%
Outpatient at government hospital	9.9%	33.4%	10.3%	15.0%	11.7%	13.8%
Outpatient at private hospital	1.1%	0.0%	1.1%	10.3%	6.7%	9.0%
Private clinic	11.0%	25.4%	11.3%	32.1%	47.8%	37.9%
Dispensary	6.7%	1.4%	6.6%	6.2%	2.0%	4.6%
Health centre	5.6%	0.0%	5.5%	2.5%	1.9%	2.3%
Drug shop	6.8%	8.9%	6.9%	10.7%	9.9%	10.4%
Pharmacy	0.2%	0.0%	0.2%	0.6%	1.1%	0.8%
Traditional healer	1.5%	0.0%	1.4%	0.4%	0.5%	0.4%
Inpatient at government hospital	0.6%	1.9%	0.6%	1.2%	1.5%	1.3%
Inpatient at private hospital	0.1%	0.0%	0.1%	1.2%	0.5%	0.9%
Other	1.5%	0.0%	1.4%	0.6%	0.1%	0.4%

Source: [9].

the norm in the health system and do little to motivate performance. The main personnel incentives are low powered, i.e. salary, training and promotion. Salaries are typically low due to the generally low tax base and competing needs of the government budget [15,25]. The evaluation system is a routine management requirement with little bearing on staff perform-ance and does not create strong performance incentives [15]. As a result, there is a high prevalence of public mistrust in the quality of services provided [26]. Informal practices such as drug misappropriation [22], corruption and dual practice are common among health providers [27]:

> Most doctors have initiated a private clinic, usually nearby the hospital. So, even if they are supposedly employed full-time in the public facility, in fact they are to be found in the clinic most of the time. They use the hospital or the public facility as a fishing-pot for new customers or, sometimes, to free-ride on expensive equipment they could not afford otherwise. User-fees were somewhat starting to change the situation, but now it is going to go back as it was before. There is also anecdotal evidence of resurgence of under-the-table payments (from Executive Secretary, Uganda Catholic Medical Bureau, extracted from [13]).

Assessment of the health system

Uganda's healthcare system faces many challenges and is suboptimal in many ways. Although health status is a function of several factors, analysis suggests that the health sector has the potential to attain better outcomes even with the current low level of resources if the areas of inefficiency in the health system could be identified and improved [28]. Even so, the financing of the system falls far below what is needed for a minimum care package to the population. Donor financing dominates the financing, now and in the future. Much of this results from the recent history of the country, which saw a breakdown of the health system, followed by restructuring led by international actors who lacked coordination and local guidance. The current distribution of care facilities and human resources exposes the rural poor to insufficient coverage and poor quality of services. Perverse organizational incentives and low salaries lead to dual practice and other informal behaviours, which are precursors of suboptimal performance within the system. Although many new interventions are being supported by global philanthropy or self-interest, the capacity of the Ugandan tax base to sustain many of these developments beyond the start-up stage is in doubt. These challenges in the provision of services have implications for HIV prevention and treatment.

The HIV epidemic

Despite these general health system challenges, Uganda has been widely held up as an African success story in its battle against HIV, with numerous countries looking to the Ugandan experience for lessons to learn in their own fight against the epidemic. Many countries from Africa and Asia have sent delegations to Uganda to investigate the technical interventions the country has initiated and study one of the world's first national HIV programmes. However, while the policies and technical interventions are important, it is equally important to understand the social, political and health systems context in which Uganda shaped its HIV response.

Uganda initiated its HIV prevention efforts in 1986, the year President Yoweri Museveni and his National Resistance Movement came to power. From early that year, Museveni prioritized HIV and AIDS as problems the country had to face, and openly addressed them as problems for all Ugandans to fight. Much has been written on the role of political leadership in HIV control [29–31], and the importance of this cannot be denied. However, Uganda's political, social and health system contexts played a large part in shaping how effective the country has been in developing and implementing HIV prevention and control strategies. Uganda has shown remarkable success in mobilizing groups across the population, both inside and outside the government, and in raising the awareness of the population. Behaviour change interventions requiring local targeting of messages have proliferated in the country accordingly. Yet, the limitations in Uganda's health infrastructure have prevented widespread implementation of more technically oriented interventions for HIV and AIDS. Therefore, to assess the Ugandan response to HIV fully, the realities of the health system and political economy of the country must be understood.

The scale of the epidemic

Uganda was described in the mid-1990s as the country worst hit by HIV and AIDS [32]. Yet, today it has seen apparent reductions in HIV prevalence unmatched in other countries. The reasons for any reduction are complex, and any changes in behaviour leading to lower HIV incidence over time are likely to have been the result of a large number of factors acting simultaneously [29,33,34]. However, the exact scale of the reduction has been difficult to assess.

Surveillance sites of pregnant women have shown declines in prevalence across the country. The most dramatic declines have been in some of the urban sites, which recorded peak prevalence around 30% at the beginning of the 1990s but had seen reductions to well below 10% by the end of the decade [35]. Some past analyses assumed that this trend was applicable to the country as a whole, but Uganda is primarily a rural country, so urban data cannot be seen as representative. Rural sites did not see nearly as high a peak in prevalence, but they, too, have seen substantial reductions over time. According to a recent UNAIDS epidemiological fact sheet, median HIV prevalence in non-urban antenatal surveillance sites declined from a peak of 13% in 1992 to 6% in 2000 [36]. In assessing the Ugandan data as a whole, Stoneburner and Low-Beer estimated that national prevalence had peaked at 21.1% in 1991, falling to 6% in 2000 [37]. Yet this estimate appears to be based on a simple arithmetic mean of surveillance data (D. Low-Beer, personal communication, 2004). Averaging figures is risky, however, as data from rural sites were limited, particularly in the earlier years, and new sites were added throughout the 1990s. Many of the non-urban sites are also located in peri-urban areas, so some downward estimation must be made if truly rural populations are assumed to have lower HIV prevalence. Nevertheless, a clear decline in serial HIV prevalence has been observed across most Ugandan sites.

There are some well-reported biases in antenatal data that make it difficult to generalize across the population as a whole, the most challenging being that fertility will decline over time in HIV-positive women, reducing their ability to become pregnant and be sampled at antenatal surveillance sites. However, the reductions in prevalence seen in Ugandan surveillance sites are corroborated by other information, including data from voluntary testing centres, sexually transmitted infection (STI) clinics, and epidemiological studies in Rakai and Masaka districts. The Masaka study is one of the few cohort studies measuring HIV incidence over time, and recently reported a declining trend in incidence for the rural population studied over the 1990s [38]. Other supporting evidence for declining incidence in Uganda comes from declining prevalence rates in younger women at surveillance sites—trends which are often seen as a proxy indicator of incidence [39]. While prevalence has decreased over time, recent studies have suggested that this involved an increase in the use of condoms combined with increased HIV-related deaths [40].

By the end of 2001, UNAIDS estimated that the Ugandan adult HIV prevalence had declined to 5%, considerably lower than many other African nations, but was still a major health threat, corresponding to 510,000 adult infections. There were an additional 110,000 children estimated to be infected at that time, and approximately 880,000 AIDS orphans. These estimates were based on surveillance mechanisms, but the number of AIDS cases reported remained low, with only 55,861 cumulative AIDS cases reported to the MoH by the end of 2001 [36].

Social mobilization and behaviour change

Much of the Ugandan success in reducing prevalence has been attributed to behaviour change across population groups. In reviewing repeated behavioural surveys, Stoneburner and Low-Beer [37] found notable changes in the average age of sexual onset, increased condom use and a 60% reduction in reported casual sexual partners. How such a large proportion of such a diverse population could have changed their behaviours is an important question to understand, and has led many to look at the specific interventions of the Ugandan government. One of the most notable features of the Ugandan response to HIV is the large number of organizations and groups involved in prevention efforts on the ground. There are hundreds, if not thousands, of non-governmental organizations (NGOs), religious groups and international actors providing HIV prevention, education and care initiatives in the country. Yet, this response evolved from the context of Uganda's political and health system in the mid-1980s. Uganda used the challenges faced by the breakdown of health services to its advantage in some ways, by encouraging donor support for HIV prevention and by allowing a large number of organizations to become involved in HIV-related activities. At the same time, the government established political structures that explicitly called for such multilateral action and maintained an overarching position in the development of the national response. The result appears to have been wide-scale social mobilization at all levels, with NGOs and religious groups tailoring messages for their own local communities. Simultaneously, international groups and donors provided support to Ugandan activities, at times through the government but also through direct assistance to NGOs.

These messages have been delivered alongside the government's own education and health promotion campaigns. The national AIDS Control Programme was established in 1986 and immediately began a mass education programme. Today, Uganda sees very high levels of awareness of HIV and ways to prevent its transmission, although this is now common in many African countries. Government programmes produced information in several languages and used multiple media, such as print, radio and travelling film shows, to reach the population. Political leaders at all levels were also called upon to speak to their constituencies about HIV and AIDS at all possible opportunities, with the President himself often including it as a subject in speeches across the country. These efforts helped to provide a base of information across the country that supported other prevention programmes.

Finally, condom promotion has been another interesting aspect of the Ugandan response to HIV. Social marketing of condoms has been a large element of the push to make them available across the country at affordable prices. International organizations have played an important role in achieving this. Yet, for many years, national policy did not discuss condoms explicitly, pursuing instead what was termed a 'quiet promotion of condoms' [41]. This appears to have been done to placate NGOs and religious groups who may have been pursuing HIV prevention in other ways and would not have responded well to a strong government dictate about the 'right' way to prevent HIV or to give strong support for condoms. The strategy appears to have worked, in that condoms are widely available, but local religious leaders appear to accept the government position, even if it differs from their own. In order to address the issue without raising conflict, some religious leaders have even been invited to participate in national condom plans. In all these ways, the government of Uganda has managed to involve and draw upon a wide range of national and international groups while enabling a diversity of approaches and messages at local level.

HIV care and treatment

The positive results seen in education- and social mobilization-based HIV interventions have helped Uganda become a model in many ways for other nations. However, not all Ugandan policies and programmes have seen such positive results. In particular, those interventions relying more on technical, biomedical interventions have struggled or proceeded more slowly in the country, despite the wide-scale political commitment to fight HIV shown by President Museveni and his government.

In general, much treatment and care of HIV-positive individuals has been difficult for the government to provide because of the limits to the health system's capacity. As a result, the most famous organization providing support to those affected by HIV is The AIDS Support Organization (TASO), which was established outside the government by families directly affected by HIV. TASO is a model for counselling and support that many other countries are attempting to emulate, yet it was distinctly non-governmental in its origins.

In terms of treatment, currently antiretroviral drugs are provided through public hospitals and private clinics. By September 2004, an estimated 35,000 people were receiving antiretroviral treatment (ART). The private clinics tend to be run by international agencies or NGOs such as TASO, Uganda Cares and Médecins Sans Frontières.

Syndromic management of sexually transmitted infections

A common strategy recommended for low-income countries internationally for the prevention of HIV is the control of STIs through a regimen of syndromic management. Such a process involves training health staff to identify signs of STIs in patients and providing drug treatment based on a standardized algorithm. This is done instead of the clinical aetiological diagnosis and precise treatment common in other areas with more developed health systems.

Uganda has included syndromic management in its policies and priorities for HIV prevention for many years, with specific World Bank support for STI control since the early 1990s [42]. However, the implementation of the policy has been limited, with recent reports finding problems with health staff's knowledge of protocols [43], limitations on the number of trained health workers, poor delivery systems for drugs, and supply chain difficulties [44]. The limitations within the health system appear to have led to difficulties in implementing this technically oriented intervention for HIV prevention and, indeed, authors have found that most Ugandans use the private sector to obtain treatment for STIs, rather than government health centres [45].

Antiretroviral therapy

Finally, one of the most important technical interventions against AIDS is the delivery of ART to those with HIV. While Uganda has been prolific in getting prevention messages across the country, ART has spread much more slowly. Unfortunately, Uganda's underdeveloped health infrastructure has meant that, as with syndromic management of STIs, ART has so far only been provided to an estimated 35,000 individuals out of an estimated 114,000 who need it. Where there are long queues or shortages of services, private payments have often determined access to care. While the government and its non-state partners have made much health information and promotion widely available across the country, the provision of expensive and complex ART regimens has been much more difficult to achieve. Antiretrovirals were first delivered to a small number of individuals in 1992, when the Joint Clinical Research Centre (JCRC) in Kampala began to administer zidovudine (AZT) to patients who could afford treatment. Other drugs were added over the following years, but treatment remained limited to this one centre for most of the 1990s.

In 1998, the international Drug Access Initiative (DAI) was launched by UNAIDS in several resource-poor settings—including Uganda, through the MoH—in an attempt to scale up ART. ART was established in other centres outside the JCRC, first in and around the capital, Kampala, and, by 2003, in over 20 facilities across Uganda [45]. However, as mentioned earlier, NGOs and international organizations have taken the lead in provision of ART. Currently there are two models of drug delivery being used by these organizations. Most provide the drugs through clinics in health facilities. However, the US Centers for Disease Control and Prevention (CDC) is evaluating a home-based provision model in Tororo and Busia districts. In this approach, medication is provided in people's home, while members of the household who are eligible are encouraged to enrol for HIV testing and counselling.

A major factor in increasing the number of patients receiving ART in Uganda has been the government's importation of generic drugs, in particular from India, and the large price cuts in patented brand drugs that occurred in 2000 alongside the importation of generics. According to one Oxfam report, the JCRC increased the number of patients on ART from 962 in 2000 to 3000 in 2001, quoting the director of the JCRC as saying that over half their patients could not continue treatment without the importation of generic drugs [47].

There is a national policy to provide ART to HIV-infected mothers free of charge in order to prevent mother-to-child transmission [46], although it is unclear exactly how many eligible women actually undertake this treatment. The initiative was to be scaled up from an initial three districts in the country in 2000, with plans to reach all 56 districts by 2005 [48]. For most HIV-infected patients, however, drugs are not offered free, although some subsidies are available, ostensibly for the least well off. The government admits that universal coverage cannot be obtained at present due to 'limited physical access' [46]. As a result, many individuals do not yet have access, and those who do must often pay out-of-pocket. Oxfam has reported that the majority of HIV-infected Ugandans cannot afford to pay for treatment, even with generic drugs available [47].

Currently, the government of Uganda estimates that 114,000 out of the estimated 350,000–880,000 HIV-infected individuals need ART. In order to meet this challenge, Uganda received funds from the Global Fund to Fight AIDS, Tuberculosis and Malaria to treat the 35,000 people currently receiving ART. The US government has given Uganda funds to cover treatment for an additional 60,000 by 2006. In both funding streams, the health providers will be from both government and the private sector. In the private sector, the main providers will be NGOs and research programmes. As a whole, ART is limited in Uganda, but there are numerous plans to scale up and increase its use. Despite global philanthropy towards HIV and AIDS, the stewards of the national economy are concerned about the huge inflows of foreign support, fearing the negative impacts these could have on the foreign exchange rate and potentially harming Ugandan exports. The government has imposed budget ceilings for each sector, implying that additional grants beyond the ceilings would be offset by a reduction in the budget. As a result, the attractiveness of new, externally funded vertical programmes has been greatly reduced in the eyes of health officials.

Conclusion

While Uganda has been widely praised for its political response to the HIV pandemic, and has seen substantial reductions in its HIV prevalence across the population, the roles of the political environment and health system must be assessed to understand what happened in the country. Emerging from a civil conflict that had devastated the country's public health infrastructure, President Museveni and his government drew upon a wide range of non-governmental actors to provide services for HIV prevention, while slowly building a national response as well. Progress has been more noticeable in interventions to change behaviour, as such changes require a wide diversity of approaches consistent with extensive NGO involvement. Progress on more technical medical interventions, such as syndromic management of STIs and ART, has been slower. In both these cases, policies are in place to support their use, but system constraints have resulted in limited achievements. However, the government's continuing engagement with NGOs and international donors is helping to build its ability to deliver technical and drug-based interventions.

A key challenge now facing Uganda is how to develop a health system that is currently characterized by drug shortages—seen for treatments as simple as chloroquine—and difficulties in delivering relatively simple interventions such as immunizations, in order to deliver complex, resource-intensive, high-tech services such as management of opportunistic infections, voluntary counselling and testing, ART and prevention of mother-to-child transmission programmes. As currently planned, the scaling-up of HIV and AIDS programmes risks displacing other essential, but underperforming, priority areas such as reducing maternal mortality and morbidity and improving childhood nutrition. To seize the opportunity of global goodwill for these efforts, Uganda needs to invest strategically in strengthening the health system as a whole—macroeconomic threats notwithstanding. By building capacity for motivated human resources, pro-poor service delivery mechanisms and structures for sustained and equitable financing, Uganda may be in a position to take full advantage of the support it receives and build a more sustainable structure for future provision of all services. This will require a broader strategy for health system building than focusing on quick-fix solutions or bypassing under-resourced establishments that have characterized many health developments in the last two decades in Uganda.

References

1. Dodge CP, Wiebe PD, eds. (1985). *Crisis in Uganda: The Breakdown of Health Wervice*. Oxford: Pergamon Press.

2. Macrae J, Zwi A, Birungi H. (1993). *A Healthy Peace? Rehabilitation & Development of the Health Sector in a Post-conflict Situation: The Case of Uganda*. London: London School of Hygiene and Tropical Medicine and Makerere University.

3. Chazan N, Lewis P, Mortimer R, Rothchild D, Stedman SJ. (1999). *Politics and Society in Contemporary Africa*. Boulder: Lynne Rienner Publishers, Inc.

4. Uganda Ministry of Health. (2003). *Health Sector Strategic Plan 2000/01–2004/05. Midterm Review Report*. Kampala: Uganda Ministry of Health.

5. Jamal V. (1991). Inequalities and adjustment in Uganda. *Development and Change* 22:321–37.

6. Uganda Bureau of Statistics. (2001). *Uganda Demographic and Health Survey 2000–2001*. Entebbe and Maryland: Uganda Bureau of Statistics and ORC Macro Calverton.

7. Talisuna A. (2001). *The Health Management Information System in Uganda: Is it Tailored to the Requirements for Monitoring the Health Sector Strategic Plan?* Kampala: Uganda Ministry of Health.

8. Uganda Ministry of Health. (2001). *Ministry of Health Statistical Abstract*. Kampala: Uganda Ministry of Health.

9. Uganda Bureau of Statistics. (2000). *Uganda Household Survey 1999/2000*. Entebbe: Uganda Bureau of Statistics.

10. Uganda Bureau of Statistics. (2002). *Uganda Census 2002, Preliminary Report*. Entebbe: Uganda Bureau of Statistics.

11. UNDP. (2001). *Uganda Development Report 2000: Attacking Poverty*. Kampala: United Nations Development Programme.

12. Uganda Ministry of Health. (2002). *Ministry of Health Statistical Abstract*. Kampala: Uganda Ministry of Health.

13. Uganda Ministry of Health. (2001). *A Feasibility Analysis of Social Health Insurance in Uganda*. Kampala: Uganda Ministry of Health.

14. Uganda Ministry of Health. (2001). *Health Financing Strategy for Uganda (Draft)*. Kampala: Uganda Ministry of Health.

15. Mathauer I. (2001). *Institutional Pluralism and Interorganizational Relations in Local Health Care Provision in Uganda: Institutionalised Pathologies or Healing Organizations?* London: London School of Economics and Political Science, Development Studies Institute.

16. Uganda Ministry of Health. (2001). *Draft Public Private Partnership Policy*. Kampala: Uganda Ministry of Health.

17. World Bank. (2003). *Traditional Medicine Practice in Contemporary Uganda*. Washington, DC: The World Bank.

18. Uganda Ministry of Finance Planning and Economic Development. (2001). *Poverty Eradication Action Plan (2001–2003) Volume 1*. Kampala: Uganda Ministry of Finance Planning and Economic Development.

19. Foster M, Mijumbi P. (2002). *How When and Why Does Poverty Get Budget Priority: Poverty Reduction Strategy and Public Expenditure in Uganda*. Overseas Development Institute.

20. Hanson K, Atuyambe L, Kamwanga J, McPake B, Mungule O, Ssengooba F. (2002). Towards improving hospital performance in Uganda and Zambia: reflections and opportunities for Autonomy. *Health Policy* 61:73–94.

21. Ssengooba F, Atuyambe L, McPake B, Hanson K, Okuonzi S. (2002). What could be achieved with greater public hospital autonomy: comparison of public and PNFP hospitals in Uganda. *Public Administration and Development* 22:414–28.

22. McPake B, Asiimwe D, Mwesigye F *et al.* (1999). Informal economic activities of public health workers in Uganda: implication for quality and accessibility of care. *Social Science and Medicine* 49:849–65.

23. Ablo E, Reinikka R. (1998). *Do Budgets Really Matter? Evidence from Public Spending on Education and Health in Uganda*. SIDA.

24. Uganda Ministry of Health. (1999). *Health Sector Strategic Plan: 2000/01–2004/05*. Kampala: Uganda Ministry of Health.

25. Smithson P. (1993). *Financial Constraints to Health Sector Sustainability in Uganda*. Save the Children Fund, UK.

26. Birungi H. (1998). Injections and self-help: risk and trust in Ugandan health care. *Social Science and Medicine* 47:1455–62.

27. Mugaju J. (1996). *The Road to Collapse*. Kampala: Fountain Publishers.

28. Knowles J, Hotchkiss D. (1996). *Economic Analysis of the Health Sector Policy Reform Program Assistance in Egypt*. Bethesda, MD: Partnership for Health Reform.

29. Monico SM. (2003). *Fighting AIDS in Uganda: What Worked*. Statement to the Foreign Relations Committee Subcomittee on Africa. 2003, United States Congress, 19/05/2003. Washington, DC: Global Health Council.

30. Karim QA, Tarantola D, Sy EA, Moodie R. (1997). Government responses to HIV/AIDS in Africa: what have we learnt? *AIDS* 11:143–9.

31. Berkley SF. (1994). Public health measures to prevent HIV spread in Africa. In: Essex M, Mboup S, Kanki PJ, Kalengayi MR, eds. *AIDS in Africa*. New York: Raven Press, p473–95.

32. Boahene K. (1996). The IXth International Conference on AIDS and STD in Africa. *AIDS Care* 8: 609–616.

33. Serwadda D. (2003) Beyond abstinence. *Washington Post*, 16/05/2003, pA29.

34. Parkhurst JO. (2001). The crisis of AIDS and the politics of response: the case of Uganda. *International Relations* 15:69–87.

35. Uganda AIDS Control Programme. (2001). *HIV/AIDS Surveillance Report*. Kampala: Uganda Ministry of Health.

36. UNAIDS. (2002). *Uganda: Epidemiological Fact Sheet on HIV/AIDS and Sexually Transmitted Infections: 2002 Update*. Geneva: UNAIDS.

37. Stoneburner RL, Low-Beer D. (2004). Population-level HIV declines and behavioural risk avoidance in Uganda. *Science* 304:714–8.

38. Whitworth JAG, Mahe C, Mbulaiteye SM *et al.* (2002). HIV-1 epidemic trends in rural south-west Uganda over a 10-year period. *Tropical Medicine and International Health* 7:1047–52.

39. Williams B, Gouws W, Wilkinson D, Karim SA. (2001) Estimating HIV incidence rates from the age prevalence data in epidemic situations. *Statistics in Medicine* 20:2003–16.

40. Wawer MJ, Gray R, Serwadda D *et al.* Declines in HIV Prevalence in Uganda: Not as Simple as ABC. Presented at the12th Conference on Retroviruses and Opportunistic Infections, Boston, MA, 23 February 2005. Oral Presentation 27LB. Available at: http://www.retroconference.org/2005/cd/Abstracts/25775.htm (accessed 4 July 2005).

41. Condom Coordination Unit. (1999). *Draft Overview of Condom Situation in Uganda*. Entebbe: Uganda Ministry of Health.

42. World Bank. (2003). *Sexually Transmitted Infection Project, Uganda*. Washington, DC: The World Bank.

43. Weissman E, Sentumbwe O, Mbonye AK, Kayaga E, Kihuguru SM, Lissner C. (1998). *Uganda Safe Motherhood Programme Costing Study: Draft Final Report*. World Health Organization.

44. Government of Uganda, Uganda AIDS Commission, UNAIDS. (2000). *The National Strategic Framework for HIV/AIDS Activities in Uganda: 2000/1–2005/6*. Kampala: Government of Uganda.

45. Walker D, Muyinda H, Foster S, Kengeya-Kayondo J, Whitworth J. (2001). The quality of care by private practitioners for sexually transmitted diseases in Uganda. *Health Policy and Planning* 16:35–40.

46. Uganda Ministry of Health. (2003). *Antiretroviral Treatment Policy for Uganda*. Kampala: Ministry of Health.

47. Smith MK. (2002). *Generic Competition, Price and Access to Medicines: The Case of Antiretrovirals in Uganda*. Oxfam International.

48. Uganda Ministry of Health. (Undated). *Prevention of Mother to Child HIV Ttransmission: Scale-up Plan: 2001–2005*. Kampala: Uganda Ministry of Health.

Chapter 18

Cambodia

Guy Morineau[*], Maurits H van Pelt, Frédéric Bourdier and R Cameron Wolf

Background

The emergence of HIV in Cambodia occurred at a time when the health system was in great need of reinforcement following the devastation of civil war and collapse of the government and health infrastructure. Health system institutions had to be rebuilt, strengthened or even created anew. Financial resources appeared rapidly and massively through donors, international aid and humanitarian assistance. Cambodia welcomed these resources and the attached foreign experts, embarking on the creation of a functional health system. The Ministry of Health's absorptive capacity was quickly stretched to its limits, while the international response to the HIV epidemic created and continues to create new channels of foreign aid to deal with the AIDS emergency, often in vertical systems. This has ultimately led to the situation today, where Cambodia has had some key successes in dealing with HIV prevention while struggling to contend with a mature AIDS epidemic as the health system is still being built.

The Kingdom of Cambodia, with 13.4 million people in 2005, is mostly Theravada Buddhist and ethnically Khmer. Cambodia is gradually recovering from a 30-year period of war and destruction. The country's ratio of tax revenue to gross domestic product (GDP) could remain exceptionally low, at just 8.4% in 2001, because of the flow of external aid provided by a multitude of countries and agencies. Foreign assistance significantly exceeded domestic financing between 1996 and 2001 [1]. This trend continues to the present; the health sector, including HIV programming, is largely financed through foreign aid. The international community meets the Royal Government annually to discuss progress and make new pledges.

Still predominantly a rural society, with more than 80% of the population living in villages, Cambodia's population is growing at 1.8% annually (Fig. 18.1). Every year an estimated 200,000 young people enter the labour market, but no more than 20,000 jobs can be created in the formal sector per year [2]. Economic growth and foreign direct investment are not currently sufficient to relieve this situation. The nation became a member of the World Trade Organization in September 2003. However, it is too early to say whether one day Cambodia will reap the benefits from membership. Cambodia endorsed the strict intellectual property framework suggested by the World Intellectual Property Organization (WIPO), which seriously threatens access to affordable essential drugs, specifically for antiretrovirals. Fortunately, this treaty does not have to be applied to drug procurement and production, including generics, until 2016.

* Corresponding author.

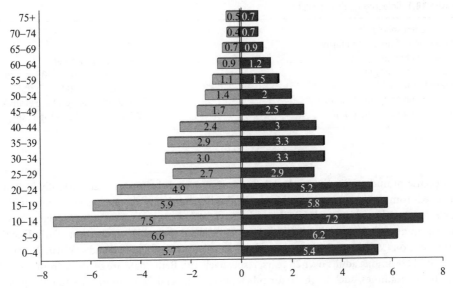

Fig. 18.1 Population pyramid, 2004. Source: Cambodia inter-censal survey 2004.

Over the past decade, several national surveys addressing demographic, health and socio-economic issues have been carried out in Cambodia, but interpreting the data in order to give a comprehensive picture of the health status in the country is a challenge, due to differences in methodologies and coverage of these studies. The service sector now occupies 40% of the GDP, matching that of the agricultural sector with a GDP per capita of US$320 in 2003. One-third of the population lives below the poverty line, as is evident by the average income of US$0.46 per day in rural areas [3]. The Gini indicator, which is related to inequality, has been rising sharply. Investigations show that healthcare-related costs play a prominent role among the direct causes of poverty [4]. Although the diseases primarily responsible for this economic burden have yet to be identified, chronic diseases are likely to play a prominent role due to their recurrent need for health services.

In the 2000 Cambodia Demographic and Health Survey, life expectancy at birth was 54 years for men and 58 years for women [5]. Maternal mortality was high at 437 maternal deaths in 100,000 live births [5]. Additionally, 20% of the children under 5 years of age were severely stunted. While qualitative surveys have shown that weaning habits and food taboos may play an important role in malnutrition, no one can deny that poverty and social inequalities are also critical factors that contribute to the persistence of malnutrition, associated with 54% of childhood deaths [6]. Other key demographic and health indicators are shown in Table 18.1.

The majority of Cambodians have little or no education, with females considerably less educated than males [5]. Gender issues appear to lie at the root of many of the Cambodian society's inequalities and health disparities, as revealed by one of the lowest gender development indices in Asia [7]. Moreover, while the burden of labour falls disproportionately on women [8], they are paid less and are treated as second-rate employees, more prone to be manipulated and socio-economically exploited. Cambodian women also lack power in reproductive decision making.

Table 18.1 Selected health indicators

Average household size	5.4
Percentage of unplanned births	32%
Total fertility rate	4 children per woman
Maternal mortality rate	437 deaths per 100,000 live births
Infant mortality rate	89 deaths per 1000 live births
Under-5 mortality rate (urban)	92.6 deaths per 1000 live births
Under-5 mortality rate (rural)	126 deaths per 1000 live births

Source: [5].

Because of underutilization and under-reporting, no reliable picture can currently be constructed from public service statistics on Cambodia's burden of disease. Many *ad hoc* studies have been conducted in Cambodia that strive to provide some indication on particular diseases in the country. One example is with diabetes, which was the subject of a recent World Health Organization (WHO) study that showed high prevalence rates in a rural and semi-rural area, at 5% and 11% among adults over 25 years, respectively [9]. Better data are available from vertical health programmes, such as those for tuberculosis (TB) and HIV voluntary counselling and testing (VCT). The 2002 national TB survey found a prevalence of 270 smear-positive cases per 100,000 population.

Rebuilding the Cambodian public health system

The Cambodian public health system was loosely modelled after the Vietnamese example during the 1980s. It virtually collapsed during the early 1990s and only started to receive the kind of international governmental development assistance it is currently getting after the 1993 elections, which were held under the auspices of the United Nations.

The gradual erosion of civil servants' wages, including health workers' salaries, has forced the latter to develop individual coping strategies that sharply reduce access of the poorest to education, health and other services. Besides asking for unofficial fees from patients at the public hospital or health clinic, government health workers have started to run private clinics. The percentage of out-of-pocket expenses for healthcare is among the highest in the world at 75–85%. They are a result of direct negotiation between the patient and the drug seller or the health staff, which takes place in an unregulated environment. As a consequence, the poor face important financial obstacles when they need to access health services, and poverty is frequently caused by illness [10]. Healthcare accounts for 30% of all household expenditures, and 45% of the recent landless in Cambodia lost their land because of illness of a family member [11]. A healthcare demand survey found that the average cost for treatment at a hospital was US$65 in 1996 and that 45% of patients had to borrow money to meet the expense [12]. The military and the police have their own health systems, which suffer from the same systemic deficiencies that wreak havoc on the civilian health system. The ensuing conflict of interest at the point of treatment undermines effective delivery of public health services. As a consequence, the majority of the Cambodian people choose to seek healthcare in the unregulated private sector.

As early as 1989, non-governmental organizations (NGOs) working in the health sector established a coordination and information platform that advocates on Cambodian health issues [13]. Since 1993, the Ministry of Health has gone through a series of ambitious health sector reform projects. Coordination of donor-driven projects has continued to pose a particular challenge for Cambodia. For example, more than 100 NGOs have joined in the largely donor-funded fight against HIV. Today, international NGOs continue to deploy significant resources to improve health service provision, although their role is increasingly being shared by Cambodian organizations as the civil society develops. To address the health problems caused by TB, malaria, dengue, sexually transmitted infections (STIs) and HIV, and to improve mother and child health, the Ministry of Health's vertical programmes have received considerable direct donor support and funding, using a variety of disease control strategies. Multiple bilateral and multilateral agencies lobby to influence the policy process serving a variety of agendas, perhaps more preoccupied with obtaining short-term results for their own political goals and objectives than the longer-term developmental goals of the country.

In 1996, the government approved its first overall framework for channelling the bulk of financial and technical assistance for the health sector based on the Operational District model. The Operational District is a decentralized health management unit covering 100,000–200,000 people. The Operational District consists of a network of health centres, each serving around 10,000 people, that provide first-level integrated curative and preventive care, called the Minimum Package of Activities, and a referral hospital of 120 beds or more that provides the so-called Comprehensive Package of Activities. Cambodia's provinces have been re-mapped into 75 Operational Districts using population and geographical rather than administrative criteria, and this system is gradually replacing the three-tier system of provincial hospital, district hospitals and commune clinics with a two-tier system of referral hospital and health centres nationwide.

Since the Operational District model became official, it has been the basis for several donor investments in health. It can be safely argued that, compared with unassisted areas in the country, these projects show spectacular improvements in utilization of key health services, provided the staff underpayment issue is addressed through salary supplementation and an effective management system is put in place. In these reformed settings, the certainty and predictability of stable user-fees and services have actually helped reduce poverty by decreasing household health expenditure by 40% in some cases [14]. The tertiary sector remains concentrated in Phnom Penh, with six national hospitals including specialized services. Patients needing hi-tech or even basic care continue to go to neighbouring Vietnam and Thailand.

The Health Sector Strategic Plan (HSSP) for 2003–2007 contains the main strategies for the coming years. Simultaneously, the National Poverty Reduction Strategy planned for the period 2003–2005 is in line with the HSSP, adding 'pro-poor' targets. However, there are no mechanisms for monitoring whether or not targets are pursued with effective actions. Both these ambitious strategies lack corresponding programme budgets for effectively tracking implementation.

Public expenditure and effectiveness of the health system

Despite the considerable aid effort, utilization of public facilities remains low at 0.3 annual contacts per person, with provincial variation between 0.1 and 0.8 contacts per person. Government facilities are used for only one-fifth of all illnesses and injuries. This proportion increases to one-third in the case of serious illness or injury, where public facilities are the choice of last resort. Self-treatment purchased over-the-counter is common, even for children under the age of 5 [15], and approximately half of these treatments have been evaluated as potentially hazardous [16]. Data from the Cambodian health information system showed a marginal increase in outpatient and child consultations from 1995 to 2003. The number of contacts remains around 0.5 contacts per child per year, far below the targeted two contacts per year.

The three main reasons behind these failures to deliver lie mostly outside the Ministry of Health's direct control: the extremely low health worker remuneration, which is causing insufficient motivation and unequal geographical distribution of human resources; the way the health budget is being managed; and the health system's lack of accountability to the ultimate users.

Human resources in particular are unevenly distributed within the health sector. Nearly 85% of people live in rural areas, but only 13% of health professionals live in these areas [7]. Given the low incentives, taking up a position in a rural area is simply not attractive to most health workers. Salaries account for just 10% of the Ministry of Health's expenditure, a proportion that ranks it among the lowest in the world [17,18].

The Ministry of Economy and Finance not only spends the capital budget for health [19], it also manages the funds for much of the recurrent part of the health budget. The Treasury is not yet computerized. Accounting continues to be done by hand, thus increasing the potential for irregularities. The government health budget often arrives late and incomplete when it finally reaches public health facilities [19]. In this context, health managers can hardly be expected to perform. New financial management mechanisms have been introduced, but these recent regulations seem to have caused fragmentation of budget management over different systems and intermediaries. No improvement occurred after the World Bank Public Expenditure reviews in 1998 and 2003. The Treasury's current handling of health budgets remains an important obstacle to the functioning of the public health system [18,19].

Until recently, there was no experience with health insurance systems in Cambodia, and it remains to be seen if and how this will develop. German bilateral cooperation started pilot programmes with social insurance in two provinces in 2004, and a plan was formally approved in 2005 by the Ministry of Health. Another phenomenon intent on reducing the excesses caused by the health market failure is the still experimental 'Equity Fund' run by Cambodian social institutions mandated to pre-identify the poor and purchase health-care on their behalf, mostly at the referral hospital level. So far, initiatives in nine provinces, including deprived areas in Phnom Penh, show rapid improvement of access to service for the poor, suggesting a potential to protect poor households against the above-mentioned phenomenon of 'poverty caused by illness'. With the official health budget caught up in a spider web of intractable threads, the steady financing source directly related to service outputs gives the service provider an incentive to perform his duty. For this simple reason, equity funds may well prove to be a cost-effective remedy to the service access problem, at least for the time being [20,21].

The HIV epidemic

Epidemiological surveillance and impact of preventive measures

The first Cambodian HIV infection was reported in 1991 by the national blood bank. HIV spread very quickly in Cambodia, as revealed by modelling of the epidemic, which shows that HIV prevalence was greater than 1% in the adult population only 4 years later [22]. Starting in 1997, international donors supported an HIV surveillance system that included regular rounds of both biological and behavioural surveys conducted on nationally representative samples of sex workers, women attending antenatal care (ANC) clinics, and occupational male groups that served as proxies of clients of sex workers due to their higher rates of reported sex with sex workers. Thanks to the large amount of nationally representative data using comparable sampling methodologies and standard data collection procedures, the Cambodian HIV surveillance system is one of the finest in Asia.

The 1997 HIV sero-survey reported a prevalence of 3.2% among women attending ANCs, which suggested a large-scale HIV epidemic threatening the Cambodian general population. Methodological improvements, as well as the performance of quality control testing of blood samples from previous rounds, have since led researchers to reduce HIV prevalence estimates from the sero-survey rounds from 1997 up to 2003. Despite the 20% downward readjustment based on the improved surveillance methods, HIV prevalence among adults aged 15–49 remained among the highest in Asia at an estimated 1.9% in 2003. Although the highest number of Cambodians suffering from AIDS was reached in 2002, the peak of AIDS mortality is yet to come (Fig. 18.2).

Current analysis of the epidemiologic trends in Cambodia now estimates that the HIV prevalence among Cambodian adults peaked at 3% in 1997 and had declined to 1.9% by 2003. This decrease is most probably due to a reduction of HIV transmission among sex workers and their clients between 1996 and 2000, as supported by a two- to threefold decrease in the prevalence of STIs [23]. This reduction in STI prevalence took place despite a limited coverage of STI services for sex workers, and men's persistence in seeking STI care at pharmacies [24]. However, brothel-based sex workers' use of medical services at last episode of discharge

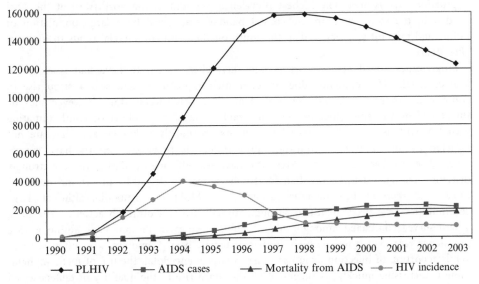

Fig. 18.2 Dynamic of the HIV epidemic in Cambodia. Source: NCHADS.

increased from 36% in 1997 to 70% in 2003 [25]. As a result, both the 100% condom use programme, which provides compulsory monthly check-ups of sex workers, and behaviour change among sex workers and clients have contributed to reducing the incidence of HIV. Between 1997 and 2001, the proportion of men reporting having visited sex workers in the past 3 months had halved, from a 50% baseline to 25%, but increased again to 35% in 2003. In addition, reported levels of consistent condom use in paid sex increased from 40–50% in 1997 to 90–95% in 2003, as reported by both sex workers and their clients. Nevertheless, brothel-based sex workers remain extremely vulnerable. About one-third report that they initiate sex through the sale of their virginity, often without using condoms. Cambodian brothel-based sex workers are also characterized by a high turnover, since 70–80% had sold sex for the first time within the past 2 years [25]. HIV prevalence among brothel-based sex workers reached a high of 44% in 1997 and dropped to 27% by 2003.

Cambodia is experiencing a generalized epidemic, which has shifted from a predominantly male epidemic led by clients of sex workers, to a more feminine epidemic, with women infected through their husbands, who had visited sex workers, and with children of these couples infected through perinatal transmission as a result. While prevalence is decreasing among men as the result of both an increase in AIDS mortality and an overall decrease in incidence of HIV, the incidence in women is still rising. As a result, women's proportion of the epidemic rose from 36% of infections in 1997 to 47% in 2003. Approximately 9000 HIV-infected women were pregnant in 2003. However, with less than one-third of women using ANC services in Cambodia, and only about 900 health centres providing ANC services throughout the country, setting up effective programmes aimed at reducing mother-to-child-transmission (MTCT) of HIV remains a challenge.

The epidemic is not evenly distributed across the country. The distribution of HIV prevalence among women at ANCs follows a pattern of mobility for employment and economic opportunities. The north-east is less affected by HIV, probably due to mountainous terrain, lower population density and poor quality roads that limit mobility of the population in this area. The highest prevalence is found in the north-west at the Thai border, in the south-west on the coastal band characterized by a large population of sailors and migrant workers, and in the south on the main commercial roads to Vietnam (Fig. 18.3).

Programmes aimed at sex workers and their clients seem to have had a successful impact on the HIV epidemic due to fewer men exposed to paid sex, a steep rise in condom use in paid sex, and the control of STIs. This success story, however, may be threatened by the emergence of new vulnerable groups. The cohort of youth initiating sexual activity is large, their sexual behaviours are mostly unknown and they are not targeted by any large-scale education programme, as prevention efforts have mainly targeted sex workers and clients. Men who have sex with men (MSM), who are strongly discriminated against in Cambodian society, have been neglected by prevention interventions until recently. Few data are available for MSM in Cambodia, although large communities have been identified through surveillance and outreach activities. In 2000, a sero-survey conducted among MSM at public venues in Phnom Penh found a 15% prevalence rate, which was as high as that of female beer-promoters, who often sell sex. While reporting of injection drug use remains largely anecdotal, the use of methamphetamine is increasing quickly, as suggested by the sharp rise in the quantity of tablets seized in Cambodia.

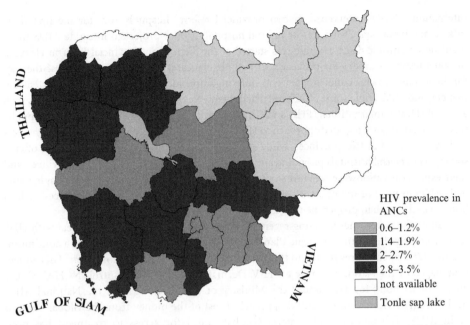

Fig. 18.3 Cambodia 2003: HIV prevalence among pregnant women at ANCs. Source: NCHADS.

National and international response

As soon as the epidemic became a concern in the early 1990s, international and local NGOs quickly developed health-related activities. However, modelling of the HIV epidemic suggests that the incidence of HIV started decreasing in 1994, before the implementation of large-scale prevention programmes [22]. Multiple interventions were introduced by bilateral and multi-lateral donors to address the emergency posed by HIV, while the health system lacked the capacity, including material and human resources, to address the emerging threat to the country. These actors focused on short-term objectives for prevention of HIV and the provision of care for infected people, rather than on longer-term development. Still, without the inter-national support, Cambodia would never have been able to address its HIV epidemic. Successes have included: the extension of anonymous counselling and testing centres, with about 100 centres being set up in 2005; increased involvement of people living with HIV (PLHIV) [26]; and skills training for providers. However, there is a very real challenge for coordination, collaboration and sustained support.

While considerable effort has been made to provide HIV programmes, infants and adults are still dying because of lack of treatment for common and easily treated pathologies. The balance of funding, which favours HIV over other morbidities, would be more acceptable if the whole health system benefited. In the absence of a more integrated approach, HIV funds may appear dispro-portionate to public health planners, given the other health concerns of the country.

Vertical and integrated approaches to HIV treatment

Apart from drugs available in private and informal sectors, the first antiretroviral drugs were officially distributed in 2000 by Médecins du Monde and Médecins Sans Frontières. These international NGOs intervened in two provincial referral hospitals and, for the first time, in a rural Operational District at its referral hospital. A pilot project to integrate AIDS treatment into a chronic diseases clinic was started at the Siem Reap Provincial Referral Hospital in 2002, testing a model for provision of ambulatory care, including antiretroviral therapy, for the steadily growing cohorts of patients suffering from chronic diseases such as hypertension, diabetes and HIV. While some NGOs restricted themselves to clinic-based activities, others such as Family Health International (FHI) and CARE International chose to work closely with public services to adopt an integrated approach to HIV, which included both medical and social aspects and was launched in two provinces, while encouraging participation and mobilization of civil society. The referral hospitals providing antiretrovirals are still restricted to a few provinces, and their expansion nationwide remains slow. As a result, the increasing number of people living with AIDS in need of medical treatment are still more likely to receive basic services such as home-based care than proper medical follow-up that includes antiretrovirals.

In 2000, the government, having received substantial external resources to deal with HIV, reinforced its policy with a Strategic Plan for HIV that included prevention and a continuum of care [27]. Expenditures related to this plan amounted to US$6.5 million a year. This budget is managed by the National Centre for HIV, Dermatology and STD Control (NCHADS), the main official body for HIV under the Ministry of Health along with the National AIDS Authority (NAA), in a multisectoral approach. Most of the money from the Global Fund to Fight AIDS, Tuberculosis and Malaria (Global Fund) for access to treatment has been channelled through NCHADS. The plan is to increase the number of people receiving antiretrovirals to 10,000 by the end of 2005, up from the 6000 who were already receiving them at the beginning of the year.

Key challenges of the HIV programme in Cambodia

When considering HIV programmes as a whole, many challenges remain. The proportion of MTCT among HIV cases is increasing. Clearly, this is an area that needs to be accorded more focused, integrated programming between enhanced antenatal care and HIV counselling and testing [28]. The 2000 Demographic and Health Survey reported that a minority of Cambodian women are in a position to deliver their babies in the limited numbers of hospitals in the country. Furthermore, few of these facilities provide single-dose nevirapine to reduce the possibility of transmission. In addition, protocols of paediatric treatments are not available, and many children have no option but to receive unsuitable adult therapies. Problems in preventing and treating HIV among mothers and children are exacerbated because prevention of MTCT, within the vertical maternal and child health programme, is not well linked under the Ministry of Health to NCHADS.

A related issue is that children of HIV-infected parents, including orphans, are largely neglected by current prevention, care and treatment efforts. These children confront both poverty and the trauma related to familial illness, death and loss from HIV. They are discriminated against by society and face increased challenges for their future. Cambodia does not currently guarantee the legal rights of these children for inheritance. Moreover, there is a lack of adequate protection for PLHIV or patients with any illness in dealing with health professionals.

HIV-related care and treatment should be patient- and family-focused in order to improve adherence to, and acceptance of, treatment. Quality of care, including basic clinical management and the control of pain and symptoms, needs to be assessed more rigorously. Social and psychological factors should be taken into account in order to provide a continuum of care that attracts patients through all stages of disease. The negative image of the public health system is so widespread that it will not be easy for the government to alter the cultural perception unless a drastic and explicit improvement in quality of care takes place.

Although some of the Cambodian people living with HIV have, since 1997, managed to come together to forge their own organizations under the sponsorship of UN agencies and NGOs, they need to have a stronger voice in determining health services throughout the country. Their contribution to promoting the feasibility of adequate and universal access to treatment is essential. Despite recent successes in providing ART in some regions, AIDS-related stigma and discrimination are still rampant in Cambodia among health staff and in society at large [25].

Provision of antiretroviral therapy is a dynamic process, in terms of both advances in medical treatment and the availability and quality of drugs. Until recently, antiretroviral drugs were purchased by six NGOs. Now, most antiretroviral drugs will be purchased through the Global Fund via the Ministry of Health procurement office. The Global Fund's recipients cannot order drugs without mid-term planning, which implies critical management and financial accountability. The need to adjust treatment in cases of drug resistance, side effects and other unforeseen complications must be appropriately met and managed. Furthermore, the triple therapy usually recommended and provided in Cambodia is the relatively inexpensive combination of nevirapine, stavudine and lamivudine, which costs US$350 per year per person and is recommended by the WHO. Some infectious disease specialists maintain that, while the recommended combination is generally biologically accepted by the patients, providers must be prepared to diversify therapy in the near future. Tackling this issue will require an expanded treatment policy that also specifies second- and third-line regimens.

Donor-driven vertical programmes may function in isolation. The TB programme, under the auspices of WHO, is a good example; the internationally criticized directly observed treatment (DOT) protocol [29] has been condemned in Cambodia for its failure to address co-infection with HIV appropriately. Until recently, according to the standard TB guidelines, co-infected individuals could not receive TB preventive therapy because they were considered ineligible; AIDS treatment sites would not begin antiretroviral treatment until the TB was addressed. HIV has gradually been rising among TB patients, from 2.5% in 1995 to 8.4% in 2002 [30]. While more than 60% of HIV-infected people are co-infected with TB [31], they had not been able to receive TB treatment because of inadequate guidelines. The integration of community-based programmes, such as home-based care and PLHIV support groups, with facility-based services is necessary in order to provide comprehensive care.

Conclusion

Donors need to have both short-term and long-term objectives and an appropriate health sector development vision. While some positive and urgently needed services have been provided to PLHIV in Cambodia, integrated strategies are vital in order to address the immediate needs for HIV prevention, care and treatment, while building a sustainable response for the future of the health system.

Beyond this shift in strategic planning, the systemic problems within the health sector outlined in this chapter must be addressed. Otherwise, access to treatment and care in the public sector may be compromised. Building a separate health system for treatment of HIV patients is one alternative, but, in the long term, that is an undesirable solution for myriad reasons. At this time, policy-makers would be wise to pay more attention to the effectiveness of public service delivery to those who need it, make resources available for integrated services, especially for the poor, and support civil society demands for more accountability and other initiatives that aim to bridge the current gap between service providers and users.

By providing funds that do not flow through regular governmental channels, the Global Fund may create fresh opportunities to make the health system perform as a whole. However, the number of different actors delivering HIV services is an unavoidable constraint to harmonization of the national HIV programme, and this may delay the implementation of an effective national policy integrating HIV as part of the global health strategy under the the Ministry of Health.

References

1. World Bank, Asian Development Bank. (2003). *Report No.25611-KH*. Manila: World Bank and Asian Development Bank.
2. Sok Hach, Sarthi Acharya. (2002). *Cambodia's Annual Economic Review 2002*. Phnom Penh: Cambodia Development Research Institute.
3. Council for Social Development. (2002). *National Poverty Reduction Strategy 2003–2005*. Phnom Penh: Council for Social Development.
4. Bloom DE, River Path Associates, Sevilla J. (2001). *Health, Wealth AIDS and Poverty—The Case of Cambodia*. Manila: Asian Development Bank.
5. National Institute of Statistics, Directorate General for Health (Cambodia) and ORC Macro. (2000). *Cambodian Demographic and Health Survey 2000*. Phnom Penh, Cambodia, and Calverton, Maryland, MD: ORC Macro.
6. Ministry of Health of Cambodia. (2003). *Analysis of Slow Progress in Child Mortality Reduction: Benchmark Report for the Consultative Group*. Phnom Penh: Ministry of Health.
7. United Nations Development Programme. (2003). *Human Development Report 2003: Millennium Development Goals: A Compact Among Nations to End Human Poverty*. New York: Oxford University Press.
8. Asian Development Bank. (2001). *Participatory Poverty Assessment: Cambodia*. Manila: Asian Development Bank.
9. King H. (2005). *Cambodia Diabetes Survey 2005*. Manila: World Health Organization.
10. Rose G. (2001). *Phnom Penh Intra-urban Health Survey*. Manila: World Health Organization.
11. OXFAM Great Britain. (2000). *Health and Landlessness; The Cambodia Land Study Project*. Vol. 4. Phnom Penh.
12. National Public Health and Reasearch Institute, World Health Organization, Gesellschaft fur Technische Zusammenarbeit. (1998). *The Demand for Health Care in Cambodia*. Phnom Penh: National Institute of Public Health.
13. Medicam. Medicam organisation and profile. Available at: http://www.bigpond.com.kh/users/medicam/organisationprofile.htm. Accessed May 2005.
14. Bhushan I, Keller S, Schwartz B. (2002). Achieving the twin objectives of efficiency and equity: contracting health services in Cambodia. In: *ERD Policy Brief 6*. Manila: Asian Development Bank.

15. National Institute of Public Health. (1999). *National Health Survey 1998*. Phnom Penh: National Institute of Public Health.

16. Vickery C, Rose G, Dixon S *et al.* (2002). *Private Practitioners in Phnom Penh: A Mystery Client Study*. Manila: World Health Organization.

17. Van Lerberghe W, Conceicao C, Van Damme W. (2002). When staff is underpaid: dealing with the individual coping strategies of health personnel. *WHO Bulletin* **80**(7).

18. World Bank and Asian Development Bank. (2003). *Integrated Fiduciary Assessment and Public Expenditure Review (IFAPER): Cambodia Enhancing Service Delivery Through Improved Resource Allocation and Institutional Reform*. Report No 25611-KH. Manila: World Bank and Asian Development Bank.

19. World Bank, Asian Development Bank. (1999). *Cambodia Public Expenditure Review: Enhancing the Effectiveness of Public Expenditure*. Manila: World Bank and Asian Development Bank.

20. Meessen B. (2003). Iatrogenic poverty. *Tropical Medicine and International Health* **8**:581–584.

21. Hardeman W, van Damme W, van Pelt M *et al.* (2004). Access to health care for all? User fees plus a Health Equity Fund in Sotnikom, Cambodia. *Health Policy and Planning* **19**(1):22–32.

22. Cambodian working group on HIV/AIDS projection. (2002). *Projection for HIV/AIDS in Cambodia: 2000–2010*. Phnom Penh: FHI/USAID.

23. National Center for HIV/AIDS Dermatology and STDs. (2002). *2001 Cambodia STI Survey*. Phnom Penh: FHI/USAID.

24. National Center for HIV/AIDS Dermatology and STDs. (1998). *Behavioral Surveillance Survey 1997*. Phnom Penh: FHI/USAID.

25. National Center for HIV/AIDS Dermatology and STDs. (2004). *Behavioral Surveillance Survey 2003*. Phnom Penh: FHI/USAID.

26. Mullemwa J, Vutheary K. (2004). *Greater Involvement of People Living with, and Affected by, HIV and AIDS (GIPA) Project in Cambodia: An Evaluation Report*. Phnom Penh: UNV/UNAIDS.

27. Ministry of Health of Cambodia. (2000). *Strategic Plan for HIV/AIDS and STI: Prevention and Care 2001–2005*. Phnom Penh: Ministry of Health.

28. UNAIDS Cambodia. (2004). *An Overview of the HIV/AIDS/STI Situation and the National Response in Cambodia—Country Profile*, 5th edn. Phnom Penh: UNAIDS.

29. Farmer P. (1998). *The Modern Plague: Infections and Inequalities*. Berkeley: University of California Press.

30. Ministry of Health. (2003). *International Symposium on TB Prevalence in Cambodia, 25–02–2003*. Phnom Penh: Ministry of Health.

31. Dye C, Scheele S, Dolin P *et al.* (1999). Global burden of tuberculosis: WHO global surveillance and monitoring project. *Journal of the American Medical Assocation* **282**:677–86.

Chapter 19

People's Republic of China

Ma Shao-Jun, Sheila Hillier[*], Zhang Kong-Lai[*], Jay
J Shen, Lu Fan, Liu Min and Jin Cheng-Gang

Background

China is the world's most populous nation and the largest and most powerful communist state. Over the last 20 years, the country has been experiencing two major transitions: China has been moving from a command economy to one based upon the market while remaining communist controlled, and from a largely rural society to an urban, industrialized one that has seen enormous economic growth, with a fourfold increase in per capita income.

Transitions of this magnitude can produce potential problems. These include insecurity in employment, relentless poverty, a poorly developed social security structure, inequalities, instability, unchecked internal migration and rising health costs [1]. All of these have occurred in China, but it has managed so far to avoid major instability and collapse. To a large degree, the population has responded and adjusted to the changes as far as they have gone; the transition is by no means complete. Political reform has lagged behind economic reform, and the legal system to cope with a developing market economy is immature.

Macroeconomic policies have had an impact on the delivery of healthcare, and the sector has benefited less than other key areas. Preventive healthcare systems have been a particular casualty. Although an efficient and effective health system should correctly be regarded as part of societal and state infrastructure, during this transitional period the health sector has been treated as a vestige of the command economy in need of the reform that would transform it into a proper market player. Although the system certainly required updating and alteration, partly to cope with a variety of new health challenges, there have been unanticipated side effects, misdirection and difficulties in problem recognition. Solutions have been subject to delays arising from the need to achieve political and administrative consensus within China's government structures.

These drawbacks, which might be regarded by the leadership as a necessary price to pay for rapid development, have undermined China's former international reputation as an impressive producer of health gains. During its first 30 years, the People's Republic of China (PRC) significantly improved the health of its people by alleviating poverty, improving literacy and producing a healthcare system that carried out extensive preventive programmes and provided a low-cost system of medical care to its huge rural population. Currently, it is fair to say that China is facing difficulties in providing good quality, affordable and equitable health services to

[*] Corresponding authors.

the majority of its rural population, and its urban and rural poor. Particular threats are posed by chronic disease and the spread of AIDS.

Important shifts are now taking place in China. The rapid pace of growth, although it may have improved long-term prospects overall, has revealed social problems—poverty and ill health—that now require attention. There are new leaders in China who will continue to push the economic reforms forward, but who must also manage the social, economic and political problems that go with them [1]. Increasingly, they will need to be aware of a variety of emerging interest groups. Chinese society has changed and become fragmented, more unequal and less homogeneous. Many of its citizens have either grown up or will come of age in a market-oriented system. They will have different experiences, demands and priorities from those of their parents

The Communist Party of China (CPC) is the central and leading political power in China. Its structure, organization, activity and future remain a source of fascination to Western scholars. They argue about the extent to which the Party represents a rational bureaucracy, with slow and guarded movement up and down the hierarchy, and the degree to which it resembles more of an arena of competing factions at the highest level. Elements of both these styles can be observed in the workings of the Party, military and government structures. What is in no doubt is the CPC's control of all the major power structures in the country.

The standing committee of the Politburo, some 25–35 top leaders with one paramount leader, has been the highest level of power in the PRC. The Politburo oversees the State Council, which is the premier governmental body responsible for national policies. It controls the activities of 29 ministries, including the *Weishengbu*, the Ministry of Public Health.

Since the mid-1980s, provincial governments have enjoyed greater independence from the centre and exercised control over their own budgets. Directly below the provincial government is that of the *xian*, or county. With reforms in local government and population changes accompanying urbanization, the number of counties has changed slightly, now standing at around 2000. The *xian* is largely a rural seat of government, but a corresponding urban structure is the city government. Independent city governments were developed in the 1980s to promote the more efficient administration of large urban centres by separating them from their provincial governments. County-level administration has traditionally exercised authority over the tier below, which is the township, but, since the administrative and economic reforms of the 1980s, townships have become more autonomous. Although county and provincial administrations set broad strategic objectives, local townships have a lot of control over resources [2]. The basic administrative unit is the village.

Provincial populations range from 1.9 million in Tibet to 100 million in Sichuan. Typically, a province will contain about 70 counties, each of which may have a population of about 350,000. A typical county will contain about 25 townships with anything from 16,000 to 50,000 inhabitants. There are about 45,000 townships in China. A township will be administratively associated with about 14–16 villages in which the population can range from several hundred to several thousand. The number of villages is around 700,000. In cities, the situation is quite similar, with neighbourhood and street committees that resemble the township–village structure.

Seventy-five per cent of China's population lives and works on the land, but some of the traditional rural–urban distinctions are becoming blurred as areas surrounding towns become increasingly urbanized. This percentage is also declining as many young and middle-aged rural people leave to seek temporary work in towns, although they are still registered as rural residents.

The health system

The health system in China displays remarkable historical continuity. China was committed to State medicine as part of the modernizing movement following the revolution of 1912, when the Chinese Republic was formed [3–5]. The nationwide hierarchical structure of hospitals and preventive health services evolved from the early 1920s and became more highly developed in the years after the communist revolution of 1948 [6]. To this day, it retains many original features and replicates the pyramidal structures of government administration. This structure, especially when expanded throughout the rural areas in the 1960s, brought important health gains to China and greatly improved the lives of rural citizens by providing low-cost, collectively financed healthcare, and vertically organized, locally run systems of epidemic control and maternal and child health.

At the apex is the Ministry of Public Health, accountable to the State Council. At each level below, there is a system of 'dual control' comprising control by the government (and, by implication, political) unit and line management by professional health staff. Each tier, down to county level, has a department of public health. At the base, a 'three-tier' organization linking county or municipality, township and village has been designed to act as a referral chain from primary to secondary care and a means of technical assistance from county health department to the villages.

The Ministry of Public Health is responsible for specific areas of work, including medical research and medical schools, and controls some national disease programmes including, most recently, HIV. Provincial capitals usually contain major, modern hospitals of 500–600 beds. The public health department of the province is supposed to manage policies for maternal and child health down through the counties and the three-tier network. The executive level is the County Health Department, which also manages the 300-bed county hospital. Training of doctors can take place at provincial, county and township level, with the lower two levels training short-course rural doctors or traditional doctors, or village health workers. These individuals staff the small 20-bed township hospitals and village clinics.

This template of organization, training and delivery of healthcare, whilst still the major form nationally, has undergone many changes since the macroeconomic transformation in China began in the early 1980s [7–9]. A major problem described then was in rural healthcare. The decline of the communes and introduction of individual methods of household production of grain and other foodstuffs led to a collapse in the collective revenues that had formed a major part of the financing of rural healthcare. The cooperative medical system (CMS), a fund to which households contributed with matching amounts from village welfare funds, disappeared. Fees for services performed became the norm. Rural hospitals had to become self-supporting and therefore raised prices. The 'barefoot doctors' left or became private practitioners. Inequalities in health began to increase; between 1981 and 1990, the ratio of rural to urban infant mortality rates increased from 1.67 to 1.75 [10].

In the cities, too, with the removal of government subsidy, hospitals became profit oriented. Overuse of expensive technologies and excessive drug use were the inappropriate means of raising revenue to which many organizations resorted. There were also difficulties with the national schistosomiasis programme and a slowing of overall improvements in health. Inequalities in health began to worsen. Existing insurance systems were limited to a small portion of the population and worked inefficiently. The number of health workers declined, especially at the basic levels. Many people were by then paying for healthcare.

The health system, 1990–2003

In the last decade of the twentieth century, both ministers and local health authorities were aware that village medical teams were weak, township hospitals were closing, there was a severe shortage of medical personnel and infectious diseases were on the rise [11]. China had received assistance from the World Bank, the World Health Organization (WHO) and UNICEF in keeping maternal and child health (MCH) programmes going and supporting some healthcare experiments in rural clinics. China was involved in the WHO's worldwide 'Health for All by 2000' initiative and set forth a number of objectives. The chief of these was that in the next 10 years, all rural counties must be at a basic standard and 10% of them would reach that standard ahead of time [12–16].

The spring and summer of 1989 saw a wave of protests in China, culminating in the Tiananmen events in June, when these protests were suppressed. Leaders realized that the movement towards economic reform had brought something much larger in its wake. The changes in the rural areas had brought increased productivity and wealth, and there was little desire to alter rural activities by more central interventions. There was to be no intervention to prevent the decline of rural healthcare. This, together with the pressures to reform the large state enterprises, meant that the focus in healthcare switched to a consideration of systems for financing urban healthcare and ridding the State of the burden of supporting hospitals and insurance systems that were deemed outdated and expensive.

Therefore, throughout the early 1990s, two trends were observed in relation to rural health. The first was a 'laissez-faire' natural experiment to let rural people pay for healthcare themselves and observe the outcome. The second was a long series of experiments with various forms of rural health insurance that were carefully monitored by government health administrators and university departments of public health. Results were published and conferences held, but on the ground, moves towards establishing a sound method for supporting rural healthcare were slow indeed.

Rural health services

Meanwhile, evidence of the failings in rural healthcare had become apparent. In one survey, 50% of farmers complained that medical expenses made them poor, and one-third of rural families claimed that their poverty was caused by illness [16]. Ministry estimates showed that costs for outpatient and inpatient visits to rural hospitals had increased almost threefold between 1993 and 1998 [17]. Essentially, nearly all rural dwellers were paying directly for healthcare and had done so for over a decade.

Commentators now seem to regard the 1970s, when the situation was very different and over 90% of China's rural dwellers had access to low-cost healthcare at village and township levels, as a 'golden age'. It was not. The cooperative medical system (CMS) was an important innovation, but it often failed [6]. To ignore the reasons why only ensures the failure of future systems for the rural areas. The funds were inadequate or used up by demands for expensive hospital treatments. These demands were reinforced by the poor levels of training of some 'barefoot doctors'. The system often worked preferentially in favour of those with political power in the village [17]. In the mid-1980s it covered only about 5% of villages [19].

There was some improvement in the early 1990s, when CMS coverage roughly doubled and a government pilot project took a detailed look at the workings of the CMS in 14 rural counties [20]. The new experimental programmes were more varied in style, with a number of payment options suited to the different economic levels of villages. Some required a small basic down-payment for which participants then got a price reduction on village and township services; some had a risk pool to cover big medical expenses; and, in others, a certain proportion of outpatient and inpatient costs was reimbursed—in both cases with contributions from the village and township governments [17,20].

The research findings point to the important fact that a moderate to high income within an area is necessary for these programmes to work. In 1998, the CMS covered 22% of the population in richer areas but only 2% in poor areas [21]. They do not solve the problem of providing affordable healthcare for the 30 million 'extreme poor' and the 60 million 'marginal poor' in the rural areas. Even in prosperous areas, in the studies above, coverage was limited. The reasons people gave for not taking up the scheme were that the benefits were small, accounting and entitlement systems were not transparent, quality of treatment was poor, or that they were healthy and did not need access [17,20,22].

The most senior organs of government, including the State Council, stated their intention to reinstate the CMS in some form in 1991, 1994 and 1997, yet a viable system still remained beyond reach in 2000 [23–25]. Organizational barriers include difficulties over collecting payments and variable skills in administration and accounting at township and village levels. The emphasis on decentralization has given local governments a lot of freedom in how they interpret the guidelines, and, through the development of village and township industries, they control resources. The fact that they are not rushing to reinstall the CMS in rural areas suggests that many of the above problems remain unsolved and township governments are reluctant to commit their resources towards what is perceived as an unproductive sector of subsidized healthcare.

Bloom notes that 'the Chinese government spends little on rural health by international standards' [1]. Localities below county level have always had to generate their own funds with little central assistance. Most of the provincial health budget goes towards paying salaries of personnel at the higher levels. There has been an increased capital building programme over the decade, but this has not solved the problems of accessibility and quality of rural healthcare.

China's 48,000 township hospitals, mostly located within half an hour's walk of the populations they serve (WHO's criterion of accessibility), are struggling. Usage rates have fallen to between 40 and 50%, and government contributions are between 10 and 15%. Much of the problem relates to quality of care, which many feel is more assured at a county-level hospital. For less serious illnesses, the private doctors in village clinics win out on accessibility. Not only are township hospitals squeezed between competitors, but poorer ones cannot retain the most skilled staff members, who leave for higher salaries elsewhere. Less than one-third of their employees have a professional medical qualification [26]. Their relationship with township governments is not well managed [27]. Though townships supply the financing, finance systems are often incoherent. In the poorest townships, over 80% of the hospital budget is spent on salaries and pensions [28].

Over the last decade, somewhere between 80 and 90% of rural dwellers have been paying fees for services [29]. Sixty-five per cent of rural patients could not go to hospital for necessary treatment and, of those who could, more than half left prematurely [29]. Two developments have contributed to the growing cost of healthcare. Of the 690,000 village health stations, about half are privately owned, and there is no healthcare subsidy. The *Peoples' Daily* acknowledged that 'the uncontrolled increase in the price of medicines and the spread of fake and low-quality medicines caused by careless supervision have created barriers for poor farmers' [30]. Medical costs have risen higher than farmers' salaries. At the same time, hospitals at all levels, given the high cost to the institutions of pensions and salaries, need to raise fees and sell services to survive. Doctors make up income from drug sales and—although these are not so common in rural areas—by overuse and misuse of advanced health technologies such as ultrasound and computed tomography (CT) scanning [31]. Some studies estimate that 65% of hospital revenues come from drug sales [32]. Government pricing policy allows a 15–30% mark-up on sales.

Rural areas are experiencing growing variation in wealth and greater diversity in enterprise. There is intra-rural inequality as well as the more commonly reported rural–urban inequality in accessibility and utilization of healthcare services. Wide variations have also been detected in mortality and morbidity, with the poorest counties experiencing higher levels of infant mortality and infectious disease. Infant mortality figures vary from 27.3 per 1000 to 72 per 1000 [33].

Urban health services

As Liu has pointed out, the distinction between rural and urban is becoming less clear, particularly in those areas surrounding cities and large towns [34]. Yet, it is still useful for understanding differences in China. Urban hospitals are better equipped and staffed than their rural counterparts, and are more accessible. Most importantly, until recently, urban dwellers, who were more likely to be employed by State enterprises or by the government, enjoyed a generous system of healthcare benefits. These were dispensed through two main insurance schemes, the Government insurance scheme, *gongfei yiliao* (GIS) and the Labour insurance scheme, *laobao yiliao* (LIS). These schemes covered both medical expenses and pensions. LIS covered about 43% of the urban population and GIS about 7%. This was a highly inequitable system, since over 60% of healthcare costs were expended on about 14% of China's population.

In the cities, because costs were kept fairly low, even the uninsured could afford care. Throughout the 1990s, however, there were strenuous and successful attempts to reform these insurance plans and make people contribute to them instead of simply laying the costs at the door of the enterprise. Typically, at the beginning of the 1990s, LIS represented about 9% of an enterprise's payroll costs [35].

Enterprises experienced a 20% increase in medical costs in the early 1990s [36]. Rises in costs occurred in urban hospitals for the same reasons they did in rural areas. Government financing was cut to cover less than 30% of expenditures, and hospitals were expected to be self-sufficient. Since there was also a cap on the fees they could charge, hospitals made up the extra revenue by drug sales and by charging for the use of magnetic resonance imaging (MRI) and CT scanners. The cost to patients of these new technologies was very high, resulting in perverse incentives and consequent overuse. At present, Beijing has more CT scanners than the whole of the UK [31]. According to World Bank figures, 75% of health spending in China goes on hospital care and 60% of that goes on drugs [31]. Nearly half the drugs bought are antibiotics [37].

A number of experiments in different types of insurance, where employees share a proportion of the costs, have been undertaken. In Zhenjiang city, Liu [33] and colleagues evaluated a new insurance scheme that covered urban residents, irrespective of their employment status, and to which they directly contributed. The study showed increased utilization, a move from inpatient to outpatient care and decreased healthcare expenditures, especially those related to the use of expensive technologies. In 1998, these new schemes were implemented across China's cities, and the two old systems were incorporated into one. Each city had a two-tier programme with contributions to individual medical savings accounts and a city-wide community health fund. Retirees and those entitled to pensions still enjoy those benefits.

In general, it can be argued that urban health reforms have had some success in cost containment and extending coverage to the uninsured. However, some difficulties remain:

- economic changes have swelled the population of cities with both legal and illegal migrants. Special Economic Zones, where private enterprise flourishes, have been a particular magnet;

- the growing number of small enterprises with fewer than 100 employees, which have traditionally been excluded from the LIS system, are rarely in a position to cover healthcare costs; this is an important source of intra-urban inequality [38], with about half the urban population left uninsured;

- although private schemes exist, at a cost of around US$600 per annum they are beyond the reach of all but the wealthy [39];

- many State enterprises, which have low productivity and are often less competitive, find themselves bankrupt and unable to pay salaries, let alone health insurance premiums.

Prevention

China has benefited from the earliest days from vertically managed preventive health programmes, in particular in relation to vaccination, immunization and epidemic control. These were located and managed largely at county level under provincial direction. Executive responsibility for execution lay largely at county level. The county was also in charge of the MCH programmes. At township and village levels, the public health departments were responsible for the delivery of vaccinations, care of pregnant women and family planning, using village health workers. These workers were also crucial in mobilizing people for the mass health campaigns to clean up the villages. After the introduction of the production responsibility system, where farmers' income was linked directly to output from their fields, they were unwilling to spare time for such activities, and village doctors turned to the more lucrative possibilities of treating acute illness.

Economic reforms put the delivery of preventive services under strain at every level by withdrawing previous levels of government support and requiring the public health department to charge for services that had previously been free. Fifty cents is a basic fee for a measles vaccination. Unsurprisingly, the demand for these services declined.

Early worries about the possible health consequences led to a retreat from the wholesale encouragement of a 'market for prevention' and the investment of some US$350 million to establish disease control in poor areas. By 2001, there were 4065 sanitation and anti-epidemic agencies compared with 3618 in the middle of the previous decade. In contrast, the specialized and lower-level prevention clinics had decreased from 1872 to 1839, or fewer than one per county, and MCH centres from 2857 to 2598 [40] between 1994 and 2001.

China has the second highest number of people with tuberculosis (TB) in the world; 130,000 die every year, and 1.5 million are suffering from TB infection. Yet, this disease is controllable by properly managed programmes—a recent World Bank programme providing free treatment in 13 provinces produced a 36% decrease in incidence [41]. There are threats from HIV, with a predicted 10 million cases over the next decade. Maternal mortality is still at worryingly high levels in the rural areas. Most strikingly, the recent epidemic of severe acute respiratory syndrome (SARS) struck almost as the situation was improving organizationally. This focused attention on the importance of preventive measures, and the SARS epidemic, which could have proved embarrassing for China internationally, was 'turned' successfully by massive, swift and concentrated action from the centre. Strong quarantine measures were introduced, and SARS 'bounties' were paid to help in contact and case finding. The Health Minister was sacked and epidemic monitoring systems tightened up. The government quickly found US$165 million to pay for treatment costs and promised to put more into the public health structure within a year [42].

The HIV epidemic

Epidemiology

The earliest cases of AIDS in mainland China were recognized in 1985. At that point, there was little understanding of the potential threat posed by the spread of HIV; it was seen as a disease of 'foreigners'. Even when, some years later, the epidemic surfaced among injecting drug users (IDUs) in the south-west border province of Yunnan, its association with minority peoples and heroin addicts led many in the leadership to believe that the problem was of limited extent [43].

Around 1994, the numbers of reported HIV cases were small. Then, in 1996, the numbers began to rise (Fig. 19.1). The rise coincided with the discovery of many HIV-infected people in China's central province of Henan. These rural people had sold their blood and, in order to increase the number of donations, had been re-transfused with pooled and infected blood after plasma extraction. By 1998, when the government enacted new laws to control commercial blood donation, it was already too late for many people. By 2001, official estimates of the number of HIV-infected people rose to 600,000, of whom 100,000 had developed AIDS [44].

By 2002, the government had over 850,000 HIV notifications, but even official sources admitted that this was likely to be an underestimate. It is now thought that the actual number of people with the virus is somewhere between 1 and 1.5 million and that there may be 200,000 cases of AIDS. Since 1985, there have been 150,000 AIDS deaths [45]. Whilst some of the increase is almost certainly due to better reporting systems and more people coming forward for treatment, the prediction of 10 million infected over the next decade *in the absence of effective measures* is a generally accepted figure. The extent of the problem was highlighted at the UNAIDS 16th Bangkok conference, which placed China's AIDS problems in an Asian regional context. The conference stressed the need for leadership at the highest level to tackle the problems [46].

We have documented some of the changes and challenges in China's healthcare system. The management of the HIV epidemic will throw those responses into the starkest relief. There is strong evidence that until relatively recently, the threat of epidemic was not taken seriously. Accurate epidemiological information is still lacking, due in part to a reluctance of officials to

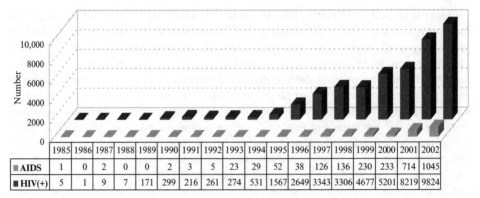

	1985	1986	1987	1988	1989	1990	1991	1992	1993	1994	1995	1996	1997	1998	1999	2000	2001	2002
■AIDS	1	0	2	0	0	2	3	5	23	29	52	38	126	136	230	233	714	1045
■HIV(+)	5	1	9	7	171	299	216	261	274	531	1567	2649	3343	3306	4677	5201	8219	9824

Fig. 19.1 Annual reported cases of HIV and AIDS, 1985–2002. Source: MoH Centre for HIV/AIDS Prevention and Control.

speak out and to a poor reporting structure. We shall consider the current approaches in terms of their strengths and weaknesses. In particular, there is a need to focus on how transmission within the general population may be contained and a social climate created where those who come forward for treatment are free from stigmatization and discrimination in education, jobs and healthcare.

Vulnerable populations

Injecting drug users

So far, the known cases of HIV transmission in China have been mainly due to injected drugs. Somewhere between 1 and 2 million IDUs, located mainly in the border provinces of Yunnan, Xinjiang and Guangxi, make up between 63 and 70% of all HIV cases in China [47]. Rates of infection in certain towns and villages are as high as 80% and generally almost 50% [48]. Use of contaminated needles is common; one survey showed 45% of users use non-sterile injecting equipment [49]. Although the potential health threat had been known for more than a decade, the problem was not tackled. Policies towards drug users tend to be severe. A 3-month mandatory sentence usually follows arrest. In rehabilitation camps, IDUs are started on a methadone maintenance programme, combined with exercise and education. Some needle exchange programmes have been started and show positive results. Debates about the 'soft' treatment of a criminal activity continue, but at present the government attitude is pragmatic.

Plasma donors

In the early 1990s, many poor villagers found that selling blood was a quick and apparently harmless way of earning money. This method of transmission now accounts for about 9% of all infections [47]. The extent of HIV infection in some villages in the central provinces of Henan, Honan and Shaanxi is between 80 and 90% of the general population. Some estimate that there are a million HIV-infected people in Henan alone. These villagers have suffered the highest death rates and have also passed the infection on to their children [50]. Harmful practices by itinerant blood collectors are blamed, but there are many background factors, including poverty, a government drive to obtain more blood supplies, and the poor state of rural healthcare. In some villages, officials connived in these practices and, even quite recently, discussion of the extent of the harm and the disquiet among villagers who cannot receive treatment has been met with official disapproval [51]. It is now agreed that the problem is not limited to the central provinces [52]. The public health infrastructure has been the recipient of US$100 million to improve the capacity for surveillance and disease control in these poor border areas and among minority peoples [47]. The latter are most severely afflicted with HIV.

In 1998, State Council legislation set limits on commercial blood donation, stressing the importance of voluntary donation but recognizing the extent of the problem by enforcing an 85% target for legal blood products [53]. The 1998 law also sought to ensure the safety of supply. In 2001, China invested over US$272 million to establish or upgrade 459 blood banks in the central and western regions. Much of the training and infrastructure to ensure safe blood supply is linked to the planned improvements in rural healthcare [22], and local governments are being forced to produce almost matching funds.

Migrant populations

There are over 130 million migrant labourers in China's rural and urban areas, their movement fuelled by economic growth and rural poverty. Most of them (65%) are under 20 years of age. Life is hard, with little access to education and healthcare. Migrants lack social support and are likely to engage in high-risk sexual behaviour [54], which spreads infection along migrant routes to the major urban centres [55,56]. Economic pressures to migrate are unlikely to alter and will probably increase. A project in Guangxi to promote condom use among long-distance truck drivers almost doubled use, from 15% to 28%, in the intervention group. Most drivers reported not knowing how to use condoms or where to obtain them [57].

Sex workers

The sex industry has been thriving since it re-emerged at the beginning of the1980s; sex workers (SWs) are often women, migrants from less-developed economic areas with both poor education and a lack of awareness of HIV. It is estimated that there are between 4 and 6 million SWs in China. In 2000, high infection rates (10%) were found in Yunnan and Guanxi [5,7], but the overall prevalence of HIV infection among this high-risk group was lower than 5%, with a national average of 1.3% in 2000 [58]. However, considering the still relatively low rates of condom use amongst SWs (only 60% in a recent survey used condoms with all partners, commercial and personal) [43] and the extremely high rate of sexually transmitted infection (STI) that has been noticed in some parts of the country [59], it is expected that SWs will play a decisive role in the HIV epidemic.

Figure 19.2 indicates that about 40% of female sex workers report never using a condom. Recently, a series of pilot programmes to promote 100% condom use was launched, together with education and STI check-ups [60]. These are still small-scale and need rapid expansion to have a real impact. In Shanghai alone, 65% of HIV infection is related to heterosexual transmission. Although sex workers may be unregistered migrant workers, their clients, as well as other migrant workers such as construction workers and miners, are also middle-class officials and businessmen. These individuals are powerful and can insist that sex workers engage in high-risk unprotected sex. The sex industry itself is estimated to be worth about US$3.6 billion. Devising policies to control both the supply and consumption of sexual services will be a challenge [61].

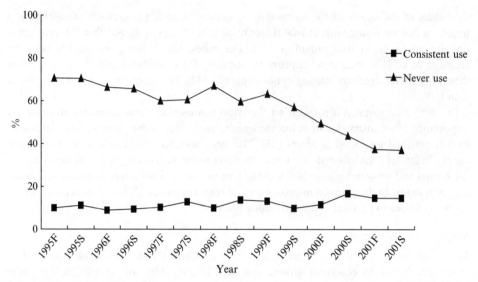

Fig. 19.2 Percentage of condom use among female sex workers, 1995–2001. F = first 6 months; S = second 6 months. Source: MoH Centre for HIV/AIDS Prevention and Control.

Men who have sex with men

The information about men who have sex with men (MSM) in China had long been limited and vague. Recent data have clearly shown that HIV has already spread rapidly among this vulnerable group, which numbers an estimated 18 million people [43,47]. Surveys have shown that many MSM engage in unsafe sex with multiple partners, putting them at a high risk of becoming infected with HIV. Male SWs in particular are ignorant about AIDS and self-protection. They are offered more money to engage in high-risk sexual activities [62]. MSM in China are still unwilling to reveal their sexual orientation publicly and are afraid of being identified by their relatives, friends and colleagues as 'aberrant'. As a consequence, they commonly get married—64% according to recent study [63]—in effect, leading a 'double life'. They are thus likely to serve as a 'bridge' population to the spread of HIV among the general population [64].

General population

Recently, many international organizations have worked with government departments to carry out interventions targeting different vulnerable populations. Large-scale campaigns have been aimed at educating the general population about the risks of HIV, mainly concentrated around World AIDS Day. Although these campaigns have succeeded in raising awareness about HIV in urban areas, people largely remain ignorant of the main modes of transmission and prevention [65]. Their actual impact on behaviour change in curbing the growth of the epidemic has been limited. Discrimination against people living with HIV (PLHIV) is still extremely commonplace, a fact which limits the impact of both education and prevention campaigns. Control of infection needs to be set against respect for human rights. New draft regulations are under discussion to protect rights to education, employment and privacy [66].

The response to the epidemic

Financial inputs

The central government's earliest response to the HIV epidemic was to establish a national coordinating committee on HIV and STIs in 1995, with the aim of coordinating the activities of 33 ministries with respect to HIV. The committee is chaired by a Vice Premier, demonstrating strong commitment from the central government.

With the rapidly growing number of HIV-infected people in the late 1990s, the central government has further reinforced legislation and increased budget allocations for HIV efforts. The long- and medium-term plans for HIV prevention and control (1998), as well as the 5-year plan of action (2001) and the Law on Blood Donation, are examples of these efforts. The National Centre for HIV/AIDS, concerned with research and development of prevention and control mechanisms, was also established in 1998.

Despite a positive change in recent years, investment in curbing the spread of HIV in China remains insufficient. In 2001, the budget allocation for combatting HIV was increased from 15 million RMB (US$1.8 million) in 2000 to 100 million RMB (US$12 million) annually. In 2004, China made a decision to provide free HIV tests for its 1.3 billion people [67]. Free treatment is offered to those living 'in poverty', although an exact definition of poverty has not been specified. At the end of 2003, the government initiated a strategy called Four Frees and One Care: free drugs to poor rural and urban citizens; free education to orphans affected by AIDS; free testing; free drugs to women to prevent vertical transmission; and provision of care to HIV patients.

Treatment

In the beginning of 2002, after a lengthy period of negotiation with international pharmaceutical companies, the Chinese government succeeded in reducing the cost of annual antiretroviral treatment from around US$10,000 to US$4000–5000. Considering that annual income for most Chinese people is less than US$1500, this was still far from affordable, while the availability of drugs was another matter of concern. In 2002, local pharmaceutical companies were approved to produce antiretroviral (ARV) drugs, including zidovudine (AZT), didanosine (ddl), stavudine (d4T) and nevirapine (NVP), which were not under patent protection in China. There are, however, still outstanding difficulties with ARV drug patent issues in China [68]. Significant price reductions have been achieved since 2003 due to the policy of localizing ARV drug production, bringing the annual cost of triple therapy as low as 3600 RMB (US$400). Although the ability of traditional Chinese medicine (TCM) to destroy HIV is still in doubt, there seems to be evidence that it can increase the immunity of PLHIV so as to prolong and improve the quality of their lives. Evidence still needs to be collected and evaluated. Many Chinese have confidence in TCM and appreciate its low cost. In some areas where free antiretroviral drugs have been distributed, around 20% of patients have stopped taking them because of side effects and have turned to traditional medicine instead [52].

Outstanding challenges and future developments

In 2002, the Ministry of Public Health [40] stated that it aimed to provide basic medical services to everyone. Treatment of AIDS is only one of the many challenges facing the system, as has been described.

Need for overall health system investment

China has become richer, but has it become healthier? The most dramatic health gains were made over 20 years ago, and some would suggest that economic improvements have brought a worsening of health, at least in the short term [69]. China is also experiencing an epidemiological transition. HIV is only one of the new challenges facing the health system. Cancer is the major cause of death in urban areas, comprising one-quarter of all deaths, followed by cerebrovascular disease (21%) and heart disease (18%). In rural areas, the figures are not greatly different: respiratory disease accounts for 23%, followed by cancer (18%) and cerebrovascular disease (18%). These conditions also carry major disability and have implications for the future style and direction of health services. At the same time, major infectious diseases such as hepatitis and HIV continue to pose problems. Despite many positive changes and an increased response to the HIV epidemic, mainland China has still not managed to slow the transmission of HIV.

The challenges are many, but without a well-designed health system, plans for development will be slowed, epidemics will remain uncontrolled, money will be wasted and social divisions, already apparent, will deepen. There is continued need for investment. The proportion of government funding spent on health places China a long way down the 'fairness list' according to the WHO. There is an urgent need for an accurate detection and monitoring system for disease outbreaks and more effective coordination between provinces and the centre. A redirection towards prevention as a health priority is essential, both to control current problems and to limit the transmission of HIV. At present, 75% of health spending goes to hospital care.

In the rural areas, there is a need to convince people of the value of cooperative systems and provide proper accounting to support them. Training of China's 1.2 million basic-level health workers to an acceptable standard is essential, especially if primary and preventive healthcare is to be carried out at the grass roots. These workers will need incentives both to retrain and to turn away from a lucrative curative role. Regenerating township hospitals may be an important part of improving accessibility to quality services in rural areas and help to reduce the pressures for the provision of higher-level hospital treatment. It is clear that funding to support the treatment of AIDS will have to have central support, even if local authorities can be persuaded to make a contribution.

In the urban areas, it will be necessary to continue to control costs and waste by more sophisticated co-payment schemes and improve coverage for itinerant and migrant workers as well as that of small enterprises. It is worth considering whether single, city-wide or province-wide fund-pooling systems might reduce administrative costs and provide more protection for the disadvantaged in the long run. Again, without specialist funding, it is clear that AIDS patients will still be competing with others who are not stigmatized and deemed to be 'more deserving'.

Need for accessible HIV facilities and specially trained staff

In China, there are fewer than 50 HIV specialists experienced in AIDS treatment working in fewer than 20 hospitals and institutes, almost all of which are located in big cities. Preventive efforts are still organized in a top-down way and, being city-based, cannot reach 80% of those infected in rural areas. The rural areas also lack skilled health workers. Misdiagnosis, fear of infection [70] and unsafe injection practices—up to 30% in one study [71]—all lower the quality of care.

It is estimated that there are more than half a million symptomatic and asymptomatic HIV-infected individuals currently needing treatment in China [72]. Unfortunately, the large gap between the number of confirmed HIV infections and the number of estimated infections indicates that the majority of those infected do not know their HIV status. The US Centers for Disease Control (CDC) has estimated that up to 90% of those infected are unaware of the fact [73]. Even for those who know their HIV status, the high price of antiretroviral drugs, combined with poor access, limits treatment. By the end of 2003, there were an estimated 8000 patients being treated with antiretroviral therapy according to WHO/UNAIDS. Results from one pilot study showed that out of 29 HIV patients who were under hospital-based medical care in Beijing's You-An hospital in December 1999, 22 (75.9%) paid for treatment themselves and five (17.2%) were reimbursed by state health insurance. The data for two were unknown. Of those 29 patients, most were infected through sexual transmission and had better education and higher incomes [74].

Need for comprehensive HIV medical and behavioural programmes

The first therapeutic intervention programme of its kind, targeting 300 HIV-positive individuals, was launched in Yunnan Province in December 2002. Antiretroviral therapy is being provided free of charge for all 300 participants during the first 3-year phase of the programme [75]. A similar programme for 30,000 people is proposed in Guandong Province [76], where it is estimated that 90% of counties have HIV carriers [77].

Recognizing the importance of comprehensive behavioural and medical approaches, the Chinese government launched the China CARES (Comprehensive AIDS Response) Programme in early 2003, through which 100 county-based sites ('Demonstration Sites of Comprehensive HIV/AIDS Prevention and Control') are to be established over the next 3 years. Fifty-one counties in 11 different provinces have been involved in the first round of the programme.

International best practices will be implemented in these sites, including peer education among high-risk populations, condom promotion among SWs, needle social marketing and STI management. Voluntary counselling and testing (VCT) will be provided at hospitals and in maternal and neonatal healthcare and family planning services. Antiretroviral treatment will be used to reduce the risk of perinatal transmission of HIV from mother to child. Methadone maintenance treatment programmes among IDUs will be carried out in a pilot phase in some sites.

Strengthening local involvement in prevention and education

Improving the overall quality of health services is one of the main objectives for the project sites in the CARES Programme. Local health authorities will both strengthen support and services for PLHIV, and improve management across all healthcare sectors in order to reduce the risk of HIV infection. China has also embarked on a 5-year programme to educate all Chinese about HIV, since high levels of ignorance and stigma still exist [65].

Conclusion

Overall, the government must:

1. Initiate strong programmes of health promotion throughout China, using all the sophisticated means of communication available. These must be implemented at local level and be responsive to the standards, values and mores of the locality. *They must be strongly supported from the centre, and continuously maintained.*

2. Promote cross-ministry cooperation with joint planning groups at each level, with an emphasis on the involvement of civil society, non-governmental organizations and local businesses in health planning.

3. Increase the overall investment in health from its current 5.3% of GDP and place it mainly in *training* and *preventive health*. For AIDS in particular, specialist training is required. Whilst supporting decentralization of funding, strong policy direction and regulation from the centre must be ensured [78]. Although 2010 might seem a reasonable target date for accomplishing all this, it is several years away and much could go wrong before then. Reforms have been attempted since the early 1990s, but progress to date has been very slow. The social repercussions of failing on the health front could be grave indeed.

4. Improve the legislative framework and protection of patients. There is no clear framework for dealing with medical malpractice, and little redress for patients. In the case of AIDS, which remains heavily stigmatized, human rights and the patient's right to treatment must be protected.

As Finkelstein and Kivlehan [2] have argued, the 'fourth generation' of Chinese leaders faced a daunting set of tasks. After years in which the emphasis of the whole economy was on 'getting rich', official rhetoric now endorses the concept of 'a fair society'. In order for that to come about, attention will have to be directed towards the underlying causes—financial, economic, social and historical—of healthcare problems so that they may be more fully understood and acted upon successfully.

References

1. Bloom G. (2001). China's Rural Health System in Transition: Towards Coherent Institutional Arrangements? Presented at the Conference on Financial Sector Reform in China, September 2001.
2. Finkelstein D, Kivlehan D, Kivlehan M. (2003). *China's Leadership in the 21st Century*. Armonk, NY: ME Sharpe.
3. Ferguson M. (1970). *China Medical Board and Peking Union Medical College 1914–1951*. New York: China Medical Board of New York.
4. Bullock MB. (1980). *An American Transplant: The Rockefeller Foundation and Peking Union Medical College*. Berkeley: University of California Press.
5. Lucas A. (1982). *Chinese Medical Modernisation*. Westport, CT: Praeger.
6. Hillier S, Jewell JA. (1983). *Health Care and Traditional Medicine in China 1800–1982*. Oxford: Routledge/Taylor & Francis Group Ltd.
7. Hillier S, Xiang Z. (1991). Township hospital and village clinics in China. *China Information* 2:51–61.
8. Xiang Z, Hillier S. (1995). The reform of the Chinese health care system: county level changes—the Jiangxi study. *Social Science and Medicine* 41:1057–64.
9. Hillier S, Shen J. (1996). Health care systems in transition in People's Republic of China. *Journal of Public Health Medicine* 18:258–65.
10. Huang Y, Liu Y. (1995). *Mortality Data of the Chinese Population*. Chinese Population Press.
11. *Jian Kang Bao* (Health News). (1989). Speeches by Li Peng Cheng Minzhang. August, 13 1989.
12. *Jian Kang Bao* (Health News). (1989). April 9, 1989.
13. *Jian Kang Bao* (Health News). (1989). April 13, 1989.
14. *Jian Kang Bao* (Health News). (1989). May 7, 1989.
15. *Jian Kang Bao* (Health News). (1989). May 12, 1989.
16. *Jian Kang Bao* (Health News). (1989). July 7, 1989.

17. Ling Zhu. (2001). Preferences of Farmers in Making Choices on Health Programmes with Insurance Components. Unpublished paper of Economics Institute Chinese Academy of Social Sciences.

18. *China Daily.* (1995). Rural medical co-ops effective. July 1995.

19. Feng Xueshan, Tang Shenglan, Bloom G, *et al.* (1995). Co-operative medical schemes in contemporary rural China. *Social Science and Medicine* **41**(8):111–8.

20. Carrin G, Aviva R, Yang Hui, *et al.* (1999). The reform of the rural co-operative medical system in the People's Republic of China: interim experience in 14 pilot counties. *Social Science and Medicine* **48**:961–72.

21. Zhongguo Weisheng Nanjian (China Health Yearbook). (1999). Renmin Weisheng Chubanshe. 396, 410, p168–9.

22. Bloom G, Tang SL. (1999). Rural health pre-payment schemes in China: towards a more active role for government. *Social Science and Medicine* **48**:951–60.

23. State Council. (1991). *A Report on the Reform and Strengthening of Rural Health Work.* Beijing, State Council. January 17, 1991.

24. Zhu Baoxia. (1995). State wants all Chinese to have health care within the next decade. *China Daily.* January 18, 1995.

25. State Council. (1997). State Council's Policy for health care reform and development. January 15, 1997, www.schinfo.net.

26. *China Daily.* (2002). Reform to hit rural doctors clinics. November, 21 2002.

27. Tang S. (1999). Adaption of Township Health Centres in the Poor Areas of China to Economic Reform. Unpublished PhD thesis 49–1244. University of Sussex.

28. Zuo X. (1997). China's fiscal decentralisation and financing of local services in poor townships. *IDS Bulletin* **28**(1):81–91.

29. World Health Organization. (2002). *World Health Report 2001.* Geneva: WHO.

30. *People's Daily.* (2001). China strives to ensure medical care of rural people. 28 June 2001.

31. World Bank. (2001). Curing China's ailing health system. *World Bank Transition Newsletter.* April–June 2004, p9.

32. Strand M and Chen A. (2002). Rural health cases in North China in an area of rapid economic growth. URL: www.yale/china.org.publication/healthjournal.

33. Liu G, Cai R, Zhao Z, *et al.* (1999). Urban health care reform initiative in China: findings from a pilot experiment in Zhengjiang city. *International Institute of Economic Development.* 1:504–25.

34. Liu G, Wu X, Peng C, Fu AZ. (2003). Urbanisation and health care in rural China. *Contemporary Economic Policy.* **21**(1):11–24.

35. State Statistical Bureau. (1991). *Chinese Population Statistics Yearbook.* Chinese Statistical Press.

36. Yuen P. (1996). Reforming health care financing in urban China. *International Journal of Public Administration* **19**:211–32.

37. *Economist.* (1998). Overdosed. November 5, 1998.

38. Wong B, Gabriel SJ. (1999). The influence of economic liberalisation on urban health care access in the Peoples Republic of China. Maryland: Johns Hopkins—Nanjing University Center/Mt Holyoke College. URL: http://mtholyoke.edu/courses/gabriel/health.htm.

39. William S. (2003). China's high cost health care. *BBC News* April 1, 2003.

40. Ministry of Public Health. (2002). *Outline for the Development of Primary Healthcare in Rural Areas.* Beijing: Ministry of Public Health, April 27, 2002.

41. Forney M. (2003). China's failing health system. *TIME Asia*, p19. May 19, 2003.

42. *People's Daily.* (2003). Chinese government pays huge SARS treatment costs. June 25, 2003.

43. Zhang KL, Ma SJ. (2002). Epidemiology of HIV in China. *British Medical Journal* **324**:803–4.

44. *People's Daily.* (2002). China vows to contain increasing spread of AIDS. October 16, 2002.

45. China AIDS Survey. (2003). Monterey, California, URL: http://casy.org/overview.htm.

46. United Nations Secretary General Kofi Annan's Speech to XV International AIDS Conference, Bangkok, July 15, 2004.

47. Ministry of Public Health. (2003). *Report of the 2002 HIV/AIDS Epidemic Situation and the Development of Prevention and Control in China.* Beijing: Ministry of Public Health.

48. Lu Fan. (2003). National Centre for AIDS/STD Prevention and Control Chinese CDC HIV/AIDS Surveillance in China. Beijing.

49. Park A. (2003). China's secret plagues. *TIME Asia* December 15, 2003.

50. Wang L, Zheng X, Li D, (2001). The survey of HIV prevalence among children 0–7 years in one county in China. *Chinese Journal of Epidemiology* 22:1.

51. Xiao Y, Yan J. (2003). Chinese health official arrested for leaking AIDS secrets. *Agence France Presse,* August 19, 2003.

52. *Agence France Presse.* (2004). China turns to traditional medicine to treat AIDS. May 3, 2004.

53. State Council. (1998). *Document 38. Control, Prevention and Treatment of AIDS: Action Plan for China 2001–2005.*

54. Zhang KL, Beck EJ. (1999). Changing sexual attitudes and behaviour in China: implications for the spread of HIV and other sexually transmitted diseases. *AIDS Care* 11:581–9.

55. Cohen M, Henderson GE, Aiello P, Zheng H. (1996). Successful eradication of sexually transmitted diseases in the People's Republic of China; implications for the 21st century. *Journal of Infectious Diseases* 174(S2):223–9.

56. Ministry of Public Health/United Nations Theme Group. (1997). *China Responds to AIDS—The HIV/AIDS Situation and Needs Assessment Report.* Beijing.

57. Liu Wei. (2000). A study of promotion of condom use among long distance truck drivers. *Guangxi Preventative Medicine Journal* 6(1):4–8.

58. Qi X. (2002). *HIV AIDS Epidemiology and China's 5-year Action Plan and Research.* Department of Disease Control. Beijing: Ministry of Public Health.

59. Van den Hoek A, Yuliang F, Dukers NH *et al.* (2001). High prevalence of syphilis and STD among sex workers in China: potential for fast spread of HIV. *AIDS* 15:753–9.

60. Ma S, Dukers NH, van den Hoek A, *et al.* (2002). Decreasing STD incidence and increasing condom use among Chinese sex workers following short-term intervention: a prospective cohort study. *Sexually Transmitted Infections* 78:110–4.

61. Lu M. (2004). Anonymous workers in a non-existent industry. *Shanghai Star* May 27, 2004.

62. *Shanghai Star.* (2003). Hazards of male prostitution. August 21, 2003.

63. Kyung-Hee Choi, Hui Lui, Yaqui Gao *et al.* (2003). Emerging HIV epidemic in China of men who have sex with men. *Lancet* 361:2125–6.

64. Zhang B. (2003). Current situation of MSM in China and HIV intervention. *Yu Lang Yixue Xin Xi Zazhi (Journal of Preventative Medicine)* 19.

65. Manchester T. (2002). *Attitudes HIV/AIDS in China.* Futures Group China/Horizon Research Group.

66. *China Daily.* (2002). New rules to control HIV/AIDS. October 16, 2002.

67. Watts J. (2004). China's shift in HIV policy marks turnaround in health. *Lancet* 363:1370–1.

68. China-United Kingdom HIV Prevention and Care Project. (2003). Development of anti-HIV/AIDS drugs and their use in China. *Hand in Hand* 6.

69. Liu Y, Hsiao WC, Eggleston K. (1999). Equity in health and health care: the Chinese experience. *Social Science and Medicine* 49:1349–1356.

70. Zhu B, Chen QF. (2002). Problems in depressed areas. *Jiankang Bao (Health Daily)* December 21, 2002.

71. Wang K. (2003). Implementing safe injection practices comprehensively. *Chinese Journal of Epidemiology* **24**:5.

72. Xu R, Zhao W. (2003). Assessment of current needs for anti-HIV drug treatment of HIV-infected cases in China. *Chinese Journal of AIDS/STD* **9**.

73. *Reuters Health.* (2004). Few in China may be aware they may be HIV positive. 2 March 2004.

74. Yang H, Li J, Wu Z, Xu L, Wang K. (2003). Study on the Utilisation of Health Services and cost of hospital-based medical care for 29 patients with HIV/AIDS in China. *Chinese Journal of Epidemiology* **24**:5.

75. Zheng L. (2002). Joint efforts of Sino–US programme to fight against AIDS. *China Daily.* 22 December 2002.

76. *People's Daily.* (2004). Guangdong to offer free HIV/AIDS treatment. June 1, 2004.

77. *Xinhua.* (2004). 90% of Guangdong Counties have HIV carriers. April 20, 2004.

78. Fuenzalida-Puelma F. (2002). *Dealing with Four Elements of Post Communist Health Systems.* Geneva: World Bank Group.

Chapter 20

India

R Priya[*], N Kumarasamy, I Qadeer, AK Ganesh,
S Solomon and SM Crowe

Background

India is the world's largest democracy, a nation of over a billion people, of whom 675 million are adults over 18 years of age and voters exercising their right to select their political representatives. In 1951, after 200 years of colonial rule, the Constitution of an independent India ensured the right to life, free speech, voting, choice of religious practice and property ownership. Covering an area of 3,287,590 km^2, India has a relatively young population that by 2004 had grown to over 1.3 billion. It is a confederation, administratively divided into 29 states and six union territories.

India is distinctive in its geographical and social diversity. Although there are no specific cultural differences between northern and southern India, there is traditionally less discrimination against women in the south compared with the north. In recent decades, western and southern India have been the focus of industrial development and growth of the service sector, leading to marked cultural changes in both rural and urban areas. Northern India has also experienced these changes, but at a slower pace.

The majority (81%) of the population practises the religion that was named 'Hinduism' only during British colonial rule, and which is in reality a conglomeration of diverse philosophical streams. Muslims constitute 12% of the population, Christians 2%, Sikhs 2%, and others 3%, including Buddhists and Jains. India has 22 constitutionally recognized languages. Distinguished by cultural pluralism, Indian society has evolved many cultural means to encourage people belonging to diverse religious, regional and ethnic backgrounds to live together harmoniously. The most negative distinguishing feature of Indian society is its caste-based stratification with an entrenched tradition of discrimination against the lower castes. This partly explains class differences and a range of inequalities that constitute India's most undemocratic face. Thus, opposing pressures of pluralism and assimilation, as well as collective stigmatization of specific groups, all co-exist.

To illustrate further the country's diversity and contradictions, India has trained some of the most sought-after software professionals in the world, while almost half its population cannot read or write. Approximately 30% of the Indian population now lives in an urban location, and sharp differences exist between urban and rural dwellers. Income levels are low, with 44% of households living on less than US$1 purchasing power parity (PPP) per capita per day [1]. Similarly, the disparity between the top 10% and the bottom 10% of incomes is low compared

* Corresponding author.

with most other countries [1]. Yet, extreme wealth is also not uncommon in urban areas. Indeed, the slums of Mumbai, whose residents barely earn the equivalent of US$1 per day, are located within a city that claims the largest number of millionaires in the world. India's corporate hospitals are sophisticated facilities that offer patients world-class care, in sharp contrast to some rural hospitals that frequently run out of aspirin and have little else to offer.

India, home to the ancient cradle of civilization, the Indus Valley, is also home to protected tribes who remain untouched by technology and other advances in social and basic sciences. India, the land of the Kama Sutra—an ancient discourse on human sexuality—is today unable even to discuss this subject with its adolescents. The land where goddesses govern wealth, education and power is also witness to the oppression of women in every stratum of society.

The health system

History and development

After independence in 1947, a conscious effort was made by government to invest in education and health services. However, India's regional and economic diversity, complex social structure and extremes of poverty and wealth made publicly funded health planning a challenging task.

Constitutionally, health services are the responsibility of the provincial states and territories. The central government defines policies, some national strategies and financial arrangements, provides services for people crossing international borders and for government employees, and regulates medical education. Districts are the operative healthcare and public health delivery units within states. Each district serves a population of about 1.3–1.5 million, with a district hospital at the apex of a three-tier pyramidal network of peripheral health institutions. Generally, primary healthcare centres are located in larger villages, intermediary care facilities are located in the administrative headquarters of a political district, and so, too, are the district hospitals. Referral hospitals are located in state capitals or larger cities, although occasionally, smaller villages may have exceptionally large health facilities established by non-governmental organizations (NGOs) or by missionary groups. These might have capacities that are on a par with, or exceed, those of the district hospitals

Tertiary care is provided through institutions chiefly located in cities. Consistent with the 'mixed economy' approach to development, the private sector was very much a part of the health services after independence, and private sector hospitals were often co-located with public sector general or multi-specialty hospitals.

Public health sector planning post-independence had two major thrusts: first, to build an infrastructure to provide basic medical care, maternal and child health (MCH) services, health information, education and referral services free of cost and with a focus on the rural areas; and secondly, to develop specific national health programmes to control communicable diseases, provide family planning services (FPS) and control severe forms of nutritional deficiency.

In the 1950s and 1960s, critical measures to control smallpox and malaria through vertical programmes took precedence. Yet, epidemiological and social research was pioneered in nutrition and tuberculosis (TB), and an infrastructure for general health services was also established in the public sector, which included health workforce development, health information and monitoring, drug and equipment production, and research. In the late 1960s, population control efforts started gaining momentum and overshadowed disease control programmes.

Pressured by the poor outcomes of its vertically oriented public health programmes, in the mid-1970s India integrated its malaria and population control programmes with the general district health services. As a result, the malaria and population control programmes had direct access to general health services' resources and undermined programmes such as TB control, MCH and nutritional services. Learning from these experiences, India signed the World Health Organization's Alma-Ata declaration in 1978 with a view to protecting its general primary health services.

By the end of the 1980s, a substantial health service infrastructure had been developed, reducing the populations served by community and primary health centres and health sub centres to 100,000, 30,000 and 5000, respectively. The medical schools and specialized hospitals located in the urban areas had also increased in number and size along with municipal services, and substantial numbers of professional and paramedical personnel had been trained.

In addition to these changes, providers of traditional medicine such as *Ayurvedic* and *Unani* dispensaries and a few hospitals had also been established as a part of the government healthcare infrastructure. The *Ayurvedic* system of medicine originated in ancient India, and the *Unani* system of medicine was incorporated into Indian society from Greek traditions. Both focus on strengthening the innate resistance of the body to infections and promoting its self-healing capacities through the use of herbal and animal remedies together with advice on healthy lifestyles.

However, although the health infrastructure had expanded, problems such as regional inequities, poor outreach and functional inadequacies remained. The 1980s saw the private sector expand much faster than the public sector. India's grand plans for health sector development were compromised by the priority given in that period to growth-centred, industry-driven economic development. They were distorted further when market fundamentalism started taking root in the mid-1980s. Premised on a 'trickle down' theory of economic growth, this economic philosophy resulted in the expansion of cities, leaving the vast rural hinterlands behind. Thus, while the annual economic growth rate rose from 2.8% in 1961–1966 to 5.7% in 1980–1985, regional disparities worsened significantly.

Since the 1980s, pressures for change in health services have come from different quarters. Increasing economic aspirations of the population have created pressures for better healthcare coverage and improved facilities. The emerging middle class has lobbied for 'hi-tech' hospitals that conform to their concepts of international standards of healthcare.

Simultaneously, international pressures for health sector reform left their mark on India's public healthcare sector. While the allocation of government funds to health remained low, the main aspects of the International Monetary Fund- or World Bank-inspired reforms were further cuts in health sector investments, opening up medical care to the private sector, the introduction of user-fees and private investments in public hospitals, and application of technocratic public health interventions. These policies harmed comprehensive primary healthcare (CPHC), which was already being undermined by a weakening food security system, massive unemployment and loss of subsistence income for many Indians. Failure to put in place mechanisms to ensure the quality and standards of treatment and access to services further compounded the problem. Ultimately, this shift served the purpose of promoting medical technologies, but there is evidence that it failed to improve overall public health [2].

By the mid-1980s, the weaknesses of the extensive public sector infrastructure for health services, which had evolved to provide modern healthcare to the majority of the population after independence, were being widely debated. However, instead of tackling these weaknesses, the proposed reforms actually increased them, leading to the decline of public health and healthcare infrastructure. Peripheral services were annexed to the vertical disease control and family planning programmes, detracting from the delivery of integrated, comprehensive services and quality care. Financing and quality of service delivery further declined over the 1980s and 1990s.

The decline in quality of publicly financed health services, together with the introduction of user-fees in the public sector, led to a major shift in utilization of services, from the public to the private sector. The National Sample Survey showed that the percentage of the population receiving outpatient treatment from public institutions decreased from 26% in 1986–1987 to 19% in 1995–1996. Admissions for inpatient care declined similarly, from 60% to 45% of the Indian population. The proportion of the population not accessing care at all due to financial constraints also increased from 10% to 20% in rural areas and from 15% to 25% in urban areas [3]. The rate of untreated ailments increased by 40% in the poorest decile of the population in expenditure terms. However, utilization of public sector inpatient care by the poorest 40% increased to 60% of all admissions by 1995–1996 [4]. This breakdown of public ambulatory care resulted in overcrowding in some institutions and the underutilization of others, depending upon the level of infrastructure, drug availability, physical access and the attitude of personnel.

The reduction in publicly financed care beyond overstretched public hospitals has encouraged the proliferation of a private sector that includes a range of service providers: from the informal practitioner with minimal formal professional education and training, perhaps with paramedical experience or degrees in *Ayurveda* or homeopathy, to the general practitioner, fully trained in modern medicine; from nursing homes and polyclinics with groups of doctor-proprietors, to a range of hospitals, some of which are part of large corporate ventures [5]. The private sector also offers services on contract to government institutions. Irrational medical practices, such as prescription of drugs via injection when oral medicine is as effective, exist in both public and private sectors, but studies show that they are much more common in the latter [6,7]. Weakening of public sector monitoring and regulatory institutions within health services, and of state controls in the economy, has furthered market forces and limited the possibility of formal regulation of the private sector [8]. Despite these drawbacks, the public perceives the private sector to be quick and, in the long run, worth paying for.

Cost and effectiveness

Unfortunately, there are substantial inequities and inefficiencies in the Indian public health system. For example, instead of focusing on poverty-related infectious diseases through comprehensive strategies, government attention has shifted to new priorities identified by international experts. Thus, non-communicable diseases were added to the list of control programmes, despite the fact that infectious diseases continued to flourish due to increasingly hazardous working conditions and the social and economic pressures of survival. Control strategies overemphasized individual lifestyle changes, failing to recognize that these cannot realistically be changed by at least 44% of the population who live below the poverty line. Secondly, the emphasis on therapeutic services for non-communicable diseases promoted the drug and equipment industry at the expense of sensible, efficient public health measures. As one might guess, these policy changes have had an adverse impact on HIV control programmes.

Furthermore, vertical and technology-intensive approaches to communicable diseases gained primacy over epidemiologically and socially informed approaches. The Indian government's reliance on a purely biomedical approach ignored the social and economic conditions in which people lived, which were the main causes of the bulk of health problems. Cost cutting, rather than maximizing population coverage, became the driving force of healthcare planning. Spending on HIV, malaria and tuberculosis has been at its highest since the mid-1990s, but with little impact on public health as reflected by unchanging mortality and morbidity attributable to the major infectious diseases [9]. The present approach, therefore, is not truly cost-effective.

A study of the Revised National Tuberculosis Control Programme (RNTCP) by the UK Department for International Development (DFID) highlighted some of these difficulties. The study in 1993–1994 showed that in four urban pilot projects, coverage only ranged between 5 and 30% of the expected case load [10]. It further showed that only half the patients diagnosed with TB in Delhi were given treatment. Those excluded were either unable to meet the demands of directly observed treatment (DOT), refused treatment because they found the behaviour of members of the clinical team unacceptable, or were migrants. Pre-selection of patients to make their clinical management easier left out those who were recent migrants, homeless or without ration cards—in other words, under the RNTCP, those most in need of help were those most often excluded [11].

Despite these administrative and budgetary obstacles, overall demographic and health indices in India slowly but steadily improved until 1999. However, the mortality differentials between classes indicate that India cannot afford to focus on the welfare of its middle class and elite alone. Also, the crude death rate and infant mortality rate fell more slowly during the 1990s compared with the 1980s. These statistics call for reforms to tackle the known weaknesses in the public health response, rather than the ones put in place in the 1990s. Losing sight of the social determinants of health and the complexity of disease causality cannot be conducive to improving health indices or controlling disease, particularly HIV infection, which is so interwoven with cultural and socio-economic status.

The HIV epidemic

Trends, prevalence and risk groups

The first reported case of HIV in India was from Chennai in 1986 [12], and early reports suggested that the epidemic primarily affected female sex workers, truck drivers and patients attending sexually transmitted infection (STI) clinics [13]. Subsequently, HIV infection was described among Indian women attending antenatal clinics, and married women [14–16]. Since the early 1980s, injecting drug use has been common among young people living in both urban and rural areas in the north-eastern states of Manipur, Mizoram and Nagaland. HIV infection was subsequently recognized within this risk group in the early 1990s, associated with drug trafficking from the Golden Triangle [17].

The early epidemic evolved, initially by expanding in large urban areas such as Chennai and Mumbai. By 2000, a substantial epidemic was established in much of southern India, with the estimated prevalence of HIV over 1% in the general adult population of Tamil Nadu, Andhra

Pradesh, Karnataka and Maharashtra [18]. Subsequently, the epidemic expanded beyond urban populations, and there is evidence that many of the rural parts of southern India now have an advanced epidemic [19]. A report from a voluntary counselling and testing (VCT) centre in central India described a seropositivity rate of 20% in 2003, with the highest prevalence in the 25–29 year age group [20].

There has also been an exponential increase in the number of cases in northern India. For example, among adult patients admitted to a tertiary care hospital in New Delhi with *Mycobacterium tuberculosis* infection, HIV seropositivity rose from less than 1% in 1994–1999 to 9% of those admitted between 2000 and 2002 [21]. Although they only comprise 3% of India's population, the north-eastern states (Manapur, Mizoram and Nagaland) have been estimated to have approximately 25% of HIV-infected people [22], with the prevalence of HIV infection in injecting drug users (IDUs) in this region reported to range from 57 to 75% [17,23,24]. The prevalence of HIV infection among IDUs in other parts of India is reported to range from 2 to 30% [25].

The regional diversity of the HIV epidemic in India is reflected in the varying prevalence of infection across the country (Table 20.1). Predictably, the epidemic, which was largely hidden for the first several years, has now become highly visible in some regions, with an ever-increasing morbidity and mortality due to AIDS. While the sentinel surveillance system has its weaknesses, it provides data relating to the current level of demand for services and medications required for managing HIV-infected people. The diversity of the Indian HIV epidemic also suggests that implementing a single approach to preventing or treating HIV infection in India is unlikely be optimal.

The early years of the epidemic gave rise to the popular notion that HIV was a disease confined to sex workers, truck drivers and IDUs. This prejudice increased both the vulnerability and the marginalization of these populations. Yet, heterosexual contact has been a major risk factor in HIV transmission in the western and southern areas [28,29], with sex work being a high-risk occupation [30]. Low socio-economic status and illiteracy have also been associated with an increased risk of infection in some studies [31], although risky sexual behaviour is also common among middle-class professionals [32]. Elevated prevalence rates in antenatal clinics [14] have confirmed the spread of HIV to the heterosexual population.

The majority of the married monogamous women in India with HIV infection have acquired HIV from their husbands [16,33]. Despite this, condom use is rare among sexually active women in a marital relationship [34]. In a study of the level of acceptance by women and support from their husbands of HIV testing of pregnant women, there was high acceptance, with 68% of women in the delivery room and 83% of women in the antenatal clinic agreeing to counselling and testing [35]. Other reports highlight the tacit sanction within the community of marital violence: 'Given the choice between the immediate threat of violence and the relatively hypothetical specter of HIV, women often resign themselves to sexual demands and indiscretions that may increase their risk of HIV acquisition' [36].

Amongst healthcare workers, including medical students, there is a high incidence of procedure-related needlestick injuries, with over two-thirds caused by re-sheathing the needle [37]. A high level of occupational exposure among healthcare workers has been reported in a recent study in rural northern India, with a mean of 2.3 percutaneous injuries per year in two-thirds of study participants [38]. In hospitals and clinics in Delhi, few needlestick injuries are reported; in most cases, the source patient is not tested for blood-borne infections, and few healthcare workers are aware of post-exposure prophylaxis [39]. A recent study also showed

Table 20.1 Distribution of the HIV-infected and AIDS cases across Indian States, 2003

Type of HIV epidemic[*]	States in India	% of national population[**]	% of reported HIV-infected people and AIDS cases[*]
Combined generalized and concentrated epidemics (ANC >1%, STD/IDU >5%)	Andhra, Goa, Karnataka, Maharashtra, Manipur, Tamil Nadu, Nagaland	29.6	79.9
Concentrated epidemics (ANC <1%, STD/IDU >5%)	Gujarat, Haryana, Himachal, Kerala, Rajasthan	16.4	8.8
Low-level epidemics (ANC <1%, STD <5%)	Arunachal, Assam, Andaman and Nicobar Islands, Bihar, Delhi, Daman and Diu, Jammu and Kashmir, Madhya Pradesh, Orissa, Punjab, Sikkim, Uttar Pradesh, West Bengal, Meghalaya, Mizoram, Tripura	54.0	11.3

ANC = antenatal cases: STI/IDU = sexually transmitted disease/injecting drug user cases.
[*]Based on National AIDS Control Organization's sentinel surveillance data published in Sen, 2003 [27].
[**]Computed from Census of India data.
Source: [26].

that disposable syringes may be thrown into drains or outside a village after use [40]. Unfortunately, complacency and a lax attitude also affect issues such as blood safety and harm reduction approaches. The lack of rational treatment for HIV-infected people encourages rampant mushrooming of 'magic cures'.

Molecular analysis of the viruses that are spreading in India shows that the main HIV-1 subtype is C, although most of the other known subtypes of HIV-1 have also been reported [41]. In a recent study of 125 samples in New Delhi, the predominant HIV-1 subtype was C (78%), followed by B (9%), A (2%) and E (2%) [42]. Recombinant strains have been reported [43]. HIV-2 infection is also present in India, accounting for 1% of all infections [19,44]. HIV-2 subtype A has been identified in individuals from different regions within southern India, both as the sole infecting retrovirus as well as in dual infection with HIV-1 [45]. Five strains of HIV-2 identified in people in Calcutta were closely related to the Senegalese HIV-2 Rod sequence [46].

By 2003, India had officially reported 5.1 million cases of HIV infection [47,48], with a cumulative total of 60,000 AIDS cases reported to the National AIDS Control Organization (NACO) by the end of that year [49]. More recent estimates suggest that there are now 5.13 million HIV-infected individuals in India, while the WHO/UNAIDS country statement for India gives the estimated range for probable HIV prevalence levels as 2.2–7 million. A wide spectrum of opportunistic infections have been documented in people living with HIV (PLHIV). The most common AIDS-defining illnesses are:

- pulmonary TB (49%; median duration of survival, 45 months);
- *Pneumocystis jirovecii* pneumonia (6%; median duration of survival, 24 months);
- cryptococcal meningitis (5%; median duration of survival, 22 months);
- central nervous system toxoplasmosis (3%; median duration of survival, 28 months) [50].

Almost 30% of the global burden of TB is within India [51], and, given the higher risk of TB in HIV-infected people and the failure of India's TB control programmes prior to the appearance of the HIV epidemic, there is growing concern about management of this public health challenge [52]. In Vellore and New Delhi, nearly 10% of all patients with TB are HIV-infected [21,53]. Opportunistic infections often co-exist in India and are associated with a 2.6-fold increase in risk of mortality [95% confidence inteval (CI), 0.95–7.09] compared with those without evidence of opportunistic infection [50].

The response to the HIV epidemic

We have previously referred to the relatively disorganized, multi-component and poorly regulated medical care and public heath system that now serves India. HIV services, including scale-up of treatment with antiretroviral drugs, have to be introduced in this context. Given the magnitude of the population and the evidence that HIV has already taken a firm hold in India, the country's response to this epidemic will probably greatly influence the outcome of the HIV pandemic. Peter Piot, Executive Director of UNAIDS, remarked that, 'The future of the global epidemic is really at stake in India' [54].

Evolution of the response

The response of the Indian government to the burgeoning AIDS epidemic has generally reflected its strategies for controlling other infectious diseases, and with similar outcomes. In response to the first cases of AIDS in the mid- to late 1980s, a high-powered committee was constituted under the Ministry of Health and Family Welfare. Subsequently, a National AIDS Control Programme (NACP) was launched in 1987 to monitor the epidemic in India and to plan prevention programmes. A surveillance system had been set up by the central government's Directorate General of Health Services in 1986 in cooperation with state governments, initially covering 13 states and increasing to 32 states by 1991. The data on HIV seropositivity generated by this system showed a rapidly growing epidemic in several parts of the country, which led to the First Acceleration Phase of the National AIDS Control Programme (NACP Phase I) in 1992, largely funded by the World Bank. The national body for HIV/AIDS control, the NACO, was also formed in 1992. As a result, there was a policy shift and an increase in the scale of the response. A national blood safety policy was implemented, and education and condom distribution programmes targeted sex workers in the red-light districts of various cities. In 1999, each state formed its own State AIDS Control Society, with a Project Director supported by technical staff.

In addition to the initiatives by NACO, hundreds of local, state, national and overseas NGOs began to work on HIV-related issues. Projects included general awareness campaigns, care and support of PLHIV, care for AIDS orphans and working with the marginalized populations most vulnerable to HIV infection, such as sex workers, truck drivers, migrant labourers, men who have sex with men and IDUs.

Despite these efforts by government, along with significant NGO and other civil society initiatives, India witnessed a phenomenal increase in infection rates among high-risk populations. Infection among Mumbai's sex workers rose from 1% to 51% in 5 years (1993–1998), with a similar increase from 1% to 52% among IDUs in Manipur during the same period [49].

There are many reasons for the relative failure of the government programme. The NACP focused on surveillance and prevention, but in a manner that did not optimally utilize the social, cultural and service resources available locally, dependent as it was on international expertise. For example, instead of initially focusing on blood safety alone, the NACP might have prevented much of the iatrogenic spread of HIV by promoting universal precautions to medical care providers through the use of sterilizable or disposable needles and syringes. Integrating the NACP into the general health services would have sensitized the whole service system to the issues involved in tackling the epidemic. Instead, the NACO created a management structure that paralleled the one already in existence, at high cost. The poor success of Indian programmes in the control of TB and HIV infection are examples of the negative effects of strategies that neglect general health services. Poor general health services make control of these diseases more difficult and, at least in the case of HIV, contribute to its spread.

India today has a large public sector investment in healthcare. Government and federal institutions across India own and manage tertiary care centres throughout the states, and these centres have traditionally made expensive treatments such as cancer chemotherapy and organ transplantation available to the community. However, with cuts in the healthcare share of the government budget, a decline of publicly financed health services, and the doubtful value of antiretroviral therapy (ART) in its initial years, the HIV programme focused on prevention alone.

The delayed implementation of ART in India appears to have been due primarily to a general apprehension that the large numbers of people eligible for treatment, coupled with evidence of a large number of new infections each year, would place an unacceptable burden on public funds. Moreover, despite early recommendations for linking prevention and treatment for HIV-infected people [55], there was a long delay in making treatment a component of HIV services, thereby delaying development of an effective national response to HIV.

It was not until the end of 2003 that the Union Minister for Health and Family Welfare announced a policy and programme commitment for providing ART to 100,000 HIV-infected patients, free of cost, starting in April 2004. According to this programme, the Government of India provides free ART in government hospitals in the six high-prevalence states of Andhra Pradesh, Karnataka, Maharashtra, Tamil Nadu, Manipur and Nagaland. This programme initially prioritized treatment for HIV-infected mothers who had participated in the programme to prevent mother-to-child-transmission (MCTC); infected children below the age of 15; and people with AIDS seeking treatment in government hospitals [26,47]. However, it is now theoretically available to all who need it.

Prevention of MTCT (PMTCT) of HIV is an important aspect of control of the HIV epidemic. There are 27 million live births a year in India, and, with a 1% prevalence of HIV infection among pregnant women, it is estimated that about 216,000 HIV-infected women deliver each year. The issue of PMTCT was not addressed until January 2000, when a pilot study was initiated in 11 antenatal clinics to assess the feasibility of administering zidovudine for this purpose. A subsequent study of nevirapine was initiated in October 2001 in the same 11 clinics. The option of breastfeeding was left to the mothers. It is clear that with increasing HIV infection among antenatal women in certain high-prevalence states in India, paediatric AIDS will undoubtedly become an increasingly important public health problem. In the second round of funding from the Global Fund to Fight AIDS, Tuberculosis and Malaria, India received US$100 million to step up PMTCT and provide antiretroviral drugs, if needed, to mothers as part of its PMTCT programme.

Even though this programme has as yet had minimal impact on access of other patients to ART, it has prompted recognition of the need for therapy as well as exposing the intricacies associated with diagnosis, counselling and follow-up of HIV-infected people

The Indian government has been working with the International AIDS Vaccine Initiative (IAVI) since 2000 to develop and evaluate a vaccine to prevent or ameliorate HIV infection based on the HIV subtype (C) most appropriate for testing in India. A vaccine has also been developed at the Indian Council for Medical Research, and a phase I safety trial is planned by the National AIDS Research Institute in Pune. However, based on the current status of other HIV vaccines in development, it seems unlikely that any HIV vaccine will be available within the next decade.

HIV treatment and care

Treatment began in Chennai, Mumbai, Delhi, Pune and Ahmedabad in the mid-1990s, mostly through the efforts of individual physicians and NGOs. In those early years, most of the drugs used had to be imported. Only about 2% of patients could afford treatment, and many patients stopped and started therapy depending on their financial state. When generic manufacturing of antiretrovirals began in India, the imported brand drugs were progressively withdrawn. The affordability of generic drugs and, more importantly, the convenience of fixed-dose combinations that generic manufacture made possible have changed the landscape of treatment in India and in the rest of the world. Indian pharmaceutical companies began manufacturing antiretrovirals both as a business opportunity and altruistically as a means of increasing the numbers of patients receiving ART. Generic antiretroviral drugs available in India are zidovudine (AZT), lamivudine (3TC), stavudine (d4T), didanosine (ddI), abacavir (ABC), nevirapine (NVP), efavirenz (EFV), ritonavir (RTV), indinavir (IDV) and nelfinavir (NFV). AZT/3TC, d4T/3TC, AZT/3TC/NVP and d4T/3TC/NVP are available as fixed-dose combinations within a single pill. These antiretroviral drugs are manufactured by the Indian pharmaceutical companies Cipla, Ranbaxy, Aurobindo, Hetero, Emcure and Alkem.

However, the decline in the cost of drugs attributable to local manufacturing capability has not been enough, by itself, to allow for a large treatment programme across the country. Although India now has the second largest burden of HIV in the world next to South Africa, the number of individuals who have commenced ART under the WHO/UNAIDS '3 by 5' programme is very small. For example, as late as 2003, a report from the largest tertiary HIV referral centre in southern India showed that only 29% of the patients in a cohort of 5000 had received any ART [50]. By December 2004, fewer than 10,000 Indians had begun ART. Currently, only some public hospitals, a few NGOs and a few employers provide ART free of charge.

There are other reasons for the relatively slow development of the Indian HIV treatment programmes aside from fears about the direct cost of treatment. The complexity and costs of monitoring ART were neither appreciated nor adequately planned for at a governmental level. As a result, the trained personnel and infrastructure needed to provide assessment and treatment, as well as to monitor toxicity and sustain adherence, were never in place in either the public or private sectors. In fact, it remains a matter of great concern that antiretrovirals continue to be available in pharmacies that neither have a role nor an inclination to identify or rectify suboptimal prescriptions for ART. Even today, few patients on therapy are adequately monitored. This omission is likely to encourage the emergence of antiretroviral-resistant HIV strains.

Studies in India have confirmed international data showing that ART for patients with low CD4 lymphocyte counts markedly improves their odds of survival (odds ratio, 5.37; 95% CI, 1.82–15.83) [50]. The safety, tolerability and effectiveness of generic, Indian-manufactured antiretrovirals have been found to be equivalent to those of proprietary drugs [56]. The cost of combination ART for an individual treated in India starts at about US$300 per year, and the cost of monitoring is around US$600 per year. Low-cost manual assays to measure CD4 and HIV viral load are being introduced into India to reduce the cost of monitoring infection [57].

In the Indian public hospital system, the process of beginning therapy is relatively straightforward. Patients who wish to be assessed for ART in government hospitals first register with the centre. A CD4 count is performed, and if it is less than 200 cells/l, the individual is registered to receive first-line therapy with either zidovudine or stavudine in combination with lamivudine and nevirapine. In some centres, individuals are admitted to monitor for toxicities of the drugs. In other centres, individuals are given treatment, return after 2 weeks of therapy and, if there are no side effects, are given drugs to last 1 month. Individuals on therapy are reviewed monthly.

In India, despite government programmes, most HIV-infected patients still pay for their ART. The lack of widespread availability of life-prolonging ART, due to its unaffordability, poses major public health challenges to India. It remains to be seen if the government's recently announced provision of free ART at selected public centres around the country will be implemented effectively.

One of the more successful local responses to the HIV epidemic is that of YRGCARE, a non-profit Indian NGO based in Chennai. Since its inception in 1993, YRGCARE has responded to the needs of the surrounding community, providing a continuum of HIV services from education and VCT to support ranging from nutrition, clinical care and research, to arranging marriages among HIV-infected individuals. Today, YRGCARE cares for over 8000 individuals with HIV. Interestingly, YRGCARE was among the first institutions to give ART to patients in 1996.

Financing HIV treatment

There is a general perception that the financial resources needed for management of PLHIV are too high for universal access to be possible. On these grounds, the International AIDS Economics Network has examined three different options for integrating HIV prevention and ART in India [58]. Free provision of antiretrovirals exclusively to those below the poverty line was estimated to be the most cost-effective treatment strategy. Provision of therapy exclusively to HIV-infected women and their partners, detected through antenatal clinics, was less cost-effective and provision of, and efforts to help patients adhere to treatment, such as strengthening of laboratory services and provision of monetary incentives for patient monitoring to both public and private providers without social criteria for exclusion, were the least cost-effective. While considering more health service issues than are usually included in calculations of cost-effectiveness, this study ignored lessons from past public health experience. For instance, analysis of the experience of targeting social services to the poor, and using incentives to make health workers perform, shows that this generally results in poor-quality services for the targeted groups. In addition, these strategies have a potentially coercive, anti-democratic thrust [59,60].

The argument that a public programme providing universal access to ART for PLHIV is unaffordable is questionable [26]. The National AIDS Control Programme had a budget of Rs.1.8 billion (US$41 million) for the year 2001–2002. To treat all those reported to the public health system—or 45,000 people with AIDS—about half of this amount would have been needed at Rs.20,000 (US$455) per person per year. This figure represented about 3% of the total budget allocation for health and family welfare in 2001–2002. Since then, costs per patient per year have fallen to around Rs.15,000 (US$340).

Of course, as treatment becomes available through the public system, more HIV-infected people are likely to come forward and more funds will be needed. However, additional costs might be defrayed, for example, by optimizing existing services and by adopting appropriate low-cost laboratory tests to assist with monitoring and treatment decision making. Rational and efficient use of existing facilities [26] might include the integration of the management and delivery structures for TB, AIDS, leprosy, and reproductive and child health programmes with general health services. This would be most cost-effective from the institutional perspective [61] and appropriate from the users' perspective. Body weight and white blood cell counts may crudely substitute for CD4 lymphocyte counts in assessing the impact of treatment in low-resource settings [62]. A CD4 lymphocyte count by flow cytometry is currently priced at Rs.500 (US$11) in public hospitals and Rs.1300 (US$30) in private laboratories, while a total white blood cell count is routinely performed for Rs.50 (US$1.14) or less. Measuring viral load by molecular assays is prohibitively expensive. Manual or semi-automated assays for monitoring CD4 and viral load costing approximately one-fifth to one-tenth the price of conventional assays are currently being evaluated.

Conclusions

The provision of prevention and treatment services for HIV-infected people through NGOs or the private sector is not an adequate solution in the Indian context. The scale of operations required, the social, religious, economic and geographical heterogeneity of India and the low income of the majority of India's citizens mean that the only solution to effective prevention and treatment of HIV infection is to develop public systems linked with community support structures.

While the private sector is currently the major provider of outpatient medical services, the public sector remains crucial for providing inpatient care to the poor and for developing standards and optimal regimens, thereby having a regulatory effect on the private sector. Given the cost of drugs and tests and the long-term nature of treatment, private providers are likely to cut corners to tailor expenditure to what patients can afford [63]. One enzyme-linked immunosorbent assay (ELISA) HIV test instead of three for diagnosis will give high false positives; ART with one or two drugs instead of three, or periodic discontinuation by the patient, will increase the prevalence of HIV strains in the community resistant to antiretroviral drugs—a highly undesirable outcome.

The poor can have access to good quality care only if there is universal access. Medical need should be the only basis on which ART should be allocated. Attempts to target public resources to those below the poverty line will not be effective and will serve to marginalize those most in need by giving them inferior care.

The most important justification for universal access to treatment is experience with other diseases, such as TB during the 1950s and 1960s, which showed that effective and timely intervention on the basis of health need reduces stigma. Once stigma becomes entrenched, it is difficult to dislodge, despite availability of treatment. This was the case with leprosy, which highlights the urgency of providing treatment and support for all those living with HIV.

In addition, any HIV prevention and treatment programme needs to be able to work alongside well-functioning general public health services. The quality of personnel and the appropriate choice of management approach, technologies, delivery system and support structure are all crucial. Different systems for HIV service delivery need to be designed for diverse epidemiological and health service situations. Finally, in order to evaluate the options in real life settings, there is an urgent need for operations research to help devise optimal systems based on a holistic public health perspective [64].

The support network for people with HIV—social workers, counsellors and networks of HIV-positive people—should be incorporated into the formal structure of any HIV prevention and treatment programme as facilitators for patients and as monitors of the quality of service provision. Organizations of people affected by HIV can be important resources in the process of designing and testing systems for HIV care and support. Community organizations should also be encouraged to provide support and ensure that PLHIV are treated responsibly by society.

A popular answer to the dilemma of developing contextually appropriate systems is decentralization. However, decentralization is no panacea for the ills of the healthcare system, which also requires appropriate public health measures, state support and efficient personnel. For decentralization to succeed in the Indian context, it has to be a process of devolution of power and not just delegation of responsibilities by the centre to the periphery. Devolution will simultaneously require strengthening of grass-roots democratic institutions, such as the

Panchayati Raj Institutions of local self-governance, defining their role in controlling health services and building their capacities to do so effectively. Similarly, decentralization of a vertical programme for something like AIDS control is not, in itself, a solution.

Although current Indian HIV policies are clearly not ideal, there are signs of beneficial change. Recent changes within NACO resulting in the moblilization of resources and development of training programmes for doctors and other paramedical staff are welcome. The introduction of antiretroviral therapy with the support of the WHO/UNAID high-profile '3 by 5' programme has had additional benefits in reducing popular fear of AIDS as a fatal disease, thereby decreasing the stigma associated with infection. It is to be hoped that the new response will include opportunities for more contact between those living with HIV and the rest of the population. This will help heal the wounds that HIV inflicts on social relationships.

References

1. United Nations Development Programme. (2003). *Human Development Report: Millennium Development Goals: A Compact Among Nations to End Human Poverty.* UNDP New Delhi: Oxford University Press, p1–3.

2. Qadeer I, Viswanathan N. (2004). How healthy are health and population policies: the Indian experience. In: Castro A, Singer M, eds. *Unhealthy Health Policy: A Critical Anthropological Examination.* Lanham, MD: Altamira Press, pp 253–279.

3. Iyer A, Sen G. (2000). Health sector changes and health equity in the 1990's. In: Raghuram S, ed. *Health and Equity-effecting Change.* Bangalore: HIVOS, p15–55.

4. Peters D, Yazbeck AS, Sharma RR, Ramana GNV, Prittchett LH, Wagstaff A. (2002). In: *Better Health Systems For India's Poor: Findings Analysis and Options.* Human Development Net Work: Health, Nutrition and Population Series. Washington, DC: World Bank, p7.

5. Ashraf A, Rodrigues M. (2002). *Private Health Sector in India.* Mumbai: CEHAT (Monograph).

6. Phadke A, Mane P, Fernandes A, Sharda L, Jesani A. (1995). *Study of Supply and Use of Pharmaceuticals in Satara District.* Pune: FRCH.

7. Uplekar M, Ranjan S. (1999). *Tackling T.B.: The Search for Solutions.* Mumbai: FRCH.

8. Qadeer I. (2000). Health care systems in transition III. The Indian experience part I. *Journal of Public Health Medicine* 22:25–32.

9. Sagar A, Qadeer I. (2004). Community health and sanitation—a vision for hunger-free India. In: Swaminathan MS, Medrano P, eds. *Towards Hunger-free India—From Vision to Action.* Madras: East West Books, pp 145–160.

10. Singh V, Jaiswal A, Porter JDH *et al.* (2002). TB. Control, poverty, and vulnerability in Delhi, India. *Tropical Medicine and International Health* 7:693–700.

11. Priya R. (1999). Public health, ethics and tuberculosis. *Indian Journal of Tuberculosis* 46:273–8.

12. Simoes EA, Babu PG, John TJ *et al.* (1987). Evidence for HTLV-3 infection in prostitutes in Tamil Nadu (India). *Indian Journal of Medical Research* 85:335–8.

13. Solomon S, Anuradha S, Ganapathy M, Jagadeeswari. (1994). Sentinel surveillance of HIV-1 infection in Tamilnadu, India. *International Journal of STD and AIDS* 5:445–6.

14. John TJ, Bhushan N, Babu PG, Seshadri L, Balasubramanium N, Jasper P. (1993). Prevalence of HIV infection in pregnant women in Vellore region. *Indian Journal of Medical Research* 97: 227–30.

15. Gangakhedkar RR, Bentley ME, Divekar AD *et al.* (1997). Spread of HIV infection in married monogamous women in India. *Journal of the American Medical Association* 278:2090–2.

16. Newmann S, Sarin P, Kumarasamy N et al. (2000). Marriage, monogamy and HIV: a profile of HIV-infected women in South India. *International Journal of STD and AIDS* 11:250–53.

17. Sarkar S, Panda S, Sarkar K et al. (1995). A cross-sectional study on factors including HIV testing and counselling determining unsafe injecting practices among injecting drug users of Manipur. *Indian Journal of Public Health* 39:86–92.

18. Ministry of Health and Family Welfare, National AIDS Control Organization. (2000). *Combating HIV/AIDS in India 2000–2001*. Delhi: Ministry of Health and Family Welfare.

19. Solomon S, Kumarasamy N, Ganesh AK, Amalraj RE. (1998). Prevalence of and risk factors of HIV-1 and HIV-2 in urban and rural areas in Tamil Nadu, India. *International Journal of STD and AIDS* 9:98–103.

20. Anvikar AR, Chakma T, Rao VG. (2005). HIV epidemic in Central India: trends over 18 years (1986–2003). *Acta Tropica* 93:289–94.

21. Sharma SK, Aggarwal G, Seth P, Saha PK. (2003). Increasing HIV seropositivity among adult tuberculosis. *Indian Journal of Medical Research* 117:239.

22. Mirante E. (1993). Drug injecting in Manipur, India. The Burma connection. *AIDS Society* 4:4.

23. Panda S, Bijaya L, Sadhana Devi N et al. (2001). Interface between drug use and sex work in Manipur. *National Medical Journal of India* 14:209–11.

24. Eicher AD, Crofts N, Benjamin S, Deutschmann P, Rodger AJ. (2000). A certain fate: spread of HIV among young injecting drug users in Manipur, north-east India. *AIDS Care* 12:497–504.

25. Panda S, Saha U, Pahari S et al. (2002). Drug use among the urban poor in Kolkata: behaviour and environment correlates of low HIV infection. *National Medical Journal of India* 15:128.

26. Priya R. (2003). Health services and HIV treatment: complex issues and options. *Economic and Political Weekly*, December, 13 2003, p5527–32.

27. Sen S. (2003). High HIV prevalence states: an analysis of the HIV/AIDS scenario. *Health for the Millions* 28:28–30.

28. Kumarasamy N, Solomon S, Jayaker Paul SA, Venilla R, Amalraj RE. (1995). Spectrum of opportunistic infections among AIDS patients in Tamil Nadu, India. *International Journal of STD and AIDS* 6:447–449.

29. Misra SN, Sengupta D, Satpathy SK. (1998). AIDS in India: recent trends in opportunistic infections. *Southeast Asian Journal of Tropical Medicine and Public Health* 29:373–6.

30. Reed KD. (2001). A tale of two cities: brothel based female commercial sex work, spread of HIV, and related sexual health care interventions in India, using Bombay and Delhi as examples. *Journal of Family Planning and Reproductive Health Care* 27:223–7.

31. Pandhi D, Kumar S, Reddy BS. (2003). Sexually transmitted diseases in children. *Journal of Dermatology* 30:314–20.

32. Bhattacharjee J, Gupta RS, Kumar A, Jain DC. (2000). Pre-and extra-marital heterosexual behaviour of an urban community in Rajasthan, India. *Journal of Communicable Diseases* 32:33–9.

33. Bhattacharya G. (2004). Sociocultural and behavioral contexts of condom use in heterosexual married couples in India: challenges to the HIV prevention programme. *Health Education Behavior* 31:101–17.

34. Ananth P, Koopman C. (2003). HIV/AIDS knowledge, beliefs, and behaviour among women of childbearing age in India. *AIDS Education and Prevention* 15:529–46.

35. Shankar AV, Pisal H, Patil O et al. (2003). Women's acceptability and husbands' support of rapid HIV testing of pregnant women in India. *AIDS Care* 15:871–4.

36. Go VF, Sethulakshmi CJ, Bentley ME *et al.* When HIV-prevention messages and gender norms clash: the impact of domestic violence on women's HIV risk in slums of Chennai, India. *AIDS Behaviuor* 7:263–72.

37. Varma M, Mehta G. (2000). Needle stick injuries among medical students. *Journal of the Indian Medical Association* 98:436–8.

38. Kermode M, Jolley D, Langkham B, Thomas MS, Crofts N. (2005). Occupational exposure to blood and risk of bloodborne virus infection among health care workers in rural north Indian health care settings. *American Journal of Infection Control* 33:34–41.

39. Wig N. (2003). HIV: awareness of management of occupational exposure in health care works. *Indian Journal of Medical Science* 57:192–8.

40. Anand K, Pandav CS, Kapoor SK. (2001). Undergraduate Study Team. Injection use in a village in north India. *National Medical Journal of India* 14:143–4.

41. Lole KS, Bollinger RC, Paranjape RS *et al.* (1999). Full-length human immunodeficiency virus type 1 genomes from subtype C-infected seroconverters in India, with evidence of intersubtype recombination. *Journal of Virology* 73:152–60.

42. Sahni AK, Prasad VV, Seth P. (2002). Genomic diversity of human immunodeficiency virus type-1 in India. *Journal of STD and AIDS* 13:115–8.

43. Tripathy SP, Kulkarni SS, Jadhav SD *et al.* (2005). Subtype B and subtype C HIV type 1 recombinants in the northeastern state of Manipur, India. *AIDS Research and Human Retroviruses* 212:152–7.

44. Pfutzner A, Dietrich U, von Eichel U *et al.* (1992). HIV-1 and HIV-2 infections in a high-risk population in Bombay, India: evidence for the spread of HIV-2 and presence of a divergent HIV-1 subtype. *Journal of Acquired Immune Deficiency Syndrome* 5:972–7.

45. Kannangai R, Shaji RV, Ramalingam S *et al.* (2003). HIV-2 subtype circulating in India (south). *Journal of Acquired Immune Deficiency Syndrome* 33:219–22.

46. Bhanja P, Mandal DK, Jana S, Bhattacharya SK, Chakrabarti S. (2004). Detection and characterization of HIV type 2 in Calcutta India. *AIDS Research and Human Retroviruses* 20:101–4.

47. NACO. (2003). *Combating HIV/AIDS in India 2000–20001, Ministry of Health and Family Welfare.* National AIDS Control Organization.

48. WHO/UNAIDS. (2004). *Country Update: India.* Epidemiological Fact Sheets on HIV/AIDS and Sexually Transmitted Infection. Geneva: WHO/UNAIDS. Available at: www.WHO.INT/GlobeAtlas/PDFFactory/HIV/index.asp.

49. NACO. (2004). *Annual Report 2003–2004.* New Delhi: National AIDS Control Programme, Ministry of Health and Family Welfare.

50. Kumarasamy N, Solomon S, Flanigan TP, Hemalatha R, Thyagarajan SP, Mayer KH. (2003). Natural history of human immunodeficiency virus disease in southern India. *Clinical Infectious Diseases* 36:79–85.

51. Chaudhury RR, Thatte U. (2003). Beyond DOTS: avenues ahead in the management of tuberculosis. *National Medical Journal of India* 16:321–7.

52. Pathni AK, Chauhan LS. (2003). HIV/TB in India: a public health challenge. *Journal of the Indian Medical Association* 101:148–9.

53. Ramachandran R, Datta M, Subramani R, Baskaran G, Paramasiva CN, Swaminathan S. (2003). Seroprevalence of human immunodeficiency virus (HIV) infection among tuberculosis patients in Tamil Nadu. *Indian Journal of Medical Research* 118:147–51.

54. Arora P, Cyriac A, Jha P. (2004). India's HIV-1 Epidemic. *CMAJ* (171)11: 1337–1338.

55. Priya R. (1994). AIDS, public health and the panic reaction, part II. *National Medical Journal of India* 7:288–291.

56. Kumarasamy N, Solomon S, Chaguturu SK *et al.* (2003). The safety, tolerability and effectiveness of generic antiretroviral drug regimens for HIV-infected patients in south India. *AIDS* 17:2267–9.

57. Balakrishnan P, Dunne M, Kumarasamy N *et al.* (2004). An inexpensive, simple, and manual method of CD4 T-cell quantitation in HIV-infected individuals for use in developing countries. *Journal of Acquired Immune Deficiency Syndrome* 36:1006–10.

58. Over M, Heywood P, Kurapati S *et al.* (2003). *Integrating HIV Prevention and Antiretroviral Therapy in India: Costs and Consequences of Policy Options.* International AIDS Economics Network.

59. Krishnan, TN. (1999). Hospitalization insurance: a proposal. *Economic and Political Weekly* April, 13 1999, p944–6.

60. Banerji D. (1985). *Health and Family Planning Services in India: An Epidemiological, Socio-cultural and Political Analysis and Perspective.* New Delhi: Lok Paksh.

61. Government of India. (2002). *National Health Policy 2002.* New Delhi: Department of Health, Ministry of Health and Family Welfare.

62. WHO. (2002). *Scaling Up Antiretroviral Therapy in Resource-Limited Settings—Guidelines for a Public Health Approach.* Geneva: WHO.

63. Centre for Health Research & Development (CHRD) and Maharashtra Association of Anthropological Science (MAAS). (2003). *Investigating Private Sector Delivery of Services for the Management of Adult HIV Patients in Pune-City, India.* Pune: CHRD, MAAS.

64. Banerji D. (1992). *Combating AIDS as a Public Health Problem in India.* New Delhi: Voluntary Health Association of India and Nucleus for Health Policies and Programmes.

Chapter 21

Indonesia

Suriadi Gunawan[*], Soewarta Kosen and Chris Simms

Background

Indonesia typifies the 'success' of the East Asian economic miracle. Between the mid-1960s and mid-1990s, the country experienced impressive economic growth, quadrupling per capita income, reducing poverty by two-thirds and making enormous advances in human welfare indicators.

In the late 1980s, the first AIDS cases began to appear, first among homosexuals, and later in population groups with high-risk behaviours, such as sex workers and their clients, and injecting drug users (IDUs). From these groups, HIV infection started to spread to the general population, such as housewives and pregnant women. The HIV epidemic entered the concentrated phase in 2000. Review of the country's healthcare system shows that failure to prioritize public health adequately and failure to meet the needs of vulnerable populations are among the constraints that may undermine the Government of Indonesia's response to the HIV crisis. Furthermore, economic and political shocks and their aftermath over the last 10 years—most notably the East Asian financial crisis, the fall of the New Order government under President Soeharto in 1998 and the decentralization of government—have, to date, thwarted the full-scale implementation of HIV prevention and control programmes. Nevertheless, the rise in democracy and human rights and the decline in centralized authority may create a more conducive environment in which to launch an effective response to the HIV epidemic [1].

The Republic of Indonesia, which consists of over 17,000 islands, is the largest archipelago country in the world, lying between the Asian continent and Australia. It is a heterogeneous country with more than 250 ethnic groups, each with its own language, customs and culture. Bahasa Indonesia is the official language and is widely spoken and understood in all parts of the country.

Population

Indonesia consists of 33 provinces, each of which is subdivided into districts (*kabupatens*) and municipalities (*kota*). At present, there are 302 districts and 89 municipalities. The next level is comprised of subdistricts (*kecamatans*) and villages (*desa* in a rural area and *kelurahan* in an urban area). There are 4918 subdistricts and 70,460 villages in all. According to the 2000 Population Census, the population was 205.8 million and projected to reach 215 million in

---

* Corresponding author.

2003. This makes Indonesia the fourth most populous country in the world. An estimated 44% of the population lives in urban areas. Due to a successful population and family planning programme, the population growth rate has declined from 2.0% in 1980–1990 to 1.5% in 1990–2000 (Table 21.1).

The age structure is as follows: 0–14 years, 30%; 15–24 years, 20%; 25–49 years, 36%; and over 50 years, 14% [2]. Population density varies significantly between different regions. The island of Java, which has only 7% of the land area, is inhabited by 59% of the population. West Java has a population density of 1009/km^2, while the national average is 112/km^2. Around 85% of the population is Muslim; other religions are Christian (10%), Hindu (2%), Buddhist (1%) and Confucian (1%).

Economic trends

Indonesia experienced steady economic growth between the mid-1960s and mid-1990s. Economic transformation progressed from the green revolution in rice to the development of labour-intensive industries, followed by trade liberalization, which led to the development of export-based manufacturing industries. Gross domestic product (GDP) grew by an average 6–7% a year. Per capita income grew from US$50 in 1965 to US$1124, with purchasing power parity of US$3000 in 1996, while the population in poverty declined from 60% to below 20%. All of these successes ended in 1997, when the Asian economic crisis started. Between 1997 and 1998, inflation surged from 6% to 78%, the value of the *rupiah* plummeted from Rp. 2250 to Rp. 12,500 per US$, while real wages fell by around one-third, unemployment rose and the proportion of people living below the poverty line jumped from 18% to 24% with a consequent reduction in their access to healthcare services. [3]

Welfare indicators

An important achievement of the Government of Indonesia during the period 1970–1998 was the improvement of welfare provision by ensuring the availability of adequate food, clothing and more equitable education and health facilities. Sixty per cent of married women are currently using contraceptives. The most commonly used methods are injectable hormones (28%), the birth control pill (13%) and the intrauterine device (6%) (Table 21.2). Use of condoms for male contraception is only 0.9% [4].

Table 21.1 Demographic indicators of Indonesia, 1990–2002

Indicator	1990 census	2000 census	2002 projection
Population (million)	179.4	206.3	211.1
Growth rate (%)	1.98	1.49	1.25
Density (population/km^2)	93	109	112
Percentage urban	31	42	44
Crude birth rate	28	23	22
Crude death rate	9	8	10
Life expectancy			
Male	57.9	63.3	64.3
Female	61.5	67.3	68.2

Source: [2].

Table 21.2 Selected welfare indicators for Indonesia, 2002

Literacy rate (10 years and older)	91%
Age of first marriage for females	23 years
Total fertility rate	2.6
Current use of contraception by women	60%
Infant mortality rate	35 per 1000
Maternal mortality ratio	305 per 100,000
Place of delivery	
Home	60%
Health facility	40%
Assistance during delivery	
Midwife	50%
Traditional birth attendant	30%
Relatives	12%
Doctor	5%
Immunization (by 12 months)	
BCG	82%
DPT 3	55%
Polio 3	63%
Measles	63%
All	44%
No vaccination	11%

Source: [4].

The infant mortality rate (IMR) declined from 142 per 1000 live births in 1969 to 35 per 1000 live births in 2002. IMR is higher in rural compared with urban areas: 52 and 32 per 1000 live births, respectively. The highest IMR is found in Gorontalo and West Nusa Tenggara (77 and 72 per 1000, respectively), while the lowest is in Bali (14 per 1000) [4]. Results of the 2001 National Health Survey showed that the leading causes of mortality for all ages were cardiovascular diseases (26%), infectious and parasitic diseases (23%), respiratory diseases (13%), digestive diseases (7%), neoplasms (6%) and injuries (6%). Maternal deaths represent 14% of all deaths of women aged 15–49, and the Indonesian Demography and Health Survey (IDHS) of 2002–2003 estimated the maternal mortality ratio at 305 per 100,000 live births for the period 1998–2002, a decrease from 390 per 100,000 live births for the period 1990–1994.

Impressive as these improvements in health indicators are, they are not commensurate with the country's economic position. For example, Indonesia's IMR of 35 per 1000 live births compares poorly with rates in Thailand at 30, Malaysia at 9, and Sri Lanka at 18. The maternal mortality ratio of 305 per 100,000 live births is high compared with 175 in the Philippines, 170 in Vietnam, 35 in Thailand, 30 in Malaysia and 10 in Singapore.

The health system

Law Number 23/1992 provides a legal basis for the health sector's activities. It stipulates that every person has the right to an optimal health status and the duty to participate in the efforts to maintain and promote the health status of individuals, families and communities. The government has the duty to provide equitable health services that are affordable for the community and increase the health status of the population [5]. In 1999, a new health paradigm was introduced that focuses health development on health promotion and prevention, rather than curative and rehabilitative services. The new vision for the health sector is reflected in the national goal, 'Healthy Indonesia 2010' [6]. To achieve the national goal, the Ministry of Health (MoH) has developed strategies in the following areas: health-oriented national development; professionalism; decentralization; and social health insurance.

Since the 1970s, through an annual Presidential Decree, Indonesia has developed an extensive network of 7237 Community Health Centres (*Puskesmas*), linked to 21,267 health subcentres and 6392 mobile clinics. Participation of the community is channelled through some 240,000 integrated service posts (*Posyandu*) run by volunteers, 33,083 village maternity posts (*Polindes*) run by village midwives, and 12,414 village drug posts (*Pos Obat Des*) (Table 21.3) [7].

Expenditure, financing and access

The level of public health expenditure is modest compared with other countries in the region. During the period 1996–1998, 0.6% of the GDP went to public health expenditure compared with 1.3% in Malaysia, 1.7% in Thailand, 0.7% in China and an average of 2.2% for all developing countries [3]. The government health budget is around 4% of total government

Table 21.3 Health expenditure and real resources, 2002

Resource/facility	
Health centres	7237
Health subcentres	21,267
Mobile clinics	6392
Integrated service posts	240,000
Village maternity posts	33,083
Village drug posts	12,414
Hospitals	1212
Government	420
Private	602
Company	78
Armed forces	112
Bed capacity	130,214
Bed population ratio	1:1650
Doctors	42,000
Nurses	75,000
Midwives	80,000
Pharmaceutical companies	198
Pharmacies	6058
Drug stores	4743
Government health expenditure	US$5/capita
Total health expenditure	US$15/capita
% of GDP	2.2%
Coverage by health insurance	20%

Source: [6].

expenditure. This is still far from the 15% target of the MoH. If public and private health expenditure is combined, approximately US$15 per capita per year is spent on health, only 30% of which is provided by the government. This is around 2.2% of GDP and still below the 5% minimum recommended by the World Health Organization (WHO) to be spent on health [7]. A law for national health insurance is being drafted by Parliament. Various governmental and private health insurance schemes, including insurance for government employees (*Askes*) and employees of private companies (*Jamsostek*), cover less than 20% of the population [7].

Analyses of access to effective healthcare in Indonesia [8,9] show that, from a historical perspective, the country's health system has never advanced beyond the initial investment stage of primary healthcare (PHC). Until the Indonesian government embarked upon the establishment of a robust and integrated network of services in the early 1980s, the public component of Indonesia's health system was minimal. Based on the WHO 'Health for All' framework, the labour-intensive, preventive approach emphasized field workers targeting both the poor and non-poor across a large geographical area. While utilization of the public health system increased significantly throughout the 1980s, the rates peaked by the early 1990s, with about one-third of the population seeking outpatient care using public facilities. By 1995, utilization rates had fallen below 30% and, by 1998, below 20%. In contrast, the private healthcare system has flourished: between 1989 and 1997, bed days in publicly run general hospitals increased by less than 1% annually compared with 5% in privately owned facilities.

Two factors may explain these trends. First, because the health system was underfunded, the government was forced to tolerate user-fees and permit government workers to provide healthcare on a private basis. This compensation strategy created systematic and perverse incentives within government health facilities. Secondly, the government imposed strong guidance and control mechanisms on health staff and, while these were intended to ensure predictable delivery of quality services, they led to micromanagement, which reduced the effectiveness and appropriateness of services [8,9].

From a more current perspective, several pieces of evidence suggest that the stress of economic crisis and the political and social transition of recent years have magnified historical weaknesses in the system and further reduced access to effective care for ordinary Indonesians. For example, although public health spending quadrupled between 1985 and 2000, at current levels it remains about US$5 per capita, compared with US$10 in the Philippines, US$27 in Thailand and US$49 in Malaysia. A recent analysis estimated that in order to make a substantial impact on health indicators, spending levels would have to increase fivefold [8]. The detrimental effect of underfunding is exacerbated by misallocation of scarce resources. Between 1997 and 2000, the government reduced per person PHC spending by 20%, while spending on hospital care increased by about 30% (Table 21.4).

Reports of poor quality of care seem to have been confirmed by low utilization and patient dissatisfaction [11]. During the period 1995–1999, there was a sharp fall-off in use of services such as *posyandu* (–4.7%), health subcentres (–40%), clinics (–26%) and primary health centres (–26%), which are most likely to be used by low-income households. On the other hand, utilization of services that tended to be used by the higher-income people, such as hospitals and private providers, only fell between 3 and 13% (Table 21.5).

The economic crisis and its after-effects have shown that healthcare financing in Indonesia is at risk. Private healthcare expenditure in Indonesia accounts for about two-thirds of total spending, with about 75% of the total being made in cash. The purchase of drugs contributes

Table 21.4 Real public expenditure[*] on primary healthcare and hospital care, 1997–2000

	1997	1998	1999	2000
Primary care spending				
per person (thousand rupiah)	10.3	9.6	8.5	8.2
Hospital spending per person (thousand rupiah)	4.1	4.4	4.6	5.3

[*]Amounts shown are in constant 1993 Indonesian rupiahs: US$1 = 2095. Source: [10].

Table 21.5 Contact rates by type of provider, 1995–1999

Provider	1995	1997	1998	1999	% change, 1995–1999
Posyandu	0.19	0.20	0.12	0.10	−47%
Traditional healer	0.73	0.63	0.43	0.40	−45%
Health subcentre	1.69	1.66	1.01	1.01	−40%
Clinic	0.42	0.39	0.34	0.31	−26%
Primary health centre	4.66	4.31	3.25	3.46	−26%
Private doctor	3.01	3.14	2.84	2.63	−13%
Public hospital	0.64	0.60	0.64	0.59	−8%
Paramedical practitioner	2.82	2.93	2.80	2.70	−4%
Private hospital	0.40	0.41	0.40	0.39	−3%

Source: [12].

significantly to private healthcare expenditure, and cash payments account for about 80% of the total pharmaceutical expenditures. Between 1996 and 1999, there was a 25% drop in real spending that corresponded to price increases of about 170% caused by massive devaluation of the rupiah during the financial crash. Set against a background of severe economic crisis and falling incomes, these high rates of cash payments obviously put health financing at risk. User-fees have become an impenetrable barrier to service utilization by the poor, and the cross-national evidence shows that exemptions from fees rarely work as intended, especially for the poor and vulnerable. On top of standard outpatient user-charges, informal charges are usually substantial [13].

Assessment [13,14] of changes in access to quality healthcare associated with the government's decision to decentralize the system presents a mixed picture. It suggests that, despite poor planning and implementation, this process has gone surprisingly well: a household survey shows that more than 50% of the people believe that services overall have improved or not deteriorated; utilization of healthcare services has remained stable overall due in part to maintenance of social service delivery spending. Although a deterioration in the management of communicable diseases and of the cold chain for immunization services has been observed, there has been no major interruption in services.

However, the utilization of modern public health facilities since 1999 has decreased (Table 21.6), on top of the sharp fall-off experienced during the period 1997–1999. While data that describe changes in utilization by provider type or by level of income are not yet available, a 55% increase since January 2001 in per capita monthly private out-of-pocket health expenditure, due primarily to increased cost recovery, is noteworthy. The implications of this trend for access to effective healthcare by low-income households have yet to be investigated.

Table 21.6 Use of health services by provider, 1997–2002

	1997	1998	1999	2000	2001	2002
Modern provider	12.8	10.5	10.6	9.0	9.6	9.8
Public	6.7	5.0	5.3	4.2	3.8	4.5
Private	6.7	6.2	5.9	5.4	5.8	5.8

Source: [9].

Identified threats to the success of decentralization that would have an impact on the fight against HIV in the future include the lack of clarity in the assignment of functions across levels of government, which is needed for local accountability and is key to the design of a government fiscal system that provides regions with sufficient funds to meet assigned responsibility. Minimum standards of service for obligatory functions will also need to be set by central government in order to clarify what the community can expect from local governments. The poor capacity of local governments to deliver services efficiently is worsened by the limited role of the province, the creation of many new provinces, districts and municipalities, and a lack of clarity in civil service reform. The new government financial resource allocation is highly unequal, since the richest local government area receives 50 times more revenue per capita than the poorest, with the poorest unlikely to be able to fund public services at acceptable standards. Inequalities in the old system are compounded by the unequal distribution of income and taxes from natural resources in the new system.

The HIV epidemic

Epidemiology

The first confirmed AIDS case was in Bali in 1987. The number of reported AIDS cases increased slowly until 1999, after which it increased rapidly, especially among IDUs. By December 2003, a total of 1371 AIDS cases and 2720 HIV infections had been reported to the MoH [15] (Fig. 21.1).

For the whole country, the rate of AIDS cases is 0.6 per 100,000 population. The highest proportion of cases was found in the 20–29 age group (42%) and 30–39 age group (31%), while only 1% was found in the 1–4 age-group. The male to female ratio was 4:1. The highest AIDS rates are found in Papua (22.8 per 100,000 population), Jakarta (4.1 per 100,000), Bali (1.5 per 100,000), Riau (1.07 per 100,000) and North Sulawesi (1.06 per 100,000).

The routes of transmission of cumulative reported cases were heterosexual (52%), homosexual (10%), IDU (25%), perinatal (0.3%), blood transfusion and use of blood products (0.2%). The proportion of IDU and perinatal transmission has been increasing since 2000.

A study of opportunistic infections among AIDS patients in Jakarta found the following pattern in descending order of frequency: oral or oesophageal candidiasis, tuberculosis, cytomegalovirus, recurrent pneumonia, toxoplasma encephalitis, *Pneumocystis carinii* pneumonia, herpes simplex, cryptosporidiosis, histoplasmosis and *Mycobacterium avium* complex [16]. Kaposi's sarcoma, cerebral lymphoma and cervical carcinoma were the most frequent opportunistic cancers.

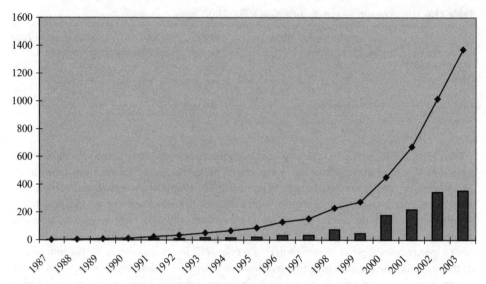

Fig. 21.1 AIDS cases reported to the Ministry of Health, 1987–2003. Source: [15].

Reporting of AIDS cases is based on an instruction of the MoH in 1988 and is not based on law. The 1371 reported cases are an underestimate, and the real number of AIDS cases is estimated to be around 10,000. Periodic surveys of HIV prevalence among sex workers have been conducted since 1987, initially with negative results. However, in 1992, the first cases of HIV infection were found among female sex workers (FSWs) in Surabaya (East Java) and Merauke (Papua). Sentinel surveillance was started in 1994 and is now operating in 22 provinces. The population groups covered are FSWs and, recently, IDUs and prisoners.

The prevalence of HIV started to rise in 1999. For example, among FSWs, a prevalence of 8% was found in Tanjung Balai Karimun (Riau), 26% in Merauke (Papua), 7% in Bali, 6% in West Java, 6% in West Kalimantan, 4% in Central Sulawesi and 4% in North Jakarta.

A new phenomenon in HIV transmission appeared in 1999, when HIV infection among IDUs began to rise. A prevalence of 18% was found among IDUs treated at the Jakarta Drug Dependence Hospital, and it rose to 40% in 2000 and to 41% in 2001. The prevalence among IDUs treated at Cipto Mangunkusumo Hospital, Jakarta, in 2000 was 33%. HIV prevalence among IDUs who were prisoners was 22% in Jakarta, 20% in Bogor, 2% in Lampung, 1% in West Sumatra, 40% in Bali and 0.5% in South Sulawesi [15].

Among transvestites (*waria*) in Jakarta, HIV prevalence rates rose from 6% in 1997 to 21% in 2002. A 2002 survey found an HIV prevalence of 3% among men who have sex with men (MSM) in Jakarta [17]. The prevalence of HIV infection among pregnant women in 2000 was 0.35% in Riau and 0.25% in Papua. In Jakarta, the rate of HIV infection among women who came for voluntary counselling and testing (VCT) was 1.5% in 2000 and rose to 2.7% in 2001. HIV infection in blood donors also started to increase: it was found in 2 per 100,000 in 1992 and rose to 16 per 100,000 in 2000, while in Jakarta it was 20 per 100,000 in 2000 [18]. It can be concluded that since 2000, Indonesia has become a country with a concentrated epidemic among IDUs and sex workers.

Studies of the genetic characteristics of Indonesian HIV cases from 1993 to 2000 show that subtype B virus was dominant in 1993–1994; however, by 1996, subtype E had become dominant and remains the major circulating subtype. Subtype E is dominant in Papua, while subtype B remains the most prevalent in Bali. Subtype B and subtype E are equally distributed in Jakarta. Only HIV-1 was found in the studies [19].

The exact number of HIV infections is not known, but a group of Indonesian and international experts made an estimate that there were 80,000–130,000 HIV-infected people in 2002 [20] (Table 21.7), an estimate which had increased to between 53,000 and 180,000 in 2003, according to WHO/UNAIDS.

Risk factors

An important risk factor that increases vulnerability to HIV infection is sexually transmitted infections (STIs), which are prevalent in Indonesia. The prevalence of STIs in pregnant women is considerable: 5–7% for chlamydia, 1–4% for trichomoniasis, 1% for gonorrhoea and 0.5% for syphilis. Prevalence of STIs among FSWs is even higher: 10–25% for chlamydia, 10–20% for gonorrhoea and 2–10% for syphilis [22]. The prevalence is particularly high in younger FSWs. Around 50% of STI patients do not go to health facilities but self-treat by purchasing over-the-counter antibiotics. As a result, considerable rates of antibiotic resistance have been found.

Several rounds of a high-risk Behaviour Surveillance Survey (BSS) have been conducted since 1996. The latest round was carried out in 2002–2003 in 13 provinces [23]. The BSS and other surveys show that knowledge of AIDS and how it is transmitted has increased. The IDHS of 2002–2003 shows that the percentage of never-married women and currently married men who had heard of AIDS and who believed there was a way to avoid HIV or AIDS increased from 51% in 1997 to 59% in women and 73% in men in 2002 [4]. The BSS among vulnerable groups, including sex workers and their potential clients, IDUs and MSM, indicates that knowledge of

Table 21.7 Estimate of people living with HIV, 2002

	Population size	Estimated HIV prevalence	People with HIV
IDUs	159,389	26.76	42,749
Partners of IDUs	121,389	8.92	10,830
SWs	233,039	3.59	8369
Clients of SWs	8,222,253	0.40	32,922
Regular partners of clients	6,113,833	0.07	4457
MSM	1,149,809	0.87	10,021
Male sex workers	2500	4.02	100
Female partners of male SWs	1182	1.50	18
Transvestites/*waria*	11,272	11.84	1334
Clients of *waria*/SWs	256,488	2.37	6085
Regular partners of *waria*	3050	5.48	167
Prisoners	73,794	11.99	8851
Street children	70,872	0.08	59
Total	16,013,508	0.69	110,800

Source: [21].

HIV and how it is transmitted is fairly high, but this apparently has little impact on risk behaviour.

Other contributing risk factors are a highly mobile population, high rates of urbanization, expanding injecting drug use, and the aftermath of the economic crisis in terms of increasing poverty, prostitution and children or families living on the streets.

Response to HIV

In 1985, the School of Medicine of the University of Indonesia and Cipto Mangunkusumo National Central General Hospital in Jakarta established a study group on AIDS (*Pokdisus AIDS*) and, in 1986, the MoH established a working group on AIDS based at the National Institute of Health Research and Development (NIHRD) in Jakarta.

After the detection of the first confirmed case of AIDS, diagnosed in a foreign tourist in 1987, the MoH established a National AIDS Commission (NAC) under the chairmanship of the Director General of Communicable Disease Control-Environmental Health (CDC-EH). Based on the Instruction of the MoH, AIDS was included among obligatory reported diseases in 1988. When the first indigenous transmission of HIV was detected among FSWs in 1990, the NAC was reorganized to include more representatives from other sectors and ministries.

A short-term plan (STP) and a medium-term plan (MTP) for AIDS control and prevention were implemented in 1988–1994 and supported by the WHO Global Programme on AIDS (GPA). The STP and MTP focused on the training of health personnel; the establishment of testing facilities; initiation of surveillance; knowledge, attitude and practices studies (KAP); and information, education and communication (IEC) activities. With assistance from the Ford Foundation, more than 30 studies were conducted to understand risk behaviours and disseminate information through the printed as well as electronic media [24]. By decree of the MoH in 1992, testing of blood before transfusion became mandatory. The Director General of CDC-EH issued a circular on the policy of 100% condom use in brothels or other sex establishments in 1992. The policy, however, had little effect, as enforcement and operational guidelines were lacking.

The 'Abstain, Be faithful, use Condoms' (ABC) message does not seem to be effective yet. Among men with mobile occupations—truck drivers, sailors, migrant workers—around 50% still engage in risky behaviour or extramarital sex, and condom use is still very low at around 10%. Even among men who have experienced STIs, condom use remains very low, even though condoms are well distributed in places where people can buy sex. Most FSWs know that condoms can prevent HIV and STIs, but condom use with all clients in the last week was only 12%, while condom use with the last client was 40%. The most frequent reason for not using a condom was that clients did not want to. Other reasons given were non-availability, high price of condoms and a belief that some clients and sexual partners were uninfected.

Almost all IDUs know that HIV is transmitted through the use of contaminated needles, but, nevertheless, 85% had used someone else's needle in the previous week and had passed their needles on to others. Most IDUs are afraid to carry their own needles, and the reason given is fear of arrest. Over two-thirds of IDUs were sexually active, 48% reported multiple partners and 40% had bought sex from an FSW in the last year. Consistent use of condoms was reported by only 10% [25].

The percentage of male senior high school students aged 16–19 years in Jakarta who reported ever having had sex was 9%, while among female high school students it was 4% in 2000. Around 5% of the male students had had sex with FSWs. In Surabaya, the percentage of male senior high school students who had ever had sex was 8% in 1997 and 11% in 2000. Among female students, the percentages were 2% in 1997 and 4% in 2000 [26].

The first non-governmental organization (NGO) to deal with AIDS, the Pelita Ilmu Foundation, was established in 1989, and this was followed by many others in major cities and provinces in which HIV cases were found. Established NGOs in the area of health, family planning, medicine, social welfare and religion became active in HIV prevention. Spiritia Foundation is a support group for people living with HIV (PLHIV) established in 1995 and has developed a national network of PLHIV. At present, more than 200 NGOs are active in HIV prevention, care, treatment and support. The Indonesian AIDS Society, the Indonesian Association of AIDS Care Physicians and the Communication Forum for HIV/AIDS NGOs were established in 1996 during the first National AIDS Conference.

In 1993, HIV projection studies were made using the Interagency Working Group-AIDS model, and it was estimated that Indonesia would have from 375,000 to 1 million HIV-infected people by the year 2000 if an effective HIV prevention programme was not implemented. This projection, which was an overestimate, and the awareness that AIDS is a development problem expedited the formation of a multisectoral NAC in 1994, by presidential decree. The Commission was chaired by the Coordinating Minister for People's Welfare, while the Minister of Health was one of the vice chairs. The presidential decree also required the formation of provincial and district AIDS commissions. Technical working groups operating under the national as well as local AIDS commissions include representatives of NGOs and affected communities.

The NAC formulated the first National AIDS Strategy and the first Five Year Program Plan for AIDS Control and Prevention 1995–2000 as part of the Sixth National Development Plan. The plan did not receive the necessary funding due to the emerging economic crisis, but attracted the interest of international donors such as USAID, AusAid, World Bank, KfW (German Development Bank), the European Union and UN agencies, which contributed almost US$60 million for AIDS projects in Indonesia in the period 1994–2000. The government budget for AIDS and STIs in the same period amounted to around US$20 million. As a result of this, in spite of the economic crisis, most activities for HIV prevention could be maintained.

Indonesia signed the Declaration of Commitment of the UN General Assembly Special Session (UNGASS) on HIV/AIDS in June 2001. This has led to a number of new policy initiatives. The establishment of the Global Fund to Fight AIDS, Tuberculosis and Malaria expedited the formulation of a strategic plan for HIV prevention and control (2003–2007) by the MoH in 2002 [27]. The plan required around US$20 million per year, or US$100 million over 5 years, with resources coming from the various donor agencies and the Indonesian government.

At a special Cabinet meeting on HIV on 28 March 2002, the Cabinet decided to give HIV a higher priority, improve inter-sectoral coordination, revitalize the NAC and start a national AIDS movement. In August 2002, the NAC developed the new multisectoral National AIDS Strategy, and this was launched on 9 May 2003. The National Strategy sets out the following principles to guide the HIV responses:

1. Take religious and cultural values and social norms into account and strive to maintain and strengthen family welfare and cohesion;

2. Give due attention to the vulnerable groups of the society, including marginalized groups;

3. Respect human rights and give due attention to justice and gender equity;

4. Prioritize prevention through information, education and communication (IEC) and the use of other effective methods;

5. Promote multistakeholder involvement based on the principle of partnership with the government taking a steering and guiding role;

6. Treat HIV as a social problem;

7. Ensure that the response is firmly based on scientific facts and data;

Seven programme priority areas were identified:

1. HIV prevention (including condom use and harm reduction);

2. Care, treatment and support for PLHIV;

3. HIV and STI surveillance;

4. Research and development;

5. Creating a conducive environment for HIV prevention (legislation, advocacy, civil service capacity and elimination of discrimination).

6. Multistakeholder coordination;

7. Sustainable response;

The roles and responsibilities of the parties involved were clearly set out, including government agencies at central and local levels, NGOs, and the private sector and business community [28].

The UN system also responded to the UNGASS Declaration by formulating a UN Joint Action Programme for HIV 2004–2007. The overall objectives of this programme are to support the NAC in implementing the National Strategy 2003–2007 and to create a supportive environment for the Indonesian response.

The UN agencies in Indonesia follow globally agreed-upon lead roles for joint UN action according to their comparative expertise: the International Labour Organization, workers; the United Nations Development Programme, governance and development; UNESCO, education; the United Nations Population Fund, young people and reproductive health; UNICEF, orphans and vulnerable children; WHO, health sector response, care and support and prevention of mother-to-child transmission; and the World Bank, evaluation of national programmes and financing.

Bilateral donors such as USAID and AusAID, which were active in the 1995–2000 period, have started phase II of their assistance projects. USAID, through Family Health International, developed the Aksi Stop AIDS (ASA) project with the MoH. This was a 5-year project (2000–2004) with a total budget of US$36 million and activities in 10 provinces. AusAID, through GRM International Pty Ltd, developed the Indonesia HIV/AIDS Prevention and Care Project Phase II. This is also 5-year project (2003–2007), with a total budget of A$34 million (or US$21 million) covering activities in six provinces. The Global Fund to Fight AIDS, Tuberculosis and Malaria agreed to fund a project, 'Prevention and Alleviation of HIV Impact in Indonesia', in four provinces with a total budget of US$7 million for 2 years starting in July 2003.

Cheaper antiretroviral drugs have been made available since 2001 through a special arrangement between a drug company in India and the AIDS Study Group (*Pokdisus*) of the School of Medicine of the University of Indonesia and Cipto Mangunkusumo Hospital in Jakarta. The project is supported by the MoH and Indonesian Food and Drug Administration, and was providing antiretroviral therapy (ART) to around 1300 PLHIV in 2003 at a cost of about US$70 for a monthly package of three drugs [29]. By October 2003, the WHO/UNAIDS estimated number of PLHIV receiving ART was 2500 out of an estimated 11,500 thought to be eligible. A state-owned pharmaceutical company, Kimia Farma, started producing five different antiretrovirals at a cost of US$50 for a monthly package of three drugs in December 2003. National guidelines on care, treatment and support of PLHIV, including the use of antiretrovirals, were launched in December 2003. In 2004, the MoH started subsidizing the purchase of antiretrovirals at US$25 per patient per month. Since the government introduced the policy of providing free ARVs in 2005, the number of PLHIV receiving ART has risen to 5000.

An important step for implementing the national strategy was the signing of a memorandum of understanding (MOU) between the Chief of National Police, Chair of the National Narcotics Agency, and the Coordinating Minister for People's Welfare, Chair of NAC, to collaborate in HIV prevention and control. This will enable the NAC to undertake pilot projects of harm reduction, including needle exchange and methadone substitution, in designated areas without interference from police.

Lessons learned

Not all activities in response to the HIV epidemic have been successful, but some lessons and some good practices can be learned from the Indonesian experience.

Epidemiological, social and behavioural surveillance, as well as research, were carried out from the early stages of the epidemic. This was useful in documenting the spread of HIV and identifying risks that increase vulnerability to the epidemic. Estimates based on projections made by national and international experts helped make policy-makers aware of the potential damage that HIV might cause if prevention efforts were not made immediately or adequately.

The government considered the epidemic an important issue of national development, calling for a multisectoral approach and partnership with NGOs at a relatively early phase. The political commitment at national level was demonstrated through the formation of the NAC in 1994 and annual special sessions of the Cabinet on HIV since 2001. The decision to launch a national AIDS movement was appropriate but did not become very strong due to a lack of leadership.

Community-based organizations have been involved in HIV prevention since the beginning of the epidemic. A broad-based NGO effort has emerged, with over 200 organizations representing specific groups such as the health professions, youth and adolescents, transvestites, homosexuals, SWs and PLHIV. Efforts to educate the press by organizing regular courses for journalists have been important in spreading reliable information and countering false beliefs, stigma and discrimination. Efforts to involve religious leaders, e.g. the Council of Ulamas, were partially successful, for instance, in decreasing formal opposition to the use of condoms.

The formulation of clear strategies and plans, beginning in the early 1990s, attracted the interest of international donors, and Indonesia was able to maintain most of its activities in HIV prevention and control both during and after the economic crisis.

Blood safety was ensured by a decree of the MoH in 1992 that all blood for transfusion should be tested for HIV by the Indonesian Red Cross, with the government providing the necessary reagents and antigens.

Another lesson learned was the successful importation of generic antiretroviral drugs from India and the production of antiretrovirals by a national pharmaceutical company, both of which make treatment more affordable. The government, however, will not provide treatment free of charge, although it subsidizes the costs.

Conclusion

Since the first case of AIDS was detected in 1987, the HIV epidemic had been growing slowly, until 1999, when a rapid increase in HIV prevalence was found in several provinces, especially among sex workers and IDUs. Since 2000, Indonesia has had a concentrated epidemic, and the total number of HIV cases is estimated at around 110,000 (range 53,000–180,000), about 10,000 of whom have progressed to AIDS, while over 16 million people are at increased risk of getting HIV.

The launch in May 2003 of the new National AIDS Strategy for an expanded response in line with the global AIDS strategy of UNAIDS was a significant step to ensure a broader multi-sectoral response. Central government ministries and local governments in partnership with NGOs have to translate the strategy into realistic action plans. The substantial resources from donor agencies such as the Global Fund, USAID, AusAID and the UN agencies have to be well coordinated to be used to implement activities under the national strategy [18].

Special issues which are formidable challenges to an effective programme are:

- low coverage of vulnerable groups such as IDUs, sex workers and their clients, MSM and the partners of these groups;
- low levels of condom use and resistance from certain religious groups to condom promotion;
- high levels of contaminated needle use among IDUs;
- widespread community stigma and discrimination;
- limited facilities for VCT and ART;
- limited facilities for STI management;
- existing legislation which criminalizes drug users and constrains harm-reduction approaches for IDUs;
- low capacity of health personnel;
- limited government funding and dependency on foreign assistance;
- inadequate leadership at national and local levels;
- a newly instituted process of health system decentralization still creating some confusion.

Various efforts of government, NGOs and international donors, and adequate funding compared with other health programmes, have not been effective enough, as shown by the increasing numbers of HIV infections, especially among IDUs in urban areas and the general population in Papua. Although knowledge of HIV transmission has increased significantly, there has been no measurable behaviour change. Condom promotion and needle exchange programmes to prevent the use of non-sterile needles among IDUs remain contentious issues.

An expanded government, donor and community response is needed to prevent further spread of the epidemic as stated in the National Strategy [18]. The main challenges to effective implementation are closely related to leadership and capacity building of government institutions and NGOs, as well as scaling up more effective projects. The NAC needs to be strengthened by a full-time secretariat to make it more effective. Above all, the people themselves ought to be empowered and actively participate in preventing the growth of this catastrophic epidemic.

Good strategies on paper alone are not sufficient. What is needed is to translate strategies into actions. All the activities of the various government agencies, NGOs and international donors should be well coordinated and mutually supportive if present conditions are to be improved.

References

1. United Nations. (2001). *Common Country Assessment for Indonesia.* Jakarta: UN Indonesia.

2. BPS-Statistics Indonesia. (2003). *Statistical Year Book of Indonesia 2002.* Jakarta: BPS (in Indonesian).

3. BPS-Statistics Indonesia. (2002). *Welfare Statistics 2002.* Jakarta: BPS (in Indonesian).

4. *Indonesia Demographic and Health Survey 2002–2003.* (2003). Jakarta: BPS-BKKBN-MoH-ORC Macro.

5. Law of the Republic of Indonesia No. 23/1992 on Health. Jakarta: Bureau of Legal Affairs and Public Relations, MoH (in Indonesian).

6. Ministry of Health. (1999). *Health Development Plan Towards a Healthy Indonesia 2010.* Jakarta: MoH (in Indonesian).

7. Ministry of Health. (2003). *National Health System.* Draft 07-08-03. Jakarta: MoH (in Indonesian).

8. World Bank. (2003). *Indonesia: Maintaining Stability, Deepening Reforms.* 25330 IND. World Bank Brief for Consultative Group on Indonesia. Jakarta: World Bank Indonesia.

9. World Bank. (2003). *Indonesia: Selected Fiscal Issues in a New Era.* Sector report 25437 IND. Poverty Reduction and Economic Management Unit, East Asia and Pacific Region. Jakarta: World Bank Indonesia.

10. Lieberman S, Yuwono M, Marzoeki P. (2001). Government health expenditures through December 2000. In: *Watching Brief,* issue 6. Jakarta: World Bank Indonesia.

11. Asian Development Bank. (2000). The Economic Crisis and Health and Nutrition in Indonesia. Presented at the Ninth Meeting of the Consultative Group on Indonesia, February 2000, Jakarta.

12. Pradhan M, Sparrow R. (2000). *Indonesia Health Sector Analysis: Changes in Health Indicators Collected in the 1995, 1997, 1998, and 1999 SUSENAS Household Surveys.* Jakarta: Central Bureau of Statistics.

13. World Bank. (2000). *Indonesia: Health Strategy in a Post-crisis, Decentralizing Indonesia.* Sector report 21318. Jakarta: World Bank Indonesia.

14. World Bank. (2003). *Indonesia: Decentralizing Indonesia, a Regional Public Expenditure Review.* Overview Report 26191 IND, June 2003, Poverty Reduction and Economic Management Unit, East Asia and Pacific Region. Jakarta: World Bank Indonesia.

15. Directorate General CDC-EH/MoH. (2003). *Quarterly Report of HIV/AIDS Cases as of 31 December 2003.* Jakarta: DG CDC-EH/MoH (in Indonesian).

16. Zubairi Djoerban. (2003). *HIV/AIDS in Indonesia: The Present and the Future.* Inaugural lecture. December 20, 2003. Jakarta: Medical Faculty University of Indonesia (in Indonesian).

17. National AIDS Commission. (2002). *The Threat of HIV/AIDS in Indonesia is Increasingly Evident and Calls for More Concrete Measures to Prevention.* Report to the Special Cabinet Session on HIV/AIDS, November 2002. Jakarta: NAC/ASA-FHI.

18. National AIDS Commission. (2003). *Country Report on Follow-up to the Declaration of Commitment on HIV/AIDS (UNGASS) 2001–2003.* Jakarta: NAC/UNAIDS Indonesia.

19. Listianingsih E, McArdle J, Graham R *et al.* (2003). Genetic and Demographic Characterization of Indonesian HIV/AIDS Cases from 1993 to 2000. Abstract. 6th Asia Pacific Congress of Medical Virology, Kuala Lumpur, Malaysia, 7–10 December 2003.

20. DG CDC-EH/MoH and WHO. (2002). *Report on the STI, HIV and AIDS Epidemiology and Consensus on HIV-cases Estimation of Indonesia.* Jakarta: DG CDC-EH/MoH.

21. DG CDC-EH/MoH. (2003). *National Estimates of Adult HIV Infection, Indonesia 2002.* Workshop Report. Jakarta: DG CDC-EH/MoH.

22. Miller P, Otto B. (2001). *Prevalence of Sexually Teansmitted Infections in Selected Populations in Indonesia.* Jakarta: Indonesian HIV/AIDS Prevention and Care Project.

23. Sub-directorate for AIDS and STD. (2003). Risk Behaviour Surveillance in Indonesia. Presented at the Workshop on the results of BSS 2002–2003, 29 October 2003, in Cisarua/Bogor. Jakarta: DG CDC-EH/MoH.

24. JEN (National Epidemiology Network). (1993). *AIDS in Indonesia (Executive Summary of 32 Studies Undertaken in 1992).* Jakarta: JEN/Ford Foundation.

25. Pisani E, Dadun, Sucahya PK, Kamil O, Jazan S. (2003). Sexual behaviour among injection drug users in 3 Indonesian cities carries a high potential for HIV spread to non-injectors. *Journal of Acquired Immune Deficiency Syndrome* 31:403–6.

26. Centre for Health Research University of Indonesia. (2001). *BSS Among Female CSWs, Adult Males, Students, Transvestites, and IDUs in Jakarta, Surabaya and Manado 1996–2000.* Jakarta: Centre for Health Research University of Indonesia (CHRUI)/ HIV/AIDS Prevention Project (HAPP)/USAID.

27. MoH/DG CDC-EH. (2002). *Strategic Plan for HIV/AIDS Prevention and Control in Indonesia (2003–2007).* Jakarta: MoH/DG CDC-EH (in Indonesian).

28. National AIDS Commission. (2003). *National HIV/AIDS Strategy 2003–2007.* Jakarta: Office of the Coordinating Minister for People's Welfare/National AIDS Commission.

29. Djauzi S, Rachmadi K. (2003). *From Small Steps Towards a Giant Leap. Experiences of the Working Group on HIV/AIDS. UI Medical School is improving access to generic ARV drugs in Indonesia.* Jakarta: Special Working Group on AIDS, University of Indonesia Medical School and Cipto Mangunkusumo Hospital (POKDISUS AIDS FKUI/RSCM) and Indonesian Perspective Group.

Chapter 22

The Philippines

Ofelia T Monzon* and Roderick E Poblete

Background

The Philippines, reeling financially from the effects of a 20-year dictatorship, experienced the sudden appearance of HIV in the mid-1990s. Through the initiative and commitment of healthcare workers, and in the absence of available resources, a series of activities was immediately launched, laying the foundation for the prevention and control programme in this country. This chapter describes how the healthcare system responded to the challenge of HIV.

Government and demography

The Philippines is an archipelago consisting of 7000 islands located in South East Asia. It is bounded by the Pacific Ocean on the east, the Celebes Sea on the south and the South China Sea on its northern and western borders. The country has three main islands: Luzon, a centre of robust economic activity where 57% of the population resides; the Visayas, comprising 19% of the population; and Mindanao, with 24% of the total population, and home to most of the country's Muslims.

The country has a population of around 82 million [1] with an annual growth rate of 2.3%. Fifty-one per cent of the population is between 15 and 49 years of age, with a slightly larger male population. Youth between the ages of 15 and 24 years make up 20% of the population. The average number of people per household is six.

The Philippines is divided into 16 administrative regions, two of which are autonomous: the Cordillera Autonomous Region (CAR) in northern Luzon, and the Autonomous Region of Muslim Mindanao (ARMM) in the southern part of the Philippines. There are 79 provinces headed by governors. These provinces are further divided into 115 cities, areas of rapid expansion and economic growth; 1497 generally rural municipalities led by mayors; and 41,595 *barangays* (villages), the smallest units of government, headed by *barangay* captains [2]. Work opportunities are found primarily in large cities, causing population migrations from agricultural to urban areas.

The Republic of the Philippines is a democracy with a presidential form of government composed of three separate and equal branches: the executive, with different departments and bureaus; the legislative, comprising the Senate and the Lower House of Congress; and the judiciary, with the Supreme Court as the highest judicial body dispensing justice. The President, as chief executive, heads the Cabinet and provides health policy direction through

---

* Corresponding author.

the Department of Health. The President, Vice President and Members of the Senate are elected nationally every 6 years. Representatives from the Lower House of Congress, Provincial Board Members and City and Municipal Councillors responsible for national and local legislation, together with the Provincial Governors, City and Municipal Mayors and *barangay* captains, are elected every 3 years. This disparity in the terms of office plays a major role in shaping the economic and socio-political policies and programmes of the government; various programmes, including those related to AIDS, are affected by changes in tenure of both officers in charge and higher-level officials.

The country has a literacy rate of 94%, which is higher in urban areas where people have greater access to education. Filipino and English are the main languages of instruction in educational institutions. Because of its geographical, cultural and ethnic diversity—a mix of Spanish, Chinese, Malay, Indian and American, with some indigenous minorities—the Philippines is home to about 100 different dialects. These differences underscore the challenges of delivering messages on reproductive health behavioural change that are culturally and ethnically sensitive and appropriate to the target audience.

Eighty-three per cent of the population is Roman Catholic, with the remainder of the population being Muslims, Protestants, Iglesia ni Cristo, Aglipayans and others. Religion, in particular the Roman Catholic Church, is perceived to be a major stumbling block in communicating reproductive health and HIV prevention messages because of its perceived opposition to these programmes. Debate on the control of the Church over its followers seems to have a substantial influence over the country's political leaders, and on the determination and implementation of its policies.

Socio-economic trends

In 2001, the country's gross national product (GNP) grew by 3.7%, while the gross domestic product (GDP) increased by 3.4%. For the same year, GNP per capita was Philippine Peso (Php) 13,088 (US$262) and GDP per capita Php12,317 (US$246). The main sources of growth were the agricultural and service sectors. Unemployment was at 11%, with a workforce of approximately 31 million Filipinos and 8 million overseas workers. In 2002, a total of 800,000 Filipinos were employed abroad, surpassing the number of newly employed workers in the country for the same year. The remittances of the overseas Filipino workers (OFWs) accounted for US$7 billion.

Poverty was around 28% in the year 2000, as measured by the proportion of families with per capita incomes below the poverty threshold. The annual per capita poverty threshold is calculated as the minimum amount required to satisfy basic food and non-food needs. The proportion of the population living below the poverty line rose from 33% in 1997 to 34% in 2000, indicating that 26.5 million Filipinos, or 4.3 million families, representing over one-third of the population in the year 2000, were trying to make ends meet. The incidence of those living below the poverty line in urban areas remained stable at 15% between 1997 and 2000, while in rural areas it rose slightly, from 40 to 41%, in the same period.

Poverty appears to create a delicate tension between development and peace. This is particularly the case when the ruling elite, in the name of development, appears to play political power games in order to maintain control over resources, oppress the people and corrupt the systems and structures designed to protect the general welfare. In the Philippines, a growing segment of the marginalized population is resorting to extra-constitutional means, such as mass action, to seek social justice, transparency and accountability, and this could undermine peace and security.

The prevailing poverty and the perception of deteriorating security might partly explain the tendency of some of the population either to move from the countryside to urban areas within the country or to choose to work abroad in search of better economic opportunities. Approximately one-quarter of the 8 million OFWs are immigrants seeking permanent resident status abroad. Another 20% of Filipino migrant workers are undocumented and working illegally, risking their personal safety and security in adverse conditions in order to improve the welfare of families left behind.

The prevailing economic hardship, coupled with the lure of a better-paying job and improved living conditions, is also driving trained nurses and other health professionals to work abroad. An increasing number of physicians are taking up nursing courses as a strategy to increase their chances of overseas employment. Eventually, this will have an impact on the severely over-extended healthcare systems and may limit HIV responses in the event of an explosive epidemic. Should the rate of growth in health professional migration continue, responses to reduce the vulnerability of the population to HIV and related issues will be adversely influenced.

Health

The average life expectancy is 69 years, with Filipino men having a shorter life expectancy of 67 years compared with women with 72 years (Table 22.1). Diarrhoeal diseases and respiratory infections are the leading causes of morbidity in the country (Table 22.2). Cardiovascular diseases, pneumonia, malignant neoplasms and accidents are the leading causes of mortality (Table 22.3).

Table 22.1 Health indicators

		Year
Life expectancy at birth (years)	69.6	2002
Crude death rate (per 1000 population)	5.8	2002
Crude birth rate (per 1000 population)	26.2	2001
Infant mortality rate (per 1000 live births)	35.3	1998
Maternal mortality rate (per 1000 live births)	172.0	1997

Sources: National Statistics Office (NSO); Family Health Services Information System (FHSIS); World Health Organization (WHO); National Demographic Health Survey (NDHS).

Table 22.2 Ten leading causes of morbidity, 2002

Rate per 100,000	Number	Rate
Diarrhoeal disease	866,411	1134.8
Bronchitis	700,105	917.0
Pneumonias	632,930	829.0
Influenza	502,718	658.5
Hypertension	279,992	366.7
TB respiratory	126,489	165.7
Diseases of the heart	52,957	69.4
Malaria	50,869	66.6
Chicken pox	35,306	46.2
Measles	23,287	30.5

Source: [1].

Table 22.3 Ten leading causes of mortality, 1998

Causes	Number	Rate
Diseases of the heart	55,830	76.3
Diseases of the vascular system	41,380	11.7
Pneumonia	33,709	46.1
Malignant neoplasms	32,090	43.9
Accidents	29,874	40.8
Tuberculosis (all forms)	28,041	38.3
Chronic obstructive pulmonary diseases and allied conditions	14,228	19.5
Diabetes mellitus	8819	12.1
Other diseases of respiratory system	7516	10.3
Nephritis–nephrotic syndrome and nephrosis	7453	10.2

Source: [1].

The health system

Facilities

There are 1708 hospitals around the country, 640 of which are public hospitals run by the national and local governments, while 1068 are privately owned institutions. Complementing these are 2045 rural health units (RHUs), each staffed by a doctor, a nurse and some midwives, and 13,096 *barangay* health stations (BHS) manned by volunteers from the community and at least one midwife.

The majority of health practitioners are located in urban areas. The situation is complicated further by the fact that a great number of physicians, trained nurses and other health-related personnel are seeking opportunities to work abroad, thus endangering the fragile health infrastructure of the country.

Organization

Responsibility for disease control and other public health programmes was centred in the Department of Health until the passage of the Local Government Code in 1992. Local governments have since delivered health services, although at the national level the Department of Health has continued to provide policy and technical assistance. Socio-political differences between national and local governments therefore influence local implementation of policies and health programmes formulated at the national level [3,4].

Access to and affordability of healthcare continue to be major issues in the country's health delivery system. It is perceived that private hospitals provide better healthcare services, which are largely unaffordable for the general population without social health insurance. Thus, public hospitals are overwhelmed, aggravating existing harsh conditions caused by inadequate basic hospital facilities, including lack of beds, water and electricity supply, medical and other care-related needs. Most of the hospitals run by the national government are located alongside local government hospitals and other facilities in urban areas. The result is an overlapping of tertiary services, which are already concentrated in these areas due to the presence of private hospitals offering the same services. Although primary care services are also provided by most government hospitals, the bulk of essential health services delivery is mostly left to ill-equipped and understaffed district hospitals and primary healthcare units run by the government in rural areas. Curative services are usually paid for out-of-pocket by patients.

In 1998, together with the government's health sector reform agenda of further decentralizing health programmes and services, the Department of Health embarked on a *Sentrong Sigla* (centres of health and wellness) quality assurance programme to set and raise the standards of health at all levels of the system. The aim of this programme is to increase coverage of the marginalized and indigent population through the government's social insurance programme, managed by the Philippine Health Insurance Corporation (Phil-Health).

The healthcare system is currently insufficient for the country's needs, but, through continuous reforms, it appears to be making progress toward its health and development goals.

Expenditure and financing

The share of GNP spent on health decreased from 3.3% in 1998 to 3.1% in 2001, significantly below the standard of 5% set by the World Health Organization for developing countries. Expenditure on personal healthcare services increased from 74% to 76% of the total health expenditures between 2000 and 2001 due to a rise in out-of-pocket expenditures and increased coverage from health maintenance organizations. An increase in social health insurance from 7.1% of the total health expenditure in 2000 to 7.8% in 2001 was noted. As of June 2003, PhilHealth had already covered 7.3 million indigent Filipinos under the government's social health insurance programme, an increase from a baseline of 2.4 million members in 2002, although this was still short of the 8 million targeted by the government. For the first half of 2003, the agency registered 3.7 million urban poor families, surpassing the 500,000 family yearly target. Much has yet to be accomplished in shifting the burden of health financing to social insurance. Furthermore, there is a need to improve the quality of healthcare services provided as well as increasing the number of people gaining access to those services.

Government spending on health fell 2% short of the 40% target share of total health expenditure set for the year 2002. Forty-four per cent of total government health expenditure was spent on personal care, as opposed to 35% spent on public health. The health budget of Php9.3 billion (US$186 million) accounted for 1.5% of the Php609.6 billion (US$1.22 billion) total government expenditure [5]. Seventy per cent of the Department of Health budget went to personal healthcare delivery such as the maintenance of hospitals and centres, while public health programmes received about 14%.

In 2003, the Php15 million (US$300,000) budget for HIV was about 0.16% of the government's total health budget, or about 0.025% of total government expenditure. External resources fund most of the responses to HIV. It is estimated that a total of US$8.5 million will be needed every year to implement adequately the comprehensive response indicated in the Third AIDS Medium-Term Plan for the Philippines. The country has submitted a US$5.5 million HIV proposal for the third round of the Global Fund to Fight AIDS, Tuberculosis and Malaria for the period 2004–2008. Assuming that the proposal will be funded, there will still be unmet needs of US$2.7 million annually.

In terms of government expenditure, the Department of Education receives the biggest appropriation of all the agencies, followed by the Department of National Defence, the Department of Public Works and Highways, and the Department of the Interior and Local Government, respectively. The health budget ranks fifth in order of priority among government agencies. It should be noted that there continues to exist a persistent lag in the provision of basic social services such as classrooms, teachers, textbooks and farm-to-market roads despite the allocation of resources. A significant part of government expenditure goes to foreign debt servicing, which is approximately 26% of the national budget.

Local government (provincial, city and municipal) is the biggest spender on public health, of the order of Php24.9 billion (US$49.8 million) in 2001, or about 21% of the country's total expenditures for health. The rural health units run by local municipal governments are the principal outlets for delivering the national public health programmes and services.

The HIV epidemic

The recognition of two HIV deaths in 1984, the testing and detection of HIV infection among female sex workers (FSWs) and men who have sex with men (MSM) in 1985 [6], and the institution of a national HIV reporting system in 1986 all led to increasing awareness of the presence of the disease in the country. The histories obtained from the early cases of AIDS indicated that their HIV infection had been acquired overseas. By 30 June 2003, a cumulative total of 1892 HIV patients had been reported to the AIDS Registry of the National Epidemiology Centre of the Department of Health [7]. Most of the cases were reported from Metro Manila cities, where the bulk of testing is done either as a requirement by overseas employers or by two government HIV referral institutions. HIV-seropositive cases have gradually increased since the institution of reporting (Fig. 22.1).

The gender distribution by age is shown in Fig. 22.2. Early cases were mainly found among FSWs in the 20–29 age group and probably reflected the fact that initial investigations centred on that population. A reversal of gender distribution was seen in more recent studies, which included more population groups. The current male to female ratio is 1.6:1. The peak prevalence among females was between the ages of 20 and 29 and among males between the ages of 30 and 39. Of note is the increasing number of HIV infections in OFWs observed since the detection of the first HIV-infected seafarer in 1990. To date, 32% of the total number of HIV-infected individuals are OFWs; 75% of these were men and 39% were seafarers.

The predominant mode of transmission among all reported cases was sexual, with infected blood, injecting drug use or perinatal transmission in other cases. No exposure category was known in 12% of cases (Table 22.4).

Except for the initial detection of seven HIV-positive anonymous samples taken from FSWs near a military base north of Manila in 1985, HIV infection was rarely observed prior to the institution of regular surveys. From 1985 to 1993, one out of a total of 1000 FSWs tested during

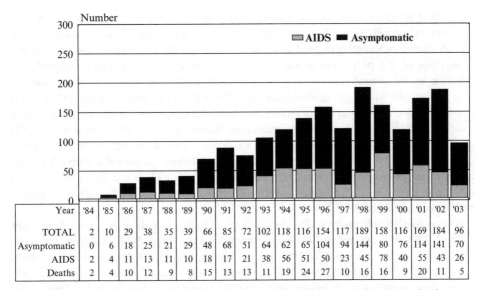

Fig. 22.1 HIV-seropositive cases by year, January 1984–June 2003 (*n* = 1892). Source: [7,8].

that period was HIV-positive (O. Monzon, unpublished data). A definite trend in rising HIV infection is now being noted in data from the annual national surveillance of four sentinel groups in 10 sentinel sites (1993–2002) [8]. Groups tested were FSWs, MSM, males attending sexually

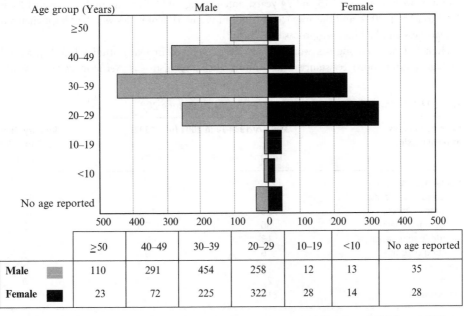

Fig. 22.2 HIV-seropositive cases by gender and age group, January 1984–June 2003 (*n* = 1892). Source: [7,8].

transmitted infection (STI) clinics and injecting drug users (IDUs). Examination for HIV infection and syphilis as an STI marker, and behavioural information were obtained. The Lot Quality Assurance Sampling method was used to detect an HIV prevalence of 1% or more in a sample size of 300 people per group. Early surveillance data revealed rarely observed HIV infection among sentinel subjects (0–1 per sample). By 2002, a prevalence of 1% or more was seen among FSWs in nine of the 10 sites, among MSM in four of 10 sites, and among STI patients in two of 10 sites. Behavioural data showed a wide gap between knowledge and behaviour, with less than 30% condom use, and needle and syringe sharing in 77% of IDUs. An increase in STI signs or symptoms was reported in 18–24% of FSWs, 7% of MSM and 5% of IDUs. Rising resistance to antibacterial agents and poor health-seeking behaviours were also found. The same investigation showed that, of 420 seafarers, 36% had had sex with FSWs and 1% had had sex with other men. The number of people living with HIV (PLHIV) was estimated by WHO/UNAIDS to be 9000 in December 2003.

Studies on HIV subtypes revealed the development of genetic diversity. In the first study, three HIV isolates collected in 1989 were characterized as subtype B [9]. A subsequent study of 51 strains isolated from 1987 to 1996 revealed that the majority of the strains seen belonged to subtype B (72%) [10]. Subtypes E, A, C and D were identified among the remaining strains. No recombinant strains were seen. A recent report on 46 samples isolated from 1998 to 2000 showed an expansion of genetic diversity, with 74% subtype B or C and the remainder recombinant strains [11]. These changes will influence future polymerase chain reaction (PCR)-based investigations, antiretroviral resistance and the development of suitable vaccines.

Many factors affect the spread of HIV. By 2005, 42% of the population was between the ages of 15 and 39 years. The Young Adult Fertility and Sexuality Study report for 2002, based on youth between the ages of 15 and 24 years, noted rising rates of pre-marital sex, from 18% in 1994 to 23% in 2002, and the absence of condom use in 31% of males who had been clients of sex workers and had had symptoms of STIs [12].

High STI rates among sex workers have been reported in many studies [13–15], as well as high antimicrobial resistance rates among such organisms as *Neisseria gonorrhoea* and

Table 22.4 Reported modes of transmission, January 1994–June 2003

Reported modes of transmission	January 1994-June 2003 (n = 1892)		January–June 2003 (n = 96)
	Total	%	Total
Sexual transmission			
Heterosexual contact	1192	63.0	72
Homosexual contact	336	17.8	18
Bisexual contact	96	5.1	6
Blood/blood product	13	0.7	0
Injecting drug use	6	0.3	0
Needlestick injuries	3	0.1	0
Perinatal	27	1.4	0
No exposure	219	11.6	0

Source: [7,8].

Chlamydia trachomatis [16]. Thus, HIV-related trends of concern in this country include increasing poverty and increased mobility of some population groups, a continuing increase in the number of HIV-infected overseas workers, a persisting knowledge gap in all groups studied, low condom use, use of contaminated injection equipment, high STI prevalence and rising antimicrobial resistance.

Demographic, economic and health system impact

Current data show a slowly rising HIV prevalence and do not yet show significant impact on the general population. However, although the total known numbers are low, some observations indicate that the effect on economic and health systems will be considerable as HIV infection increases. In 1994, the Department of Health Research Institute for Tropical Medicine (DoH-RITM) studied 50 HIV-infected patients [17]. A clinical classification using the presence or absence of symptoms was utilized for cost analysis. An average lifetime of 7 years with an asymptomatic stage of 5 years and an AIDS stage of 2 years was observed. Twelve patients received zidovudine (AZT) monotherapy. These patients formed part of a group of 106 HIV-infected patients found to have an average of six infections during their AIDS stage [18]. Total direct costs amounted to Php196,420 (US$3928) per patient, and total indirect costs varied depending on any resulting loss of employment or life. Income loss ranged from Php5,956,389 (US$119,128) to Php8,543,925 (US$170,878). Premature mortality resulted in a lifetime income loss of Php13,085,289 (US$261,706). Increased indirect costs reflected the fact that more than half of the cases were previously employed in other countries and had earnings considerably higher than earners in the local setting.

A complex interplay of such factors as poverty, increased mobility, personal behaviour and insufficient resources will ultimately have a considerable and adverse impact on the demography, economy and healthcare system of the Philippines

Prevention

Health education, promotion and HIV prevention measures were initially conducted in 1986 by the Department of Health to targeted groups in Metro Manila. Distribution of information, education and communication (IEC) materials, telephone hotlines, counselling, condom promotion and various multimedia approaches were carried out intermittently thereafter. This programme has undergone three revisions and expansions of medium-term plans (1988–1993, 1994–1999 and 2002–2004).

Other early responses included health education programmes for health workers [19], overseas workers [20], youth [21] and FSWs [22]. Ongoing Department of Health programmes include annual training of medical technologists performing HIV tests (1987), accreditation of HIV testing laboratories (1988), promotion of voluntary blood donation and HIV testing of donated blood (1988), upgrading of STI clinics (1990) and training of core groups of HIV healthcare workers in 74 government and private hospitals throughout the islands (1999). These trained teams are expected to provide primary HIV care at their respective hospitals as well as providing guidance to other hospital personnel in the management of HIV. These programmes were mostly implemented in collaboration with external partners.

Other government departments have participated in prevention activities through integration of HIV information at the middle school (Grades 5–6) and high school levels, the creation of the Philippine National AIDS Council (PNAC) in 1993 followed by local government AIDS councils, and AIDS in the workplace programmes.

Involvement of non-governmental organizations (NGOs) from around 1990 has made an important contribution to the National AIDS Prevention and Control Program of the Philippines. Most NGO activities were initially aimed at improving knowledge, attitudes, behaviours and practices of groups, but have since expanded into other aspects of AIDS programmes, including healthcare.

A comprehensive AIDS Prevention Law enacted by Congress and signed into law by President Fidel V Ramos in 1998 has provided a legal framework for AIDS prevention in the country [23]. The Act dealt with Education and Information, Safe Practices and Procedures, Testing, Screening and Counselling, Health and Support Services, Monitoring, Confidentiality, Discriminatory Acts and Policies, and the legal creation of the PNAC as the central advisory planning and highest policy-making body for AIDS prevention and control. The council is composed of 26 members: high ranking members of government offices, health professionals, NGOs involved in AIDS prevention and a representative of an organization of PLHIV. The law also strengthens the ethical guidelines on AIDS investigations prepared in 2000 by the AIDS Society of the Philippines [24] in collaboration with PNAC, thus providing sturdy signposts for the protection of infected individuals.

Innovative prevention approaches include an ongoing partnership between an NGO and top-level trimedia representatives [25] and workshops conducted in various regions of the country. Activities include the dissemination of accurate information and discussion of legal and ethical considerations.

In relation to prevention of mother-to-child transmission, the HIV/AIDS Registry of the Department of Health has reported a total of 27 perinatal cases. Under a collaborative programme of the San Lazaro Hospital (SLH) and the Obstetrics Department of the Philippine General Hospital initiated in 1999, seven mothers and children received the recommended AZT therapy [R Tactacan-Abrenica, personal communication]. A pharmaceutical company provided AZT for the first 2 years, with the patients shouldering the costs. None of the infants became infected.

Treatment and care

Initial responses to HIV had consisted of the testing of sex workers by the DoH-RITM [6] and US Naval Medical Research Unit II in 1985. The DoH-RITM response was carried out through the voluntary participation of healthcare workers and without budgetary support from the government. In addition to sex workers, DoH-RITM also tested multiply transfused patients. HIV test supplies were donated by several diagnostic companies and scientists from Japan. Outpatient and inpatient care was then provided by DoH-RITM, and subsequently by SLH. These two government hospitals continue to serve as referral hospitals providing primary to tertiary care of HIV-infected patients. In addition, outpatient care is now being provided by the STI/AIDS Cooperating Clinical Laboratory (SACCL). Few patients have been seen at private and provincial clinics and hospitals, although eventually these patients are referred to the two major referral hospitals for AIDS care. Patients unable to travel to Manila for long-term care are referred to infectious disease specialists on their island.

At referral hospitals, baseline studies include routine blood and radiological examinations. Counselling of patients and family members is provided as part of a management protocol. Follow-up visits are scheduled every 3–6 months as their medical conditions require.

To assist healthcare professionals in their management of HIV disease, a 5-year study on the natural history and prognostic markers for HIV infection was conducted at DoH-RITM from 1991 to 1995 [26]. The most frequent serious infections seen were due to mycobacteria, cytomegalovirus and *Pneumocystis carinii* pneumonia (PCP).

Antiretroviral therapy

Monotherapy with AZT was given to a few patients shortly after the drug became locally available in 1987, but was irregularly prescribed thereafter in the absence of adequate patient resources. Triple or quadruple antiretroviral therapy (ART) has been given in recent years. Locally obtained antiretroviral drugs are available but cost more than generic combinations purchased from another Asian country. An organization of HIV-infected people has purchased the generic drugs and made these available to patients. A total of 68 patients were on ART at RITM, SLH and SACCL in 2003, and that number had risen to 87 at the time of writing.

Treatment of opportunistic infections

Prophylactic and curative treatment of opportunistic infections such as PCP and tuberculosis (TB) is based on recommended CD4 counts and radiological findings. Cotrimoxazole is commonly administered for PCP, and anti-TB drugs such as isoniazid, ethambutol, pyrazinamide and rifampicin are given for TB. Other, less frequent opportunistic infections are treated based on the offending microorganism.

Financing of treatment and care

The costs of managing HIV are shouldered partly by the government and partly by patients or by NGOs. Thus, such routine procedures as blood counts, urinalyses, blood chemistries and chest X-rays may be supported by government budgets, whereas viral load and CD4 count costs are usually the patient's responsibilities or are covered by grants.

RITM patient costs are as follows: complete blood count (CBC) and blood chemistries, Php2000 (US$40); urinalysis, Php60 (US$1.20); viral load, Php8000 (US$160); CD4 count, Php5000 (US$100); and chest X-ray, Php280 (US$4). Optimally, such routine examinations for patients on ART are performed every 3 months for a total of US$1220 yearly [R Ditangco, personal communication, 2004].

Table 22.5 shows the financing sources of 68 patients currently receiving ART. Seventy-one per cent was patient-financed, and the remainder came from NGO contributions. Antiretroviral triple generic drugs purchased from another country cost either Php1900 (US$38) for 3TC–nevirapine–stavudine (d4T) combination, or Php2400 (US$48) for lamivudine (3TC)–AZT–nevirapine combination monthly. The yearly cost may be either US$456 or US$576, respectively [R Ditangco, personal communication]. Treatment of opportunistic infections has been intermittently supported by government budgets. At RITM, a 5 year study grant from the Japanese Foundation for AIDS Prevention covered drug costs from 1990 to 1995 [O Monzon *et al.*, unpublished data]. Subsequently, needs were met through grants

Table 22.5 Financing of antiretroviral treatment by centre ($n = 68$)

Sources	RITM ($n = 56$)	SLH ($n = 5$)	SACCL ($n = 7$)	Total ($n = 68$)
Patient-financed	41 (60%)	1 (1.5%)	6 (9.0%)	48 (71%)
NGO contributions	15 (22%)	4 (6.0%)	1 (1.5%)	20 (29%)

Source: Department of Health (DoH) National Epidemiology Center (NEC) 2003.

from a quasi-governmental agency, the Philippines Charity Sweepstakes office (PCSO). In 2002, the government budget for RITM for all HIV-related care, including medications, was Php800,000 (US$16,000), and PCSO's contribution was Php1,500,000 (US$30,000). Prophylactic treatment for PCP usually requires the administration of cotrimoxazole at a daily cost of Php2.40 (US$0.05), or Php312 (US$6.24) monthly. Quadruple anti-TB treatment (isoniazid, rifampicin, pyrazinamide and ethambutol), a common need among Filipino patients, costs Php10 daily or Php300 (US$6.00) monthly [R Ditangco, personal communication]. At SLH, the government allocation for 2002 was Php1,500,000 (US$30,000) [R Tactacan-Abrenica, personal communication]. Small contributions for supportive therapy by some NGOs have provided less than optimal coverage for opportunistic infections for about 25% of SLH patients.

As part of the effort to reduce expenses, DoH-RITM investigated the use of pooled sera for HIV screening in 1990 [27]. This procedure, reported to be cost-effective and technologically accurate when testing batches of five samples in low-prevalence settings, was utilized in the annual surveillance programme. Quality control safeguards were part of the procedure.

Conclusion

Based on the AIDS Registry numbers, the Philippines remains a country with low HIV prevalence with a seroprevalence rate of 0.01% concentrated among vulnerable populations. This can be attributed to early recognition by the government, complemented by strong community interventions by NGOs and the strategic infusion of external resources from partners and donors. Collaboration among stakeholders led to sound policy formulation and comprehensive responses to HIV. Thus, although the current health system is insufficient to meet the needs of the country as it continues to undergo reforms, it has, nevertheless, been able to cope with the challenges of managing a relatively small number of affected individuals in partnership with local NGOs and external organizations.

On the other hand, a number of observations suggest the potential for an explosive epidemic unless the national prevention programme is strengthened further. A more aggressive and sustained health education programme, together with involvement of more community sectors, is vital in the face of ominous findings of rising HIV prevalence in specific groups, a high STI prevalence in these groups, evidence of unchanged risky behaviour, a fast-growing young population, increasing mobility and continuing poverty. More money is needed to improve the health services necessary to meet the current needs and cope with increasing demands associated with rising HIV infection rates. Realistically, inadequate health services will continue as resources for improving the health system remain scarce and other government priorities come ahead of health.

Given the threat that the epidemic could easily grow, the PNAC is continuing to address and improve the framework of needed prevention programmes. Consideration of cultural and religious nuances, which influence acceptance, need to be built into many education programmes, together with the committed collaboration of religious and other community groups. Unfortunately, the sustainability of successful activities that are highly dependent on the availability of external resources continues to be a challenge

Of utmost importance is the continued recognition of the importance of HIV prevention by officials concerned with budgets and by donors looking at prevalence figures as indices for financial priority. The lessening of the economic impact of HIV through prevention cannot be overemphasized. The strong external partnerships seen in the country's early responses need to continue in order to maintain current low prevalence levels. The approval of the Philippines' proposal to the Global Fund to Fight AIDS, Tuberculosis and Malaria may meet some of the future health expenditure needs. However, with decentralization, it remains imperative to ensure effective application of health policies at the community level.

Acknowledgements

We thank the following for the valuable information and assistance they provided in producing this chapter: Assistant Secretary Austere Panadero (Department of Interior and Local Governments), Cesar Montances (Division Chief, Office of Public Assistance, Office of the Secretary, Department of Interior and Local Governments), Dr Carlos Calica (President, AIDS Society of the Philippines), Dr Socorro Lupisan (Assistant Director, Department of Health Research Institute for Tropical Medicine), Dr Rossana Ditangco (Head, DoH RITM AIDS Research Group), Dr Rose Aplasca-de los Reyes (Head, Clinical Medicine, DoH RITM), Dr Dorothy Agdamag (Chief, STD-AIDS Cooperating Central Laboratory), Dr Rosario Tactacan-Abrenica (San Lazaro Hospital AIDS Unit), Dr Isabel Melgar (Ateneo de Manila University and AIDS Society of the Philippines), Dr Dominic Garcia (Program Manager, AIDS Society of the Philippines) and Ms Arlene Ruiz (Chief, Economic Development Specialist, National Economic Development Authority).

References

1. National Statistical Coordination Board. (2003). *Philippine Statistical Yearbook 2002.* Republic of the Philippines.
2. Health Action Information Network, Philippine National AIDS Council, Joint United Nations Programme on HIV/AIDS. (2003). *HIV/AIDS Country Profile Philippines 2002.* Philippines.
3. National Statistical Coordination Board. (2003). *2001 Philippine National Health Accounts.* Republic of the Philippines.
4. Republic of the Philippines General Appropriations Act. (2003). Philippines.
5. Taguiwalo M, Poblete, RE. (2001). *Assessing the Vulnerabilities to HIV/AIDS in Selected Cities in the Philippines.* Philippines: Philippine National AIDS Council.
6. Monzon OT, Capellan JM, Balis A, Sotocua E, Costa C, Florentino V. (1989). Risks for HIV infection in a low prevalence country. *Philippine Journal of Microbiol Infect Dis* 18:5–9.
7. The Department of Health National Epidemiology Center. (2003). *HIV/AIDS Registry.* Philippines: DoH.

8. The Department of Health National Epidemiology Center. (2003). *The 2002 Technical Report of the National HIV/AIDS Sentinel Surveillance System. Status and Trends of HIV/AIDS in the Philippines.* Philippines: DoH.

9. Tsuchie H, Saraswathy TS, Sinniah M. (1995). HIV variants in South and Southeast Asia. *International Journal of STD and AIDS* 6:117–20.

10. Paladin FJE, Monzon OT, Tsuchie H, Aplasca MRA, Learn GH Jr, Kurimura T. (1998). Genetic subtypes of HIV-1 in the Philippines. *AIDS* 12:291–300.

11. Espantaleon A, Kageyama S, Bernardo MT. (2003). The influence of the Expanding HIV genetic diversity on molecular diagnosis in the Philippines. *International Journal of STD and AIDS* 14:125–31

12. Raymundo CM. (2002). *Sexuality and Reproductive Health of Filipino Youth.* Young Adult Fertility and Sexuality Study. Population Institute, University of the Philippines, p1–5.

13. Monzon OT, Santana RT, Paladin FJE. (1991). The prevalence of sexually transmitted diseases and human immunodeficiency virus Infection among Filipino sex workers. *Philippine Journal of Microbiol and Infect Dis* 20(2):41–44.

14. Abellanosa IP, Manalastas R, Ghee AE. (1995). Comparison of STD prevalence and the behavioral correlates of STD among registered and unregistered female sex workers in Manila and Cebu City. In: *Proceedings of the Second National Research Forum on AIDS in the Philippines.* p56.

15. Klausner JD, Aplasca MR, Mesola VP, Bolan G, Whittington WI, Holmes KK. (1999). Correlates of gonorrhea among female sex workers. *Journal of Infectious Diseases* 179:729–33.

16. Aplasca MR, Pato-Mesola V, Klausner JD *et al.* (2001). A randomized trial of ciprofloxacin versus cefixime for treatment of gonorrhea after rapid emergence of gonococcal ciprofloxacin resistance in the Philippines. *Clinical Infectious Diseases* 38:1313–8.

17. Aplasca MR, Monzon OT, Mapua CA, Tan-Torres T, Romano E, Solon O. (1996). An analysis of the direct and indirect costs of HIV infection/AIDS in the Philippines. XI International Conference on AIDS, Vancouver. Abstract Book 1:256–257.

18. Monzon OT. (1994). Clinical manifestations of HIV infections/AIDS in the Western Pacific Region. Official Proceedings to the Fourth Western Pacific Congress on Chemotherapy and Infectious Diseases. *Journal of the American Medical Association Southeast Asia* 10(Supplement)(3):145–6.

19. Santana RT, Monzon OT, Mandel J, Hall TL, Hearst N. (1992). AIDS education for hospital workers in Manila: effects on knowledge, attitudes, and infection control practices. *AIDS* 6:1359–63.

20. Arciaga RS, Monzon OT, Romano EM *et al.* (1990). Development and evaluation of an innovative AIDS education strategy for Filipino overseas workers. In: *Annual Report, Research Institute for Tropical Medicine (RITM).* Alabang, Muntinlupa City, Philippines.

21. Aplasca MR, Siegel D, Mandel JS. (1995) Results of model AIDS prevention programme for high school students in the Philippines. *AIDS* 9 (Supplement 1):57–513.

22. Monzon OT, Bagasao MTP, Santana RT. (1992). Meeting the challenges of a health education/intervention program on AIDS/STDs for commercial sex workers in Manila, Philippines. Proceedings of the Third Western Pacific Congress on Chemotherapy and Infectious Diseases, Indonesia, p205–208.

23. Republic of the Philippines. (1998). Republic Act 8504: The Philippine AIDS Prevention and Control Act of 1998.

24. The AIDS Society of the Philippines and the Philippine National AIDS Council. (2000). *Ethical Guidelines in AIDS Investigations in the Philippines,* p1–26.

25. Garcia D. (2001). AIDS Media Awards: making media a proactive partner in the fight against AIDS. Sixth International Congress on AIDS in Asia and the Pacific, Melbourne, Australia. Abstract Book p132.

26. Monzon OT, Aplasca MRA, Santana-Arciaga, Paladin FJ. (1994). Clinical picture of HIV infection among Filipinos. Proceedings of the National Research Forum on AIDS in the Philippines, p10–11.

27. Monzon OT, Paladin FJE, Dimaandal E, Balis AM, Samson C, Mitchell S. (1992). Relevance of antibody content and test format in HIV testing of pooled sera. *AIDS* 6:43–8.

Chapter 23

Thailand

Viroj Tangcharoensathien[*], Wiput Phoolcharoen, Sombat Thanprasertsuk and Chutima Suraratdecha

Background

Thailand is a lower middle-income country in South East Asia. Prior to the financial crisis in 1997, Thailand had had a remarkable economic performance for a decade, from the mid-1980s to the mid-1990s. Gross domestic product (GDP) per capita increased from US$861 in 1986 to a peak of US$3060 in 1996. In 2000 and 2001, per capita GDP dropped to the 1992 level of US$1846. GDP growth in 1997 and 1998 was negative, at −1.7% and −10.8%, respectively. However, there have been promising signs of economic recovery since 2002. GDP per capita growth was 4.7% in 2002 and 6.1% in 2003. The economic crisis has had a major impact on the social sector but less impact on the health sector, despite government fiscal constraints (see Box 23.1) [1].

As a result of major political reform in 1997 and a new Constitution, Thailand has become an advanced democratic society in South East Asia, in which check-and-balance mechanisms are in place to foster good governance in the public and private sectors. Political accountability, good governance and active citizen participation have significantly influenced the health sector's performance and facilitated reforms such as universal coverage and decentralization.

Burden of disease

Thailand has gone through a rapid process of epidemiological transition, from communicable to non-communicable lifestyle-related diseases. A double burden of disease has been observed. HIV is one of the major communicable diseases, while morbidity and mortality due to non-communicable diseases such as hypertension and diabetes have increased.

Studies of the burden of disease (BOD) in 1999 [2] indicated that the total BOD among the Thai population, measured in terms of disabled adjusted life years (DALYs) loss, was 5.6 million DALYs among men and 4 million among women. The top 10 leading causes accounted for 52% of the total national burden among men and 44% among women (Table 23.1).

The three leading causes of DALY loss among men are HIV, traffic injury and stroke, while among women they are HIV, stroke and diabetes. More than half of these causes are preventable by primary reduction of risks, notably through safer sex, traffic injury prevention and control of tobacco consumption.

Three major risks that contributed to the BOD were unsafe sex, alcohol and tobacco among men [3], and unsafe sex, high blood pressure and obesity among women (Table 23.2). Though we are seeing a decreasing trend in tobacco use due to a successful public campaign and tough law

* Corresponding author.

Box 23.1 **Thailand's profile**

Human development profile.

2002 Human Development Index (HDI) 0.768;
HDI trends: 1975, 0.613; 1980, 0.651; 1985, 0.676; 1990, 0.707; 1995, 0.742;

Demographic parameters

Population 62.2 million;
Life expectancy 69.1 years;
Total fertility rate (2000–2005) 1.9.

Economic performance

GDP per capita US$7010 purchasing power parity 2002, growth rate 2.9% (1990–2002);
Income distributions, richest 10% to poorest 10% 13.4, richest 20% to poorest 20% 8.3, Gini
coefficient (0–1) 0.43.

Education

Adult literacy rate, 92.6%;
Public education expenditure, 5% of GDP, total government expenditure 31%, of which
primary 42.3%, secondary 20.5%, tertiary 21.7 (1999–2001).

Health (2002)

Infant mortality rate 24, under 5 mortality rate 28, adjusted maternal mortality rate 44
(2000), reported maternal mortality rate 36 (1985–2002);
One year old fully immunized against measles, 94%;
Birth attended by skilled health staff 1995–2002, 99%;
Physician per 100,000 population, 1990–2003, 30;
2001 total health expenditure: public 2.1% of GDP, private 1.6% of GDP, per capita US$254
purchasing power parity;
2003 people living with HIV adult 15–49, 1.5% (0.8–2.8).

Source: [1].

enforcement, high prevalence of tobacco consumption in past decades made tobacco the third and
fourth contributing factor to the BOD in men and women, respectively, in 1999.

Alcohol consumption is the second largest contributory risk factor for BOD among men.
Alcohol abuse leads not only to domestic violence, but also to disability, loss of income and loss
of life. Recent campaigns on drunk driving were not very successful, and tougher law enforcement
is required. Since October 2003, the government has started to regulate on-air advertising of
alcoholic beverages, aiming to curb consumption among teenagers and young adults.

The health system

Organization

In Thailand, the public sector has long played a major role in health service provision. In 2000,
67% of all hospitals were owned by the Ministry of Public Health (MoPH), 7% by other

Table 23.1 Top 20 conditions in DALYs, 1999

Rank	Men	DALY	%	Women	DALY	%
1	HIV	960,087	17	HIV	372,947	9
2	Traffic accidents	510,907	9	Stroke	280,673	7
3	Stroke	267,567	5	Diabetes	267,158	7
4	Liver cancer	248,083	4	Depression	145,336	4
5	Diabetes	168,372	3	Liver cancer	118,384	3
6	Ischaemic heart disease	164,094	3	Osteoarthritis	117,994	3
7	COPD (emphysema)	156,861	3	Traffic accidents	114,963	3
8	Homicide and violence	156,371	3	Anaemia	112,990	3
9	Suicide	147,988	3	Ischaemic heart disease	109,592	3
10	Drug dependence/harmful use	137,703	2	Cataracts	96,091	2
11	Alcohol dependence/harmful use	130,654	2	COPD	93,387	2
12	Cirrhosis	117,527	2	Deafness	87,612	2
13	Lung cancer	106,120	2	Lower respiratory tract infections	84,819	2
14	Drowning	98,464	2	Low birth weight	83,879	2
15	Depression	95,530	2	Dementia	70,191	2
16	Osteoarthritis	93,749	2	Anxiety disorders	66,992	2
17	Tuberculosis	93,695	2	Schizophrenia	60,800	2
18	Deafness	93,497	2	Tuberculosis	60,643	2
19	Low birth weight	91,934	2	Birth trauma and asphyxia	57,488	1
20	Anaemia	87,610	2	Nephritis and nephrosis	55,258	1
	Total top 20	3,926,813	70		2,457,197	62
	Total national	5,600,000	100		3,980,000	100

Source: [2].

ministries and 26% by the private sector. In terms of hospital bed share, the MoPH owned 64%, the private sector 22%, and 14% belonged to other ministries such as Education (teaching hospitals). Nevertheless, private hospital bed share increased from 13% in 1991 to 22% in 2000.

Table 23.2 Attributable risks for top 12 burden of disease conditions, 1999

Rank	Men	DALY	%	Women	DALY	%
1	Unsafe sex	883,087	9.3	Unsafe sex	344,686	3.6
2	Alcohol	465,000	4.9	High blood pressure	225,694	2.4
3	Tobacco	458,193	4.8	High body mass index	231,063	2.4
4	Non-use of crash helmet	329,149	3.5	Tobacco	171,782	1.8
5	High blood pressure	260,239	2.7	Malnutrition	94,640	1.0
6	High body mass index	119,019	1.2	Cholesterol	92,113	1.0
7	Less fruit and vegetable (low fibre diet)	114,553	1.2	Non-use of crash helmet	74,064	0.8
8	Malnutrition	106,738	1.1	Physical inactivity	60,126	0.6
9	Cholesterol	106,606	1.1	Less fruit and vegetable (low fibre diet)	48,085	0.5
10	Air pollution	50,863	0.5	Alcohol	38,935	0.4
11	Physical inactivity	42,310	0.4	Water sanitation	32,288	0.3
12	Water sanitation	29,342	0.3	Air Pollution	28,374	0.3

Source: [3].

Since the fifth 5-year National Socio-Economic Development Plan (1981–1986), MoPH policy has focused on service expansion at the district level through the construction of 10- to 90-bed district hospitals in all districts and subdistrict health centres to cover at least 5000 patients. By the seventh National Socio-Economic Development Plan (1991–1996), healthcare infrastructure had very high geographical coverage.

In 2001, there were 92 hospitals in 75 provinces besides Bangkok (25 regional and 67 general hospitals), 720 district hospitals in 795 districts (91% coverage) and 9738 health centres in 7255 subdistricts (100% coverage). These health facilities are the backbone of preventive, health promotion and curative services throughout the country. Interestingly, while the MoPH has been strong in service expansion, locally elected governments, especially municipalities, have done far less in terms of service provision in urban settings.

The three levels of healthcare are organized to promote a rational use of resources and foster referral systems. Health centres provide mainly primary services and focus on prevention and promotion services. District hospitals staffed by 2–6 general practitioners, 1–3 pharmacists, one or two dentists and a cadre of professional nurses provide secondary care, including ambulatory, basic surgery and inpatient services. Provincial general hospitals staffed by specialists provide high-level sophisticated tertiary services and sub-specialties. MoPH regional hospitals and teaching hospitals provide most of the super-specialty care on referral.

The private hospital sector has focused its service expansion in more affluent areas, such as provincial cities and metropolitan areas. A symbiotic relationship between public and private hospitals has been observed. Public doctors are permitted to have out-of-hours private practices either in their own private clinics or in private hospitals.

Thailand is self-sufficient in health workforce production; almost all health professionals are trained at public expense. Compulsory rural health service by all new medical graduates, which has been enforced since 1972 and has subsequently been applied to nurses, pharmacists and dentists as well, has had a major impact on health development in rural areas.

Expenditure and financing

Table 23.3 shows the trend in financing healthcare between 1995 and 2000, as compiled by the World Health Organization (WHO) [4]. Total health expenditure ranged from 3.4 to 3.7% of GDP between 1995 and 2000. Government expenditure on health as a percentage of total health expenditure increased from 48.9% to 57.4% in a 6-year period, with a converse reduction in private expenditure.

Through the strong political will of a major party-led coalition government, Thailand achieved universal healthcare coverage (UC) by October 2001. Previous governments had employed a piecemeal targeting approach by gradually increasing coverage for specific populations [5], beginning with a tax-financed Social Welfare Scheme (SWS) targeting means-tested low-income households and later expanded to cover individuals over 60 years of age and children under 12. Eventually, all socially disadvantaged groups were covered by the SWS.

A voluntary health card scheme (VHC) covered the borderline populations who were not eligible for the SWS. This scheme did not perform well in terms of coverage expansion and financing viability. The voluntary nature of the scheme resulted in adverse selection whereby the sick participated and the healthy opted out. This ended up being financially non-viable in spite of more than 50% government financing and stagnant coverage expansion.

Table 23.3 National expenditure on health, and sources, 1995–2000

	1995	1996	1997	1998	1999	2000
Total health expenditure (THE) % GDP	3.4	3.6	3.7	3.9	3.7	3.7
Government expenditure on health (GGHE) % THE	48.9	51.1	57.2	61.4	58.3	57.4
Private expenditure on health (PvtHE) % THE	51.1	48.9	42.8	38.6	41.7	42.6
GGHE % general government expenditure	8.1	9.6	10.9	13.3	11.4	11.4
Social security expenditure on health % GGHE	26.5	27.9	30.2	25.8	26.3	26.4
External resources funded expenditure on health % GGHE	0.2	0.6	0.5	0.7	0.9	0.9
Private pre-paid plans expenditure on health % PvtHE	7.6	7.8	8.6	9.7	9.7	9.6
Net out-of-pocket spending on health % THE	44.7	42.6	36.9	32.7	35.3	36.2
THE per capita at exchange rate (US$)	97	110	93	71	73	71
GGHE per capita at exchange rate (US$)	47	56	53	44	43	41
THE per capita at international dollar rate	210	237	242	228	229	240
GGHE per capita at international dollar rate	103	121	138	140	133	138

Source: [4].

Private sector employees are covered by the Social Security Scheme (SSS), a tripartite contributory scheme. Its coverage gradually expanded from private enterprises employing more than 20 workers, to 10, five and finally to one employee by April 2002. Unfortunately, the only beneficiaries are the workers themselves. To date, no serious efforts have been made by the social security administration to expand its healthcare coverage to the workers' spouses and dependants, despite huge surpluses in the social security fund. The employer-funded Workmen Compensation Scheme runs in parallel to cover work-related illnesses, injuries, disabilities and death compensation among the same private sector employees.

A generous tax-financed Civil Service Medical Benefit Scheme (CSMBS) covers current public employees, retired officials and their dependants, including spouses, parents and up to three children under the age of 20. Government policy on downsizing the public sector has resulted in limited potential to increase coverage of this scheme.

Despite efforts made during the past 20 years, prior to October 2001, almost 30% of the population was not covered by any scheme [6] (Table 23.4). During the last 10 years, experience was gained in insurance management, and lessons were drawn from strengths and weaknesses in terms of efficiency, quality under different provider payment methods and, notably, fees-for-services and capitation. Once the 'piecemeal' approach to coverage reached its expansion limit, Thailand adopted a policy of universal healthcare.

Table 23.4 Insurance coverage before October 2001

Health insurance schemes	Coverage (%)
Social Welfare Scheme	38
Voluntary Health Card Scheme	12
Civil Servant Medical Benefit Scheme	11
Social Security Scheme	9
Private insurance	~10
The uninsured	~30
Population million people	61.46

Source: [5].

Table 23.5 Household non-food expenditure on health(%) 1996–2002

Percentage of non-food expenditure on health	Percentage of households			
	1996	1998	2000	2002
0–0.5	31.9	33.2	34.5	41.2
0.5–10	51.3	51.5	50.8	48.1
10–25	11.9	10.9	11.0	7.6
25–50	3.5	3.6	3.1	2.5
>50	1.4	0.8	0.7	0.5
Total households	100.0	100.0	100.0	100.0

Source: National Statistical Office 1996, 1998, 2000 and 2002.

Catastrophic illnesses are considered a serious social problem because they destroy household financial stability. Households with catastrophic illnesses are those spending more than 25% of their non-food consumption expenditures on healthcare. Analysis of the 1996–2002 socio-economic survey conducted by the National Statistical Office (NSO 1996, 1998, 2000 and 2002) indicated that the proportion of households facing catastrophic health spending decreased from 4.9% in 1996 to 3% in 2002 (Table 23.5). This was a result of government policy to provide safeguards against financially catastrophic illnesses through health insurance expansion, especially the implementation of the VHC.

The treatment costs for opportunistic infections (OIs) for people living with HIV (PLHIV) can be catastrophic to their households on several grounds: first, the high cost of medicine; secondly, the high incidence of hospital admission; and thirdly, income loss due to illnesses. Fortunately, all OI treatment costs are now subsidized under all the health insurance schemes that together provide universal coverage. However, income loss due to illnesses remains a serious problem for households.

The HIV epidemic

HIV is the leading contributor to the BOD, now surpassing traffic injuries, cardiovascular diseases and cancer. In 1984, the first case of AIDS was reported in Thailand [7]. Since then, the HIV epidemic has grown from a handful of infections to become a major national threat, with wide-ranging medical, social and economic consequences. Responses to prevent HIV infection and mitigate negative effects of the epidemic have gradually evolved. This section highlights key programmes that have been developed and built into the national effort on HIV prevention and alleviation.

Surveillance of HIV infection and AIDS

Soon after the first case of AIDS was reported, a national HIV and AIDS reporting system was established. Based on the national epidemiological surveillance network, all hospitals and healthcare facilities were required to report AIDS cases and HIV infection. However, in 1991, it was determined that the reporting of HIV infection had no epidemiological value and it was discontinued. The case definition of AIDS for Thailand was adapted from the AIDS case definition for surveillance of the US Centers for Disease Control and Prevention (CDC) and the WHO Case Definition of AIDS. Reporting systems for AIDS required demographic data, risk factors and indicative disease information. Cases were then reported using a unique code to avoid repeated reports, without any personal identification data [8].

In 1989, a national sentinel surveillance system for HIV infection was launched to monitor the changes in rates of HIV infection among various population groups [9]. Target groups in the system were female sex workers (FSWs), male sex workers (MSWs), injecting drug users (IDU)s, men attending sexually transmitted infection (STI) clinics, pregnant women at antenatal clinics (ANCs) and blood donors. Surveys to collect point prevalence of HIV infection were conducted twice yearly between 1989 and 1995, and after that the surveys were carried out each June. In each group, a sample size of 100–200 was required. The survey had participating sites in 14 provinces in the first survey in June 1989 and gradually expanded to cover all 76 provinces after the third survey in June 1990. Blood from randomly selected subjects in each target group was sent for testing using a standard method at provincial hospitals or regional centres where HIV serology tests were available. All screening tests used in the sentinel surveillance programme were well controlled by the standardized methods of the Thai Food and Drug Administration. A repeated positive result in two screening tests was counted as positive to estimate the HIV seroprevalence rate. The average national rate was derived from the median value of provincial estimate rates.

In addition to the sero-sentinel surveillance programme described above, HIV seroprevalence rates among military recruits were also monitored systematically beginning in 1989 [10]. Surveys were carried out twice a year, and the results helped provide a comprehensive understanding of the spread of HIV in the country. These surveys are still being carried out today.

Epidemiology

Based on the results of the surveillance programme, it can be said that HIV was first introduced in the late 1980s. Men who have sex with men (MSM) were among the first group of patients reported in the first few years. However, during 1988–1989, the HIV epidemic in Thailand gained its first foothold in the drug-injecting community [11], where an explosive outbreak in Bangkok was observed. At almost the same time, in 1989 and onward, HIV infection among FSWs increased alarmingly [12] and subsequently spread with frightening speed to the population at large.

A long-term follow-up of HIV infection rates in various groups in the surveillance programme, as well as data from reporting systems on AIDS, indicate that the HIV problem among IDUs has not been resolved. The rate of infection in this group is still sustainably high at approximately 40–50% throughout the course of the epidemic [13]. HIV infection rates for the rest of all targeted groups declined after reaching their peak around the mid-1990s (Figs 23.1 and 23.2).

A projection of AIDS and HIV infections based on available demographic, epidemiological and behavioural information, and using a well-conceptualized method demonstrated that in the early 2000s, twice as many men as women were HIV-positive, but this imbalance is projected to level out as transmission occurs from clients of sex workers, who may not be aware of their seropositivity, to their wives, girlfriends and children [14].

The projection also illustrated that Thailand has achieved significant success in controlling the spread of HIV, with new infections falling from 143,000 cases in 1991 to 23,000 in 2002

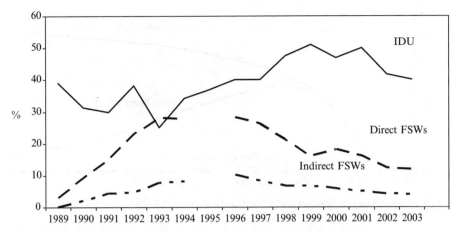

Fig. 23.1 HIV seroprevalence rates in IDUs and direct and indirect female sex workers (FSWs) in Thailand, 1989–2003. During 1989–1994, HIV seroprevalence surveys in these three groups were conducted twice a year in June and December. From 1995 onward, the survey was done once every year in June. Data presented in this figure illustrate HIV seroprevalence rates only from the June survey of each year. Direct FSWs are those who work in brothel settings; indirect FSWs are those who work in other settings such as bars, nightclubs, massage parlours, etc. The HIV seroprevalence survey among FSWs in 1995 did not distinguish between direct and indirect FSWs. Source: Bureau of Epidemiology, Department of Disease Control, Ministry of Public Health, Thailand.

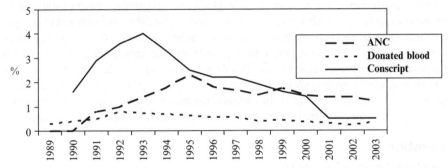

Fig. 23.2 HIV seroprevalence rates among pregnant women, blood donors and military conscripts, 1989–2003. During 1989–1994, HIV seroprevalence surveys among pregnant women were conducted, and data on HIV seroprevalence rates among blood donors were collected, twice a year in June and December. From 1995 onwards, the survey was done and data were collected once every year in June. Data presented in this figure illustrate HIV seroprevalence rates only from the annual June survey. Data among military conscripts were collected in May and November of each year. Only data from May surveys are presented in this figure. Sources: Bureau of Epidemiology, Department of Disease Control, Ministry of Public Health; and Royal Thai Army, Ministry of Defense, Thailand.

(Fig. 23.3). However, in 2003, the country still had as many as 635,057 people living with HIV. Approximately 398,369 people have already died from the disease since the beginning of the epidemic. It is estimated that 50,000 people will die from the disease each year during the period of the ninth National Economic and Social Development Plan (2002–2006). Ninety per

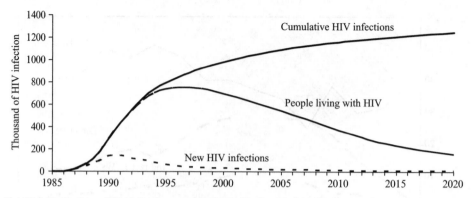

Fig. 23.3 Projection of HIV infections and PLHIV in Thailand, 1989–2020.

cent of the cases will be people 20–44 years of age, who constitute the main workforce of the country. This points to serious consequences for the country in terms of the increased burden on medical and socio-economic systems, affecting not only HIV-infected people, but also their families.

Active epidemiological assessment efforts began fairly early in response to the epidemic. Data have been systematically and regularly collected and disseminated, which has been helpful in addressing the extent of the HIV epidemic, identifying potential risk factors, determining ongoing prevention programme directions and needs, and demonstrating the effectiveness of prevention programmes on a national scale [15]. The widespread dissemination of this information, especially to high-level policy-makers such as the Prime Minister and the Cabinet, Parliament, national planners and provincial governors, has led them to favour strong advocacy and resource mobilization in response to the needs and has convinced civil society of the benefits of an aggressive response to HIV. This demonstrates how Thailand has been successful in translating timely epidemiological evidence in to policy and programming designs in response to the changing epidemics. In addition, the health system's capacity to deliver HIV programmes relies on adequate human and financial resources for a successful response.

Prevention

Promoting the use of condoms

An important breakthrough in the fight against AIDS in Thailand was the 100% condom use programme launched in 1989, targeting sex workers and their customers [16]. Two years later, this programme was approved by the National AIDS Committee as one of the priority programmes in an effort to prevent sexual transmission of HIV and was expanded nation-wide. Under this programme, government-subsidized condoms are distributed free of charge to FSWs and MSWs. Educational activities to promote condom use, including door-to-door visits to all brothels and sex service establishments, have been implemented throughout the country. The increase in condom use at sex-related establishments was assessed by various methods. Based on a simple interview method, it was found that rates of condom use among direct and indirect FSWs were greater than 95% and 90%, respectively, in recent years [17].

After the implementation of the 100% condom use programme, the incidence rates of sexually transmitted diseases among FSWs and MSWs observed in the governmental STI clinics were reduced, and HIV seroprevalence rates among FSWs subsequently fell (Fig. 23.1). This success stemmed from strong political commitment, collaboration between local authorities and establishment owners, availability and accessibility of quality condoms, availability of STI care, and frequent monitoring and evaluation activities.

As the sexual behaviour of the general population changed and casual sex with less condom use [18] was found to be a potential route of HIV and STI, public campaigns promoting condom use were initiated and organized regularly. Affordably priced condoms are available on the shelves of most convenience stores and supermarkets as well as in drug stores throughout the country. However, surveys of condom use have identified obstacles to accessing condoms among youth due to their shyness about buying them, despite the perception that condoms prevent HIV/STI and pregnancy. In order to improve accessibility to condoms, vending machines of quality condoms at low prices are now being promoted [19].

Sex education and life skills for youth

Generally, HIV infection rates are high among people aged 15–24. This is a global phenomenon. Engaging in casual sex is more common among young adults. Unprotected sex is not uncommon, along with a lack of awareness of possible HIV/STI infection. As the problem is increasing rapidly among Thai youth, the Ministry of Education and the MoPH, together with many non-governmental organizations (NGOs) working with youth, have developed an effective communication approach to reach young people, including sex education and life skills for youth both in and out of schools [20,21]. Furthermore, education on HIV, sex and family life has been adopted in the normal school curriculum, beginning at the primary level and through secondary level, and in to vocational training and university levels [22,23].

Prevention of mother-to-child HIV transmission (PMTCT)

Since 1995, voluntary HIV counselling and testing (VCT) for pregnant women has been gradually implemented throughout Thailand. A study on the use of a short course of zidovudine (AZT) conducted in Thailand between 1995 and 1998 demonstrated a reduction of perinatal HIV infection from 19% to approximately 8% [24]. The short course of AZT was soon introduced on a wider scale for HIV-positive pregnant women during the antenatal period until delivery, together with AZT syrup and breast milk substitutes for newborns. It is expected that this will reduce transmission from mother to child by two-thirds. This intervention has been shown to be cost-effective, even at less than 5% HIV prevalence among pregnant women.

Data gathered in 2002 found that all of the 559,702 pregnant women who came for antenatal care had been approached for VCT and almost all (97%) were tested for HIV. Of these, 6336 (1%) were found to be HIV-infected. Of all identified HIV-infected women, 4882 (77%) received a short course of AZT [25]. At least 1 year of breast milk substitution was provided free of charge by the government to all babies born to HIV-positive mothers.

A follow-up study on the babies born to HIV-infected mothers and whose mothers received the prophylaxis treatment revealed an infection rate of 5% [26]. The MoPH is planning to improve the coverage of VCT for pregnant women and the accessibility of antiretroviral agents for the prevention of HIV transmission from mother to child. Consideration is being given to adding one more antiviral (nevirapine) in to the course of drugs to improve PMTCT on the basis of recent research.

Harm reduction and outreach programmes for IDUs

During the early years of the epidemic, an intensive educational programme to train IDUs on the use of bleach and to avoid sharing injection equipment was carried out nationwide. Drug treatment centres of the Bangkok Metropolitan Administration and the MoPH now provide methadone services for IDUs seeking treatment, and selected centres provide short (21-day) in-patient drug detoxification regimens. Methadone maintenance treatment is provided for IDUs who are unable to stop using heroin.

However, based on the available data, it seems the dynamic of HIV transmission among IDUs is more complicated than previously thought. A substantial number of IDUs use different types of drugs; for instance, it has been found that approximately 16–17% of amphetamine users inject the drug intravenously [27]. There is also insufficient information available regarding use of contaminated injection equipment and related behaviours. Recognizing that IDUs still have low access to HIV prevention programmes, new efforts in harm reduction and outreach activities are currently being undertaken.

Blood safety

Since 1989, screening of all blood for the HIV antibody prior to use has been strictly practised [28]. Hospital and blood bank personnel are trained in the importance of screening policy and practice, and all blood bank services are equipped with the necessary machines for HIV screening. Voluntary, non-remunerated blood donation is encouraged and promoted, while paid donation is not considered acceptable. A donor deferral programme has been widely implemented. Approximately 800,000 units of blood are donated each year, and sentinel surveillance has found that approximately 0.1–0.3% of donated blood is HIV-infected. Infected blood is discarded and destroyed.

Universal precaution and post-exposure prophylaxis for health personnel

The MoPH has developed a guideline on universal precautions for health personnel [29,30]. All health personnel receive training in the practice of universal precautions for care and service provision as if all patients were infected with HIV. The use of appropriate protective apparatus is advised and emphasized. In addition, a counselling and reporting system for healthcare workers who are accidentally exposed to contaminated blood or body fluid has been established to provide them with confidential psycho-social and medical care. Antiretroviral agents for post-exposure prophylaxis are stored in all healthcare settings for essential health personnel.

AIDS vaccine

The current National Plan for Prevention and Alleviation of HIV (2001–2005) emphasizes the participation of all sectors (private, public and communities) in solving the AIDS problem. The National AIDS Committee of Thailand, at the instigation and with the cooperation of the WHO and the Joint United Nations Programme on HIV/AIDS (UNAIDS), has prioritized the development of an HIV vaccine and implemented the National Plan for HIV/AIDS Vaccine Development. Established in 1993, this was the first vaccine initiative aiming to foster and facilitate collaboration on HIV vaccine research and technology transfer among national and international organizations. By 2003, there were 11 HIV vaccine clinical trials under way, including the first phase III trial of AIDSVAX B/E gp120 vaccine in a developing country. However, phase III trials in both the USA and Thailand proved gp120 by itself to be completely incapable of preventing or ameliorating HIV-1 infection [31].

Besides engendering cooperation, collaboration and technology transfer among national and international scholars, Thailand, with a long-standing commitment to stem the AIDS epidemic, has strongly supported the identification, building and strengthening of national capacity in the areas of regulatory and policy support, pre-clinical and laboratory networks, preparation of cohort networks, clinical trial networks, data management networks, national repository networks for biomedical products related to HIV vaccine trials and evaluation, public relations networks, and manufacturing, licensing and accessibility networks.

While progress has been made in clinical sciences, Thailand also challenges the best efforts in policy research on HIV vaccines to improve knowledge of potential markets and demand, define future financing and pricing mechanisms for vaccine adoption, and assess the delivery infrastructure and the potential use of vaccines in addition to other preventive measures [32]. Several proactive policy steps in preparation for a potential HIV vaccine have been taken or are planned.

Continuum and comprehensive care for people living with HIV

PLHIV have to confront physical, psychological and socio-economic problems affecting not only themselves but their families as well. Early in the epidemic, the MoPH developed and implemented a comprehensive continuum of care on a national scale. Comprehensive care includes medical care, emotional support, social services and rights protection. The continuum of care is translated through the networks and linkages among institutions, community, family and self-care [33].

The services for treatment of opportunistic infections and prophylaxis of selected common opportunistic infections are provided at all levels of the health system. Integration of treatment into the universal healthcare coverage also ensures availability of care.

HIV pre- and post-test counselling services are provided in all hospitals. Long-term counselling for HIV-infected individuals is delivered in anonymous counselling clinics in hospitals. Counselling for related issues, such as tuberculosis (TB), STI and reproductive health, has gradually been integrated in to the HIV counselling programme. More recently, counselling has become an important component in the antiretroviral therapy (ART) programme, as it aims to support and ensure adherence to treatment.

The comprehensive care service system for HIV patients has been developed on the basis of maintaining strict patient confidentiality. Networks of care among tertiary, provincial, district and subdistrict healthcare providers, as well as local NGOs available in each locality, have been strengthened in order to provide a complementary service for patients. Only patients who wish to do so are referred to the nearest HIV care unit for follow-up.

Treatment

The availability of antiretroviral drugs has greatly reduced the mortality and morbidity of PLHIV and AIDS patients in industrialized countries. Thailand has a programme to make antiretrovirals available through different mechanisms. The national guideline on the clinical management of HIV in children and adults, which advises the use of antiretrovirals, was developed in 1992 and has been revised regularly since then [34]. Initially, monotherapy was the only choice available. In order to maximize the efficiency of the programme and to ensure quality, consistency and equity to PLHIV, antiretrovirals were provided under the clinical research network programme.

The cost of antiretrovirals has been the main obstacle to providing them on a large scale, but the government has recently taken steps to make them affordable to the health system through generic drug production and resource mobilization. In 2002, the government provided highly active antiretroviral therapy (HAART) to 13,000 HIV-infected individuals and AIDS patients through an access-to-treatment programme, and expanded this to 36,000 in 2003 and to 50,000 in 2004. This programme also aims to strengthen capacity building for healthcare workers and provide a laboratory network with standard quality assurance, a counselling network with referral and consultation system, a stock management system and a monitoring system. It should be noted that ART is only one component of a comprehensive and continuum of care programme for HIV patients to improve their quality of life. During the transition phase of scale-up, in which there was rationing of HAART, it was generally agreed that low CD4 count and readiness of PLHIV to comply with ART were two major criteria for access.

Conclusion

Conceptual framework for policy and health system responses to HIV

Information and evidence played a very significant role in influencing overall HIV policy as well as shaping specific programmes for different population groups. The trends in condom use rates based on sero-sentinel and sexual behaviour sentinel data have been crucial to informing both policy formulation and monitoring of interventions. Likewise, clinical evidence on the outcome of vertical transmission interruption has had a major impact on the scale-up of PMTCT.

National capacity in analysis and advocacy has led to a paradigm shift in programme interventions, from targeting high-risk groups to targeting individual behavioural risks and social vulnerability. Ultimately, AIDS is a product of social inequity, in which the health of the poor, and of young women in particular, is exploited through the sex industry.

Good health infrastructure and financing of health services are the backbone of HIV programme implementation. HIV services were able to be piggybacked onto the existing extensive geographical distribution of healthcare services, from subdistrict health centres to district and provincial hospitals. The rapid 100% scale-up of PMTCT in 2 years is a classic demonstration of the capacity of the resilient Thai health system to accommodate an additional nationwide programme in a short period of time. Fortunately, Thailand's AIDS programme was able to access adequate resources, since Thailand spent 3.4–3.7% of GDP on the health of the population between 1995 and 2000.

Universal health coverage has had a major impact on access to care by the poor, who are generally the people mostly affected by HIV and AIDS. Universal access to ART is also expected to have a major impact on the number of lives saved and on cost savings from the reduction of opportunistic infections in the future.

Lessons learned

The Thai experience has provided several lessons on how the health system and health policy need to respond to the dynamic of HIV epidemics. The country's capacity to collect, analyse and disseminate information and translate this information into policy and programme design, as well as the skill and capacity to influence policy-makers, is a major factor in any effective health policy response to HIV. A strong political will ensures the adequate financing and delivery of programmes. Furthermore, an extensive geographical coverage of healthcare infrastructure and adequate numbers of qualified staff are key to effective programme implementation.

However, AIDS is more than a health system problem. Its multisectoral nature requires effective and genuine collaboration across the public and private sectors and civil society. All these activities are addressed through governmental and non-governmental partnerships; there is a crucial role for government to play as steward and coordinator of these challenging national endeavours.

The final lesson concerns the role of donors. The AIDS programme in Thailand was mainly driven by national policy interests. Recent studies of the National AIDS Accounts indicate that programme financing was dominated by local resources, with a very small proportion coming from external donors. Having less reliance on donor funding protects the programme from a donor-driven agenda, which at times can result in programme fragmentation.

Acknowledgements

The authors wish to acknowledge the Thailand Research Fund for its institutional grant to the Senior Research Scholar Programme in Health Systems and Policy Research, and to the Health Systems Research Institute for its support of the International Health Policy Programme.

References

1. United Nations Development Programme (UNDP). (2004). *Human Development Indicators.* UNDP.
2. The Thai Working Group on Burden of Disease and Injuries. (2002). *Burden of Disease and Injuries in Thailand.* Bangkok: Ministry of Public Health, Bureau of Health Policy and Planning.
3. The Thai Working Group on Burden of Disease and Injuries. (2003). *Attributable Risk for Burden of Disease in Thailand. A Preliminary Report.* Bangkok: Ministry of Public Health, Bureau of Health Policy and Planning.
4. World Health Organization. (2002). *National Health Expenditure Thailand.* Geneva: World Health Organization.
5. Tangcharoensathien V, Teokul W, Chanwongpaisal L. (2003). *Social Welfare System in Thailand: A Challenge from Targeting to Universality.* A paper presented at United Nations Research Institute for Social Development (UNRISD) workshop on Social Policy in a Development Context: Transforming the Developmental Welfare State in East Asia June 30–July 1, 2003. Bangkok, Thailand.
6. Tangcharoensathien V, Srithamrongswat S, Pittayarangsarit S. (2001). Overview of health insurance systems. In: Thammathat-aree J, ed. *Health Insurance Systems in Thailand.* Health Systems Research Institute. Bangkok: Desire publisher.
7. Limsuwan A, Kunapa S, Siristonapun Y. (1986). Acquired immunodeficiency syndrome in Thailand: a report of two cases. *Journal of the Medical Association of Thailand* 69:164–9.
8. Division of Epidemiology. (2000). *Definition of AIDS and Symptomatic HIV infection for Surveillance,* 4th Revision. Bangkok: Ministry of Public Health, Permanent Secretary Office, Division of Epidemiology.
9. Division of Epidemiology. (1990). *Guideline on the National Sentinel Sero-prevalence Surveillance for HIV Infection in Thailand,* Revised Version. Bangkok: Ministry of Public Health, Department of Communicable Disease Control.

10. Torugsa K, Anderson S, Thongsen N *et al.* (2003). HIV Epidemic among Young Thai Men, 1991–2000. Emerging Infectious Disease. URL: http://www.cdc.gov/ncidod/EID /vo19no7/ 02-0653.htm.

11. Vanichseni S, Sakuntanaga P. (1990). Results of three seroprevalence surveys for HIV in IVDU in Bangkok. *International Conferece on AIDS* 6(2):116 (abstract no. FC105).

12. Thanprasertsuk S, Ungchusak K, Chokevivat V *et al.* (1992). Report on the third survey of the sentinel surveillance for HIV infection in Thailand, June 1990. *Thai AIDS Journal* 4(1): 1–13.

13. Plipat T, Sangwanloy O, Phokhasawat K, Chemnasiri T. (2004). *Results of HIV Sero-Surveillance, Thailand 1989–2003.* Bangkok: Ministry of Public Health, Department of Disease Control, Bureau of Epidemiology.

14. The Thai Working Group on HIV/AIDS Projection. (2001). *Projections for HIV/AIDS in Thailand: 2000–2020.* Bangkok: Ministry of Public Health, Department of Communicable Diseases Control, Division of AIDS.

15. Bureau of Epidemiology. (2004). Reported cases of AIDS and symptomatic HIV infection in Thailand, January 31, 2004. *Weekly Epidemiological Surveillance Report* 35(6):94–6.

16. Rojanapithayakorn W, Hanenberg R. (1996). The 100% condom program in Thailand. *AIDS* 10(1):1–7.

17. Pinprateep P. (1992). Model Development of Increasing Condom Use Rate Among Service Girls by the Owners of Sex-work Places to Reduce Sexual TRansmitted Diseases and Acquired Immune Deficiency Syndrome in Phitsanulok Municipality. The Second National Seminar on AIDS (May 20–22, 1992), p40.

18. Suttachana S, Nuntee S, Chemnasiri T, Plipat T. (2004). *Results of Behavioral Surveillance System Among Male Conscripts, Thailand 1995–2003.* Bangkok: Ministry of Public Health, Department of Disease Control, Bureau of Epidemiology.

19. Assavanonda A. (2000). Condom Machines to Be Fitted [in Thailand]. *Bangkok Post Online.* URL: www.bangkokpost.com.

20. Saritaphiluk S, Imami N, Trakulwongse B, Keawkarnkha B. (1994). Efficacy of AIDS Prevention Education Program in Grade 12 Student School in Petchaburi Province. Presented at the Fourth National Seminar on AIDS (27–29 July 1994), p53–54.

21. Nopkesorn T, Mastro TD, Teppa T, Buadit N, Sornlump R and Shinvorasophak V. (1994). Peer Education Activity in Vocational Students. Presented at the Fourth National Seminar on AIDS (July 27–29, 1994), p65–66.

22. Siraprapasiri T, Ratanavaraha J, Kaewruamwong N. (1996). AIDS Intervention-linked Research in Three Vocational Schools. Presented at the XI International Conference on AIDS, Vancouver (7–12 July 1996): PubD 1367.

23. Division of Non-formal Education Development. (1994). *AIDS Curriculum, Primary School level (1 Volume) and Secondary School level (2 Volumes).* Bangkok: Ministry of Education, Department of Non-formal Education.

24. Shaffer N, Chuachoowong R, Mock P *et al.* (1999). Bangkok Collaborative Perinatal HIV Transmission Study Group. Short-course zidovudine for perinatal HIV-1 transmission in Bangkok, Thailand: a randomized controlled trial. *Lancet* 353:773–80.

25. Bureau of AIDS, TB and STIs. (2003). Follow-up to the Declaration of Commitment on HIV/AIDS (UNGASS), Country Report Format, Reporting period: January–December 2002. Bangkok: Ministry of Public Health, Department of Disease Control.

26. Chantasiriyakorn S, Sangwanloi O, Limpakarnjanarat K *et al.* (2002). Preliminary result of perinatal HIV outcome monitoring system implementation in 4 pilot provinces, 2001. *Monthly Epidemiological Surveillance Report* 33:51–60 (in Thai).

27. Vanichseni S, van Griensvan F, Suntharasamai P *et al.* (2002). The Emergence of Midazolam Injection and its Association with Needle Sharing Among Injecting Drugs Users (IDUs) in Bangkok, Thailand. Presented at the XIV International AIDS Conference, Barcelona, July 7–12, 2002, p435 (ThOrC1396).

28. Ministry of Public Health and Thai Red Cross. (1989). *National Policy on Blood Services.* Bangkok: Ministry of Public Health, Department of Communicable Disease Control, AIDS Division.

29. Task Force on the Revision of Guideline on Prevention of Infection from Medical and Public Health Service. (1995). *Guideline on Prevention of Infection from Medical and Public Health Service (Universal Precautions),* Second Revision. Bangkok: Ministry of Public Health, Permanent Secretary Office, Nursing Division.

30. Sirisreetreerux R, Rojnapithayakorn W, Phoolcharoen W. (1998). Practice of Universal Precautions in Health Care Workers in Thailand, 1987–1997. Presented at the XII International AIDS Conference, Geneva, 28 June–3 July, 1998: 23345.

31. Cohen J. (2003). AIDS vaccine still alive as booster after second failure in Thailand. *Science* 302:1309–1310.

32. Akaleephan C, Tangcharoensathien V, Tanprasertsuk S, Tiemchai V, Suraratdecha C. (2004). *Policy Framework for the Adoption of and Demand Forecast for an HIV Preventive Vaccine in Thailand.* Nonthaburi: International Health Policy Program.

33. The Committee for Development of the Comprehensive and Continuum of Care. (2002). *Comprehensive and Continuum of Care Guideline for Persons Living with HIV/AIDS.* Bangkok: Ministry of Public Health, Department of Communicable Disease Control, AIDS Division.

34. Bureau of AIDS, TB and STIs. (2003). *Guideline on the Implementation of Antiretroviral Treatment and Monitoring Program for People with HIV/AIDS.* Bangkok: Ministry of Public Health, Department of Disease Control.

Chapter 24

Barbados

E R Walrond[*] and T C Roach

Background

Barbados is a small island in the southern Caribbean. The islands in the Caribbean were colonized from the time of the arrival of Columbus in the New World and were used as plantations and as trans-shipment ports between South America and Europe, with labour provided primarily by slaves brought in from Africa. Barbados was a British colony from the early seventeenth century through to its independence in 1966. Ninety-five per cent of the population reflects the predominantly African roots of the plantation workers, whilst the distribution of wealth is still skewed to the British ownership and management structure of the plantations and other business interests of the colonial period.

The religious beliefs of the population reflect the island's colonial heritage, with Anglican (Episcopalian) and other Protestant faiths predominating. The constitution of the country guarantees freedom of religion, and about 8% of the population is Catholic, with smaller and more recent immigrant groups of Muslims and Hindus. There are no indigenous African religious practices left, as they were either incorporated into Christian rites or banned by law in the colonial period. Most Barbadians express conservative religious views on issues such as abortion, contraception and homosexuality, although the population does not practise such conservatism in their daily lives. It was in this atmosphere that the society received the news of AIDS as a fatal disease among men who have sex with men (MSM) and, as in many other places, dubbed it the wrath of God against homosexuality.

The country is a parliamentary democracy in which the head of state represents the Queen of the British Commonwealth. However, the executive power lies with the Prime Minister and the Cabinet as long as they enjoy the support of a parliamentary majority. The laws of the country largely reflect the common law position existing in Britain at the time of independence, but subsequent governments have not adopted many of the changes in law in Britain, even though the final court of adjudication remains the British Privy Council. For example, sodomy remains illegal, and that law is fiercely defended even by those who hold allegiance to the British Anglican Church, which appears to have embraced the repeal of that law in Britain. This attitude to homosexuality has led to a negative outpouring of sentiment when such matters as allowing the use of condoms by prisoners are discussed [1].

Culturally, there is a rich mix of indigenous forms of Afro-Caribbean music and dance, and the wide canvas of American popular culture with its largely sexual themes. The population of some 270,000 people occupies the 166 square mile area of the island primarily along its

---

* Corresponding author.

Table 24.1 Population structure, 1980 and 2000

Age group (years)	1980		2000	
	Percentage of the population	Approximate population	Percentage of the population	Approximate population
<15	30	75,600	21.5	56,850
15–29	30.5	76,850	23.5	62,150
30–44	15	37,500	24	63,450
45–64	15	37,500	19	50,250
65 and over	9.5	23,950	12	31,700

Sources: [2,3].

Caribbean coastline, making it one of the most densely populated countries in the world. In addition, there is a good network of roads and a high proportion of private vehicles, making the population very mobile.

Improvement in the country's economic situation is illustrated by the increase in gross national product (GNP) from US$530 in 1965, the year before independence, to US$4200 in 1984 and US$6370 in 1999. This increase occurred in spite of severe recessions in the middle of the 1970s and the beginning of the 1990s. The economy, which was traditionally based on agriculture, went through a phase of growth in light manufacturing after independence, but is now dominated by tourism and services related to that industry.

Barbados has been able to keep its population growth under control by significantly lowering its birth rate through the absorption of messages related to contraception and the economic benefits of small family size. However, it is acknowledged that men frequently have several sexual partners and some women have children by several men. Therefore, the country has the sexual behaviour patterns conducive to the spread of HIV. Although the population has not grown significantly, the population pyramid has changed markedly in the last two decades, with an increasing percentage of elderly inhabitants and a current average life expectancy of 75 years. Because of a reduction in the proportion of children, the increasing number of elderly has not increased the dependency ratio, which was 0.4:1 in 1980 and 0.3:1 in 2000 (see Table 24.1).

The health system

History

At the beginning of the twentieth century, Barbados was described as the unhealthiest place in the British Empire; at the beginning of the twenty-first century, it is considered amongst the healthiest of developing countries. The sorry state described at the beginning of the last century can be traced back to the social, economic and political state of the country after the abolition of slavery in 1834. Governance and political representation remained with the property owners, who had no further direct interest in the healthcare of their former slaves. The majority of the population lived in deplorable conditions as regards housing and sanitation, and received meagre incomes.

The Barbados General Hospital was established in 1834 as a public institution to serve the entire population. Ten per cent of the hospital beds were private beds, but only the most destitute chose to use the public wards, for it was thought that the authorities and the doctors cared only for the private patients. Similar statements are still made today about the public wards of the Queen Elizabeth Hospital (QEH), which replaced the Barbados General Hospital in 1964. It was to these wards and a generally poor attitude to public patients that the cases of AIDS had to be admitted for care, with all the stigma and fear that the disease carried. Patients were often left unattended, even to the point where no one wanted to remove the utensils with which they ate.

The changes in the health status of the population of Barbados over the years is reflected in the infant mortality rate, which was 400 infant deaths out of every 1000 live births at the turn of the twentieth century, and had reached 10.5 in every 1000 by 1993 [4,5]. Infectious diseases had raged at the beginning of the twentieth century, and the social and racial differences in the prevalence of disease were recorded by the authorities in the 'white, black and mixed' populations. At the time, protests from the few available doctors about health conditions were ignored by the authorities to the extent that help offered by the Rockefeller Foundation for the provision of public health services was rejected. No progress was made for the general population until a wave of riots swept through the Caribbean in the late 1930s. As a response to these riots, the British government sent out a commission that recorded the poor social conditions and state of health, which lay reported but not acted upon both in the local files and at the Colonial Office in London. Following the end of the Second World War in 1945, the Moyne Commission produced its report proposing a version of the social model that was envisaged for post-war Britain, i.e. provision of health services for the whole population free at the point of delivery and funded by taxation.

Thereafter, progress in improving health conditions was brought about by a combination of a change in political representation based on universal adult suffrage and a series of changes in education, public health services and the provision of improved hospital services with the construction of the QEH in 1964. Free secondary education was instituted in the early 1960s, and public education became available at the primary, secondary and tertiary levels, and became compulsory for all children up to the age of 16.

Education has provided the essential basis for improvement in health. Better education has led to better economic opportunities and the ability of the majority of the population to take advantage of the basic tools of good health, such as adequate housing with safe sanitary disposal, access to potable water, adequate nutrition and safe food storage. This is probably best seen in the success of family planning and population control. With a literacy rate of 99%, education has also released the energies of women, who have been the main caregivers as well as care users. The change in education that had the most direct impact on health service provision was the opening of the University of the West Indies (UWI), which started training doctors in 1948. Medical school trainees are now predominantly young women rather than men, as had been the case for most of the first three-quarters of the twentieth century. Training of doctors for the region expanded to Barbados in 1967 and ensured the increase in the medical workforce that has been an essential ingredient in improving healthcare. The trends in the health workforce following independence in 1966 are shown in Table 24.2.

By the time the first indigenous case of AIDS had been diagnosed in Barbados in 1984, there was enough expertise to deal with the condition. However, most of the health personnel exhibited the same fear and stigmatization that affected the general population and had to be educated about HIV and AIDS and re-educated about their legal and ethical obligations as well as the importance of observing universal precautions in the workplace. Table 24.2 shows

Table 24.2 Number of healthcare staff, total population and ratio of number of health professionals per population (   ), 1968–1999

Health personnel	1968	1984	1990	1999
Physicians	121 (2,040)	225 (1120)	294 (886)	288 (918)
Graduate nurses	429 (575)	774 (325)	836 (307)	882 (300)
Nursing auxiliaries	172 (1,440)	390 (646)	502 (512)	273 (968)
Pharmacists	71 (3480)		131 (1988)	188 (1406)
Social workers			8 (32,561)	8 (33,050)
Laboratory technicians	25 (9880)	48 (5426)	32 (8262)	
Estimated total population	246,840	252,000	260,490	264,400

Sources: [2,3,6–8].

that the health sector workforce has stagnated in the last decade, particularly in nursing personnel, social workers and laboratory staff. This raises the concern as to whether there might not be sufficient personnel in future to deal with the epidemic and its growth.

Financing

The employees of most large companies, including government workers, are enrolled in private health insurance schemes. However, unemployment rates generally vary between 10 and 15%, and the vast majority of the working population is made up of unskilled workers or artisans who are not usually covered by private health insurance. Therefore, the public system is predominantly used by the jobless, the elderly, small entrepreneurs such as market vendors, and employees of small enterprises. Thus there is a 'mixed' healthcare system, with private financing—both personal and through insurance—of both hospital and primary care services. The existing private hospital has a 35 bed capacity in comparison with the 550 beds of the QEH. Government allocates 10–15% of its budget to the Ministry of Health, with a per capita expenditure of about U$500 per annum. Nevertheless, the services provided by government remain overcrowded in both the hospital and primary care sectors.

Public health services

In the early part of the last century, public health services were largely neglected. Infectious diseases, particularly the enteric fevers and malaria, were rampant, and malnutrition among children was the norm. The Moyne Commission recommended improvements to health services in 1945, and in 1953 the first rural public health centre was opened. More of these centres were built over the years, and Barbados can now boast modern public health and primary care facilities in eight polyclinics that serve the entire population.

The health centres were crucial in the mass immunization of children in the wake of a polio outbreak in the early 1960s. All children born since then have been protected against tetanus, diphtheria, whooping cough, poliomyelitis and now measles, and a child is not allowed to enter primary school without such immunization. Nevertheless, health challenges remain, for while the infant mortality rate has for some years been reduced to 10.5 per 1000 live births and most of the infectious diseases are not major problems, inadequate vector control has left the population vulnerable to dengue fever. Changing nutritional habits and more sedentary occupations have resulted in an epidemic of obesity, diabetes and hypertension.

In the early response to the HIV epidemic, nurses in the polyclinics were trained as counsellors and educators and have played a crucial role in education in the community and in the schools, in pre-test counselling of pregnant women and others, as well as the domiciliary care of those affected.

Primary care services

Until the time of independence, general practitioners provided first contact medical care as well as acting as public health and hospital doctors. Primary care was and is provided predominantly in the private sector, but government had also provided such services for those indigent people who were unable to pay, through district medical officers and now through the island-wide system of polyclinics, which are free to any citizen or resident who chooses to use them. There is no means test to use the publicly provided services, and people choose to use the public sector for varying reasons. In addition, many people use the emergency department in the hospital for primary care services. One of the polyclinics houses a joint government/UWI Family Practice Clinic that provides undergraduate and postgraduate training in the discipline.

Government support for postgraduate family practice training was given at a time when it was proposed to organize general practitioner services along the lines of the British National Health Service (NHS), and legislation to this effect was passed in 1980. However, the representative body of doctors, forced by government to unionize in order to negotiate on behalf of the profession, rejected the government's proposals by an overwhelming vote, and service provision has remained a mixture of private general practitioners and government services provided through polyclinics. General practitioners, with some notable exceptions, do not get involved in the management of HIV patients beyond the provision of testing for insurance, US immigration and diagnostic purposes. Most symptomatic HIV patients are referred to the AIDS Management Team (AMT) first established at the QEH, and now at a separate unit at the Ladymeade Reference Unit.

The Barbados Drug Service

At the time of the proposed NHS, a proposal by doctors for improvements in the health services was adopted by government, and the Barbados Drug Service was introduced in 1980 as the first phase of an NHS. The service provides drugs free at the point of delivery to the elderly, the chronically ill and children. With the advent of HIV, the National Advisory Committee on AIDS (NACA) recommended the provision of zidovudine (AZT) to AIDS patients through the Drug Service. Although this proposal was not approved at the time, limited supplies were made available from 1995 onward for use in the prevention of mother-to-child transmission (PMTCT). Since 2001, the Drug Service has been mandated to provide antiretroviral drugs in the expanded response for the management of AIDS patients.

Hospital services

The Barbados General Hospital (BGH) was built in 1834, when slavery was abolished, to provide services for the island's population. However, at the hospital's centennial, the Chief Medical Officer remarked that the 'high percentage' of private beds (10%) meant that the authorities were more concerned with the treatment of 'poor sick whites'. In the two decades after the Second World War, with the increased output of doctors from the UWI, things started to improve for the majority of the population. Trained specialists became available but were still a rarity. In 1964, just before independence, the 550 bed QEH was opened as a replacement for the BGH. Even so, in the new hospital there were frequently two or three malnourished children to a cot, particularly around Christmas and during the crop season when mothers were out in the fields at work.

Hospitals also had to deal with the tragic consequences of 'slip and slide' abortions carried out or started by nurses, orderlies and druggists, which contributed significantly to the maternal mortality rate. For those who could afford it, there were doctors who provided a safer, albeit illegal, abortion service. This dangerous plight of young women changed dramatically in the last two decades with the introduction of the Termination of Pregnancy Act in 1983. Since then, the maternal mortality rate has dropped to zero in some years. This Act provided an option for HIV-positive pregnant patients that few used when efforts to reduce MTCT were introduced.

Although the QEH was designed as an upgraded version of the old BGH, it has developed to provide far more modern healthcare. Within 3 years of its opening it became a teaching centre of the UWI. The specialist staff has expanded from four when the hospital was opened, to more than 50, serving 550 beds and providing all specialist services, including open-heart surgery, neurosurgery and renal dialysis. Teaching has expanded to include specialist training and continuing education for practitioners on the island and those in the Eastern Caribbean. Unfortunately, the hospital's capacity appears to exceed the resources available to run it, since some of the services are underutilized or are out of commission, whilst the wards are overcrowded. On the other hand, over the years, some facilities have been upgraded and some new services introduced. The QEH, which employs the largest and most diverse work-force of any workplace in the island, has more beds than any hotel on the island and consumes the largest share of the Ministry of Health budget. The hospital appears to move from crisis to crisis and has recently been placed under a separate board of management in the expectation that the absence of micromanagement by the Ministry of Health will improve the management systems and styles, which are currently more appropriate to the middle of the twentieth century.

Other institutions, such as St. Michael's Geriatric Hospital, have been refurbished, upgraded and renamed to try and remove the stigma of their origins as almshouses, yet that hospital does not meet the demands for care of the elderly. The Psychiatric Hospital is also one of those vital but stigmatized public institutions that have served the community's health needs for more than a century. Attempts at reforms in mental health services have included the reduction of custodial care, the development of a community psychiatric service, halfway houses, a drug rehabilitation unit and a psychiatric ward at the QEH.

Private institutions with fewer facilities and less expertise than the public institutions have caught the attention and favour of the public, for the legacy of the twentieth century is the popular view that anything private must be better than a public service. However, the public hospitals have provided more services and expertise than the private sector has. Despite this, public services are associated with poor access, long waiting times, lack of comfort and poor staff attitudes, including a sense of a lack of confidentiality, even for those who are paying for services. These deficiencies tend to overshadow in people's minds the improvements in the quality and quantity of health services that are provided in the public service.

The HIV epidemic

The response

When HIV struck, Barbados was a community no longer accustomed to coping with major infectious diseases. In the period immediately after the first case was diagnosed in 1984, AIDS patients were feared, stigmatized and poorly cared for. This poor attitude towards AIDS patients was an important stimulus to the first institutional response to the epidemic, the establishment of an AIDS Task Force by the Barbados Association of Medical Practitioners in 1985, 6 months after the first indigenous case of AIDS had been diagnosed.

In spite of the deficiencies in the public sector described above, the HIV response was predominantly crafted in the public sector, and Barbados has many notable achievements to its credit. In 1987, the Ministry of Health, responding to the lead of the World Health Organization (WHO) through the Global Programme on AIDS, established the first NACA. The NACA was charged with the task of advising the Ministry on measures to reduce the transmission of the virus and to reduce the mortality and morbidity of the disease. It was a broadly based committee comprising the medical personnel who showed the greatest interest in dealing with this problem: a nursing sister in charge of the ward to which most of the cases were admitted, the chief social welfare officer, a counsellor from the Ministry of Education, a representative from the Youth Council, an advertising executive and a journalist nominated from the Association of Media Practitioners.

The NACA acted swiftly to produce the Report of the National Advisory Committee on AIDS in 1988, which was adopted by government as a policy document [9]. The report was a seminal publication in the battle against this disease, as it drew the attention of the government of the day to the destructive potential of HIV. In this document, the routes of transmission—sexual, blood contact and mother-to-child—were clearly defined, measures to protect the blood supply were identified, and the importance of counselling in the management of the disease was emphasized. Despite the view that HIV was primarily a health problem, the importance of the protection of human rights was recognized at this early stage and was acknowledged in the government's responses. An AMT was established at the hospital and, apart from the medical management, the team incorporated counsellors, social workers and an education officer who concentrated on training the hospital staff in both the technical aspects of the disease and the attitudes of health workers through an exploration of the legal and ethical issues related to the affected patients. An AIDS information centre was established, and within it was incorporated a telephone hotline service.

From the recognition of the first case of AIDS, strenuous efforts were made to record the cases presenting at the QEH. Surveillance of the disease was facilitated by several factors:

- blood testing for HIV (by enzyme-linked immunosorbent assay) was performed only at the QEH laboratory;
- a single pathologist was responsible for the analysis and collation of the tests, thus multiple test requests coming from different sites could be identified and avoided, and confidentiality maintained;
- virtually 100% of patients presenting with AIDS-defining illnesses were seen at the QEH, for only a handful of individuals with AIDS had the necessary financial resources to seek treatment privately or abroad;

◆ the institution of the centralized, QEH-based AIDS Management Team ensured that accurate statistics and quality diagnostic skills resulted in a focused surveillance system.

Table 24.3 shows the number of AIDS cases diagnosed from 1984 to 2002. Analysis of the statistical reports reveals several trends that characterized the HIV epidemic in Barbados. Similar trends have been reported from several of the English-speaking Caribbean countries [10]:

1. The early years of the epidemic saw the majority of AIDS cases being reported among MSM. However, by 1990, the Caribbean Epidemiology Centre (CAREC) reported that 53% of cases were transmitted by heterosexual contact [11].

2. Injecting drug use has never been a major mode of transmission for the Caribbean, with the exception of Puerto Rico, where 80% of cases have been reported in injecting drug users (IDUs), and a smaller number reported in Bermuda.

As noted in other countries, the 20–44 year age group accounted for the majority of cases, although recent figures have indicated a disturbing trend of increased infection in older men and younger girls [12]. The estimated number of HIV-infected people in 2003 was 2500, or 1.5% of the population.

Confidence in these statistics is based on the vast majority of AIDS cases presented at the QEH, the adequacy of diagnostic facilities and the reluctance of most private practitioners to deal with these patients, who were therefore referred to the QEH. This allowed the trends in AIDS cases to be recorded and forecast, and the public to be warned about what to expect in the absence of treatment for HIV. Nevertheless, in 1990, a doctor working in a single polyclinic and relying on interviews about the sexual habits of the patients seen over a period of a few weeks projected that 'within ten years, half of the population between the ages of 10 and 60 will be at risk of dying from AIDS'. This prediction caught the imagination of the press and the public. The health authority's estimate, based on Global Programme on AIDS (GPA) models, of a 2% risk to the population at that time went largely ignored, with columns appearing in the press claiming that HIV could be spread by mosquitoes and in food [13]. On the other hand, knowledge, attitude and behaviour surveys done at that time showed a high level of accurate knowledge about transmission routes for HIV among school children and the general population [14]. The high level of knowledge among school children at that time is reflective of the educational system and the efforts made to educate children as well as the general public about HIV.

Table 24.3 Cumulative total number of AIDS cases diagnosed and deaths reported, 1984–2002

Year	Male		Female		Unknown		Annual total		Cumulative total	
	Cases	Deaths	Cases	Deaths	Cases	Deaths	Cases	Deaths	Cases	Deaths
1984–1989	89	62	21	11	0	0	109	83	281	196
1990–1999	792	658	291	203	3	1	1086	862	6242	4947
2000–2002	251	166	131	68	7	1	389	235	4367	3325
Years unknown	7	0	2	0	0	0	13	0	1597	1180
Total	1139	886	445	282	10	2	1597	1180	12487	9648

Source: Ministry of Health.

Between 1985 and 1994, the following was achieved in response to the epidemic:

1. Universal screening for HIV of all donated blood was instituted in May 1985, 2 months before such practice was implemented in the USA.

2. The importance of counselling and informed consent before HIV testing was emphasized and has remained a cornerstone in all subsequent programmes. Training of counsellors was initiated as one of the first programmatic responses.

3. Confidentiality in all medical and social matters pertaining to HIV has remained paramount, in spite of many contrary professional and lay perceptions.

4. An AIDS information centre was established, and extensive public education programmes were conducted utilizing all forms of media—radio, television and print—thereby insuring that the public was acquainted with the latest developments and advances at that time. The programme established a presence at all cultural events, including forming a costumed band in the local 'Crop Over' festival, which won prizes for best small band and best message.

5. An AIDS Hotline was established and manned by trained volunteers.

6. Every effort was made to ensure that disadvantaged groups such as inmates or orphans were included and specifically addressed in the education and awareness process.

7. Care and support of the HIV-infected were mainly focused on the QEH, and to this end a multidisciplinary clinical team, the AMT, was established in 1990. The team comprises medical experts in the areas of internal medicine, paediatrics and obstetrics, as well as ward nurses, community and antenatal nurses, a social worker and health educator. Notable achievements of the AMT have included the HIV education of all hospital staff, the establishment of a counselling clinic for outpatient management of HIV-positive patients, the establishment of a food bank, the implementation of an occupational exposure protocol for healthcare workers, the initiation of the PMTCT programme and the development of a support group called CARE.

8. Members of the NACA played crucial regional and international roles in the response as members of the management team of the Global Programme on AIDS and in the activities of the Caribbean Epidemiology Center, which was mandated through PAHO/WHO to coordinate the response in the Caribbean region.

Although the Ministry of Health coordinated most activities, there were significant developments within the community. The most important of these was the establishment of the AIDS Society of Barbados (ASOB) in 1990, the first AIDS-related non-governmental organization (NGO) to be established in Barbados. ASOB has made a major contribution to AIDS awareness and support for the HIV community over the years by providing education, counselling and financial support for people with HIV.

In 1996, NACA was given a new mandate to establish a broader-based, multisectoral response to the HIV epidemic in keeping with the UNAIDS programme that had replaced the Global Programme on AIDS, indicating a change in thinking on the national responses to HIV and a desire to attract more partners in the ongoing battle against the epidemic.

This second NACA was as successful as the first, and the period 1996–1998 saw many significant advances. In the care and support areas, a hostel for homeless people living with

HIV—the Elroy Philips Hostel, named after the first AIDS patient who agreed to be identified in public before his final illness—was established and the PMTCT programme was initiated.

Prevention of mother-to-child transmission

Barbados is among the developing countries where PMTCT of HIV received high priority early in the course of the epidemic. Antenatal voluntary counselling and testing (VCT) has been a part of routine antenatal care since 1988. Patients are offered such options as termination of pregnancy and Caesarean delivery, and are advised against breastfeeding and supplied with baby formula. Antenatal HIV screening has increased from just over 20% in 1992 to over 80% since 1997 [15], and a recent study has shown that less than 3% of pregnant women refuse HIV testing after counselling [16].

Following the publication of the results from the AIDS Clinical Trials Group (ACTG) 076 study in 1994, the PMTCT programme with antiretrovirals was launched in 1996. From 1996 to 2000, free AZT was provided for all HIV-infected pregnant women during the second half of their pregnancy and during labour, and to the newborn for the first 6 weeks of life, using a modified ACTG 076 protocol. Huge success was reported with this programme, with the reduction of perinatal HIV transmission to 6% as compared with 27% in a control group studied retrospectively between 1992 and 1996. This corresponded to a reduction of 80% in MTCT [17].

In the late 1990s, the efficacy of single-dose nevirapine (NVP) during labour was reported and its economic advantage and single-dose regimen attracted worldwide attention. In late 2000, the decision was made to switch from AZT to NVP for PMTCT. From 2000 through 2002, all HIV-infected pregnant women received a single dose of NVP during labour, and their newborns received one or two doses of NVP in the first 2 days of life. An interim analysis demonstrated that NVP was effective, although less efficacious than the use of peripartum AZT [18].

The PMTCT of HIV has been a huge success story in Barbados. The national commitment and a comprehensive surveillance system, together with the country's excellent pre-existing antenatal care have all contributed to this success. However, there is still room for some fine tuning and examination of some of the programme's weaknesses in order to make it more efficacious. For example, fathers have not been informed of their child's condition, and 21% of HIV-positive women have repeated pregnancies after they have been diagnosed, most with different fathers [19].

Treatment of HIV

Until the 1990s, Barbados concentrated on education, counselling and protection of the blood supply in order to prevent the spread of HIV. In Western countries, there was significant progress in the development of medical treatment for HIV infection; however, the cost of such drugs remained out of the reach of developing countries such as Barbados and others in the Caribbean. The worldwide recession in the early 1990s further emphasized the disparity in the resources available for treatment as well as education and other control measures. For example, the government-owned television station required payment from the NACA to carry its advertisements. It is therefore unsurprising that the government did not approve the recommendation of the NACA for the provision of antiretrovirals to treat AIDS patients at this time, though other drugs for the treatment of AIDS-defining illnesses were made available. It was therefore a significant advance that AZT was approved for an MTCT programme in Barbados in

1996. Although this programme was to be very successful, it addressed only a limited part of the problem of transmission and the specific treatment of HIV infection.

The initial disappointments in the use of single-agent antiretroviral therapy (ART) were re-evaluated, and initial trials reporting the success of multiple drug therapy were reported at the VIII International AIDS Conference in Vancouver in 1996 [20]. The cost of such treatment was prohibitive to all but the most affluent nations, and at that time the cost to Barbados of 1 month's highly active antiretroviral therapy (HAART) was US$800 per patient. Despite the expense, it became increasingly apparent that such therapy was very beneficial to those able to access it, with decreased hospitalizations and, in many cases, the ability to return to work. Thus, there were economic benefits to be derived from the use of such expensive drugs. Meanwhile, economic analyses in the region showed that, with the predominance of young adults dying from the disease, declines in economic activity could already be demonstrated in terms of reduced productivity, loss of skills and dependency costs in the absence of treatment.

The HIV epidemic had been on the agenda of the Caribbean Conference of Ministers of Health since 1988, and there was a realization that a broader multisectoral effort was required, an effort that could only be catalysed by the heads of government. After many years of trying, HIV was placed on the agenda of the Caribbean Heads of Government Conference hosted by Barbados in October 2000. The Prime Minister, who was also the Minister of Finance, announced that Barbados' HIV programme was to be shifted from the Ministry of Health to be administered by the Office of the Prime Minister. This has subsequently resulted in a significantly expanded response by government to the epidemic. The stated goals of the expanded programme were to reduce mortality from HIV by 50% by 2004, and to reduce the incidence of HIV by 50% by 2006. Eight key government ministries are involved: Health; Education, Youth Affairs and Culture; Social Transformation; Labour and Sports; Tourism; Home Affairs; and the Ministry of the Civil Service.

To coordinate the expanded response, a 16-member National HIV/AIDS Commission (NHAC) with an expanded secretariat has replaced the NACA. The Commission has the responsibility to advise government on HIV policy, to advocate for the effective involvement of all sectors and organizations in implementing programmes and strategies, to monitor the implementation of the strategic plan for 2000–2005 and to create and strengthen partnerships for an expanded response among all sectors. The NHAC is responsible for policy decisions and also for monitoring and evaluating the programmes that are instituted by government minis-tries. In addition, the Commission has been mandated to mobilize resources internationally and locally for the implementation of the National HIV/AIDS Programme and to recommend appropriate research. Its further responsibilities are to ensure that the various ministries are fully 'AIDS aware' and that each ministry has an HIV development plan plus a core group responsible for its implementation. The NHAC also seeks to encourage the private sector to contribute to the fight against HIV.

Following decisions made in October 2000, the government of Barbados embarked on negotiations with the World Bank and secured a US$15.15 million loan to assist in its expanded response. The resulting Government of Barbados/International Bank for Reconstruction and Development HIV/AIDS (GOB/IBRD/HIV/AIDS) Prevention and Control Project is to assist in:

+ prevention and control of HIV transmission;
+ diagnosis, treatment and care of people living with HIV (PLHIV);

- management and institutional strengthening.

The anticipated outcomes are:

- reduction in the incidence rate of HIV infections;
- improvement in the quality of life and life expectancy for PLHIV;
- enactment of the appropriate anti-discriminatory legislation;
- establishment of sustainable institutional arrangements for managing the epidemic.

The conditions for the loan have been met, and the project officially started in February 2002. The majority of the loan (US$9.45 million) was set aside for the purchase of antiretroviral medications, with a US$8.3 million matching fund from the government; these expenditures can be compared with the expenditure of US$12 million for other drugs in the Drug Service. This was the first time the World Bank had offered financing for the provision of therapy for a medical condition throughout the world; previous loans had been confined to infrastructural development and specific development projects.

There have been several developments since the GOB/IBRD project began, starting with a significant reduction in the price of ART from US$800 per month to US$192 per month. This reduction has been achieved through negotiations by the Ministry of Health with the established pharmaceutical companies rather than a move to use generic drugs as has happened in Brazil. However, these prices remain out of step with prices of less than US$50 per month offered elsewhere. With the assistance of the Clinton Foundation, the Pan Caribbean AIDS Initiative (PANCAP) is trying to negotiate further reduction in prices, as the cost of ART is the major hurdle for all the developing countries in the region.

In order to expand access to medication, the treatment infrastructure has been improved. The Ladymeade Reference Unit has been established by the refurbishment of two buildings in an area close to the QEH. One of the buildings houses a clinic and the other a state-of-the-art laboratory capable of performing the necessary CD4 and viral load tests for monitoring therapy, and the result has been a big increase in the services provided to the HIV-positive community. Patients are now able to access domiciliary care, community care, a complete range of antiretroviral drugs, laboratory monitoring with CD4 and viral load estimations, post-exposure prophylaxis for both occupational accidents and sexual assault, and an expanded VCT service.

Since the institution of the HAART treatment programme in 2002, there has been a reduction in the mortality of AIDS patients from 80% to 43% and a corresponding jump in the numbers of AIDS patients alive and on treatment. However, compliance with the treatment regimen and the emergence of drug resistance are concerns that will have an impact on the overall costs and effectiveness of the treatment programme.

Conclusion

Achievements

Barbados has had a record of achievement in health, education and economic progress that is outlined in the history, social, economic, religious, education and health services background of the country and its people. This background is important in understanding how the epidemic took hold in the country, the advantages and impediments in trying to control the spread of

HIV, and the professional and government responses to the epidemic thus far. Although the responses of the professions and the government were swift and their efforts have held the epidemic in check, the economic depression of the early 1990s and the negative societal reaction to people affected by HIV have probably hindered a decline in HIV prevalence.

However, by March 2003, when the expanded response had been running for 1 year, a review of the project stated that:

> The Barbados Programme is to be commended. During the past year, Barbadian society has progressed in its HIV/AIDS-related knowledge, attitudes and beliefs. Public sector partners have embarked on their new responsibilities, some even with zeal and creativity. NGOs and CSOs have done the same. Private sector partnerships have been solicited and initiated. The level and extent of HIV/AIDS care and treatment available in Barbados would surpass many industrialized nations around the globe. After only one year 150 patients with HIV are now accessing antiretroviral therapies free of charge, thanks to this programme. The NHAC has been established upon the goals of multisectoral participation from all walks of life. Its Directorate is there to assist, whenever possible, in making sure these partnerships are empowered for action [21].

Challenges

Despite such a glowing accolade, there are still challenges to overcome. Foremost is the question of sustainability. The World Bank loan has been instrumental in establishing the expanded HIV response, but such funding is a temporary measure and the government of Barbados must seek to establish the mechanisms necessary to continue funding the programme. Without a reduction in new HIV infections, the number of patients requiring ART, as well as its attendant costs, will continue to grow. Scientific methods must therefore be employed to monitor the HIV epidemic and put the programme in a position to respond appropriately.

The problem of stigma and discrimination continues to be an obstacle to progress. HIV-positive individuals in the Caribbean have experienced significant discrimination in the work-place and in the community from healthcare workers, the general public and in the insurance sector. Stigma and discrimination are fuelled particularly by homophobia and its reinforcement by some in their interpretation of religious texts, and by the retention of sodomy laws. This is compounded by the lack of legislation in many areas; although legislation will not stop these problems overnight, it is important to make progress in this area as soon as possible. Recently, the Attorney General sought a consultation on these issues and the resulting legal initiatives are eagerly awaited.

Support and advocacy for HIV-positive individuals is not as widespread as it should be, and further development and empowerment of the fledgling support groups should be a priority of the expanded programme if those who may be HIV-infected are to be encouraged to come forward and be diagnosed. However, there are many well-meaning people involved in these efforts who have little training or expertise and may, therefore, be counterproductive to the aims of the programme.

Whilst continuing surveys have shown that knowledge of HIV is good, there is little evidence that such knowledge has translated into the behaviour changes that were achieved in the early efforts of the NACA. Research elsewhere has shown that existing legislation is often a barrier to high-risk groups empowering themselves with safer practices. A national campaign with a focus on every Barbadian learning his or her HIV status, coupled with expanded awareness of safe sex practices and an emphasis on each individual assuming responsibility for their sexual health, needs to be instituted, but is unlikely to succeed in the absence of appropriate legislative changes.

The recent priority in the areas of care and support for the HIV-positive community has been the provision of ART. However, it is important that Barbados continue to seek reduced prices for these drugs and to effect meaningful reduction in HIV prevalence.

Barbados is in a strong position from which to move forward further, based on the foundation of a committed government, a relatively well-developed infrastructure, dedicated human resources and, with the help of World Bank resources, the development of a model HIV treatment programme that may be considered as an example for others to follow.

References

1. Howe G, Cobly A, eds. (2002). *The Caribbean AIDS Epidemic*. UWI Press.

2. PAHO/WHO. (1970). *Health Conditions in the Americas 1965–8*. No. 207, Vol. 11, p174–5.

3. PAHO/WHO. (1986). *Health Conditions in the Americas 1981–4*. No. 500, Vol. 11, p150–3.

4. Colonial Medical Service. (1923). *Report of the Public Health Inspector*. Barbados.

5. Health statistics from the Americas. (1998). *PAHO Scien. Pub.* **567**:29.

6. PAHO/WHO. (1994). *Health Conditions in the Americas 1994*. No. 547, Vol. 1, p369.

7. Ministry of Health, Barbados. (1995). *CMO Report 1991–92*.

8. Ministry of Health, Barbados. (2000). *CMO Report 1997–98*.

9. Walrond ER, ed. (1988) *Report of the National Advisory Committee on AIDS*. Barbados: Ministry of Health.

10. CAREC surveillance reports 1986–1992.

11. CAREC surveillance reports. (1990). Vol. 16, No. 5.

12. Ministry of Health. (2004). *Statistical Update on HIV/AIDS in Barbados 1984*. Barbados: Ministry of Health.

13. Howe, G. (2000). Press and public reactions to HIV/AIDS in Barbados since 1984. In: Howe G, Cobley A, eds. *The Caribbean AIDS Epidemic*. University of the West Indies Press, pp 42–56.

14. Walrond E, Jones F, Hoyos M, Souder M, Ellis H, Roach T. (1992). An AIDS-related knowledge, attitudes, beliefs and practices survey among schoolchildren in Barbados. *Bulletin of the PAHO* 26(3):208–19.

15. Kumar A, St. John MA. (2002). Trends in HIV Seroprevalence Among Pregnant Women and Perinatal HIV Exposure to Infants in Barbados. Presented at the XIV International AIDS Conference, July 2002, Barcelona, Spain.

16. Kumar A, Rochester E, Gibson M, Gibson T, Robinson H, Forde S. (2004). Antenatal voluntary counselling and testing for HIV in Barbados—success and barriers to implementation. *Rev Panam Salud Publica* 14(4):242–8.

17. St. John MA, Kumar A, Cave C. (2003). Reduction in perinatal transmission and mortality from human immunodeficiency virus after intervention with Zidovudine. *Pediatric Infectious Disease Journal* 22:422–6.

18. St. John MA, Kumar A, Cave C, Carmichael K, Abayouri A. (2003). Efficacy of Nevirapine Administration on Mother to Child Transmission of HIV Using a Modified HIVNET 012 Regimen. Presented at the 48th Caribbean Health Research Council annual conference, Bahamas.

19. Kumar A, Bent V. (2003). Characteristics of HIV-infected child bearing women in Barbados. *PAHO Public Health* 13(1):1–9.

20. NIAID AIDS Agenda. (1996). *New Findings Bring Hope to Vancouver AIDS Conference.* September 1996. Available at http://www.niaid.nih.gov/ publications/agenda/0996/page1.htm. Accessed 10/3/2004.

21. Gayle JA. (2003). *HIV/AIDS Prevention and Control Project. Year One Progress Review.* Government of Barbados/International Bank for Reconstruction and Development.

Chapter 25

Cuba

M I Lantero Abreu[*], J Waller, J Joanes Fiol, J Perez Avila, R Torres Peña, M Santín Peña, R Ochoa Soto and G Estevez Torres

Background

Cuba is the largest of the Caribbean islands, with over 11 million inhabitants [1]. The Spanish conquistadors wiped out the original Carib peoples in the early sixteenth century, and the island was repopulated by waves of principally Spanish immigrants and, to a lesser extent, West African slaves. The Cuban nation grew out of the extensive intermarriage and cultural inter-mingling of their descendents. The leading religious practice, for instance, is Santeria, an amalgam of animistic Yoruba beliefs and Catholicism. Since 1959, the values of socialist humanism have become deeply rooted.

Decades of revolutionary nationalist struggle eventually overthrew the Spanish colonial power at the very end of the nineteenth century. However, the US military intervention in the final stages of the war turned the newly independent Cuba into a *de facto* US colony, which oscillated for nearly 60 years between military and civilian rule. The revolution of 1959 was met with great hostility from the US government, which instituted a total economic embargo against the island in 1962 [2]. The Cuban government turned to the Soviet Union for support, and Cuba became part of the Soviet trading bloc, the Council for Mutual Economic Cooperation (COMECON), trading principally sugar, nickel and citrus fruits for oil, manufactured goods and some foodstuffs, with prices fixed at 1962 levels, which were generous to Cuba. Almost the entire economy was state-run.

The Soviet Union's collapse in 1991 plunged Cuba into a profound economic crisis, which it terms the 'Special Period'. The gross domestic product (GDP) dropped by 35% between 1991 and 1993, and external trade by 75%. This was exacerbated by the US Congress passing laws that sought to internationalize the trade embargo and create a full economic blockade of Cuba. Since 1994, there has been a slow economic recovery based principally on the rapid expansion of mass international tourism, and the development of diversified trade and foreign investment from Western Europe, Canada and Latin America in particular. The state remains by far the dominant economic actor, but with important new players such as foreign enterprise and local small businesses. These capitalist economic elements have generated disparities in wealth, with the government seeking to redistribute that wealth through taxation and spending policies.

* Corresponding author.

The health system

History

1959–1991

Before 1959, private health provision catered to the well off in the capital, Havana, whilst a self-financing insurance-based system gave some coverage to 20% of the population [3]. Health indices were those typical of a poor country.

Since 1959, the government has assumed full responsibility for its citizens' healthcare. Funds come almost entirely from the state budget, private provision has ended, and the service is universal and free at the point of access, except for modest prescription charges in primary care. Structurally, a single agency, the Ministry of Public Health, is responsible for coordinating everything related to preventive and curative healthcare.

Healthcare provision has gone through several distinct phases since 1959 [4]. Many doctors left for the USA in the early 1960s, prompting the government to begin a rapid training programme for doctors and nurses. The emphasis was on providing a doctor-led service rather than training community health workers or 'barefoot doctors'. Nurses had a role, but with limited clinical autonomy.

The focus was on mass childhood immunization, quality care and safe hospital delivery for pregnant women, and public health measures such as clean water, improved sanitation and the elimination of vectors to infection. This was accompanied by profound socio-economic changes in employment, housing and land tenure, as well as improved access to food implemented through a ration book system. Great efforts were made to bring health workers and medical facilities to the rural areas where 75% of the population then lived.

From the mid-1960s to the mid-1980s, a full healthcare system was put in place. Primary care was provided by a nationwide system of polyclinics, each serving some 25,000–30,000 people. These provided one physical location, under one organization, for general medical care, paediatrics, gynaecology, psychology, dentistry, optometry and many laboratory, environmental and related social services. Remote rural polyclinics also had inpatient facilities for routine childbirth and admissions of simple cases.

A major hospital building programme brought about an extensive secondary care sector throughout the island, as well as medical schools in each of the 14 provinces. Specialist centres for tertiary care were developed in Havana and the larger provincial capitals.

Facing public criticism over poor continuity of care in the polyclinics, the Ministry initiated its Family Doctor programme in 1984 [3]. Under a new national medical curriculum, Cuba began to train a new generation of doctors to be practitioners and, potentially, specialists in 'integral' general medicine [5]. Integral meant integrating individual pathology with the economic, social and family determinants of ill health. Each doctor lives in a neighbourhood and, together with a nurse, provides medical care to a registered population of 600–700 people [6]. This includes systematic monitoring of people with, or at risk of developing, chronic disease. There is now 100% coverage of the population, and family doctors are also placed in large workplaces, schools, nurseries and homes for the elderly.

A strong emphasis on selecting candidates with a record of community involvement [7], plus free medical education, has helped develop a medical workforce that, in terms of gender, race and class background, reflects the Cuban nation.

The introduction of family doctors as an additional service allowed the polyclinics to shift their role partially to become small groups of specialists providing postgraduate training, support and point of first referral for the family doctors. A group of about 15 family doctors has the support of a team comprising more experienced doctors, a senior nurse, a psychologist and a social worker. Aside from the permanently resident specialists, consultants in many other fields such as orthopaedics, dermatology, cardiology and psychiatry hold regular outpatient clinics at the polyclinics. All polyclinics now provide a 24-hour on-site emergency service for minor illness and injury, and one-third have a more extensive casualty unit.

Meanwhile, Cuba has strived to improve its secondary and tertiary care with a number of national or regional referral centres that can undertake the vast majority of procedures known to modern medicine, including, for instance, all forms of transplant surgery.

The blockade: effects and response

Since 1991, secondary and tertiary care and, to a lesser degree, primary care have been badly hit by shortages of medicines, supplies, machinery and spare parts. Due to the economic crisis, the Ministry's annual budget for purchases from abroad fell from US$227 million to US$70 million in the early 1990s, and, whilst under the blockade, Cuba is not legally able to purchase on the US market or from US multinationals and their subsidiaries anywhere in the world [8].

During the early 1990s, the crisis caused nutrition levels to fall by a third, and water purity declined sharply, leading to significant effects on morbidity and, to a lesser extent, mortality [9]. The year 1993 saw an epidemic of optic neuritis and polyneuropathy amongst adults, due principally to food and vitamin deficiency, whilst tuberculosis (TB) levels rose significantly. With slow economic recovery came better nutrition, and health indicators have since resumed their steady improvement, though iron deficiency anaemia in pregnant women and young children remains a problem [10]. The foreign exchange budget is now about US$140 million, but shortages of supplies and medicines continue to be a major problem, and there is close monitoring of prescribing to eliminate waste and fraud.

The Ministry has alleviated the shortages by enthusiastically promoting non-pharmaceutical approaches labelled 'green medicine', an eclectic mix of herbal remedies and traditional Chinese medicine. All family doctors now receive training in these approaches, can prescribe from a national formulary [11] and can refer on to a specialist unit within each polyclinic.

The government has also invested significant domestic finance into building up its pharmaceutical industry and, within that, a specialized biotechnology sector [12]. Cuba has made some major breakthroughs, particularly in the field of vaccines, most famously against meningococcal meningitis B. It now has the scientific expertise to produce two-thirds of the 800 medications on its national formulary, but the limiting factor is hard currency to purchase the raw materials from abroad. Donations of medicines from solidarity movements and non-governmental organizations (NGOs) have filled some gaps.

Structure and accountability

The Ministry is answerable to the National Assembly of People's Power, the Cuban system of elected representative government, with assemblies also at the provincial and municipal levels. Standards and overall policies are set nationally, but the lower assemblies have financial and administrative authority in their areas. Operational management of hospitals and polyclinics is entirely clinician-led.

Popular participation in the implementation of healthcare programmes is stimulated through the nationwide network of block-based neighbourhood Committees for the Defence of the Revolution (CDRs) plus the local branches of the Cuban Women's Federation (FMC). Local activists promote childhood immunization, cervical smears, blood donation and the clean-up of insanitary areas. They also help transmit health education material.

In 1995, amid criticism of bureaucracy in the formal structures, 'people's councils' were established at submunicipal level to bring together people in the administrative bodies and mass organizations locally. Within them are health councils, which seek creative solutions to local health problems and shortages.

Performance

Cuba, a middle-level developing nation, now has health indicators on a par with the developed world [13]. The infant mortality rate is 6.2 per 1000 live births, life expectancy at birth is over 76 years, [14] and inter-provincial differences for the various indicators are relatively small. Cubans are now more likely to die of heart disease, cancer or strokes than of malnutrition, infectious or parasitic diseases (see Table 25.1).

These remarkable achievements are partly due to the public health service, but perhaps more to wider socio-economic improvements in food distribution, education, employment, housing, sanitation, the liberation of women and egalitarian income distribution [15]. The Cuban government's ability to fund such an extensive health service in a relatively

Table 25.1 Cuban health statisitics, 1990-2001

Indicator	Year	
Population[*]	2001	11,230,000
Life expectancy at birth[*]	1995–2001	76
Infant mortality/1000 live births[*]	2001	6
Urban population as % of whole[*]	2001	75%
GDP per capita		N/A
Health expenditure as % of GDP[*]- public	1990–1998	8.2%
- all	1990–1998	9.1%
Crude birth rate/1000 people[**]	2001	12.4
Crude death rate/1000 people[**]	2001	7.1
Direct maternal mortality/100,000 live births[**]	2001	29.6
% Low birth weight babies[**]	2001	5.9%
% Live births in hospital[**]	2001	99.9%
Family doctors[**]	2001	30,726
All doctors[**]	2001	67,128
Doctor:patient ratio[**]	2001	1:67
Nurse:patient ratio[**]	2001	1:33
Health budget per capita—Cuban pesos[**]	2001	169.0
Health foreign exchange budget per capita–US$[**]	2001	12.5
Facilities[**]- hospitals	2001	267
- polyclinics	2001	444
Beds/1000 population[**]- medical care	2001	5.0
- social care	2001	1.3

[*]Source: [14]; [**]source: Ministry of Health annual health statistics 2001.

poor country relies on the country's socio-economic structure, which is based on a high 'social wage' that everybody receives, and low personal wages. This makes doctors extremely cheap to train and employ, permitting Cuba to have an exceptionally high doctor–patient ratio of 1:167.

The current primary care-led system has significantly reduced the demand for more expensive hospital care and has kept waiting times to see a specialist down to a few weeks at most [16]. The annual hospital admission rate peaked in 1985 at 16 per 100 people and by 1999 was down to 12 [1]. In 1980, hospitals dealt with 80% of emergency care, and polyclinics, 20%. By 1999, the figures were hospitals 45% and polyclinics 55%, and the emergency attendance rate per person was 15% lower. Family doctors and nurses are providing a 'hospital at home' service, and polyclinic-based day surgery is expanding quickly.

The impact of Cuban healthcare has also been felt abroad. Since 1960, the government has provided over 50,000 volunteer health workers to 91 poor countries in Latin America, Africa and Asia.

Future developments and challenges

Dramatically improved socio-economic opportunities for women, together with free family planning and abortion, have caused a major decline in the crude birth rate, from 35 per 1000 people in 1963 to 12 per 1000 in 2001. This, combined with the large increase in life expectancy, means that the Cuban population is in rapid transition to a developed-world age structure. Currently, 10% of the Cuban population is over 65 years of age, but the World Bank projects this to rise to 14% by 2015 and to 19% by 2030 [1]. How to ensure that healthy living accompanies longevity is perhaps the largest single challenge facing the Cuban health service, since the elderly make the most demands on healthcare.

The principal focus of Cuban healthcare now and in the future is on non-communicable chronic illness, together with education about healthier lifestyles. However, communicable diseases have not been forgotten. Currently, 99% of Cuban children receive immunization against 13 diseases [17], of which six are now effectively eradicated from the island. Malaria was also eradicated in the 1960s, and, in 2002, a nationwide public health campaign virtually eliminated the breeding places for the mosquito that carries dengue fever.

The systems for epidemiological surveillance are rigorous, aided now by Infomed, a national health Intranet. Consultations and patient records remain paper-based, but every hospital, polyclinic and pharmacy now has basic computers attached to the Internet for email communication and access to medical databases and learning resources.

The US government's economic blockade seems set to continue for the immediate future, so the Ministry will have to continue with strategies that, amongst other things, contain foreign exchange costs. This includes extending 'green medicine', pharmaceutical development and the increasing transfer of personnel, training and diagnostic equipment to primary care settings [18]. Resources have to be spent carefully, but since 2000, work has begun on major repairs to, and re-equipping of, hospitals and polyclinics that for 10 years had received almost no maintenance. More problematic is the importation of high-cost equipment. The Ministry's approach is initially to import one item, assess its costs and benefits and take centralized decisions about numbers to purchase and geographical allocation.

Financing will remain overwhelmingly from the state, but since the early 1990s, Cuba has made its advanced health facilities available for a fee to non-Cubans. Currently, several thousand per year are taking advantage of this 'health tourism'. The proceeds contribute to the free treatment of both Cubans and some foreign nationals; for example, 19,000 child victims of the Chernobyl nuclear disaster have received free curative and rehabilitation therapy at a special hospital.

Wages for individual health workers are an issue. A key element of the economic recovery has been the legalization of the US dollar in 1993. Cuba now operates a complex two-currency economy. This has brought in crucial foreign exchange, but fostered a two-tier economy where those who receive dollar payments, tips or production bonuses are significantly better off than those, such as all health workers, who are paid only in Cuban pesos. Some health workers have left their profession to earn more money in the tourist industry [19], though the great majority have remained committed to their work.

Doctors' peso wages were boosted significantly in 2000, but the main short-term strategy is to keep training new recruits, especially now in nursing. There remains a surplus of doctors, and the Ministry has used part of its medical training capacity to set up the Latin American School of Medicine and a programme to train, for free, 10,000 young people from the poorest communities throughout the Americas to be doctors [20].

Cuba has the training capacity and research expertise to keep abreast of cutting-edge developments in medicine and surgery. It has pioneered a treatment for vitiligo and a surgical procedure for the eye condition retinitis pigmentosa. Vaccine development remains its forte, however, and work is under way on therapeutic vaccines for some forms of cancer [21], as well as a candidate AIDS vaccine.

The HIV epidemic

Incidence and prevalence

Cuba's current HIV epidemiological situation is favourable. There is a virtual absence of infantile AIDS cases, transmission through blood transfusions or through injecting drug use. From 1986 to the end of 2004, 6025 HIV-infected people were detected, of whom 2535 have developed AIDS and 1222 have died. Of all cases, 80% are men and 20% are women. The estimated prevalence rate of people living with HIV (PLHIV) in the 15–49 age group is 0.07% [22].

The first known cases were individuals who had contracted the infection in African countries where Cuba was providing civil and military collaboration. They later infected their sexual partners in Cuba, a phenomenon that initiated the spread of the infection within the nation. Another route of infection, particularly for those with bisexual or homosexual preferences, was via Cubans who had visited the USA and other Western countries [23].

During 1986–1987, the people diagnosed with HIV were mostly heterosexual. By 1988–1989, when other sectors of the population began to be tested, the first evidence of male-to-male sexual transmission was found [23]. Men who have sex with men (MSM) are now the most vulnerable group, representing 86% of all reported male cases [22] (see Fig. 25.1). There have been only 17 reported cases of vertical transmission and 20 of parenteral transmission [22]. Sexual transmission accounts for 99% of all cases.

Through voluntary testing in different sectors of the population, the epidemiological sur-veillance programme has continuously monitored the prevalence among diverse population groups. Cumulative prevalence at the end of 2004 was 0.005% among pregnant women and 0.014% in blood donors. Among those diagnosed with other sexually transmitted infections

(STIs), 0.07% were also infected with HIV, with a prevalence of 0.04% among individuals with multiple sexual partners [22]. Services offering anonymous testing have been available since 1998, complementing the epidemiological surveillance.

The cumulative incidence of HIV in Cuba has remained highest in the western and central regions of the island, with over half of all reported cases in the country's capital, Havana [22].

The early response

At the beginning of the 1980s, the Working Group for Confronting and Fighting AIDS (GOPELS) was created, presided over by the Ministry of Public Health and comprising representatives from the most important state and non-governmental organizations (NGOs). This group was responsible for establishing, directing and comprehensively evaluating all control and preventive policies [23,24]. The first measures aimed at preventing the spread of the disease were adopted in 1983 and began with a comprehensive, multidisciplinary study of HIV.

The importation of human blood products, as well as any other plasma products processed in foreign countries, was strictly prohibited. Additionally, a total of 20,000 potentially infected containers were destroyed. Other international suppliers were found, and local production of these items was begun in response to national demand [23,24]. In October 1983, an Epidemiological Surveillance Programme was initiated in all of the nation's hospitals. Cases such as pneumonia, potentially indicative of *Pneumocystis carinii* pneumonia (PCP), and dermatological lesions, suggestive of Kaposi's sarcoma, had to be reported for subsequent review [24]. By the end of 1985, the necessary funding was made available to purchase the medical equipment and supplies required to diagnose samples at all of the nation's blood banks. Fifty laboratories were constructed throughout the country, including a National Referral Laboratory [24]. Simultaneously, the development of local diagnostic tests and procedures was begun.

The health system then started to test for HIV all Cubans who had been abroad since 1981, resulting in the detection of the first HIV-positive individuals in the country [23,24]. Every seropositive individual had detailed contact tracing of sexual partners, all of whom were

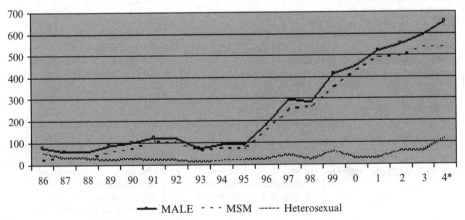

Fig. 25.1 HIV-positive males by sexual preference, 1986–2004. Source: National HIV/AIDS Programme. *Preliminary data.

contacted and screened [25]. At the same time, the first Programme for the Prevention and Control of HIV was initiated, comprising four components: epidemiological surveillance; education and prevention; care and support; and research [23].

By 1986, all of the blood donated in Cuba was being tested for HIV antibodies, and in 1987, other population groups such as pregnant women, individuals diagnosed with STIs and in-patients, among others, were similarly tested [23,24].

The principal measures taken were aimed at preventing sexual transmission, since blood transfusions, injecting drug use and perinatal transmission were considered largely avoidable forms of infection in Cuba. The experience of syphilis and gonorrhoea control programmes, in effect since 1972 [27], also influenced the new HIV strategies, which included:

- developing a wide-reaching health education programme aimed at the general population;
- conducting blood tests on sectors of the population;
- performing a full medical examination of all infected individuals and notifying and testing their sexual partners, with the aim of identifying the probable source of infection and potential secondary cases;
- admitting all HIV-infected individuals into specialized healthcare centres (sanatoria) [23,24].

Figure 25.2 provides an overview of HIV testing, and treatment and care protocols.

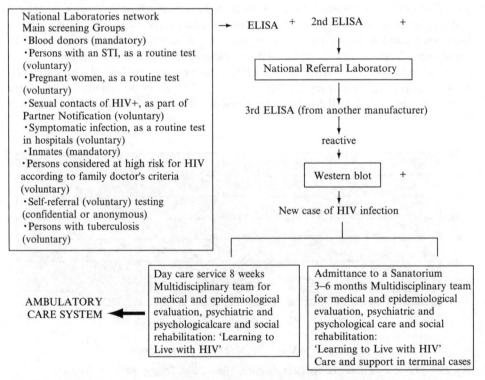

Fig. 25.2 HIV infection diagnosis algorithm and mode of care of PLHIV. Source: [26].

Care and support

To guarantee a high quality of care for those infected with HIV, a national network of sanatoria was established in 1986, providing medical, epidemiological, psychological and social services. Housing, treatment and diets to satisfy individual requirements are provided in environments more akin to hospices than hospitals [23,28].

The sanatorium policy generated a lively and controversial debate in medical journals about its human rights implications [29]. Did seeking to control the spread of an incurable and ultimately fatal communicable disease justify the—at the time—compulsory care of PLHIV in sanatoria? Aviva Chomsky, in the chapter entitled 'Health and revolution in Cuba: the threat of a good example', wrote: '. . . the opinion of US medical experts who have studied Cuba's AIDS policy is virtually unanimous in arguing that Cuban policies toward AIDS are absolutely consistent with its policies toward other diseases and epidemics and with its health care system as a whole' [30].

The relative isolation of HIV cases during the period 1986–1988 has, since 1989, been progressively replaced by a closer relationship with the community. Through public education, community fears had to be addressed in order to avoid hostility toward, and stigmatization of, PLHIV who were returning to their communities.

Developing a thorough programme of social integration was key to the approval, in 1993, of an outpatient care system [24]. PLHIV were then able to receive specialized care whilst living at home after 3–6 months of comprehensive care at a sanatorium, including an interactive course in 'Learning to Live with HIV', which instructed them in the care of their own and others' health.

At the end of 2004, 61% of the 4693 PLHIV were using the ambulatory care option [22]. Since 1998, an alternative 8-week day hospital service at a specialized centre has been offered to newly diagnosed HIV-positive individuals [24].

The care and support offered to PLHIV now comprises three levels: a primary level, through a family doctor and nurse; a secondary level, offered by the country's network of provincial hospitals and sanatoria; and a tertiary level, offered at the Pedro Kourí Institute of Tropical Medicine. This institution also serves as a national reference centre for HIV medical care.

All PLHIV retain full rights to their jobs or studies and can return to them after a period of institutional care if they wish. Many HIV-positive individuals, including doctors and nurses, have become health promoters in the national effort to minimize the impact of the epidemic on the population. All services offered at every level are free and include access to highly active antiretroviral therapy (HAART).

Treatment

The first therapeutic methods employed in 1986 consisted of the use of domestically produced immune modulators. Zidovudine (AZT) therapy was introduced into Cuba's healthcare system in 1987.

Steep prices and other numerous limitations imposed on Cuba by the USA through its trade embargo made it virtually impossible to have ready access to the antiretroviral drugs available in the international market during the 1990s [31,32], and in 1996, 93 AIDS patients died due to lack of antiretroviral treatment. It was the solidarity shown by individuals and organizations supporting Cuba through their donations that made it possible in 1996 to offer triple therapy to 100 HIV-infected Cubans. Though more substantial donations were made in the years to follow, there remained unmet need in the population [32].

From 1997 to 2001, while the domestic production of AIDS drugs was still at the research phase, the Cuban government paid international prices to acquire all of the medication needed to offer triple therapy to mothers and children who were HIV-positive. From 2001 onward, more antiretroviral agents were manufactured domestically and became increasingly available in Cuba, which resulted in a 100% level of coverage for HAART by December 2002 [33]. Currently, four reverse transcriptase inhibitors (zidovudine, stavudine, didanosine and lamivudine) and one protease inhibitor (indinavir) are being produced in Cuba. Following international recommendations, these drugs are offered free of charge to anyone in need of them [33]. Other domestically manufactured drugs, allowing for new combinations and other therapeutic alternatives for treating the phenomenon of viral resistance, will soon be available to Cubans [34]. The current treatment regimen is summarized in Box 25.1.

Research and its results

Some of the nation's most prestigious research centres have collaborated in a large research project in response to the demands of the national HIV programme. Among these are: the Centre for Immune-Assay, the Centre for Genetic Engineering and Biotechnology, the National Reference Laboratory, the Pedro Kourí Institute and the NOVATEC Laboratory [34]. The results of this collaboration include: the use of Cuba's own Ultra Micro Analytic System technology in all of the country's blood banks and laboratories, as well as reagents employed in testing and confirming a diagnosis; and the development of Cuba's own medications and the progress made towards developing a vaccine against HIV [34].

Health promotion and prevention

Health promotion and prevention measures are developed by the Ministry of Public Health and implemented at the community level with the participation of other ministries, including the Ministries of Education, Radio and Television, and the Ministry of Trade and Tourism, and most especially with organizations such as the FMC and the CDRs. The most important measures include:

- training of family doctors and nurses, social workers, teachers, professors, community leaders, health promoters, volunteers and health educators, and familiarizing them with methods and procedures that promote positive behaviours regarding the prevention of HIV;
- information and education campaigns, and their subsequent evaluation through nationwide surveys;
- encouraging the distribution of condoms;
- encouraging the participation of PLHIV in strategies for health promotion and prevention;
- educating the public on safer sexual practices, particularly among adolescents and young adults;
- training health promoters for educational work with vulnerable groups;
- employing the mass media as part of these strategies [24].

The initial educational strategies were directed toward young people and the general population without focusing attention on specific vulnerable groups such as MSM and sex workers. The preponderance and growth of new cases among MSM can be partly attributed to the relative delay in adopting a strategy that targeted them. An intervention strategy specifically for MSM has now been developed with the active participation of MSM themselves.

Box 25.1 HIV treatment regimen

Complete clinical and immunological evaluation which includes:
   CD4 count and %
   Viral load
   Chest X-ray
   PPD skin test
   Toxoplasmosis serology (IgG)
   Gynaecological evaluation with Pap smears and pelvic exam
   Complete blood count
   Serum chemistry
   Hepatitis serology (B and C)
   CMV, HSV IgG
   Lipid profile
   Syphilis serology
   Others: glycaemia, sputum Gram stain
Follow-up according to clinical stage:
   AIDS cases: weekly appointments
   Mild symptomatic: every 15 days
   Asymptomatic: once a month
Evaluation by other medical specialties if necessary
Treatment of HIV infection and AIDS:
   Treatment of opportunistic infections and cancer
   Antiretroviral treatment
Submission to tertiary level:
   Tropical Medicine Institute
   Other hospital for surgery

Source: [26].

All educational activities now take place in the context of the challenges posed, since 1992, by the economic shortages and the new social conditions of Cuba. These conditions have led to the re-emergence of large-scale prostitution attracted by the opportunity to earn US dollars from overseas tourists.

Impact of the response

Cuba's response to the HIV epidemic has had a decisive influence on the current state of the epidemic in the country. Slowing the spread of the epidemic, keeping perinatal transmission and infection through blood transfusions to a minimum and early detection of the infection are some of the achievements of this response. The scope and quality of antenatal care offered by Cuba's healthcare system have facilitated routine testing of all pregnant women at their first antenatal consultation and the provision of specialized care throughout pregnancy of all those who, having tested HIV-positive, have decided to bear children [28].

Of over 3 million pregnant women tested for antibodies to HIV, only 0.0031% has tested positive. A combined strategy including prophylaxis through AZT therapy for both mother and

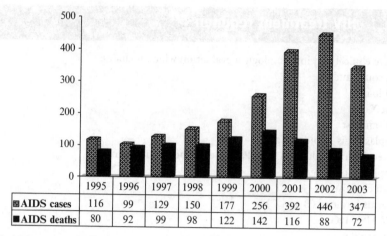

	1995	1996	1997	1998	1999	2000	2001	2002	2003
▦ AIDS cases	116	99	129	150	177	256	392	446	347
■ AIDS deaths	80	92	99	98	122	142	116	88	72

Fig. 25.3 AIDS cases and AIDS deaths per year, 1995–2003. Source: National HIV/AIDS Programme.

child, elective Caesarean section procedures and bottlefeeding of newborns has reduced the risk of transmission to 10% [22].

Universal and free access to HAART since 2001 has had an impact on mortality, which decreased by 18% in 2001, 23% in 2002 and 20% in 2003, with a global reduction in the period 2001–2003 of 44%. Average survival time in patients with HAART has also increased [33] (see Fig. 25.3).

Other results of the treatment programme include a reduction in the numbers hospitalized and the length of their hospitalization, improved well-being and weight gain resulting from treatment, and more people returning to their work or studies [33].

Progress has been made in the educational component of Cuba's strategy, which has also meant an increase in the sale of condoms in the last 5 years. Over 90 million were sold in 2004 [22]. The percentage of people using condoms in their last sexual intercourse with a non-regular partner increased from 22% in 1996 [35] to 54% in 2001, whilst the number of individuals informed about STIs and HIV and aware of preventive and prophylactic methods has grown steadily [35,36].

Conclusion

Cuba has had considerable success in limiting the spread of HIV and in caring for those infected by the virus. Much of this achievement is rooted in the nature of, and the broader achievements of, Cuban healthcare and Cuba's socialist system.

1. Crucial factors in the response to the epidemic have included universal and free healthcare; the priority given to the population's well-being by Cuba's government; the tradition of intersectoral collaboration in solving the population's health problems; and strong organizations and a civil society that is used to participating in health-related issues [29].

2. The family doctor and nurse network, through direct medical and health education services offered to the general public, and the sophisticated epidemiological surveillance and reporting systems have played a decisive role in supporting the HIV programmes.

3. The experience the country had already gained from successfully dealing with other critical epidemics, such as dengue fever, facilitated the prompt implementation of measures to prevent HIV from posing a serious problem to the general health of the population [28,29].

4. A deeply rooted trust and respect for the health service in the community provided the background societal consent for a programme of large-scale HIV testing.

5. The government's pre-investment in a sizeable pharmaceutical research capacity committed to seeking solutions for the nation's most pressing health problems has been crucial in making high-quality treatment and testing financially possible.

The greatest future challenges will be sustaining epidemiological control in a different economic and social context from that of the 1980s, particularly with respect to strengthening the educational interventions in vulnerable social groups. A further challenge under the economic hardships imposed by the US embargo will be to maintain and improve the national production of medicines and reagents to support the excellence of medical care for PLHIV and their universal access to HAART.

References

1. Ministry of Public Health. (1999). *Annual Health Statistics Report.* Havana, Cuba: National Health Statistics Bureau.

2. Krinsky M, Golove D, eds. (1993). *United States Economic Measures Against Cuba.* Northampton, MA: Aletheia Press.

3. Gilpin M. (1991). Update-Cuba: on the road to a family medicine nation. *Journal of Public Health Policy* 12:83–103.

4. Macdonald TH. (1999). *A Developmental Analysis of Cuba's Health Care System Since 1959.* New York: Edwin Mellen Press.

5. Ministry of Public Health. (1991). *Cuba's Family Doctor Programme.* Havana: Ministry of Public Health.

6. Waller J. (2001). A day in the life of a Cuban family doctor. *British Journal of General Practice* 51:244–5.

7. Macdonald TH. (1999). Selection for medical schools in Cuba. *Student British Medical Journal* 7:70–1.

8. Kirkpatrick A. (1996). Role of the USA in shortage of food and medicine in Cuba. *Lancet* **348**: 1489–91.

9. American Association of World Health. (1997). *Denial of Food and Medicine: The Impact of the US Embargo on Health and Nutrition in Cuba.* Washington, DC.

10. Garfield R, Santana S. (1997) The impact of the US embargo on health in Cuba. *American Journal of Public Health* **87**:15–20.

11. Ministry of Public Health. (1993). *Plantas Medicinales.* Havana: Comision Tecnica Fitomed II.

12. Bravo EM. (1998). *Development Within Underdevelopment: New Trends in Cuban Medicine.* Havana: Editorial Jose Marti.

13. Pan American Health Organization. (1999). Cuba: basic country health profile. *Epidemiological Bulletin* 21:No.4.

14. World Bank Development Indicators. (2001).

15. Susser M. (1993). Health as a human right. *American Journal of Public Health* 83:418–26.

16. Waller J. (2002). Cuban health care: healing by primary intention. *Health Matters* 47:17.

17. Waitzkin H, Wald K, Kee R, Danielson R, Robinson L. (1999) Primary care in Cuba: low and high technology developments pertinent to family medicine. *Journal of Family Practice* 45: 250–8.

18. Castro F. (2003). The basic idea is to make primary care services more accessible to the public. Speech published in *Granma International*. 7 April. Havana, Cuba.

19. Veeken H. (1995). Cuba: plenty of care, few condoms, no corruption. *British Medical Journal* 311:935–7.

20. Interreligious Foundation for Community Organization. (2002). *Health Care in Cuba: A Health Care System Dedicated to Health and Healing in Cuba and Throughout the World.* New York.

21. Pilling D. (2001). Cuba's medical revolution. *Financial Times.* January 13. London. p10–11.

22. Cuban Ministry of Public Health. (2004). *Programme for the Prevention and Control of HIV/AIDS: Periodical Informs.* Havana City: Ministry of Public Health, p1–18.

23. Cuban Ministry of Public Health. (1997). *Programme for the Prevention and Control of HIV/AIDS.* Havana City: Ministry of Public Health, p3–27.

24. Cuban Ministry of Public Health. (2002). *National Strategic Plan for the Prevention of HIV/AIDS/STI.* Havana City: Ministry of Public Health, p9–18.

25. Hsieh Y, Arazoza H. (2002). Estimating the number of Cubans infected sexually by human immunodeficiency virus using contact tracing data. *International Journal of Epidemiology* 31: 679–83.

26. Ministry of Public Health. (2002). *National AIDS Programme Annual Report 2002.* Havana: Ministry of Public Health.

27. Cuban Ministry of Public Health. (1995) *Programme for the Prevention and Control of Sexually Transmitted Infections.* Havana City: Ministry of Public Health, p13–8.

28. Farmer P. (2001). Health achievements in perspective: infectious disease in Cuba and Haiti. In: *Seminar on Cuban Health System: Its Evolution, Accomplishments and Challenges.* The David Rockefeller Center for Latin American Studies. Paper No. 02/03-4: A13–16.

29. Scheper-Hughes N. (1993). AIDS, public health, and human rights in Cuba. *Lancet* 342:965–7.

30. Chomsky A. (2000). Health and revolution in Cuba: the threat of a good example. In: Jim Y, Joyce V. Millen A, John G, eds. *Dying for Growth: Global Inequality and the Health of the Poor.* Monroe, ME: Common Courage Press, p320–2.

31. Kuntz D. (1994). The politics of suffering: the impact of the US embargo on the health of the Cuban people: report to the APHA of a fact-finding trip to Cuba. *International Journal of Health Services* 24:161–79.

32. Dalia Acosta. (2001). *Health-Cuba: Guaranteeing Treatment for HIV/AIDS patients.* Inter Press Service. URL: http://www.ips.org/ (accessed August 2003).

33. Pérez J, Pérez D, Gonzalez I, Diaz Jidy M, Orta M. (2004). *Approaches to the Management of HIV/AIDS in Cuba: Case Study.* Geneva: World Health Organization.

34. Castellanos J, Guzmán G. (2001). The production of medicines and Cuba's biotechnology sector. In: *Seminar on Cuban Health System: Its Evolution, Accomplishments and Challenges.* The David Rockefeller Center for Latin American Studies. Paper No. 02/03-4: A26–32.

35. National Statistics Office and Cuban Ministry of Public Health. (1996). Periodical inform. In: *Cuban Populations Sexual Behavioral Survey.* Havana: Ministry of Public Health.

36. National Statistics Office and Cuban Ministry of Public Health. (2001). Periodical inform. In: *Cuban Populations Sexual Behavioral Survey.* Havana: Ministry of Public Health.

Chapter 26

Haiti

Antoine Augustin, Daniel W Fitzgerald* and Jean William Pape

Background

Haiti is a country of 8 million people and 10,000 square miles, sharing the Caribbean island of Hispaniola with the Dominican Republic. Its population is made up primarily of descendants of African slaves, with a small minority of people of European and Middle-Eastern origins. It is the oldest republic in the Western Hemisphere after the USA, and celebrated 200 years of independence in 2004, the result of a successful slave rebellion.

Haiti has a distinguished history of helping establish self-determination for the people of the Americas by first participating in the War of Independence of the USA, then by abolishing slavery on its soil through the first successful slave revolt in the history of the world, by ousting the French from its borders, and by giving military support to Simon Bolivar in his fight against the Spanish. Its own history, however, is one of succeeding dictatorships that have done little to improve the lives of its own citizens. This continued instability has had a major impact on the economic development of the country and on the effectiveness of its health system.

Today, Haiti is mired in poverty, with a gross national product (GNP) that has remained essentially unchanged over the past 20 years at around US$4 billion, while the population has grown by 60% [1–3]. Close to 4% of the GNP, or about US$160 million, is spent on health, with 15% of that amount spent by the public sector. Haiti occupies 153rd position in the UN's Human Development Index [4], and its annual per capita income is estimated at US$450. In constant 1988 dollars, the per capita income fell between 1960 and 2000 [1–3].

The majority of Haitians earn their livelihood directly or indirectly from agriculture, which comprises 22% of the GNP. Tourism, once a thriving industry, is in severe recession. The assembly industry, which provided over 70,000 jobs in the formal sector, was hard hit by the economic embargo that followed the military coup of 1991 and has not fully recovered. In spite of these bleak prospects, Haitians have managed to reduce the level of malnutrition in the country, and mortality rates have fallen in the face of increased poverty.

The health system

Whether the performance of the public health sector can account for these positive changes is a matter of debate. Haiti's health system is divided into three sectors: public facilities accounting

* Corresponding author.

for about 40% of service delivery; private not-for-profit facilities and programmes accounting for another 40%; and private for-profit providers (medical clinics and hospitals) accounting for 20%. As in most countries, the Ministry of Health (MoH) oversees the entire system, licensing practitioners and facilities, promulgating treatment norms, overseeing the sale of pharmaceuticals and defining priorities. In recent years, the Ministry has significantly improved its capacity for overall health sector governance by decentralizing its authority, by elaborating, issuing and disseminating norms of care, by providing strong leadership in the fight against major health priorities such as HIV and tuberculosis (TB), and by improving care at public facilities, leading to their increased utilization. A Charter of Partnership between Public and Private Sectors negotiated by the MoH governs relationships between the private and the public sectors, and efforts have been made through the progressive organization of local health systems to network primary, secondary and tertiary facilities more rationally.

The country has a long way to go to ensure appropriate coverage and equity of care. Nowhere is this more evident than in the issue of maternal health. Close to 60% of the population lives in the countryside [3], and approximately 75% of deliveries take place at home, performed by traditional birth attendants [5]. The major reason for this is the concentration of maternity hospitals, wards and obstetricians in large cities. When an obstetric emergency occurs in a remote village, it is likely to result in death.

Constitutional guarantees notwithstanding, access to services is hindered by a variety of factors, including distance, the direct and opportunity costs of visiting health facilities, as well as user-fees. This translates into low coverage levels for childhood vaccination, with only 34% of children under 1 year completely vaccinated; low rates of contraception, with only 25% of women in union using a modern method of birth control; and low hospital occupancy rates in the face of a dearth of hospital beds. Only a minute segment of the population is privately insured, although all 50,000 government employees are covered. There are 1850 physicians and 1013 nurses in the country. There are only seven hospital beds per 10,000 people, and the national ratio of two physicians per 10,000 people is misleading since most work in the capital city of Port-au-Prince and other large towns. Thus, in some provinces, the ratio of physician to population is 1 per 67,000 people [5]. Services offered by private for-profit physicians, clinics and hospitals vary widely in quality, as regulatory mechanisms are weak. Hospitals run by non-government organizations (NGOs) are generally well supplied and well attended. Public hospitals tend to suffer from limitations in personnel, equipment and supplies, and this has a significant impact on the quality of services provided.

Recent and current developments

During the past decade, the major policy initiative of the Ministry of Health has been to set up approximately 60 local health units in the country (*Unité Communale de Santé*, or UCS), of which 10 are currently functioning according to the norms established by the Ministry. These UCSs were conceived as self-contained units able to provide the majority of services that patients would require. Each local health unit has a referral hospital with the four basic medical specialties (medicine, surgery, obstetrics and paediatrics) and a network of primary care centres equipped mainly for ambulatory care. The major drawback that has significantly slowed down actual implementation of this structure has been a lack of finance. Disbursement of funds from a major loan agreement with the Inter-American Development Bank (IDB) signed in 1997 was held up until recently because of a political stalemate about contested elections between the government of Haiti and various opposition parties. The IDB has since begun the process of releasing funds.

The slow progress in setting up local health systems did not preclude the implementation of major programmes in the areas of nutrition, TB, integrated management of childhood illnesses (IMCI) and HIV. This was made possible through the intensive collaboration of private and public sectors, with major programming and implementation responsibilities assigned by the MoH to various NGOs, including CARE, Catholic Relief Services (CRS), Save the Children (nutrition), International Child Care (TB), Population Services International [PSI–promotion of oral rehydration therapy (ORT)] and Cornell/GHESKIO (*Groupe Haïtien d'Etude sur le Sarcome de Kaposi et les Infections Opportunistes*) (HIV). Haiti was also awarded a grant by the Global Fund to Fight AIDS, Tuberculosis and Malaria (Global Fund). Activities are overseen by a Country Coordination Commission made up of public sector ministries, NGOs, delegates representing church groups, the media, socio-professional organizations, as well as bilateral and multilateral organizations including USAID, French Cooperation, the World Health Organization (WHO), UNICEF, the United Nations Development Programme (UNDP) and the United Nations Fund for Population Assistance (UNFPA). Funds from the Global Fund are being disbursed through an innovative grant management system that employs the services of a foundation affiliated with the biggest bank in Haiti as well as the UNDP.

Performance

Haiti is considered by the UN Food and Agriculture Organization (FAO) to be the third most 'food insecure' country in the world [6]. Ten years ago, Haiti occupied 11th place in the FAO ranking [1]. Yet, between the years 1990 and 2000, levels of childhood malnutrition fell (Table 26.1).

During the same period, the prevalence of a number of diseases seems to have decreased: diarrhoea prevalence fell from 42% in 1995 to 26% in 2000, and the prevalence of acute respiratory infections similarly fell. Child mortality rates fell from 204 per 1000 in 1975–1980 to 119 per 1000 in 1995–2000, and infant mortality declined from 137 per 1000 to 80 per 1000 in the same periods [8,9].

Many factors contributed to these decreases, including the organization of a number of localized, population-based health systems where the entire population is registered and followed prospectively according to a pioneering model initially developed at the Albert Schweitzer Hospital. That model has been adopted by close to 40 other institutions, with catchment areas varying from 50,000 to 200,000 people. Another reason may be the continuing availability of Title II PL480 resources, food donated by the US Government that is either sold for cash to finance various development projects or distributed in kind to various beneficiaries.

Table 26.1 Nutritional status of children under 5 years of age, 1990–2000

	1990	1995	2000
Percentage with chronic malnutrition	34	32	23
Percentage with acute malnutrition	5	8	4.5
Percentage underweight	27	28	17

Source: [7].

For the past 20 years, the programme has provided the country with between 60,000 and 100,000 tons of concessional food per year, distributed through community and institutional channels to vulnerable populations.

Another important intervention has been the use of ORT for children evaluated for dehydration and diarrhoea. Initiated at the State University Hospital (*Hôpital de l'Université d'Etat d'Haïti*), the country's largest hospital, by the Cornell-GHESKIO team, this intervention led to a decrease in the in-hospital case fatality rate for diarrhoea-associated dehydration from over 45% during the decade 1969–1979 to less than 1% after the first year of the project. From 1979 to 2000, over 160,000 children were treated and 13,000 health personnel trained throughout the country. As parents stayed with their hospitalized children, they took part in their care and were trained to prepare ORT. They were taught to recognize early signs of dehydration and instructed in the proper methods to avoid contaminated water. Convinced parents have become the best promoters of ORT. From over 9000 children per year admitted in the early years, which amounted to three times the total number of children admitted in paediatrics, fewer than 200 were admitted in the year 2000, and the unit was closed that same year.

Future developments

The progress of the local health systems (UCSs) illustrates a major challenge faced by the Haitian health system in its attempt to increase coverage and decrease mortality and morbidity. The system still looks somewhat like a mosaic, with high-coverage areas adjoining low-supply zones. Many, but not all, of the high-coverage programmes are run by NGOs that are privileged in that they receive grants from bilateral donors, principally, while other areas have to depend on meagre public resources. To match the level of expenditures found in these donor-aided programmes, the MoH would need to augment its budget by at least 50% and assign this increase exclusively for this purpose. For the foreseeable future, this seems an unlikely prospect.

The challenge to identify a proper mix of financing strategies for the health sector is hampered by the deep, pervasive poverty of Haitian households. Many Haitians might be able to afford to finance cost recovery schemes along the lines of the Bamako Initiative, i.e. through the setting up of village-based fee-for-service payment schemes to support health centres, if payments were limited to low-cost interventions and essential drugs. However, out-of-pocket payments for more complex care, including hospitalization, are beyond the financial capacity of most people. Preliminary indications are that some type of local area community-based financing schemes might be more appropriate than a national centrally run system. Currently, the procurement of essential drugs is based on a revolving fund strategy whereby drugs are bought on the international market by a central processing facility and then sold to service delivery institutions with a small mark-up. These institutions, in turn, sell drugs to their customers. The proceeds of sales keep the system going.

The public–private mix in the provision of health services is likely to continue, but one may anticipate a strengthening of public sector facilities with the resumption of multilateral donor agency funding, particularly from the IDB. Barring unforeseen developments such as a major change in public policy as to how healthcare should be provided, the private non-profit sector is likely to continue receiving funding from bilateral organizations. Under the US President's Emergency Plan for AIDS Relief (PEPFAR), allocation of funds to this sector should increase significantly and contribute to an expansion of the fight against HIV.

The use of market incentives may be important in the for-profit sector, where a number of small hospital facilities, many offering lower-cost services, have multiplied in large cities. This phenomenon affects only a limited segment of the population, the one capable of paying the requisite fees. However, for certain commodities such as condoms and oral rehydration salts, a social marketing approach will continue whereby goods subsidized by donors are sold to the public and some of the costs are recovered from consumers.

In terms of technology, Haiti has been a leader in the field of HIV. Over the next few years, one would expect new developments in the application of diagnostic and therapeutic tools within the context of resource-poor settings. Haitian researchers will explore new rapid testing algorithms for HIV, as well as new, simple, rapid and inexpensive tests using whole blood for syphilis, a major cofactor for HIV infection, simpler determination of viral load and new vaccines against HIV.

These new developments are designed to strengthen the capacity of individual institutions to improve the standard of services they offer and link institutions within efficient referral networks across various localized health systems. In the limited number of sites where the UCSs are functioning well, access to healthcare has generally improved. Within this context, the setting up of community health councils is slated to make health providers more accountable to the population. This aspect of the implementation of the UCS programme has lagged behind, but there are indications that it will pick up again as IDB funds become available to set up additional local health systems.

The HIV epidemic

The HIV epidemic in Haiti was recognized soon after the first cases of AIDS were reported in the USA by the US Centers for Disease Control and Prevention (CDC). A retrospective review of autopsy reports and pathology specimens documented the first case of AIDS in Haiti to be a 19-year-old man who died of toxoplasmosis of the brain in 1978. Haitian physicians reported the first description of patients with AIDS in a tropical developing country in 1983 [10].

Haiti has a generalized HIV epidemic, with approximately 3% of the adult population infected. It has the highest rates of HIV infection in the Americas and the highest rates anywhere outside Africa. A 1985 sero-survey showed that HIV infection was associated with men who reported exchanging sex for money with male tourists to the island [11–13]. In this 1983 survey, 65% of all men with AIDS reported a history of sexual contact with men. HIV quickly spread to the urban heterosexual population, and the male-to-female ratio approached 1:1 by 1990 [13,14]. For heterosexual men, the greatest risk for HIV was through contact with a female sex worker. In 1987, 65% of female sex workers on the streets were HIV-infected. For heterosexual women, the greatest risks were exchanging sex for money, sexual contact with a partner with AIDS, and a history of blood transfusions. Forty per cent of women infected with HIV early in the Haitian epidemic reported receiving a blood transfusion from a commercial blood bank, which was closed in 1986. The first AIDS cases occurred among people living in Port-au-Prince, and particularly Carrefour, a neighborhood with a large red-light district. In the early 1990s, the epidemic spread to rural Haiti, with prevalence rates in some rural areas approximating those in urban areas. The rapid spread of HIV in the urban and rural heterosexual population was accelerated by high rates of other sexually transmitted infections

(STIs), including syphilis, gonorrhea and chlamydia [15]. In 2000, it was estimated that 65% of HIV-infected people lived in the West department, where the capital is located.

Heterosexual transmission rates from sexually active HIV-infected adults to their spouses have been reported at 5.4 infections per 100 follow-up years [16]. Vertical HIV transmission from HIV-infected mothers to their children is estimated at 30 infections per 100 live births [17]. Recent national seroprevalence studies suggest that national rates of HIV have declined from levels around 6.2% in 1993 to 3.1% in 2003 [18], although the WHO/UNAIDS estimates for 2003 ranged between 2.5 and 11.9%. The same surveys showed a similar decrease in serological syphilis. In 2000, Haiti had an estimated 250,000 people living with HIV (PLHIV) and 50,000 deaths each year from HIV [19]. An estimated 4000 newborns are infected with HIV annually, and there are 200,000 AIDS orphans in Haiti. The latest WHO/UNAIDS estimates varied between 120,000 and 600,000 HIV-infected people alive.

HIV disease in Haiti has progressed rapidly and is associated with high rates of TB and other tropical co-infections. A prospective cohort study was conducted in Port-au-Prince of 42 adult patients with documented dates of HIV seroconversion [20]. Patients were treated for bacterial, mycobacterial, parasitic and fungal infections, but antiretroviral therapy (ART) was not available at the time of this study. Among the 28 people who developed AIDS, the AIDS-defining illnesses were TB in nine (32%), wasting syndrome in eight (28%), a CD4 count less than 200 in four (14%), candida oesophagitis in two (7%), chronic diarrhoea from enteric spore-forming protozoa in two (7%), and other opportunistic infections in three patients. The median time to AIDS (CDC category C) was 5.2 years, and the median time from infection to death was 7.4 years. HIV disease progression in Haiti was nearly twice as fast as progression observed in the USA in the pre-antiretroviral era. It was postulated that rapid HIV disease progression in Haiti was due to malnutrition and interactions between HIV and TB or other tropical co-infections.

Prospective cohort studies of children born to HIV-infected mothers before antiretroviral prevention and therapy demonstrated a similar rapid disease progression in HIV-infected children. The median survival of newborns infected with HIV in Haiti was less than 6 months, with HIV-infected children frequently dying of a sepsis syndrome of unknown aetiology [17,21,22].

The HIV epidemic has had important effects on the economy: because Haitians were branded as a special risk group by the CDC, this contributed to the destruction of the tourism industry in the early 1980s. Because so many Haitians are unemployed, it is difficult to assess the effect of the epidemic on the supply of labour. Similarly, it is difficult to assess to what extent the epidemic strained the resources of the health system as a whole, although, for specific families that were affected, the disease meant financial ruin, either because of the expenses the family incurred for the treatment of the infected individual, or because many breadwinners succumbed to the disease.

The health system response

The HIV epidemic was recognized and defined very early in its course in Haiti, and a coordinated public and private response was quickly mounted. For example, a local non-governmental research institution, GHESKIO, recognized that HIV infection in Haiti was associated with receiving a blood transfusion from a for-profit blood bank and informed the Haitian Ministry of Health in 1986. The Ministry closed all for-profit blood banks and placed the blood supply under the control of the Haitian Red Cross. Based on evidence of more recent sero-surveys, receiving a blood transfusion in Haiti is no longer a risk for HIV.

There have been many other examples of private and public partnerships in Haiti. A large national education campaign by the public and private sectors increased public knowledge of HIV. The programme began in the mid-1980s and is ongoing. Today, 95% of Haitian adults have heard of AIDS. Condom availability has increased through social marketing, with condom sales increasing from less than 1 million units in 1992 to over 15 million in 2002. National syndromic treatment algorithms for STIs were developed based upon local data, and thousands of public and private healthcare workers were trained in their use. Religious leaders conducted AIDS education through church organizations. This early public–private response to the epidemic may explain why prevalence rates for HIV decreased between 1993 and 2003, when many experts had predicted a doubling of the prevalence rate. The existence of public–private partnerships culminated in the receipt of a Global Fund award of US$67 million in 2002. The country coordinating mechanism (CCM) has representatives from government, civil society, non-governmental service providers, academic centres, religious groups, donor agencies and people with AIDS.

The process of setting up UCSs throughout the country will result in an expansion of integrated HIV care and prevention services. These services should include HIV voluntary counselling and testing (VCT); HIV care, including ART; prevention of mother-to-child transmission (PMTCT); management of sexually transmitted diseases; screening and treatment for TB; and reproductive health services. Such models of integrated HIV services, including provision of highly active antiretroviral therapy (HAART), have already been successfully developed in Haiti [23]. Funds from the Global Fund, PEPFAR and various donors (Canada, France, IDB, etc.), as well as multilateral contributions from various UN agencies, will cover the costs of programme expansion, at least for the next 5 years.

A Haitian HIV training network has been formed. The GHESKIO centre in Port-au-Prince, in partnership with the MoH, is providing training in integrated HIV prevention and care services to public and private health centres in each of Haiti's 10 health departments. These departmental 'centres of excellence' will then supervise other primary care centres in their geographical areas. To date, there are 76 VCT sites, 55 sites offering PMTCT and 21 sites providing HAART. This expansion of HIV care and prevention services is being coordinated with public education and awareness campaigns to mobilize communities and encourage people to seek HIV services. Again, diverse members of the public and private sectors are involved in this public campaign, including government officials, artists, journalists, PLHIV and religious leaders. This training network will allow rapid scale-up of services. It will also provide a systematic way for guidelines to be updated and implemented at a national level.

Existing resources (Global Fund, PEPFAR, the Canadian International Development Agency (CIDA), French Cooperation, the Inter-American Development Bank, the Pan American Health Organization (PAHO), WHO, UNICEF, UNFPA and UNDP) are being used to finance activities in prevention and to develop a pilot model for case management of patients with AIDS in a selected area of Haiti (the Central Plateau). These activities are guided by a National Strategic Plan to Fight AIDS, adopted in 2001. The plan focuses on three components: the reduction of the risk of HIV infection; the reduction of vulnerability to HIV; and the reduction of the impact of HIV.

Under risk-reduction, programmes to change behaviour, encourage safe sex and distribute condoms nationwide have been set up by most agencies involved with HIV in Haiti. PSI has received significant support from the Global Fund and USAID to promote and sell condoms. Most health facilities are now able to treat STIs, while some offer services to prevent MTCT, currently reaching about 20% of pregnant women, with funding from CDC, USAID, UNICEF and UNFPA. As noted above, GHESKIO, with Global Fund and USAID resources, set up 27 VCT centres around the country, and Partners in Health, six new rural centres. To these should be added centres that were made operational by the MARCH Foundation, PSI and other organizations, so that by the end of 2004, over 40 VCT sites were operational. Finally, high-risk groups such as female sex workers and men who have sex with men have been targeted for interventions. In 2003, close to US$18 million was spent on HIV in Haiti, and this figure rose to US$40 million for fiscal year 2004–2005. Taking into account planned donor contributions, there will be an estimated gap of US$90 million between available resources and what is needed over the next 4 years. At this time, it is difficult to see how this gap can be filled from domestic resources. The country's annual health budget does not exceed US$30 million.

Vulnerability reduction activities focus primarily on factors that could lead youth and women, and especially young women, to unsafe sex. These include economic factors, inadequate capacity for sex negotiation and emotional immaturity. A number of organizations such as FOSREF (*Fondation pour la Santé Reproductive des Femmes*) and VDH (*Volontariat pour le Développement d'Haïti*) (youth); the MARCH Foundation (young women); *Konesans fanmi* (women and families); and *Promoter Zero Sida* (POZ) (PLHIV) have empowerment programmes for young women, income generation activities and peer-to-peer support networks. Over 500,000 youth are now being reached.

The impact reduction component comprises activities in treatment, mitigation and stigma reduction. Four centres now offer combination ART: GHESKIO, the Cange Hospital in the Central Plateau of Haiti, the MARCH Foundation and the Salvation Army medical centre. Almost 3000 patients were under combination ART as of October 2004 out of an estimated 42,000 needing therapy according to WHO/UNAIDS. These centres also offer comprehensive community-based support services for these patients as well as for other HIV-infected individuals, and their efforts are complemented by those of other NGOs such as CARE, POZ, the Albert Schweitzer Hospital and some PLHIV organizations such as the Boucicault Foundation, GIPA (Great Implication of People with AIDS) and ASON (*Association Nationale des Personnes Vivant avec le VIH*).

HIV activities are being monitored and evaluated through a variety of mechanisms: periodic seroprevalence surveys of pregnant women seen at sentinel sites, the last one in 2003; periodic behaviour surveys, the most recent one conducted in 2003; routine service statistics provided by HIV service providers, many of them audited by an independent technical review organization, the *Institut Haïtien de l'Enfance* (IHE); and ongoing proactive site visits and data collection performed by IHE at all PMTCT sites.

Conclusion

There is much that can be learned from the experience in Haiti that is relevant both to the HIV epidemic response and to broader health issues in other similar countries. Haiti has demonstrated that effective services can be implemented despite political unrest and limited financial support. Haiti has had 14 governments in 18 years, but the political commitment to fight HIV has been a constant: the HIV epidemic was recognized and defined very early in its course in Haiti, and a coordinated public and private response was quickly mounted. This response would have been unsuccessful were it not for the effective participation of the private health sector and the recognition of the importance of public and private philanthropic partnerships. This was evidenced by Haiti's successful Global Fund application, which was the result of close collaboration between the public and private sectors in Haiti

Early on, the design of interventions was based on locally available data. This highlights the importance of having local research capacity to inform decision making. For example, epidemiological data in 1985 about blood banks and their role in HIV transmission led to effective measures in this regard. Also, epidemiological data from GHESKIO indicated that risk factors among Haitians with AIDS were comparable with those among similar patients in the USA, prompting the CDC to remove Haitians from the '4 H category' (homosexuals, heroin addicts, haemophiliacs, Haitians) in 1985 [24]. The GHESKIO research infrastructure made it possible to provide antiretroviral care to patients through the availability of viral load testing, CD4 counts and culture for mycobacterium, including the BACTEC™ method.

The association of Haitian centres with foreign institutions (USA, France, and Canada) provided capacity building for research and training. Aside from the association of GHESKIO with Cornell University and the French Fondation Rodolphe Mérieux, one could also note that of Partners in Health/Zanmi Lasanté with Harvard University and that of the MARCH Foundation with Tulane University. These three institutions have implemented innovative service delivery approaches worth replicating, including the following:

1. The hub concept of coordinated care, the hub being a central facility offering VCT and antiretroviral services, as well as technical, referral, logistical, managerial and clinical support to satellite facilities that may be health facilities, youth centres, centres for female sex workers, etc. The hub is linked to other hubs via the Internet to exchange information, compare notes and keep abreast of new developments. At present, only one hub is functional, that of Partners in Health/Zanmi Lasanté (PIH/ZL) in the Central Plateau.

2. DOT/HAART. Building on its directly observed therapy (DOT) protocol for TB, PIH/ZL used funding from the Global Fund to apply this experience to combination ART. This successful experience is being replicated in other parts of rural Haiti.

3. Mobile VCT. The MARCH Foundation has developed a successful model of bringing VCT services to remote populations that would be unlikely to seek such services at fixed facilities because of the distance. Rapid tests are used, and test results given on the spot. This experience is being replicated in other areas of Haiti where road access to fixed facilities is problematic.

4. The use of clinical algorithms to treat and follow patients on combination therapy. GHESKIO has developed useful clinical algorithms to simplify and facilitate the treatment of advanced HIV disease based on signs and symptoms and readily available laboratory tests such as the lymphocyte count. The algorithms will be validated further and disseminated.

These innovations and other advances rely on an appropriate level of training capacity. In Haiti, the GHESKIO centres piloted a successful programme to prevent MTCT. After documenting the success of this model, GHESKIO was able to train thousands of healthcare workers across the country in its application. Training is an integral part of GHESKIO's mission. Over 7000 people, including 4000 health personnel, have been trained in HIV prevention and care. GHESKIO training and research capabilities have helped in the development of national training guidelines for HIV prevention and care.

It is also important to elicit the participation not only of health workers, but also of organized groups of individuals, such as religious leaders and PLHIV. Haiti has had several dynamic religious leaders who have worked with churches across the country to strengthen churches' roles in HIV care and prevention. In a country with a paucity of infrastructure, all influential organizations need to be working together against the epidemic. As for PLHIV, they constitute a group of committed soldiers in the fight against AIDS. They are now beginning to organize, and their effectiveness will grow as more join these organizations.

Finally, Haiti is not unique in showing that HIV care and prevention must work together. While some view HIV care and HIV prevention as opposing programmes vying for limited resources, Haiti's stated policy is that prevention and care are synergistic and, forged together, will be a powerful weapon in the fight against AIDS in Haiti and in many other developing countries.

References

1. Augustin A, Van Bokkelen A *et al.* (1992). *Haiti: Nutrition and Food Security.* CAPS. Port-au-Prince: Editions de l'Enfance.

2. Banque de la République d'Haïti. (2003). *Rapport Annuel 2003.*

3. Institut Haïtien de Statistiques et d'Informatique. (2003). *Recensement Général de la Population, Résultats Préliminaires.*

4. United Nations Development Programme. *Human Development Index, 2004.*

5. Ministère de la Santé Publique et de la Population. (2004). *Plan Stratégique National pour la Réforme du Secteur Santé (Octobre 2003–Septembre 2008).* Port-au-Prince: MoH.

6. Demographic and Health Survey. (2001). *Enquête Mortalité, Morbidité et Utilisation des Services (DHS) 2000.* Institut Haïtien de l'Enfance. Port-au-Prince: ORC Macro.

7. Demographic and Health Survey (1995; 2000). *Haiti's Nutrition Situation, 1990.* Port-au-Prince: DHS.

8. US Centers for Disease Control and Prevention, Institut Haïtien de l'Enfance, Ministère de la Santé Publique et de la Population, Pan American Health Organization and United States Agency for International Development. (1993). *Haiti's Nutrition Situation in 1990.* Port-au-Prince.

9. Food and Agriculture organization (FAO). (2004). *L'Etat d'Insecurité Alimentaire dans le Monde 2003.* Rome: FAO.

10. Enquête Mortalité, Morbidité et Utilisation des Services (DHS) 1995. (1995). Institut Haïtien de l'Enfance. Port-au-Prince: ORC Macro.

11. Pape JW, Liautaud B, Thomas F *et al.* (1983). Characteristics of the acquired immunodeficiency syndrome (AIDS) in Haiti. *New England Journal of Medicie* 309:945–50.

12. Pape JW, Liautaud B, Thomas F *et al.* (1986). Risk factors associated with AIDS in Haiti. *American Journal of Medical Science* 291(1):4–7.

13. Pape JW, Stanback ME, Pamphile M *et al.* (1990). Prevalence of HIV infection and high-risk activities in Haiti. *Journal of Acquired Immune Deficiency Syndrome* 3:995–1001.

14. Pape J, Johnson WD. (1993). AIDS in Haiti: 1982–1992. *Clinical Infectious Diseases* 17(Supplement 2): S341 – 5.

15. Behets F, Desormeaux J, Joseph D. (1995). Control of sexually transmitted diseases in Haiti: results and implications of a baseline study among pregnant women living in Cité Soleil shantytowns. *Journal of Infectious Diseases* 172:764–1.

16. Fitzgerald DW, Behets F, Roberfroid D, Lucet C, Fitzgerld JW, Kuykens L. (2000). Economic hardship and sexually transmitted diseases in Haiti's Artibonite Valley. *American Journal of Tropical Medicine and Hygiene* 62:496–501.

17. Deschamps MM, Pape JW, Hafner A, Johnson WD. (1996). Heterosexual transmission of HIV in Haiti. *Annals of Internal Medicine* 125:324–30.

18. Ministère de la Santé Publique et de la Population, Institut Haïtien de l'Enfance, Centres GHESKIO, US Centers for Disease Control and Prevention. (2004). *Etude de Séroprévalence par Méthode Sentinelle de la Prévalence du VIH, de la Syphilis, de l'Hépatite B et de l'Hépatite C chez les Femmes Enceintes en Haïti 2003/2004.* Port-au-Prince.

19. UNAIDS. Haiti: Epidemiological fact sheet. Accessed at www.unaids.org January 2003.

20. Deschamps MM, Fitzgerald DW, Pape JW, Johnson WD Jr. (2000). HIV infection in Haiti: natural history and disease progression. *AIDS* 14:2515–21.

21. Pape JW, Johnson WD Jr. (1989). Perinatal transmission of the human immunodeficiency virus. *Bulletin of the Pan American Health Organization* 23:50–61.

22. Jean SS, Pape JW, Verdier RI. (1999). The natural history of human immunodeficiency virus 1 infection in Haitian infants. *Pediatric Infectious Diseases* 18:58–63.

23. Jean SS, Reed JW, Verdier RI, Pape JW, Johnson WD Jr, Wright PF. (1997) Clinical manifestations of human immunodeficiency virus infection in Haitian children. *Pediatric Infectious Diseases* 16:600–6.

24. Ministère de la Santé Publique et de la Population. (2004). *Manuel de Normes de Prise en Charge Clinique et Thérapeutique des Personnes Vivant avec le VIH.* Port-au-Prince: MoH.

Chapter 27

Jamaica

Robert Carr[*], J Peter Figueroa and Peter R Carr

Background

Jamaica is an island nation located in the Caribbean Sea approximately 90 miles south of Cuba and 100 miles west of Haiti. It is the largest of the English-speaking countries in the Caribbean, with a total area of 11,244 km^2. Rugged mountainous terrain, running the length of the island, accounts for approximately 80% of its surface area. A large proportion of the population lives on the plains, and most of the main economic activities occur in the coastal areas. Jamaica is subject to flooding that follows torrential rains, hurricanes and frequent tropical storms, and is vulnerable to earthquakes.

Jamaica's natural environment is rich in resources such as bauxite, although it is not an oil-producing country. The island has one of the largest selections of native flora and fauna in the world and is renowned for the physical beauty of its beaches and mountains. The country has a good network of roads, allowing for easy communication and mobility. This is supported by air transport to important population centres within the country. Physical infrastructure, including roads and water supply, continues to receive priority attention from the government. Many communities in both urban and rural areas still experience occasional disruptions in the electricity and water supply. Jamaica has a vibrant culture and is known internationally for its music, art, drama and cuisine as well as for its world-class athletes and high-quality professionals.

A former colony of Britain, Jamaica gained its independence in 1962 and is governed through a Westminster-style parliamentary system, with a Senate and House of Representatives. The central government is responsible for health, education, defence, security, justice, monetary and fiscal policy as well as development planning. The local government system, administered by councils in each of 13 administrative units called parishes, shares responsibility with the central government for roads and works, water supplies, public health, relief for the poor, and fire brigade services.

In 2001, the population of the island was 2.6 million, with an annual growth rate of 0.6% reflecting a high rate of migration, with 21,700 people leaving Jamaica in that year. The population of Jamaica is equally distributed between urban and rural areas, with approximately 43% of the population living in the capital city and its environs, the Kingston Metropolitan Area (KMA). The increase in urbanization can be attributed to better economic and social conditions and opportunities, lower rates of poverty and greater access to economic opportunities in the KMA, coupled with a decline in rural agricultural production.

* Corresponding author.

As a result, Kingston has a number of 'slum' areas in which migrants from rural areas as well as inner-city people live in harsh conditions, and sometimes extreme poverty.

According to the *Jamaica Survey of Living Conditions 1998*, which included a special module on poverty, the private poverty line 'has tended to fall within the third consumption quintile', meaning that some three-fifths of the country's population are classified as poor [1]. The 2002 *Survey* cited the incidence of absolute poverty at 19.7% of households in Jamaica, with absolute poverty defined as the inability to achieve regular consumption of a minimum nutritional food basket per person per household [2]. This means that in 2002, an estimated 20% of Jamaicans were unable to meet their basic nutritional needs, an increase from 17% in 2001. On the whole, poverty in Jamaica is also consistently greatest in rural areas [2]. As a measure of inequality at the national level, the Gini coefficient (0–1) for 2002 was 0.3986, up from 0.3843 in 2001, marking an increase in societal inequality for the period. The 2002 *Survey* reported that since 'persons in the lower deciles account for [increasingly] less of national consumption, it becomes harder for the poor to achieve the minimum consumption level required to exit poverty' [3]. In absolute terms, in 2001, the wealthiest 20% of the population spent over 50 times more on items that provide relatively indirect benefits than the poorest 20% of the population [3].

The demographic profile of the population has seen some changes over the last three decades. The proportion of children under 14 years of age fell from 34% of the total population in 1991 to 31% in 2001. By 2020, the under-14 population is projected to fall to 23%. There was also a rise in the number of elderly in the population, though Jamaica remains essentially youthful, with 62% of its population aged 15–64 years. State agencies such as the Planning Institute of Jamaica and the Statistical Institute of Jamaica report a general aging of the Jamaican population [2].

Migration is an important reason for the changing demographic profile of the island. Migration brings both negative and positive consequences for the country, such as the loss of skilled workers and professionals. Of particular concern has been the impact of migration for children whose parents go abroad. On the one hand, substantial remittances to care for those children left behind bring positive financial gains to the country; on the other hand, migration may also have an adverse impact on family cohesion, which may result in emotional or material deprivation of children who may subsequently become wards of the state. These children may exhibit antisocial behaviours such as drug abuse and irresponsible sexual or criminal behaviours. Some of these negative consequences are also seen in response to internal migration, which usually manifests itself as a steady movement of unskilled or semi-skilled labour to urban areas, in search of economic opportunities.

Jamaica is very dependent on tourism as its main source of income. Bauxite, agriculture and light manufacturing play smaller but important roles in the country's economy, which has seen slow growth since the first half of the 1990s. In 2001, real gross domestic product (GDP) grew by 1.7% and increased another 1% in 2002 [4]. However, the island has had single-digit inflation since 1997, with the rate at 7% in 2002—down from a high of 77% in 1992—the longest single-digit inflation run since the 1960s. On the other hand, the country has experienced high interest rates, declining real revenues and a rapidly growing public, largely internal, debt. The public debt rose to 147% of GDP at the end of 2002, 60% of which was domestic debt. Debt servicing accounted for 36% of GDP in 2002, down from 42% in 2001. Despite the adverse economic climate, government continues to place priority on health and education services.

Between 1995 and 1999, expenditure in the health and education sectors increased by 26% and 40%, respectively. In real terms, however, per capita spending on health increased marginally, from J$1531 (US$43) in 1995/1996 to J$1864 (US$45) in 1999/2000. During the same period, per capita spending on education also increased from J$3387 (US$95) in 1995/1996 to J$4593 (US$110) in 1999/2000. For its size and stage of development, this represents a sizeable investment in education and health by Jamaica. In fiscal year 2001/2002, the government allocated 11% of its budget to education and 7% to health. Government spending is skewed to the secondary and tertiary provision of both healthcare (67%) and education (50%), reflecting the traditionally high cost of providing services at these levels.

The national data show that in the academic year 2001/2002, the gross enrolment rates in the public education system for the pre-primary (3–5 years) and primary (6–11 years) levels were 92% and 97%, respectively. Enrolment at the secondary level was 89%, and at the post-secondary (community colleges, vocational schools, etc.) and tertiary (university) levels combined was 15% [4]. The adult literacy rate was 80% in 2000, up substantially from 47% in 1975 and 68% in 1987 [5,6].

According to 2002 data, the labour force participation averaged 73% for men compared with 55% for women [4]. As these data take into account only people looking for work, the bleakness of the labour market becomes evident. Unemployment for women (21%) was almost double that of men (11%). This shows up in the analyses of living conditions, where the majority of households living in poverty were headed by women, and women-headed households showed consistently low levels of per capita consumption [2]. This is despite the fact that women make up 71% of university students, dominating every discipline except engineering (85% male) and agriculture (59% male) in 2000. Women earn less than men do, partly because more women have lower-paying jobs and partly because they are paid less than men for the same job [6]. Women who are poor perceive that high female unemployment results in greater dependency on a man for income and that increased dependency increases domestic violence [7].

Almost half (46%) of all working-age youth are unemployed, with the highest unemployment rates among those who did not complete their secondary education. Teenagers who are out of school and out of work have few skills, and many are illiterate [8] and more vulnerable to antisocial behaviours, violence and drug abuse.

Although the levels of crime and violence are high, the crime rate is in fact declining. While the solution rate for crime overall was 80% in 2001, the annual murder rate remains very high at 43 per 100,000 [9]. Violence is primarily concentrated in low-income urban areas, with 72% of all murders taking place in the KMA, and 98% of those arrested for major crimes are men [4]. Violence also results in large numbers of wounds that require hospital care.

Health indicators have been reasonably stable over the past 5 years [10]. In 2001, the crude birth rate was 21.2 per 1000 population and the crude death rate 6.6 per 1000 population. Life expectancy at birth was 72 years. The maternal mortality rate was 111 per 100,000 live births, and the infant mortality rate was 24.5 per 1000 live births. The leading causes of death in 2001 were cardiovascular diseases, followed by cancer. In ambulatory care, respiratory tract infections, hypertension and diabetes were among the leading reasons for visits.

The health system

Structure and organization

The health system comprises a public and private health sector, with the private sector focusing more on ambulatory care and pharmaceutical and diagnostic services, while the public sector has 90% of the hospital beds and a vast network of health centres strategically located throughout the country. The current public health system is the product of a health reform process that was started in 1972 and continues. The system is hierarchical, with primary care delivered at the lowest level of the system, secondary care at hospital level, and tertiary care at the specialized hospital level. At present, public primary care services are provided through a network of approximately 345 health centres scattered across the country. Secondary care services are provided in 24 public hospitals that deliver different levels of care depending on the facility type: at the lowest level, there are 11 'type C' hospitals, strategically located in parishes outside the capital, which provide basic hospital services; these are supported by four 'type B' hospitals that provide a more comprehensive level of hospital care and act as referral centres for the type C hospitals; the highest level of hospital care is provided at three 'type A' hospitals, and these are supported by six specialist hospitals that offer specialist services for children, mentally ill patients, chest conditions, rehabilitation, palliative care and those in need of obstetric services. One of the type A hospitals is the University Hospital of the West Indies, which provides the advanced care feasible at a training institution for medical doctors and other health professionals.

Decentralization of government healthcare services is a major component of the health reform programme and has resulted in the establishment of four health regions responsible for the delivery of health services within their geographical areas. In each of these regions, a Regional Health Authority (RHA) has been established, managed by a Regional Board, with responsibility for human, material and financial resources in the region. Each health region consists of a group of parishes that make up the geographical boundaries of the local government system; these parishes report to the RHA for that region. The network of hospitals that fall within each region is under the authority of its respective RHA. However, within the parishes, the hospital and health centre services are integrated under the management of a parish manager. All public health facilities remain the property of the government of Jamaica.

Currently, the Ministry of Health is responsible for setting policy and standards, strategic planning, negotiating finances for the health sector and contracting with the RHAs to provide specific services for the population in the regions they serve. Responsibility for the day-to-day administration of health services, as well as supervision and the maintenance of standards and delivery of services, is contracted to the RHAs.

Moving from a centrally managed system in which the Ministry of Health was funder, purchaser and provider of public health services, with centralized control over financial management, human resource management and healthcare delivery, to a system in which the provider functions are now under the control of four RHAs has resulted in a profound change in the role and function of the Ministry. The emphasis at central level is now on governance of the health system and playing a steering role. This involves national policy and planning issues, quality assurance programmes and protocols to guide the delivery of services, and establishment of standards and regulations for both the public and private health sectors.

It has also resulted in the development and implementation of Annual Service Agreements with each RHA to guide the provision of health services to the public and the establishment of management and technical audit systems to monitor the quality and quantity of services delivered.

In keeping with the present health profile of the country, the state's emphasis is increasingly on health promotion and preventive care at the primary care level, with a strong emphasis on healthy lifestyles to address widespread chronic diseases such as diabetes, hypertension and obesity. The Ministry of Health is responsible for setting national goals and targets as well as attracting funds from external sources. It also formulates strategic plans to guide the development of the health sector, and a range of strategic plans for each programme area has been developed. Notable among these is the HIV/AIDS/STI National Strategic Plan (2002) and the Strategic Mental Health Plan 2001–2006.

Financing

The financing of the health system was one of the major factors pushing the health reform process and remains a challenge today. The RHAs came into being with a debt burden they were obligated to manage and a budget allotted to them by the Ministry of Health on the basis of Annual Service Agreements. As Jamaica's economy experiences marginal growth and costs for healthcare escalate, there is increasing pressure on the RHAs to collect user-fees at the point of service to meet targets set under these service agreements. Cost recovery through user-fees increased from a little more than 1% at the beginning of the 1990s to approximately 10% of the health budget in 2000 [10]. A means test is used to determine whether clients of the system are able to pay, but there are reports from both staff and patients that this system is not functioning as intended and that some who cannot afford to pay are being denied service, whereas those who can afford to pay are able to access care at a very nominal fee.

Issues such as coverage and quality of service remain a challenge at RHA level, given the high standards that are set for the health services centrally. In some instances, decentralization has resulted in more immediate attention to the demands of the public than was previously the norm. At the same time, the RHAs face challenges meeting the needs of the public within budget while maintaining Ministry standards, and struggle to finance themselves and manage their debt. Budgetary constraints at the level of central government contribute to the pressure on the RHAs to collect more revenue in user-fees while ensuring that no one is denied service because of inability to pay.

Human resources

At present, there are approximately 11,600 people employed in the government health system. This includes a wide variety of professional staff such as medical specialists, medical doctors, registered nurses, midwives, pharmacists, radiographers and health administrators. The Ministry of Health spends approximately 75% of its budget on salaries. All these professional staff are certified and accredited by the appropriate legal organization to function within the health services of Jamaica. These professionals are distributed throughout the government health system, with specialist staff located at the hospital levels and a network of registered nurses, medical doctors, midwives and others staffing the public health clinics across the island. Nevertheless, human resource management remains a major challenge for the health services, particularly in relation to the attraction and retention of professional staff (Table 27.1). For example, in March 2004, there were 2237 posts for registered nurses, of which 355 (16%) were vacant; of 552 posts for midwives, 227 (41%) were vacant; of 1069 posts for enrolled assistant nurses, 392 (37%) were vacant; and of 122 pharmacist posts, 64 (52%) were vacant [11].

Medical specialists in the public sector have the right to private practice, which at times may be located within the same institution in which they are employed. Clients accessing public services may face long waiting lists for some specialist appointments and elective surgery due to the heavy patient load, and various bottlenecks due to limited staff and facilities or inadequate equipment and supplies. Fully paying private clients are able to avoid the waiting lists and be treated more promptly during the time that the medical specialists have assigned for private practice.

The HIV epidemic

Epidemiology

Between 1982 and 2002, 7027 AIDS cases were reported in Jamaica. It is estimated that 1.5% of the adult population is HIV-positive. UNAIDS estimated that the number of people living with HIV (PLHIV) aged 15–49 rose from approximately 14,000 in 2001 to 22,000 in 2003. Although the epidemic affects the entire country, the cumulative AIDS case rates range from a low of 97 per 100,000 in the parish of Manchester to a high of 601 per 100,000 in the parish of St. James (see Fig. 27.1). AIDS is a leading cause of death in children aged 1–4 years and among young women aged 20–29 years. HIV infection rates among pregnant women in the parishes range from 0.5 to 2.7%, with the highest infection rates recorded in the 25–29 age group. The age group hardest hit by AIDS is the 20–49 year olds, the most productive age group in the society (see Fig. 27.2). The HIV seroprevalence rates were estimated to be as high as 20% among men who have sex with men (MSM) and 25% among female sex workers (FSWs), according to studies undertaken in the 1990s [12]. AIDS cases occur in all occupational groups and social classes, and 33% of cases report a previous sexually transmitted infection (STI). The main mode of transmission is heterosexual, with an adult male-to-female ratio of 1.5:1 in 2002.

If the epidemic's current trends continue, an increasing number of people aged between 20 and 30 years will be infected, especially young women, and there will be a growing problem of AIDS orphans. The Ministry of Health has begun an aggressive prevention of mother-to-child transmission (PMTCT) programme through the antenatal clinics run by RHAs. Antiretroviral drugs are provided free to HIV-positive pregnant women and their newborns. However, antiretrovirals are not otherwise available in the public sector for the treatment of AIDS unless the patient can purchase them privately. Although prices have continued to come down, access to antiretroviral drugs remains unaffordable for most of the population seen in the public health system and in non-governmental organizations (NGOs) working with HIV-positive people. Given the widespread poverty in Jamaica, many working-class people face difficult choices between drugs, food, sending children to school or paying rent. A grant from the Global Fund to Fight AIDS, Tuberculosis and Malaria enabled the government to establish a public access programme for antiretroviral treatment (ART) of people with AIDS in 2004 [12].

Table 27.1 Approved positions and vacancies for selected categories of staff by health region, March 2004

Category of Staff	Western Region		North-East Region		South-East Region		Southern Region		Total posts	Total net vacancies
	Approved post	Vacant	Approved post	Vacant	Approved post	Vacant	Approved post	Vacant		
Registered nurse	219	0	327	96	1306	218	385	41	2237	355
Midwife	154	96	94	0	188	72	116	59	552	227
Enrolled assistant nurse	245	98	138	41	556	253	130	0	1069	392
Medical doctor	55	0	55	0	288	0	75	0	473	0
Public health inspector	105	28	75	5	155	43	76	10	411	86
Pharmacist	11	0	17	9	71	35	23	20	122	64
Dental auxiliary	57	34	21	5	66	0	26	0	170	39
Dentist	11	3	8	0	31	10	8	1	58	14
Radiographer	12	0	5	0	45	15	11	3	73	18

Source: Ministry of Health, Personnel Department. Unpublished Report, March 2004.

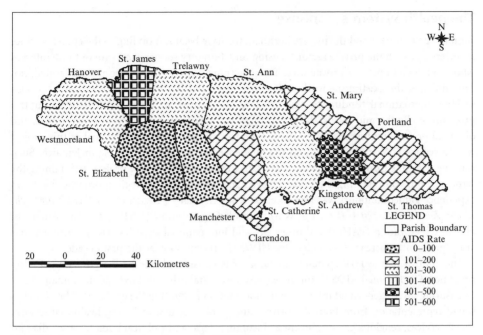

Fig. 27.1 Cumulative AIDS cases by parish, 1982–2002. Source: [13].

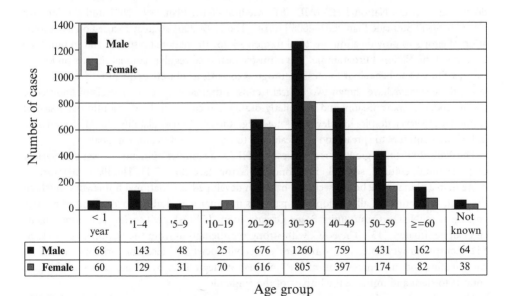

	< 1 year	'1–4	'5–9	'10–19	20–29	30–39	40–49	50–59	≥=60	Not known
Male	68	143	48	25	676	1260	759	431	162	64
Female	60	129	31	70	616	805	397	174	82	38

Fig. 27.2 Distribution of AIDS cases by age group. Source: [13].

The health system's response

Both the government and the private health sector have been responding to the epidemic since its inception, with the private sector focusing on laboratory services and care of those infected who can afford to pay for private care. The government's response has been multifaceted, not only utilizing the existing network of health centres and hospitals to provide care, but also seeking international funding to support a comprehensive national HIV/AIDS/STI control programme. By the mid-1980s, the government was developing prevention programmes, and obtained project funding from USAID in 1988 to fight the epidemic. The goal of this project was to reduce HIV transmission and the incidence and prevalence of STIs in Jamaica. Such funding has gone through more than one project cycle, with each new project maintaining the same goal but consolidating the gains achieved and adding new strategic approaches based on experience gained. Support was also received from Germany's *Deutsche Gesellschaft für Technische Zusammenarbeit* (GTZ), the World Health Organization (WHO), the Pan American Health Organization (PAHO) and other UN and international agencies. The government has also significantly increased its budget for HIV/STI prevention over the past decade.

The control of the HIV epidemic in Jamaica is considered one of the government's top priorities. The National AIDS Committee (NAC) was established in 1988 and has remained key to ensuring inter-agency and intersectoral coordination in fighting the epidemic. The NAC has broad representation from both the private and public sectors, including health, education, social services, religious groups, business, insurance, legal and political bodies, the media and NGOs. Since 2002, the government has secured a US$15 million loan from the World Bank to continue the fight against HIV/STI.

The main strategic approaches used by the government over the past decade have been documented in the National HIV/AIDS/STI Medium-Term Plan 1997–2001 and the Jamaica HIV/AIDS/STI Strategic Plan 2002–2006 [10,14]. The 1997–2001 strategy focused on a combination of efforts to provide a multisectoral framework for the national response and to build the capacity of the National Programme. The Ministry instituted regular national surveys on knowledge, attitudes and behaviour to measure progress towards its objectives quantitatively. Over the years, these surveys have shown two critical trends: a dramatic increase in levels of knowledge about modes of transmission; and a similarly dramatic increase in the distribution and sale of condoms. However, despite high levels of knowledge and condom availability, the AIDS epidemic in Jamaica continues to spread and is threatening to undermine development goals.

The 2002–2006 Strategic Plan recognizes that HIV is a complex epidemic driven by a variety of behavioural, cultural, societal and economic factors (see Box 27.1). The Plan, therefore, is more than a plan for the health sector; it has been developed as a 'national framework in which the work and actions of all development partners in Jamaica, including government ministries and agencies, NGOs, Community Based Organizations (CBOs), civil society and donor agencies can be situated' [15]. The NAC, with strong representation from the National HIV/AIDS/STI Control programme, line ministries and civil society, is also the primary means of coordinating the implementation of the National Strategic Plan by all the actors working in concert to stem and mitigate the impact of the epidemic.

The guiding principles enunciated by the government for implementing the HIV/AIDS/STI Strategic Plan include the following [15]:

1. HIV is a developmental issue and not just a health problem, and as such is a national priority.

2. HIV must be normalized so that it becomes a part of the customary public discourse.

Box. 27.1 Factors affecting the spread of HIV in Jamaica

Behavioural factors

Early sexual activity—median age of initiation for boys is 13 years and for girls is 14 years
Multiple sexual partners
Inconsistent use of condoms
Commercial sex—19% of all reported AIDS cases
Lack of perception of personal risk
Use of crack cocaine—7% of all cases

Economic factors

Slow economic growth and poverty
High levels of unemployment—21% in 2002
Tourism and population movement
Economic importance of drugs and commercial sex

Socio-cultural factors

Stigma and discrimination associated with HIV and AIDS, as well as homophobia, drive the
epidemic underground
Gender roles—male dominance
Transactional sex is common and takes varied forms
Lack of high-level commitment

Social services

Limited access to specialty care and antiretroviral drugs
Inadequate attention to HIV and AIDS in the education sector

Source: [15].

3. The rights and dignity of every individual, including those who are socially marginalized, should be recognized.

4. PLHIV must be involved in the national response.

5. There must be support for individual and community empowerment to prevent the spread of HIV.

6. Prevention and care are synergistic components of one strategy. Each is dependent on and enhanced by the other.

7. Responses must be multidimensional and multisectoral.

8. Policies must be formulated on the basis that HIV transmission is preventable, through an understanding of the nature of the epidemic.

The National HIV/AIDS/STI Programme, based on the current Strategic Plan (2002–2006), has the following main objectives:

♦ to develop and implement an effective multisectoral response to the epidemic, including private, public and community-based sectors;

- to reduce individual vulnerability to HIV infection through an effective behaviour change programme and the distribution of affordable and accessible condoms to the sexually active population;
- to reduce transmission of new HIV infection;
- to improve care, support and treatment for PLHIV.

The Programme calls for strengthening of existing health facilities, including laboratory services, to cope with the epidemic and for considerable training of health and other personnel to provide the quality of services and care needed. It also includes support for the development of policies and programmes in five Ministries (Education, Tourism, Labour, National Security and Local Government), the strengthening of the NAC and a mechanism to provide support to NGOs and community-based organizations.

Effect of the response

In analysing the response of the government to date in dealing with the epidemic, one sees that significant infrastructure and programmes have been put in place. The blood supply is safe, although the majority of people giving blood continue to be replacement donors. An HIV reference laboratory has been established. Facilities for the treatment of STIs have been expanded and the number of STI/HIV contact investigators/counsellors increased. Syphilis testing has been decentralized and rapid HIV tests introduced for pregnant women. Computerized information systems have been developed for the surveillance of HIV and other STIs. A considerable number of training programmes have been conducted for health providers and others in the public, private and NGO sectors with respect to counselling, care and treatment, syndromic management of STIs, behaviour change, universal precautions, stigma reduction and programme management. Condoms are widely available in both the public and private sectors.

PLHIV may seek care with a private practitioner or at any government health centre or hospital. Most PLHIV gravitate to a limited but growing number of private practitioners who have developed expertise in HIV and AIDS treatment, or to the health centres with specialist STI/HIV services, or to hospital outpatient departments. Government policy mandates that no person in need, including PLHIV, should be refused treatment. However, there are reports from time to time of HIV patients not being treated with the required dignity and confidentiality, resulting in discrimination by some staff and visitors to the hospital. While instances of stigma and discrimination associated with HIV in the health services—and in society as a whole—have been declining, such reports remain too frequent. Programmes to actively combat this problem are ongoing.

The experience of HIV control in Jamaica shows that a comprehensive programme that includes targeted interventions may begin to slow down the epidemic. The emphasis on STI control has resulted in a significant decline in syphilis, congenital syphilis, gonorrhoea and ophthalmia neonatorum. The numerous and varied education, intervention and outreach programmes, including mass media, person-to-person interaction and cultural approaches, have resulted in a significant increase in condom use, a small decline in the proportion of men with multiple sex partners, and a small increase in the proportion of women abstaining from sex. Condom use among sex workers is very high. Social stigma is declining, and more sectors of society are recognizing that they need to play a part in the response to the AIDS epidemic. These changes may begin to reduce the number of new cases.

Conclusion

For the future, the National Programme in Jamaica remains committed to strengthening the response to the epidemic, including better financial and technical support for multisectoral strategic responses as well as concrete support for the inclusion of NGOs in the process. The challenge of providing public ART, which began in 2004, is one of the main priorities of the National Programme. This requires ongoing training of medical professionals in care and treatment of HIV-positive patients, the dissemination of treatment protocols, strengthening laboratory capacity to monitor patients adequately, as well as extensive consumer education and counselling in the importance of adherence. Other major challenges include the need to combat the stigma and discrimination associated with AIDS more effectively as well as to intensify and scale up comprehensive prevention and intervention programmes to turn the tide of the HIV and AIDS epidemic.

References

1. Planning Institute of Jamaica and Statistical Institute of Jamaica. (1999). *Jamaica Survey of Living Conditions 1998.* Kingston, Jamaica: Statistical Institute of Jamaica/Planning Institute of Jamaica.

2. Planning Institute of Jamaica and Statistical Institute of Jamaica. (2003). *Jamaica Survey of Living Conditions 2002.* Kingston, Jamaica: Statistical Institute of Jamaica/Planning Institute of Jamaica.

3. Planning Institute of Jamaica and Statistical Institute of Jamaica. (2002). *Jamaica Survey of Living Conditions 2001.* Kingston, Jamaica: Statistical Institute of Jamaica/Planning Institute of Jamaica.

4. Statistical Institute of Jamaica. (2003). *Economic and Social Survey of Jamaica 2002.* Kingston, Jamaica: Statistical Institute of Jamaica.

5. JAMAL Foundation, Jamaica. (1988). *National Literacy Survey 1987.* Kingston, Jamaica: JAMAL.

6. Planning Institute of Jamaica. (1998). *Labour Market Information Newsletter.* No. 28.

7. Moser C, Holland J. (1997). *Urban Poverty and Violence in Jamaica.* Washington, DC: World Bank.

8. Statistical Institute of Jamaica. (2000). *Labour Force Survey, 1990–1999.* Kingston, Jamaica: Statistical Institute of Jamaica.

9. Planning Institute of Jamaica. (2002). *Economic and Social Survey of Jamaica 2001.* Kingston, Jamaica: Planning Institute of Jamaica.

10. Ministry of Health. (1997). *1997–2001 Medium Term Plan.* Kingston, Jamaica: Ministry of Health.

11. Ministry of Health Personnel Department, 2004. Unpublished report.

12. Jamaica's Country Coordinating Mechanism for HIV/AIDS Response. (May 2003). *A Proposal to Scale Up HIV/AIDS Treatment, Prevention and Policy Efforts in Jamaica.* Available at: http://www.the-globalfund.org/search/docs/3JAMH_661_0_full.pdf.

13. Ministry of Health. (2003). *National HIV/AIDS/STI Control Programme.* Kingston, Jamaica: MoH.

14. Figueroa, JP. (2001). Health trends in Jamaica: significant progress and a vision for the 21st century. *West Indian Medical Journal* 50(Supplement 4):15–22.

15. Ministry of Health, Jamaica. (2002) *Jamaica HIV/AIDS/STI National Strategic Plan 2002–2006. Time to Care. Time to Act.* Kingston, Jamaica: Ministry of Health.

Chapter 28

Argentina

Gabriela Hamilton[*], Carlos Falistocco, Pedro Cahn
and Carlos Zala

Background

Argentina is the second largest country in South America, with a total area of 2,766,890 km^2. It borders the Atlantic Ocean between Chile and Uruguay. In 2002, the population within its 23 provinces plus Buenos Aires City was 38 million, most of whom lived in urban areas: Buenos Aires City (2.8 million), Province of Buenos Aires (8 million), Cordoba (1.3 million), Rosario (1.2 million) and Santa Fe (0.5 million). Ninety-seven per cent of the population in the country is Caucasian, mostly second- or third-generation Spanish, Italian and other European immigrants, among others. Over 90% of the inhabitants are nominally Roman Catholic, and the Catholic Church has historically influenced Argentinian culture [1].

Economic and social context

In the 20 years since its last military government, Argentina's healthcare indicators have improved steadily and remarkably. For example, the infant mortality rate declined from 26% in 1985 to 16% in 2001 [2]. Unfortunately, by the end of 2001, the political and economic instability that has characterized the Latin American region led Argentina to an institutional breakdown that touched every single civil institution, including the healthcare system.

Argentina is currently struggling to emerge from the deepest socio-economic crisis in its history. In the 1990s, Argentina began a structural process that promised to reverse economic stagnation and stabilize the economy by balancing public accounts, privatizing state-owned companies, deregulating economic activities and opening up markets [3]. By the end of 2001, Argentina was in such political turmoil that the elected President was forced to resign. The country was then governed by a succession of presidents elected by Congress, while it defaulted on its external debt payments. This was followed by the devaluation of the local currency, rapid inflation and the most serious economic, financial and institutional crisis ever faced in Argentina. The economic crisis was characterized by:

- high unemployment rates;
- progressive cuts in the financing of the social security system;
- a substantial increase in the price of medical and non-medical supplies as a result of currency devaluation, leading to interruptions in supply;
- an increasing number of people seeking assistance at public hospitals.

* Corresponding author.

In 2002, as economic recession continued, inflation skyrocketed to 70% in the first quarter of the year. Between 1995 and 2003, the proportion of the population in poverty increased from 29% to 58%, resulting in new and greater demand for social and health services. Rates of unemployment rose from 7.3% in 1990 to 21.5% in 2002 [4], forcing people previously enrolled in the social security and private healthcare plans to seek medical assistance in already overcrowded public hospitals, where they are cared for by underpaid healthcare workers. Along with the rest of the population, people living with HIV (PLHIV) have had to face the consequences of this downturn. In the absence of a welfare plan to mitigate the impact of the crisis, little could be done for the increasing number of marginalized HIV-infected individuals unable to reach a hospital to get their medications in a timely manner.

In this socio-economic context, the Ministry of Health declared a National Health Emergency in 2002 in order to prevent the total breakdown of the health system. Under Decree 486/02, the following programmes were given top priority:

- a primary care programme to protect the health of pregnant women;
- a mass vaccination programme for children;
- the optimization of the National AIDS Programme (NAP).

The health system

How much does Argentina spend on health?

In 2001, only 1.2% of the total government budget, or 0.2% of gross domestic product (GDP), was allocated to the Ministry of Health. However, if public and private health spending as a percentage of GDP is considered, a significant portion (8–9%) of Argentina's economy was allocated to the healthcare system compared with other countries in the region (Table 28.1). In 2002, per capita spending on health was US$200. This figure is over twice the average for Latin America, but significantly lower than that of industrialized countries [5].

Organization

Argentina's healthcare system is divided into three sectors according to source of funding: the public sector; social security; and the private sector (Table 28.2). This structure has allowed the medical needs of most of the population to be covered [7].

Table 28.1 Health spending in Argentina between 1995 and 2001 (in current US$)

Year	Expenditure in billions	% of GDP	Per inhabitant
1995	7.1	8.6%	206.84
1996	7.2	8.2%	205.12
1997	7.7	8.1%	212.40
1998	7.9	8.2%	220.37
1999	8	8.7%	220.80
2000	7.8	8.5%	212.53
2001	7.1	8.2%	198.12

Source: [6].

Table 28.2 Structure of the Argentinian health system

System	Users	Source of financing
Public	Universal. However, it assists mainly low-income people	Tax revenues or public resources. Implemented by the government at the three jurisdictional levels (national, provincial and municipal)
Social security	Middle-income sector, part of employees' terms of employment	Social contributions transferred to social services, national, provincial, municipal or others belonging to, for instance, universities, the army, Congress, etc.
Private	High-income sector that acquires services through direct hiring or health insurance	Private spending or family spending. Direct payment or voluntary quotas

Source: [7].

The public sector

The public sector comprises 8000 beds in 1200 hospitals and more than 5700 institutions for outpatient treatment. Medical care at public institutions is free of charge to anyone without either private or social security coverage. Administration of the public sector is organized on three levels: national, provincial and municipal. The Ministry of Health is the highest authority on health issues; it coordinates, regulates, provides technical and financial support and establishes programmes and guidelines that enable the coordination of activities within the different sectors. However, decision making at the level of the Ministry is limited by the autonomy of the provinces, which implement their own health policies and programmes. There are regular meetings between the national Ministry and provincial ministries in order to analyse and define policies. The *Consejo Federal de Salud* (COFESA), Argentina's federal health council, sets out the respective responsibilities of national and provincial authorities.

Over the last few years, demand for public health services has soared. The reasons for this increase include:

- a sustained increase in unemployment since the mid-1990s, which has led many workers and their families to lose their social security coverage or to quit private healthcare plans;
- growth of the informal economy;
- new working conditions that do not provide health insurance, compelling workers to pay for more of their own medical services than in the past.

Social security

The social security system provides medical assistance to enrolled workers and to their immediate families. Within this scheme, each employee allocates a fixed proportion of income to a selected healthcare plan. Because the choice of healthcare plans is broad, workers have the freedom to choose a plan according to their preferences and needs. The social security institutions are regulated by the state through the Health Services Superintendence. A similar scheme is in place for employees of provincial governments and universities. People enrolled in this system are entitled to receive a Minimum Care Package (*Programa Médico Obligatorio*).

The private sector

The private sector comprises health insurance companies, a small group of private health service providers and independent professionals that provide ambulatory and hospital services. These organizations and individuals generally sign agreements with the social security sector in order to provide their services to workers enrolled in social security plans and are obliged to provide the Minimum Care Package.

Coverage in the three sectors

An overview of services provided by the three sectors between 1997 and 2001 shows an increase of 18% in the population that used only public sector services. These are services provided under the National Health Emergency Plan. Table 28.3 shows the pattern of use of the three healthcare sectors for that period.

Around 20 million people, or just over half the population, reported some insurance coverage, through either social security or private health plans. Some received benefits from both. Between 1991 and 1995, there was a drop of 10% in the number of beneficiaries covered by social security. Nevertheless, because of the number of people subscribing to both systems, there was no significant change in the absolute number of people covered. This overlap in medical coverage was reduced in the early 1990s and had almost disappeared by 2001. In 1991, 4.5 million people had more than one type of medical insurance, plummeting to 0.4 million in 2001 (Table 28.3).

The data show that most of Argentina's population has some kind of coverage (52%). Social security plans cover most of the needs of workers and their families (50%), and the growth in unemployment seems not to have affected social security coverage as much as might be expected. Some workers are able to maintain their coverage through their spouse.

The HIV epidemic

Since the *Programa Nacional de Lucha contra los Retrovirus del Humano, SIDA y ETS* (National Programme against Human Retroviruses, AIDS and STIs) was launched in 1989, its activities have been widespread. There has been a clear political will to solve HIV-related issues, even during the worst of Argentina's economic and financial crisis in 2001. Prevention and medical care management for PLHIV are considered major and ongoing priorities. In accordance with these priorities, the health system response has included all three health system components: the public, social security and private sectors.

Table 28.3 Use of the healthcare system by financing source, 1991–2001

| Year | 1991 | | 1997 | | 2001 | |
	Millions	%	Millions	%	Millions	%
Social security only	13.2	40.3	17.9	50.2	16.9	46.5
Private health insurance	1.5	4.6	2.8	7.9	3.3	9.0
Social security and private health insurance	4.5	13.9	1.5	4.2	0.4	1.0
Public services only	13.4	41.2	13.4	37.7	15.8	43.5
Total population	32.6	100.0	35.7	100.0	36.3	100.0

Source: [8].

By October 2003, nearly 26,000 AIDS cases and approximately 14,402 AIDS-related deaths had been reported to the Ministry of Health [9]. It is estimated that 120,000 people are currently living with HIV across the country, but only 35% are aware of their sero-status. Figure 28.1 shows the annual rates of AIDS and AIDS deaths. Most new infections occur within vulnerable groups, including sexually active youth from underserved areas, patients without private health insurance, adolescent females, pregnant women and newborns.

The AIDS epidemic has remained an urban disease with limited spread to rural areas. The highest prevalence of HIV infection and AIDS cases reported is in cities with more than 1 million inhabitants. Of those, the city of Buenos Aires and its suburbs, Rosario and Cordoba, account for 79% of the total AIDS cases reported in the country [10].

Since the beginning of the epidemic, the gender and age of the affected population have changed over time. The first AIDS cases in Argentina were identified among homosexual males with a history of overseas travel, and injecting drug users (IDUs). Five years into the epidemic, heterosexual transmission of HIV had emerged as the main route. The male-to-female ratio changed from 15:1 in 1988 to 3:1 in 2003 due to an increase in the number of women infected through heterosexual transmission (Fig. 28.2).

The proportion of HIV-infected women rose from none in 1985 to 23% of the total reported cases in 2003 (Fig. 28.3). By March 2004, most AIDS cases were aged between 25 and 34 years. In this epidemiological context, pregnant women and their newborns have become the populations most vulnerable to HIV infection. Prevalence of HIV infection in pregnant women from selected areas of Buenos Aires is currently above 1%, and the rate of paediatric cases has remained among the highest in Latin America, accounting for 7% of the total cases of AIDS reported in the country.

A number of local studies have attempted to characterize the main risk factors associated with vertical transmission of HIV. However, retrospective design and limited resources allocated to programmes targeting HIV-infected pregnant women and their newborns have limited the interpretability of the data collected [10]. Given the availability of healthcare services that provide voluntary counselling and testing (VCT), antiretroviral drugs and trained physicians, it

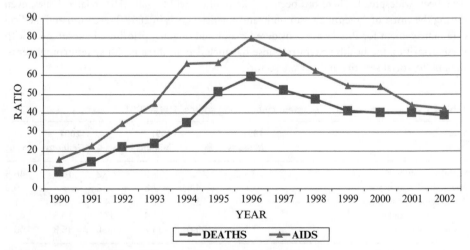

Fig. 28.1 AIDS cases and AIDS deaths in Argentina, 1990–2002.

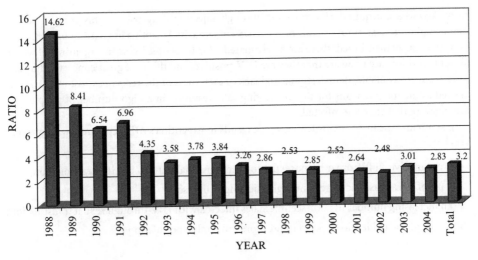

Fig. 28.2 Male/female ratio of AIDS cases, 1982–2002.

remains a puzzle why, in some areas of the country, the number of HIV-infected children is so high. Nevertheless, most caregivers and experts in the field agree that inadequate antenatal care, failure to implement family planning programmes and late access to antiretroviral therapy (ART) are the main reasons for a high rate of paediatric infection in the country.

The educational background of the individuals being diagnosed with HIV has also changed during the last decade. While middle- to upper-class, well-educated males were affected at first, HIV infection has now rapidly spread to the poorest, least educated and most marginalized individuals. Recent data from the Ministry of Health indicate that 36% of the adults suffering

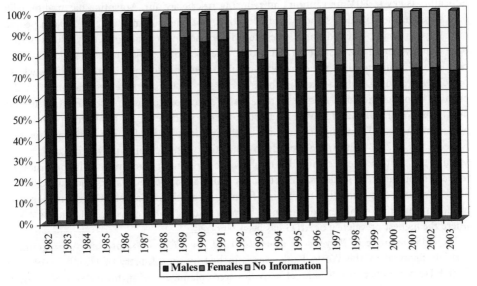

Fig. 28.3 AIDS cases by gender, 1982–2003.

from AIDS have acquired HIV infection through injecting drug use. In this complex socio-demographic context, future trends of the AIDS epidemic in Argentina are hard to predict.

As previously mentioned, there are an estimated 120,000 people living in Argentina, of whom about two-thirds are unaware that they are HIV-positive, and this is of great concern. Although VCT is widely available, denial, stigma and lack of awareness of the risks of exposure to HIV are viewed as the main reasons for the low testing rate, resulting in a high number of people who are unaware that they are infected.

In summary, the main socio-demographic trends in Argentina's AIDS epidemic within recent years are:

+ a progressive shift from a homosexual to a heterosexual pattern of HIV transmission;
+ 34% of AIDS cases acquired through injecting drug use;
+ an increasing number of adolescent females infected with HIV through sexual transmission;
+ a shift of the epidemic to poorer and more vulnerable populations.

The response

The public sector has handled most of the burden of the epidemic, while the private sector and the social security system have shown little commitment to fighting HIV. Private healthcare administrators have generally been reluctant to develop strategies for prevention among their own clients and their families or to become actively involved in community programmes to raise awareness about prevention and care issues. In contrast, several non-governmental organizations (NGOs) and civil society organizations have responded with commitment and solidarity in fighting the AIDS epidemic and helping those in need.

Health education

Education is key to HIV prevention and reducing risk behaviour. Argentina has traditionally been distinguished by high standards of education, boasting a literacy rate of 97% in people over 10 years of age. Unconditional access to primary, secondary and university education has been proudly viewed as a basic civil right. However, educational programmes in Argentina have been strongly influenced by the conservative opinions of the Roman Catholic Church, whose principles regarding human sexuality have led to the exclusion of sex education from the primary school curriculum. In spite of this, health education concerning sexually transmitted infections (STIs), AIDS and related issues such as reproductive health has been implemented with some success. Following an initiative by the Ministry of Health, the National Congress passed a law in 2003 concerning reproductive health issues, including prevention and care of sexually transmitted diseases and HIV, to allow the training of teachers and the provision of relevant information to students. Unfortunately, while advocates, educators and public health officers welcomed the initiative, complaints from the Argentinian Catholic Church managed to block implementation of sex education at private schools in the province of Buenos Aires, where the highest prevalence of AIDS has been reported.

The LUSIDA project (*Proyecto de Control del SIDA y ETS*), a comprehensive programme partially financed by the World Bank, was launched by the Ministry of Health in 1997 to fight HIV. A number of educational activities were planned during the 1998–1999 period, including a training programme for school teachers and community leaders that was implemented in the three locations most affected by the AIDS epidemic: Buenos Aires, Córdoba and Santa Fe. Overall, the programme reached 1744 schools—11% of the schools located within the target area. Unfortunately, these activities were not fully evaluated due to changes in the Ministry of Health that followed a change in government in early 1999.

The LUSIDA project has recently been integrated into the National AIDS Programme (NAP) launched in 1992 by the Ministry of Health in response to the AIDS epidemic. While the initial goals of the NAP were to provide diagnosis, treatment and monitoring of HIV disease across the country, it subsequently assumed responsibility for surveillance, education and prevention activities as well. More recently, the NAP has been involved in the development of an HIV prevention and control project funded by the Global Fund to Fight AIDS, Malaria and Tuberculosis.

In addition to the above-mentioned prevention programmes, mass media campaigns to raise awareness about HIV were developed through both the Ministry of Health and several NGOs. Lack of sustainability and disagreement among health officials, NGOs and the community at large about the messages being conveyed have been the main criticisms and reasons cited for the failure of these campaigns to reduce sexually acquired HIV infections. Despite a strong commitment from many organizations, it has been hard to develop a coordinated plan to tackle the lack of awareness about HIV in the population as a whole. From this perspective, the efforts of several NGOs along with the Ministry of Health to sustain public awareness about HIV transmission have been remarkable and fruitful.

With regard to prevention of mother-to-child HIV transmission, the Ministry of Health has recently implemented a number of measures. Outstanding among them is a law recently passed by the National Congress for the provision of VCT for all pregnant women as part of their antenatal care. In addition, a number of initiatives in the area of operational research and prevention have recently been established through cooperative projects funded by the US National Institutes of Health (NIH) and the Global Fund to Fight AIDS, Tuberculosis and Malaria, respectively. Among them, an observational study on pregnant HIV-infected women and their exposed newborns was implemented in 2002 at three public hospitals in Buenos Aires under the sponsorship of the NIH. The Global Fund has also recently been involved in the development of prevention, care and support projects for people living with HIV.

HIV-related health care

In the early days of the AIDS epidemic, from 1985 to 1992, care of HIV-infected individuals presenting with advanced disease was restricted to three or four hospitals located in the largest cities. As the epidemic grew, patients overflowed from tertiary hospitals to suburban hospitals and clinics. Although this helped respond to the needs of more patients, decentralization also led to a wide variation in the quality of clinical management, depending on the training and resources of physicians and institutions.

Voluntary counselling and testing

Voluntary counselling and anonymous testing have become widely available at public hospitals and private clinics across the country. Within the public health system, an HIV-positive screening test is further confirmed by western blot at a reference laboratory. More recently, rapid testing is being offered to pregnant women presenting in labour with no antenatal controls at sentinel sites. Once an HIV diagnosis is confirmed, patients can choose a clinical care setting for follow-up within the public, social security or private systems.

Antiretroviral therapy

Antiretroviral therapy (ART) is currently provided free of charge to all HIV-infected individuals at public and private institutions within their assigned medical coverage and according to local therapeutic guidelines. In 1990, the National Congress passed a law by which the Ministry of Health guaranteed diagnosis, care and treatment of HIV-infected individuals through the provision of ART and drugs for the treatment of AIDS-related conditions, including opportunistic infections. In 1995, the law was extended to include health services provided by the social security system and, later, private health insurance companies. In 2004, the public sector, social security and private insurance companies were covering 70%, 25% and 5%, respectively, of the approximately 30,000 HIV-infected individuals receiving therapy. However, the proportion of people being treated in these three sectors has shifted due to the recent socio-economic situation. Data from the National Institute of Statistics and Surveys (INDEC) indicate that medical coverage through social security and private insurance in the Province of Buenos Aires declined from 52% to 39% between 1991 and 2002.

The guaranteed Minimum Care Package covers quarterly HIV RNA testing, CD4 cell count, safety laboratory and triple combination therapy, including either a non-nucleoside analogue reverse transcriptase inhibitor (NNRTI) or a protease inhibitor plus two nucleoside analogue reverse transcriptase inhibitors (NRTIs). Patients with a CD4 cell count below 200 cells/mm^3 are eligible for prophylaxis with cotrimoxazole. Patients with a count of less than 50 CD4 cells are also eligible to receive azithromycin for primary prophylaxis of *Mycobacterium avium* complex disease. In March 2002, 75% of HIV-infected individuals receiving ART were fully covered by the National AIDS Programme. The remaining 25% are entitled to receive the Minimum Care Package through social security or private insurance. Because HIV care and treatment provided by both the social security healthcare services and private insurers are subsidized by the national government, equity in access to treatment and monitoring across all three sectors is financially and legally guaranteed.

Trends in the use of antiretroviral therapies

Monotherapy with zidovudine (AZT) was first available in Argentina in 1987. In 1995, soon after the results of the ACTG 175 trial were released, dual combination therapy with AZT plus either didanosine (ddI) or zalcitabine (ddC) was introduced in clinical practice. Later, in 1997, triple combination therapy including a protease inhibitor became the standard of care. Currently, 14 antiretroviral drugs are available in Argentina: five nucleosides [AZT, ddI, ddC, lamivudine (3TC), stavudine (d4T) and abacavir (ABC)], two NNRTIs [nevirapine (NVP) and efavirenz (EFV)] and six protease inhibitors [saquinavir (SQV), indinavir (IDV), ritonavir (RTV), nelfinavir (NFV), amprenavir (APV) and lopinavir (LPV)].

The pattern of use of ART in Argentina has closely followed therapeutic guidelines issued by international expert panels, including the International AIDS Society [11]. In 1997, the Ministry of Health gathered a team of key local experts to advise on treatment strategies for the use of antiretrovirals. This technical group has recently been expanded to include PLHIV. Local therapeutic guidelines are continually reviewed by experienced physicians from local scientific societies such as the Argentinian AIDS Society and the Argentinian Society for Infectious Diseases. They provide input to the technical group in order to update therapeutic guidelines following medical breakthroughs and the availability of new drugs. Table 28.4 shows the number of patients on ART from 1994 to 2003.

Table 28.4 Number of patients on ART, 1994–2003

Year	Number of patients
1994	2543
1995	2908
1996	3605
1997	4296
1998	6701
1999	10,104
2000	14,500
2001	14,984
2002	15,220
2003	17,153

Source: Ministry of Health.

AZT is widely available to HIV-infected pregnant women at obstetric clinics according to the ACTG 076 protocol. According to local guidelines, HIV-infected mothers are strongly discouraged from breastfeeding their newborns. A number of public and private programmes make feeding formula available through obstetric services and outreach clinics.

Treatment and prophylaxis for AIDS-related opportunistic infections have been in place since the beginning of the epidemic. Diagnosis of opportunistic pathogens can be microbiologically confirmed at a referenced microbiology laboratory, and regular measurement of CD4 cell counts by flow cytometry is used to guide prescription of prophylaxis and assessment of response to ART.

Financing of antiretroviral therapy

ART and laboratory monitoring for 84% of the HIV-infected individuals currently on treatment are financed through the Ministry of Health. The remaining 16% is covered by a subsidized social security plan (14%) or private health insurance companies (2%). Purchase and delivery of antiretroviral drugs for patients seeking care in the public system are centralized at the NAP, which pays for antiretroviral drugs and laboratory testing.

National legislation allows for the use of generic drugs, which in many cases are manufactured by local pharmaceutical companies following the importation of active ingredients. Since 1999, widespread availability of generic drugs within the Argentinian market has resulted in substantial price reductions, in the range of 10–99% for 80% of purchases [12]. Figure 28.4 shows that the price falls between 1999 and 2003 for most of the antiretrovirals available through the NAP.

The Ministry of Health encouraged market competition among multiple suppliers of generic and brand antiretrovirals to obtain drugs at a lower price within the local market. This strategy succeeded in reducing the cost of triple combination therapy by more than 60% in 2003 alone (Table 28.5). It was estimated that such a price reduction would allow a saving of US$17.5 million, enough to provide treatment to 25,000 HIV-infected people.

In addition, at a summit held in Peru in 2003, health authorities from 10 Latin American countries—Argentina, Bolivia, Colombia, Chile, Ecuador, Mexico, Ecuador, Peru, Uruguay and Venezuela—and leaders of multinational drug companies discussed strategies for differential

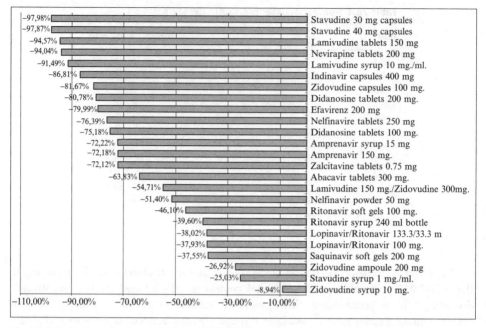

−97,98%	Stavudine 30 mg capsules
−97,87%	Stavudine 40 mg capsules
−94,57%	Lamivudine tablets 150 mg
−94,04%	Nevirapine tablets 200 mg
−91,49%	Lamivudine syrup 10 mg./ml.
−86,81%	Indinavir capsules 400 mg
−81,67%	Zidovudine capsules 100 mg.
−80,78%	Didanosine tablets 200 mg.
−79,99%	Efavirenz 200 mg
−76,39%	Nelfinavire tablets 250 mg
−75,18%	Didanosine tablets 100 mg.
−72,22%	Amprenavir syrup 15 mg
−72,18%	Amprenavir 150 mg.
−72,12%	Zalcitavine tablets 0.75 mg
−63,83%	Abacavir tablets 300 mg.
−54,71%	Lamivudine 150 mg./Zidovudine 300mg.
−51,40%	Nelfinavir powder 50 mg
−46,10%	Ritonavir soft gels 100 mg.
−39,60%	Ritonavir syrup 240 ml bottle
−38,02%	Lopinavir/Ritonavir 133.3/33.3 m
−37,93%	Lopinavir/Ritonavir 100 mg.
−37,55%	Saquinavir soft gels 200 mg
−26,92%	Zidovudine ampoule 200 mg
−25,03%	Stavudine syrup 1 mg./ml.
−8,94%	Zidovudine syrup 10 mg.

Fig. 28.4 Antiretroviral price reductions, 1999–2003.

pricing of HIV drugs for the region. As a result, a substantial price reduction of up to 90% in selected brand drugs was agreed upon by governments and companies. Figure 28.5 illustrates a hypothetical scenario comparing the cost of triple combination therapy using only generics versus using only brand drugs, based on prices quoted to the NAP in September 2003.

Impact of antiretroviral therapy

The initial response to the AIDS epidemic in Argentina was late and ineffective. However, in 1992, the Ministry of Health established the NAP, which made universal VCT and free ART available to all HIV-infected individuals, including HIV-infected pregnant women and their newborns and visitors from neighbouring countries. A positive impact from this intervention has already emerged. According to the Ministry of Health, the number of newly reported AIDS cases since the introduction of highly active ART (HAART) has dropped by 50%, from 2750 cases in 1996 to 1070 cases in 2002. Although limited information is available regarding

Table 28.5 Savings in purchases of triple antiretroviral regimens during 2003

Regimen	Annual percentage price reduction	Annual savings in US$
AZT + 3TC + Efavirenz	63.7	4,635,216
AZT + 3TC + Nevirapine	76.7	4,718,696
AZT + 3TC + Indinavir	63.1	4,352,118
AZT + 3TC + Nelfinavir	51.3	3,794,427
Average saving	63.1	17,500,457

Source: National AIDS Programme, 2003.

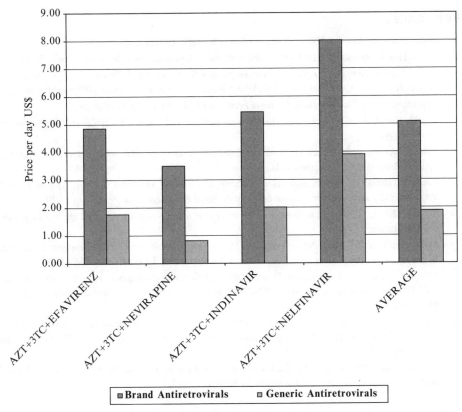

Fig. 28.5 Likely cost of generic versus brand antiretroviral drugs for triple combination therapy in Argentina.

hospital admission of HIV-infected patients, utilization of drugs for the treatment of AIDS-related opportunistic infections has significantly declined. A reporting procedure for new HIV infections has recently been implemented. Limited information from sentinel serological surveys suggests a declining trend in the number of newly HIV-infected pregnant women and injecting drug users. Confirmation of these trends warrants further evaluation.

Conclusion

The HIV epidemic in Argentina has changed substantially in demographic and socio-economic terms. These changes have challenged the ability of public health officials and the community at large to deal with the consequences of this devastating disease. Furthermore, the political and economic instability that characterized the region during the last 10 years has hampered the design and implementation of sustainable action to fight HIV. In 2002, Argentina faced one of the most difficult periods in its history. These crisis conditions created a favourable environment for the transmission of HIV. Optimizing existing resources and improving access to the public healthcare system for vulnerable populations remain our most important outstanding tasks.

References

1. Wikipedia Encyclopedia. (2004). URL: es.wikipedia.org/wiki/Argentina.
2. World Health Organization (WHO). Health Indicators, Argentina. Available at www3.who.int/whosis.
3. World Bank Poverty Report. (2000). *Poor People in a Rich Country. A Poverty Report for Argentina.* Report No. 19992 AR. Washington, DC: World Bank. Available at www.wbln0018.worldbank.org.
4. Argentina. Economic Indicators. In: *Latin Focus.* Available at www.latin-focus.com.
5. World Health Organization. Key health expenditure indicators. Available at www3.who.int/countries/arg/en.
6. Tobar F, Ventura G, Montiel L and Falbo R. (2002). *El Gasto en Salud en la Argentina y su Método de Cálculo.* Buenos Aires: Ediciones ISALUD número 5.
7. Tobar F (2003). Financiamiento del sistema de salud en la Argentina. In: Mera J and Bello J. *Organización y Financiamiento de los Servicios de Salud en la Argentina.* PAHO, pp 83–91.
8. Tobar F (2003). *Cambios en la Población Cubierta por el Sector Salud Argentina.* Program a Remedian MSAN. Mimeo.
9. Ministry of Health. (2003). *Boletín sobre el SIDA en la Argentina.* Buenos Aires: Ministerio de Salud de la Nación, Programa Nacional de Lucha control los Retrovirus del Humano, SIDA y ETS.
10. Ceballos A, Pando MA, Liberatore D *et al.* (2002). Efficacy of strategies to reduce mother-to-child HIV-1 transmission in Argentina, 1993–2000. *Journal of Acquired Immune Deficiency Syndrome* 31:348–53.
11. Cahn P, Zala C, Gun A *et al.* (1998). 1996 IAS-USA recommendations in clinical practice in Argentina: one year after. In: *Program and Abstracts of the 5th Conference on Retroviruses and Opportunistic Infections.* Chicago, IL.
12. Hamilton G. (2003). Accesibilidad a los tratamientos ARV de alta eficacia: hacia la sustentabilidad económica de las terapias. *Actualizaciones en SIDA* 11:124–7.

Chapter 29

Brazil

Maya L Petersen[*], Claudia Travassos, Francisco I Bastos, Mariana A Hacker, Eduard J Beck and José Carvalho de Noronha

Background

The early days of the HIV epidemic in Brazil occurred during a period of transition in Brazil's social and political institutions. After two decades of military dictatorship, the 1980s were a time of democratization and reform in Brazil. A wide range of social movements led to increased freedom of speech and civil rights. Public health was considered a fundamental component of civil rights and social equality, and was advocated for by individuals and non-governmental organizations (NGOs). In 1988, Brazil adopted a new Constitution guaranteeing universal and equitable provision of healthcare to all Brazilians.

The first case of HIV was diagnosed retrospectively in Brazil in 1980. As HIV emerged as a growing public health problem, both the social will and an institutional framework to fight the epidemic were in place. The political climate of the time helped to ensure that advocacy by the public health sector and by social activists played a fundamental role in shaping the nation's early response to the epidemic. This included lobbying successfully for universal free access to antiretroviral drugs.

The early inclusion of antiretroviral therapy (ART) in the Brazilian HIV programme played a major role in its success, and sets Brazil apart from most other developing countries. However, implementation of an integrated and truly universal HIV treatment and prevention programme in Brazil remains a challenging and unprecedented task. Brazil has one of the most unequal distributions of wealth in the world [1], as well as one of the largest populations, and the geographic regions of Brazil have strikingly different degrees of urbanization, economic development and access to healthcare infrastructure [2].

Income disparities, geographical diversity and sheer size have all complicated the Brazilian response to HIV. Universal access to ART quickly became a reality in major metropolitan areas served by well-functioning local health systems. The logistics of drug delivery and patient monitoring were more complicated in remoter regions of the country, and development of adequate infrastructure in these regions required significant investment, which took longer to achieve [3].

Collaboration between the Brazilian Ministry of Health, NGOs and international organizations has characterized the Brazilian response to the HIV epidemic throughout its evolution. While dispensing and monitoring treatment remain the responsibility of public healthcare

* Corresponding author.

providers and is financed by the federal government, NGOs play a key role in the delivery of prevention services. Financing of Brazil's HIV prevention strategy is the result of collaboration between the federal government and international organizations, including the World Bank [4].

Brazil's size, geopolitical and economic importance, and the uniqueness and relative success of its HIV programme suggest that Brazil's experience confronting the HIV epidemic may offer important insights to other nations struggling against the epidemic. In this chapter, we provide a brief description of Brazil's geography, demographics and political economy. We describe the Brazilian healthcare system, and how that system has shaped and been shaped by the nation's response to HIV. We focus on the collaborative roles played by NGOs and international institutions, and provide an in-depth discussion of the antiretroviral programme in Brazil.

Geography and political economy

Brazil is the fifth largest country in the world, occupying over 8 million km^2, including 7367 km of Atlantic coastline. It shares a border with all South American countries except Chile and Ecuador. The majority of Brazilians live along the coastline, primarily in the south-eastern states of São Paulo, Rio de Janeiro and Minas Gerais.

The Brazilian population is a mixture of various cultural and ethnic groups, and the proportion of the population with a mixed ethnic background continues to increase. In addition to indigenous peoples and the Portuguese, Brazilians count among their ancestors Africans brought to Brazil via the slave trade, European immigrants and, more recently, Japanese immigrants to the state of São Paulo. Portuguese is spoken throughout Brazil, although a few Indian groups retain their indigenous languages.

Brazil is a federal republic divided into 26 states and one federal district. As of 2000, the states were divided into 5561 municipalities. A president is directly elected every 4 years and governs with the assistance of freely designated ministers of state. The National Congress, composed of the Chamber of Deputies and the Federal Senate, exercises legislative power at the federal level. A governor and a legislative assembly are elected every 4 years to govern each state. A directly elected mayor and local council administer each municipality. The judiciary is composed of several institutions at the three different tiers. At the federal level, the highest court is the Federal Supreme Court, with 13 ministers named by the President following approval by the Senate.

Brazil lived under military rule from 1964 until 1985. Beginning in 1985, political parties became free to organize. In 2002, for the first time in Brazilian history, a candidate from the Left, and with no higher education, won the presidential elections.

Brazil has a diversified economy. Prior to the mid-1990s, Brazil was a primary producer and exporter, but it has subsequently evolved into a fairly industrialized country. In 2002, secondary production accounted for 34% of the gross domestic product (GDP), and the tertiary sector for 56% [5]. Following the Second World War and until the late 1970s, Brazil experienced a very high rate of economic growth, with industrial production growing by 10% annually for several years. Agriculture's share of the GDP declined over this period. Manufactured and semi-manufactured goods had replaced coffee as the main Brazilian export by 2000, accounting for 74% of exports [6].

After the oil and debt crises of the late 1970s, the country underwent a period of stagnation and inflation with low growth rates (Fig. 29.1). Inflation declined sharply as a consequence of

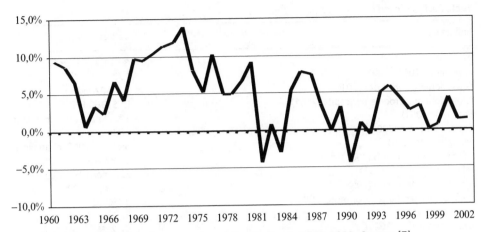

Fig. 29.1 Gross domestic product annual growth rate, Brazil, 1960–2002. Source: [7].

economic measures associated with the establishment of a new currency, the Real, in 1996. However, economic growth has not resumed at the pace anticipated. Interest rates have remained very high and were over 16% in December 2003; external debt reached US$228 billion in 2002, and total debt accounted for 55% of the GDP by mid-2003 [7].

Brazil ranked sixty-fifth in the Human Development Index (HDI) published by the United Nations Development Programme (UNDP) in 2001. Brazil's HDI ranking is relatively low given its per capita GDP, partly due to the high level of inequity in distribution of income [8]. In 1999, 40% of the national income was controlled by the wealthiest 10% of the population, while only 12% was controlled by the poorest 50% [9]. Ten per cent of the population, or more than 17 million people, have incomes lower than US$1 a day, and 24% have incomes lower than US$2 a day [8].

Demography and health

Brazil has experienced dramatic demographic changes during the last 50 years. Basic demographic and health indicators are summarized in Table 29.1. The population grew from 41 million inhabitants in 1990 to over 170 million by 2000. Population growth was accompanied by rural-to-urban migration; by the year 2000, 81% of Brazilians lived in urban areas. During this period, fertility rates declined by 60% to a birth rate of 2.2 children per woman of childbearing age in 2001. However, the fertility rate of women aged 15–19 years, particularly those living in poor and rural areas and those with less education, increased slightly during this period [10,11].

Infant mortality also declined steadily in Brazil during the twentieth century, from 158 deaths per 1000 live births during the 1930s to 29 per 1000 by 2000 [12]. Despite this decrease, Brazil's infant mortality rate remains one of the highest in Latin America [16]. Life expectancy at birth increased by 25 years between 1940 and 1991, and in 2000 was 73 years for women and 65 years for men [14]. Although Brazil remains a young country, the decrease in fertility rate and the extended life expectancy have resulted in an aging population. During the last 40 years, the population over the age of 60 has grown by 500% [17].

Table 29.1 Basic indicators, Brazil

Indicators	Values
Area[*]	8,514,215.3 km^2
Population (2001)[*]	172,385,776
Gross domestic product (2001)[+]	US$502 billion
Gross domestic product per capita (2001)[†]	US$7360 PPP
Birth rate (2001)[*]	19.89 per 1000 inhabitants
Total fertility rate (2001)[*]	2.18
Mortality rate (2001)[*]	6.68 per 1000 inhabitants
Life expectancy at birth (2001)[*]	68.82 years
Infant mortality rate (2001)[*]	32.7 per 1000 live births
Maternal mortality rate (1998)[‡]	126.8 per 1000 live births
Population aged 60 years or more (2001)[*]	9.1%
Adult literacy rate (2001)[*]	87.7%
Urban population (2000)[*]	81.25%
Physicians (2001)[‡]	2.08 per 1000 inhabitants
Hospital beds (2002)[‡]	2.7 per 1000 inhabitants

PPP = purchasing power parity.
Sources: [*][12], [+][13], [†][8], [‡][14], [§][15].

Cardiovascular diseases are the leading cause of death in the country, as in all South American countries. During the 1980s in Brazil, deaths due to 'external causes of injury and poisoning' increased from the fourth to the second most common cause of death [18], reflecting a dramatic increase in deaths due to road accidents and violence. External causes are the main causes of death between 5 and 39 years of age [14]. Deaths from violence are steadily increasing, particularly among young boys and male adolescents [19]. Cancer is the third most common cause of death in Brazil. Deaths due to infectious diseases, including HIV, are declining but in 1999 were still responsible for 5% of all deaths [20].

Despite improvements, levels of health in Brazil remain below those observed in countries with a similar per capita GDP (Table 29.2). Mortality and morbidity vary by region (Table 29.3). In 2001, life expectancy at birth varied from 72 years in the southern state of Rio Grande

Table 29.2 Life expectancy at birth and GDP per capita in US$ PPP, selected countries, 2001

Country	GDP per capita	Life expectancy
Venezuela	5670	73.5
Mexico	8430	73.1
Libya	7570	72.4
Colombia	7040	71.8
Bulgaria	6890	70.9
Paraguay	5210	70.5
Turkey	5890	70.1
Peru	4570	69.4
Thailand	6400	68.9
Brazil	7360	67.8

PPP = purchasing power parity.
Source: [8].

Table 29.3 Population size and selected health indicators by region, 2000

Region	Population in millions	Fertility rates	Infant mortality rates (per 1000 live births)	Life expectancy at birth (years)	% births in women less than 19 years old
North	12,901	3.09	28.9	68.5	30.7
Northeast	47,742	2.64	44.9	65.8	26.5
Southeast	72,412	2.08	19.1	69.6	20.2
South	25,108	2.09	17.1	71.3	21.3
Midwest	11,638	2.11	21.9	69.4	26.2
Brazil	169,799	2.32	28.3	68.6	23.5

Source: [15].

do Sul to 63 years in the north-eastern state of Alagoas. Infant mortality rates vary from 118 deaths per 1000 live births in some municipalities in the north-east, to eight deaths per 1000 live births in some southern municipalities [20].

The health system

Health reform

Prior to the Constitution of 1988, the Brazilian healthcare system relied on social security, and most healthcare services were accessible only to formally employed people and their families. The poorer members of society had access to limited care through state or local services. In response to this system, 'reforma sanitária', or health reform, became a prominent issue in Brazil in the late 1970s. Reform efforts during this era focused on fighting inequalities in living and health conditions, and on access to healthcare.

With the return of democracy in 1985, social policies rose up the federal policy agenda. Healthcare delivery was among the major issues in the so-called 'New Republic'. A National Health Conference was called by the President and held in Brasilia in 1986, the culmination of over a year of nationwide technical and political debate. It brought together more than 5000 people, including health professionals, healthcare providers and consumers [21]. The conference focused the healthcare policy agenda on pursuing equity, assuring universal entitlement to services, increasing funding for healthcare, unifying and integrating various services and providers—preventive and curative, federal, state and municipal—and empowering people to exert more control over healthcare delivery [22].

The new Constitution adopted in 1988 explicitly incorporated the right to healthcare, stating in its chapter on health (Article 196) 'Health is a basic right, and it is the duty of the state to ensure that right through social and economic policies aimed at reducing the risk of disease and other hazards, and through universal and equitable access to the activities and services necessary to promote and protect good health' [23]. The Constitution formally entitles every Brazilian citizen to free healthcare at the point of delivery.

Most reform efforts thereafter were directed towards implementing universal access to services and integrating healthcare sectors managed by different levels of government. Regulations were passed that defined new roles for each tier of the health administration, and decentralization of responsibilities to local government became a key piece of the reform.

In September 1990, the current Brazilian public healthcare system, called the *Sistema Único de Saúde* (SUS or Unified Health System), was established. The SUS formally distributes responsibilities for healthcare delivery between federal, state and municipal governments. The federal government is responsible for the following healthcare functions: development of national policies; regulation of the national health system; development of nationwide technical norms; financing and technical cooperation with states and municipalities; regulation of private–public relationships; evaluation of trends in national health indicators; monitoring and evaluation of health system performance; support of scientific and technological development and the development of human resources; regulation of research ethics; regulation of medical products; and nationwide coordination of the Health Information System. Each tier of government has a health council responsible for policies at its respective level. The councils are composed of consumers, health workers, and public and private healthcare providers. Every 4 years, a National Health Conference, preceded by municipal and state conferences, is held to set the direction of major health policies.

Healthcare delivery

The Brazilian health system is two-tiered. The richest 25% of the population uses mostly private services, financed through indemnity and group health plans, and obtained from fee-for-service doctors. Private insurance coverage declines with decreasing income (Table 29.4). The majority of the Brazilian population uses the publicly financed SUS [21].

Public and private facilities often provide different standards of care; cutting-edge medical technology is available in the private hospitals of Rio de Janeiro and São Paulo, while nearby public services may be lacking the most basic medical devices. Access to health services is also highly unequal between socio-economic levels. Among sick people, the richest income group uses services at a rate 53% higher than the poorest income group [2]. However, although inequalities in healthcare delivery remain, there are indications that these inequalities did not increase between 1989 and 1997 [25].

A mix of public and privately owned facilities provide care to the SUS. Private providers deliver most of the inpatient care (70%) to patients covered by the SUS. In 1998, there were 14.4 million hospital admissions (9.12 per 100 inhabitants), of which 25% were financed privately, mainly by health insurance plans [26]. Private providers are reimbursed by the

Table 29.4 Private insurance and health plan coverage by income group, 1998

Family income group	Private coverage (%)
Up to 1 minimum wage	2.56
1–2 minimum wages	4.83
2–3 minimum wages	9.36
3–5 minimum wages	18.58
5–10 minimum wages	34.72
10–20 minimum wages	54.03
20+ minimum wages	76.18
Total population coverage	24.45

Source: [24].

SUS using a prospective system similar to diagnosis-related groups (DRGs), with fixed reimbursement determined on the basis of a list of diagnoses weighted by severity. The average payment per hospital admission was about US$120.00 [about US$275.00 purchasing power parity (PPP)] in the first quarter of 2003. Since 1996, state or local governments have been responsible for reimbursing healthcare facilities for services delivered at the state or local level, respectively [20].

Ambulatory care is provided mainly through public and teaching institutions. Primary care is generally delivered by the municipalities, either through health centres and posts or through the Family Health Programme (PSF) that has been widely expanded since 1996. In 2002, SUS paid for 1.12 billion primary care procedures, or 6.42 per capita, of which 22% were medical consultations, 582 million specialized diagnostic and therapeutic ambulatory care procedures, or 3.33 per capita, and 134 million tertiary ambulatory care procedures, or 0.77 per capita. Ambulatory care is reimbursed by the SUS according to the volume of services performed. Private facilities delivering secondary ambulatory care and laboratory and other diagnostic and therapeutic services accounted for approximately 30% of total procedures and almost 50% of federal payments in 2002 [21].

In 2002, there were 65,343 health facilities in Brazil, of which 7397 provided inpatient care with a total of 471,171 beds. Sixty-five per cent of the facilities providing inpatient care and 24% of those providing only ambulatory care, excluding diagnostic and other ancillary services, were private. Eighty-three per cent of private beds were allocated to general public care sponsored by the SUS. The ratio of beds per 1000 inhabitants varied from 1.59 in the state of Amazonas in the north to 3.4 in Rio de Janeiro in the south-east [15]. The country has a relative scarcity of nurses, with four doctors to every nurse. The distribution of health services and professionals among the various regions is unequal, with services concentrated in the more economically developed regions and in state capitals. Fifty-eight per cent of the nation's physicians are located in south-eastern Brazil, which has 2.8 physicians per 1000 inhabitants, while northern Brazil has 1.1 physicians per 1000 inhabitants [15].

It is estimated that Brazil spends about 8% of its GDP on health. Although this represents a relatively large share of GDP, per capita healthcare spending is low compared with other, wealthier countries in the Americas (Table 29.5). Inequity in healthcare expenditures is striking. Assuming total annual spending of US$267 per capita, as observed in 2000 [27], the richest 20% of Brazilians spend an average of approximately US$890 per capita, while the remaining 80% spend an average of US$110.

Anticipated developments

Infant mortality in Brazil will probably continue its decline, and the Brazilian population will continue to age and become increasingly concentrated in urban areas. In response to these demographic changes, services for children should become more focused on perinatal care, and the availability of complex health procedures and social services to assist the elderly should be expanded. Trauma care will remain a major healthcare priority for the foreseeable future.

Pressure for more public financing of healthcare will also grow as Brazilian healthcare reform focuses on providing universal coverage free of charge. Current income distribution places a ceiling on the size of the private insurance market. Some expansion of private coverage may be expected as the country resumes its economic development, provided that growing indebtedness and interest payments do not overshadow the government's capacity to develop inclusive

Table 29.5 Total health expenditure per capita and share of GDP, selected American countries, 2000

Country	US$ PPP per capita	Share in GDP (%)	Government share in total health expenditures (%)
Peru	238	4.8	59.2
Mexico	483	5.4	46.4
Colombia	616	9.6	55.8
Brazil	631	8.3	40.8
Chile	697	7.2	42.6
Canada	2534	9.1	72.0
USA	4499	13.0	44.3

PPP = purchasing power parity.
Source: [27].

social policies that equalize income distribution. Growing regulation of private markets is due to occur as congressional legislation from the late 1990s is implemented. Health technology evaluation in Brazil is at an early stage of development, but there is a growing concern that indiscriminate use of inappropriate diagnostic and therapeutic devices and procedures may impose an unbearable financial burden on the expanding healthcare system. Primary healthcare should grow as the Family Health Programme expands its coverage to larger urban areas. Primary care will almost certainly be delivered by public providers.

Current mechanisms for public accountability, such as health councils and national health conferences, are important safeguards of the constitutional principles underlying the Brazilian health system. Health-related issues are constant subjects of media scrutiny, and growing access to the Internet is giving the public a greater awareness of their rights. Public attorneys are increasingly taking part in the protection of citizen's rights in health matters.

The HIV epidemic

Epidemiology

Estimates suggest that there were approximately 600,000 people living with HIV (PLHIV) between the ages of 15 and 49 years in Brazil at the end of 2001 [28,29], resulting in an overall HIV prevalence among adults of 0.7%. While AIDS prevalence in Brazil is moderate in comparison with many global populations, Brazil's population of over 170 million individuals increases the scale of the epidemic. By September 2003, 277,154 AIDS cases had been reported to the Brazilian Ministry of Health [29], making Brazil's AIDS epidemic the fourth largest in the world. AIDS incidence in Brazil has stabilized at around 14 new cases per 100,000 inhabitants in recent years, and since 1998 has declined slightly [28]. This trend has not been uniform across Brazil, however, and AIDS incidence among both men and women continues to increase in the southern part of the country [30].

AIDS-related mortality has also declined in recent years. Between 1984 and March 2002, a total of 105,000 cumulative deaths due to AIDS were reported to the Brazilian Ministry of Health [31]. AIDS mortality began to decline among men living in major metropolitan areas beginning in 1991 [32]; however, after the introduction of universal access to ART in 1996, AIDS mortality began to fall for both men and women and in all regions of Brazil [33]. Trends in adult AIDS incidence and mortality in Brazil are summarized in Fig. 29.2.

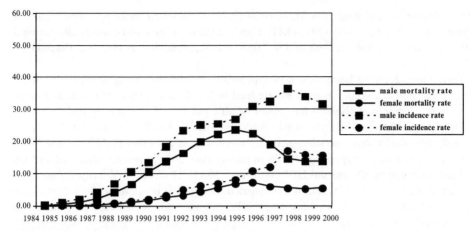

Fig. 29.2 AIDS incidence and mortality rates per 100,000 inhabitants for adults aged 15–54 years, 1984–2000. Source: Brazilian Ministry of Health (SIM & SINAN-AIDS data banks).

The HIV epidemic in Brazil began primarily among relatively affluent men who had sex with men (MSM) and recipients of contaminated blood products living in Brazil's major metropolitan areas. The epidemic subsequently spread to injecting drug users (IDUs), their sexual partners and MSM living in urban areas throughout Brazil. More recently, HIV is increasingly transmitted heterosexually, resulting in growing numbers of HIV infections among women [32,34]. As in many countries, HIV in Brazil is also increasingly affecting poor residents of smaller municipalities. The proportion of newly diagnosed AIDS cases among unemployed and unskilled workers, and among individuals with no more than a primary school education grew dramatically over the last two decades [35–37]. Sentinel sero-surveillance suggests that the prevalence of HIV among pregnant women has remained below 1% since 1990. Mother-to-child transmission (MTCT) accounts for approximately 3% of all AIDS cases [31]. Although fewer surveillance data are available for specific high-risk groups, HIV prevalences as high as 18% and 40% were reported in 1998 among sex workers and IDUs, respectively [28,38,39].

HIV prevention

Both mass media and targeted education and information campaigns have been launched by the Brazilian Ministry of Health (BMH) as part of its HIV prevention programme. Mass media campaigns using the radio, television and newspapers have focused on raising awareness about risk factors for HIV transmission, including drug use and unprotected sex, and about decreasing stigma and fostering support for PLHIV. Campaigns targeting specific risk groups, including pregnant women, youth, IDUs, MSM and sex workers, have also been launched by both the government and private NGOs.

Surveys conducted by the BMH suggest that AIDS knowledge and awareness in Brazil are quite high. In 1999, 98% of the adult population could name at least two acceptable methods of protection from HIV infection, and 83% could correctly identify misconceptions about AIDS transmission and knew that a healthy-looking person could transmit AIDS [28]. While the impact of education campaigns on preventive behaviours is difficult to assess, the percentage of men in Brazil who reported using condoms for all sexual intercourse increased from 25% in 1993 to 37% in 1996 [40,41]. Condom sales also increased dramatically during the 1990s; 53 million condoms were sold in Brazil in 1992, 70 million in 1993 and 350 million in 2000 [42].

Brazil has adopted a harm reduction approach to prevention among IDUs. Both purchase and possession of injecting equipment are legal in Brazil. The number of needle and syringe exchange programmes (NSEPs) has grown steadily since the first NSEP opened in Brazil in 1994, financed by the BMH, the World Bank and local NGOs. By the end of 2002, approximately 100 NSEPs were operating in Brazil, more than in any other middle- or low-income country [43]. Studies suggest that NSEPs in major urban areas have successfully reduced rates of contaminated needle use and HIV prevalence [39,44]. However, HIV transmission among IDUs in the south of Brazil continues unabated, despite the presence of the nation's largest NSEP in that region [45]. In addition, NSEPs in some regions of Brazil continue to face substantial local opposition.

HIV treatment

In 1991, zidovudine (AZT) was in use in Brazil but was not widely available [3]. Over the next 5 years, there was intense lobbying by individuals and NGOs for improved treatment for PLHIV, including a lawsuit brought against the federal government for failure to provide treatment to all Brazilians with AIDS. In response to this pressure, a federal law guaranteeing universal free access to ART was passed in 1996. This law states that: 'HIV-infected people and/or people living with AIDS are entitled to receive from the National Health System, at no cost, all medicines necessary for their treatment' [46].

In 2003, approximately 125,000 people were being clinically managed with ART in Brazil [47]. This represents approximately 20% of the estimated 600,000 PLHIV [29]. Under Brazilian treatment guidelines, any HIV-infected person with symptoms or a CD4 count below 200 cells/mm^3 is eligible to receive free ART, while individuals with CD4 counts of 200–350 cells/mm^3 are monitored closely and considered for treatment [48]. The number of HIV-infected individuals meeting these criteria in Brazil is unknown.

Currently, 15 antiretroviral drugs, including nucleotide reverse transcriptase inhibitors, protease inhibitors and non-nucleotide reverse transcriptase inhibitors, are distributed by over 500 dispensing units throughout Brazil. ART in Brazil is publicly administered and financed; only public health services can be accredited by the federal government to dispense ART drugs. Public outpatient services, clinics and hospitals can all apply for accreditation, which requires previous experience working with PLHIV, demonstration of sufficiently trained staff, and basic pharmacy and laboratory capabilities [41].

Responsibility for distribution and monitoring of ART is shared between municipal, state and federal levels of government, in accordance with the delegation of healthcare responsibilities under the SUS. Antiretroviral drugs are dispensed at primary care centres administered by municipalities. Primary care doctors are responsible for the day-to-day treatment and follow-up of PLHIV, including prophylaxis and treatment for opportunistic diseases, both prior to and following AIDS diagnosis. If medical complications arise, an individual can be referred to secondary or tertiary care centres, most of which are jointly supervised and run by the federal government, universities and research centres. The federal government is responsible for setting national treatment standards and guidelines, accrediting primary, secondary and tertiary care units for the treatment of AIDS and maintaining national networks for AIDS case notification, patient monitoring and tracking of prescription drugs [48].

The existence of national treatment standards and national networks for patient monitoring has been crucial in ensuring universal access to quality ART despite significant regional disparities in the availability of resources, laboratory capacity and trained staff. While nation-wide laboratory networks provide ongoing patient follow-up, including CD4 counts and viral loads, and track drug prescriptions, these regional disparities have complicated the effective implementation of such networks. In addition, although referral centres in major urban areas are linked via the Internet, dispensing units in other regions of Brazil are not accessible via telephone lines, and their only link to national networks is by mail. Also, delays in the return of laboratory results vary from region to region and may be considerable. The Brazilian AIDS epidemic remains primarily urban, simplifying the task of delivering care and services. Seventy-four per cent of adult and 91% of paediatric cumulative AIDS cases from 1980 to 2000 lived in urban municipalities [20].

The emergence and transmission of HIV strains resistant to antiretroviral drugs have often been cited as potentially disastrous consequences of expanded access to ART in resource-limited settings [49,50]. Evidence available to date suggests that resistant HIV is a growing problem in Brazil, as it is in the USA, Europe and other settings in which ART is widely available [51,52]. However, the prevalence of resistance among both treated and treatment-naïve populations observed to date in Brazil remains no higher than the prevalence observed in high-income nations [53–55].

Financing prevention and treatment

HIV prevention activities in Brazil are financed by one of the World Bank's largest loan programmes [56]. The federal government matches funds provided by World Bank loans. Between 1994 and 2002, the World Bank approved loans of approximately US$325 million, and a third loan agreement was approved in November 2003. The World Bank loans have not been used to fund the production, procurement, delivery or monitoring of ART in Brazil.

In 1998, the total government budget for HIV was approximately US$600 million (PPP), or about US$4 (PPP) per capita [57]. This constitutes about 1% of Brazil's total health expenditure [55]. Fifty-six per cent of government expenditure on HIV went directly toward the purchase of antiretroviral drugs [57].

The Brazilian government has adopted several strategies to reduce the costs of ART. Before 1997, Brazil had no legislation prohibiting the generic domestic production of drugs still under patent protection in other nations. As the Brazilian capacity for domestic drug production increased, Brazil came under increasing pressure from international governments and pharmaceutical companies to adopt laws protecting drug patent rights. Consequently, in 1997, a law was passed to protect drugs patented after that date from generic production. However, drugs patented before 1997 are not similarly protected, despite continuing pressure from the pharmaceutical industry to prohibit their generic production.

This legal framework allowed Brazil to begin producing local versions of antiretroviral drugs still under patent in other countries. Brazil currently produces generic versions of eight antiretroviral drugs, accounting for 50% of all antiretroviral drugs consumed in Brazil [42]. In addition, Brazil has succeeded in negotiating differential pricing agreements and joint ventures with international pharmaceutical companies, ensuring substantial discounts on the purchase of drugs not produced in Brazil [4].

Antiretroviral drugs fall under Brazil's three-tiered drug classification system. Brand name antiretroviral drugs are classified as 'reference medicines' and certified by the BMH. Generic versions of antiretroviral drugs are also certified by the BMH after rigorous evaluation, including bioequivalence testing, and are used interchangeably with their equivalent reference medications. Mandatory bioequivalence testing and additional quality control measures have helped to ensure the quality of Brazil's generic drug supply. Finally, *similares* (similar medicines) have similar active products and formulas to reference drugs, but their bioequivalence is not certified by the BMH; *similares* are sold under brand names, with differential packaging. All antiretrovirals have passed bioequivalence tests in Brazil, so currently all antiretrovirals delivered in the country are either reference medicines or generics.

These strategies have allowed Brazil to contain the price of ART. In 2001, antiretroviral drugs were provided at an annual cost of US$2530 per patient, compared with the previous cost of over US$4860 in 1997 [42]. It is estimated that costs would increase by 32% in the absence of generic drug production [58]. Although most of the monies used for the HIV programme come from public sources, overall expenditures are financed from a variety of sources (Table 29.6).

Evaluating the Brazilian HIV programme

Evidence suggests that the Brazilian prevention and treatment strategy for HIV has reduced AIDS-associated morbidity and mortality and stabilized the growth of the HIV epidemic (Fig. 29.2). Median survival following AIDS diagnosis increased from 5 months in the early 1980s to 18 months in 1995, and 58 months in 1996 [33]. The proportion of AIDS cases presenting with tuberculosis, candidiasis, *Pneumocystis carinii* pneumonia and other opportunistic diseases has also declined over the past two decades [59].

It is difficult to attribute Brazil's apparent success in controlling the HIV epidemic to any one aspect of its comprehensive treatment and prevention strategy. However, the fact that the Brazilian government made the containment of their HIV epidemic a high political priority enabled a broad and comprehensive programme to be developed and sustained. It seems clear that the introduction of universal access to ART in 1996 contributed to population-wide reductions in AIDS mortality, as has been observed in other countries [60,61]. Universal access may also have contributed to the subsequent stabilization observed in AIDS incidence by decreasing HIV transmission, since it is hypothesized that ART decreases the relative infectivity of HIV-infected individuals, provides increased incentive for HIV testing and decreases the stigma surrounding HIV infection [62,63].

Few data are available about the effectiveness or efficiency of specific prevention initiatives in Brazil. The World Bank estimates that preventive interventions averted 38,100 new HIV infections between 1994 and 2000, at a cost of US$9600 per HIV infection avoided [64,65]. Assuming each HIV-infected person causes an average loss of 20 discounted disability-adjusted life years (DALYs), this is equivalent to 353,029 DALYs saved, at a cost of US$481 per DALY. Alternative estimates suggest even greater efficiency: US$83 per DALY gained, or US$1600 per HIV infection averted [66].

Estimated gains achieved as a result of both prophylaxis against opportunistic diseases and ART are even greater. Declines in AIDS-associated morbidity and mortality are estimated to

Table 29.6 Sources of expenditure for HIV service provision in 12 South American countries, 2000

Country	Total expenditure on HIV/national expenditure on health	Public expenditure on HIV/public expenditure on health	Public expenditure on HIV/total expenditure on health	Private expenditure* on HIV/total expenditure on HIV	Out-of-pocket expenditure on HIV/total expenditure on HIV	External expenditure on HIV/total expenditure on HIV
Argentina	0.7%	ND	68.5%	31.35%	23.92%	0.06%
Bolivia	ND	ND	2.36%	24.21%	24.15%	73.38%
Brazil	1.38%	2.60%	79.70%	19.51%	15.10%	0.75%
Chile	0.68%	0.73%	55.03%	43.73%	22.15%	1.18%
Costa Rica	ND	ND	ND	ND	ND	ND
El Salvador	2.25%	ND	78.34%	11.75%	3.53%	6.02%
Guatemala	1.38%	ND	72.30%	18.00%	14.67%	9.63%
Mexico	0.55%	1.01%	90.20%	9.49%	10.85%	0.27%
Nicaragua	ND	ND	39.00%	23.00%	20.88%	37.63%
Panama	ND	ND	88.62%	8.15%	5.82%	3.21%
Paraguay	1.25%	0.56%	29.64%	70.36%	42.22%	50.03%
Peru	ND	ND	22.79%	74.70%	74.10%	2.49%
Dominican Republic	ND	ND	ND	ND	ND	ND
Uruguay	0.85%	0.64%	37.99%	62.00%	40.96%	0.00%
Average	1.13%	1.11%	55.37%	33.02%	24.86%	15.39%

Source: Sidalac, National Accounts.
*Includes private insurance and out-of-pocket expenditure; ND = not declared.

have saved 234,000 hospitalizations between 1996 and 2001, resulting in estimated savings of over US$1 billion [4,28]. These estimates do not incorporate any indirect benefits of treatment resulting from prevention of new HIV cases. Overall, the analyses performed so far are fairly crude, and few detailed analyses have been performed on the use, cost and outcome of HIV service provision in Brazil.

The impacts of the HIV treatment and prevention programme have been felt throughout Brazil and among all sectors of society [33]. However, an equitable distribution of treatment and prevention benefits remains to be achieved. Geographical disparities in the number of and accessibility to ART dispensing units persist; the urban south-east (72 million people) has over 200 antiretroviral dispensing units, while the vast Brazilian north (13 million people) is served by only 12 units [30]. While this distribution is appropriate relative to the scale of the HIV epidemics in the respective regions, it implies significant geographical barriers to access for PLHIV in northern Brazil because of its widely dispersed population.

Counselling, testing and other preventive services are also concentrated in the south and south-east regions of Brazil [3]. Surveillance data for some hard-to-reach populations, including sex workers and migrant labourers, remain extremely sparse. Surveillance data available for IDUs living in southern Brazil and for poor women living in *favelas* (slums) suggest that HIV transmission continues unabated in these vulnerable populations. Although antenatal care and voluntary testing and counselling are widely available in Brazil, an HIV prevalence of 3–6% has been reported in the south among women who do not regularly access antenatal care, the majority of whom are poor and have little education [66].

Conclusion

Brazil's reforms in the 1980s produced a healthcare system based on the principle that care should be delivered according to need rather than ability to pay. This commitment to equity played a major role in shaping the nation's response to the HIV epidemic, as is particularly evident in Brazil's provision of universal free ART. However, dramatic disparities between socio-economic groups and geographical regions in Brazil remain a challenge to the realization of this ideal, both within the HIV programme and across the Brazilian health system more generally. Vulnerable populations, including the poor, women and IDUs, are increasingly bearing the brunt of the HIV epidemic. Access to both treatment and prevention services should be increased in remote regions of Brazil, and marginalized populations targeted more effectively. Expanded access to ART may result in increased risk behaviours and the emergence and transmission of resistant strains of HIV [3,54], though it could increase the incentive to be tested. Expanded clinical, behavioural and laboratory monitoring should be coupled with efforts to improve patient adherence to medications and clinical follow-up, and direct prevention services toward individuals receiving treatment.

Clearly there are challenges still to be met. However, the accomplishments of the Brazilian HIV programme in providing reasonably equitable care to an extremely disparate population are impressive. AIDS mortality has fallen nationwide and among both sexes, and incidence is declining in most regions. Although it is too early to draw definite conclusions about future trends in ART resistance, data on both adherence to medications and transmission of resistant HIV strains are hopeful.

The HIV programme can be seen as a successful first step in Brazil's ambitious national project to achieve equity in healthcare. Many sectors of the Brazilian healthcare system, however, are neither as well funded nor as well organized as the HIV programme. As the country recovers from the hard economic legacy of the early 2000s, the coming years offer an important opportunity for other sectors of the health system to benefit from the experience of the HIV programme. The provision of free ART for all in need should be taken as a model for expanding access to other essential medicines. To date, the HIV programme has largely been built up vertically from a minimal foundation. Horizontal integration with the larger Brazilian health system would both improve HIV care and extend the gains of the HIV programme to other areas of the health system.

Brazil's achievement among low- and middle-income countries was to provide universal access to ART at an unprecedented early stage in its epidemic. Much of the developing world faces more severe resource and infrastructure limitations than Brazil. However, it may be possible for these nations to form regional networks to make the production of generic drugs, negotiation of bulk discounts and provision of laboratory follow-up financially and logistically feasible.

The Brazilian HIV programme has successfully implemented a wide range of treatment and prevention activities, drawing on the organizational and financial resources of state and national governments, NGOs and donor organizations. It is hoped that this model can be applied in other resource-limited settings where the HIV epidemic continues unabated.

References

1. Szwarcwald CL, Andrade CL, Bastos FI. (2002). Income inequality, residential poverty clustering and infant mortality: a study in Rio de Janeiro, Brazil. *Social Sciences and Medicine* 55:2083–92.

2. Almeida C, Travassos C, Porto S, Labra ME. (2000). Health sector reform in Brazil: a case study of inequity. *International Journal of Health Services* 30:129–62.

3. Bastos FI, Kerrigan D, Malta M, Carneiro-da-Cunha C, Strathdee SA. (2001). Treatment for HIV/AIDS in Brazil: strengths, challenges, and opportunities for operations research. *AIDScience* 1(15). URL: www.aidscience.org.

4. Galvao J. (2002). Access to antiretroviral drugs in Brazil. *Lancet* 360:1862–5.

5. ECLAC–Economic Commission for Latin America and the Caribbean. (2003). *Statistical Yearbook for Latin America and the Caribbean 2002*. Santiago: ECLAC.

6. Abril Editora. Balança comercial brasileira. A exportação brasileira. In: Brasil. Economia. Almanaque Abril. URL: http://almanaque.abril.uol.com.br.

7. Instituto de Pesquisa Econômica Aplicada (IPEA). (2003). Sinopse Macroeconômica. Ipeadata. URL: www.ipeadata.gov.br. Accessed 13 August 2003.

8. United Nations Development Programme (UNDP). (2003). *Millennium Development Goals: A Compact Among Nations to End Human Poverty*. Human Development Report. New York: Oxford University Press.

9. Instituto de Pesquisa Econômica Aplicada (IPEA). (2003). Renda—parcela apropriada. In: Temas: Indicadores Sociais. Ipeadata. URL: http://www.ipeadata.gov.br.

10. Instituto Brasileiro de Geografia e Estatística (IBGE). (2000). *Revista do Censo* 9:8.

11. Camarano A. (1998). Fecundidade e anticoncepção da população jovem. In: *Comissão Nacional de População e Desenvolvimento (Org.). Jovens Acontecendo na Trilha das Políticas Públicas*, Vol. I. Brasília: Ministério do Planejamento e Orçamento, p109–33.

12. Instituto Brasileiro de Geografia e Estatística (IBGE). (2003). *Síntese de Indicadores Sociais 2002. Estudos e Pesquisas Informação Demográfica e Socioeconômica*, no. 11. Rio de Janeiro: IBGE.

13. The World Bank. (2003). World Development Indicators 2003. Washington, DC. http:// www.world-bank.org/data/wdi2003/.

14. Melo Jorge MH, Gotlieb SL, Laurenti RA. (2001) *Saúde no Brasil: Análise do Período 1996 a 1999.* Brasília: Organização Pan Americana da Saúde.

15. Ministério da Saúde, Brasil. (2003). Indicadores e Dados Básicos, Brasil, 2002. IDB–2002. In: Informações de Saúde. Datasus. URL: http://datasus.gov.br.

16. Simões CCS, Monteiro CA. (1995). Tendência secular e diferenciais regionais da mortalidade infantil no Brasil. In: Monteiro CA, ed. *Velhos E Novos Males Da Saúde No Brasil.* São Paulo: HUCITEC/ NUPENS/USP, p153–6.

17. Editorial. (2003). *Cadernos de Saúde Pública* 19(3):700–1.

18. Swarcwald CL. (1987). Mortalidade por Causas Externas nas Capitais e Grandes Regiões Metropo-litanas Brasileiras, 1977–1985. São Paulo: II Congresso Brasileiro de Saúde Coletiva. São Paulo (mimeo).

19. Souza ER. (1994). Homicides in Brazil: the major villain for public health in the 1980s. *Cadernos de Saúde Pública* 10(Supplement 1):45–6.

20. Ministério da Saúde, Brasil. (2003). Informações de Saúde. Datasus. URL: http://datasus.gov.br.

21. Noronha JC, Levcovitz E. (1996). Brazil. In: Hurrelmann K, Laaser U, eds. *International Handbook of Public Health.* Westport, CT: Greenwood Press, p66–84.

22. Ministério da Saúde, Brasil. (1986). *Anais da 8ª Conferência Nacional de Saúde.* Brasília: Ministério da Saúde.

23. Constitution of Brazil. (1988) *Constituição. República Federativa do Brasil.* Brasília: Senado Federal (literal translation).

24. Brazilian Institute of Geography and Statistics (IBGE). (1998). National household survey (PNAD). URL: http://www.ibge.gov.br.

25. Travassos C, Viacava F, Fernandes C, Almeida C. (2000). Social and geographical inequalities in health services utilization in Brazil. *Ciência e Saúde Coletiva* 5(1):133–49.

26. Brazilian Institute of Geography and Statistics (IBGE). (2000). *Acesso e Utilização de Serviço de Saúde: 1998.* Rio de Janeiro: IBGE.

27. World Health Organization (WHO). (2002). *The World Heath Report 2002: Reducing Risks, Promoting Healthy Life.* Geneva: WHO. Annex, Table 5.

28. UNAIDS. (2002). *Report on the Global HIV/ AIDS Epidemic.* Geneva: UNAIDS.

29. Szwarcwald CL, Carvalho MF. (2001). Estimated number of HIV-infected individuals aged 15–49 years in Brazil, 2000. In: Ministério da Saúde Brasil, *Boletim Epidemiológico* XIV(1), January–March 2001.URL: www.aids.gov.br.

30. Hacker MA, Petersen ML, Enriquez M, Bastos FI. (2004). Highly active antiretroviral therapy in Brazil: the challenge of universal access in a context of social inequality. *Rev Panam Salud Publica* 16(2):78–83.

31. Ministério da Saúde, Brasil. (2003). URL: www.aids.gov.br.

32. Lowndes CM, Bastos FI, Giffin K, Reis ACGV, d'Orsi E, Alary M. (2000). Differential trends in mortality from AIDS in men and women in Brazil, 1984–1995. *AIDS* 14:1269–73.

33. Marins JR, Jamal LF, Chen SY *et al.* (2003). Dramatic improvement in survival among adult Brazilian AIDS patients. *AIDS* 17:1675–82.

34. Szwarcwald CL, Bastos FI, Castilho EA. (1998). The dynamics of the AIDS epidemic in Brazil: a space–time analysis in the period 1987–1995. *Brazilian Journal of Infectious Diseases* 2:175–86.

35. Fonseca MG, Bastos FI, Derrico M, Andrade CL, Travassos C, Szwarcwald CL. (2000). AIDS and level of education in Brazil: temporal evolution from 1986 to 1996. *Cadernos de Saúde Pública* 16(Supplement 1):77–87.

36. Fonseca MG, Szwarcwald CL, Bastos FI. (2002). A sociodemographic analysis of the AIDS epidemic in Brazil, 1989–1997. *Revista de Saude Publica* **36**:678–85.

37. Fonseca MG, Travassos C, Bastos FI, Silva N, Szwarcwald CL. (2003). The social distribution of AIDS in Brazil according to participation in the labour market and socio-economic status of cases, from 1987 to 1998. *Cadernos de Saúde Pública* **19**(5):1351–63.

38. Caiaffa WT, Mingoti SA, Proietti FA *et al.* (2003). Estimation of the number of injecting drug users attending an outreach syringe-exchange program and infection with human immuno-deficiency virus (HIV) and hepatitis C virus: the AjUDE–Brasil Project. *Journal of Urban Health* **80**:106–14.

39. Mesquita F, Kral A, Reingold A, Bueno R, Trigueiros D, Araujo PJ. (2001). Trends of HIV infection among injection drug users in Brazil in the 1990s: the impact of changes in patterns of drug use. *Journal of Acquired Immune Deficiency Syndrome* **28**:298–302.

40. Chequer P, VanOss Marin B, Paiva L *et al.* (1997). AIDS and condoms in Brasilia: a telephone survey. *AIDS Education and Prevention* **9**:472–84.

41. Ministério da Saúde, Brasil. (2001). Implementation and Monitoring Report—AIDS II- December 1988–May 2001. World Bank Loan BIRD 4392/BR, 2001. URL: www.aids.gov.br.

42. Levi GC, Vitoria MA. (2002). Fighting against AIDS: the Brazilian experience. *AIDS* **16**:2373–83.

43. Mesquita F, Doneda D, Gandolfi D *et al.* (2003). Brazilian response to the human immunodeficiency virus/acquired immunodeficiency syndrome epidemic among injection drug users. *Clinical Infectious Diseases* **37**(Supplement 5):S382–5.

44. Hacker MA, Friedman SR, Telles PR *et al.* (2005). The role of 'long-term' and 'new' injectors in a declining HIV/AIDS epidemic in Rio de Janeiro, Brazil. *Substance Use and Misuse* **40**(1): 99–123.

45. Bastos FI, Malta M, Hacker MA et al. (2006). Assessing needle exchange operations in a poor Brazilian community. *Substance Use and Misuse* (in press).

46. Ministério da Saúde, Brasil. (2000). *Brazilian Legislation on STD and AIDS*. Brasilia: Ministério da Saúde.

47. Ministério da Saúde, Brasil. (2003). *National Response to the HIV/AIDS Pandemic in Brazil*. National STI/AIDS programme.

48. Ministério da Saúde, Brasil. (2002). Recommendations for Anti-retroviral Therapy in HIV-infected Adults and Adolescents. URL: www.aids.gov.br.

49. Harries AD, Nyangulu DS, Hargreaves NJ, Kaluwa O, Salaniponi FM. (2001). Preventing antiretro-viral anarchy in sub-Saharan Africa. *Lancet* **358**:410–4.

50. Popp D, Fisher JD. (2002). First, do no harm: a call for emphasizing adherence and HIV prevention interventions in active antiretroviral therapy programs in the developing world. *AIDS* **16**:676–8.

51. Grant RM, Hecht FM, Warmerdam M *et al.* (2002). Time trends in primary HIV-1 drug resistance among recently infected persons. *Journal of the American Medical Association* **288**:181–8.

52. Little SJ, Holte S, Routy JP *et al.* (2002). Antiretroviral-drug resistance among patients recently infected with HIV. *New England Journal of Medicine* **347**:385–94.

53. Tanuri A, Soares MA, Brindeiro RM *et al.* (2002a). Brazilian network for drug resistance surveillance: results from the first national survey. Presented at the XIV International AIDS Conference. Barcelona, Spain, July 7–12.

54. Hart S, Shafer R, Tanuri A *et al.* (2003). Global Mapping of HIV-1 drug resistance patterns. Presented at the 10th Conference on Retroviruses and Opportunistic Diseases. Boston, Massachusetts, February 10–14. Abstract 622.

55. Tanuri A, Caridea E, Dantas MC *et al.* (2002). Prevalence of mutations related to HIV-1 antiretroviral resistance in Brazilian patients failing HAART. *Journal of Clinical Virology* **25**:39–46.

56. Bastos FI, Petersen M, Kerrigan D, Boily MC. (2004). Prise en charge du VIH-sida et ses facteurs psychologiques et sociaux: perspectives d'une expérience brésilienne. In: Levy J, ed. *Les Antirétroviraux: Expériences et Défis*. Québec: Les Presses de l'Université du Québec.

57. Izazola-Licea J, Avila-Figueroa CA, Aran D *et al.* (2002). Country response to HIV/ AIDS: national health accounts on HIV/AIDS in Brazil, Guatemala, Mexico, and Uruguay. *AIDS* 16(Supplement 3):S66–75.

58. Guimaraes MD. (2000). Temporal study in AIDS-associated disease in Brazil, 1980–1999. *Cadernos de Saúde Pública* 16(Supplement 1):21–36.

59. Palella FJ, Delaney KM, Moorman AC *et al.* (1998). Declining morbidity and mortality among patients with advanced human immunodeficiency virus infection. *New England Journal of Medicine* 338:853–60.

60. Pezzotti P, Napoli PA, Acciai S *et al.* (1999). Increasing survival time after AIDS in Italy: the role of new combination antiretroviral therapies. *AIDS* 13:249–55.

61. Blower SM, Farmer P. (2003). Predicting the public health impact of antiretrovirals: preventing HIV in developing countries. *AIDScience* 3(11). URL: www.aidscience.org.

62. Garnett GP, Bartley L, Grassly NC, Anderson RM. (2002). Antiretroviral therapy to treat and prevent HIV/AIDS in resource poor settings. *Nature Medicine* 8:651–4.

63. The World Bank. (1998). *Project Appraisal Document on a Proposed Loan in the Amount of US$ 165 Million Equivalent to Brazil for a Second AIDS and STD Control Project*. Human and Social Development Group, Brazil Country Management Unit, Latin America and the Caribbean Region; July 31, 1998: World Bank.

64. The World Bank. (1998). *Implementation Completion Report. Brazil. AIDS and STD Control Project (Loan 3659-BR)*. Brazil Country Management Unit, Human Development Sector Management Unit, Latin America and the Caribbean Regional Office; December 21, 1998.

65. Bastos FI, Lowndes KM. (2002). *A Critical Review of the Brazilain AIDS Program: Lessons for Others*. Paper commissioned for The Department for International Development (DfID) America and Transitional Economies Regional Health Meeting, Fortaleza, Brazil, April 17–19.

66. Bastos FI, Derrico M, Veloso VG *et al.* (2002). Risk Factors for HIV Among Late-presenting Pregnant Women in Porto Alegre (POA), Southern, and Rio de Janeiro (RJ), South-eastern Brazil. Presented at the XIV International AIDS Conference, Barcelona, Spain, 7–12 July.

Chapter 30

Costa Rica

Jessica Salas Martínez and Ignacio Salom Echeverria[*]

Background

Demography and health

Costa Rica covers an area of 51,100 km², with an average population density of 75 people per km², a total population of 3.8 million at the 2000 census, of whom 49.9% were men and 50.1% women, and an annual growth rate of 2.8% (1984–2000 intercensal period).

Ninety-six per cent of Costa Ricans identify themselves as white or *mestizo*; 2% as Afro-Costa Rican; 1.7% as belonging to one of the various indigenous groups, including the Chorotegas, descendents of both Mayan and Aztecs, and the Borucas, Bribri, Cabecar and Ngobe, more akin to other South American indigenous groups; and 3% identify themselves as 'other'. Ninety per cent of Costa Ricans are Roman Catholic, the official state religion. Costa Rica has a literacy rate of 95%, and the unemployment rate is below 6.2% in urban areas.

Costa Rica enjoys relative economic prosperity when compared with its neighbours in the region. The lack of military expenditure results in increased expenditure on health and education.

Health indicators

Life expectancy at birth during the census year 2000 was 77.5 years, with men enjoying a life expectancy of 75.4 years and women, 80.1 years, equivalent to many high-income countries (Table 30.1). Literacy reached 95%, representing an increase of 2% since the 1984 census.

Table 30.1 Health and demographic indicators, 2000

Indicators	Year 2000
Total population	3,810,179
Gross birth rate	19.9 per 1000 mid-year population
Infant mortality rate	10.2 per 1000 births
Gross death rate	3.8 per 000 mid-year population
Life expectancy at birth (males)	75.4 years
Life expectancy at birth (females)	80.1 years
Total fertility rate	2.35 children
Population growth rate	1.61% per year
Percentage foreign-born population	7.8%
Estimated net annual immigration	20,000–30,000 people

Source: [1].

* Corresponding author.

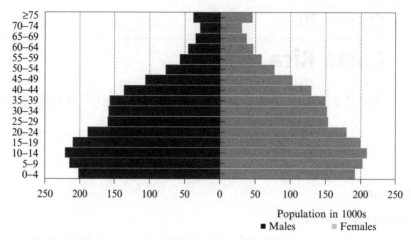

Fig. 30.1 Population structure by age and gender, 2001. Source: [1].

Table 30.2 Principle causes of mortality , 2001 (rate per 10,000 inhabitants)

Major cause groups	Number	Rate
Total	15,809	38.8
Diseases of the circulatory system	4884	12.1
Neoplasms	3416	8.5
Supplementary classification of external causes	1766	4.4
Diseases of the respiratory tract	1554	3.9
Diseases of the digestive tract	1008	2.5
Other causes	2979	7.4

Source: [1].

The Costa Rican population pyramid (Fig. 30.1) shows dramatic changes over the last 50 years, with a slow but steady aging of the population corresponding to a decline in mortality and fertility, as well as an increase in international migration over the last two decades (Table 30.1). These factors have substantially altered the population's epidemiological profile and demand for services (Table 30.2). In the last 10 years, it has become evident that the Costa Rican population has crossed the threshold into a process of relative aging, which will continue for the foreseeable future [2].

Over a period of 11 years (1990–2001), the infant mortality rate declined from 15.3 to 10.8 per 1000 live births, achieving the proposed target rate of 11 per 1000 or less in the last 2 years of the period. Over the last 10 years, maternal mortality has been 2.56 per 10,000 live births. The principal causes of death are described in Table 30.2.

The health system

Concern for public health has been a historical constant in Costa Rica since the mid-1800s. In 1973, the General Health Law and the Statutory Law of the Ministry of Health (*Ministerio de*

Salud) were proclaimed. This legislation made the Ministry of Health responsible for defining national health policy, as well as the organization, coordination and ultimate direction of the country's public and private health services. This constituted the basic legal foundation for the development of its leadership role in the country's healthcare system.

In the 1990s, as a part of the health sector reform process and further to the Law on Public Sector Financial Equilibrium (No. 6955, February 24, 1984), the Structural Adjustment Programme III (PAE) and obligations under Law 7374 (January 19, 1994) regarding financial operations between the Government of Costa Rica and the Inter-American Development Bank, the Ministry of Health assumed effective control of the health sector, while at the same time transferring activities directly related to healthcare provision to the Social Security System (*Caja Costarricense de Seguro Social*, or CCSS).

In its role of maintaining and improving the population's health, the Ministry of Health has four strategic functions: health surveillance; strategic planning; scientific research and technological development; and health services regulation. Currently, the Ministry's role provides opportunities for organizations within civil and political society to identify health problems and design interventions in response. This process implies a consolidation of the close relationships with community organizations, municipalities, educational institutions, private enterprise, public and private health centres, government agencies, non-governmental organizations (NGOs) and other public institutions, as well as all local, national and international organizations that participate in health-related activities [3].

The National Health System

The public National Health System (NHS) was first created at the end of 1993. However, it was deemed necessary to involve other sectors, so a new law was enacted that incorporated other health-related institutions into the system. As a result, health is no longer solely the responsibility of the health sector; rather, it involves different community actors and social institutions that influence the health of social groups in a specific population. The general objectives of the institutions that make up the health sector are to provide integrated care for the population, health promotion, rational utilization of resources and meeting the mission goals and principles of the NHS in order to preserve health and foster good quality of life for citizens.

The current NHS is the result of numerous activities carried out in response to social demands, a specific epidemiological profile and the state's social policies. Each institution within the NHS has a discrete role in ensuring the health of the Costa Rican population. The Ministry of Health is responsible for overseeing the health and social welfare system as a whole. The CCSS is the healthcare provider for all insured citizens and also provides care for the indigent. The National Insurance Institute (*Instituto Nacional de Seguros*) provides occupational and rehabilitation services for all workplace injuries. The Costa Rican Institute for Aqueducts and Water Services is responsible for ensuring the availability of potable water throughout Costa Rica and for treatment of all household and industrial water. The universities are engaged in health research, education and social action programmes. Private health establishments share similar objectives in integrated medical care, and treatment and diagnostic services. Some private health service providers use some of their profits to develop social programmes.

Together with other social and economic factors, the public health system has allowed the country to achieve health indicators that make Costa Rica stand out among countries with similar or higher levels of economic development.

Health expenditure and financing

In 2001, national health expenditure totalled ¢405,702 million colons (US$1.275 billion), or 7.4% of the gross domestic product (GDP) (Table 30.3).

Public social expenditure includes health, education and housing, as well as targeted poverty reduction programmes. Public resources for healthcare come primarily from payroll deductions to the CCSS and not from specific or general taxes collected by the government. Workers, employers and the state are the main contributors to the CCSS.

Increases in health expenditure mainly reflect expenditure in tertiary care. Despite enjoying universal healthcare with a tripartite programme, the percentage of private expenditure continues to increase. Furthermore, there has been an overall decrease in public social expenditure, including health. Table 30.4 compares expenditures among the different institutions that make up the public health sector, clearly indicating that the CCSS dominates spending.

Table 30.5 shows the trends in public insurance coverage under the CCSS since 1960. Voluntary insurance was designed for self-employed workers and employers, with the contribution rate for an unskilled or semi-skilled worker set at 4.8% of earnings on 70% of the minimum wage for his or her category of work. The state subsidizes a further 3.2%, and in this way the total system contribution is 8%. Public social security predominates, so that a universal compulsory contributory scheme covers a significant proportion of the country's labour force. It functions as insurer, financer and health service provider.

Organization and operation of healthcare services

The public sector

The CCSS is responsible for administering hospitals, clinics, and health areas and regions, as well as provision of services. The National Insurance Institute is responsible for providing

Table 30.3 Health expenditure, 1991–2001

Year	Per capita (US$)	% GDP	Composition (%) Public	Private	Health as % of public social expenditures
1991	156.7	6.9	76.8	23.2	32.3
1992	171.6	6.5	75.3	24.7	30.0
1993	194.5	6.7	76.2	23.8	29.4
1994	218.8	7.1	76,0	24.0	29.2
1995	238.5	7.1	74.8	25.2	30.1
1996	238.1	7.2	75.1	24.9	28.9
1997	250.0	7.2	73.5	26.5	27.3
1998	256.1	6.8	73.7	26.3	28.3
1999	269.9	6.6	72.7	27.3	29.7
2000	286.7	7.1	71.8	28.2	29.0
2001	295.6	7.4	71.0	29.0	28.5

Source: Análisis Sectorial de Salud de Costa Rica; Gasto y Financiamiento de la Atención de la Salud.

Table 30.4 Percentage distribution of public expenditure on health, 1991–2001

Year	Ministry of Health (%)	CCSS (%)	Institute for Aqueducts and Water Services (%)	National Insurance Institute (%)	University of Costa Rica (%)	Total (%)
1991	9.8	74.5	8.2	6.2	1.3	100
1992	9.1	74.0	9.3	6.2	1.4	100
1993	8.0	74.3	9.3	7.1	1.3	100
1994	8.1	75.9	8.8	6.1	1.1	100
1995	8.5	74.9	8.6	7.0	1.0	100
1996	7.9	74.0	10.1	6.7	1.3	100
1997	7.6	73.3	11.7	6.0	1.3	100
1998	6.6	77.1	10.8	4.1	1.4	100
1999	6.0	80.7	9.2	2.8	1.2	100
2000	5.5	80.2	9.5	3.6	1.2	100
2001	5.1	82.1	7.8	3.9	1.1	100

Source: Análisis Sectorial de Salud de Costa Rica; Gasto y Financiamiento de la Atención de la Salud.

rehabilitation and medical services for the population covered by Occupational Hazard Insurance and Obligatory Vehicular Insurance, which are compulsory for employers and vehicle owners, respectively.

The CCSS administration is divided into central, regional and local levels. The central level primarily fulfils a political, regulatory, investigative and financial function; the regional level coordinates services, and supervises and trains staff; and the local level delivers services. Care structure is subdivided into primary, secondary and tertiary levels. The primary level covers basic health services, which include health promotion and disease prevention, curative health services and less complicated rehabilitation. Activities are oriented towards individuals and their health- or environment-related behaviours. The secondary level supports the primary level by providing preventive, curative and rehabilitation services of varied complexity and specialization. Care is provided in both hospitals and health centres such as health posts, regional hospitals, temporary shelters and convalescent homes (*Casa de Salud*).

Table 30.5 CCSS insurance coverage by type, 1960, 1970, 1980, 1990 and 2001 (% of population)

Type of insurance	1960	1970	1980	1990	2001
Employee-obligatory	7.6	11.7	19.3	18.0	18.4
Voluntary insurance	–	–	3.8	6.0	5.1
Covered family member	7.7	35.1	47.9	40.9	42.1
State-paid coverage	–	–	–	9.2	12.4
Retirees	0.1	0.2	3.0	4.6	6.2
Family member of retiree	0.0	0.2	1.7	3.3	3.4
Not insured	84.6	52.8	24.3	18.0	12.5
Total	100.0	100.0	100.0	100.0	100.0
Coverage rates	15.40	47.15	75.70	81.95	87.50

Source: Dirección Actuarial y de Planificación Económica 1960, 1970, 1980, 1990 and 2001.

Tertiary-level care comprises highly specialized and complex preventive, curative and re-habilitation services. These services are provided by national or central hospitals and specialized hospitals that serve large populations

The goal of the system is integrated healthcare. The three tiers of care services are obliged to collaborate, so they are closely tied to each other with a view to providing efficient and coordinated care. The aim is to ensure that the population receives timely, integrated and continuous care under the guiding principles of universality, solidarity and equity.

The private health sector

Private health providers offer both general and specialized health services in private offices and hospitals, as well as offering dental care, clinical laboratories and diagnostic services in exchange for payment. Some private health service providers have entered into contractual agreements with the CCSS to provide primary health services. The Ministry of Health also oversees private healthcare providers and is responsible for their accreditation and compliance with national healthcare standards.

Utilization of health services

With regard to the type of care required, 67% of patients seek generalist medical care and 22% require specialized medical care. Seventy-eight per cent of the population utilizes the CCSS service network, 57% in the EBAIS (Basic Integrated Health Care Teams) and clinics, and 21% in hospitals. Those who are uninsured can either pay for services at the CCSS or seek private healthcare services. Emergency services are offered to all without regard to their ability to pay.

Human resources

This is a neglected area of health policy that requires prompt attention. Table 30.6 shows the increase in the number of professional members registered in the different professional colleges.

Currently, there are 2832 registered medical specialists in Costa Rica. The most common specializations are paediatrics, internal medicine, obstetrics and gynaecology, anaesthesiology and general surgery, since these are basic to hospital operation. It is worth noting that there may significant under-reporting of the number of nurses in the country, since this table includes only those registered in the nurses' college, a professional association.

Table 30.6 Registered professionals by college, 1999 and 2002

Colleges	1999	2002
Total	13,363	19,596
Physicians and surgeons	6788	7015
Microbiologists and clinical chemists	1092	1255
Pharmacists	1289	2199
Dentists	1594	2086
Nurses	2600	4781
Social workers	n/d	1465
Veterinarians	n/d	795

Source: 1999 data, *Observatorio de Recursos Humanos*, and Survey data, 2002.

Table 30.7 Medical specialists by citizenship and specialization, 2002

Specialization	Nationals	Aliens	Total
Total	1328	146	1474
Allergology and clinical immunology	24	1	25
Anaesthesiology	187	5	192
General surgery	143	19	162
Obstetrics and gynaecology	224	39	263
Communicable/infectious diseases	11	2	13
Internal medicine	239	37	276
Paediatrics	418	39	457
Public health	82	4	86

Source: College of Physicians and Surgeons, 2002.

Equity in the health system

In a recent study of health indicators conducted for the Ministry of Health, the Pan American Health Organization (PAHO) and the World Health Organization (WHO), Dr Marcelo Bortman found improvements in all the health indicators studied in terms of life expectancy at birth, years of potential life lost, mortality, mortality due to uterine cancer and infant mortality, but with the exception of maternal mortality. However, this could be due to a substantial under-reporting problem [4]. The study, which covered the period 1980–2001, found that differences among groups had decreased with regards to the indicators studied. This suggests that strategies targeting the most vulnerable social groups have been successful. While differences persist when comparisons are made between *cantones* (townships), overall a high degree of homogeneity has been achieved in terms of access to health services. The challenges that remain include maintaining the level of equity attained thus far, continuing programmes targeting the most vulnerable groups, and making quality of care a priority.

The HIV epidemic

According to data provided by the AIDS Control Unit (*Unidad de Control del Sida*) [5], the total cumulative number of AIDS cases between 1983 and August 2003 was 2455. Adding the cases with HIV infection, the total climbs to 4307 cumulative and confirmed cases in a population of 4 million inhabitants. The estimated number of people living with HIV (PLHIV; 0–49 years) varies between 6000 and 21,000. According to these data and world standards, Costa Rica has a low-prevalence epidemic. Furthermore, it is an epidemic that is concentrated among vulnerable groups, predominantly men who have sex with men (MSM), though there is a growing trend towards transmission among heterosexuals. The case reports for AIDS show an upward trend from 1983 through to the end of 1997, when the antiretroviral treatment (ART) programme began, with a definite impact in reducing the number of cases (Fig. 30.2) [6].

Once ART became available to the infected population, the number of HIV-infected people continued to increase while the number of AIDS cases declined (Fig. 30.3). This can be attributed to the fact that people infected with HIV are currently seeking treatment from health services earlier in their infection, before developing AIDS. Currently, the incidence of HIV appears to be steady.

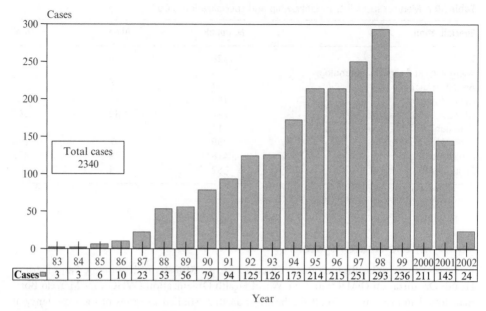

Fig. 30.2 AIDS cases per year, 1983-July 31, 2002. Source: [5].

In Costa Rica, HIV infection has been predominantly a male problem. During the 1980s, infection in women was practically non-existent, and it was only in the 1990s that infections began to appear among females. Different studies carried out in Costa Rican hospitals show a male predominance of 87% [6], with the greatest prevalence among MSM at 44%, followed by heterosexuals at 25% and bisexuals at 16%. The remaining 15% is made up of haemo-philiacs, children, injecting drug users, recipients of blood transfusions or people for whom there is no information [7]. It is worth noting that 40% of the cases occur among heterosex-uals and bisexuals, which partly explains the rising risk of infection among women.

The concentration of the largest number of cases (59%) can be seen in San José Province, where the capital and the majority of the country's inhabitants are located [7]. However, if the

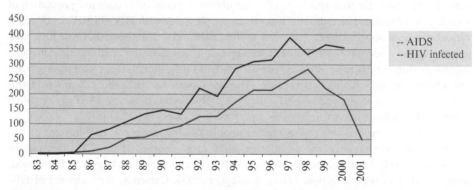

Fig. 30.3 Annual trends in HIV and AIDS cases, 1983–2001. Source: [5].

burgeoning problems of poverty and drug addiction in the ports are not addressed, these sites, which are also highly attractive for sex tourism, may see an increasing incidence of cases in the coming years. By the end of July 2002, the ports of Puntarenas and Limon presented a prevalence of 5% and 4%, respectively, of the total number of cases in the country [7].

In line with worldwide epidemiological reports, HIV in Costa Rica is prevalent among young, sexually active individuals, and this has been the main route of infection. Among people aged 25–44 years, 69% of cases, infection was probably acquired 5–10 years prior to virological diagnosis.

Between 1997 and 2000, mortality decreased as a direct result of the initiation of ART and levelled off at around 150 patient deaths per year. According to estimates, the country has approximately 550 new HIV cases per year either visiting health facilities for highly active ART (HAART), seeking treatment for opportunistic infections or seeking information on their immune system and virological status.

According to one study presented in 1998 [8], HIV infection in pregnant women had a prevalence below 1% and the epidemic still had not spread amongst children. Fewer than 50 HIV patients are currently being treated at the National Children's Hospital [HIV Clinic (2003), National Children's Hospital, CCSS, personal communication].

The health system's response to the HIV epidemic

History of the response and influence of the existing health system

The 1980s

In 1983, the first cases of HIV were detected in Costa Rica. In keeping with the country's healthcare structure, most of these patients were referred to tertiary care centres. Three hospitals in the San José metropolitan area took charge of caring for the sick. At that time, the aetiological origin of AIDS, its transmissibility, as well as the pathways for infection, were unknown, and fear of contagion predominated. Apprehension on the part of health staff slowly diminished as knowledge of the disease grew, and it became evident that AIDS was caused by HIV and that its potential for non-sexual transmissibility was not as great as initially feared.

Throughout the 1980s, all of the AIDS patients arriving at the hospital for consultation died within 2 years of their first admission. The average survival time after diagnosis was 8 months, according to reports from the AIDS Clinic at México Hospital in San José and studies done worldwide at the time [9].

Because of the health system's characteristics, any sick person who required emergency consultation or hospitalization had access to treatment. During this period, all of the sick received medical care, even if it was not of the quality and level of compassion that patients and their families would have desired.

The early 1990s

Hospitals became progressively better organized and were able to provide more humane and scientific care for HIV patients by the beginning of the 1990s, when some of the centres opted to treat HIV patients using interdisciplinary teams made up of several professionals. Team consolidation was very important to the handling of HIV-related opportunistic infections and neoplasms as well as the management of patients and families in their preparation for the process of dying.

The health system continued to be fully accessible during this period (1990–1997), and relationships between health personnel and patients improved to some degree, although survival rates remained unchanged. At this stage, the CCSS still had not incorporated mono- or dual ART into its basic drug formulary.

A new stage: the advent of HAART

Supported by a number of physicians, informal groups of PLHIV as well as NGOs began lobbying the CCSS to purchase the antiretroviral drugs used in triple or more combination therapy (HAART). At the end of 1997, the Constitutional Court advised the CCSS of its obligation to provide antiretroviral drugs to all HIV patients requiring them throughout the country. From that point on, three tertiary care hospitals in the San José metropolitan area were designated to provide ART and suitable follow-up with immunological and virological evaluation. At least two of these hospitals had interdisciplinary teams of care providers in place for these patients, which contributed significantly to the progress of HAART.

Since November 1997, HIV patients in Costa Rica have been treated with HAART whenever they show a CD4 count below 350 cells/mm^3, a viral load above 55,000 copies of RNA/mm^3, are symptomatic carriers of HIV or present with AIDS. Morbidity and mortality have decreased as a consequence of better hospital organization and more effective treatment, with figures similar to those reported in the literature worldwide. The first study of HIV-positive patients carried out by the Integrated Care AIDS Clinic at México Hospital [6] found that over 70% of patients had undetectable viral loads after 1 year of triple treatment.

A systematic response to the AIDS epidemic was organized by the National Commission on AIDS, made up of representatives from the different health institutions involved in HIV care. Coordinated by the Minister of Health, the National Commission recently took its first steps toward resolving the serious deficiencies in the areas of epidemiological surveillance and prevention that have characterized the response to the epidemic in Costa Rica. On a more positive note, the National Law on HIV was passed in May 1998 to protect patients' rights to quality healthcare, confidentiality and the right to work and education, which had been abrogated in the early years of the epidemic [10].

Prevention

Costa Rica has had preventive measures related to the HIV epidemic since the 1980s. Those first years were characterized by uncertainty, ignorance, prejudice and repression. Some preventive measures, which, fortunately, have now disappeared, included seeking—unsuccessfully—to close the borders to seropositive individuals wishing to enter the country, HIV testing of all public employees, and closing clubs frequented by MSM. Mass media campaigns contributed to the creation of the popular conception of the disease, linking it to death, sex, promiscuity and homosexuality, causing stigma that remains today and making it more difficult to implement effective prevention campaigns for both the general population and the groups at greatest risk of infection.

During those first years, however, there were also important public health measures that contributed to a significant reduction in the advance of the pandemic. For instance, pharmaceutical companies producing blood-derived products were required to provide certification from recognized national and international health agencies for the quality of their manufacturing process and HIV negativity. In 1985, enzyme-linked immunosorbent assay (ELISA) antibody testing became mandatory for all blood donors in the country, thus curtailing transmission by this route.

NGOs were also very important in those early years of the epidemic, providing education campaigns that targeted the groups at highest risk for HIV infection.

Studies done by the México Hospital AIDS Clinic have shown that while the adult population was aware of the risk of sexual transmission of HIV [11], at the same time patients acknowledged that they engaged in unprotected sexual relations, avoiding condom use for a variety of reasons [K Chacón and I Salom (2003), unpublished data].

Antiretrovirals and treatment of opportunistic diseases

Between November 1997 and August 2003, the México Hospital AIDS Clinic evaluated some 700 patients, approximately 460 of whom are currently undergoing treatment. The other three metropolitan hospitals that are managing HIV-positive patients show similar survival proportions. By 2004, the total number of patients treated had reached approximately 2000. Unfortunately, there are no data to confirm exactly how many of them were still alive, but there is a 15% annual mortality rate. As mentioned previously, the National Children's Hospital has fewer than 50 HIV-positive patients, all of whom have access to ART.

México Hospital receives an average of 120 new HIV patients per year, with an average mortality of 20 during the same period, mainly the very sick who are late in reaching the health system and present with very advanced opportunistic or neoplastic diseases. The second-tier hospitals are capable of caring for different problems that patients present with, except for providing ART. When a patient's condition is very serious or warrants special laboratory and imaging facilities, the service network also allows them to be referred to third-tier hospitals for management.

In general, the system provides the necessary conditions for handling the most frequent causes of infection by opportunistic organisms or neoplasms related to HIV. Within the basic drug formulary, there are about eight different antiretroviral drugs, including nucleoside reverse transcriptase inhibitor (NRTI) analogues, non-nucleoside reverse transcriptase inhibitor (NNRTI) analogues and protease inhibitors (PIs). It is also possible to purchase other inhibitors directly in those cases showing viral resistance and when the physicians opt for rescue treatment.

Case follow-ups allow for CD4 cell and viral load counts as well as routine examinations for all patients on ART or awaiting CD4 cell counts to fall below 350 cells/mm^3, which is the limit for starting ART according to the protocol. In special cases, patients under treatment may obtain genotype determinations to assist in salvage therapy, even though this is a procedure carried out under a research protocol, with extra-institutional funding, and for very few patients.

Initially, the antiretroviral drugs used in Costa Rica were proprietary, but, in recent years, in view of their cost, most of the products purchased are generics. Most come from India or from Costa Rican companies.

The number of patients receiving ART is continuously growing. Every patient who meets the criteria for treatment will receive it from the CSSS through the third-tier hospitals previously mentioned. In spite of the increase in the number of patients receiving ART, the budget for HIV drugs has declined as a proportion of the CCSS' total drug budget since 2000. In 2002, 6% of the total institutional drug budget was used to treat 1598 HIV-positive patients, compared with 10% for 937 patients in year 2000 [12]. This is related to a decrease in drug prices caused by the availability of generics and price reductions by pharmaceutical companies.

In general, the health system has sufficient human and material resources for diagnosis and management of patients with opportunistic infections associated with HIV. When the patient responds satisfactorily to treatment for an opportunistic infection in a second-tier hospital, he or she is later referred to a third-tier hospital to commence ART. This type of treatment is carried out exclusively by physicians specializing in immunology and infectious diseases.

Treatment is available for all seropositive pregnant women and their children. There are approximately 70,000 pregnancies per year in Costa Rica, with fewer than 1% being seropositive [8]. The screening programme for women with HIV is fairly recent and still does not adequately cover examination requests for this population, despite the existence of sufficient reagents for this purpose. A survey currently under way at México Hospital indicates that an AIDS test was requested during pregnancy for 60% of the women hospitalized for childbirth [7].

In summary, under the CSSS, ART, drugs for managing opportunistic infections and neoplasms, and treatment for seropositive pregnant women are fully guaranteed for the population with social insurance.

Conclusion

Achievements

Costa Ricans have been concerned about the country's health indicators since the nineteenth century, but more particularly since the so-called Law on Social Guarantees was passed at the end of the 1940s. This interest contributed to the development of social rights and institutions, which, in turn, led to the creation of an organized healthcare system covering almost 80% of the population. It is because the healthcare system was built on the principles of solidarity, in which everybody contributes according to their income but only those requiring services use the health facilities; universality, by which everybody can benefit from health coverage; and equity, through which all those requiring healthcare have the same opportunity of access and treatment, that the country has managed to care for all HIV patients, whether they are hospitalized or outpatients.

In 1983, when the first AIDS case was diagnosed in Costa Rica, the healthcare system was at least prepared to treat these patients for their opportunistic infections. In many cases, the patient's condition was terminal, but all were treated, regardless of their insurance status within the social security healthcare system. In this context, patients often survived for a few months only to return to hospitals to die, either from a recurrence of the same opportunistic infection or from new AIDS-related infections.

The country's most important achievement in dealing with the epidemic thus far has been ensuring access to affordable antiretroviral drugs for all patients who need them. It must be remembered that Costa Rica is a developing country with limited resources to spend on services, and yet it prioritized and managed this problem as though it were part of the wealthier, industrialized world—and did so without any foreign financial support. What made this possible was the size of the epidemic: by the time HIV patients started receiving HAART (November 1997), there were no more than 400 patients requiring it.

As soon as they appeared, antiretrovirals were purchased as generics, with optimal results in terms of CD4, viral load and health recovery. It should also be noted that the decision of some pharmaceutical companies to decrease the price of their proprietary products helped health authorities to manage the budget for HIV drugs.

Challenges

While Costa Rica was able to deal with the treatment aspect of HIV, it was not fully prepared to deal with prevention and epidemiological surveillance, nor was it ready to overcome the prejudices, stigma and myths that together conspired against taking control of the HIV epidemic. These are serious issues in Costa Rica that very urgently need to be addressed as the epidemic evolves and increasingly affects the broader community.

Costa Rica recently obtained a loan from the Global Fund to Fight AIDS, Tuberculosis and Malaria to support prevention activities targeting groups at highest risk of infection. It will be years before the results of such a programme appear. National funds have also been raised, pending a decision from Costa Rican health authorities, for mass media campaigns directed at adolescents and housewives. Without such activities, the epidemic will continue to grow and the HIV treatment programme will be at risk.

References

1. National Statistics and Census Institute. (2000). *2000 Census.* Costa Rica: Instituto Nacional de Estadística y Censos, INEC.
2. Ministry of Health. (2002). *Análisis Sectorial de Salud Costa Rica. Análisis Demografico y Epidemio-logico.* San José, Costa Rica. Section 1, p35–81.
3. Ministry of Health. (2002). *Memoria Anual.* San José, Costa Rica: Ministry of Health.
4. Bortman M. (2002). Indicadores de Salud. San José, Costa Rica : Organizacion Panamericana de la Salud.
5. AIDS Control Unit. (2003). *Annual Inform.* San José, Costa Rica: CCSS.
6. Salom I *et al.* (1998). HIV Patients' Response to HAART at México Hospital in Costa Rica. Presented at the LXth National Medical Congress, Costa Rican College of Surgeons and Physicians, Costa Rica.
7. Salas J, Vives M, Salazar H. (2003). *HIV/AIDS: A Public Health Problem in Costa Rica.* San José, Costa Rica: Ministry of Health.
8. Víquez A, Elizondo J. (1998). *Epidemiological Projections. HIV/AIDS in Costa Rica. Current Situation and Projections for the Future.* San José, Costa Rica: Ministery of Health, CCSS. p13.
9. New York State Department of Health. (1991). *AIDS in New York.* Albany: Department of Health.
10. General Law on HIV/AIDS. (1998). In: *General Law of Public Administration No. 7771.* San José, Costa Rica: Government of Costa Rica.
11. Salom I, Leon MP, Brenes M *et al.* (2001). Knowledge about HIV Infection in Young Adults in Costa Rica. Presented at the Xth Congress of the Pan American Association of Infectology.
12. CCSS, Department of Pharmacology. (2000). *Annual Inform.* San Jose, Costa Rica: CCSS.

Chapter 31

France

Yves-Antoine Flori, Céline Moty, Edith
Patouillard, François Dabis[*] and Roger Salamon

Background

As of January 1, 2004, Metropolitan France had 59.3 million inhabitants, and increasing at
0.4% per year, making it the third most populous country in the European Union (EU).
The Overseas Departments have 1.7 million inhabitants. At the 1999 census, there were 2.4
million foreign-born people living in France [1], about half of whom (1.6 million) came from
former African colonies. France's female life expectancy of 83 years is the fifth highest in the
world [2]. France's gross national product (GNP) totalled €1,520.8 billion (US$437.7 billion),
or €24,837(US$23,480) per capita [1]. After several years of rapid expansion (1997–2001), the
French economy entered into a period of slow growth of 1.5% in 2003, but reached a growth
rate of about 2% by the beginning of 2004 [1].

The health system

In order to better manage public expenditures as a whole, since the 1990s, France has implemented reforms with the aim of ensuring that all stakeholders contribute to controlling and
improving the effectiveness of healthcare spending [3–6]. Initiatives such as decentralization and
new budget framework legislation should permit society to meet the fiscal challenge posed by
population aging, while retaining high levels of service. However, up to now, these measures have
had a real, but limited, impact on the overall rise in spending. Initiatives to modify incentives
and behaviour have either been insufficient or slow in implementation. The overall social
security deficit reached 3.4% of the GNP in 2002 due to a 6.4% deficit in the health insurance
programme [7,8], while total health spending was around 10% of GNP (Table 31.1).

To better understand how the French healthcare system works, it is useful to look at the
French health insurance system, the provision of care, and the overall advantages and drawbacks of the system.

Health insurance and access to care

The public health insurance programme, one of the social security system's entitlement
programmes, was set up in 1945. Coverage was gradually expanded over the years to include
all legal residents, and now covers 99% of the population [9].

---

[*] Corresponding author.

Table 31.1 Health expenditure and sources of financing

Total	1995	2000	2001	2002
Total health expenditure as % of GNP	9.5	9.3	9.5	9.5
Public expenditure as % of total	76.0	76.0	75.8	76.0
Social security expenditure as % of total public	75.7	73.5	75.4	75.7
State and local administration as % of total	1.1	1.2	1.3	1.0
Supplementary insurance as % of total	11.5	12.0	12.4	12.7
Household (out-of-pocket) as % of total	11.7	11.4	11.0	10.6
Total	100.0	100.0	100.0	100.0
Hospital				
Hospital expenditure as % total health expenditure	48.2	45.5	44.9	44.7
Acute beds per 1000	7.0	6.9	6.7	6.5
Social security as % of total hospital expenditure	91.6	91.2	91.2	91.5
Supplementary insurance expenditure as % of total hospital expenditure	3.2	3.7	3.9	4.1
Household expenditure as % of total hospital expenditure	4.2	3.9	3.6	3.6
Outpatient care (physician services)				
Physician expenditure as % of total health expenditure	13.0	12.7	12.4	12.5
Social security expenditure as % of total physician expenditure	65.3	63.9	64.1	64.0
Supplementary insurance as % of total physician expenditure	20.3	20.7	20.7	21.0
Household expenditure as % of total physician expenditure	15.1	14.3	13.8	13.8
Pharmaceuticals				
Pharmaceutical expenditure as % of total expenditure	19.0	20.9	21.3	21.0
Social security expenditure as % of total pharmaceutical expenditure	54.9	57.9	58.6	59.7
Supplementary insurance expenditure as % of total pharmaceutical expenditure	19.7	18.5	18.8	19.4
Household expenditure as % of total pharmaceutical expenditure	24.4	22.3	21.3	19.9

Source: Health Accounts (*Comptes de la santé*), 2002.

The funding and benefits of the French public health insurance system (PHIS), much like Germany's, were originally occupationally based. The main fund covers 80% of the population; two other funds cover the self-employed and agricultural workers (16%). In 2001, disparate reimbursement rates were replaced by uniform rates across all funds. The funds are financed by employer and employee contributions, as well as personal income taxes. The latter's share of the financing has been ever-increasing in order to compensate for the relative decrease in wages, limit price distortions in the labour market and more fairly distribute the system's financing among all citizens.

Most health insurance funds are jointly managed by employers' federations and unions, and are under the State's supervision. Joint labour and management control has always sown discord within the funds' boards, as well as between the boards and the State. As a result, the responsibilities of the various actors in the system are not always shared in the most coherent manner. For example, since 1996, Parliament's budget provisions have determined how much public money will go to health expenditure (National Objective of Health Expenditure, or ONDAM), the Cabinet decides reimbursement rates and sets the level of contributions earmarked for the funds, while the funds themselves negotiate with healthcare professions to set fees designed to ensure the system breaks even. Responsibilities are frequently redefined, but never to the satisfaction of all those involved. Consequently, the ONDAM is never fully implemented [7,8].

The PHIS covers about 75% of total health expenditure. Half of the balance is covered by patients' out-of-pocket payments, and the other half is paid by private health insurance companies. These supplementary health insurance policies can be taken out by individuals or groups (Table 31.1). Approximately 85% of the population holds such policies. An important feature of the funds is that they cover a very wide range of goods and services, including, for example, stays in thermal spas. In the hope of curbing consumption and expenditure, co-payments were implemented and have increased over time. These co-payments are relatively high for many outpatient services; for instance, patients pay 30% of the social security charge for a physician's visit. Co-payments are also high for dental prostheses and eyewear. This has tended to deter the poorest citizens, few of whom have supplementary insurance, from seeking care.

Many experts advocate a change in the way health insurance covers care. In principle, it would be more efficient and equitable to clearly define a set of essential goods and services that would be available to everyone and 100% publicly financed [10–12]. The remaining goods and services would be available to those who desired and could afford them, with or without private insurance.

Access to care through the PHIS is not rationed; patients can see as many physicians as they like, as often as they like. Patients do not need referrals to see specialists, and, in general, there is no gatekeeping system of any kind. Doctors can freely prescribe brand-name drugs without restriction. This may partly account for the World Health Organization's high ranking of France's healthcare system in 2000; the rating system emphasized system responsiveness, a measure of patients' freedom and flexibility—a quality the French system provides, though undeniably at the expense of overall efficiency [13].

Provision of care

Hospitals

In France, hospitals have always been the core of the healthcare system. This probably accounts for the extremely specialized, technical, curative nature of our care, arguably to the detriment of prevention and community services. The number of hospital acute beds has decreased over time: it currently stands at 6.4 per 1000 inhabitants, which is close to the European average [14]. Hospital expenditure accounts for 45% of national health expenditure, and social security covers more than 90% of the costs [15] (Table 31.1).

Hospitals can be roughly divided into two categories: public and private for-profit. The state has an important role in managing the system. Three-quarters of all beds are in public hospitals, accounting for two-thirds of hospital spending, and public hospital staff has the status of civil servants. Public hospitals are funded out of global budget appropriations that are set annually by the authorities and allocated every month by the health insurance funds. Modest payments by patients top up these budget appropriations. Up to now, the appropriations have been set on the basis of the historical operating costs of hospitals, with modest allowance made for their actual level of activity, the average case mix and the specific costs of treating certain diseases and expensive drugs. Private clinics are paid on a fee-for-service basis. A uniform hospital information system has been implemented to monitor the activity in the various establishments. In future, all public and private establishments are expected to gradually switch to a prospective, diagnosis-related group (DRG) payment system.

Health professionals

There are currently about 200,800 physicians licensed to practise in France, or 3.3 doctors per 1000 population. In the last 30 years, the number of physicians has tripled, but the rate of increase is now very slight. Indeed, since 1971, the Ministry of Health has limited the number of medical students, a measure that, along with the retirement of currently active doctors, will result in a decrease in the number of physicians in the near future.

Half of all physicians are specialists. Health professionals account for 12% of the total health expenditure, of which social security pays around 64%. Supplementary insurance covers 21% of these expenditures and reduces the effect of co-payments (Table 31.1).

In France, physicians and other professionals generally work in either public hospitals or private practice. Twenty-five per cent of physicians work in public hospitals; another 11% work in other types of public establishments. They are in essence public servants and are paid an amount that is fixed by the government. Today, many physicians feel that the prestige of working in a hospital does not compensate for the trying working conditions.

Fifty-six per cent of physicians work in private practice and are paid on a fee-for-service basis. The relative reimbursement rate for different procedures is set by expert panels, and prices are negotiated between physicians' unions and the public health insurance funds. Since the creation of social security, the relationship between private practice physicians, the state and public insurance funds has always been strained. An agreement setting the general regulatory framework and the remuneration of the profession is supposed to be signed every 5 years by the physicians' unions. The root of the current problem is that private practice physicians are strongly opposed to the capping of outpatient expenditure. They have always had a great deal of freedom over where and how they practise and what they prescribe compared with their counterparts in other countries. Yet the bulk of their income (64%) is paid by public funds. This contradiction becomes more glaring as concerns about soaring health expenditure grow.

Pharmaceuticals

The pharmaceutical supply is regulated [16], but demand is not, since co-payments are relatively low for a large share of the population. This is reflected in per capita consumption of pharmaceuticals: in 1996, France had the second highest level of pharmaceutical consumption in the world after Japan, and the highest in Europe. Pharmaceuticals account for 21% of the total health expenditure, and the cost is still growing. Roughly 60% of drug expenditure is reimbursed by social security. Again, supplementary insurance reduces the co-payment effect for patients (19%) (Table 31.1).

Supply is regulated through incentives offered to drug companies and pharmacists. An agreement was concluded between the government and the pharmaceutical industry in July 1991, with a strong emphasis on administrative control and quantified targets for consumption in each therapeutic class. These targets were set so as to be consistent with the national targets for health insurance expenditure (ONDAM). This agreement has opened the way to subsequent arrangements between individual drug companies and the government. Each arrangement contains undertakings by the signatory laboratory as to the level of sales, refunds due in the event of target overruns, reduction of promotional expenditure and development of generic drugs. In 2003, 138 drugs were 'de-selected' and can now be bought without a prescription.

Advantages and drawbacks of the system

The system is perceived to be satisfactory . . .

The population seems to be satisfied with the healthcare system. Surveys such as the Euro-barometer show relatively high opinion ratings for the French system, with two-thirds of the population being fairly satisfied as compared with 40% in the UK and 20% in Italy [17]. The population appears to be happy with a system that combines freedom of choice, swift service delivery and a high quality of care delivered with a comparatively extensive use of modern medical technology and practice.

France also performs very well among OECD countries in terms of health and mortality indicators. For example, in 2001, female life expectancy at birth (83 years) was second only to Japan (83.8 years). Old-age disability is on a marked downward trend, particularly for men, in line with trends in the USA and Japan [18–21]. The same is true for infant mortality, which is very low and, at 4.6 per 1000 live births in 2001, only slightly higher than the rates in Scandinavian countries (Table 31.2). The high early mortality for men compared with the OECD average is nonetheless disquieting. Life expectancy at birth for men is relatively low at 75.5 years. Reports on public health show, however, that this is due to factors that have little to do with the functioning of the health system proper and is caused by the high number of violent deaths from suicides and road accidents, as well as an incidence of AIDS well above the European average and comparable with that of other Mediterranean countries such as Spain and Italy [22]. Another factor is high tobacco and alcohol consumption, with its attendant consequences of higher rates of cancer of the lung and of the upper respiratory and digestive systems. This shows the need for a broad-based, coherent approach to public health, which is beginning to emerge.

The cost is high . . .

A healthcare system with which the population is very satisfied and which delivers good outcomes does not come cheap. It is thus not surprising that the French system is relatively expensive by international standards. The share of health expenditure rose from 7.6% of GDP in 1980 to 8.9% in 1990 and 9.5% in 2001 (Table 31.1). On this indicator, France ranks fourth in the world, behind the USA, Germany and Switzerland [14,15].

On average, working households spend 20% of their gross income on health, including supplementary insurance contributions. Given the weight of social contributions in the cost of labour, modifications have been made to the way in which healthcare is financed, with, in particular, the introduction of a more broadly based contribution in 1991 (*contribution sociale*

Table 31.2 Health data 1998–2001

	1998	1999	2000	2001
Female life expectancy at birth	82.4	82.5	82.7	83.0
Male life expectancy at birth	74.8	75.0	75.2	75.5
% of population aged 65 years and over	15.9	16.1	16.4	16.9
Infant mortality per 1000 live births	4.6	4.3	4.6	4.6

Source: OECD CREDES (Centre de Recherche et de Documentation en Economie de la santé), 2003.

généralisée), and its gradual extension in order to finance the health insurance schemes. However, as Ventelou said, the growth of health expenditure is, in France, a '*maladie d'amour*' [23].

Inequalities remain...

In order to ensure greater equity in access to healthcare, universal health insurance (*couverture médicale universelle* or CMU) has been available since January 1, 2000 to the neediest members of society [24]. The first part of CMU provides basic coverage to all those legally residing in France, irrespective of their employment situation or insurance contribution record. In this regard, as an equitable nationwide scheme, CMU represents a considerable step forward. However, households whose incomes are too low to allow them to contribute to a supplementary insurance scheme, but too high for them to qualify for universal health insurance, have to pay a substantial part of their healthcare themselves, particularly for services that are poorly reimbursed, such as dental and optical care. It can also be a problem for them to have to pay in advance [25]. Also, access to certain types of care is relatively expensive, given that a quarter of the medical profession in the ambulatory care sector is free to charge extra fees not reimbursed by social security on the basis of having higher qualifications, and supplementary insurance schemes reimburse only a small part of the cost of private beds and treatment by hospital doctors.

There are also instances of geographical inequity [26,27]. Different arrangements contribute to inequalities in access to care between regions and even within regions. For example, there are significant disparities in ambulatory care supply, doctor density being highest in the Ile de France and the Mediterranean regions [19]. Where hospitals are concerned, despite centralized decision-making procedures, there are sizeable differences in resource allocation between regions in terms of beds, hospital medical staff, equipment and funds. In some localities, waiting times for non-life-threatening conditions are considered to be excessive [e.g. positron emission tomography (PET) scan examinations for cancer]. The authorities have therefore embarked on a policy of progressive equalization that should ultimately reduce these inequalities between regions [28].

A weak public health policy...

Until recently, French public health policy suffered from shortcomings that are only just starting to be addressed [29]. These shortcomings have become more visible in recent years as past burdens accumulate [30]. Public health has historically occupied a minor place in the French decision-making and training system. Specialist training in public health during the internship phase of medical studies has only recently been made available. Teaching and research structures, though well developed, are still well behind those in anglophone countries. A national body (*Haut Comité de la Santé Publique*) was set up in 1990 to coordinate public health policy, and tools for monitoring public health have been particularly strengthened by the creation of a disease monitoring centre (*Institut de Veille Sanitaire*), which replaced the former National Public Health Network.

Lastly, for the past 10 years, the government has been steadily creating independent agencies under the aegis of the Ministry of Health for drug evaluation, blood supply management, food safety, and medical accreditation and evaluation. Despite this progress, France still does not have an explicit health policy with global health objectives and measures to achieve a better balance between prevention and care.

On balance...

In many respects, France has a healthcare system that other OECD countries might envy: the health status of the population ranks among the best in the industrialized countries; public spending is generous; patients have great freedom of choice between healthcare providers; patients generally do not have to queue for treatment; and considerable resources are allocated to healthcare, by international standards.

However, health sector reform does remain a priority. The French experience shows that purely economic measures are insufficient to contain costs and improve efficiency. There is need for a new definition of the roles of the main actors and of what should be financed by public insurance versus private funds either by households, private insurance or others, so as to meet the challenges posed by an aging population and higher pharmaceutical costs, while retaining high levels of service.

The HIV epidemic

As in other developed countries, the efforts of scientists, clinicians, activists and public administrations have succeeded in influencing the HIV epidemic in France since its onset. Human resources, drugs and time were allocated to both treatment and prevention of HIV infection. In France, this fight against the epidemic led to innovation in prevention, patient care and health policy. Historically, as noted by Rosenbrok *et al.* [31], the treatment of AIDS has moved from exceptionalism to normalization.

In the first 'exceptional' phase of the epidemic (1985–1991), the occurrence of AIDS opened up a window of opportunity [32] for implementing new public health policies prompted by the emergence of new public health actors such as non-governmental organizations (NGOs) and social scientists. In the context of fighting stigmatization, this produced innovations, some of which went beyond the boundaries of the conventional health system, such as:

- the *Pacte Civil de Solidarité* (PACS), a civil contract for all types of couples;
- The National Council on AIDS, whose aim is to protect the rights of people living with HIV (PLHIV);
- A ban on discrimination against PLHIV in the workplace.

Other measures were related to new prevention concepts, such as:

- the creation of the *Agence Française de Lutte Contre le SIDA* (AFLS);
- the coordination of research studies with the creation of the *Agence Nationale de Recherche sur le SIDA* (ANRS);
- new forms of care coordination, such as care networks.

Efforts were made to ensure that all these components were linked together, as in all European countries. However, the implementation of this new form of response was challenging, since it relied, on the one hand, on the official health policy structures that had existed prior to the epidemic—which were medically dominated, not always efficient and unskilled in the new ways of working needed—and, on the other, on emerging coalitions formed between the gay community NGOs such as AIDES, Act UP, ARCAT SIDA, SOL en SI and social scientists, which generated new prevention concepts and pointed to uncomfortable incompatibilities between prevention and discrimination.

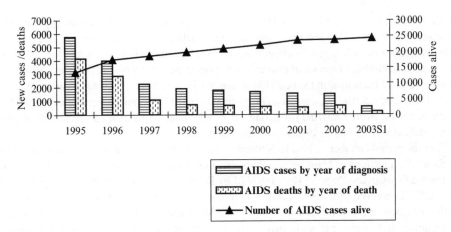

Fig. 31.1 Evolution of the AIDS epidemic. Source: Institut National de Veille Sanitaire (INVS) 2004.

Since 1996, the management of AIDS has become normalized, making it similar to other chronic diseases. 'Exceptionalism' ended for the following reasons: first, the worst-case scenario did not occur—the number of HIV-positive people remained stable; secondly, there was a declining interest in the issue of HIV, mainly because other health issues grabbed the attention, such as, for example, bovine spongiform encephalopathy (BSE); and, finally, and very importantly, the availability, with limited restrictions, of highly active antiretroviral therapy (HAART), which resulted in the reintegration of HIV policy into the mainstream of the health system, along with hospital leadership in care and resource allocation.

Epidemiology

AIDS

In France, it is mandatory to report every new AIDS case to the *Institut National de Veille Sanitaire* (INVS), which collects and analyses these data. Since March 2003, it has also been mandatory to report every HIV infection. On December 31, 2003, 24,606 people were estimated to be living with AIDS (Fig. 31.1). The number of new AIDS cases was 1641 in 2001, 1575 in 2002 and 1364 in 2003, with women making up half of new cases. So a decrease in the annual number of new cases continues to be observed, but this decrease is now less than 5% per year. The cumulative number of AIDS deaths since the beginning of the epidemic was estimated at the end of December 2003 at 33,841 [33].

With 581 deaths in 2001, 669 in 2002 and 492 in 2003, AIDS mortality is now stable (Fig. 31.1). The number of new AIDS deaths each year is lower than the number of new cases. The total number of PLHIV and acquiring AIDS is increasing by 6% per year. The dramatic fall in new cases and deaths after 1996–1997 is directly linked to knowledge of HIV status and HAART. Between 1996 and 2001, the number of new AIDS cases among people seeking treatment was reduced by 79%, transforming AIDS in France into a chronic disease [33].

Annual statistics on new AIDS cases by transmission group show that heterosexual transmission has been the most frequent mode of transmission since 1997. In 2003, this transmission mode accounted for 53% of all new HIV cases, compared with transmission among men who have sex with men (MSM) and injecting drug users (IDUs), which accounted for 21% and 3%, respectively. Transmission modes categorized as 'other' or 'unknown' accounted for 23% [33]. The same distribution of modes of transmission is observed among new AIDS cases. Since 1998, mother-to-child transmission (MTCT) has accounted for less than 0.5% of AIDS cases (Fig. 31.2) [33]. The rate of infection among pregnant women between 1991 and 2000 remained stable. Due to antiretroviral treatment (ART), the number of HIV-infected women completing their pregnancy increased from 500 in 1992 to 1200 in 2000 [33].

Over the period October 1, 2002 to September 30, 2003, the rate of new AIDS cases was 24 per million HIV infections in Metropolitan France and Overseas Departments, with the highest rate in the Antilles-Guyane Region (124), followed by Ile de France (59) and Provence Côte d'Azur (31) [33]. Transmission patterns are different from one area to another. Ile de France is the region with the highest rate of sexual transmission among MSM and among heterosexuals in the African community. IDU transmission is predominant in Provence Côte d'Azur, and heterosexual transmission predominates in Antilles-Guyane. More than eight out of 10 transmissions among heterosexuals come from African or Caribbean communities [33].

HIV

The epidemiological monitoring system for HIV infection was considerably delayed. The mandatory notification system was set up in March 2003. France appears to be very late in terms of implementation of its monitoring system compared with other European countries. The number of HIV-positive people was estimated to be between 70,000 and 120,000 in 1997. According to the French Ministry of Social Affairs, HIV infection affected 110,000 people in France in 1999, 92,100 of whom were treated in hospital [33–36]. In 2003, 1301 new HIV infections had been reported by September 30 [33], contributing to the estimated 120,000 PLHIV in December 2003. It appears that the epidemic is now under control thanks to the availability of HAART, but it remains alarming in Overseas Departments and African communities.

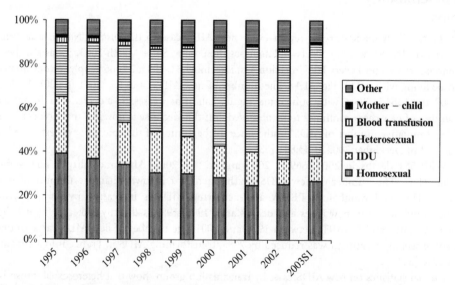

Fig. 31.2 Transmission patterns. Source: Institut National de Veille Sanitaire (INVS) 2004.

Prevention

1989–1999

Policies of prevention and risk reduction can be split into two phases: before and after 1999. The strategy implemented in the first phase of the epidemic (1989) had two objectives: first, to reduce the risk of transmission; and, secondly, to prevent discrimination against MSM, PLHIV and AIDS patients. The approach was to present AIDS as a disease that should concern everyone equally.

This policy of promoting individual rights produced new prevention tools. At the beginning of the 1990s, the *Agence National de Lutte Contre le SIDA* created a toll-free call-in line, '*SIDA info service*', to provide information anonymously regarding HIV infection, with at least one free and anonymous testing centre (*Centre de diagnostic anonyme et gratuite*, or CDAG) in each department. This agency, in collaboration with the French committee for health education (CFES), also launched information campaigns directed toward the general population. For example, information activities were conducted in schools. This policy produced good results in terms of non-stigmatization of HIV-infected people and knowledge of transmission modes, but its impact on the incidence of HIV infection is not known. Possible adverse effects such as potentially influencing the initiation of sexual activity among young people were not evaluated.

The CDAG system also facilitated the testing of the French population, but without investigating their risk group. For pregnant women, the non-mandatory testing system facilitated treatment and continuation of pregnancy. At the same time, however, action targeting IDUs was delayed, and the infection rate did not decrease as rapidly in this risk group as in others [37,38]. The incidence of AIDS among this group only decreased in the late 1990s, thanks to the availability of needle exchange programmes [38]. CDAG was closed in 1993, and the CFES became the National Institute for Prevention and Education on Health (INPEIS) in 2002.

Current policy

Since 1999, the government's information and prevention policy has aimed to reduce the epidemic within risk groups (MSM, IDUs and in Overseas Departments) as well as within the general population, and to deal with inequalities. The latest plan (2001–2004), prepared in collaboration with NGOs and implemented by the Ministry of Health, gave a high level of autonomy to local administrations [39]. The policy comprised specific campaigns towards risk groups, in collaboration with NGOs, as well as general information campaigns.

With the advent of HAART, these campaigns remain crucial. Even if some signs of improvement in risk behaviours among MSM [40] and youth [41] were observed in the late 1990s, there are growing problems among immigrant populations, the rate of STI has increased in the Paris area, mostly among MSM, and the use of condoms among young people has decreased. Moreover, the number of tests carried out by CDAG remained stable at 45,000 per year between 1998 and 2001 [33,36]. The rate of HIV has increased mostly within the African community.

In the context of current budget restrictions, there is a great risk that the funding devoted to prevention will be reduced. The target of information campaigns should be redefined in order to focus on risk groups.

Treatment and care

Organization

The hospital is at the heart of HIV care in France, and only a small number of physicians treat HIV patients outside the hospital network [42]. To facilitate hospital care and moderate expenditure, some innovations emerged in the 1980s. First, in each region, a centre for information and care of HIV (*Centre d'information et de Soins de l'Immuno-Déficience Humaine*, or CISIH) was created—there were 31 of these by 2002—to gather information about patients, participate in clinical investigation and coordinate care with the hospital care networks created in 1989. Their networks are the link between hospitals and outpatient care, to promote continuity of care and development of outpatient care. There were 92 of these networks in 2000. To support this effort, the French Ministry allocated special budgets to the CISIHs to recruit practitioners and technicians, and to invest in materials. Since they were established, some 630 physicians and 6400 technicians have been recruited.

Secondly, hospitals were reorganized. Evening outpatient clinics were created to enable working people to come in for consultations, and NGOs were allowed to work inside these departments.

Thirdly, the *Direction de l'Hôpitalisation et de l'organisation des soins* (DHOS) and the *Institut national de la santé et de la recherche médicale* (INSERM) created a database called DMI2, the Medical Dossier on Human Immunodeficiency (version 2), which gathers patient-specific clinical and socio-economic information from public hospitals treating HIV-infected individuals. To date, 68 hospitals have collected data producing epidemiological results, allowing the monitoring of patient characteristics, hospital activity and evaluation of costs and resource utilization.

The final innovation was the publication of HIV infection management recommendations in 1997, revised in 2002 [34,43]. These widely disseminated reports were produced by a group of experts and representatives of medical associations, and provided updated information on best practice treatment for HIV patients.

Trends in treatment and care

Most of the data about hospital care come from the DMI2 database [36,44], which provides a large amount of information regarding the number and types of patients seeking hospital care, the volume of care and treatments. In 2001, 92,100 HIV patients were being treated at hospitals. The number of patients treated increased by 43% between 1995 and 1999 and now remains stable. From 1997 to 2001, the rate of patients with a CD4 count greater than 200 and a viral load greater than 500/ml rose from 23 to 53% (Table 31.3).

The pattern of hospital care changed between 1995 and 2001, with a shift from inpatient to ambulatory care, either day hospitalization or outpatient visits. The availability of HAART reduced the rate of inpatient stays by 65% for all patients—and by 68% for AIDS patients—due to the decrease in opportunistic infections and deaths. In the same period, the length of stay was reduced by 19%, from 13 days in 1995 to 10 days in 2001. The rate of day hospitalization was reduced by 20% between 1995 and 1999 and now remains stable (Table 31.3).

Between 1995 and 2001, the proportion of patients receiving antiretroviral drugs grew from 61% to 86%. Of these, 70% were on triple therapy, 20% on quadruple or more therapy, and 8%

Table 31.3 Trends in treatment and care of HIV patients

	1995	1996	1997	1998	1999	2000	2001
Percentage of patients with CD4 >200 and viral load <500	n/a	n/a	22.7	40.4	47.4	50.2	53.5
Number of patients followed-up							
AIDS + HIV (24 hospitals)	10,820	11,902	12,785	14,610	14,798	15,820	15,580
HIV (23 hospitals)	6943	7801	8428	10,155	10,677	10,574	10,177
AIDS (23 hospitals)	2810	2895	3161	2860	3152	3194	3211
Inpatient hospital discharge rate per 1000 patients							
HIV + AIDS	277	237	111	124	117	117	88
AIDS	715	629	252	308	294	290	206
HIV	102	90	59	73	65	67	51
Hospital visits rate per 1000 patients	1029	1164	1043	1070	1116	1100	1110
Day hospitalization rate per 1000 patients	1306	1262	1122	942	790	800	786
Length of stay (days)	12.7	12.2	9.3	9	9.9	9.6	10
Patients eligible for antiretroviral treatment (%)							
Treated	61.1	72.3	80.8	86.2	87	87.6	85.6
Untreated	38.9	27.7	19.2	13.8	13	12.4	14.4
Antiretroviral combination							
Monotherapy	68.5	15.5	2	0.9	0.7	0.5	0.6
Dual therapy	31.5	66	46.6	29.2	16.5	11.8	9.2
Triple therapy	0	18.2	47.6	60.5	70.4	70.9	70.2
Four or more drugs therapy	0	0.3	3.8	9.4	12.4	16.8	20

Source: French Ministry of Health, 2003, key statistics.

remained on double combination therapy (Table 31.3); 39% of the combination therapy included a non-nucleoside reverse transcriptase inhibitor (NNRTI). The two most frequent combinations prescribed in 2001 were zidovudine (AZT) + lamivudine (3TC) + nevirapine (6.2%) and AZT + 3TC + efavirenz (5.9%) [34,36].

On a given day in 2000, among the 3526 HIV patients in one hospital, 43% were consulting a physician in an ambulatory ward; 20% were in inpatient wards—two-thirds of them AIDS patients; 18% were in day hospitalization; and 8% were in long-term care [36]. The use of hospitals appears to be linked not only to health status, but also to socio-economic status. On a given day in 1999, more than 50% of HIV patients attending hospital in France were unemployed, 20% were on disability benefits, 7% on unemployment benefits and 6% were earning at the minimum wage level. These figures reflect the changing patterns of the epidemic, with more and more poor people infected and thus making proportionately high use of hospitals [45].

In France, patients with social security insurance are fully covered, therefore they do not pay for either drugs or visits, and are well treated. However, such is not the case for patients without social security or those with the CMU, which only provides basic healthcare coverage. For these growing numbers, as tests and treatments are delayed, opportunistic infections and new AIDS cases increase.

Financing

As previously noted, in France, 75% of healthcare costs, and over 80% of hospital costs, are financed by social security, with a small additional budget from the Ministry of Health. It is not easy to calculate exactly how much is spent on HIV prevention, testing and care, and how this is financed, as available information is from an aggregated budget. What follows are some rough estimates of the expenditures and how they are financed.

In the Ministry of Health budget, the allocation for HIV testing, prevention and communication was €73 million (US$69 million) in 1999 and €65.2 million (US$61.6 million) in 2000 and 2002 [36,44]. Since 1990, HIV care has been financed through both the main hospital budgets and a special Ministry of Health budget. The amount of this supplementary budget is based on the number of patients treated. The Ministry of Health allocates this special budget as a global amount by region, and then local authorities, in turn, allocate the resources to each hospital. Between 1990 and 1996, this special budget was used to finance both hospital care and drugs. In 1997, antiretrovirals were removed as part of the normalization of the HIV response and are now financed by the social security drug budget. Between 1995 and 2002, expenditure from hospital budgets decreased from €602 million (US$569 million) to €461 million (US$436 million) due to both a reduction in admissions and lengths of stay, and a shifting of pharmaceutical expenditure out of hospital budgets [36].

A 2001 survey by the Ministry of Health estimated that hospital antiretroviral expenditure totalled €302.8 million (US$286.2 million) in 2000 (Ministry of Health, personal communication). It should be noted that since 1997, antiretrovirals can be bought in either pharmacies or hospitals in France. A recent detailed survey carried out by social security showed a total reimbursement of €147.4 million (US$139.3 million) for HIV care in 2000, with drugs bought in pharmacies accounting for €98 million (US$92.6 million) [46]. This represents a cost of €12,404 (US$11,727) per insured infected person, a figure close to that arrived at by Yazdanpanah et al. [47]. Based on these figures, we can roughly estimate that the total health expenditure for treating insured HIV patients was €969.4 million (US$916.4 million) in 2000, or 0.9% of the health expenditure for that year (Table 31.4).

Table 31.4 HIV expenditure in France in 2000

Category	Amount in millions €	Amount in millions of US$
Testing and prevention	65.2	61.6
Hospital care (excluding drugs)	454	429.2
Hospital pharmaceuticals	302.8	286.2
Social security expenditure for HIV care, including ambulatory expenditure, including pharmaceuticals bought from pharmacies	147.4	139.3
Total	969.4	916.4
Total as % of the total health expenditure	0.9%	0.9%

Source: French Ministry of Health, 2003, key statistics.

Conclusion

France's response to HIV has involved many actors—government, NGOs, clinicians and social scientists, among others—and produced innovations in terms of access to care and the protection of patients' rights. As in other European countries, the availability of HAART has led to a significant reduction in mortality as well as improvement in the health status of all HIV-infected patients. As a result, HIV is considered to have moved from an acute to a chronic disease in France. The fact that most patients have been covered by social security has been a key factor in effective treatment efforts. However, transmission pathways are changing, and the epidemic is increasingly affecting poor and vulnerable populations that have inadequate health coverage; risky behaviours also appear to be on the rise. Sustaining and strengthening existing policies and programmes in the face of budget constraints calls for maintaining prevention programmes targeting groups at high risk, coordinating care and extending health insurance coverage to all vulnerable populations. A good system for monitoring utilization and cost is also needed. If all this can be done without increasing expenditure, equal access to care and prevention will truly be available for all.

References

1. Institut National de la Statistique et des Sciences Economiques (INSEE). (2003). *France in Figures*. Paris: INSEE. URL: www.insee.fr.

2. World Health Organization. (2003). *The World Health Report 2003. Shaping the Future*. Geneva: WHO. URL: www.who.int/whr/2003/en.

3. Imaï Y, Jacobzone S, Lemain P. (2000). *The Changing Health System in France*. OECD Economic Working Paper No. 269. Paris: OECD.

4. OECD. (2003a). *Economic Survey of France 2003. Policy Brief, July 2003*. URL: www.oecd.org/dataoecd/46/12/3220451.pdf.

5. OECD. (2003b). *Economic Outlook 2003*. Paris: OECD. URL: www.oecd.org/.

6. Institut National de la Statistique et des Etudes Economiques (INSEE). (2003). *Comptes Nationaux 2003*. Paris: INSEE.

7. Commission des Comptes de la Sécurité Sociale. (2003). Les comptes de la Sécurité sociale. Paris: Government of France. URL: www.social.gouv.fr/htm/zctu/secu/compters/index-comptes.htm.

8. Cour des Comptes. (2002). *La Sécurité Sociale*. Paris: Les Editions du Journal officiel.

9. ADECRI. (2003). *The French Social Protection System*. Saint Etienne: ADECRI. URL: www. adecri.org/publications/documents/The_French_Social_Protection_System.pdf.

10. Bureau D, Plassart A. (1999). *Comment Réguler les Dépenses de Santé?* Paris: Les Cahiers Français, No. 292 (Emploi et Protection Sociale).

11. Johanet G. (1998). *Sécurité Sociale, l'Échec et le Défi.* Paris: Le Seuil.

12. Mougeot M. (1999). *Régulation du Système de Santé.* Rapport du Conseil d'Analyse Economique, No. 13. Paris: Editions La Documentation Française.

13. World Health Organization. (2001). *World Health Report 2000—Improving Performance.* Geneva: WHO. URL: www.who.int/whr2001/2001/archives/2000/ en/index.htm.

14. OECD. (2003). *Health Data.* Paris: OECD.

15. Commission des Comptes de la Santé. (2003). Les comptes de la santé. Paris: Government of France. URL: www/sante.gouv.fr/drees/etude-resultat/er-pdf/er246.pdf.

16. Jacobzone S. (2000). *Pharmaceutical Policies in OECD Countries: Reconciling Social and Industrial Goals.* Labour Market and Social Policy Occasional Papers No. 40. Paris: OECD.

17. Mossialos E. (1997). Citizens' view on health systems in the 15 member states of the European Union. *Health Economics* 6:109–16.

18. Jacobzone S, Cambois E, Robine J-M. (2000). Is the health of older persons in OECD countries improving fast enough to compensate for population ageing? *OECD Economic Studies* No. 30, 2000/ I:149–90.

19. Vilain A, Niel X. (1999). Les inégalités régionales de densité médicale. *DREES, Etudes et Résultats* No. 30.

20. OECD. (2001). *ECO-SANTE 2001—Analyse Comparative de 30 Pays.* Paris: OECD et CREDES.

21. OECD. (2002). *Measuring Up. Improving Health System Performance in OECD Countries.* Paris: OECD.

22. Haut Comité de la Santé Publique. (1998). *La Santé en France 1994–1998.* Paris: Editions La Documentation Française.

23. Ventelou B. (1999). Les dépenses de santé des Français: une maladie d'amour? *Revue de l'OFCE* No. 71. Paris.

24. Sénéquier H. (1999). La couverture médicale universelle. *Regards sur l'Actualité.* Paris, November.

25. Dourgnon P, Grignon M. (2000). *Le Tiers Payant Est-il Inflationniste?* Etude de l'inflation du tiers payant sur la dépense de santé. CREDES report No. 1296. Paris.

26. Mesrine A. (1997). Les inégalités de mortalité par milieu social restent fortes. *La France, Portrait Social.* Paris: INSEE.

27. Mormiche P. (1997). Inégalités de santé et inéquité du système se soins. In: Jacobzone S, ed. *Economie de la Santé, Trajectoires du Futur.* Paris: INSEE Méthodes/ Economica.

28. Cour des Comptes. (2000). *La Sécurité Sociale.* Paris: Les Editions du Journal Officiel. URL: www.comptes.fr/.

29. Dab W. (1997). Crises de santé publique et crise de la santé publique. *Revue Française des Affaires Sociales,* December. Paris.

30. Morelle A. (1996). La défaite de la santé publique. *Forum.* Paris: Flammarion.

31. Rosenbrock R, Dubois-Arber F, Moers M, Pinell P, Schaeffer D, Setbon M. (2000). The normalization of AIDS in Western European countries. *Social Science and Medicine* 50:1607–1629.

32. Kingdon J. (1984). *Agendas, Alternatives, and Public Policies.* Boston: Little, Brown & Company.

33. Institut National de Veille Sanitaire (INVS). (2004). La notification obligatoire du VIH, une priorité de santé publique, un engagement de tous. *Bulletin Epidémiologique Hebdomadaire* 24–25:101–8.

34. Delfraissy JF *et al.* (2002). *Prise en Charge Thérapeutique des Personnes Infectées par le VIH.* Paris: Ministère de l'emploi et de la solidarité, Médecine-Sciences Flammarion.

35. Costaliola D, Lievre L, Mary-Krause M. (2002). Caractéristiques de l'infection à VIH en 2001. In: Pons G, Tréluyer JM, Blanche S *et al.*, eds. *Médicaments du SIDA de l'Enfant et de l'Adulte*. Paris: Springer Verlag, p1–9.

36. Ministère de la Santé. (2003). *Les Chiffres Clés: Sida et Hépatite*. Paris: Flammarion Médecine-Science. URL: www.sante.gouv.fr/htm/publication/dhos/vih_vhc/index.htm.

37. Lert F. (2000). Drug use, AIDS and social exclusion in France. In: Moatti JP, Souteyrand Y, Prieur A, Sandfort T, Aggleton P, eds. *AIDS in Europe*. London: Routledge.

38. Moatti JP, Souteyrand Y. (2000). Editorial: HIV/AIDS social and behavioural research: past advances and thoughts about the future. *Social Science and Medicine* 50:1519–32.

39. Ministère délégué à la santé. (2001). Plan national de lutte contre le VIH/Sida – 2002/2004. Paris: Government of France. URL: www.sante.gouv.fr/htm/dossiers/sida02/1sida2.htm.

40. Adam P. (2002). Baromètre gay 2001: résultats du premier sondage auprès des clients des établissements gays parisiens. *BEH 2002* 18:77–9. URL: www.invs.sante.fr/beh/2002/18_beh_2002.pdf.

41. Gremy I, Beltzer N, Vongmany N *et al.* (2001). *Les Connaissances, Attitudes, Croyances et Comportements au VIH/SIDA en France*. Paris: Observatoire Régional de Santé d'Ile-de-France.

42. Obadia Y, Souville M, Morin M, Moatti JP. (1999). French general practitioners' attitudes toward therapeutic advances in HIV care: results of a national survey. *International Journal of STD and AIDS* 10:243–9.

43. Dormont J *et al.* (1999). *Prise en Charge Thérapeutique des Personnes Infectées par le VIH*. Paris: Ministère de Emploi et de la Solidarité, Médecine-Sciences Flammarion.

44. Ministère de l'Emploi et de la Solidarité. (2000). *Les Chiffres Clés: Sida et Hépatite C*. Paris: Flammarion Médecine-Science.

45. De Peretti C, Wcislo M, Nadal JM. (2001). *Les Patients Soignés pour Infection à VIH en 1999 dans les Services Hospitaliers de Court Séjour*. Paris: DREES, Etudes et Résultats 2001, p1–7. URL: www.sante.gouv.fr/drees/etude-resultat/er-pdf/er149.pdf.

46. Silvera R. Revue médicale de l'assurance maladie (in press).

47. Yazdanpanah Y, Goldi SH, Losina E *et al.* (2002). Lifetime cost of HIV care in France during the era of highly active antiretroviral therapy. *Antiviral Therapy* 4:257–66.

Chapter 32

Italy

Francesco Taroni, George France*, Andrea Tramarin*, Emma Conti, Andrea Donatini and Fernando Antonio Compostella

Background

Italy is a parliamentary republic with a population of about 58 million, divided into 20 regions. The Constitution distinguishes between 15 'ordinary' and five 'special statute' regions, of which one is divided into two autonomous provinces, with responsibility for a number of policy areas. Regions are extremely varied in terms of size, ranging from 25,000 km² for Piedmont to a mere 3000 km² for Valle d'Aosta, with Lombardy having 16% of the total national population and Val d'Aosta less than 1%, and with gross domestic product (GDP) per capita 32% higher in Lombardy and 39% lower in Calabria than the national average.

Italy has the most elderly population in the European Union (EU): in 2000, there were 126 people aged 65 years or older for every 100 people of 14 years or younger, against an EU average of 99. Again, there are wide inter-regional differences—the proportion of people 65 years or older is 23% in Liguria compared with 13.5% in Campania.

In 2001, 1,464,000 people of foreign origin were officially resident in Italy, of whom just under 1 million were non-EU citizens.

The health status of Italians, as judged by traditional proxy measures such as life expectancy and infant mortality, is among the best in the world and continues to improve [1]. Life expectancy at birth was 76.5 years for males and 82.5 years for females in 1999, compared with 74.4 and 80.8, respectively, in 1995, while infant mortality was 4.3 per 1000. These national averages mask substantial inter-regional variation. There is a clear-cut north–south divide in demographic terms: nationally, 19% of the population is over 65, but in the northern regions of Liguria and Emilia-Romagna it reaches 25%, and the two largest southern regions, Puglia and Campania, each register 14%. There is also an epidemiological divide: infant mortality in Italy in 2000 stood at 4.5 per 1000, but was 6.2 per 1000 in Sicilia. Finally, per capita health expenditure in the north was €1900 compared with €1400 in the south.

The National Health Service

In 1978, Italy established a National Health Service (*Servizio Sanitario Nazionale*, or SSN) loosely modelled on the British National Health Service (NHS). This replaced a system of over

---

* Corresponding authors.

100 health insurance funds that covered different segments of the workforce [2]. Each insurance fund had its own regulations, benefits package and contribution rates, and was affiliated with different physicians and facilities. About 7% of the population lacked coverage altogether. The system was characterized by organizational fragmentation, compartmentalization across levels of care, unnecessary duplication of services and red tape. Regional disparities were superimposed on those between social groups, the wealthier northern regions being better endowed than the southern part of the country. The towering financial debt of the health insurance funds in addition to the increasing power of the regions created a window of opportunity for the creation of the SSN, an idea born during the Second World War [3].

The SSN is organized according to the principles of universality, comprehensiveness of coverage and public financing. Although it has undergone several major reforms in its 27 years, its fundamental principles are still widely popular.

The 1978 reform envisaged that the SSN would gradually move to an integrated system of financing based on progressive taxation. Instead, compulsory social health insurance contributions remained the main source of funding for a long time. The chief threat to contributive equity posed by social health insurance lay in its regressive rate structure; contributions declined with earnings and varied very considerably depending on type of occupation and health insurance scheme.

Social contributions were only abolished in 1998 and were replaced by a regional business tax, which accounts for approximately 40% of regional health funding. This is supplemented by a National Equalization Fund, financed from Value Added Tax (VAT) revenues, aimed at ensuring that the poorer regions have sufficient resources to guarantee adequate healthcare provision to their residents [4].

Thus, the SSN today is financed through taxation and, to a very small degree (3%), by patient co-payments for specialist ambulatory service. The state and the regions share responsibility for healthcare. The former is responsible for defining the core benefits package (*Livelli Essenziali di Assistenza* or LEA) to which all residents throughout the country are entitled, while the regions have shared legislative powers, limited fiscal autonomy and virtually exclusive responsibility for the administration and organization of healthcare. The LEA includes inpatient and outpatient acute care, coverage for drugs included in the National Formulary, and long-term residential and home care. Wide inter-regional differences still exist in terms of healthcare facilities, their public–private mix and expenditure (Table 32.1).

Financial resources are allocated to the regions according to a formula based on population size, weighted by national age and gender utilization rates of hospitals, drugs and specialist

Table 32.1 Selected indicators of inter-regional diversity

	Minimum	Maximum	Italy
Population (×1000)	120	9029	57,613
>65 years (%)	13.5	24.6	17.8
GDP (000s US$), per capita	9.9	21.4	16.1
Public health expenditure, per capita (000s US$)	0.94	1.4	1.0
Hospital beds (% inhabitants)	3.9	6.2	5.1
Private beds (%)	–	35.4	18.4

Sources: [1,5].

ambulatory care services, with each region's standardized mortality rate as a proxy for health-care need. The formula has been modified frequently, leading to substantial annual variation in the level of funding that each region receives.

The SSN owes much of its present organization to reforms in 1992, which were only marginally modified by reforms in 1999 [5]. Regional governments are responsible for ensuring the LEA through a network of Local Health Enterprises (LHEs), which provide comprehensive care to a geographically defined population of around 500,000 inhabitants. In addition, some 100 major hospitals, most of which are affiliated with universities, are semi-independent Hospital Enterprises. LHEs and Hospital Enterprises have substan-tial organizational and financial autonomy, and their activities are regulated by civil rather than public administrative law. Both types of enterprise are headed by a Chief Executive Officer, appointed by and responsible to the region, on a 5-year performance-based contract.

Under the SSN, Italians have considerable freedom to choose from a wide array of public and private providers, including hospital and ambulatory care delivered by facilities managed directly by the LHE, Hospital Enterprises, research hospitals, and non-profit and for-profit providers under contract with the SSN. Private hospitals operating under contract to the SSN in 2000 accounted for 17% of inpatient cases, with wide inter-regional variation [6]. Primary care is provided by independent general practitioners, paid mainly on a capitation basis, while hospital specialists are salaried and a small number of independent specialists provide ambu-latory care on a fee-for-service basis.

Expenditure

In 2002, the SSN spent €62.2 billion(US$58.8 billion), 6.4% of GDP, while private health expenditure was €20.3 billion(US$19.1 billion), 2% of GDP [7]. Approximately 13% of families supplement their coverage under the SSN with private health insurance at a cost of about € 724 million(US$684.4 billion). Most recent data on private health expenditure estimate that 44% was spent on drugs, 32% on doctors' services and 24% on hospital care, mostly for obstetrics and minor surgery. Private healthcare therefore basically complements public care and plays no role in dealing with major health risks, including HIV. In addition, HIV patients are completely exempt from co-payments both for drugs and for outpatient specialist care. This means that out-of-pocket expenses are not a barrier to access to healthcare.

Outputs and organization

Public healthcare provision is dominated by the hospital sector, which accounts for about 46% of total healthcare expenditure. For many years, policy focused on reducing SSN bed capacity, and beds per 1000 inhabitants fell from 13 in 1975 to five in 2001 [4]. The 1992 reform introduced a prospective payment system based on diagnosis-related groups (DRGs), replacing payment per patient-day for contracted private hospitals and full cost financing for public hospitals [8]. According to this system, hospitals are funded in terms of their number of admissions, with payment levels calculated using a specific tariff for each of around 500 distinct diagnostic groups. The idea of basing hospital funding on DRGs originated in America, but Italy changed the incentives for a payment system that would be expected simply to encourage hospitals to increase admissions towards one that increased throughput and substituted inpatient care with day cases or outpatient care. This was done by exploiting the incentives of the new payment system to reduce length of stay and to manage case mix better in order to improve appropriateness of hospital utilization. Most regions were slow to adopt DRGs due to the shortcomings of existing hospital information systems, inadequate patient-based data on hospital costs and lack of appropriate technical expertise [8].

Future developments

Italy's National Health Service today is at a crossroads. Regional autonomy has increased over the years, especially in terms of expenditure. This greater independence was given formal recognition with a constitutional amendment in 2001 that assigned the state exclusive responsibility for setting national standards and gave the regions virtually exclusive power in organizing and administering the health services in their territory.

The National Equalization Fund was also given constitutional status with the aim of guaranteeing the resources necessary to provide the LEA entitlement in the poorer regions. The current government, elected in early 2001, has submitted legislation for further devolution and plans to cede additional revenue sources to the regions, while at the same time pledging respect for the key principles of the SSN. The government also claims that its plans for further devolution will be neutral in terms of their effect on the healthcare budget.

However, even before these latest proposals were announced, many observers were expressing doubts about the capability of the state to enforce national standards regarding coverage, the LEA. Their constitutional basis notwithstanding, the LEA will prove difficult to enforce: the virtually unconditional transfer of revenues to the regions planned by central government means that it will lack any real financial leverage over the regions. Indeed, there is a fear that the SSN could fragment into 21 distinct regional health services, each applying different co-payment rates and setting different eligibility rules for use of regional facilities by patients from other regions. Regions may also develop different policies regarding delisting and supplementary private insurance for services not covered by the public system. However, this should not have a negative impact on access to services that are already part of the LEA package, such as those for HIV patients, since the package will continue to be defined nationally. Inter-regional differences in how services are organized could instead have negative implications for continuity of care, which is already a problem given the high mobility of such patients.

Finally, difficulties could arise with inter-regional coordination, for example in planning and financing supra-regional facilities. Existing inter-regional differences in levels of care provided and in health status are significant. It is premature, moreover, to predict neutral budgetary effects from devolution. For example, considerable additional transaction costs can be expected for the SSN as a result of a marked rise in jurisdictional disputes between regions and the state. New mechanisms for intergovernmental negotiation will be required to prevent this, but these will also generate additional transaction costs. Moreover, there will be extra costs for public healthcare as a whole if individual regions duplicate facilities in an attempt to reduce inter-regional mobility of patients. Nevertheless, the central government tends to regard devolution as the principal instrument for ensuring the financial sustainability of an SSN built on the principles originally established in 1978.

The HIV epidemic

The first Italian AIDS patient was diagnosed in 1982. As in several other countries, gloomy predictions of the spread of the disease prompted an intense political, institutional and professional debate on how best to prepare an adequate societal response to the looming epidemic. The development of the epidemic turned out to be much slower than anticipated, and the fact that the SSN is required to provide universal access to comprehensive care, which is largely free at the point of use, helped in the organization of an effective healthcare response without overwhelming the system.

Epidemiology

Italy has the third highest prevalence of AIDS in Europe. Between 1982 and mid-2003, almost 52,000 AIDS cases were diagnosed, of which 33,350 (65%) have died [9]. Seventy-eight per cent of AIDS cases were reported among males, and 1% were paediatric cases. The mean age at diagnosis of AIDS has increased over time for both sexes, from 29 years for men and 24 years for women in 1995 to 40 and 36 years, respectively, in 2003. The total number of HIV-infected individuals is unknown, as large-scale anonymous testing is not allowed in Italy. Estimates using regional registries place the number of HIV-positive individuals in the range of 95,000–125,000.

Injecting drug users (IDUs) have been, and still are, the largest population infected with HIV (Table 32.2). In 1985, when the HIV test became available, as many as 50% of IDUs were found to be HIV-positive in large metropolitan areas such as Milan, Genoa and Rome. It is estimated that about 70% of the prison population, about 50,000 people, are drug users, and 7000 of these are either HIV-positive or have fully developed AIDS [10].

An important route of transmission in the early years of the HIV epidemic was blood transfusion. There are over 1.2 million blood donors in Italy, 70% of whom are regular donors. Infection reached a peak between 1983 and 1984, but testing of blood for HIV began in 1985 and infection through this route fell dramatically, with only 12 cases recorded in 1986 [9]. Another transmission route is via illegal immigrants from North America and Latin America who, in order to survive financially, turn to prostitution and crime. This source of HIV is becoming increasingly important. For example, in the region of Lazio, where Rome is located, foreign-born cases as a proportion of total cases increased from 16% in 1995 to 25% in 2000 [11].

Table 32.2 Reported AIDS cases: distribution by risk groups (%) and years

Risk group	Pre-1993	1993–1994	1995–1996	1997–1998	1999–2000	2001–2002	2003	Total
MSM	16.0	15.4	14.9	15.9	17.9	17.2	18.0	15.9
IDU	67.4	63.2	60.0	50.7	41.0	37.0	36.6	58.8
IDU/MSM	2.5	2.0	1.6	1.3	0.5	0.7	0.2	1.8
Haemophiliacs/ transfusion	2.4	1.4	1.3	0.6	0.8	0.5	0.2	1.5
Heterosexual	10.7	16.2	20.0	22.6	34.4	38.5	41.1	19.0
Other	1.0	1.8	2.3	8.8	5.5	6.1	3.9	3.0

Source: [9].

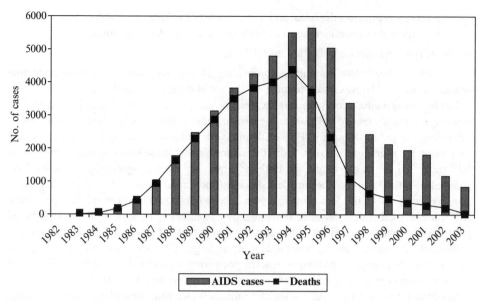

Fig. 32.1 Distribution of new AIDS cases and mortality per year. The incidence is corrected for the delay in reporting.

The peak of the AIDS epidemic occurred in the mid-1990s (Fig. 32.1), and the number of new cases decreased by 30% between 1997 and 2001. The distribution of AIDS cases by risk group has also changed over time (Table 32.2). While IDUs accounted for 63% of all cases in 1993, this had fallen to 37% by 2003, and heterosexual transmission rose from 16% to 41% over the same period. The proportion of AIDS cases among heterosexuals with no history of drug use is now equal to that for IDUs. A change in the pattern of the epidemic is emerging, with a shift away from the traditional high-risk group of IDUs to the large, low-risk general population exposed in the main through heterosexual transmission [11–13].

The social and institutional response

The main responses to the AIDS epidemic were the creation of the AIDS Operations Centre (AOC) within the National Institute of Health, the technical arm of the SSN, and the establishment of the National Aids Commission (NAC), which was given the responsibility of mobilizing and coordinating the multisectorial national response to the epidemic. The AOC has operational responsibility for developing a national AIDS surveillance system and actively investigating the disease, promoting and conducting clinical and basic research on AIDS and implementing a national educational programme, focusing on healthcare workers and school teachers.

The NAC has a multidisciplinary advisory board, chaired by the Minister of Health and composed of 40 people including epidemiologists, infectious disease physicians and researchers, ethics scholars and journalists. The NAC has an extremely broad mandate:

- to develop a national strategy for basic and clinical research and an effective healthcare policy;
- to inform the public and prevent the spread of HIV;

- to protect and promote the social and human rights of people with AIDS or HIV infection, such as the right to confidentiality and protection against discrimination;
- to propose and oversee legislation on HIV issues.

In 1989, a consultative committee comprising 20 representatives of non-governmental organizations (NGOs) was set up to focus on the social dimensions of the epidemic.

The first mass media information and advertising campaign was initiated in 1988, using TV, newspapers, magazines and billboards. The annual nationwide campaigns had the dual goal of informing the public about the HIV epidemic, with the aim of combating ignorance and preventing the stigmatization of and discrimination against those infected, and of preventing HIV transmission in high-risk groups. Both the targets and the messages of the campaigns have changed over time and have become less shocking and aimed more at the vulnerable groups. The main message of the first campaign was, 'If you know AIDS, you avoid it; if you know AIDS, it won't kill you', and was accompanied by a frightening TV spot depicting an infected person surrounded by a violet silhouette, implying that HIV was an inconspicuous but dangerous killer loose among the population at large. This was followed by a series of provocative photographs by Oliviero Toscani portraying a person dying of AIDS. The most recent messages are no longer intended to shock; they simply say: 'Stop AIDS'.

In addition to general campaigns, specific initiatives targeting particular groups or settings were developed, usually in collaboration with regional governments or led by voluntary organizations. A typical example is the special educational programme for teachers and school principals, aimed at promoting sex education in schools.

Some 20 NGOs have been active in counselling and supporting HIV-infected people [10]. The most active on a national scale have been ANLAIDS (The National Association for the Fight Against AIDS), LILA (Italian League for the Fight Against AIDS), ARCI-Gay and Positifs. ANLAIDS is a fund-raising organization that supports educational campaigns and clinical and basic research. LILA is more of a grass-roots organization, a federation of regional and local activist agencies involved in education, helplines and practical support for HIV-infected people. ARCI-Gay is a national gay organization dealing with broad social issues and gay rights, while Positifs has mainly focused on lobbying for the rapid approval of new drugs to be added to the national drug formulary and their early adoption.

The main achievement of the NCA was a law, passed in 1990, which set in motion a number of medium-term initiatives: constructing or restructuring infectious disease wards, with over 7000 additional hospital beds initially envisaged; recruiting additional medical, nursing and technical staff; mandating professional training and refresher courses for hospital staff; and developing residential, home care and hospice care for terminally ill patients. The law also contained rules to protect and promote the social and human rights of people with AIDS and HIV, such as the right to confidentiality, protection from discrimination in the workplace and in public places such as bars and restaurants, and the obligation of healthcare workers to treat HIV-positive people.

The national AIDS research programme, with annual funding averaging over US$10 million, is considered to have produced good results in terms of high-quality scientific publications, preparation of young researchers and accelerating the adoption of clinical and technological innovations. The research programme also led to an experimental AIDS vaccine, which was recently tested. However, it has also been accused of a bias in funding, with an excessive emphasis on basic research and inadequate attention to clinical and social questions, all of which prompted a major restructuring in 1997 [14].

The response of the healthcare system

Initially, the SSN was slow in responding to the epidemic. First diagnoses of the disease tended to be made when it was already at an advanced stage and when the presence of opportunistic infections had already reduced the effectiveness of care [15]. Hospitalization was excessive and stays lengthy due to the lack of alternative services. The use of azidothymidine (AZT) treatments was limited, and the same was true for programmes to prevent opportunistic infections, especially *Pneumocystis carinii* pneumonia (PCP). Finally, and above all, there was great variation between hospitals with regard to which patients were managed, and how.

The situation improved rapidly, however. The initiatives of the NAC set the pace, pressing for uniformity in the adoption of new therapies and the development of new organizational frameworks, mainly through setting and disseminating clinical and administrative guidelines. Care for people with HIV came to be provided along a comprehensive continuum, embracing home, community, outpatient and inpatient facilities. This continuum included clinical management, counselling, social support and, to some extent, palliative care [16,17]. Voluntary organizations, mostly church-based, focused primarily upon support and care, contributing to the spread of home and hospice care financed by public funding.

The litmus test for the new organizational arrangements was the clinical community's response to the challenges posed by the availability of highly active antiretroviral therapy (HAART), which became widely adopted in 1996. This caused a dramatic decrease in opportunistic infections and deaths, a shift of resources from inpatient to outpatient services for the management of HIV-related conditions, and a substantial reduction in total direct costs for inpatient care of HIV-positive patients, accompanied by a significant increase in the cost of drugs [18,19].

Data from the national AIDS registry, however, show that by 2002, only 35% of newly diagnosed AIDS cases had received one course of antiretroviral treatment (ART) and only 37% had received triple combination therapy [9]. This varied according to risk group: start-up of HAART was tardy for 87% of IDUs compared with 38% of those infected through heterosexual transmission. This confirms earlier data showing that people with AIDS in the lower socio-economic classes have double the risk of dying compared with those in the highest socio-economic class, and that survival is significantly shorter for women and IDUs [20]. Problems with access to healthcare, despite the universal coverage offered by the SSN, and with clinical management of the complex HAART protocol, including patient adherence to prescribed therapy, are some of the reasons why the SSN has failed to maximize the potential benefits of the new HAART regimens.

Assessing the response to the healthcare needs of IDUs, who constitute the main vulnerable population of the Italian HIV epidemic, is a much more complex matter. Italy already possessed a well-funded network of public and privately contracted services for drug users, providing psychological support, counselling, blood testing, education and prevention. These services are available in schools and prisons. However, competing values seem to have been operating. On the one hand, some services—mainly publicly managed—run risk-reduction programmes such as needle and syringe exchange schemes and methadone substitution treatment; on the other hand, 'therapeutic communities' run by voluntary organizations, most of which are church-based but financed mainly by the state, promote a policy of strict abstinence. These differences are both the consequence and the cause of an ideological battle—still in progress—over methadone maintenance and needle exchange programmes. Although the success of some risk-reduction programmes has been demonstrated—for example, in Rome only 10% of IDUs were estimated to have used contaminated needles in 1992 compared with 90% in 1985–1986 [12,21]—these services are periodically threatened with closure [22].

Conclusions

The HIV epidemic has presented Italian society and its healthcare system with a series of complex political, ethical, organizational and technical issues. The fact that the SSN is supposed to work on the basis of the key principles of universal access to comprehensive care free at the point of delivery should, in theory, have spared Italy the problems of access faced by people with HIV infection in other countries. In practice, however, the availability of a highly effective therapy such as HAART has created disparities between different socio-economic classes and risk groups for timely access to effective care and, therefore, for survival.

The structural fragmentation of the SSN and the turmoil provoked by the launching of a major health reform when the AIDS epidemic was at its peak produced serious coordination problems within the service and between the healthcare system and other sectors. The exclusive reliance, during the first phase of the epidemic, on inpatient hospital care and the lack of other services as alternatives to hospitalization increased costs and reduced timeliness of access to good quality care. Furthermore, HIV prevention strategies had to be coordinated across a spectrum of policy sectors with few or no previous linkages. Initiatives ranged from sex education in schools and for drug users, sex workers and prison inmates, to counselling of HIV-infected mothers and enforcing safer standards in the blood and organ donation system. More generally, Italy is a country with a strong Catholic tradition, and the response to the HIV epidemic has been affected by controversies over issues that were, and still are, easily politicized. Good examples of this are the legitimacy of public policies focusing on private behaviour and personal lifestyles, including sexuality and drug use, HIV testing in the workplace, and the right of health workers to refuse treatment to people with HIV because of the perceived potential risks to themselves.

The debate on public policy in relation to HIV was complicated further by the particular nature of the epidemic in Italy, where two-thirds of cases were IDUs, prison inmates, sex workers and illegal immigrants operating in the sex industry. These groups were socially marginalized, easily stigmatized and lacked the ability to lobby for, or support, public policy in their favour and organize self-help, educational and behavioural change initiatives common in gay communities in Italy and elsewhere. This helps explain the distinct role of the voluntary sector in Italy in the fight against AIDS, where NGOs concentrated on supporting long-term residential and home care and on promoting and funding research [10,23].

In addition, the HIV epidemic posed the challenge of developing new models of public health intervention to address high-risk populations, based on proximity and outreach strategies by mobile teams of peers, which fell more naturally into the field of social work than traditional public health. Clinical care also had to be modernized, with staff training, development of protocols for the new, complex therapies and provision of residential and hospice care for the terminally ill.

This thrust to modernize was stymied by three events. The first was the serious economic crisis that hit Italy in 1992, which forced it to leave the European Monetary System and led to a drastic cutback in public funding of healthcare. The second event, previously cited, was a sweeping reform of the SSN, with a major transfer of power to the regions and the transformation of local health authorities and major hospitals into semi-independent public health enterprises. Finally, financial scandals in the highest ranks of the SSN had a negative impact on funding for the fight against AIDS. Nevertheless, the perception of the gravity of the AIDS crisis and the need for immediate action was strong enough to overcome most traditional barriers to change, such as the fragmented nature of the SSN and the 'atrophy' of public administration. Policy change was bolstered further by the strong leadership of the NAC by Elio Guzzanti, a highly respected figure in the Italian public health community, who subsequently became Minister of Health.

The NAC programme for HIV research, care and training received quite generous funding, and this was ring-fenced, buffering NAC activity from the financial crisis then hitting the SSN. In the field of AIDS policy, the regions did not use the considerable autonomy the 1992 reform granted them in the organization and delivery of health services. Rather, they first ratified and then joined in the implementation of the NAC action plan and did the same from 1997 onwards with the AIDS projects contained in the National Health Plan prepared by the Ministry of Health.

On the whole, regional initiatives tended to focus on the problem of drug addiction, for which a tried and tested network of services was already in place. Community-based outreach risk-reduction programmes, such as syringe and needle exchange, methadone maintenance and free condom distribution, produced good results locally. These programmes, however, led a troubled existence due to political conflict over the issue of risk-reduction versus abstinence, as well as tensions between the regions and the municipalities, which, in Italy, have responsibility for social programmes.

On a more positive note, during the HIV epidemic, Italy invested in a major programme of hospital renovation, staff training and development of home and hospice care aimed at modernizing poorly equipped infectious disease departments and making them better able to cope with the rapidly growing number of HIV patients. The epidemic prompted the adoption of standardized treatment protocols made necessary by the rapid development of complex and costly medical therapies and the involvement of the medical sector in an unusually wide-ranging attempt to coordinate care and standardize treatment. In addition, with the risk of HIV transmission through medical procedures and the spread of drug resistance, the prevention of nosocomial infection and protection of staff assumed a renewed urgency [24]. Furthermore, the HIV epidemic moved public health from the margins of the medical system and made it the centre of political attention.

More than 20 years after the diagnosis of the first case of AIDS, the pattern of the AIDS epidemic in Italy has significantly changed. HAART has altered the natural history of HIV, bringing a reduction in mortality and morbidity and, in a sense, transforming it from the acute and devastating disease of the early epidemic into a chronic condition. This has been the case in all countries able to afford the costly new therapy. A particular feature of the Italian case is that heterosexual transmission has been increasing, mainly as a result of sexual contact with IDUs. This reflects the fact that, despite a number of local success stories, Italy has not been successful in preventing the spread of HIV infection both among and from IDUs. This is in the main attributable to problems in information and risk-reduction programmes targeting the IDU population. There have been reports of a resurgence in risky sexual behaviour, and the pendulum seems to be swinging back in favour of policies for drug abstinence [22]. This suggests that the HIV epidemic will remain a serious public health problem for Italy, but in a different form.

References

1. Istituto Centrale di Statistica. (2003). Health for all. Italy. URL: www.istat.it/DATI/.
2. Brown LD. (1984). Health reform, Italian-style. *Health Affairs* 3:75–101.
3. France G, Taroni F. (2005). The evolution of health care policy in Italy. *Journal of Health Politics Policy and Law* 30:1–29.
4. Donatini A, Rico A, Lo Scalzo A *et al.* (2001). *Health Care in Transition—Italy*. Copenhagen: European Observatory on Health Care Systems.
5. Sistema Informativo Sanitario. (2001). Annuario Statistico del SSN—2001. URL: http://www.ministerosalute.it/.
6. OECD. (2003). *OECD Health Data 2002*. Paris: OECD.
7. Taroni F. (2000). Devolving responsibility for funding and delivering health care in Italy. *Euro Observer* 2:1–2.
8. Benigni M, D'Ambrosio MG, Simon G *et al.* (2000). Adozione e impatto del sistema di pagamento a prestazione degli ospedali nelle regioni italiane. *Politiche Sanitarie* 1:77–86.
9. Istituto Superiore di Sanità. (2003). Aggiornamento dei casi di AIDS notificati in Italia al 30 Giugno 2003. Notiziario dell'Istituto Superiore di Sanità 16 Supplement 1.
10. Baron C. (1999). HIV/AIDS Policies and the Role of the Voluntary Sector: A Comparative Report of Sweden, Germany and Italy. URL: www.lse.ac.uk/collections.
11. Porta D, Perucci CA, Forastiere F, De Luca A. (2004). Temporal trend of HIV infection. An update of the HIV surveillance system in Lazio, Italy, 1095–2000. *European Journal of Public Health* 14:156–60.
12. Brancato G, Perucci CA, Abeni DD, Sangalli M, Ippolito G, Arcà M. (1997). The changing distribution of HIV infection: HIV surveillance in Lazio, Italy, 1985 through 1994. *American Journal of Public Healt* 87:1654–8.
13. Ippolito G, Galati V, Serraino D, Girardi E. (2001). The changing picture of the HIV/AIDS epidemic. *Annals of the New York Academy of Sciences* 946:1–12.
14. Biggin S. (1997). AIDS research. Program funding, Italian style. *Science* 276:191.
15. Taroni F, Anemona A. (1993). L'assistenza ospedaliera ai pazienti con AIDS in Italia. *Giornale Italiano AIDS* 4:2–15.
16. Tramarin A, Milocchi F, Tolley K *et al.* (1992). An economic evaluation of home-care assistance for AIDS patients: a pilot study in a town in northern Italy. *AIDS* 6:1377–83.
17. Tramarin A, Tolley K, Campostrini S, de Lalla F. (1997). Efficiency and rationality in the planning of health care for people with AIDS: an application of the balance of care approach. *AIDS* 11:809–16.
18. Torti C, Casari S, Palvarini L *et al.* (2003). Modifications of health resource-use in Italy after the introduction of highly active antiretroviral therapy (HAART) for human immunodeficiency virus (HIV) infection. Pharmaco-economic implications in a population-based setting. *Health Policy* 65:261–7.
19. Tramarin A, Campostrini S, Postma MJ *et al.* (2004). The Palladio Study Group. A multicentre study of patient survival, disability, quality of life and cost of care among patients with AIDS in northern Italy. *Pharmaeconomics* 22:43–53.

20. Rapiti E, Porta D, Forastiere F, Fusco F, Perucci CA. (2000). Socioeconomic status and survival of persons with AIDS before and after the introduction of highly active antiretroviral therapy. *Epidemiology* 11:496–501.

21. Davoli M, Perucci CA, Abeni DD *et al.* (1995). HIV risk-related behaviors among injection drug users in Rome: differences between 1990 and 1992. *American Journal of Public Health* 85:829–32.

22. Davoli M, Ferri M, Perucci CA, Liberati A. (2002). Health policies on drug dependence must be based on scientific evidence. *British Medical Journal* 324:1338.

23. Steffen M. (2004). AIDS and health-policy responses in European welfare states. *Journal of European Social Policy* 14:165–81.

24. Ippolito G, Puro V, De Carli G. (1993). The risk of occupational human immunodeficiency virus infection in health care workers. Italian Multicenter Study. *Archives of Internal Medicine* 153:1451–8.

Chapter 33

The Russian Federation

J Stachowiak[*], A Peryshkina and S Lessof

Background

The capacity of the Russian Federation to respond to the threat of HIV and AIDS is enormously constrained by the burden of its Soviet inheritance and the recent traumas of transition. The strengths and, more tellingly, the weaknesses of its health system can best be understood therefore in light of the Soviet 'Semashko' model of healthcare delivery; the attitudes to health engendered by the Soviet system; and the cutbacks in finance and erosion of organizational capacity that followed the break-up of the USSR. It is also important to bear in mind that the way the Russian Federation copes with any health challenge is mediated by its colossal size. It covers over 17 million km^2, 10 time zones, and includes 89 'federal entities', a mix of *oblasts* or regions, republics, autonomous territories and federal cities, as well more than 100 registered national minorities. It would be difficult in these circumstances to manage a consistent and equitable response to HIV, even without the very considerable upheavals of transition.

The health system

The *Semashko* model and its consequences for the Russian health system

The Soviet Union included what is now the Russian Federation plus a further 14 Soviet Republics that achieved independence at the start of the 1990s. It was highly centralized, with a huge amount of power concentrated at the pan-Union level in Moscow. Just as importantly, a comprehensive and all-embracing set of norms operated across the whole USSR. They ensured harmonization of education, employment policy, housing design and rent, and, of course, health services.

The health system followed what was known as the *Semashko* model. It vested responsibility for health in the government, guaranteed free healthcare at the point of use, proliferated norms to govern provision across the USSR and was tax-based [1]. The taxes that supported health services were largely derived from enterprises and rental income generated by different tiers of government. Individual taxation played a much less significant role. The Ministry of Health in Moscow determined how many hospital beds and staff were 'needed' by a given number of people and mandated all subordinate levels of local government to deliver uniform territorial services as specified, as well as negotiating the appropriate budget allocation with the Ministry of Finance.

* Corresponding author.

There were layers of provision, based in rural communities at health posts or *feldsher/* midwife stations, the first point of health system contact for populations of up to 4000. A *feldsher* is a kind of nurse practitioner or public health nurse working relatively autonomously in a rural setting. In urban areas, non-specialist *'therapeutists'* were housed in polyclinics and acted, at least in theory, as the primary care providers for their local population. The services they offered were basic and included little more than screening and immunization, sickness certification and treatment of minor ailments. Health centres covered rural populations of up to 7000, while dispensaries and larger polyclinics played an equivalent role in urban settings. It was commonplace for specialists providing ambulatory care to be located in health centres and polyclinics alongside primary care staff. This tended to blur the boundaries between the two modes of care, and, with no effective gatekeeping or filter system, patients often referred themselves directly to specialists. In larger towns, there were also specialist paediatric and obstetric/gynaecology polyclinics, again mixing primary and secondary services and allowing patients to bypass primary care in accessing secondary services.

The secondary, inpatient sector was overlarge because it was designed to cope with mass hospitalization in the event of major epidemics. The fear of epidemics related to experiences of civil and global war. Further excess bed capacity was added in the 1970s to allow extensive annual screening of the population for potential health threats. This sector consisted of hospitals at the *uchastok* (local), *rayon* (district) and *oblast* (regional) levels. The first were very small, totalling some 50 beds and offering few services; the second had between 100 and 700 beds and offered a fairly full range of general and surgical services; and *oblast* hospitals served whole provinces and were larger and even more specialized. Above these there were Republic-level and All Soviet centres of excellence often linked to research institutions, the latter normally based in Moscow and serving the whole Soviet Union.

In addition, there were a large number of work-based clinics offering primary care and limited specialist ambulatory services, reflecting the very close link between employment and entitlement in the USSR. All 'healthy' adults were obliged to work in the Soviet era, and work was provided for everyone. There was no unemployment, and the workplace and trade unions acted as a transmission belt for many non-monetary benefits. There was an extensive set of parallel health systems funded by, and serving, the staff of the Ministries of Defence, Railways, Interior, and so on, as well as a series of special hospitals reserved for members of the *nomenklatura*, the political elite. Finally, there was a large network of rehabilitative clinics and hospitals offering non-medical care, physical therapy and 'curative' baths that ranged from prestigious hotels to more ordinary sanatoria. Many were linked to the trade union movement or the Party, and the use of them was often seen as a part of a worker's compensation package.

The impact of this model is still clearly observable today across the Russian Federation. The most obvious and most tangible legacy is the huge physical infrastructure, which, despite efforts to close beds and facilities, persists today. The healthcare network is of recognizably Soviet proportions, even though public funding, following a series of crises up to 1998 and pressures from the International Monetary Fund (IMF), cannot maintain facilities or services. The sustained growth of recent years, the improvement in real wages and disposable incomes, and falling unemployment [2] have not fundamentally altered the picture, not least because of weakness in establishing the country's tax base. There are simply insufficient resources to cover the demands arising from the scale and the dereliction of the health system (Table 33.1) [3].

Some health facilities in rural areas are without running water or reliable electricity supplies. This makes it difficult to respond to emerging health threats such as HIV, and although the government has invested heavily in testing, insufficient funds have been made available to address treatment and counselling needs. There are also real problems in terms of maintaining best practices in hygiene, health and safety standards.

The demands on the health system are exacerbated by the high staffing levels, which were the norm in the Soviet Union and have only altered marginally since 1991. Since then, the number of qualified physicians has actually increased, although the numbers of nurses have fallen somewhat. Traditionally, the numbers of doctors and nurses were high, at least in part because of state policy of full employment and low labour costs (Table 33.1). The health sector had even fewer constraints on staff numbers than other employers because staff were relatively poorly remunerated since they were deemed unproductive compared with industrial workers. This low pay also possibly reflected the fact that the health workforce was overwhelmingly female. Even before the break up of the USSR, this had created dissatisfaction and a sense of being undervalued, which contributed to the erosion of humanity of care and a tolerance of 'gratitude payments', or under-the-table cash gifts to medical staff.

The economic collapse following 1991 devastated public sector wages, and these have never recovered in value. The result is that today's workforce is extremely poorly paid and under-resourced, and is struggling with difficult physical conditions. Staff do not have the facilities or the supplies they need to deliver a quality service and are financially insecure. This creates immense stresses on the workforce and destroys motivation and commitment. It also re-inforces the proliferation of under-the-table or informal payments that are now normal practice [4]. All this militates against sensitive, professional responses to people living with HIV (PLHIV) and is likely to create barriers to access for populations at risk, both in terms of staff attitudes and because patients are likely to be asked for money to meet the cost of their treatment.

A further legacy of the Soviet era that impedes appropriate responses to HIV is a latent conservatism in management, which stems from the extensive use of norms and the highly judgemental culture of the past that had little tolerance for individualism or failure. There was,

Table 33.1 Indices for the Russian healthcare system

Health system data	1991	1993	1995	1997	1999	2001	2003
% GDP on health	3.0	3.0	2.2	–	2.8	–	–
Total health expenditure PPP$/capita	207.9	148.5	96.6		209.2		
Doctors/100,000	404.6	397.2	385.9	415.5	422.6	420.3	–
Nurses/100,000	845.0	835.7	816.8	820.8	817.5	793.0	809.2
Acute hospital beds/100,000	1036.9	1002.7	974.3	924.5	903.7	911.7	–
Average length of acute stay (days)	13.7	13.6	13.6	14.3	13.7	13.2	–
Outpatient contacts/person/year	9.0	9.2	9.1	9.1	9.3	9.5	–
Inpatient admissions/100	21.8	21.8	21.3	20.5	21.0	22.5	–

Source: [13].
Data exclude out-of-pocket expenditure (formal or informal) and spending in parallel health systems, which together are estimated by WHO, the World Bank and others to bring the percentage of GDP devoted to health to something approaching 7%.

it is true, always an informal system shadowing formal structures, whereby individual managers used a range of enterprising strategies to overcome the shortcomings of the official sphere. However, there was no tradition of integrating innovation into the workplace or of managers building their own coping skills into mainstream organization. This makes it difficult now for institutions, and indeed for local authorities, to contemplate and execute locally tailored responses to particular needs, for example in areas with high prevalence of injecting drug use, or to particular users such as injecting drug users (IDUs).

Soviet attitudes to health and their ongoing influence

Just as the stultifying effect of the *Semashko* system norms still inhibits change by managers, so do Soviet attitudes to health continue to influence the way in which the health system is able to address HIV. The system was premised on the idea that the state could and should provide the full spectrum of a citizen's needs. It did little to foster a sense that people had real responsibility for their own health and well-being. Although state domination of society is ebbing, Russians still have a powerful tendency to regard healthcare issues as being the responsibility of the 'authorities', and this acts against efforts both to prevent HIV infection and to allow PLHIV to manage their health and their treatment themselves. What is more, many Soviet citizens had a profoundly jaded response to government exhortations to behave in particular ways, and this cynicism persists in undermining the efforts of health promotion agencies to spread health education messages.

There was also within Soviet culture a profound intolerance of difference and a tendency to be highly prescriptive and judgemental. Sexually acquired infections were viewed as indicative of social deviance, and there was a huge amount of prejudice against gay men. There was official denial of injecting drug use and of the extent to which men having sex with men (MSM) was normal both in prisons and in the army. On top of this, health services played what was, in effect, a punitive role, often enforcing long periods of compulsory hospitalization for sexually transmitted infections (STIs). This reflected the fear of epidemics, the perceived need to oversee treatment and the distaste for individuals who 'stepped out of line'. These attitudes have not disappeared with the fall of communism, and none of them makes it easy to work effectively with vulnerable individuals and groups and with PLHIV. Amongst vulnerable groups, there is also an enduring suspicion of health services, which encourages the concealment of symptoms, avoidance of medical help, and self-treatment with the help of pharmacists and friends.

Economic and political transition and impact on the Russian health system

The break-up of the USSR meant the collapse of a centrally planned economy and enormous economic, physical and emotional dislocation for Russian society. Industry declined, employment levels plummeted, and there were no adequate welfare systems or unemployment benefits in place to cushion the population. The initial upheaval, the rampant inflation of subsequent years and the effects of radical economic reforms, or 'shock therapy', adopted to achieve a rapid shift to a market economy together helped trigger a crisis in health status and undermined the coping strategies of individuals, with disastrous consequences for life expectancy and for the survival of middle-aged men in particular [5]. There were also huge pressures on the young, some of whom had become involved in commercial sex work, maladaptive coping strategies and injecting drug use. The health system was of course profoundly affected, facing additional demands and overwhelming budget constraints, and in many respects it has still not fully recovered. There is a traditional Russian focus on and preoccupation with children, and there has been considerable public panic about their health status. This concern does not, however, extend to young adults, who tend to have been neglected as a group.

The crisis prompted efforts to decentralize, to shift the funding base of the system and to re-engineer the role of primary care vis-à-vis hospitals, all of which had an impact on the response to HIV. Attempts to decentralize were somewhat desperate and were bound up with the need to signal tangible and symbolic change. They often led to responsibilities being passed to local government before there was sufficient local management capacity or funding to cope.

The Ministry of Health in Moscow was also stripped of a number of powers somewhat arbitrarily, and not all of these have been picked up by other authorities. Some *rayons* and *oblasts* are coping well, but in many there is simply a lacuna in leadership and management in which health services wallow. This bodes ill for responsiveness to HIV, particularly in poorer areas, and has allowed enormous inequalities to open up between regions [6–8]. There has also been a breakdown in the formerly highly centralized public health service or San Epid system that was responsible for surveillance, and this has led to a dearth of data and gaps in understanding about what is actually happening in parts of the country, and, again, this is problematic in terms of tackling HIV.

Financing was also reformed early on, with changes introduced throughout the early 1990s in an attempt to capture more monies for healthcare. A mandatory social health insurance element was introduced to supplement the tax-based elements. A payroll levy of 3.6% is paid by employers, while local government is meant to contribute for the non-working population. The insurance payments, which represent about 16% of total financing, are then meant to flow from the Territorial Mandatory Health Insurance Funds to Branch Funds and insurance companies that are then expected to contract with providers on behalf of the population covered. In practice, some areas have no insurance companies, and there is no real notion of strategic purchasing. Neither pooling nor risk-bearing are properly established, and branches and companies do little more than process paperwork, simply asking territorial funds to reimburse providers retrospectively without challenging them on the volume or quality of services provided.

This social insurance funding stream runs alongside tax-based revenues that are paid by local government directly to providers. These make up some 40–45% of total financing and are not geared in any way to create incentives for better performance. The reforms have failed to secure extra resources or lever extra efficiency or responsiveness and leave patients to provide some 34% of finances out-of-pocket. They may have helped create some sense of cost consciousness and encouraged managerial skills, but they are not creating a platform for specialist service agreements, which might allow third party payers to secure appropriate packages of care for PLHIV. Furthermore, the idea of limited entitlement created by social health insurance is worrying in a society with a huge grey economy, particularly as at-risk populations are often involved in the informal sector [9–11].

The reforms following 1991 also sought to develop primary care and shift the balance from secondary and tertiary care. There are several pilots that use per capita payments and build on fund-holding models to increase efficiency and responsiveness, as first tested in the Soviet *Kemerovo* experiment with fund-holding group practices. However, these have not changed prevailing attitudes to general practitioners (GPs), who are less highly regarded than specialists, and hospitals continue to dominate the health sector. Nor are there suitable settings for newly trained GPs to implement a family medicine approach. There continues to be a powerful attachment to the notion that specialist paediatricians should care for children, while obstetricians and gynaecologists provide reproductive health services and general physicians care for other adult health needs. Indeed, the idea of families as the unit for care is resisted, which makes integrated approaches to HIV prevention and treatment less feasible [12].

Health system weaknesses and their implications for the HIV response

Health system reforms prompted by transition have fractured services and funding flows, created considerable chaos, particularly in poorer regions, and allowed immense inequalities to appear. Major facilities are still almost invariably owned by the relevant branch of local government, but many enterprise-based clinics have closed down and sanatoria have also suffered badly, reducing access to care. Data on non-mainstream services, including parallel health systems, are scarce, but it does seem that the services for staff of ministries such as Defence or Railways have been cushioned from the worst effects of transition and are still relatively well resourced. Provision of care and technology has become increasingly patchy, and there are shortages of supplies in some areas; this clearly impedes efforts to tackle HIV consistently. Perhaps most tellingly of all, there is extensive reliance on out-of-pocket payments in all areas. These include formal charges for pharmaceuticals and dental care, both now in the private sector, and informal, under-the-table payments for all other services, both of which constitute real barriers to access.

Reform has been so overwhelming and traumatic that the scope for positive innovation and for a change in attitudes and approaches has been lost. Services are still delivered in a disjointed fashion and with little consideration for the whole patient, the context or family they live in or their individual needs, while STIs, injecting drug use and HIV continue to be stigmatized. As long as resource constraints operate to the degree now being experienced, the system itself will militate against more holistic or humane approaches to care and the types of respect, confidentiality and sensitivity that have been linked to success in preventing and treating HIV in other countries.

There is, of course, hope, and the Russian economy is experiencing rapid and sustained growth. Nonetheless, the Russian population is aging and fertility rates are falling, which raises the spectre of a smaller, economically active population sustaining a large, inactive population. So there may not be any respite from the kinds of pressure the health system now experiences. Reforms of the early 1990s, such as decentralization and social insurers as purchasers from separate providers, have failed to promote efficiency savings or create incentives for better quality care. The market is confined to small pockets of privatized services and to what individual physicians can charge their patients informally, and, since payments are far from transparent, no real market pressures apply. Nor does cost containment offer the answer, since the funding issue is more about a lack of resources than of their misuse—a problem linked to the failure of civil society to generate either tax revenues or a culture of compliance with tax regimes. Real change, then, is uncertain, and without change both in the resource base of the system and in its attitudes towards patients and to accountability, there is little prospect of an appropriate response to the HIV epidemic.

The HIV epidemic

Socio-economic context

The health system may be ill-equipped for change, but it desperately needs to respond to the threat of HIV across the Russian Federation. The transition from communism to an emerging capitalist economy has been accompanied by a dramatic downturn in the health of the population (Table 33.2). Currently, male life expectancy at birth is 59 years. Much of this is due to premature mortality from homicide, suicide, accidents and alcohol-related deaths. The epidemic of tuberculosis (TB) is also extremely serious, with an estimated 130,000 cases diagnosed and 30,000 deaths per year (Table 33.2). In addition, the population of the Russian Federation is aging. Birth rates are below replacement level, at 1.2 per woman. Early mortality, low birth rates and emigration are resulting in the loss of approximately 700,000 citizens each year [13]. At current levels, even optimistic projections point to a population numbering only 100 million by 2050, down from a national population of 140 million today [13].

HIV was introduced into the Russian Federation at almost the same time as the huge upheaval caused by the break-up of the Soviet Union and the turbulent years that preceded and followed it. Although there are many factors leading to the vulnerability of the population to HIV, many of them can be directly traced to the economic and societal breakdown discussed above. The Russian Federation is only now beginning to rebuild itself, and economic transition must be seen as one of the primary causes of sex work and drug use. Experts have identified many additional contributing factors to the HIV epidemic in the Russian Federation, including: rapid diffusion of IDU; population migration and mixing; modes of drug production, distribution and consumption; declines in public health revenue and infrastructure; and political, ideological and cultural transition [14,15]. Other factors include changing gender roles, sexual mixing patterns, a poorly controlled private medical sector and growth of self-medication, problems of alcohol abuse, and increased opportunity for travel and migration within and outside the Russian Federation [16–18].

What is more, drug injection in the country has risen to unprecedented levels, and addicts are estimated to have increased 12-fold in the past decade, with one recent survey estimating that one-half of Russian college students had injected drugs [19]. Today, there are an estimated 3–4

Table 33.2 Russian health indicators, 1991–2003

Health indicators	1991	1993	1995	1997	1999	2001	2003
Mid-year population (millions)	148.3	148.2	147.8	146.9	145.9	144.4	143.2
Life expectancy at birth (years)	69.2	65.1	64.7	66.9	66.0	65.3	–
Male life expectancy at birth (years)	63.4	58.9	58.3	61.0	60.0	59.1	–
Female life expectancy at birth (years)	74.3	71.9	71.7	73.0	72.5	72.3	–
TB incidence/100,000	34.0	43.3	65.9	83.1	92.6	92.2	–
Syphilis incidence/100,000	7.2	34.1	178.3	277.7	187.2	144.1	–
Diphtheria incidence/100,000	1.3	10.4	24.3	2.8	0.58	0.63	–
Cigarette consumption/person/year	–	–	–	1836.0	2018.0	–	–
Litres of pure alcohol/person/year	5.9	6.2	8.9	7.5	8.8	8.7	–

Source: WHO Regional Office for Europe, Health for All databases.

million IDUs in the Russia Federation, out of a total population of 140 million [20]. These numbers are supported by reports from individual cities [21,22] and represent a higher percentage of the population than anywhere else in the world [23].

AIDS-related deaths are looming on the horizon. To date, there have been just over 3500 reported deaths from AIDS, but those diagnosed 6–8 years ago will soon begin to be symptomatic, especially given the current dearth of treatment. As in most other countries, almost everyone with HIV is under 35 years of age, which, given the above demographic statistics and the epidemic of premature male mortality, is especially alarming.

Epidemiology

It is difficult, if not impossible, to characterize the epidemic using official statistics. Because of the reliance on a case-finding system to determine HIV cases, apparent infection trends are influenced by the geographic availability and demographic determinants of the use of test kits. However, these are the statistics that drive the Russian government's response to HIV. To date, there is no sentinel surveillance system in place that would provide more accurate numbers and greatly reduce the costs of testing.

By April 2004, according to the Russian Federal AIDS Centre, the official number of HIV-infected individuals in the Russian Federation was 274,808. Eighty per cent of the new HIV cases had been reported in the previous 3 years. This sharp upward trend has led UNAIDS to state that Russia has the fastest-growing epidemic in the world [24,25]. Both Russian and international experts agree that the official prevalence is a severe underestimate of the true numbers; they have ventured guesses of the true prevalence ranging from four to 10 times the official statistics [13,26–28]. The WHO/UNAIDS estimates for PLHIV in Russia at the end of 2003 ranged between 420,000 and 1.4 million. However, even the higher estimates are still in the range of 1–2% of the total population, making the epidemic only low to medium prevalence by global standards. On the other hand, given the aforementioned demographic crisis in the population of the Russian Federation, even this rate is alarming. According to the World Bank, if current HIV trends persist, Russia's gross domestic product (GDP) in 2010 will be as much as 4% lower than it would have been in the absence of HIV. By 2020, the loss could increase to over 10% [29].

The epidemic in the Russian Federation is still concentrated among IDUs, estimated to represent 80–90% of cases [15, 30]. Beginning in 2002, Russian and international experts reported that new infections were down, especially among IDUs [31].

It is also important to point out when discussing trends such as declining proportions of people infected through injecting drug use that roughly 40% of new infections in 2001 were of undetermined route of transmission. To date, 6265 babies have been born with HIV in the Russian Federation. This represents a 400% increase since the beginning of 2002. It is unclear what this dramatic increase represents; possibilities include, among others, the entry of HIV into the general population or a testing artefact resulting from simply testing all pregnant women and therefore finding more HIV than is found among the smaller percentage of IDUs who are arrested or registered at treatment centres.

Among the very first cases of HIV found were 270 children infected in 1988–1989. These infections occurred nosocomially in birth centres in four regions, through the administration of vitamins and antibiotics with contaminated needles. Only one child was reported to have been infected through breastfeeding. Notably, 22 women were reported to have been infected through breastfeeding HIV-positive infants since 1987, a phenomenon that has not been reported in other countries. Transmission among MSM comprised 32% of the cases detected at the beginning of the Russian epidemic. According to official statistics, they now comprise only 0.4% [32].

Attention must always be brought back to the weaknesses of the official data based on case finding, as well as to the 40% of transmissions that are of indeterminate origins. In 2002, the supply of test kits to the regions by the Federal government was stopped, and many regions, unable or unwilling to purchase test kits from their own budgets, drastically reduced the number of tests run. This will undoubtedly have had an impact on reported incidence data. For example, the number of drug users tested was 524,300 in 2001, dropping to 331,100 in 2002 [32].

Russian responses to HIV

The HIV services in the Russian healthcare system are resource-poor. Despite the many dedicated government officials and healthcare workers throughout the country who are devoted to preventing HIV and helping those already infected, the budget for a country the size of the Russian Federation, with a quickly growing epidemic, is very small. The Federal budget allocation for 2003 totalled approximately 122 million roubles, or US$4 million. This is equivalent to approximately US$16 dollars per person diagnosed with HIV to date. Regional health departments all allocate money to HIV as well, but, added to the Federal budget, the total sum still comes to less than US$20 million for the entire country and includes all prevention, diagnostic and treatment costs [29].

Russian medical approaches to HIV infection differ from those used with other illnesses because, although it is incurable and chronic, it is also infectious. In order to understand Russian strategies for HIV control as well as general healthcare provision, it helps to understand the previous Soviet approach to disease control, which was characterized by a case-finding surveillance system and lengthy, mandatory inpatient treatment regimens, which, in addition to ensuring patient compliance, also isolated contagious people from society. These measures were underpinned by contact tracing, police involvement in ensuring compliance with screening and follow-up, and a patient registration system for tracking compliance with treatment and follow-up. These measures, while arguably infringing on the human rights of its citizens, did help the USSR to limit epidemics of curable and semi-acute infections such as active TB and syphilis.

Prevention

Thus, the history of the Russian HIV epidemic has been greatly affected by systems and structures that were created long before the world had even heard of HIV, and is primarily based on the Soviet approach to infectious disease control. When HIV was identified in the USSR in 1987 in a naval officer who had been stationed abroad, it served to solidify the conviction of Russian public health officials that HIV was still a foreign problem, not a Russian one. However, the aforementioned 1988–1989 outbreak of nosocomial infections among infants in four cities brought immediate action from the government. HIV was regarded as another infectious disease threat, eliciting a response that was similar to the approaches that had worked in the past for STIs and TB. Immediately a network of 89 AIDS centres was established across the country, with the mandate to screen huge numbers of citizens in order to find all cases of HIV [17]. To date, over 320 million HIV antibody tests have been performed at a rate of 140 per 1000 population, the highest in the world [29]. The vast majority of these tests were performed without the consent of the patient and on groups identified by the government [17,33,34]. These groups include those who are both low-risk, such as pregnant women, blood donors, occupational groups and hospital patients, and more vulnerable populations such as IDUs, prisoners and patients at STI clinics [35]. Although the Federal Law on HIV states that all citizens have a right to anonymous and consensual tests, according to official numbers, these tests comprise less than 0.3% of the total number of tests undertaken.

It is at this critical point that the Soviet approach to infectious disease control becomes very problematic in terms of stopping the spread of HIV, whereas it had worked with other diseases. With syphilis and TB, any cases found could then be treated and cured, thus stopping the chain of transmission. Russian health officials realized that this was not the case with HIV. So they chose to deal with the incurable nature of HIV by trying to control behaviour through legislation. Upon testing positive, a person was immediately required to sign a form stating that he or she understood that, according to Article 122 of the Criminal Code of the Russian Federation, it is illegal to put someone at risk of HIV infection. Stated in such broad terms, this has led to the prosecution of married people with HIV, as well as others in consensual relationships.

As a result, until recently, government-sponsored HIV prevention focused mainly on the compulsory testing of the population. Indeed, the case-finding method of surveillance has been the main feature of the Russian approach to the HIV epidemic. While the mission of the 89 AIDS centres established in 1989 is supposed to include prevention and care for people with HIV, they receive money primarily for testing.

In response to the explosive HIV epidemic among IDUs, the laws concerning narcotics possession were revised in 2000, making the penalties for possession of even the tiniest amount of illicit drugs extremely harsh. This has served to swell the prison population, which is already the second highest per capita in the world—exceeded only by the USA—as well as vastly increase the numbers of people with HIV in prison. In April 2002, there were thought to be 1,220,368 prisoners in Russian jails. It is estimated that between 15 and 20% of all PLHIV in the Russian Federation are in prison or detention facilities [36]. With so many HIV infections attributable to drug injection, penal codes and prison conditions are particularly important factors in the epidemic's spread. Sharply increasing rates of drug-related arrests and extended periods of pre-trial detention have crammed cells designed for 28 people with as many as 110 prisoners [37]. Health risks include multidrug-resistant TB, rape and use of contaminated injection equipment. A recent study in seven Russian prisons found that 21% of prisoners had injected drugs while detained, and 14% began injecting while behind bars [38]. Preventive efforts in prison, such as education and provision of condoms and needles, are almost completely unheard of, as the Russian Federation has not adopted the 1993 guidelines for HIV prevention and treatment in prison issued by the World Health Organization [39].

In addition to the severe penalties levied for drug possession, opportunities for prevention among drug users are made more difficult as substitution therapies for drug addiction, such as methadone and sublingual Buprenorphine, are illegal [23]. Russian authorities claim that they are simply adhering to the Single Convention on Narcotic Drugs, which concentrates on defining and limiting access to Schedule I drugs that are considered 'dangerous' narcotics with high potential for abuse and which should only be used for 'medical' or 'scientific' purposes [40]. This list contains drugs of abuse, such as heroin and methamphetamines, as well as methadone.

Though government-sponsored prevention efforts were initially concentrated on testing, followed by the imposition of legal penalties for exposing others to HIV, in recent years, the Ministry of Health of the Russian Federation has finally endorsed harm-reduction efforts as well as prevention programmes targeting sex workers [41,42].

Treatment and care

According to the Central and Eastern European Harm Reduction Network, in October 2004 approximately 2800 people in the Russian Federation were receiving antiretroviral therapy (ART) [43]. Seven hundred of these people are receiving triple therapy. It is alarming to note that, while 93% of people with HIV are former or current IDUs, only 13% of those receiving triple therapy were infected through injecting drug use [43]. In Moscow, hospital policy prevents IDUs from receiving therapy. In St. Petersburg, where registered cases of HIV exceeded 15,000 in 2002, there are only 100 people on triple therapy. None of these people were infected through injecting drug use. The majority of such patients are in Moscow, with a small percentage in St. Petersburg. Patients in other regions only rarely receive antiretroviral drugs. In one study, it was found that no triple therapy was available in two-thirds of the administrative regions surveyed [43]. Current prices for the government purchase of triple therapy are between US$9000 and US$10,000 per patient per year [44]. Currently, the Russian Federation only manufactures its own analogues of azidothymidine (AZT), called phosphazide or thymazide. In one survey, many respondents indicated that monotherapy with one of these medications was the only available form of ART [43].

Anecdotal evidence points to inconsistent use of antiretroviral medications by those who have received them, further complicating the treatment issue. This is caused by both inconsistent supplies and lack of patient adherence due to misinformation and the belief that breaks in treatment schedules are an acceptable way to relieve side effects. As previously mentioned, the Russian paternalistic medical tradition does not encourage patients' participation in their own treatment. This has led to horrifying anecdotes about inconsistent adherence to ART for those who are lucky enough to have access to them. One patient described his medication regimen as follows: 'I take them for one month, then I stop for a month. After a while, the diarrhoea goes away and I feel good enough to start taking them again. This way [the medicines] last longer too' [J Stachowiak, personal communication (2004)].

Even with the small amounts of drugs that are available, the Russian Federation lacks the infrastructure and expertise to implement highly active antiretroviral therapy (HAART), which involves a sophisticated system of diagnostics and laboratory assays to monitor viral load and CD4 cell count, consistent and reliable supplies of drugs, and an excellent level of trust and communication between patient and physician. The situation is best summed up by a patient interviewed in Penza, who said:

> When people come to the AIDS centre, they receive a diagnosis and a long list of medicines that they are supposed to buy themselves. There is no access to antiretroviral treatment except monotherapy in extreme cases. There is no bacteriological laboratory for proper diagnosis and treatment of opportunistic infections or other complications. There is no viral load testing of plasma. People have no access to medications for prevention of opportunistic infections. And they don't know where to turn [43].

Role of NGOs

Much of the response to the HIV epidemic in the Russian Federation has originated in the non-governmental sector. Non-governmental organizations (NGOs) only appeared in any number after the fall of the Soviet Union in 1991. The initial NGO response to HIV was one of trying to fill the gaps in the government healthcare system's approach to the epidemic. These activities mainly focused on the provision of preventive information to citizens, as well as current and accurate information for those working with AIDS patients.

When the epidemic exploded among IDUs in 1996, NGOs began working more intensively on targeted prevention measures, such as harm reduction programmes involving needle exchange for drug users. Simultaneously, organizations began to focus more energy on working with government institutions in order to enhance the activities of both. NGOs are currently collaborating with government institutions to improve the surveillance system, perform quality clinical and behavioural research, enhance pre- and post-test counselling, provide necessary patient and prevention materials, provide psychological support to people living with HIV, and influence policy and legislation on HIV.

There are further positive developments in Russia's fight against HIV. The Russian Federation has recently signed a US$150 million loan from the World Bank to put programmes in place to address TB and HIV. The HIV component of the loan 'will allocate $50 million to support capacity building, surveillance, programme development, and interventions for prevention and care over a period of five years' [29,45]. This represents a tripling of the resources devoted to HIV by the Federal government.

In addition, the Global Fund to Fight AIDS, Tuberculosis and Malaria has approved a grant of US$89 million to a consortium of NGOs [46]. This grant is to be spent over 5 years to increase the capacity of governmental institutions and NGOs in 10 regions. The money will go to networking and support for PLHIV; prevention and education activities among vulnerable groups such as sex workers, prisoners, drug users and youth; provision of palliative care; lobbying for and capacity building to improve access to treatment; media campaigns related to prevention of HIV transmission and stigma; human rights education and monitoring; and prevention of mother-to-child transmission.

Conclusion

To date, the Russian experience has particularly demonstrated:

◆ that Russia's infectious disease control measures not only violate human rights but are ineffective in limiting the spread of HIV;

◆ that case-finding surveillance in itself is not HIV prevention and can be misleading;

◆ that punitive legislative approaches in the absence of accurate information about the epidemic and education of people at risk serve to increase stigma, make the most vulnerable people even more difficult to reach and raise the risk of further HIV infection in these groups.

However, there has recently been some positive movement on the part of government and the international community to address the HIV epidemic in the Russian Federation in a more constructive and comprehensive manner, especially involving collaborations between NGOs and the state.

References

1. Tragakes E, Lessof S. (2003). *Health Care Systems in Transition: Russian Federation*. Copenhagen: European Observatory on Health Systems and Policies.

2. Economic Survey of the Russian Federation. (2004). *OECD Observer*. URL: www.oecd.org.

3. McKee M, Healy J, eds. (2002). *Hospitals in a Changing Europe*. Buckingham: Open University Press.

4. Afford C. (2003). *Corrosive Reform: Failing Health Systems in Eastern Europe*. Geneva: ILO/PSI.

5. Leon D, Chenet L, Shkolnikov VM *et al.* (1997). Huge variation in Russian mortality rates 1984–1994: artefact, alcohol or what? *Lancet* **350**:383–8.

6. Stoner-Weiss K. (1999). Central weakness and provincial autonomy: observations on the devolution process in Russia. *Post-Soviet Affairs* **15**:1.

7. Leitzel J. (1997). Rule evasion in transitional Russia. In: Nelson M, Tilly C, Walker L, eds. *Transforming Post-communist Political Economies*. Washington, DC: National Academy Press.

8. Chernichovsky D, Potapchik E. (1999). Genuine federalism in the Russian health care system: changing roles of government. *Journal of Health, Politics and Law* **24**:1.

9. Shishkin S. (1999). Problems of transition from tax-based systems of health care finance to mandatory health insurance model in Russia. *Croatian Medical Journal* **40**:2.

10. TACIS. Review of Russian health care financing system. URL: www.tacishf.mednet.ru.

11. Sheiman I. (2001). Paying hospitals in Russia. *Eurohealth* **7**:3.

12. World Bank. Health Reform Pilot Project, Russian Federation. URL: www.worldbank.org.

13. Fechbach M. (2003). *Russia's Health and Demographic Crises: Policy Implications and Consequences*. Washington, DC: The Chemical and Biological Arms Control Institute.

14. Rhodes T, Ball A, Stimson GV *et al.* (1999). HIV infection associated with drug injecting in the newly independent states, eastern Europe: the social and economic context of epidemics. *Addiction* **94**:1323–36.

15. Rhodes T, Stimson GV, Crofts N *et al.* (1999). Drug injecting, rapid HIV spread and the 'risk environment'. *AIDS* **13**(Supplement A):S259–69.

16. Kalichman SC, Kelly JA, Sikkema KJ *et al.* (2000). The emerging AIDS crisis in Russia: review of enabling factors and prevention needs. *International Journal of STD and AIDS* **11**(2):71–5.

17. Bingham JS, Waugh MA. (1999). Sexually transmitted infections in the Russian Federation, the Baltic States and Poland. *International Journal of STD and AIDS* **10**(10):657–8.

18. Amirkhanian YA, Kelly JA, Kukharsky AA *et al.* (2001). Predictors of HIV risk behavior among Russian men who have sex with men: an emerging epidemic. *AIDS* **15**(3):407–12.

19. Kramer J. (1991). Drug abuse in the USSR. In: Jones A, Conner WD, Powell DE, eds. *Soviet Social Problems*. Boulder, CO: Westview Press, p94–118.

20. Nosov NN, Tarasov VK. (1999). The acceptance of a strategy for decreasing the risk of contracting an HIV infection among drug abusers. *Zhurnal Mikrobiologii Epidemiologii i Immunobiologii* **1**: 96–7.

21. Fedotova TT, Zemerov VB, Efimova OS. (2003). Development of HIV infection epidemic among intravenous drug users in the Sverdlovsky region. *Zhurnal Mikrobiologii Epidemiologii i Immunobiologii* **3**:86–9.

22. Blinova O, Alekseenko N, Patokin S *et al.* (2000). An analysis of the situation with injection narcotic usage in the city of Voronezh during the development of the HIV infection epidemic in Russia. *Zhurnal Mikrobiologii Epidemiologii i Immunobiologii* **4**: 40–4.

23. Malinowska-Sempruch K, Hoover J, Alexandrova A. (2003). *Unintended Consequences: Drug Policies Fuel the HIV Epidemic in Russia and Ukraine*. New York: Open Society Institute, International Harm Reduction Development.

24. Lowndes C, Rhodes T, Judd A. (2002). Female Injection Drug Users who Practice Sex Work in Togliatti City, Russian Federation: HIV Prevalence and Risk Behavior. Presented at the XIV International AIDS Conference, Barcelona, Spain.

25. Anonymous. (2001). Russia has world's fastest growing HIV/AIDS epidemic. *IAPAC Monthly* 7(2):39.

26. Anonymous. (2003). Are former Soviet nations plodding down wrong path? Experts lack optimism for the region. *Aids Alert* 8(11):139–41.

27. Anonymous. (2003). Rapid increase in HIV rates—Orel Oblast, Russian Federation, 1999–2001. *Morbidity and Mortality Weekly Reports* 52(28):657–60.

28. United States Intelligence Council. (2000). *The Global Infectious Disease Threat and its Implications for the United States.* Washington, DC: United States Department of State.

29. US-Russia Working Group Against HIV/AIDS. (2003). On the frontline of an epidemic: the need for urgency in Russia's fight against AIDS. In: *A Report of the US-Russia Working Group Against HIV/AIDS.* New York: Transatlantic Partners Against AIDS.

30. Rhodes T, Lowndes C, Judd A *et al.* (2002). Explosive spread and high prevalence of HIV infection among injecting drug users in Togliatti City, Russia. *AIDS* 16(13):F25–31.

31. Dehne KL, Kobyshcha Iu V. (2000). *The HIV Epidemic in Central and Eastern Europe: Update 2000.* Geneva: UNAIDS.

32. Pokrovskii VI, Ladnaia NN *et al.* (2002). HIV-infection. *Information Bulletin No. 22.* Moscow: Ministry of Health, Federal Scientific-Methodological Center on HIV.

33. Russian NAMES Fund. (1999). Discrimination and human rights abuse in Russia. *Canadian HIV/AIDS Policyy & Law Review* 5(1):22–7, 29–34.

34. Russia, secret HIV testing is the norm despite new law. (1996). *AIDS Policy Law* 11(13):5.

35. Dehne KL, Kobyscha Y, Hamers F, Schwartlander B (1999). The HIV/AIDS epidemic in eastern Europe: recent patterns and trends and their implications for policy-making. *AIDS* 13(7):741–9.

36. Alexandrova A. (2003). Russia: new criminal process code promises a more tolerant incarceration policy. *Canadian HIV/AIDS Policy & Law Review* 8(1):54.

37. Stern V. (2001). Problems in prisons worldwide, with a particular focus on Russia. *Annals of the New York Academy of Sciences* 953:113–9.

38. Frost L, Tchertkov V. (2002). Prisoner risk-taking in the Russian Federation. *AIDS Education and Prevention* 14(5 Supplement B):7–23.

39. Bollini, P, Laporte JD, Harding TW. (2002). HIV prevention in prisons. Do international guidelines matter? *European Journal of Public Health* 12(2):83–9.

40. United Nations. (1961). *Single Convention on Narcotic Drugs.* New York: United Nations.

41. Dement'eva LA. (2000). The realization of the concept of harm reduction in Russia. *Zhurnal Mikrobiologii Epidemiologii i Immunobiologii* 4:58–61.

42. Onishchenko GG, Narkevich MI. (2000). New strategies in preventing the spread of HIV infection in Russia. *Zhurnal Mikrobiologii Epidemiologii i Immunobiologii* 4:5–9.

43. Harm Reduction Network. (2002). *Injecting Drug Users, HIV/AIDS Treatment and Primary Care in Central and Eastern Europe and the Former Soviet Union.* Vilnius: Central and Eastern Europe Harm Reduction Network.

44. Rühl C, Pokrovsky V, Vinogradov V. (2002). *The Economic Consequences of HIV.* Moscow: The World Bank Group.

45. Webster P. (2003). World Bank approves loan to help Russia tackle HIV/AIDS and tuberculosis. *Lancet* 361:1355.

46. Webster P. (2003). Global Fund approves grants to fight HIV/AIDS in Russia. *Lancet* 362:1729.

Chapter 34

Spain

Jesús Castilla, Isabel Noguer[*] and José Ramón Repullo

Background

Spain is a South-Western European country of half a million km^2 and some 42 million inhabitants. Population density is higher along the coast and, in the central plain, is concentrated in the capital, Madrid. A dry climate in the centre and south, and mountainous terrain are characteristics that affect economic and social conditions. Like other countries, Spain has experienced a progressive concentration of the population in urban centres and a corresponding move away from rural areas of the interior. The economy is dominated by the service sector, with large-scale tourist activity, particularly along the coasts and on the islands. Spanish is the official language of the country as a whole, and in some regions a second official language is spoken (Catalá, Galego and Euskera). There is no official state religion in Spain, yet Roman Catholicism predominates and remains an important influence in political and social spheres.

With the democratic Constitution of 1978, the administrative structure, which until then had been very centralized, began to undergo a progressive, though uneven, process of devolution of responsibilities to the 17 so-called 'Autonomous Communities' (*Comunidades Autónomas*). Responsibility for education, public health and healthcare services was transferred to the respective regional authorities, with the central government retaining the basic functions of regulation, coordination and international relations.

The growth of the Spanish population has levelled off, and it has aged in the last few decades due to a reduction in the birth rate and an increase in life expectancy to over 70 years. In 1998, the population over 60 years of age was higher than that aged 0–19. The proportion of youth within the population shrank to below 20% in 2000 [1].

Spain has had little immigration, but in the last few years the foreign-born population has been growing and now comprises 6% of the total. Approximately a third of foreign residents in Spain are from the European Union (EU), 32% come from Africa, 22% from Latin America, 8% from non-EU countries in Europe and 8% from Asia [2].

Spain is relatively less wealthy compared with other countries in the EU, with a per capita gross domestic product (GDP) 10% below the average of the 15 EU countries in 2002 (EU-15), though that gap has been narrowing in recent years.

Education is both compulsory and free until the age of 16. Since 1990, teaching programmes have included school-based health and sex education. Approximately 30% of all primary and

---

[*] Corresponding author.

secondary school students attend private schools, which are mainly linked to the Catholic Church.

The health system

Financing and expenditure

The National Health System provides free medical and hospital healthcare coverage to all residents of Spain, including immigrants. Drugs administered in hospitals are available free of charge, while those dispensed in pharmacies are 60% publicly subsidized, except in the case of old-age pensioners and the chronically ill, who receive all such medication at no cost. Antiretroviral drugs are free of charge and dispensed exclusively in hospitals. The public sector prevails, both in primary healthcare and in the nation's hospital network, although a growing percentage of the population also tends to have private medical insurance.

There are different schemes of social and private health insurance, which have evolved separately until now (Table 34.1). The Spanish National Health System (SNHS) constitutes a highly effective and modern public service, at least compared with other public services, though surveys reveal varying degrees of satisfaction among the general population [3,4]. Dissatisfaction is concentrated in the wealthier and better-educated classes [5]. Reasons for dissatisfaction vary, but those most frequently mentioned were problems such as waiting lists for chronically ill patients, lack of personalized care and poor responsiveness to patient preferences.

Spanish per capita health expenditures are 15% lower than in the other EU-15 countries. The proportion of GDP devoted to health—approximately 7.7%—has lagged behind economic growth. Less than 70% of healthcare costs are publicly financed. Therefore, Spain has a higher share of private health expenditure than other similar systems, such as the UK National Health Service (NHS). This reflects a situation in which many people complement the universal

Table 34.1 Health insurance schemes

Coverage	Type	Specific scheme	% of population covered
General health risks	Public compulsory insurance	Social security—National Health System	93%
		Civil service system covered by the National Health System	<1%
		Civil service system covered by private health insurance	>5 %
		Health insurance organized or contracted by companies for their workers	<1%
	Voluntary insurance	Private insurance (complementary to public coverage)	>10%
Labour risks	Range of mutual schemes for occupational diseases and accidents (2.3% of public health expenditure)		16 million workers

coverage of the SNHS, which focuses on severe and complex illnesses, by buying care for minor conditions and elective procedures.

Economic convergence with wealthier EU countries will probably push up total healthcare expenditure, though cost-containment policies in the public sector will constrain this to some degree. If the public system is very limited, this is likely to give rise to increased use of complementary private insurance and out-of-pocket payment, making the overall system less equitable.

Organization of provision

Provision of healthcare in the public sector is split between primary healthcare and specialist care. Catchment areas for primary health centres are between 5000 and 25,000 people on the basis that populations can access their centre in less than 30 minutes by public transport. The specialist system includes outpatient facilities in the community serviced by professionals from the general hospitals, where referrals from primary care are initially seen. Hospitals also have outpatient departments for referrals, more complex consultations and clinical tests, as well as emergency departments, inpatient services, intensive care units and new units for day care, ambulatory surgery and home care services.

General hospitals serve a 'Health Area' that covers an average of 250,000 people, and there is a referral system for more highly specialized services provided at a smaller number of centres. Spain, when compared with other developed countries, has fewer hospital beds (4.1 per 1000 inhabitants) and a lower rate of utilization (8.5 discharges per 100 inhabitants per year).

There are two different networks of providers, including hospitals: the State and social security providers. Social security, through its purchasing power, has had a gradual impact on other public providers, while creating and expanding its own network. Reforms have led to increasing integration of all public services into a single network, and to decentralization to the 19 regions (17 Autonomous Communities and two autonomous cities). Like other public and universal systems, Spain has had its successes and its problems. How to steward and regulate a highly regionalized system is one of the main challenges currently being faced [6]. It is a complex task to maintain a national standard of coverage and benefits in a system that is regionally organized and financed.

In January 2002, the process of regional devolution of all public centres and services was deemed complete, and a new financial system was put in place: Autonomous Communities receive funds from a basket of taxes, including a percentage of sales tax and income tax, with the right to modify tax rates at the regional level up to a threshold fixed by the national government. They are empowered to collect taxes to finance a specific set of decentralized services, mainly educational, social and health services.

The HIV epidemic

In Spain, the first HIV infections probably occurred around 1980. During that decade, HIV spread widely among a large number of injecting drug users (IDUs), and this mode of transmission was responsible for more than two-thirds of early infections [7,8]. Drugs held an attraction for youth, and heroin use was a nationwide problem, particularly in industrial areas. Evidence points to Spain as having one of the highest prevalence rates in Europe [9].

HIV also spread among men who have sex with men (MSM), although much less rapidly [10]. The high number of HIV-infected IDUs, most of them sexually active young adults, led to secondary transmission of HIV by heterosexual and perinatal routes. At the start of the 1990s, more than 100,000 people had already been infected with HIV, and HIV-related mortality ranked first among the major causes of potential years of life lost, making Spain the European country most heavily affected by the epidemic [9].

The seriousness of the situation alarmed Spanish society. In 1986, the Ministry of Health launched the first of a series of mass media campaigns that sought to create a social climate that would be favourable to both prevention and 'normalization' of the disease, as a point of departure for other strategies. In 1992, for the first time ever, the Ministry of Health promoted the use of condoms as an HIV prevention measure. Harm-reduction programmes targeting IDUs were expanded in the mid-1990s [7]. The number of young people engaging in injecting drug use gradually decreased [11], resulting in an aging of the active IDUs. Added to this was a trend toward replacing injecting drugs with drugs that are inhaled or smoked [11]. All these changes led to a marked reduction in the rate of new HIV infections, as has been shown by serial studies of HIV seroprevalence in IDUs [5], MSM [3] and female sex workers [10].

By the mid-1990s, the highest rates of morbidity and mortality had been reached, with more than 7000 new AIDS diagnoses and more than 5000 deaths annually [10]. Since highly active antiretroviral therapy (HAART) was introduced at the end of 1996, there has been a considerable improvement in the immune status and prognosis of HIV-infected individuals, resulting in a rapid reduction in AIDS incidence of over 60% in the next 4 years and a decline in mortality of 67% in just 2 years [10].

HIV

The available data point to a steady decline in HIV transmission rates in Spain in recent years. However, the number of new HIV diagnoses is still high (Table 34.2), and the possibility that transmission will rise again cannot be ruled out. In regions where epidemiological data on newly diagnosed cases of HIV infection are available, a reduction of over 70% has been noted since the early 1990s. In spite of this large decrease, an overall total of 60 new HIV infections per million inhabitants were diagnosed in these regions in 2002, a figure that is still high in comparison with other European countries [8].

The highest risk factors associated with HIV are, in order of importance: risky practices related to IDU; unprotected sex among MSM; and unprotected heterosexual contact with an HIV-infected partner. In spite of this, sexual transmission has been the leading cause of new infections in recent years, since this presents the most widespread exposure to risk in the population [10] (Fig. 34.1).

There have been major changes among IDUs over the years that have led to a marked reduction in the number of new HIV infections. Of these, the most important has been a steady decline in the number of youths who start injecting drugs, with a consequent decline in the risk of infection by this route [11]. At the same time, some former IDUs, mostly heroin users, have stopped using, and many others have switched from injecting to inhaling drugs [12]. While the risk of HIV infection continues to be very high among those who inject drugs, various studies have found moderate reductions in prevalence, probably due to the expansion of methadone maintenance and needle exchange programmes [11] (Fig. 34.2).

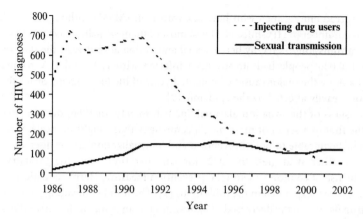

Fig. 34.1 HIV infections newly diagnosed in adults and adolescents by transmission category. Source: Elaborated by the authors with data from three regions.

Spain has been one of the European countries with the highest rates of AIDS affecting MSM [8]. HIV seroprevalence in MSM declined in the first half of the 1990s and has since remained stable at around 8% [10,13]. Recent studies have found that male sex workers and transvestites are groups especially vulnerable to HIV infection.

HIV transmission through heterosexual contact has remained an endemic phenomenon, without appreciable changes. The marked decrease in other modes of HIV transmission has caused heterosexual transmission to become the leading cause of infections in recent years, although this does not imply an increase in the number of infections by this route. The risk of HIV infection is not uniformly distributed in the heterosexual population. The data that probably best summarize this prevalence are those in women delivering a live-born child,

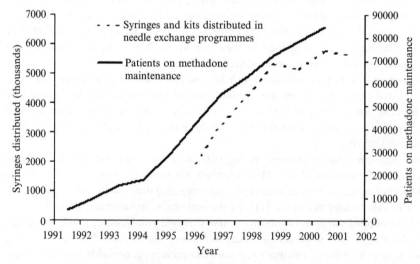

Fig. 34.2 Trends in harm-reduction programmes. Source: Observatorio Español sobre Drogas.

which ranges from one to three per 1000, although there are differences between regions [13]. The highest risk of heterosexual HIV infection is found in those with an infected sexual partner, most of whom are IDUs or ex-IDUs. Over the years, the people with an infected heterosexual partner have shown infection prevalence rates of over 5%, with no clear signs of a decrease [10].

Among women who engage in sex work, HIV seroprevalence has fallen below 2%, and injecting drug use has become an uncommon practice. While there has, in recent years, been a massive influx of female sex workers from Latin America, sub-Saharan Africa and Eastern Europe, an increase in levels of infection has not been observed to date [10].

New diagnoses of HIV infection from heterosexual transmission are stable [10], which corresponds to the lower frequency of sexual risk behaviours in the Spanish population compared with other countries and the continuous decrease in the incidence of sexually transmitted diseases during the 1990s.

As a consequence of the large epidemic among young adults, from the mid-1980s to the late 1990s Spain had the highest incidence of mother-to-child transmission (MTCT) in Europe. The effectiveness of antiretroviral therapy (ART) in reducing MTCT has virtually eliminated infections transmitted by this route, a goal for which early diagnosis of infection in all pregnant women is a prerequisite. In recent years, it is estimated that 500–1000 HIV-infected women annually have delivered a live-born child in Spain. Thanks to antiretroviral prophylaxis, the number of HIV infections and AIDS cases in children has been markedly reduced (Fig. 34.3) [14], but there is still a long way to go before complete control of this mode of transmission has been achieved.

Although immigration in Spain is a relatively recent phenomenon, this population had increased to 6% of the total Spanish population by 2003. Prior to 2002, less than 4% of AIDS cases diagnosed in Spain were residents of foreign origin, reflecting the fact that the HIV epidemic mainly affected the native-born population [14]. However, in recent years, with the gradual control of HIV transmission in the native-born population, together with a growing influx of immigrants to Spain, this is changing [14]. This may be partly attributable to the fact that some immigrants come from countries where HIV

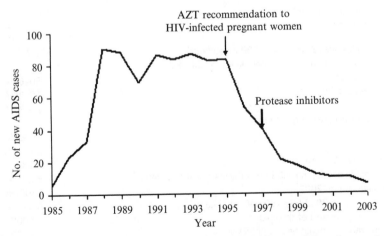

Fig. 34.3 AIDS cases in children infected through mother-to-child transmission. Source: Centro Nacional de Epidemiología.

is highly endemic, but it is likely that adverse social and economic conditions in Spain leading to greater vulnerability to HIV infection, such as sex work or drug use, as well as cultural and linguistic barriers in accessing prevention measures and health services, play a more important role [2]. Over 25% of those diagnosed with HIV infection in 2002 were immigrants, a percentage that has doubled in just 3 years [10]. The most frequent origin was Latin American, followed by sub-Saharan African and Eastern European. In general, the categories of transmission bear a relationship with those predominant in their countries of origin, except in the case of those coming from northern Africa, where IDU is one of the main transmission routes. HIV prevalence rates among immigrants who underwent voluntary testing were no higher than those found in a Spanish population of similar characteristics, except in people from sub-Saharan Africa and in men from Latin America [15].

In light of this new evidence, the Ministry of Health has developed new strategies targeting immigrant populations. For example, since 2000, the annual campaign promoting HIV testing and condom use has been waged in different languages, and prevention programmes are being culturally adapted [16].

Number and characteristics of people living with HIV

The key feature of the current epidemic in Spain is the large number of people living with HIV (PLHIV; Table 34.2). Advances in ART have improved survival and quality of life of HIV-infected people considerably but have been unable to achieve a cure, and, once started, treatment must be maintained indefinitely. HIV prevalence in the general population is approximately three infections per 1000 inhabitants, increasing to six per 1000 in the 20–39 age group [10]. In line with the general pattern of the epidemic in industrialized countries, seroprevalence in men is three times higher than in women. In mothers of newborns, rates range from one to three per 1000 in most regions [10]. Based on these seroprevalence data, it is estimated that there are between 110,000 and 150,000 PLHIV in Spain, although probably more

Table 34.2 The HIV epidemic, 2002

People living with HIV	110,000–150,000
Prevalence of HIV infection (rate per 1000 inhabitants)	2.7–3.8
Probable mechanism of infection in people living with HIV	
Injecting drug users	50–60%
Men who have sex with men	15–25%
Heterosexual risk	20–30%
Characteristics of people living with HIV	
Men	75–80%
Women	20–25%
Children (under 13 years)	<1%
Number of people developing AIDS since the start of the epidemic[*]	65,000–75,000
New AIDS diagnoses in 2002[*]	2500–3000
AIDS incidence rate in 2002 (per 100,000 inhabitants)[*]	6.3–7.5
AIDS deaths since the start of the epidemic[*]	40,000–50,000
People living with HIV–hepatitis C co-infection	60,000–80,000

[*]Estimates take into account under-reporting.

than a quarter of them have not yet been diagnosed. In recent years, the HIV-infected population has remained relatively stable, since both the number of new infections and the number of HIV-related deaths has fallen [10] (Fig. 34.4).

The epidemiological characteristics of this population depend less on new infections than on those that have accumulated over the course of the epidemic. These characteristics can be determined by studying the number of AIDS cases diagnosed in recent years or the number of patients with HIV infection reported in hospital surveys, as both figures arise directly from PLHIV. Based on either of these sources, we can estimate that a little more than half (50–60%) of HIV-infected people acquired the infection through contaminated drug injection equipment, 20–30% from unprotected heterosexual contact, and 15–25% are men who became infected through unprotected homosexual contact. The ratio of men to women is approximately 4:1, and the average age is 35–40 years and rising [10]. The high rate of injecting drug use among PLHIV in Spain explains why more than half of them are also infected with hepatitis C virus.

Treatment and care

Following the introduction of HAART at the end of 1996, there were very sharp decreases in the incidence of AIDS and related mortality (Fig. 34.5). In recent years, these decreases have become less pronounced, and the ceiling for the effectiveness of HAART may have been reached. In 2002, the lowest AIDS rates in the last 10 years were recorded, with 5.7 new AIDS cases per 100,000 inhabitants.

Patients enjoy free access to healthcare, which has steadily incorporated therapeutic advances. ART currently plays a fundamental role in preventing AIDS incidence and mortality from returning to former levels, since the number of PLHIV is still very high. The main factors hindering a greater impact of ART are: late diagnosis of AIDS, leading to delays in starting treatment; lack of patient compliance with treatment; the emergence of resistance to antiretroviral drugs; and adverse reactions requiring prescribed treatments to be withdrawn or changed.

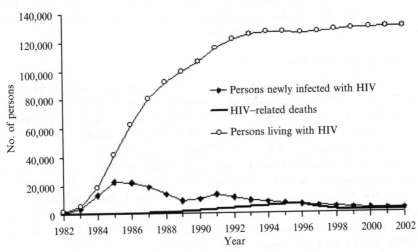

Fig. 34.4 Estimated time trends of the HIV edipemic. Source: Secretaría del Plan Nacional sobre el Sida, 2002.

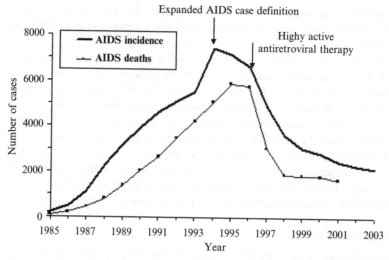

Fig. 34.5 Time trends in AIDS incidence and mortality. Source: Centro Nacional de Epidemiología.

Delayed diagnosis of HIV infection has been shown to be an important factor in reducing the impact of ART [17], and probably of preventive measures as well. Among those diagnosed with AIDS since 1998, over a third had not known they were HIV-positive, and this proportion exceeds 50% in people infected through sexual transmission.

Improved life expectancy of people living with HIV is providing the opportunity for other late-developing health problems to appear, as well as secondary effects of ART. The most notable of these is the high rate of hepatitis C infection, which is leading to an increasing incidence of chronic liver disease and cirrhosis.

The National Health System is coping with a new burden of HIV infections among immigrants, mostly originating from developing countries. Among the patients seeking hospital services due to their HIV infection, the proportion of people originating from other countries increased from 4% in 2001 to 8% in 2003 [18].

The system's response

Spain's decentralized health system structure has had a significant impact on the organizational response to HIV. Regions have a large degree of autonomy in both public health and education. However, the central government does play an important role as coordinator of national and regional policies. In 1983, the National AIDS Commission was created for the purpose of coordinating sectoral, ministerial (Public Health, Social Affairs, Education, Justice and Interior) and regional policies in which professional medical and retail pharmacist associations and non-government organizations (NGOs) also took part. The National AIDS Plan Secretariat, which comes under the Ministry of Health, is the Commission's standing body, tasked with drawing up proposals for the prevention and control of infection. The first integrated response to the epidemic came in 1996 with the HIV/AIDS Multisectoral Plan 1997–2000, whose main goals were those approved in 1987 by the World Health Assembly: the prevention of new infections, reduction of the negative personal and social impact of the epidemic, and the mobilization and coordination of the fight against HIV [19]. Epidemiological surveillance and other information systems have guided results and evaluation since the establishment of the Plan [20].

It is estimated that over €21 million(US$19.8 million) was allocated to HIV prevention in Spain in 2002 [20]. Although primary responsibility for developing the Plan belonged to the public health administration, the multisectoral nature of the epidemic created the need for strategic alliances between and amongst the educational system, social services, health services in prisons, the National Drug Plan and NGOs. To achieve its global objectives, the Plan promoted interventions of proven effectiveness aimed at the general population as well as the most vulnerable groups and individuals. In 2000, the Multisectoral Plan was renewed for the period 2001–2005 [19].

Free, voluntary HIV testing is available in primary healthcare centres, hospitals and sexually transmitted infection (STI) clinics. In Spain's larger towns and cities, voluntary, free and anonymous HIV testing and counselling are offered by specialized clinics.

HIV treatment has always been provided by specialized units at public hospitals, which have been quick to incorporate the newest therapeutic advances and guidelines. Access to ART is free of charge for all residents of Spain, including immigrants. The cost of ART in 2002 was estimated to be over €335 million(US$317 million)[20]. Advances in quality of life as a result of ART have led to a reduction in HIV-related hospitalization, from 48% in 1995 to 24% in 2002, among those seeking hospital services. In addition, AIDS patients have the right to receive a pension based on pre-established criteria [18].

In order to collaborate in the control of the HIV epidemic around the world, Spain funds cooperative programmes for prevention and access to therapies in Latin America and Africa. Concerning HIV activities, the Ministry of Health has two main areas of cooperation. The first is with the Pan American Health Organization (PAHO), with the following goals: strengthening managerial and planning capacity of national HIV/STI programmes to achieve appropriate health policy and management standards; strengthening epidemiological surveillance; developing best practice models for behavioural interventions aimed at specific target groups in the region; and developing models of care for HIV-infected individuals and AIDS patients in Latin America and the Caribbean.

A second area of cooperation consists of bilateral projects. One of the most successful examples is the Hospital AIDS network (ESTHER), which has been in place since 2001. This project involves cooperation between Spanish and Latin American hospitals in order to develop and implement best practice treatment for HIV patients.

The future of the epidemic

The HIV epidemic in Spain is on a favourable course. However, in the medium term, HIV infection is expected to continue to require substantial investment, both in prevention activities, so as to ensure an ongoing reduction in the rate of new infections, and in healthcare delivery to the large numbers of persons infected with the disease. Prevention programmes will have to lay greater emphasis on sexual transmission and target the most vulnerable groups, including immigrants, sex workers and prison inmates.

In addition, there are a number of factors that could have a negative or positive impact in the short term on the progress made to date:

1. HIV transmission appears much lower than it was in the past, but is still high. Complacency could cause new upturns in the epidemic at any time.

2. The presence of large numbers of people with undiagnosed HIV infection has implications for the course of the epidemic. Not only might they play a significant role in HIV transmission, but they also do not benefit from ART, with consequent adverse effects on AIDS incidence and mortality.

3. Treatment of HIV infection is continually evolving. Resistant viral strains could spread, with negative consequences, or the introduction of new drugs could improve therapy, with positive consequences.

4. The demographic and social changes that are occurring in Spain as a result of immigration introduce new elements to be taken into account in prevention and control of the epidemic.

Conclusion

The regional decentralization of the healthcare system contributes to a better tailoring of services to local needs but requires a greater effort to coordinate activities at different levels in a range of settings.

The National Health System has been shown to provide a framework that can respond quickly to the growing need for HIV control within the population. Its HIV-related interventions have always been based on the principles of free access, universality and equity. In order to decrease delays in HIV diagnosis, offering confidential and anonymous HIV testing and counselling as widely as possible has also proven highly effective. In particular, providing free antiretroviral drugs to all patients who can benefit from this treatment has proved to be effective in reducing AIDS, premature death, hospital admissions and length of stay due to opportunistic infections.

However, the Spanish response has weaknesses. For instance, the proportion of HIV-infected people with a diagnosis is still low. HIV outbreaks among IDUs could still occur if favourable conditions were to recur, in which case controlling the outbreak would become extremely difficult. Harm-reduction programmes among IDUs are probably the best and most practical response in the short term and must be maintained.

References

1. Gènova R. (2003). Demografía. In: *Salud Pública y Enfermería Comunitaria*, 2nd edn. Madrid: McGraw-Hill, p735–74.

2. Secretaría del Plan Nacional sobre el Sida. (2001). *Prevención del VIH/sida en Inmigrantes y Minorías Étnicas*. Madrid: Ministerio de Sanidad y Consumo.

3. INSALUD. (2002). *Memoria 1999*. Instituto Nacional de la Salud. Madrid: Ministerio de Sanidad.

4. Rico A, Pérez-Nievas S. (2001). La satisfacción de los ciudadanos con los servicios sanitarios públicos en España. Conclusiones. In: López-Casasnovas G, ed. *Evaluación de las Políticas Sanitarias Autonómicas*. Bilbao: Fundación BBVA, pp 363–450.

5. Murillo C, Calonge S, Gonzalez Y. (1997). La financiación privada de los servicios sanitarios. In: López Casasnovas G, Rodríguez Palenzuela D, eds. *La Regulación de los Servicios Sanitarios en España*. Madrid: FEDEA-AES-Civitas, pp 245–290.

6. Freire Campo JM, Infante Campos A, Rey del Castillo J. (2003). La política de Salud en el Estado de las Autonomías. In: Garde JA, ed. *Políticas Sociales y Estado de Bienestar en España*. Madrid: FUHEM, p283–318.

7. Castilla J, Bolea A, Suárez M, de la Fuente L. (2002). Spain. In: Macerate K, ed. *HIV and AIDS: A World View.* Westport, CT: Greenwood Press, p183–99.

8. European Centre for the Epidemiological Monitoring of AIDS. (2003). *HIV/AIDS Surveillance in Europe. Year End Report 2002.* Saint-Maurice: Institut de Vielle Sanitaire, No. 69.

9. European Monitoring Centre for Drugs and Drug Addiction. (1997). *Annual Report on the State of the Drugs Problem in the European Union.* Lisbon: EMCDDA.

10. Secretaría del Plan Nacional sobre SIDA. (2002). *HIV and AIDS in Spain, 2001.* Madrid: Ministerio de Sanidad y Consumo.

11. Observatorio Español sobre Drogas. (2002). Informe no. 5, Julio 2002. Madrid: Delegación del Gobierno para el Plan Nacional sobre Drogas.

12. De la Fuente L, Barrio G, Royuela L, Bravo MJ. (1997). The transition from injecting to smoking heroin in three Spanish cities. *Addiction* 92:1733–44.

13. Centre d'Estudis Epidemiològics sobre la Sida de Catalunya. (2002). *Sistema Integrat de Vigilància Epidemiològica del VIH/sida a Catalunya (SIVES). Informe Anual 2001.* Barcelona: Departament de Sanitat i Seguretat Social.

14. Centro Nacional de Epidemiología. (2003). Vigilancia epidemiológica del Sida en España. Situación a 30 de Junio de 2003. *Boletín Epidemiológico Semanal* 11:293–6.

15. The EPI-HIV Study Group (2002). HIV infection among people of foreign origin voluntarily tested in Spain. A comparison with national subjects. *Sexually Transmitted Infections* 78:250–4.

16. Castilla J, Sobrino P, de la Fuente L *et al.* (2002). Late diagnosis of HIV infection in the era of highly active antiretroviral therapy: consequences on AIDS incidence. *AIDS* 16:1945–51.

17. Secretaría del Plan Nacional sobre el Sida. (1997). *Plan de Movilización Multisectorial de lucha contra el VIH/sida en España, 1997–2000.* Madrid: Ministerio de Sanidad y Consumo.

18. Secretaría del Plan Nacional sobre el Sida. (2003). *Encuesta Hospitalaria de Pacientes VIH/sida 1995–2002.* Madrid: Ministerio de Sanidad y Consumo.

19. Secretariat of the National Plan on AIDS. (2002). *HIV infection and AIDS in Spain. Multisectoral Plan 2001–2005.* Madrid: Ministerio de Sanidad y Consumo.

20. Secretaría del Plan Nacional sobre el Sida. (2003). *Indicadores de Evaluación del Plan Multisectorial 2001–2005.* Madrid: Ministerio de Sanidad y Consumo.

Chapter 35

Ukraine

Valerya Lekhan, Volodomyr Rudiy, Ellen Nolte[*],
Jantine Jacobi, Lidia Andrushchak, Alla Shcherbinska
and Yuriy Kruglov

Background

While still relatively low compared with the rest of the world, rates of HIV infection have been rising extremely fast in many parts of Eastern Europe and the former Soviet Union (FSU). 'One out of every hundred adults walking down the streets of a city in Eastern Europe or the Commonwealth of Independent States … carries the HIV virus' [1]. The number of people in the region living with HIV has risen exponentially in just a few years, reaching 1.2–1.8 million at the end of 2003, and it has been estimated that as many as 280,000 people were newly infected with HIV in that year. Most have contracted HIV from injecting drug use, mainly affecting young people under the age of 30 [2].

Ukraine is among the countries worst hit by the epidemic, along with the Russian Federation, Estonia and Latvia, with the highest rate of new infection in Europe and the Commonwealth of Independent States (CIS). About 1% of the adult population (15–49 years of age) is estimated to be HIV-infected, and around 250,000 Ukrainians are believed to be living with HIV or AIDS, although some estimates are higher (Fig. 35.1).

The number of AIDS cases is now increasing rapidly; an incidence rate of 17.2 per million was reported in 2001, and as many as 11,000 may have died because of AIDS in the same year [4]. It has been projected that in the absence of a comprehensive response to the epidemic, over 1.4 million Ukrainians may be living with HIV by 2010, with as many as 95,000 likely to die of AIDS in that same year [4]. The country has recognized the need to step up its efforts to contain the epidemic and has successfully secured new funding for a comprehensive policy response. While a number of challenges still lie ahead, it appears that Ukraine now has in place the most crucial elements required to reverse or at least control the spread of HIV.

Economic trends

Ukraine is the second largest country in Europe, with a population of about 48.4 million, of which 78% is Ukrainian, 17% Russian, and the remaining 5% comprising a number of minority groups such as Belorussians, Moldavians, Bulgarians, Crimean Tatars, Jews and Roma [5].

[*] Corresponding author.

The views expressed in this chapter are those of the authors and are not necessarily those of the organizations they work for, unless specifically stated in the text.

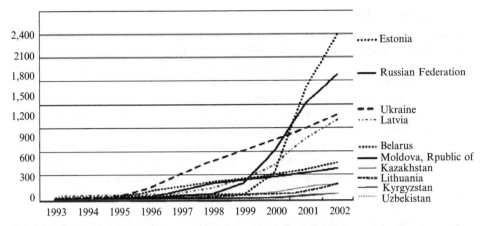

Fig. 35.1 Cumulative reported HIV infections per million population in Eastern European countries, 1993–2002. Source: [3].

Ukrainian is the official state language; Russian, Romanian, Polish and Hungarian are also spoken. The main religions are Ukrainian Orthodox and Ukrainian Catholic (Uniate), with smaller numbers of Protestants and Jews. Ukraine only became an independent state in August 1991, following the break up of the Soviet Union. Since then, the country has undergone a difficult transition towards a democratic system of governance and a market-oriented economy. This process culminated in the 'Orange Revolution' at the beginning of 2005, which was an extension of the process of democratization still taking place in the country.

Ukraine inherited substantial structural problems that made any prospect of immediate economic prosperity almost impossible, experiencing a sustained economic crisis that included the worst hyperinflation in the region. Between 1991 and 1999, the gross domestic product (GDP) fell by 62% [6]. Recovery only came in 2000, when Ukraine registered growth of 5.8% in the GDP for the first time since independence, which continued in 2001 [7]. However, despite these positive trends, in 2002, per capita GDP in Ukraine was still only 44% of the level seen in 1989 [8].

The economic crisis had a serious and long-term impact on the income and well-being of the population and resulted in a marked decline in living standards and increasing poverty. The employment rate fell from 82% in 1990 to 66% in 1999 and has remained at that level despite recent economic growth [8]. By 2001, real wages had fallen to 59% of the 1989 level. Official statistics on economic activity, however, give only part of the picture. A considerable proportion of economic activity is now taking place in the informal sector, with recent figures estimating it to comprise at least 50% of the total economy [7]. Also, many of those who are employed receive their wages late or are paid in kind. While most people in Ukraine have been affected by the economic decline, some have suffered more than others. Survey estimates suggest that in 2000, over 80% of respondents perceived themselves as poor and only 3% of households had a per capita income over 300 *Hryvnia* (UAH) per month (US$56), which is the suggested minimum income required for food, shelter and medical care [9]. This indicates that a considerable percentage of the population in Ukraine is still facing substantial economic difficulties.

Demography and health

The transition has also had a major impact on demographic and health indicators. Since Independence, Ukraine's population has fallen by 7.5%, with current estimates projecting a further decline of 1% per year over the period 2000–2005 [9]. The birth rate fell by almost 40% between 1990 and 2000, with the total fertility rate now the lowest in Europe [10]. At the same time, Ukraine experienced a severe mortality crisis in the first half on the 1990s, with male life expectancy at birth falling by 4.4 years between 1990 and 1995 and female life expectancy falling by 2.4 years. While there was some improvement after 1995, mortality rates rose again after 1998, with little subsequent indication of a reversal in this trend (Fig. 35.2). By 2002, life expectancy at birth had fallen to 62.2 years for men and 73.7 for women. The fluctuations in life expectancy in Ukraine in the 1990s were largely driven by changes in mortality from cardiovascular diseases and external causes of death affecting mainly young and middle-aged men.

As in many other parts of the FSU, smoking accounts for a considerable part of the burden of disease, particularly among men, with smoking prevalence rates of about 57% [11,12]. Recent estimates suggest that in 2000, about 100,000 deaths, or 15% of all deaths in Ukraine, may have been attributable to smoking [13]. Another important factor is excessive alcohol consumption [14].

Women have been relatively less affected in terms of mortality than men; however, their health is also compromised. Maternal mortality, while falling since 1992, remains high, at 24.7 per 100,000 live births in 2000, which is about five times the European Union (EU) average [10]. Ukraine has a very high proportion of pregnancies that are terminated through abortion, contributing substantially to maternal mortality. In 2000, about one-fifth of all maternal deaths in Ukraine were related to abortion, or 4.9 per 100,000 live births. A recent decline in abortion rates has been attributed, in part, to initiatives in reproductive health. However, abortion continues to be an important method of birth control in Ukraine, with access to modern contraceptives, despite increasing demand, remaining difficult [15].

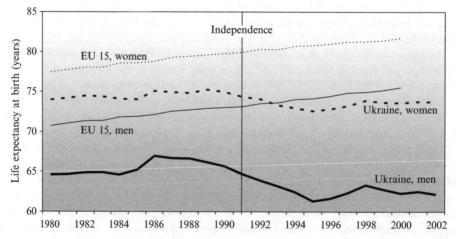

Fig. 35.2 Life expectancy at birth in Ukraine and the European Union (EU-15; before May 1, 2004), 1980–2002. Source: WHO Regional Office for Europe.

Ukraine has also experienced a resurgence of communicable diseases such as diphtheria and tuberculosis (TB) due to a combination of factors, including weakened prevention and control programmes in the early stages of independence, deteriorating socio-economic conditions, and the emergence of HIV contributing further to the already high burden of disease in the country and posing substantial challenges to the country's health system.

Health system

The process of economic restructuring since independence was accompanied by substantially reduced living standards for large parts of the population, especially retired people, the disabled and other vulnerable groups, leading to further worsening of the population's health. This increased need for healthcare took place against the background of reduced ability of the healthcare system to respond adequately. The general economic downturn has also had an impact on the resources available for healthcare at a time when the costs of running the healthcare system have increased substantially.

In Soviet times, costs for materials, medical supplies and basic services such as electricity and heating were fixed, which allowed the state to maintain an extensive network of healthcare facilities. Also, the operating costs of hospitals were comparatively low, as were the costs of pharmaceuticals, since the limited range available from production in the Soviet Union or in other socialist countries was subsidized. The transition to the principles of a market economy has resulted in soaring prices for pharmaceuticals and basic services and utilities, thereby further complicating the already difficult economic situation in the healthcare sector. In such a context, maintaining the complex, inefficient public healthcare system in Ukraine, with its unbalanced structure of health services, has resulted in a healthcare system that is highly inequitable and of poor quality.

Organization and financing

The formal healthcare system in Ukraine is supervised by the state. In theory, the Ministry of Health has responsibility for health policy. In practice, its influence is limited, as it directly manages only a few specialized facilities. Most healthcare is delivered in state-owned facilities, and managed and funded at regional and local levels by the respective tiers of government from allocations provided by the Ministry of Finance or raised locally. In practice, therefore, the scope of the national Ministry of Health is confined to issuing normative guidance and developing national health policy.

Unlike many other areas of the economy, healthcare financing in Ukraine has essentially retained the Soviet approach based on taxation, providing universal coverage, at least in theory, free of charge. Officially, the provision of free services in public health facilities is guaranteed by the 1996 Constitution of Ukraine, which also secures the right of citizens to health insurance and further requires that the state 'encourage the development of health facilities of all forms of ownership'. However, the private health sector is developing only slowly, and government budgets therefore remain the major official source for healthcare finance in Ukraine, with some 80% of financing from local budgets and the remaining 20% from the state budget.

The exact level of health expenditure in Ukraine is difficult to determine, mainly due to problems in obtaining data on healthcare spending in the informal sector. According to national data, public healthcare spending in 2001 was 2.7% of GDP [9]. This is one of the lowest proportions in the World Health Organization (WHO) European region. In absolute terms, Ukraine spends US$148 purchasing power parity (PPP, 2001) per person per year on healthcare, which is only 7% of the EU average of US$2226 PPP. Compared with other former Soviet countries, Ukraine is lagging behind Belarus (US$350 PPP) and Russia (US$243 PPP in 2000) [10].

This shortage of public funds in healthcare is increasingly leading to patients being indirectly charged for services in public facilities, disguised as 'donations' or 'voluntary cost recovery' [16]. Official user-fees appear to be of minor importance, representing about 2% of the total healthcare spending, as is the role of voluntary health insurance. However, 'under-the-table' payments for health services are very common.

Until 1996, before the introduction of official user-charges, the public share of healthcare financing in Ukraine was about 80%, falling to 66% in 2000. However, taking into account informal payments, the share of resources derived from general taxation was even lower, at 48%. At the same time, direct out-of-pocket health expenditure by the population increased swiftly, rising from 18% in 1996 to 30% in 2000; if we include informal payments, out-of-pocket expenditure on health was as high as 51% in 2000. Such heavy reliance on health financing from private sources is usually only found in low-income developing countries, although comparable figures have also been reported in Russia [17].

These developments have led to a substantial decrease in access to healthcare. A recent survey showed that 27% of households were unable to obtain necessary healthcare for any member of the family in 2002 [18]. For the majority of respondents, this was mainly because of exceptionally high costs for drugs, devices for home care and health services. Furthermore, about 9% of households were unable to consult a doctor in case of illness of household members because of financial difficulties, with another 5% being unable to obtain necessary inpatient treatment for the same reason. The study also demonstrated that 93% of hospital patients were charged for drugs, 83% for food and 64% for bed linen (64%), the very services that the state health system is by law supposed to provide. Between 1998 and 2000, user expenses for hospital treatment nearly doubled.

Certain vulnerable groups are exempt from user-charges, including patients with AIDS, who, in theory, do not have to pay for outpatient drugs; however, the quantity of available drugs is very limited. The trend of rising healthcare costs, in both absolute and relative terms, is especially worrying as family incomes fall, creating a situation whereby low-income groups delay their visits to healthcare providers for economic reasons, with consequences for their health.

Healthcare delivery

The basic principles of healthcare delivery in Ukraine have changed little since Independence, with much of the system still working according to the Soviet model. It maintains policies that stimulate further expansion of the health facilities network and an increase in capacity, particularly hospital beds and physicians, despite the simultaneous sharp reduction in the budget. This takes place against the backdrop of a society in which the majority of the population is facing substantial financial difficulties, thus aggravating the problem of healthcare accessibility and affordability. In addition, despite recent increased efforts to improve the quality of care, many healthcare facilities, especially those in rural areas, still face severe structural problems. Many buildings have become dilapidated, with run-down and outmoded equipment.

Replacement of outdated medical equipment is still progressing very slowly, with replacement rates of less than 2% per year in most facilities.

By January 2001, Ukraine had over 9000 health facilities, including multi-specialty inpatient facilities that provide both inpatient and outpatient care, independent polyclinics and ambulatories, which provide outpatient care, and over 16,000 *feldsher*-midwife aid posts (FMAPs). *Feldshers* represent a special category of middle-level health works somewhat like nurse practitioners. About 86% of these facilities are publicly owned, as the private sector has been developing slowly during the last decade. Most private health facilities have limited capacity, and their role in providing health services to the population has so far been insignificant. Further expansion of the private healthcare sector is inhibited by the low living standards of the majority of the population.

The primary healthcare (PHC) system currently in place in Ukraine is essentially that inherited from the Soviet era. There is a large network of primary-level healthcare units in rural and urban areas, comprising paediatric polyclinics or polyclinic departments in hospitals; polyclinic units of *medsanchasts*, or workplace-related clinics; women's consultation clinics; rural physicians' ambulatories; and outpatient departments in rural hospitals. The organization of primary care delivery is territorial, and the area serviced by a particular PHC unit is further divided into catchment areas (*uchastok*) with a certain number of residents. In rural areas, each physician's *uchastok* encompasses, on average, 4–5 FMAPs providing simple curative services, first aid, prescription of drugs, antenatal and postnatal care, and basic preventive activities such as immunization.

There is no strict distinction between primary and secondary care in Ukraine. Patients may seek care from a specialist directly without formal referral by their catchment area physician, and this opportunity is widely used. Secondary care is provided in polyclinics and outpatient departments of hospitals and dispensaries. Dispensaries are specialized health facilities that provide outpatient and inpatient secondary care to defined categories of patients and systematically monitor their health. Specialists in municipal polyclinics provide services both to patients referred by primary care physicians and to those who seek care directly. As at the primary care level, organization of secondary outpatient care is based on each polyclinic being assigned a defined catchment area. Area residents are entitled to full diagnostic examination and appropriate treatment, and may be referred to the tertiary level when necessary.

Public health in Ukraine remains based on the traditional and largely obsolete functions of the state Sanitary and Epidemiological Service (San-Epid), whose main ostensible objectives are the control of communicable diseases and environmental protection. However, new public health functions are now being developed, especially in response to the re-emergence of infectious diseases such as TB and newly emerging health threats such as HIV. Disease prevention and health promotion programmes are being implemented, as well as a specific programme for reproductive health.

A key feature of the medical workforce in Ukraine is the overprovision of specialists relative to physicians working at the primary care level, who constituted only 27% of the total number of active physicians in 2000. The current situation is further characterized by low remuneration of doctors and other staff; the average salary in the healthcare sector is less than half the average wage in the industrial sector. At the same time, there were about 13,000 vacant physicians' posts in 2000. Shortages are especially critical in the primary care sector and the TB service. In addition, the majority of physicians are concentrated in urban areas. The supply of nurses in Ukraine is falling steadily, which has been attributed to declining prestige of this middle-level health profession. Nurses are increasingly leaving the health sector because of low remuneration and lack of career prospects, and replacing them with new personnel is becoming more and more difficult due to the falling numbers of nurses graduating.

Healthcare reforms

Since independence, the government has been engaged in reforming the healthcare sector; however, Ukraine still lacks an integral long-term programme for reforming its national healthcare system. Instead, the country has succeeded in creating a legal framework that is characterized by fragmentation and complexity, with overlapping and often ambiguous lines of accountability and inadequate resources to meet its stated goals. Soviet-style capacity planning for public healthcare facilities continues, accompanied by state guarantees of universal and unlimited access to healthcare free of charge in the face of an acute shortage of public funds due to the difficult economic situation in the country. As a result, the drastic reduction in quality and accessibility of healthcare, with widespread unofficial payments and other forms of charging the population for health services, are likely to persist unabated.

The HIV epidemic

Epidemiology

The first HIV cases were reported in 1987, when HIV screening of population groups was introduced in Ukraine. In 1995, a sudden outbreak among injecting drug users (IDUs) occurred, mainly in southern Ukraine, with a subsequently rapid expansion throughout the country [19]. Currently, the number of IDUs in all of Ukraine is estimated to be 560,000 [20]. Although the majority of HIV infections still occur through injecting drug use, with 67% of those HIV-infected being IDUs, the number of infections through sexual transmission is on the increase, partly because a significant proportion of female IDUs are involved in sex work. Also, a growing number of women are reporting that they have been infected by a non-injecting partner [21]. It is known that the number of HIV cases registered at the AIDS centres is far lower than the estimated number of cases, for reasons such as inadequacy of surveillance and voluntary counselling and testing (VCT) services, and stigma and discrimination [22]. As shown in Fig. 35.3, there has been an increase in the number of officially registered HIV cases, with a temporary dip in 1998, when the mandatory testing policy became voluntary [23]. By 2004, only 62,365 people with HIV were registered, whereas a total of 111,102 had tested HIV-positive. The WHO and UNAIDS estimated that at the end of 2003, between 130,000 and 416,000 people were living with HIV. According to 2003 data, more than 60% of those were under 30 years of age and 43% were women [Ukrainian AIDS Centre (2004). Kyiv. Unpublished data.].

Figure 35.4 shows surveillance data obtained from seven cities for 2002, revealing that HIV prevalence rates among IDUs ranged from 17 to 58%, with the highest levels observed in the southern and eastern regions. HIV infection rates among female sex workers (FSWs) were found to be between 4 and 31%, whereas patients with sexually transmitted infections (STIs), reporting at public institutions, had HIV infection rates between 0.3 and 28%. The rates of HIV infection among IDUs, FSW and STI clients show a generally consistent pattern [24].

Ukraine was the first country of the FSU to decriminalize consensual sexual relations between adult men (1991). However, due to prevailing stigmatization, surveillance data on HIV

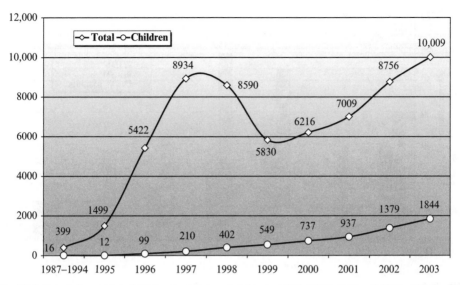

Fig. 35.3 Trends in registered HIV cases, total and children, 1987–2002. Source: Ukraine Centre for AIDS Prevention, 2003.

infection rates among men who have sex with men (MSM) are practically unavailable. Since the beginning of the epidemic, only 43 cases of HIV infection have been registered. A small study among male sex workers (MSWs) revealed that about 16% were HIV-infected [24].

The response to the epidemic

Initial response

Recognizing the global threat of the HIV epidemic, the government of Ukraine established an AIDS Prevention Centre in 1989, tasked with providing guidance to authorities and health workers and developing a legal framework. In 1990, a special government commission was created to oversee the HIV response. However, with independence from the Soviet Union in 1991 and the associated substantial political, economic and social changes outlined above, health and social services in Ukraine deteriorated, which also affected the quality of healthcare provided to people living with HIV (PLHIV) [25]. Thus, in 1992, the National Committee to fight AIDS was established under the President of Ukraine. It comprised national experts and was responsible for the development of state policies and for the planning and implementation of the national response.

Legal framework

The response to the HIV epidemic was regulated by the 1991 law on AIDS Prevention and Social Protection of the Population. The law stipulated that HIV was a state public health priority requiring a multisectoral response. It articulated the rights and duties of the state and of HIV-infected individuals, including the principles of confidentiality and access to healthcare. In 1998, this law was amended to revoke compulsory testing, in line with international standards, and to provide IDUs with protection [26]. The legal provisions particularly affecting vulnerable groups were, first, that manufacturing and distribution of illegal drugs became a criminal

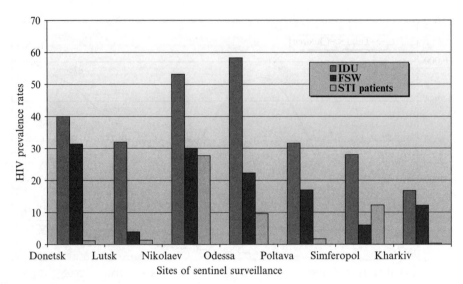

Fig. 35.4 HIV prevalence rates among IDUs, FSWs and STI patients in seven cities in Ukraine, 2002. Source: [24].

offence under the law on drug trafficking [27] and, secondly, that prostitution, which had previously been regulated by the administrative code, was to be criminalized in 2001 [28]. However, consensual sex between adult men had been decriminalized as early as 1991, and remained so.

The Cabinet issued six resolutions related to the implementation of the 1998 law, including details of how medical services were to be provided to PLHIV and solutions to other HIV-related problems. During 2000–2001, the President of Ukraine signed three decrees to extend the scope of epidemic response activities, including the announcement that the year 2002 would be the Year to Fight AIDS in Ukraine, and implement additional measures to strengthen the response to HIV, such as wider information dissemination, improved medical assistance, and involvement of civil society organizations [29].

In December 2003, Parliament held its first open hearing on HIV, addressing a range of issues concerning prevention and establishing the Interim Ad Hoc Commission of the Supreme Council of Ukraine on HIV/AIDS, Tuberculosis and Drug Use. It also led to the creation of new charitable organizations, focusing on children with HIV abandoned by their parents. This was followed by an Order by the President in August 2004, requiring the Cabinet to establish, in 2004–2005, domestic production of antiretroviral drugs and drugs for the treatment of opportunistic infections; a reference laboratory for the identification of resistant forms of HIV; and a specialized clinic for treatment of children with HIV.

National programmes

Since 1992, a total of four national HIV prevention programmes have been developed and implemented. The first three programmes focused on HIV prevention among the general population, ensuring blood safety and generating public awareness. The Second National Programme (1995–1997) allowed the development of AIDS Centres to provide healthcare services to PLHIV [4]. The third programme (1999–2000) was adopted at a time of reorganization, including the dissolution of the National AIDS Committee by order of the Cabinet and the transfer of its functions to the Ministry of Health in 1998 [4]. A National Coordination Council was established subsequently, but it was replaced after only 1 year by the National Commission on AIDS in November 2000, following Ukraine's commitment to the United Nations Millennium Development Goals to combat the spread of HIV. The National Commission is responsible for coordinating Ukraine's response to the epidemic.

The 2001–2003 countrywide programme acknowledged the HIV epidemic to be a state priority within the context of social development and health protection, recognizing the negative impact of economic instability, increasing unemployment, drug use and prostitution, and the limited coverage of prevention activities. The programme provided the political base for the development of intersectoral cooperation and paid particular attention to preventive interventions among vulnerable groups as well as treatment and care for PLHIV. Implementation was undertaken with the technical and financial assistance of the United Nations, international donors and non-governmental organizations (NGOs) [30].

The National Strategy on HIV/AIDS up to 2011 and a fifth national programme for the period 2004–2008 were adopted in March 2004 [31]. The programme recognizes the continuing contribution of the country's difficult socio-economic situation to the HIV epidemic and acknowledges the impact of the concurrent TB epidemic and the increase of STIs. However, the fifth programme is unique in stressing the need for participation of representatives from vulnerable groups, especially PLHIV, in the design, implementation, monitoring and evaluation of the programme. It also stipulates that government at all levels must lead by coordinating the actions agreed to by those implementing the programme, thereby fostering cooperation between state institutions, the private sector and NGOs. The programme underlines Ukraine's commitment to the Declaration of Commitment on HIV approved at the Special Session of the United Nations General Assembly (UNGASS) and the Millennium Development Goals.

Prevention

As noted earlier, the first three national programmes focused predominantly on prevention in the general population, in particular the prevention of HIV transmission through blood transfusion, and the provision of general information and safety measures in healthcare and related services. During this period, the production of protective consumables and testing kits was established to support the implementation of prevention programmes. However, the early programmes had yet to target vulnerable groups with specific preventive interventions [4].

Prevention programmes for vulnerable groups were only launched in 1996, almost entirely at the initiative of local NGOs and with the financial and technical support of international agencies and donors. Acknowledging the limited availability of public funds and thus the ability to provide financial backing, the government did not oppose the initiatives, and some regional centres cooperated with NGOs at the local level. Up to now, 37 HIV prevention projects for IDUs have been established in 18 of the 27 administrative regions in Ukraine, and 18 projects for FSWs in 18 regions. These projects provide information and education activities as well as training for specialists and representatives of target groups. Services include condom promotion and distribution, harm reduction for IDUs, counselling, treatment and providing supportive environments. The NGOs targeting IDUs and FSWs have established a network. In 2001, with the assistance of UNICEF and UNAIDS, the State Centre for Youth Services initiated harm-reduction services [20].

The IDU harm-reduction programmes, especially outreach services and programmes lasting over 1 year, have generally proved successful. The programmes were able to raise awareness of HIV and change practices, such as increased use of new needles and syringes, reduced needle sharing, safer methods of purchasing drugs and increased use of condoms by sex workers. At present, the different projects only cover, on average, about 15% of IDUs. This illustrates the need for additional technical and financial input to reach the agreed target of 60% in order to have an impact on HIV transmission among this population [20]. Research so far has not been able to demonstrate the effectiveness of primary drug abuse prevention interventions, whereas tertiary prevention programmes encounter serious problems due to lack of rehabilitation institutions and substitution programmes [20].

The projects targeting FSWs have raised the profile of sex work in the country. Available services are, however, still too limited in coverage and quality, and mainly focus on condom distribution and needle exchange [32,33].

With the assistance of UN agencies, a prevention programme was initiated among the armed forces in 1999, through the Education Department of the Ministry of Defence. The project has resulted in the incorporation of HIV prevention in the general training programme for new recruits, and extension of the programme to other uniformed services, including prisons, is currently being planned [34]. An extra-curricular peer education programme to train both teachers and pupils was implemented in all *oblasts* from 2000 onwards, aiming to promote healthy lifestyles, including prevention of drug use, HIV and pregnancy among school children and adolescents. The approach proved to be an appropriate methodology, and the curriculum was adopted by other partners to expand the coverage of the education programmes within schools [35].

UNICEF, together with the Ministry of Health, has implemented effective interventions to prevent HIV infection of the newborn. Currently, 91% of HIV-infected pregnant women and their infants receive a complete course of antiretroviral prophylaxis, thus reducing mother-to-child-transmission (MTCT) of HIV from 28% in 2000 to 10% in 2003 [4]. Based on the progress made, Ukraine may be able to eliminate MTCT of HIV, and its prevention programme may become an example for neighbouring countries.

To date, the government has established a network of 27 regional centres for HIV prevention and 127 centres for anonymous testing for HIV. In addition, a network of diagnostic laboratories was established to allow testing of individuals and donor blood [4].

Treatment and care

There are 224 hospital beds in seven centres assigned to provide specialized inpatient care for PLHIV. The private for-profit healthcare sector is not allowed to provide care and treatment for PLHIV, and the non-medical private sector has only been marginally involved [Ministry of Health (2002). Strategy Document. Unpublished.]. Examples of NGOs involved in service delivery include Médecins Sans Frontières (MSF), which provides prevention of MTCT (PMTCT) and antiretroviral treatment (ART). The Ministry of Health has welcomed partners as long as they demonstrate a willingness to adhere to national standards and guidelines.

Overall, however, care and treatment have been severely affected by limited public funds, resulting in a lack of medicines and equipment, an overall deteriorating quality of service provision and a reduced capacity to meet the health needs of the population. Those not aware of their HIV-positive status present their opportunistic infections and HIV-related illnesses as a general health problem and, as a result, tend to receive routine care. The health service provided at the AIDS Centres is supposed to be free of charge, assuming that drugs and supplies are available, but there are usually few drugs for the treatment of opportunistic infections in stock.

IDUs are entitled to free and confidential treatment in drug dependency treatment centres and hospital infectious and toxicological departments. However, because of potential legal consequences, IDUs face additional constraints in accessing health services for HIV- or IDU-related illnesses. In addition, relevant medical knowledge and expertise regarding the specific health needs of IDUs is relatively scarce in rural areas [20].

At present, access to, and use of, confidential VCT services is still problematic, even though the state guarantees easy access. Obstacles include inadequate public knowledge of existing services, the location and limited number of testing centres, inconsistencies in pre- and post-test counselling procedures, including the cost of testing, and inadequate supply of testing kits [Ministry of Health (2002) Strategy Document. Unpublished.].

Psychosocial support is predominantly provided by NGOs, including the All Ukrainian Network of PLHIV [Ministry of Health (2002). Strategy Document. Unpublished.]. However, there is an increasing state interest in the provision of care and support, including palliative care, and the Ministry of Health has recently requested the assistance of UNAIDS and WHO in defining care and support models for Ukraine and coordinating implementing organizations.

Ukrainian health authorities were among the first in Eastern Europe to express interest in the United Nations Accelerating Access Initiative to enhance access to antiretroviral drugs. It was estimated in April 2005 that 17,300 HIV patients were in need of ART. However, public and donor funds have been very limited so far. They have secured funding for antiretrovirals through the Global Fund to Fight AIDS, Tuberculosis and Malaria (Global Fund) of US$17.3 million for a period of 5 years [36], and the imminent World Bank Project of US$1.7 million for 5 years [25].

Ukraine aims to provide patients with antiretrovirals and strengthen its health system with the support of international agencies and NGOs. By March 2005, 1521 patients had received ART, including 173 patients in Kyiv, Odessa and Nikolaev through public funds, 172 through MSF and 700 through the Global Fund-supported programme [Ministry of Health of Ukraine (2004). Unpublished report.]. Also, through the Global Fund programme, the Ministry of Health, the All Ukrainian Network of People with HIV/AIDS (NAPC) and the International HIV/AIDS Alliance (IHAA) have, with technical support from WHO and UNAIDS, developed an antiretroviral scale-up plan for the treatment of 2100 patients in six *oblasts*, which covers 80% of patients eligible for treatment over a period of 1 year. The government also provides antiretroviral drugs to prevent HIV transmission from mother to child and will continue to do so through the above-mentioned arrangements.

Conclusion

Despite its recent independence from the Soviet Union, leaving behind a history of top-down planning and a command economy, the difficult transition towards a democratic system of governance and a struggling market-oriented economy, and the relative novelty of the HIV epidemic, the government of Ukraine engaged in numerous efforts to face the problems and respond to the epidemic, either directly or through partners and NGOs. At the same time, the country has recognized the need to step up its efforts to contain the epidemic and has successfully secured additional funding in order to do so. The biggest challenge is to scale up interventions that appear to be successful. Although some information is available, better understanding is required about the effectiveness and efficiency of interventions. While equity in preventive interventions may be less of an issue, access to comprehensive HIV care is of major concern, partly because of stigma and discrimination, but also because of substandard quality of services.

With the introduction of a national monitoring and evaluation (M&E) system, including the M&E of programme or project implementation, the government of Ukraine aims to address some of these issues. The national M&E system is to be government-based and-led, multi-sectoral, with active involvement of all stakeholders, and based on the existing system and practices. The main components of this comprehensive M&E system include second generation surveillance, which builds on epidemiological and behavioural surveillance, research in the field of behavioural and socio-economic impact, monitoring of finance and resources, and pro-gramme monitoring and evaluation.

In the meantime, support is being provided to improve health service delivery, reviews of different programmatic areas are being planned to identify and overcome obstacles, and efforts have been undertaken to work towards an enabling environment in which human rights are respected, and professionals and beneficiaries work closely together to ensure success.

References

1. United Nations Development Programme. (2004). *Reversing the Epidemic. Facts and Policy Options.* Bratislava: UNDP.
2. UNAIDS/WHO. (2002). *AIDS Epidemic Update, December 2002.* Geneva: UNAIDS.
3. European Centre for the Epidemiological Monitoring of AIDS. (2002). *HIV/AIDS Surveillance in Europe. End-year Yeport 2002.* Saint-Maurice: Institut de Veille Sanitaire.
4. United Nations Development Programme. (2003). *Ukraine and HIV/AIDS: Time to Act.* Kyiv: UNDP.
5. State Statistics Committee of Ukraine. (2002). Results of the census. http://maidan.org.ua (accessed February 2003).
6. Dyczok M. (2000). *Ukraine. Movement Without Change, Change Without Movement.* Amsterdam: Harwood Academic Publishers.
7. United Nations Development Programme. (2002). *Ukraine Human Development Report 2001. The Power of Participation.* Kyiv: UNDP.
8. UNICEF. (2003). *Social Monitor 2003.* UNICEF Innocenti Research Centre: Florence.
9. United Nations Country Team in Ukraine. (2002). *Ukraine: Common Country Assessment.* Kyiv: United Nations.
10. WHO Regional Office for Europe. (2003). *Health for All Database, January 2004.* Copenhagen: WHO Regional Office for Europe.
11. Gilmore A, McKee M, Telishevska M, Rose R. (2001). Epidemiology of smoking in Ukraine. *Preventive Medicine* 33:453–61.

12. Alcohol and Drug Information Centre Ukraine. (2002). *Economics of Tobacco Control in Ukraine from the Public Health Perspective.* Kyiv: Alcohol and Drug Information Centre Ukraine, http://adic.org.ua/adic/reports/econ/inde (accessed July 21, 2003).

13. Peto R, Lopez A, Boreham J, Thun M. (2003). Mortality from smoking in developed countries 1950–2000, 2nd edn, data updated July 15, 2003. http://www.ctsu.ox.ac.uk/tobacco/ (accessed August 4, 2003).

14. Pomerleau J, McKee M, Rose R, Balabanova D, Gilmore A. (2002). *Comparative Health Report Health Conditions and Health Behaviours. Living Conditions, Lifestyles and Health Project.* Draft report. London: London School of Hygiene & Tropical Medicine.

15. Kiev International Institute of Sociology. (2001). *1999 Ukraine Reproductive Survey.* Kyiv: Kyiv International Institute of Sociology.

16. Lakiza-Sachuk N, Burkat N, Zagaiskiy S, Pidgorna L, Voitsehivsky V. (2002). Health care financing in Ukraine: current situation and prospects for reform. In: Lekhan, V. ed. *Strategic Directions of Health Care Development in Ukraine.* Kyiv: International Renaissance Foundation, p10–36.

17. Schieber G, Maeda AA. (1997). Curmudgeon's Guide to Financing Health Care in Developing Countries. Proceedings of a World Bank Conference. March 10–11, 1997.

18. State Statistics Committee of Ukraine. (2003). *State of Public Health.* Kyiv: State Statistics Committee of Ukraine.

19. Shcherbinskaya AM, Kruglov YV, Andrushchak LI. (2000). HIV/AIDS epidemic development in Ukraine. In: *HIV/AIDS Surveillance in Ukraine (1987–2000).* Kyiv: Ministry of Health of Ukraine, Ukrainian AIDS Centre, UNAIDS, p.8.

20. Balakireva O, Varban M, Yaremenko O, Andrushchak L, Artukh O. (2003). *The Prospects for Development of HIV Prevention Programmes among Injecting Drug Users.* Kyiv: Social Monitoring Centre, UNICEF, UNAIDS.

21. Grund J-P, Bochkova L, Kruglov Y, Martsynovskaya V, Scherbinskaya A, Andrushchak L. (2002). *QUO VADIS? A Case Study of the Ukrainian HIV Case Registration System.* Kyiv: Ukrainian AIDS Centre, Ministry of Health, UNAIDS.

22. UNAIDS. (2002). *Fact Sheet 2002, Eastern Europe and Central Asia.* Geneva: UNAIDS.

23. Shcherbiaya AM, Kruglov YV, Andrushchak LI. (2000). Adequacy analysis of the operating national system for epidemiological surveillance over HIV/AIDS at the current epidemic stage. In: *HIV/AIDS Surveillance in Ukraine (1987–2000).* Kyiv: Ministry of Health of Ukraine, Ukrainian AIDS Center, UNAIDS, p.19.

24. Aleksandrina TA, Moiseyenko RA, Kalyuzhna LD *et al.* (2003). Key findings of the sentinel epidemiological surveillance of HIV infection according to the 2002 pilot survey. In: *Introduction of Second Generation HIV Epidemiological Surveillance in Ukraine.* Kiev: Ministry of Health, Ukrainian Centre for AIDS Prevention, State Committee on Family and Youth, State Institute on Family and Youth, p19–24.

25. Ministry of Health of Ukraine. (2002). Accelerating Access to Care and Support for Ukrainians Living with HIV/AIDS. A Strategic Initiative of the Government of Ukraine, the United Nations System, the Non-Governmental Organizations and the Private Sector. Strategy Document. Kyiv: Ministry of Health. Unpublished.

26. Law of Ukraine on AIDS Prevention and Social Protection of the Population. New edition. (1998).

27. Ukraine. (2001). Chapter XIII of the Criminal Code of Ukraine.

28. Balakireva OM, Bondar TV, Galustyan YM *et al.* (2001). Overview of the Ukrainian and International Legislation on Prostitution. In: *Sex Business in Ukraine: An Attempt at Scientific Analysis.* Kyiv: Ukrainian Institute of Social Research, UNAIDS, p44–45.

29. Ministry of Health of Ukraine. (2002). Materials on the Accelerated Access for PLHA to Medical Treatment. Kyiv: Ministry of Health. Unpublished report.

30. National Programme on HIV/AIDS Prevention in Ukraine for 2001–2003. (2001). Resolution of the Cabinet of Ukraine No. 790. Kyiv.

31. National Programme on HIV/AIDS Prevention, Care and Treatment of People Living with HIV in Ukraine for 2004–2008. (2004). Kyiv.

32. Yaramenko A, Balakirevo O, Artyukh O *et al.* (2003). *Cost-effectiveness Analysis: Aiding Decision-making in HIV prevention in the Ukraine.* Kyiv: Ukrainian Institute for Social Research, London School of Hygiene and Tropical Medicine, p78–86.

33. British Council. (2001). National Meeting of Sex Workers Projects. Kyiv: British Council, UNAIDS, International Renaissance Foundation. Unpublished report.

34. UNAIDS. (2003). *HIV/STI Prevention Activities in Military and Peacekeeping Settings in Ukraine.* Country report. Draft report. Kyiv: UNAIDS.

35. UNDP. (2002). Promotion of Peer Education on Healthy Lifestyle for Young People in Ukraine. Annual Project Report UKR/00/H01. Kyiv: Ministry of Education and Science, UNDP, UNAIDS. Unpublished report.

36. Government of Ukraine. (2002). Overcoming HIV/AIDS Epidemics in Ukraine. Proposal to the Global Fund for Fighting AIDS, TB and Malaria. Kyiv: Ministry of Health. Unpublished report.

Chapter 36

The United Kingdom

John Imrie[*], Sarah Dougan[*], Kimberly Gray, Michael W Adler, Anne M Johnson, Barry G Evans and Barry S Peters

Background

Political organization

The UK has an estimated population of 58.8 million (2001) and is the third most populous country in the European Union (EU) [1]. The UK is a constitutional monarchy and parliamentary democracy based on universal suffrage, with 18 as the voting age. The UK is divided into three countries (England, Wales and Scotland) and the province of Northern Ireland. Sovereignty and primary legislative powers rest with the Parliament, consisting of the Monarch, House of Lords, House of Commons and Judiciary. Recently, regional and fiscal decision making, including some aspects of health provision, has been devolved to the Scottish Parliament and National Assemblies in Wales and Northern Ireland. Local government structure varies in each country, although it is essentially based on combinations of National Assemblies, county councils and unitary urban authorities. The UK is a member of the EU, and EU legislation is an increasingly important element of government.

Demography

Table 36.1 shows the age and sex distribution and Table 36.2 the estimated ethnic composition of the UK population at the 2001 census. Women now outnumber men from age 22 onwards. Greater emigration and lower fertility rates have reduced population growth, which was 2.6% between 1991 and 2001 [2]. More than 20% of the population is over 60, and this is expected to increase during the coming decades [1,2].

The white, British-born population has declined from 95% of the total population in 1981, to 92% in 2001 [1]. The numbers of black, South Asian and Chinese people living in Britain has risen by more than 40% in the last decade, due mainly to immigration and increased numbers of political and economic refugees. The African population has increased by 240% in the decade since 1991 [4]. Some new arrivals, particularly those from sub-Saharan Africa, have been seriously affected by HIV, with attendant implications for health and social welfare systems. Fifty per cent of Britain's ethnic minority population lives in Greater London and

* Corresponding authors.

Table 36.1 Age distribution of the resident population (000s), 2001

Age group (years)	Male n	%	Female n	%	All n	%
0–4	1781	6.2	1697	5.6	3478	5.9
5–14	3901	13.6	3713	12.3	7614	12.9
15–24	3648	12.8	3579	11.8	7227	12.3
25–44	8430	29.5	8706	28.9	17,136	29.1
45–59	5520	19.3	5624	18.6	11,144	19.0
60–89	5246	18.3	6614	21.9	11,860	20.2
90+	85	0.3	291	1.0	376	0.6
Total	28,611	100	30,224	100	58,835	100

Source: [3].

other inner-city areas of England. The current policy of geographic refugee dispersal is producing small pockets of new arrivals throughout the country [1].

Economic conditions

The UK economy has grown consistently for the last 12 years. Recent growth has been below the post-war average at 2.5%, but remains consistent and ahead of most EU members [1]. Growth continues to be dominated by the service sectors, particularly telecommunications, business and financial services, with the most notable declines in manufacturing. Unemployment, at 5% or 1.5 million people in the summer of 2003, was at its lowest for 40 years. Inflation in each year since 1997 has remained close to the

Table 36.2 Estimated population by ethnic group, 2001

	Total population (million)	% of total population	Minority ethnic population (%)
White	54.2	92.1	n/a
Asian or Asian British			
Indian	1.05	1.8	22.7
Pakistani	0.75	1.3	16.1
Bangladeshi	0.28	0.5	6.1
Other Asian	0.25	0.4	5.3
All Asian groups	2.33		
Black or black British			
Caribbean	0.56	1.0	12.2
African	0.49	0.8	10.5
Other black	0.10	0.2	2.1
All black groups	1.15		
Mixed	0.68	1.2	14.6
Chinese	0.25	0.4	5.3
Other	0.23	0.4	5.0
All minority ethnic population	4.64	7.9	100.0
All population	58.79	100.0	n/a

Source: [3]. n/a=not applicable

government's target rate of 2.5% set in 1997 [5]. Average earnings have risen consistently, although private sector earnings consistently outstrip the public sector, resulting in an ever-widening pay divide. Nationally, average gross weekly pay (pre-tax) was £356(US$648) in 2002. This figure is subject to significant regional variation, with higher rates observed in London [1]. Eighteen per cent of British households, with an income below 60% of the median income, are classified as 'low-income'. Nearly two-thirds of Pakistani and Bangladeshi, one-quarter of black, Indian and other minorities are considered low-income compared with 17% of whites [6]. More young people (74%) aged 16–18 are in full-time education than at any time in the past.

The health system

Healthcare expenditure is currently 7.3% of gross domestic product (GDP), significantly below the EU average (Table 36.3). New government funding will increase spending to £109.4 billion (US$199.1 billion) by 2007–2008, or 9.4% of estimated GDP, bringing the UK in line with other EU members [1].

Coverage

The National Health Service (NHS) was created in 1948 to provide healthcare to the UK's resident population on the basis of need and not ability to pay. The NHS is the principal care provider in the UK and the largest organization in the EU, with a workforce in excess of 1 million. Less than 10% of UK residents carry comprehensive private medical coverage. NHS services include inpatient hospital care, as well as most outpatient and a significant proportion of community nursing, dental, optical, chiropody, ambulance and pharmacy services. Most services and treatment are provided free, but some incur a user-charge, such as dental care and vision tests. Prescription charges apply only to medications delivered to outpatients. They do not apply to hospital- or specialist-prescribed medications, including antiretrovirals, or to any prescriptions for those over age 60, where the cost is entirely borne by the NHS.

Table 36.3 Health indicators

Life expectancy at birth (years)	
Males	76
Females	80
Childhood mortality (<5 years) (per 1000)	
Males	7
Females	6
Total fertility rate	1.6
Adult HIV prevalence (% population aged 1–49 infected)	<0.1
No. of people living with HIV/AIDS (2001)	41,200
Total health expenditure*	US$102.7 billion
Per capita health expenditure	US$1747
Health expenditure as % of GDP	7.3
Health expenditure as % of total government expenditure	14.9

+Source: [7].
*Source: [3].

Finance and accountability

NHS service provision is met largely by central government through general taxation (78%), by employer and employee contributions through National Insurance at 12%, and only a small fraction (10%) comes from patient charges, private donations and services delivered to private patients. In 2003, increases in National Insurance were implemented to provide extra funding specifically for the NHS' modernization programme. In England, the NHS is managed by the Department of Health and is accountable to the Government's Secretary of State for Health. The Department of Health is responsible for developing and implementing policies and overall regulation and inspection of health services, both NHS and private. Under the political devolution arrangements, the Welsh Assembly Government, the Scottish Executive Health Department, and the Department of Social Services and Public Safety in Northern Ireland have similar responsibilities.

Organization

Every UK resident has a right to be registered with a general practitioner (GP) or primary care physician, usually their first point of contact with the NHS. GPs generally work in small group practices serving a local area and provide free consultations. GPs also act as gatekeepers, with responsibility for referring patients to specialist services. The only parts of the specialist hospital services that are open access and do not require GP referral are genito-urinary medicine (GUM) services.

Within the NHS in England, there is a purchaser–provider separation. NHS hospital and community services are purchased for the local population by Primary Care Trusts. NHS hospital services are separately managed by NHS Trusts. Most specialist hospital services are overseen by Strategic Health Authorities in defined geographical areas covering up to 1.5 million residents.

Specialist healthcare is overwhelmingly provided through the NHS, with only a minority of mostly elective surgery being supplied by the private sector. Demand for healthcare exceeds supply, and waiting lists exist for most conditions referred to the hospital sector. Government policy is committed to reducing waiting lists, and several innovative strategies are being implemented. The overwhelming majority of healthcare professionals are salaried employees of the NHS on national pay scales. GPs are self-employed and contracted by local Primary Care Trusts.

Restructuring and transition—the NHS plan

The NHS has often been accused of being a victim of its own success [8] and, at times, the financial limits of the NHS have necessitated restructuring or reform. The most far-reaching of these involved the introduction of a so-called 'internal market' in 1990. Through the 'internal market', some health authorities and GPs became 'purchasers', who were given budgets to buy healthcare from 'providers' (acute-care hospitals, community care, etc.) for their resident populations. The introduction of the 'internal market' had the effect of improving cost consciousness within the NHS, but at the price of creating excessive competition and, frequently, duplication of services. The Labour government, elected in 1997, brought forward a modified approach that aimed to build on what had worked previously and discard what had failed. The result was a 10-year plan set out in a white paper entitled *The New NHS. Modern. Dependable.* Implementation of the reform programme began in 2001.

The NHS Plan involves reform and investment to improve clinical performance and health service productivity. The Plan's successful implementation is to be measured against a number of key performance targets. Within each of the specific priority groups and diseases, such as children and cancer, the Plan proposes development and implementation of National Service Frameworks (NSFs) designed to set standards, raise quality, reduce geographic variation and ensure patients' smoother progression through different NHS services. At present, there are no plans to introduce an NSF in respect of sexual health or HIV.

Services for sexually transmitted infections and HIV

Services for sexually transmitted infections (STIs) were set up on a free and confidential basis in 1916 following a Royal Commission report [9]. It is remarkable that a free service was created for these conditions three decades prior to a universally free NHS in 1948. Original funding for STI services, known in those days as venereal diseases, was from central (75%) and local (25%) governments. Once the NHS was founded, central government took responsibility for funding, and clinics, many of which had previously been run as free-standing local government clinics, were incorporated into the hospital sector. The vast majority (99%) of care for patients with STIs and HIV is nowadays provided by the NHS, within infectious diseases or STI clinics (GUM Departments). Clinics, as well as being free, do not require a referral.

The first cases of HIV infection were seen in the UK in 1983 in a small number of London STI clinics. These clinics had developed special relationships and ties with homosexual men who considered staff in these clinics to be sympathetic and non-judgemental. Gay men, fearful of the new 'epidemic', used these clinics [10]. Most HIV infection within the UK is now managed both on an out- and inpatient basis either by physicians specialized in GUM/STIs or by infectious diseases specialists. The advent of HIV brought an increase in the number of clinics, staff and resources. For example, between 1985 and 1998, the number of specialists doubled [11]. Currently in the UK, there are 238 specialists (consultant physicians) in GUM, working in 268 dedicated STI and HIV clinics.

The total number of attendances at GUM clinics has doubled in 10 years, reaching 1.5 million in 2002. One in 10 of the UK population aged 16–55 has at some time been diagnosed with an STI [12]. Particular increases have been seen in cases of syphilis, gonorrhoea and chlamydia. Concern over these increases in infections led the government to develop a National Strategy for Sexual Health and HIV, published in 2001 [13]. Subsequent to this, the House of Commons Health Select Committee reviewed the approach to sexual health within England and published a very hard-hitting report in June 2003, which called the government to task for not treating STIs and HIV as a public health priority [14].

Resources for STI and HIV services

Funding for STI services prior to HIV came from central government as part of the general funding of NHS hospitals. Historically, these services had been under-resourced, with poor staff-to-patient or population ratios and premises. In 1985–1986, specially earmarked money was made available for HIV. This, in effect, meant that central government, through its Department of Health, 'ring-fenced' money with specific instructions on how it should be spent. In 1985–1986, this sum was small at £680,000 (US$1.2 million), but rose to £223.5 (US$406.8 million) for treatment and care by 2001–2002. In the first few years, ring-fenced money was spent on improving facilities and staffing levels in departments of GUM. Allocations were made on the basis of reported live AIDS patients treated. In addition to this, money was made available to local government through the AIDS Support Grant. In the first year of this initiative (1987–1988), the amount was £2 million (US$3.6 million) and was to be used to support patients in the community through social work and home care teams. In 2003, it was decided to end ring-fenced funding and mainstream all resources, adding this sum to NHS baseline allocations. In general, this was not welcomed by specialists working in the statutory or voluntary sector, who feared that it would be much harder to stop funds from being siphoned off into other services.

Antiretroviral treatment (ART) was funded through the ring-fenced special allocation, but this did not keep up with patient load. 'Persistent under-funding, combined with spiralling drug costs and the emergence of many new drugs onto the market, means that clinicians struggle to prescribe the appropriate therapies for their patients and that funds needed for other sexual health services may be diverted to pay for HIV drugs' [14].

The overall average cost of managing a patient with HIV in the UK varies from £10,000 (US$18,200) per year for patients in US Centers for Disease Control (CDC) stage A, to £20,000 (US$36,400) per year for AIDS patients (CDC stage C). Current estimates are that providers are underfunded by approximately £3000–£5000 (US$5460–US$9100) per patient per year. Given the increase in newly diagnosed HIV cases, cost pressures are bound to increase.

The Medical Foundation for AIDS and Sexual Health (MEDFASH) has suggested that by 2007, the cumulative lifetime treatment costs for those in the UK known to be HIV-infected will exceed £5 billion (US$9.1 billion) [14]. This makes all the more powerful the figure quoted in the National Sexual Health HIV Strategy and calculated by the Department of Health that preventing onward HIV transmission would save between £0.5 million (US$910,200) and £1 million (US$1.8 million) in terms of individual health benefits and treatment costs [13].

The HIV epidemic

Epidemiology

The first case of AIDS in the UK was diagnosed in December 1981, and since then there have been 61,179 HIV diagnoses, 20,096 AIDS diagnoses and 15,601 deaths in HIV-infected individuals to the end of December 2003 [15]. However, cumulative figures mask the recent rapid increases in numbers diagnosed and accessing HIV-related services, as well as the decline in AIDS incidence and deaths since the introduction of highly active antiretroviral therapy (HAART) [15–17] (Fig. 36.1). AIDS incidence peaked in 1994, declining thereafter, with deaths following a similar trend [15]. While the UK's HIV epidemic has remained relatively small compared with France, Italy and Spain [18], in 2002 an estimated 49,500 adults were living with HIV in the UK, of whom 31% were undiagnosed [19]. WHO/UNAIDS estimated that there were 32,000 (16,000–52,000) adults and children living with HIV at the end of 2003. Of the 31,000 adults, approximately 7000 were women [20]. This equates to an adult (aged 15–49) prevalence of 0.1% (0.1–0.2%).

Men who have sex with men (MSM) have been the group most affected by HIV in the UK, with 30,986 diagnoses, and with the highest HIV prevalence [15,21]. Improved survival and continuing new diagnoses make MSM the largest group accessing HIV-related services, with 13,976 attendees in 2002 [17]. MSM also remain the behavioural group at highest risk of

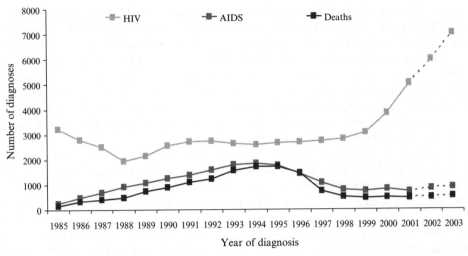

Fig. 36.1 New HIV diagnoses, AIDS case reports and deaths in HIV-infected individuals. Sources: [19], reports received by end of December 2003; 2002 and 2003 figures have been adjusted for reporting delay based on the pattern of previous years.

acquiring HIV within the UK, with substantial evidence for continuing transmission. In 2001, among MSM attending sentinel GUM clinics for syphilis serology, incidence was 3.1% in London and 1% elsewhere [22]. Most infections are diagnosed in MSM under 25 years of age and in those who previously tested negative (seroconverters) [23,24]. Diagnoses of uncomplicated gonorrhoea in MSM have risen [19], and syphilis outbreaks have occurred [25], indicative of high-risk sexual practices that have also increased [26,27]. There is a clear need to strengthen preventive work amongst MSM of all ages.

Since the explosive HIV outbreaks among injecting drug users (IDUs) in Scotland during the mid-1980s, HIV transmission through IDU has been relatively low in the UK [28]. In 2002, HIV prevalence among IDUs in contact with drug agencies was 1% [29], and in the same year, an estimated 1700 IDUs were living with HIV infection in the UK, of whom 38% were undiagnosed [19]. However, ongoing transmission among IDUs remains a threat. The proportion of IDUs using contaminated injecting equipment has risen in recent years, with continued transmission of hepatitis B [30].

Treatment of haemophilia with pooled factor VIII, mainly obtained from abroad, caused over 1200 HIV infections in the UK before the introduction of viricidal heat treatment [31]. Since the introduction of blood donation testing, only two instances of the acceptance of HIV-infectious donations for transfusion have been reported; the units were donated during the 'window' period between infection and development of HIV antibody [32,33]. Five healthcare workers have acquired HIV in the UK through work-related needlestick incidents [34,35].

Infections acquired through heterosexual intercourse have driven the rapid increase in numbers of HIV diagnoses in the UK since 1997. Of the 3419 heterosexually acquired infections diagnosed in 2002, 75% were probably acquired in Africa [15]. While infections acquired in

Eastern Africa, particularly Uganda, initially predominated over heterosexual diagnoses in the UK, by the late 1990s the focus had shifted to infections acquired in South-Eastern Africa, particularly Zimbabwe [36]. In England and Wales (2001–2002), prevalence of HIV infection among heterosexual attendees at sentinel GUM clinics was 9% in those born in sub-Saharan Africa, compared with 0.3% among those born in the UK [21]. Diagnoses of infections acquired through heterosexual intercourse in the Caribbean are increasing [37], with little impact in the UK from the Indian subcontinent's HIV epidemic as yet [38,39]. At the end of 2002, there were an estimated 24,500 adults living in the UK with heterosexually acquired HIV, 38% of whom were thought not to have been diagnosed [19].

Historically, the UK has not diagnosed HIV infection in pregnant women effectively, and preventable mother-to-child transmissions (MTCTs) have occurred [40]. In recent years, the number of births to HIV-infected women in the UK has risen, from 298 in 1997 to 686 in 2002 [2,41]. Over the same period, the proportion of maternal HIV infections diagnosed during pregnancy has increased, from approximately 32% in 1997 to 79% in 2002 [2,41]. In 2002, there were an estimated 51 infants infected, a figure that would have been substantially higher without improved diagnosis of HIV infection prior to delivery and the subsequent use of interventions [21]. By the end of June 2003, an estimated total of 3576 children of HIV-infected mothers had been born in the UK, of whom 28% were known to be HIV-infected, 48% uninfected and, for the remainder, status was unresolved or unreported [19].

Prevention

Public health responses to AIDS in the UK began in 1983–1984 with information and awareness initiatives run by voluntary organizations [10]. In 1986, government-led campaigns targeting the general population involved mass media and a national leaflet drop to every household [10,42]. By 1987, the 'tombstone' advertisements appeared, as part of the 'AIDS—don't die of ignorance' campaign. General population campaigns were associated with reduced transmission of STIs through behaviour change and heightened awareness [43]. There were campaigns specifically targeting MSM, and transmission of both HIV and syphilis fell [43]. Testing of all blood donations, introduced in October 1985, had been preceded since 1983 by calls for those with recognized risk factors for HIV to avoid donating blood. For IDUs, supplies of sterile syringes were increased and more needle exchange projects established which, along with support and outreach services, have undoubtedly contributed to the restriction of HIV spread among IDUs [42]. These early vigorous approaches to prevention probably blunted penetration of HIV within the UK, and may explain the relatively low prevalence compared with other European countries [43].

By the early 1990s, campaigns began focusing on personal testimonies: *Eastenders*, a popular television series, introduced an HIV-infected character into its storyline, and there was a series of advertisements featuring Mrs Dawson, an older lady who works in a condom factory [43]. The little known about the sexual behaviour of the British population fuelled continuing debate about the future of the AIDS epidemic, and so the first national survey into sexual practices and attitudes was implemented [44]. In the mid-1990s, health promotion became more focused [43], but the improving trends in gay sexual health indices of the mid-1980s were not sustained. Rising levels of risk-taking behaviour among MSM, along with increasing STI diagnoses in the general population, suggested that the impact of the 1980s HIV and AIDS campaigns had worn off [43].

As part of the movement toward targeting HIV prevention that occurred during the 1990s, the government-funded Community HIV and AIDS Prevention Strategy (CHAPS), led by a voluntary organization—the Terrence Higgins Trust (THT)—was launched in 1996, to develop and coordinate a multi-agency, collaborative HIV health promotion programme for MSM [45]. The programme's 'Making It Count' strategy focused on reducing HIV incidence in MSM, using mass media advertisements in the gay and 'positive' press and at gay venues, along with smaller media and face-to-face interventions [46,47].

African communities face a disproportionate burden of HIV in the UK. The THT has run campaigns specifically for black Africans, focusing on dispelling stigma against people living with HIV (PLHIV), and promoting the idea that 'It's better to know', stressing the advantages of getting an HIV test to allow improved treatment and care of HIV-infected black Africans [48]. For future prevention within African communities, the Department of Health will be publishing a National Prevention and Social Care Framework and will fund the African HIV Policy Network (AHPN), an umbrella organization that represents African community groups, to commission and manage HIV health promotion within African communities in England [49]. As yet, there is no rigorous evidence of effective HIV prevention programmes relevant to UK African communities [50].

In England, Wales and Northern Ireland, diagnoses of acute bacterial STIs increased substantially between 1996 and 2001 in the general population, with an associated rise in high-risk sexual behaviours and increases in testing for chlamydia [51]. The Second National Survey of Sexual Attitudes and Lifestyles has shown that there have been notable changes in sexual behaviour since the survey in 1990 [44], with increases in numbers of lifetime partners, lower age at first intercourse, and a greater proportion of people with concurrent partners [52,53]. While there have been no HIV prevention programmes targeting the general population in recent years, in 2002, the government's 'Sex Lottery' campaign began, aiming to halt the rises in the incidence of STIs among young people through use of condoms, which, if successful, will also reduce HIV transmission [54,55]. A series of lottery-style scratch cards with a question and answers about STIs is being used, as well as mass media advertisements.

Treatment and care

History

In the UK, the history of HIV treatment and care is not dissimilar to that of other developed countries that have had sufficient political will, access to funding, community-driven advocacy and adequate healthcare systems to address the epidemic. The use of antiretrovirals began in 1988 with zidovudine (AZT) monotherapy, which was superseded by dual therapy in the early 1990s and triple therapy or HAART by 1996.

Today there are 17 licensed HIV medications in the UK, with several more available through clinical trials or expanded access prior to probable licensing. Ultra-sensitive viral load tests (sensitive to <50 copies) were part of regular HIV care by 1999–2000, and clinicians now have access to both geno- and phenotypic assays to assist with understanding resistance patterns. Therapeutic drug monitoring is used in special circumstances, i.e. drug interactions or drug toxicities, although guidelines on optimum use do not exist in the UK.

Clinical guidelines

The British HIV Association (BHIVA) developed the first national guidelines for ART of HIV-positive individuals in 1997 [56]. They were updated in 1998 [57], 2000 [58], 2001 [59] and 2003 [60]. The BHIVA guidelines have been criticized for not adequately reflecting recent advances in the field [61], yet they have served as an invaluable tool for healthcare providers when lobbying healthcare purchasers for funding. In 2001, the first of a rolling annual programme of clinical audits produced national data on treatment patterns, and subsequent audits will evaluate the effectiveness of the BHIVA clinical guidelines [62].

The UK was criticized for lack of a coordinated response to reducing MTCT earlier in the epidemic [40,63]. This began to be addressed when the Intercollegiate Working Party [64] made recommendations that subsequently informed the government's 1999 policy geared towards reducing MTCT, with targets to increase both uptake of antenatal HIV testing to 90% and the proportion of HIV infections diagnosed prior to delivery to 80% by the end of 2002 [65]. Substantial improvements in maternal HIV diagnosis rates were seen by 2002, although there were marked variations between health authorities [21]. Guidance was also issued in Scotland and Wales on universal antenatal testing [66,67]. The UK's first guidelines for the management of HIV infection in pregnant women were published in 1999 [68] and updated in 2001 [69]. Controversy still exists over the recommendation in the guidelines to treat pregnant women who do not clinically require HAART with AZT only. Recently, the Children's HIV Association of UK and Ireland (CHIVA) was formed to promote issues affecting children infected or affected by HIV, develop standards of care and promote involvement in multicentre research trials [70].

HIV is probably unique at present in terms of the need for strict adherence to therapy in order to maintain long-term success. Paterson *et al.* showed that anything less than 95% increased the chances of treatment failure [71]. Although the BHIVA guidelines recommend that clinicians consider factors affecting adherence [72], the need was recognized for national guidelines to address the diversity of adherence services that have arisen in the UK and to 'ensure equity of service provision and benefits of HAART across the UK' [73]. A set of draft guidelines was put out for consultation to the wider HIV community [73].

Financial constraints, eligibility and access

There has been considerable debate over maintaining the specialist nature of HIV services to protect resources versus 'mainstreaming' care in the UK [74]. The debate is particularly heightened in London, where over 60% of those diagnosed in the UK are attending clinics [19]. In London, increases in new HIV diagnoses have not resulted in a corresponding increase in hospital space, staffing and support. Another issue for purchasers of HIV services is the difficulty in reconciling local budgets with patient movement across open access service. The London Regional Specialised Commissioning Group conducted a review of the current commissioning arrangements in 2003–2004, which may again bring more changes.

The availability of NHS healthcare has ensured that those in need, and who are eligible, have access to HIV treatment and care. In fact, unlike other diseases, patients do not have to pay a prescription charge for medications. However, the financial constraints of a publicly funded system can delay access to state-of-the-art technologies and treatments. In a recent audit [62], a minority of centres reported restrictions on access to HIV resistance testing and limited availability of ultra-sensitive viral load assays—both accepted as the appropriate standard of care in the UK. As HIV therapy is a rapidly developing field, new compounds are often available prior to licensing, by means of either trials or expanded access programmes. Both of these approaches are usually only available to large treatment centres, therefore creating the potential for inequity of access to newer treatments throughout the UK.

A current contentious matter in HIV funding and policy is eligibility of overseas visitors for HIV care [75]. The legislation states that visitors who have not applied to remain in the UK, or are on a short-stay visa, are not eligible for HIV treatment beyond testing and counselling or emergency treatment [76]. This policy is to discourage an influx of economic health migrants, although there are few or no data on the number of individuals who fall into this category. This raises important public health, financial and ethical issues related to definitions of essential care, prevention of long-term health costs and public health implications of HIV-infected individuals remaining outside the healthcare system. Health professionals are put in the awkward, and possibly unethical, situation of enforcing a financially driven policy instead of providing clinically relevant healthcare. These issues are compounded further with the recent policy of dispersing asylum seekers outside the London area to relieve pressure on local services [77]. This policy can result in an unacceptable disruption in HIV clinical care and treatment, particularly for pregnant women, and uncertainty regarding the availability of HIV specialist services outside major metropolitan areas [75].

A new model of treatment in future?

HIV services in the UK are highly specialized and hospital-based, since they grew out of hospital GUM services. Major HIV centres consist of multidisciplinary healthcare teams and specialist clinics to address matters such as adherence, metabolic complications, HIV-related emergencies, mental health, physiotherapy, pregnancy, paediatrics and young people, co-infection and salvage therapy. Voluntary organizations have provided much-needed treatment-related information and support to the HIV community and health services alike [48,78,79]. In addition, London-based clinics have also had to devise appropriate specialized services for African patients, such as community liaisons and interpreters, to reflect the changing demographics of the disease. Africans also continue to present to outpatient clinics at a more advanced stage of disease compared with Europeans, which has consequences for treatment efficacy and prognosis [80–82].

Today's model of HIV treatment and care through specialized HIV clinics has led to the underuse and underdevelopment of primary care services for HIV-positive people [83,84]. This raises the question of whether it is necessary for HIV patients who achieve clinical stability to continue to attend a specialist HIV clinic for routine monitoring and medication [83]. On the other hand, as HIV evolves into a manageable disease in the UK, HAART-related toxicities will become more complex and, as the patient population ages, there may be more problems to manage. This may reinforce the case for specialist services, but undoubtedly HIV services will continue to change, as will the specialties involved in the management of the disease.

Conclusions

Even with a relatively small HIV epidemic and a stable socio-political and economic position, the UK's NHS is experiencing some problems meeting increased HIV treatment and care costs. Historically, the NHS and the GUM speciality were able to provide high-quality holistic care for people with HIV and benefited from additional ring-fenced funds. Removal of the ring-fencing and 'mainstreaming' HIV services in the competition for funds creates the potential for diversion of funds into other government priority areas in order to achieve performance targets, with obvious detrimental consequences for services and PLHIV.

The UK's HIV epidemic is likely to continue to grow in the foreseeable future. Diagnoses will increase as HIV-infected individuals migrate from countries with high HIV prevalence, and HIV transmission in the UK continues among MSM. As the epidemic evolves, so, too, must surveillance systems, HIV prevention campaigns and treatment and care services.

References

1. Office of National Statistics, UK. (2002). *The Official Yearbook of the United Kingdom of Great Britain and Northern Ireland.* London: Her Majesty's Stationary Office (HMSO). Available at: www.statistics.gov.uk.

2. Hindess G. (2003). Population review of England and Wales, 2001. *Population Trends* 112:7–14.

3. Office of National Statistics. (2003). *UK Census 2003.* London: Office of National Statistics. Available at: www.statistics.gov.uk.

4. *The Guardian*, 04.09.03. London.

5. Office of National Statistics. (2003). *Work and Joblessness—August Assessment: Unemployment Falls.* London: Office of National Statistics. Available at: www.statistics.gov.uk.

6. Department of Social Security. (1998). *Family Resources Survey 1996–98.* London: DSS/HMSO.

7. Ham C. (1992). *Health Policy in Britain—The Politics and Organisation of the National Health Service,* 3rd edn. London: Macmillan Publishers.

8. World Health Organization. (2003). *Selected Health Indicators, 2003.* Geneva: WHO.

9. Adler MW. (1980). The terrible peril: a historical perspective on the venereal diseases. *British Medical Journal* 281:206–11.

10. Berridge V. (1996). *AIDS in the UK: The Making of Policy, 1981–1994.* Oxford: Oxford University Press.

11. Adler MW. (1999). Cinderella and the glass slipper: the growth and modernization of a specialty. *Sexually Transmitted Infections* 75:439–44.

12. Fenton KA, Johnson AM, McManus S, Erens B. (2001). Measuring sexual behaviour: methodological challenges in survey research. *Sexually Transmitted Infections* 77:84–92.

13. Department of Health. (2001). *The National Strategy for Sexual Health and HIV.* London: Department of Health.

14. House of Commons Health Select Committee. (2003). London: Department of Health.

15. Health Protection Agency Communicable Disease Surveillance Centre and Scottish Centre for Infection and Environmental Health. Quarterly Surveillance Tables No. 61:03/4. URL: http://www.hpa.org.uk/ infections/topics_az/hiv_and_sti/hiv/epidemiology/files/quarterly.pdf.

16. PHLS Communicable Disease Surveillance Centre and Scottish Centre for Infection and Environmental Health. (1997). Survey of Prevalent HIV Infection Diagnosed (SOPHID) Tables. Available at: http://www.hpa.org.uk.

17. Health Protection Agency Communicable Disease Surveillance Centre and Scottish Centre for Infection and Environmental Health. (2002). Survey of Prevalent HIV Infection Diagnosed (SOPHID) Tables. Available at: http://www.hpa.org.uk/infections/topics_az/hiv_and_sti/publications/sophid2002.pdf.

18. European Centre for the Epidemiological Monitoring of AIDS. (2003). *HIV/AIDS Surveillance in Europe. Year-end Report.* Saint-Maurice: Institut de Veille Sanitaire, 2003. No.68. URL: http://www.eurohiv.org/AidsSurv/Rapport_68/rapport_68.pdf.

19. Health Protection Agency, Scottish Centre for Infection and Environmental Health (SCIEH), Scottish Information and Statistics Division (ISD), National Public Health Service for Wales, Communicable Disease Surveillance Centre (CDSC) Northern Ireland and the Un-linked anonymous surveys steering group (UASSG). (2003). *Renewing the Focus. HIV and Other Sexually Transmitted Infections in the United Kingdom in 2002.* London: Health Protection Agency. URL: http://www.hpa.org.uk/infections/topics_az/hiv_and_sti/publications/annual2003/annual 2003.pdf.

20. UNAIDS. (2004). *Report on the Global AIDS Epidemic.* Geneva: UNAIDS. Available at: http://www.unaids.org/bangkok2004/report.html.

21. Health Protection Agency, Institute of Child Health, London, Scottish Centre for Infection and Environmental Health. (2003). Supplementary Data Tables of the Unlinked Anonymous Preva-lence Monitoring Programme: Data to the End of 2002. Surveillance Update 2003. URL: http://www.hpa.org.uk/infections/topics_az/hiv_and_sti/hiv/epidemiology/ua.htm#supplement.

22. Murphy G, Charlett A, Jordan JF, Osner N, Gill ON, Parry JV. (2004). HIV incidence appears constant in men who have sex with men despite widespread use of effective antiretroviral therapy. *AIDS* 18:265–72.

23. Dougan S, Brown A, Logan LE *et al.* (2004) HIV and younger people in England, Wales and Northern Ireland. *Communicable Diseases and Public Health* 7(1):47–55.

24. Gupta SB, Gilbert RL, Brady AR, Livingstone SJ, Evans BG. (2000). CD4 cell counts in adults with newly diagnosed HIV infection: results of surveillance in England and Wales, 1990–1998. *AIDS* 14:853–61.

25. Health Protection Agency, Communicable Disease Surveillance Centre. (2003). Recent developments in syphilis epidemiology. *Communicable Disease Report Weekly,* Vol. 13, No. 31. URL: http://www.hpa.org.uk/cdr/PDFfiles/2003/cdr3103.pdf.

26. Dodds JP, Nardone A, Mercey DE, Johnson AM. (2000). Increase in high risk sexual behaviour among homosexual men, London 1996–8: cross-sectional, questionnaire study. *British Medical Journal* 320:1510–1.

27. Elford J. Bolding G. Sherr L. (2002). High-risk sexual behaviour increases among London gay men between 1998 and 2001: what is the role of HIV optimism? *AIDS* 16:1537–44.

28. Madden PB, Lamagni T, Hope V, Bennett D, Goldberg D. (1997). The HIV Epidemic in Injecting Drug Users. Communicable Disease Report Review Vol 7 Review No 9:R128 – R130. URL: http://www.hpa.org.uk/cdr/CDRreview/1997/cdrr0997.pdf.

29. Health Protection Agency, Scottish Centre for Infection and Environmental Health (SCIEH), Na-tional Public Health Service for Wales, Communicable Disease Surveillance Centre (CDSC) Northern Ireland, Centre for Research on Drugs and Health Behaviour (CRDHB), and the Unlined anonymous surveys steering group (UASSG). (2003). *Shooting Up: Infections among injecting drug users in the United Kingdom 2002.* London: Health Protection Agency.

30. Hope VD, Rogers PA, Jordan L *et al.* (2002). Sustained increase in the sharing of needles and syringes among drug users in England and Wales. *AIDS* 16(18):2494–6. www.hpa.org.uk/infections/topic-s_az/injectingdrugusers/shooting_up.htm.

31. Mortimer JY, Spooner RJD. (1997). HIV infection transmitted through blood product treatment, blood transfusion and tissue transplantation. *Communicable Disease Report Review* Vol. 7 Review No. 9:R130–2. URL: www.hpa.org.uk/cdr/CDRreview/1997/cdrr0997.pdf.

32. The Serious Hazards of Transfusion Steering Group (SHOT). (2003) *SHOT Annual Report 2001/2002.* Manchester: SHOT.

33. Crawford RJ, Mitchell R, Burnett AK, Follett EAC. (1987). Who may give blood? (letter). *British Medical Journal* 294:572.

34. Heptonstall J, Gill ON, Porter K, Black MB, Gilbart VL. (1993). Health care workers and HIV: surveillance of occupationally acquired HIV infection in the United Kingdom. *Communicable Disease Report Review* Vol. 3, No. 11. URL: www.hpa.org.uk/cdr/CDRreview/1993/cdrr1193.pdf.

35. Hawkins DA, Asboe D, Barlow K, Evans B. (2001). Seroconversion to HIV-1 following a needlestick injury despite combination post-exposure prophylaxis. *Journal of Infection* 43:12–8.

36. Sinka K, Mortimer J, Evans B, Morgan D. (2003). Impact of the HIV epidemic in sub-Saharan Africa on the pattern of HIV in the UK. *AIDS* 17:1683–90.

37. Dougan S, Payne L, Brown AE *et al.* (2004). Black Caribbean adults with HIV in England, Wales & Northern Ireland: an emerging epidemic? *Sexually Transmitted Infections* 80:18–23.

38. Cliffe S, Mortimer J, McGarrigle C *et al.* (1999). Surveillance for the impact in the UK of HIV epidemics in South Asia. *Ethnicity and Health* 4(1–2):5–18.

39. Sethi G, Lacey CJ, Fenton KA *et al.* (2004). South Asians with HIV in London: is it time to rethink sexual health service delivery to meet the needs of heterosexual ethnic minorities? (Letter) *Sexually Transmitted Infections* 80:75–6.

40. Nicoll A. Peckham C. (1999). Reducing vertical transmission of HIV in the UK. *British Medical Journal* 319:1211–2.

41. Unlinked Anonymous Surveys Steering Group. (2002). Prevalence of HIV and Hepatitis Infections in the United Kingdom 2001. London: Department of Health. URL: http:// www.hpa.org.uk/infections/topics_az/hiv_and_sti/publications/hiv_ua_annual_2001.pdf.

42. Acheson D. (1993). Behold a pale horse: a view from Whitehall. *PHLS Microbiology Digest* 10(3):133–40.

43. Nicoll A, Hughes G, Donnelly M *et al.* (2001). Assessing the impact of national anti-HIV sexual health campaigns: trends in the transmission of HIV and other sexually transmitted infections in England. *Sexually Transmitted Infections* 77:242–7.

44. Johnson AM, Wadsworth J, Wellings K, Field J. (1994). *Sexual Attitudes and Lifestyles.* Oxford: Blackwell Scientific Press.

45. Weatherburn P, Dodds C, Branigan P *et al.* (2003). *Successful Measures: Evaluation of CHAPS National HIV Prevention Campaigns Targeted at Gay Men, 2001 to 2003.* London: Sigma Research.

46. Hickson F. (1998). *Community HIV & AIDS Prevention Strategy. Making it Count: a Theory, Ethics and Evidence Based Health Promotion Strategy to Reduce the Incidence of HIV Infection Through Sex Between Men in England.* London: Sigma Research.

47. Hickson F, Nutland W, Doyle T *et al.* (2002). *Making it Count: A Collaborative Planning Framework to Reduce the Incidence of HIV Infection During Sex Between Men,* 2nd edn. London: Sigma Research, Terrence Higgins Trust. Published on behalf of the CHAPS Partnership.

48. Terrence Higgins Trust. URL: www.tht.org.uk.

49. The African Policy Network. URL: www.aphn.org.uk.

50. NHS Health Development Agency. (2001). *HIV Prevention and Sexual Health Promotion with People with HIV. Professional Briefing 4.* London: National HIV Prevention Information Service.

51. Fenton K, Hughes G. (2003). Sexual behaviour in Britain: why sexually transmitted infections are common. *Clinical Medicine* 3:(3).

52. Johnson AM, Mercer CH, Erens B *et al.* (2001). Sexual behaviour in Britain: partnerships, practices, and HIV risk behaviours. *Lancet* 358:1835–42.

53. Wellings K, Nanchahal K, Macdowall W *et al.* (2001). Sexual behaviour in Britain: early heterosexual experience. *Lancet* 358:1843–50.

54. Department of Health. (2001). The NHS Guide to Sexually Transmitted Infections. URL: www.doh.gov.uk/ sexualhealthandhiv/.

55. Department of Health. (2004). New drive to tackle rise in sexual diseases: Valentine's ad campaign warns young people against playing the 'sex lottery'. Press release: Friday 06 February 2004. URL: www.info.doh.gov.uk/doh/intpress.nsf/page/2004-0043?OpenDocument.

56. British HIV Association (BHIVA). (1997). British HIV Association guidelines for antiretroviral treatment of HIV seropositive individuals. BHIVA Guidelines Co-ordinating Committee. *Lancet* **349**:1086–92.

57. Gazzard B, Moyle G. (1998). 1998 revision to the British HIV Association guidelines for antiretroviral treatment of HIV seropositive individuals. BHIVA Guidelines Writing Committee. *Lancet* **352**:314–6.

58. British HIV Association (BHIVA) Writing Committee. (2000). British HIV Association (BHIVA) guidelines for the treatment of HIV infected adults with antiretroviral therapy. *HIV Medicine* **1**:76–101.

59. British HIV Association (BHIVA) Writing Committee. (2001). British HIV Association (BHIVA) guidelines for the treatment of HIV-infected adults with antiretroviral therapy. *HIV Medicine* **2**:276–313.

60. British HIV Association (BHIVA). BHIVA 2003 Draft Treatment Guidelines. URL: www.bhiva.org/pdf/2003/guides/BHIVA-2003-draft.pdf.

61. Carey P, Lloyd J, Timmons D. (1997). British HIV Association guidelines for antiretroviral treatment of HIV seropositive individuals. *Lancet* **349**:1837.

62. Curtis H, Sabin CA, Johnson MA. (2003). Findings from the first national clinical audit of treatment for people with HIV. *HIV Medicine* **4**(1):11–7.

63. Ottewill M. (2000). Antenatal screening for HIV: time to embrace change. *British Journal of Nursing* **9**:908–14.

64. Intercollegiate Working Party. (1998). *Reducing Mother to Child Transmission of HIV Infection in the UK*. Executive summary and recommendations. London: Royal College of Paediatrics and Child Health.

65. NHS Executive. (1999). *Reducing Mother to Baby Transmission of HIV*. Health Service Circular 1999/183, London.

66. The National Assembly for Wales. (2000). *Antenatal Screening to Reduce Mother to Baby Transmission of HIV*. Cardiff: National Assembly for Wales.

67. Scottish Executive Health Department. (2002). *Offering HIV Testing to Women Receiving Antenatal Care*. Health Department Letter No. 52. Edinburgh: Scottish Executive Health Department. URL: http:// www.show.scot.nhs.uk/sehd/viewpublication.asp?PublicationID=648.

68. British HIV Association (BHIVA). (1999). Guidelines for prescribing antiretroviral therapy in pregnancy. *Sexually Transmitted Infections* **75**:90–7.

69. Lyall EG, Blott M, de Ruiter A *et al.* (2001). Guidelines for the management of HIV infection in pregnant women and the prevention of mother-to-child transmission. *HIV Medicine* **2**(4):314–34.

70. Children's HIV Association of UK and Ireland. (2003). URL: www.bpaiig.org/NEWS%20folder/CHIVA.htm.

71. Paterson D, Swindells S, Mohr J *et al.* (2000). Adherence to protease inhibitor therapy and outcomes in patients with HIV infection. *Annals of Internal Medicine* **133**(1):21–30.

72. Walsh JC, Sherr L. (2002). An assessment of current HIV treatment adherence services in the UK. *AIDS Care* **14**(3):329–34.

73. British HIV Association (BHIVA)/Medical Society for the Study of Venereal Diseases (MSSVD). (2002). Draft British HIV Association (BHIVA)/Medical Society for the Study of Venereal Diseases (MSSVD) Guidelines on Provision of Adherence Support to Individuals Receiving Antiretroviral Therapy. URL: www.aidsmap.org/about/bhiva/bhiva_adherence.asp.

74. Luger L, Carrier J, Beck E, Dalziel M. (1997). Developing the Agenda—HIV Services in the Late 90's and Beyond: Report of a Conference January 31, 1997. London: North Thames Regional Office, NHS Executive.

75. Terrence Higgins Trust (THT). (2003). Written Evidence to All-Party Parliamentary Groups on AIDS and Refugees: Inquiry into Migration and HIV. London: House of Commons/HMSO. URL: http://www.tht.org.uk/policy/policy_pdfs/migration02.pdf.

76. Department of Health. (1999). Overseas Visitors' Eligibility to Receive Free Primary Care. A Clarification of Existing Policy Together with a Description of the Changes Brought in by the New EC Health Care Form E128. Health Service Circular 018. London: Department of Health.

77. Home Office. (2002). Nationality, Immigration and Asylum Act 2002. London: Queen's Printer of Acts of Parliament.

78. National AIDS Manual. (2005). URL: www.aidsmap.com.

79. i-Base. (2003). URL: www.i-base.info.

80. Low N, Paine K, Clarke R, Mahalingam M, Pozniak AL. (1996). AIDS survival and progression in black Africans living in South London, 1986–1994. *Genitourinary Medicine* 72:12–6.

81. Del Amo J, Petruckevitch A, Phillips A *et al.* (1998). Disease progression and survival in HIV-1 infected Africans living in London. *AIDS* 12:1203–9.

82. Saul J, Erwin J, Bruce J, Peters B. (2000). Ethnic and demographic variations in HIV/AIDS presentation at two London referral centres 1995–9. *Sexually Transmitted Infections* 76:215.

83. Singh S, Dunford A, Carter Y. (2001). Routine care of people with HIV infection and AIDS: should interested general practitioners take the lead? *British Journal of General Practice* 51:399–403.

84. Smith S, Robinson J, Hollyer J, Bhatt R, Ash S, Shaunak S. (1996). Combining specialist and primary health care teams for HIV positive patients: retrospective and prospective studies. *British Medical Journal* 312:416–20.

Chapter 37

Canada

Melanie Rusch, Victor Alfonso, Catherine Hankins, Julio Montaner, Michael O'Shaugnessy and Robert Hogg[*]

Background

Canada is a large, decentralized federal state extending from the Pacific to the Atlantic to the Arctic Oceans and bordered on the south by the USA. It is governed in Westminster parliamentary tradition, with the Prime Minister as head of government and the Governor General as head of state, and comprises 10 provinces and three federally administered northern territories. Its national capital is Ottawa, and its current population is 32 million. Canada is officially a bilingual country; the majority of Canadian households are anglophone, but there is also a sizeable francophone population. Canadian society can be characterized as ethnically and culturally diverse, and as a predominantly urban society.

The Constitution Act of 1867 gave Canada autonomy from the British Empire. A federal system was adopted, with each province having legislative jurisdiction over issues of provincial importance, among them authority over the provision of healthcare and education. Federal powers include jurisdiction over direct taxation and the creation and collection of income taxes. In order to maintain a balance between responsibility to citizens and ability to finance programmes, provinces adopt federal healthcare policies in exchange for partial federal funding.

Health system

Canadians enjoy a relatively high level of health (Table 37.1). Each province is the primary provider of healthcare for its citizens, while the Government of Canada is responsible for securing and strengthening the system through the use and enforcement of the five principles of healthcare in the Canada Health Act of 1984—universality, accessibility, comprehensiveness, portability and public administration—that define the structure of medical care in Canada. The federal government promotes and protects the health of Canadians through Health Canada, with Ministry of Health-sponsored clinics and education programmes. The Ministry is ultimately accountable for the overall health of all Canadians, including, through the First Nations and Inuit Health Branch (FNIHB), the aboriginal populations of Canada. The FNIHB has a mandate to ensure accessible healthcare for First Nations and Inuit populations, assist these communities in addressing health barriers and disease threats,

[*] Corresponding author.

The views expressed in this book are those of the authors and are not necessarily those of the organizations they work for, unless specifically stated in the text.

and build partnerships with First Nations and Inuit to improve the health system [1]. Research is also a major aspect of federal healthcare funding, including research into HIV and other communicable diseases.

History

Universal healthcare in Canada grew out of provincial and federal reforms instituted shortly after the end of the Second World War [6]. Healthcare had largely been privately financed and delivered until 1947, when Saskatchewan became the first province in Canada to pass a compulsory health insurance plan, followed by the provinces of Alberta and British Columbia in 1949 [7]. Then came the 1957 Hospital Insurance and Diagnostic Act, which ensured that provinces providing a basic level of care for their residents would have their expenditure matched by the federal government as part of the 50/50 cost-sharing programme, thus creating a new emphasis on hospital care [6].

In July 1962, Saskatchewan passed the Medical Care Insurance Act, creating a government-approved fee schedule for all physicians. This sparked a month-long physicians' strike, but slowly doctors began to sign on to the new plan [6]. Shortly thereafter, in order to assess the feasibility of a nationalized universal health insurance scheme, the federal government established the National Royal Commission on Health Services: the Hall Commission [8]. In 1964, the Hall Report recommended the creation of 10 provincial health insurance systems similar to Saskatchewan's. This led to the federal Medical Care Insurance Act, 1966, which created a mandatory minimum of healthcare coverage that each province had to provide in order to receive federal funds.

By 1977, the cost-sharing programmes were replaced by Established Programme Financing (EPF), a system of federal grants to the provinces [7]. Effectively, the federal government forfeited some taxation power to the provinces and also transferred cash. However, there was no provision disallowing extra-billing by physicians, which led to the creation of the Health Services Review in 1980 [6]. The Review found that extra-billing could create a two-tiered healthcare system: one for the rich, who could afford the extra cost, and one for the poor, who could not.

Table 37.1 Healthcare expenditures and selected measures of quality of health and healthcare in Canada compared with other OECD countries

	Canada	USA	France	Spain	UK
Total health expenditure as % of GDP[+] [2]	9.1	13.0	9.5	7.7	7.3
Public expenditure as % of total[*] [2]	72.0	44.3	76.0	69.9	81.0
Private expenditure as % of total[+] [2]	28.0	55.7	24.0	30.1	19.0
Health expenditure per capita (PPP)[+] [2]	2534.0	4499.0	2335.0	1539.0	1774.0
Life expectancy (years)[†] [3]	81.9	79.5	82.9	82.6	79.9
Estimated healthy years of life lost (years) [†] [3]	10.4	10.7	9.5	9.6	9.0
HIV prevalence (%)[+] [4]	0.3	0.61	0.44	0.58	0.11
MRIs per 1 million inhabitants [5]	2.5[*]	8.1[+]	2.8[+]	4.9[*]	3.9[*]

PPP = purchasing power parity.
[+]1999.
[*]2000.
[†]2001.
Sources: [2–5].

The federal government passed the Canada Health Act in 1984, essentially amalgamating the Hospital Insurance and Diagnostic Services Act and the Medical Care Act, and including a provision to prevent physicians from extra-billing [9]. More importantly, the new act outlined the five principles of healthcare; in a sense, the Canada Health Act is the constitution of healthcare in Canada [6].

Medicare

Central to the implementation of provincial healthcare is adherence to the five principles. To meet these criteria, the 10 provinces and three territories maintain a separate, but parallel, medical insurance scheme known as Medicare [9]. Medicare must equally cover all eligible residents of a province in order to ensure universality of healthcare. To maintain accessibility, all covered medical services are paid for by Medicare and are free at point of access. Individuals may opt for private insurance for coverage of services outside Medicare; however, no third-party insurance can pay for services covered by Medicare. Most notable of these non-covered services is dentistry, although the province of New Brunswick now offers partial coverage [10].

Comprehensiveness requires that Medicare should cover all 'medically necessary' services, including hospital and physician visits. Such coverage is retained, for a minimum of 3 months, by all residents while travelling within Canada in accordance with the principle of portability. A health insurance plan must be operated by a publicly accountable agent of the provincial government on a non-profit basis, subject to audit, in order to be considered publicly administered.

Financing

Provincial healthcare budgets are drawn from general revenue. This makes progressive personal and corporate income taxes the primary financier of healthcare [8]. In British Columbia, for example, CA$4.9 billion (US$3.7 billion) of the estimated CA$9.5 billion (US$7.3 billion) spent on healthcare came from income taxes in 2002 [11].

The Canada Health and Social Transfer (CHST), an annual block grant from the federal government, which is the second largest financier of healthcare, increases over time in relation to national gross domestic product (GDP) growth. The CHST replaced the EPF in 1996 and consolidated the social programme grants into a single grant for both healthcare and social service provision, thus increasing flexibility in provincial spending [9]. As part of the grants, the federal government also lowered personal and corporate taxes in 1977, and again in 1996, transferring tax power to the provinces in order to boost provincial revenue earmarked for spending on health and social programmes. Additional funding is gained through lotteries, sales taxes, payroll levies, etc. British Columbia and Alberta are the only two provinces to impose a social insurance premium to augment healthcare funding [8].

Provision

Canadian hospitals provide primary and secondary services, and those hospitals affiliated with medical schools also conduct research and physician training. Hospitals may be run by organizations and religious groups on a not-for-profit basis, or by autonomous, government-created corporations known as Regional Health Authorities (RHAs). As of 2003, less than 3% of hospitals in Canada were privately run [12]. The breakdown of not-for-profit versus RHA-operated facilities varies by region, with the majority of foundation-supported hospitals located in large urban settings. With the exception of the province of Ontario, which did not regionalize health authorities as did other provinces, all hospitals receive provincial funds through RHAs [13]. The separation of RHAs from the governments has created a *de facto* purchaser/provider split [6].

Hospitals are funded through global budgets, separated into two categories: capital and operating budgets [8]. Capital budgets are used to purchase medical equipment, renovate or build new hospitals and pay for non-service-related hospital upgrades. Additional funding for these projects is often secured through hospital fundraisers. Operating budgets fund all healthcare services provided in the hospital, including healthcare professionals' salaries.

Primary care services are readily available through private practitioners operating on a fee-for-service basis, with direct billing to provincial Medicare plans. Patients are free to see any physician; however, a referral from a general practitioner (GP) is needed to see a specialist. Any specialist who accepts a patient without a referral must bill based on the established GPs' fee schedule, and therefore receive a smaller remuneration for the services provided [9].

The amount of coverage for supplemental healthcare services differs by province. For example, visits to chiropractors, osteopaths and podiatrists are not covered in many of the eastern provinces, while British Columbia, Saskatchewan and Ontario have varying degrees of coverage for these services, Manitoba allows up to 12 chiropractor visits per year, and Alberta includes osteopath services in its medical plan [14–18]. Coverage for ambulance, prosthetics and adult immunizations also varies by region. Some provinces, such as Manitoba and Ontario, offer travel reimbursement programmes for those living in remote areas [19,20].

Fee schedules are negotiated between medical associations and provincial governments, and they dictate the required payment for a particular service [9]. Doctors cannot request a co-payment from a patient for any service covered by Medicare, ensuring that healthcare remains free at point of access. Tertiary services are available through residential care facilities, mostly privately operated with a mix of private and public money, as well as through some hospitals.

Private care

Dentistry, pharmaceuticals, out-of-country health insurance and other healthcare services are only partially covered, or not covered at all, by Medicare in each province. Private insurance is available to cover most of these services. Eighty per cent of Canadians are covered for supplementary benefits, normally through employer-sponsored insurance programmes [21]. Unlike Medicare, private insurance requires patients to pay for services out-of-pocket and submit a claim with the insurer for subsequent reimbursement [9].

Publicly covered services accounted for 71% of the total expenditure on healthcare in 2001, at a total of CA\$79 billion (US\$60.6 billion) [22]. Private insurance and out-of-pocket payments covered the remaining 29% of health expenditure [22]. These numbers vary between provinces, but all are approximate to the 70/30 split [9]. At the time of the creation of the Canada Health Act in 1984, public health expenditure accounted for 76% of all healthcare costs [22]. This reduction in public share has been attributed, in part, to growing healthcare costs in uninsured services, including ever-increasing drug costs.

Problems of the system

Beset by increasing treatment costs and an aging population, the continuing stability of universal healthcare has been questioned [23]. Although healthcare expenditure in terms of GDP has remained relatively flat since 1990, the total cost of healthcare has risen from CA$62.5 billion in 1990 (US$48 billion), to CA$97.6 billion in 2001 (US$74.9 billion) [22]. The average cost of care of senior citizens (aged 65+) was CA$10,834 (US$8323) per capita in 2001, up from CA$8131 (US$6246) in 1990, amounting to 43% of total healthcare expenditure [22].

New, expensive drugs and emerging medical technologies are another burden on the healthcare budget. HIV medication, which can cost CA$10,000–CA$15,000 (US$7682–US$11,523) a year per patient, is fully or partially covered in all provinces. Canada trails most other OECD nations in acquiring magnetic resonance imaging (MRI) machines and other new medical technology [24].

Elective surgeries and services are stalled by waiting lists as long as 19 weeks for an MRI scan in British Columbia and a median wait of 45 weeks for cataract extraction in Saskatchewan [25,26]. Concern over access to certain procedures, specialist visits or advanced diagnostics has fuelled intense public debate over the last few years, and has led to a general dissatisfaction with the healthcare system, as indicated through a large drop in the percentage of Canadians perceiving their healthcare system to be 'excellent' or 'very good' in the 1998 Angus Reid poll [27].

A distinctive problem is the vast area over which its population is spread, resulting in a significant proportion living in sparsely populated rural and remote areas. According to Statistics Canada, approximately 22% of Canada's population is rural, defined as those living in communities with fewer than 1000 residents or with fewer than 40 people per km^2 [28]. Smaller communities face problems not only with access and institutional resources, but with attracting and retaining health professionals as well [29].

Canada is a culturally diverse country. Unfortunately, a number of communities have been identified as potentially underserved by the health system. Aboriginal populations, immigrants and refugees, visible and linguistic minorities, those with alternative sexual orientations, people with disabilities and those who are marginalized or particularly vulnerable all face possible barriers and challenges to accessing and utilizing Canada's health system [30].

Canada's aboriginal peoples—registered First Nations (North American Indians), non-registered First Nations, Métis and Inuit—make up approximately 3% of the population [30]. There is considerable cultural and linguistic diversity within the aboriginal population, making communication, cultural appropriateness and respect for traditional beliefs important aspects of healthcare provision. First Nations people living on reserves face problems similar to remote populations in terms of lack of medical resources. However, the FNIHB is responsible for providing services in these areas, which often means that primary care is more accessible and more culturally appropriate for those living on reserves as compared with the 70% of aboriginal people who have migrated to urban centres [30]. Distrust and discomfort arising from poor historical and personal experiences with the system may also create barriers to accessing healthcare [30], and financial barriers may exist for non-registered aboriginal people who are ineligible for non-insured health benefits provided by the FNIHB.

Immigrants and refugees, as well as visible and linguistic minorities, also make up a significant portion of the Canadian population. In 2001, approximately 18% of the Canadian population was foreign-born [31]. While availability of services is not generally a problem, barriers to accessing these services include financial circumstances, difficulty in navigating the system, communication and language difficulties, cultural appropriateness and acknowledgement of different health beliefs, as well as stigma and discrimination [30]. All of these points have been identified as issues requiring increased attention from the healthcare community.

Current and future reforms

Steadily increasing costs, in spite of cost containment efforts, have forced the provincial and federal governments of Canada to examine the potential impact of a future budgetary crisis. Accessibility of healthcare services has been compromised by growing waiting lists for elective surgeries. The federally mandated Romanow Report, delivered in November of 2002, made 47 suggestions to preserve public healthcare in Canada [29]. The report rejected abandoning the five principles of healthcare in favour of increased private care. Instead, the Romanow Commission recommended the creation of separate federal health transfers covering primary healthcare, home care, rural healthcare, increased drug coverage and diagnostic equipment purchases [29]. The Commission also recommends the creation of the Health Council of Canada, which would be responsible for tracking the efficiency of each provincial system.

At a First Ministers' Conference in 2003, the provinces and federal government took the first step toward implementing the Romanow reforms. On April 1, 2004, the Canadian Health and Social Transfer was split into two separate federal transfers: the Canadian Health Transfer (CHT) and the Canadian Social Transfer (CST). The CHT is now a multiyear, cash-only transfer representing 64% of the previous CHST and dedicated solely to healthcare provision in the provinces [32], thereby providing greater transparency about how, and how much, is being allocated to healthcare by the federal government.

In the wake of the severe acute respiratory syndrome (SARS) epidemic, which revealed serious communication and coordination problems in public health in Canada, the Canadian Medical Association's Naylor Report recommended the creation of a Canadian Office for Disease Surveillance and Control headed by a chief public health officer. This person would be the lead scientific voice on public health in Canada and work with provinces/territories to develop and implement a pan-Canadian public health action plan [33].

Budgetary issues will continue to affect access to essential medical services, posing a problem as Canada's population ages and requires more non-urgent surgeries. Such problems may undermine the principles of accessibility and universality if some patients in some provinces or hospitals are better able to receive care than others. Policy changes brought forward by the Romanow Commission's report to Parliament may alter inefficiencies caused by decentralized healthcare management by increasing federal power in this area. Ultimately, however, sustainable healthcare in Canada may have to abandon the five principles of the Canada Health Act and allow increased private financing of medicine for those who wish to or can pay for it.

The HIV epidemic

Epidemiology

The first case report with symptoms attributed to what would later be known as AIDS was recorded in Canada in 1979. In 1982, the Laboratory Centre for Disease Control (LCDC) in

Ontario set up surveillance for this mysterious new illness [34–36]. By November 1983, the LCDC had 51 reported cases, with the majority in the provinces of Quebec and Ontario [37]. Eighty-six per cent were male, half were homosexual and a third were Haitian immigrants [37,38]. Cases among injecting drug users (IDUs), sex workers (SWs) and blood product recipients were also observed [39].

At the end of 2002, 52,680 cases of HIV and 18,934 cases of AIDS had been reported to the Centre for Infectious Disease Prevention and Control (CIDPC) [40]. Annual reporting dropped from nearly 3000 cases in 1995 to just over 2100 in 2001, which, while indicating a general decrease, was followed by a 13% increase in 2002 [40]. Notably, more people are living with HIV disease today than ever before (see Table 37.2).

Men who have sex with men (MSM) continue to make up the majority of cases; however, HIV transmission through heterosexual contact is rising. The proportion of MSM cases decreased as the epidemic spread, from over 80% in the first few years to 44% in 1995 [40], by which time AIDS had become the second leading cause of death in Canada among men aged 25–44 [41]. The decline continued until 1998; however, recent years have seen a resurgence [40].

Infections among IDUs spread quickly in the late 1980s, reaching a peak of 47% of HIV infections in 1996 [40]. HIV infections attributable to IDU had decreased to approximately 24% in 2002 [42]. Cases among women, estimated to account for 10% of infections in the late 1980s [43], doubled by the end of the 1990s [42]. While this appears to be levelling off at around 24%, a high risk of infection remains among IDUs, who comprise approximately 54% of female cases, adolescent and young women (15–29 years of age), and aboriginal women [42].

Studies conducted in urban settings indicate that aboriginal people constitute a disproportionate number of those at high risk [43]. In Alberta, aboriginal people represent approximately 5% of the population, yet 25% of HIV cases are found in that population. From 1996 to 1999, HIV cases increased by 25% nationwide, while aboriginal cases nearly doubled, reaching 6% in 1999 [40,42].

Youth under the age of 20 represent a small proportion of total HIV infections at 1.5% [42]; however, studies among street populations and IDUs under 25 years of age have shown prevalence rates ranging from 4 to 17% [44–46]. Young adults 20–29 years of age comprise 27% of cases nationwide [42].

The availability of antiretrovirals for prevention of mother-to-child transmission (PMTCT) has enabled Canada to keep the rate of perinatal HIV infection low, with the majority of the 420 recorded paediatric HIV cases occurring early in the epidemic [40]. National estimates indicate that the number of HIV-positive pregnant women receiving antiretrovirals increased from 19% in 1992 to 90% in 2002, reflected also in the percentage of exposed infants confirmed HIV-positive, which decreased from 33% in 1994–1995 to 3% in 2002. The percentage of pregnant women screened for HIV has been increasing as well, with over 90% screened in the provinces of Alberta and Newfoundland-Labrador, and about 80% screened in the provinces of British Columbia and Ontario in recent years [47]. Comparing the proportion of infants diagnosed with HIV across ethnic groups, it is apparent that minorities, including aboriginal, Asian and African-Canadian populations, are at increased risk [40]. In the provinces of Ontario and Quebec, where over 60% of the 420 paediatric cases occurred, the majority of HIV-infected mothers indicated their risk category was being from an HIV-endemic country [47].

Table 37.2 Annual reporting and cumulative total of HIV-positive tests by province and territory[*]

Province	Pre-1996	1997	1998	1999	2000	2001	2002	Total
British Columbia	8347 (2505)	561 (120)	482 (129)	427 (100)	419 (100)	439 (36)	441 (26)	11,116 (3256)
Alberta	2759 (844)	217 (42)	135 (27)	177 (34)	185 (42)	169 (35)	174 (26)	3816 (1122)
Saskatchewan	213 (112)	42 (11)	25 (10)	30 (3)	35 (12)	40 (4)	24 (6)	409 (186)
Manitoba	573 (149)	76 (2)	71 (10)	73 (6)	57 (11)	65 (6)	68 (6)	983 (206)
Ontario	17,458 (5897)	967 (227)	996 (172)	932 (138)	897 (105)	911 (105)	1143 (85)	23,304 (7196)
Quebec	8444 (4635)	628 (191)	567 (154)	567 (103)	493 (95)	526 (55)	620 (19)	11,845 (5943)
New Brunswick	247 (111)	6 (4)	14 (6)	5 (8)	14 (2)	10 (3)	9 (0)	305 (148)
Nova Scotia and PEI	482 (231)	32 (11)	34 (11)	26 (9)	16 (6)	14 (3)	15 (4)	619 (296)
Newfoundland-Labrador	175 (56)	7 (1)	14 (6)	6 (1)	3 (2)	5 (2)	0 (0)	210 (86)
Yukon	19 (3)	2 (0)	3 (0)	1 (0)	5 (1)	4 (0)	3 (2)	37 (8)
North West Territories	29 (17)	1 (0)	1 (0)	1 (0)	0 (0)	2 (0)	1 (0)	35 (22)
Nunavut	N/A	N/A	N/A	N/A	0 (0)	0 (0)	1 (0)	1 (0)
Total	38,746 (15,716)	2539 (716)	2342 (621)	2245 (484)	2124 (427)	2185 (297)	2499 (174)	52,680 (18,469)

* numbers in brackets are AIDS cases.
PEI = Prince Edward Island.
Source: [40].

History of the government response

The National Advisory Committee on AIDS was established in 1983 in response to the AIDS crisis. Initially, CA$1.6 million (US$1.2 million) was allocated over 4 years for research regarding this emerging infection. In 1985, the Federal Government approved testing of all donated blood products. Licensing of treated blood products for people with haemophilia occurred at a slower pace in Canada than in the USA. In 1989, the Federal Government initiated the Extraordinary Assistance Program to compensate those infected through contaminated blood. Following a public inquiry, the 1997 Krever report established that inadequate action was taken during the early years of the epidemic [48,49].

In 1990, the National Strategy for HIV/AIDS was launched with a 3-year mandate to organize prevention, treatment and surveillance, and in 1993 was extended for another 5 years [50]. Rumours of discontinuation led to increased public mobilization and political support, resulting in a new national strategy [51]. Renamed the Canadian Strategy for HIV/AIDS (CSHA), the organization broadened its mandate to encourage new approaches to prevention and research into root causes of the epidemic [50]. Since 1994, an annual CSHA budget of CA$42.4 million (US$32.5 million) has funded programmes through non-governmental organizations (NGOs) and AIDS Service Organizations (ASOs), and, for research, through organizations such as the Canadian HIV Trials Network (CTN) and the Canadian Institute for Health Research (CIHR) [50].

The Ministerial Council on HIV/AIDS informs and advises the Minister of Health and the CSHA. It consists of 15 members, five of whom are HIV-positive, giving voice to those directly affected by the virus [52]. Recommendations are based on three principles: sustainability and integration; focus on high risk; and public accountability [52].

Monitoring and surveillance

Anonymous HIV testing, which places responsibility on the client to come back for their test results, is available in all provinces except Prince Edward Island and Manitoba. Non-nominal testing, in which the healthcare worker ordering the test is aware of the patient's identity but uses initials or a code to place the order, is available everywhere. In the event of a positive test, public health officials will follow up with the person ordering the test, but will not necessarily be given the name of the patient. Since 1985, anonymous testing has been offered in British Columbia through any clinic. Quebec has developed more than 60 sites since 1987. In 1992, Ontario made anonymous testing legal and has since established 33 sites. Alberta and Saskatchewan have each opened three sites since 1992–1993. The province of Nova Scotia, with one site, and New Brunswick, with seven, began anonymous testing in 1994 and 1998, respectively, while Newfoundland-Labrador offers it on request [34].

HIV and AIDS are reportable in all provinces and territories, although only since 2003 in British Columbia [42]. With the exception of having a CD4 threshold, AIDS diagnosis follows the 1993 US Centers for Disease Control (CDC) definition. National surveillance data, comprised of non-nominal HIV test information and different extents of demographic data, are unable to account for duplicate tests.

HIV strain surveillance is carried out by several laboratories and compiled by the LCDC [42]. Since 1996, the Drug Treatment Program in British Columbia has tested over 10,000 individuals for the presence of genetic markers of drug resistance in addition to typing predominant strains. The HIV strain predominantly found in North America is subtype B, while other subtypes are found in South Africa, Eastern Europe and South-East Asia. Recent reports indicate that approximately 7% of strains were non-B, the majority observed among those arriving in Canada from abroad [42].

Resistant strains of HIV among newly infected individuals are monitored by the Canadian HIV Strain and Drug Resistance Program. A jump from zero to approximately 10% primary resistance was seen between 1997 and 1998 [45]. In 2001, approximately 11% of samples had some type of resistance [42]. Resistance has shifted from nucleoside reverse transcriptase inhibitors (NRTIs), which were the first developed antiretroviral medications, to non-NRTIs, protease inhibitors (PIs) and multiple combinations.

Prevention

Injecting drug users

With IDUs representing a quarter of HIV infections in Canada, harm-reduction programmes are an important component of prevention. Vancouver was one of the first cities in North America officially to establish a needle exchange programme (NEP), providing clean needles and referrals to other services [53], and was quickly followed by CACTUS–Montreal, the first federal–provincial cost-shared NEP demonstration project, both commencing in 1989.

A recent survey of addiction services revealed 63 NEPs across Canada [54]. Methadone maintenance therapy, available in Canada since 1959 [55], was offered in all provinces except Prince Edward Island. Researchers and advocacy groups have pushed for the implementation of pilot supervised injection facilities (SIFs) and heroin prescription trials [56–60]. In 2003, Health Canada agreed to receive SIF proposals and approved a Vancouver pilot site [61]. The North American Opiate Medication Initiative (NAOMI), a North American initiative for heroin prescription, was awarded CIHR funding for three Canadian sites in 2002 [62,63].

Prisons

In 1994, Correctional Services Canada (CSC) agreed to compassionate parole for inmates in the terminal stages of a disease [64] and introduced condoms in Canadian penitentiaries following indications of high levels of HIV infection among inmates in Quebec provincial prisons [65–68]. Recommendations for NEPs in prisons were made in 1996, but at present these have not been implemented by government [69,70]. In 1998, CSC instituted methadone maintenance for federal inmates who were on a programme prior to incarceration. In 1999, expansion allowed other inmates in exceptional circumstances to join the programme, and, in 2002, the programme was opened to any inmates requesting treatment [70].

Youth

A Family Life component in the public education system introduces concepts of reproductive health and sexuality to children and adolescents. Health Canada publishes a set of guidelines for sex education programmes [71], provincial and territorial governments issue curriculum guides, and school boards establish programmes. Sex education classes begin as early as kindergarten or as late as the fifth grade [72]. In general, programmes for adolescents include approaches for both safer sex and delay of sexual initiation. Classes are not mandatory and parents may withdraw their children [71].

Antenatal testing

There are two distinct programmes at the provincial or territorial level for testing and treating pregnant women. The first includes voluntary HIV testing as part of the routine testing given to women at antenatal clinics, allowing them to opt out [73]. The second shifts responsibility, requiring doctors to offer HIV tests, including pre- and post-test counselling, and requiring patients to opt in with informed consent [73]. Supporters of the opt-out programme argue that this catches a larger portion of the population; however, opponents of the opt-out programme fear there is a lack of adequate counselling and informed choice [74,75].

Immigration

In 2002, Immigration Services Canada implemented mandatory testing of immigrants [76]. Those testing HIV-positive may be deemed too large a burden on the healthcare system and refused entry. This initiative was not supported by the CSHA [52]. Most testing is done abroad, and exceptions are made for those with resident-status family in Canada.

Accountability and impact assessment

The accountability of programmes depends largely on the agency funding them. The CSHA delivers an annual public report that includes descriptions of monies disbursed and programmes initiated [52,77]. Academic research undergoes rigorous peer review. Some provincial action plans include broad goals such as reduced incidence of new infections, but do not necessarily set goals for direct programme assessment. High-profile programmes such as NEPs and SIFs have been well studied, although conclusions are still unclear due to the variety of confounding issues surrounding these interventions. The monitoring and evaluation of HIV prevention and support programmes has waned in recent years. There is, therefore, a need for improved assessment of existing and emerging initiatives in order to focus increased support on programmes that have shown results.

Care, treatment and support

Globally speaking, Canadians have enjoyed relatively good access to HIV drugs since the introduction of AZT in 1986. The Therapeutic Products Directorate (TPD) of Health Canada, responsible for regulating new drugs [78], has been criticized for having a slower approval process than the USA.

In 1954, the Emergency Drug Release Program was initiated by the government to allow provision of pre-licensed drugs on a case-by-case basis [79]. In the 1990s, the Special Assistance Program (SAP) was launched [80]. Physicians apply for access to unlicensed drugs and may receive up to a 6-month supply for their patient(s). SAP attempts to respond within 24 hours; however, physicians may apply for anticipated use where there is an indication [80].

Provincial and territorial programmes for HIV medications range from complete coverage for all HIV-infected individuals to special coverage categories, or coverage through Pharmacare programmes with income-based deductibles. Importantly, it is left to provinces and territories to determine which HIV drugs to include in their formularies for coverage, leaving the largest budget item as a provincial responsibility. Provincial formularies range widely in the number and types of HIV drugs included. The province of New Brunswick lists only six drugs: five non-NRTIs and one PI [81]. The provinces of Alberta, Saskatchewan and Quebec list 17 or more drugs, as does the federal Non-Insured Health Benefits programme [82–85]. Two provinces—Alberta and Nova Scotia—include one of the most expensive drugs, Enfuvirtide (Fuzeon®), belonging to the newest class of HIV drugs, fusion inhibitors (see Table 37.3) [82,86].

Table 37.3 Coverage of HIV medication in each province and territory

Province	Programme	Programme entry	Co-pay	2001-2002 budget (CA$)
British Columbia	Drug Treatment Programme	Physician registration	None	37.8 million*
Alberta	Province-wide services	Physician referral	None	9.5 million**
Saskatchewan	Pharmacare: special beneficiaries	Self-application	None	<5.02 million*** ~ (1.5 million†)
Manitoba	Pharmacare: income/social assistance	Self-application	2% of family income if <15,000; 3% if greater	~3.3 million† (3.4 million‡)
Ontario	Pharmacare: trillium programme	Self-application	Prorated/quarterly deductible (maximum $1022) + max $2 dispensing fee	219 million††
Quebec	Pharmacare (if on social assistance, co-pay is covered by provincial government)	No private insurance	$8 base + 28% monthly deductible (maximum $70)+ annual premium based on age/income ($0–$460)	42.6 million† (15.2 million‡)
New Brunswick	Prescription drug programme: special benefits U plan	Self-application	None if family services client; $50 registration, 20% of drug cost (maximum $20)	2.2 million‡ (1.3 million†)
Nova Scotia	Department of Health: special funding assistance	No other insurance	Income-based deductible (33%; min $3 to max $30); max dispense fee of $9 for uninsured	0.6 million‡ (1.7 million†)
Prince Edward Island	Drug cost assistance programme	Diagnosis confirmed by Chief Health Officer	None; those with third-party insurance can submit for reimbursement	<2.67 million‡‡ (0.1 million†)
Newfoundland-Labrador	Pharmacare: income support plan	On income support or by application	None	~1.9 million‡ (0.8 million†)
Yukon	Drug programme: chronic disease	Non-native; no other insurance	$250 per annum; can apply for waiver	–
North West Territories	Extended health benefits	Non-native; no private insurance	None	–
Nunavut	Pharmacare	Non-native; no other insurance	None	
Federal	First Nations and Inuit Health Branch: non-insured health benefits	Registered First Nations, Inuit and Innu	None	<<183.7 million¶ ~ (0.5 million‡)

Estimates for HIV drug expenditures in British Columbia, Alberta and Ontario come from drug delivery programmes; all other provinces and territories are based on a variety of sources and assumptions as indicated.

* Information obtained from the Drug Treatment Programme.
** Two regional authorities dispense province-wide services: estimate comes from actual cost for Capital Health Authority (CHA) plus estimated cost for Calgary Regional Health Authority based on percentage of HIV drugs from CHA of total prescription drugs covered.
*** Amount expended by drug programme for *all* anti-infectives.
† Estimate based on the number of HIV cases in the region and average annual drug costs, assuming 30% of cases are treated.
†† Estimate from Ontario Drug Programs Branch.
‡ Percentage of total HIV drug programme expenditure, based on average percentage for HIV drugs out of total drug costs for other provinces (on average, Pharmacare programmes account for 5–6% of total healthcare programme expenditures; HIV drugs account for 3–5% of Pharmacare costs).
‡‡ Total expenditure for specified drug funding programme.
¶ Expenditure for total health insurance programme.

The location of service provision for HIV-infected individuals is another variable that changes from province to province. In Quebec, services are both hospital-based and community-based, with several large clinics in Montreal staffed by family physicians who have developed expertise in HIV treatment modalities and who participate in providing 24-hour hotline mentoring to physicians following HIV patients anywhere in Quebec. Specialty clinics offer the majority of services in Ontario due, in part, to the large number of cases in Ontario, as well as to provincial differences in the management and operation of healthcare.

Research

In 1989, the government called for a national programme to organize and initiate trials for HIV treatments. The Canadian HIV Trials Network (CTN), a collaborative effort between researchers and academics from across Canada, was officially inaugurated in 1991 [87]. Since then, 77 trials have been implemented, examining treatment for opportunistic infections, comparing antiretroviral regimens, testing the effectiveness of less stringent regimens and evaluating outcomes of treatment interruptions [88].

The first phase III clinical trial of the AIDSVAX vaccine was carried out recently with partnerships between several organizations across three countries: Canada, the USA and The Netherlands. The Canadian arm was carried out in Vancouver, Toronto and Montreal, involving close to 300 volunteers. While the vaccine was not found to be effective, demonstration of the ability to carry out an HIV vaccine trial of this size was an important step [89,90].

Approximately CA$13 million (US$9.9 Million) in CSHA funding was distributed among 91 research initiatives in 2002 [50]. Nonetheless, evaluation of population effectiveness, cost-effectiveness and acceptability of programmes are all areas requiring greater attention.

Challenges

In spite of numerous programmes, HIV continues to be a major public health concern in Canada. Old problems of access and discrimination persist, and new problems of multidrug resistance have emerged. Treatment costs continue to climb, from around CA$1 million in 1992 to CA$38 million in 2002 in British Columbia, for example. With current antiretroviral regimens, the estimated cost for treating one individual can be CA$10,000–$15,000 (US$7682–11,523); however, the introduction of a new class of drug such as Fuzeon® could increase this to CA$40,000 (US$30,730) [91,92]. Even in a universal healthcare system, care and treatment service quality continues to be unequal. Marginalized populations have less access to services, with drug use and homelessness complicating service delivery. Women, aboriginal people (e.g. on reserves), drug users and those with lower income continue to be at higher risk of infection and less likely to seek treatment [93–95]. While all regions provide coverage for primary care, specialized care centres are concentrated in urban areas.

Discrimination and stigmatization remain a problem [96]. Surveys conducted among people living with HIV in British Columbia indicated widespread feelings of discrimination [97]. A study of IDUs in Ontario found that approximately 40% required some type of medical treatment in the past year but had not sought it [98]. In British Columbia, of IDUs clinically eligible for treatment, only 40% were on therapy, and 60% of these were on suboptimal therapy [99].

For those receiving therapy, maintaining strict schedules and dealing with painful and disfiguring side effects are difficult challenges [100]. Lack of adherence has led to an increase in resistant strains of HIV. The shift towards more resistant strains among primary infections mirrors that seen in other countries with access to highly active antiretroviral therapy (HAART) [42]. The ever-changing face and increasing cost of the epidemic makes it difficult to develop appropriate, sustainable responses.

Conclusion

The Canada Health Act, with its five principles, has broadly influenced the response to the HIV epidemic. The CSHA and Health Canada provide guidelines for various HIV-related policy issues, while each province and territory develops its own response to the epidemic [101–104]. Canada's universal healthcare system has not eliminated inequity in access to treatment and care, although it is not as marked as that observed in other systems. Other problems include complacency and resurgence in the third decade of the HIV epidemic, despite prevention and education programmes, and the cost of healthcare. The pressures of costs associated with HIV are felt in the types of services deemed 'medically necessary', the availability of primary care doctors experienced in treating HIV, the availability and cost of home care services, the accessibility of expensive procedures and, above all, the availability of expensive antiretroviral treatments. System reform has begun; however, more innovative solutions must be found in order to find the balance between providing adequate care and sustaining a public system of healthcare.

References

1. First Nations and Inuit Health Branch. Mandate and Priorities. Health Canada, First Nations and Inuit Health Branch. URL: http://www.hc-sc.gc.ca/fnihb-dgspni/fnihb/mandate_priorities.htm; last updated May 21, 2001.

2. WHO. (2002). *The World Health Report 2002*. Geneva: World Health Organization.

3. WHO. (2003). *Country Indicators*. Geneva: World Health Organization.

4. Central Intelligence Agency. (2003). The CIA World Factbook. Available at: www.cia.gov/cia/ publications/factbook.

5. OECD. (2002). *OECD Health Data 2002*. Paris: OECD.

6. Brown MC. (1986). Health care financing and the Canada Health Act. *Journal of Canadian Studies* 21:111–32.

7. Attenborough R. (1997). The Canadian health care system: development, reform, and opportunities for nurses. *Journal of Obstetric, Gynecologic, and Neonatal Nursing* 26:229–34.

8. World Health Organization. (1996). *Health Care Systems in Transition: Canada*. Copenhagen: WHO, Regional Office for Europe.

9. Scott C. (2001). *Public and Private Roles in Health Care Systems*. Buckingham: Open University Press.

10. New Brunswick Department of Health and Wellness. (2003). *In-country Coverage and Claims*. Moncton: Government of New Brunswick.

11. British Columbia Medical Association. (2000). *Policy Backgrounder: Federal Transfer Payments for Health Care*. Vancouver: BCMA.

12. Canadian Institute for Health Information (CIHI). (2004). *The Canadian Management Information Systems Database.* The Canadian Institute for Health Information, 1995/96–2001/02. Ottawa: CIHI.

13. Deber RB. (2002). *Delivering Health Care Services: Public, Not-for-profit, or Private?* Discussion paper No. 17. Commission for the Future of Health Care in Canada. Ottawa: Government of Canada.

14. Saskatchewan Health. Programs and Services. URL: http://www.health.gov.sk.ca/ps_coverage_full.html; last updated 2003.

15. Alberta Health and Wellness. Health Care Coverage and Services. URL: http://www.health.gov.ab.ca/coverage/benefits/aadl.html; last updated February 13, 2004.

16. Newfoundland Department of Health and Community Services. Medical Care Plan. URL: http://www.gov.nf.ca/mcp/html/mcp.htm; last updated May 30, 2003.

17. Ministère de la Santé et des Services sociaux du Québec. Régie de l'assurance maladie du Québec. URL: http://www.ramq.gouv.qc.ca/en/citoyens/programmesetservices/servicesmedicauxdroits.sht*ml*; last updated February 23, 2004.

18. British Columbia Ministry of Health. Medical Services Plan of BC. URL: http:// www.healthservices.gov.bc.ca/msp/; last updated September 22, 2003.

19. Manitoba Health. Questions and Answers about Health Care Coverage. URL: http://www.gov.mb.ca/health/mhsip/index.html#insuredmedicalbenefits; last updated March 2, 2004.

20. Ontario Ministry of Health and Long-term Care. Health Services in Your Community. URL: http://www.health.gov.on.ca/english/public/program/ohip/ohipfaq_dt.html; last updated March 4, 2004.

21. Secretariat I. (2001). *Private Health Insurance in OECD Countries.* Compilation of National Reports. Copenhagen: OECD, p23–8.

22. Health Policy and Communications Branch. (2002). *Health Expenditures in Canada by Age and Sex, 1980–81 to 2000–01.* Ottawa: Health Canada.

23. Inglehart JK. (2000). Revisiting the Canadian health care system. *New England Journal of Medicine* 342:2007–12.

24. McDaid D. (2003). Co-ordinating health technology assessment in Canada: a European perspective. *Health Policy* 63:205–13.

25. Avery G. (2001). *Wait List Report II: Executive Summary.* Vancouver: British Columbia Medical Association.

26. Glynn P, Taylor M, Hudson A. (2002). *Surgical Wait List Management: A Strategy for Saskatchewan.* Saskatoon: Saskatchewan Ministry of Health.

27. The Angus Reid Report. *Canadians' Perspectives on Their Health Care System.* Public Policy Focus. Toronto: Angus Reid, March/April 1998: p17–25.

28. Wootton J. (1999). New Office to Focus on Rural Health Issues. *Farm Family Health* 7(1). Health Canada, Health Protection Branch-Laboratory Centre for Disease Control. (April, 1999). URL: http://www.hc-sc.gc.ca/main/lcdc/web/publicat/farmfam/vol7-1/ff7-1b-e.html.

29. Romanow RJ. (2002). *Building on Values: The Future of Health Care in Canada.* Ottawa: Government of Canada, Commission on the Future of Health Care in Canada.

30. Bowen S. (2000). Access to health services for underserved populations in Canada. (2001). In: *Certain Circumstances: Issues in Equity and Responsiveness in Access to Health Care in Canada.* Ottawa: Health Canada, p26–37.

31. Statistics Canada. (2001). *Census Canada 2001.* Canadian statistics. URL: http://www.statcan.ca/english/Pgdb/; last updated March 9, 2004.

32. Canada Department of Finance. (2003). *Canada Health and Social Transfer.* Ottawa: Government of Canada.

33. Canadian Medical Association. (2003). Viruses don't have visas. *Canadian Medical Association Interface* **4**:1. URL: http://collection.nlc-bnc.ca/100/202/300/cma_interface/2003/vol4-07/no-1.htm.

34. Archibald CP, Sutherland J, Geduld J, Sutherland D, Yan P. (2003). Combining data sources to monitor the HIV epidemic in Canada. *Journal of Acquired Immune Deficiency Syndromes* **32**:S24–32.

35. Elmslie K, Nault P. (1986). AIDS surveillance in Canada. *Canadian Medical Association Journal* **135**:780.

36. Rose DB, Keystone JS. (1983). AIDS in a Canadian woman who had helped prostitutes in Port-Au-Prince. *Lancet* **2**:680–1.

37. Handzel S. (1983). *Canada Diseases Weekly Report.* Ottawa: Laboratory Centre for Disease Control **9**:186–7.

38. Joncas JH, Delage G, Chad Z, Lapointe N. (1983). Acquired (or congenital) immunodeficiency syndrome in infants born of Haitian mothers. *New England Journal of Medicine* **308**:842.

39. Gilmore NJ, Beaulieu R, Steben M, Laverdiere M. (1983). AIDS: acquired immunodeficiency syndrome. *Canadian Medical Association Journal* **128**:1281–4.

40. Health Canada. (2003). *HIV and AIDS in Canada. Surveillance Report to December 31, 2002.* Surveillance and Risk Assessment Division, Centre for Infectious Disease Prevention and Control. Ottawa: Health Canada.

41. Schanzer DL. (2003). HIV/AIDS mortality trends in Canada, 1987–1998. *Canadian Journal of Public Health* **94**:135–9.

42. Health Canada. (2003). *HIV and AIDS Epi Updates to December 31, 2002.* Division of HIV/AIDS Epidemiology and Surveillance, Centre for Infectious Disease Prevention and Control. Ottawa: Health Canada.

43. Schechter MT, Marion SA, Elmslie K, Ricketts M. (1992). How many persons in Canada have been infected with human immunodeficiency virus? An exploration using back-calculation methods. *Clinical Investigative Medicine* **15**:331–45.

44. Alary M, Parent R, Hankins C, Claessens C, SurvIDU Working Group. (2002). Synergy between risk factors and the persistence of high HIV incidence among injection drug users in the SurvIDU. *Canadian Journal of Infectious Disease* **13**(Supplement A):49A (abstract 316).

45. Elliott LJ, Blanchard JF, Dinner KI, Dadwood MR, Beaudoin C. (1999). The Winnipeg Injection Drug Epidemiology (WIDE) Study. *Canadian Journal of Infectious Disease* **10**(Supplement B):46B (abstract 314).

46. Miller C, Tyndall M, Li K, Laliberte N, Spittal P, Schechter MT. (2001). High rates of HIV positivity among young injection drug users. *Canadian Journal of Infectious Disease* **12**(Supplement B):65B (abstract 340P).

47. Health Canada. (2004). *HIV/AIDS Epi Updates, May 2004.* Ottawa: Surveillance and Risk Assessment Division, Centre for Infectious Disease Prevention and Control, Health Canada.

48. Wainberg MA, Read SE. (1986). Public funding for AIDS research in Canada and the USA. *Canadian Medical Association Journal* **134**:109.

49. Health Canada. (1997). *Krever Commission Report.* Ottawa: Health Canada.

50. Canadian Society on HIV/AIDS. (2002). *Lessons Learned: Reframing the Response.* Ottawa: Health Canada.

51. McIlroy A. (1996). Ottawa attacked for complacency on AIDS. *Globe and Mail* July 6, pA1, A6.

52. Canadian Society on HIV/AIDS. (2002). *CSHA Ministerial Council Annual Report 2001–2002.* Ottawa: Health Canada.

53. Canadian Centre for Substance Abuse. (1994). *Syringe Exchange: One Approach to Preventing Drug-related HIV Infection.* Ottawa: CCSA National Working Group on Policy.

54. Ogborne A, Fischer B, Rosidi S. (2001). *Services for Injection Drug Users in Canada: Results of a National Survey*. Ottawa: Canadian Centre for Substance Abuse.

55. Fischer B. (2000). Prescriptions, power and politics: the turbulent history of methadone maintenance in Canada. *Journal of Public Health Policy* 21:187–209.

56. Fischer B, Rehm J, Kim G, Robins A. (2002). Safer injection facilities (SIFs) for injection drug users (IDUs) in Canada. A review and call for an evidence-focused pilot trial. *Canadian Journal of Public Health* 93:336–8.

57. Fischer B, Rehm J, Kirst M *et al.* (2002). Heroin-assisted treatment as a response to the public health problem of opiate dependence. *European Journal of Public Health* 12:228–34.

58. Martens D. (2002). Injection facilities needed to combat infection crisis, AIDS network says. *Canadian Medical Association Journal* 166:1455.

59. Wood E, Tyndall MW, Spittal PM *et al.* (2001). Unsafe injection practices in a cohort of injection drug users in Vancouver: could safer injecting rooms help? *Canadian Medical Association Journal* 165:405–10.

60. Gold F. (2003). Advocacy and activism: supervised injection facilities. *Canadian Nurse* 99:14–8.

61. Jurgens R. (2002). Supervised injection sites: Minister of Health ready to review applications for pilot research projects. *Canadian HIV/AIDS Policy and Law Review* 7:25–7.

62. Fischer B, Schechter MT, Anis A *et al.* (2002). North American Opiate Medication Initiative— Canada. Presented at the Third Network Meeting on the Medical Prescription of Heroin, Utrecht, The Netherlands, CCBH.

63. Brissette S. (2001). Medical prescription of heroin: a review. *Canadian HIV/AIDS Policy and Law Review* 6:1, 92–98.

64. Betteridge JG. (2001). Inquest into the death of a prisoner co-infected with HIV and hepatitis C: how many more will there be? *Canadian HIV/AIDS Policy and Law Review* 6:65–9.

65. Hankins C. (1994). Confronting HIV infection in prisons (editorial). *Canadian Medical Association Journal* 151:745.

66. Hankins C, Gendron S, Handley M, Richard C, Lai-Tung MT, O'Shaughnessy M. (1994). HIV and women in prison: assessment of risk factors using a non-nominal methodology. *American Journal of Public Health* 84:1637–40.

67. Hankins C, Gendron S, Handley M, Rouah F. (1991). HIV-1 infection among incarcerated men— Quebec. *Canadian Disease Weekly Report* 17-43:233–5.

68. Hankins C, Gendron S, Richard C, O'Shaughnessy M. (1989). HIV-1 infection in a medium security prison for women—Quebec. *Canadian Disease Weekly Report* 15–33:168–70.

69. Jurgens R. (2000). HIV/AIDS in prisons: more new developments. *Canadian HIV/AIDS Policy and Law Review* 5:64–8.

70. Jurgens R. (2002). HIV/AIDS in prisons: recent developments. *Canadian HIV/AIDS Policy and Law Review* 7:13–6.

71. Population and Public Health Branch. (1997). *Canadian Guidelines for Sexual Health Education*. Ottawa: Health Canada.

72. Thompson L, Hartley T. (2001). *Personal Planning K to 7/Career and Personal Planning 8 to 12: Curriculum Review Report 2001*. Vancouver: BC Ministry of Education.

73. Walmsley S. (2003). Opt in or opt out: what is the optimal for prenatal screening for HIV infection? *Canadian Medical Association Journal* 168:707–8.

74. Kenney P. (2002). Medical association calls for routine HIV testing of pregnant women. *Canadian HIV/AIDS Policy and Law Review* 7:32–3.

75. Jayaraman GC, Preiksaitis JK, Larke B. (2003). Mandatory reporting of HIV infection and opt-out prenatal screening for HIV infection: effect on testing rates. *Canadian Medical Association Journal* 168:679–82.

76. Klein A. (2002). Concerns raised about new immigration rules. *Canadian HIV/AIDS Policy and Law Review* 6:32–3.

77. Health Canada. (1998). *Canadian Strategy on HIV/AIDS. Accountability Framework.* Ottawa: Health Canada.

78. Health Products and Food Branch of Health Canada. Therapeutic Products Directorate. URL: http://www.hc-sc.gc.ca/hpfb-dgpsa/ tpd-dpt/aboutus_e.html; last updated October 2, 2003.

79. Gilron I. (1993). The emergency drug release program: regulatory aspects of new drug access in Canada. *Canadian Medical Association Journal* 148:1151–3.

80. Health Products and Food Branch of Health Canada. Therapeutic Products Directorate: Special Access Programme Fact sheets. URL: http://www.hc-sc.gc.ca/hpfb-dgpsa/tpd-dpt/sap_factsheet2002_e.html; last updated April 22, 2003.

81. Health and Wellness Prescription Drug Program. New Brunswick Prescription Drug Formulary. URL: http:// www.gnb.ca/0212/NBPDPFormulary-e.asp; last updated September 1, 2004.

82. Calgary Health Region. Paying for Drugs. URL: http://xweb.crha-health.ab.ca/clin/sac/payingfo.htm; last updated October 1, 2004.

83. Saskatchewan Health: Drug Plan and Extended Benefits Branch. Online Formulary. URL: http://formulary.drugplan.health.gov.sk.ca; last updated October 21, 2004.

84. Régie de l'assurance maladie Québec. The Public Plan—Prescription Drugs Covered. URL: http://www.ramq.gouv.qc.ca/en/citoyens/assurancemedicaments/regimepublic/medicament_general.shtml; last updated August 13, 2004.

85. Canadian Aboriginal AIDS Network. HIV & the Non-insured Health Benefits (NIHB) Program for Aboriginal People in Canada. URL: http://www.caan.ca/english/grfx/resources/fact_sheets/NIHB_english.pdf; last updated June 21, 2004.

86. Novia Scotia Pharmacare. Nova Scotia Formulary Search Selection Page. URL: http://www.gov.ns.ca/health/pharmacare/formulary.asp; last updated November 15, 2004.

87. Canadian HIV Trials Network. What is the Canadian HIV Trials Network? URL: http://www.hivnet-t.ubc.ca/ BackgroundFrame.html; last updated August 1, 2003.

88. Canadian HIV Trials Network. (2003). *Knowledge = Strength: Annual Review of the Canadian HIV Trials Network, 2001–02.* Canada: CHTN.

89. Francis DP, Heyward WL, Popovic V et al. (2003). Candidate HIV/AIDS vaccines: lessons learned from the world's first phase III efficacy trials. *AIDS* 17:147–56.

90. O'Connell JM, Hogg RS, Chan K et al. (2002). Willingness to participate and enroll in a phase 3 preventive HIV-1 vaccine trial. *Journal of Acquired Immune Deficiency Syndrome* 31:521–8.

91. Krentz HB, Auld MC, Gill MJ, HIV Economic Study Group. (2003). The changing direct costs of medical care for patients with HIV/AIDS, 1995–2001. *Canadian Medical Association Journal* 169:106–10.

92. Canadian AIDS Treatment Information Exchange. T-20 (Fuzeon) goes on sale in Canada. URL: http://www.catie.ca/aidsinfo.nsf/9d6a0a99ab2787c985256b9c005b053b?OpenView ; last updated October 28, 2003.

93. Mocroft A, Gill MJ, Davidson W, Phillips AN. (2000). Are there gender differences in starting protease inhibitors, HAART, and disease progression despite equal access to care? *Journal of Acquired Immune Deficiency Syndrome* 24:475–82.

94. Wood E, Montaner JS, Chan K *et al.* (2002). Socioeconomic status, access to triple therapy, and survival from HIV disease since 1996. *AIDS* 16:2065–72.

95. Hankins C, Lapointe N, Walmsley S. (1998). Participation in clinical trials among women living with HIV in Canada: Canadian Women's HIV Study Group. *Canadian Medical Association Journal* 159:1359–65.

96. Canadian HIV/AIDS Clearinghouse. (2002). Stigma and discrimination greatest barriers to preventing more infections. *HIV Prevention Plus* 3:1–2.

97. Kirkham CM, Lobb DJ. (1998). The British Columbia Positive Women's Survey: a detailed profile of 110 HIV-infected women. *Canadian Medical Association Journal* 158:317–23.

98. Fischer B, Gliksman L, Rehm J, Daniel N, Medved W. (1999). Comparing opiate users in methadone treatment with untreated opiate users: results of a follow-up study with a Toronto opiate user cohort. *Canadian Journal of Public Health* 90:299–303.

99. Strathdee SA, Palepu A, Cornelisse PG *et al.* (1998). Barriers to use of free antiretroviral therapy in injection drug users. *Journal of the American Medical Association* 280:547–9.

100. Heath KV, Singer J, O'Shaughnessy M, Montaner JS, Hogg RS. (2002). Intentional non-adherence due to adverse symptoms associated with antiretroviral therapy. *Journal of Acquired Immune Deficiency Syndrome* 31:211–7.

101. BC Ministry of Health, Provincial HIV/AIDS Strategy Advisory Committee. (1998). *British Columbia's Framework for Action on HIV/AIDS.* Victoria: Government of British Columbia.

102. Saskatchewan Ministry of Health, Provincial HIV Strategy Team. (2002). *At Risk: Recommendations for a Provincial Strategy on HIV, Blood-borne Pathogens and Injection Drug Use.* Saskatoon: Government of Saskatchewan.

103. Ministère de la Santé et Services Sociaux. (1997). *Stratégie Québécoise de Lutte Contre le SIDA.* Québec: Direction générale de la santé publique.

104. Manitoba Department of Health. (1996). *Manitoba Provincial HIV/AIDS Strategy.* Winnipeg: Government of Manitoba.

Chapter 38

Mexico

Jose Antonio Izazola-Licea[*], Carlos Avila-Figueroa and Sandra Gómez-Fraga

Background

The challenge posed by the HIV epidemic for the health system in Mexico is to improve the health indicators of the population through comprehensive provision of preventive and curative services. However, existing means of paying for antiretroviral therapy (ART) potentially threaten to consume limited healthcare resources to the point where the financial sustainability of other priority health programmes is at risk. Health sector reform requires achieving universal coverage by improving the public and private provision of services, strengthening the responsive capacity of public hospitals, improving the labour conditions of health workers, ensuring the quality of care, decentralizing services and generally improving the efficiency of the health system across the country.

Recent healthcare reform in Mexico is based on principles of universality, access, efficiency and quality. Its objective is to guarantee comprehensive provision of preventive and curative services. The impact of the HIV epidemic will be examined in the context of health system reform in Mexico, including new ways of financing the provision of preventive and curative services to control HIV infection.

Mexico is a federal republic with 31 states and one of the largest capital cities in the world. It occupies an area of 1,972,550 km^2 between the Atlantic and Pacific Oceans, and is bordered on the north by the USA and on the south by the Central American countries of Guatemala and Belize. A third of the population is Amerindian and speaks indigenous languages, predominantly Mayan and Nahuatl. Eighty-nine per cent of the population is reported to be Roman Catholic. Adult literacy is 91% for females and 94% for males.

The President is the head of state and is elected by popular vote for a 6-year term. Elections held in July 2000 marked the first time since the 1910 Mexican Revolution that the Opposition, in free and fair elections, had defeated the party in government. The legislative branch comprises a bicameral National Congress consisting of the Senate and the Federal Chamber of Deputies. The Supreme Court of Justice represents the judicial branch of the government, with judges appointed by the President with the consent of the Senate. Political interests are represented by several industry and employers' groups, the chamber of commerce, workers' unions and the Roman Catholic Church.

Mexico has a market economy, with a mixture of modern and outmoded industry and agriculture increasingly dominated by the private sector, which has expanded under recent

* Corresponding author.

The views expressed in this chapter are those of the authors and are not necessarily those of the organizations they work for, unless specifically stated in the text.

governments. Economic competition has become more prevalent. Ongoing economic and social concerns include low real wages, underemployment of a large segment of the population, inequitable income distribution and few advancement opportunities for the largely Amerindian population in the impoverished southern states. Forty per cent of the population lives below the poverty line, and household spending of the poorest 10% by percentage share is 1.6% compared with 41.1% for the richest 10%. The distribution of family income is unequal, and Mexico had a Gini coefficient of 0.52 in 2003 [1].

Mexico has an estimated labour force of 39.8 million, of which 20% is employed in agriculture, 24% in industry and 56% in the service sector. The urban unemployment rate is reported to be 3%. However, it is widely accepted that this is an underestimate, as there is considerable hidden unemployment due to part-time employment and underemployment [2].

A devaluation of the peso in late 1994 threw Mexico into economic turmoil, triggering the worst recession in over half a century, but the nation has made an impressive recovery. The value of Mexican currency rose from 9.1 Mexican pesos per US$ in 1998 to 11.5 in May 2004. The inflation rate based on consumer prices was 6.4% in 2002. Trade with the USA and Canada has tripled since the implementation of the North American Free Trade Agreement (NAFTA) in 1994. Mexico also implemented free trade agreements with Guatemala, Honduras, El Salvador and the European Free Trade Area in 2001, placing more than 90% of foreign trade under free trade agreements. The industrial production growth rate was 4.9% in 2002, with an oil production of 3.6 million barrels per day. Mexico's main trading partners are the USA, Canada, Japan and Germany. Based on purchasing power parity, the 2002 gross domestic product (GDP) was US$924.4 billion, with a real growth rate of 0.7% and a per capita GDP of US$8900. Thus, Mexico is considered to be a high middle-income country.

In July 2003, the population of Mexico was estimated to be 105 million, with 32% aged 14 years and under, 63% between 15 and 64 years, and the remaining 5% 65 years and over. The population growth rate was approximately 1.4% per year, the birth rate was 22 births per 1000 population, and there was a negative net migration rate of 2.7 migrants per 1000 population [3].

The health system

Mexico's healthcare system was well developed during the last century, with a large proportion of the population having quite good access to healthcare, which is reflected in the current life expectancy at birth of 72.3 years—69.3 years for men and 75.5 years for women. The 2003 mortality rate was 5 deaths per 1000 population, the infant mortality rate was of 23.7 per 1000 live births, and the fertility rate was 2.5 children per woman [4].

Morbidity due to chronic conditions and infectious diseases such as diabetes, obesity and hypertension associated with the so-called 'epidemiological transition', as well as pneumonia and diarrhoea, is prevalent in Mexico, and it is estimated that 10% of the population currently lacks effective access to the health services, mainly because of inadequate financing and mal-distribution of services. Healthcare access also remains a problem for the estimated 2 million people—2% of the population—living in remote districts. In addition, the health system faces pressures to allocate resources for prevention and treatment of infectious diseases that are emerging or re-emerging, such as AIDS, tuberculosis (TB) and malaria. Faced with this double set of pressures, the needs of the population could increase at a rate greater than the ability of the health system to respond. For example, there is increasing demand for services related to chronic conditions such as diabetes, obesity and hypertension, as well as for sophisticated medical technology to care for patients with injuries, cancer, organ failure and premature birth requiring intensive care [5].

Financing and structure

Healthcare services in Mexico are provided and financed through a mix of public and private schemes. In 2000, health expenditure was estimated to be 5% of GDP, or US$210 per capita. The public sector finances around 50–60% of the costs. As in other Latin American countries, the health sector in Mexico comprises a social security system, public hospitals and clinics for the uninsured, and private medicine. Most workers in the formal economy, or about 50% of Mexican families, are covered by the social security system.

The social security system is organized into various subsystems according to the employment status of individuals and their families. The Mexican Social Security Institute (IMSS) is the social security institution for employees of private companies, serving 40 million people; the Social Security Institute for State Employees (ISSTE) covers government employees, with 9 million people enrolled.

Approximately 50% of the population is uninsured, covered neither by social security institutions nor by private insurance, nor by the new 'Seguro Popular', described below. Of these, it is estimated that the poorest segment of society—approximately 2% of the population—lives in remote areas without any access to health services.

By law, the Mexican Ministry of Health is mandated to provide healthcare services and public health protection for the whole population as the 'provider of last resort'. However, in practice, only the poorest and those without the financial means to withstand catastrophic diseases use the Ministry of Health's services, known as the Secretaria de Salud (SSA). In 2003, there were 450 public hospitals and 12,000 primary healthcare clinics in the country providing services for the uninsured [6].

The poor and the lower middle class utilize public hospitals and health centres that collect modest user-fees and offer services perceived by users to be of low quality. The better off remainder of the uninsured population have partial or total access to health services through the private sector. The high-income population purchases private health insurance or pre-paid medical services, or simply pays out-of-pocket. Middle-income people with access to both social and private medical insurance tend to use specialized public hospitals for high-cost services; these hospitals charge user-fees that are highly subsidized by the federal government.

Recent reforms

The political changes of the past 10 years have created an environment favourable to transforming the health system through a major reform of the General Health Law. Over the years, the health sector has evolved through a slow decentralization process to a broad overhaul of financing, management and provision of health services. The main challenges to the health system were explicitly identified by a new federal government in the 2000 National Health Plan (PNS) [7] as: providing financial protection, improving the quality of care, increasing access to health services, preserving dignity and reducing socio-economic inequality in health services among the population. After 18 months of intense debate, reforms to the General Health Law received Congressional approval in April 2003. The law enshrines the principles of universality, solidarity and efficiency, while acknowledging for the first time that resources for health services are finite.

The main feature of the new legislation was the creation of the national Social Health Protection System or *Seguro Popular*. The system is designed as a social insurance scheme open to all by voluntary enrolment, as opposed to the traditional view of the public health service as a public assistance programme. Begun as a pilot project in 2002, the *Seguro Popular* aims to enrol 12 million families (52.8 million people) by the end of 2014, thereby making it the second largest insurance scheme in Mexico. The scheme is financed by federal and state governments, and by contributions levied on enrolled families. Resources transferred from the federal government to the state governments for the *Seguro Popular* relate to the number of families enrolled and are to cover the cost of an essential package of services. The states have to improve the provision, access to and quality of services in order to retain enrolees, increase the number of new enrolees and obtain additional resources. Each family receives an identification card, and its socio-economic information is kept in a database subject to government and independent audits. This information is used to determine the family's income level and establish its related financial contribution. Families classified as level 1 or 2 are in the lowest income bracket and are exempt from any contribution; families in levels 5 and 6 pay a maximum of US$5 per month. The programme is also funded by federal and state governments. The state and federal contributions come from general tax revenues, thus allowing for cross-subsidy from rich to poor, from healthy to sick, and from working adults to children and the aged. By the end of 2004, only 2 years after the programme was launched, there were 2 million families, or 7.8 million people, enrolled in the *Seguro Popular*, receiving health services in 29 of 32 states across the country.

The new system now guarantees access to an explicit list of medical services. This requires the government to implement a package of benefits with explicit limits built upon prioritization criteria. Thus, the reforms focus on guaranteeing utilization of appropriate and timely services.

Defining an essential package of services

The goal of the recent health reforms and the establishment of the *Seguro Popular* was to improve the health status of the most vulnerable segments of Mexico's population by guaranteeing access to a minimum package of essential services. These were defined as the cost-effective interventions affordable within available resources. Historically, the decisions about what should be included in benefits packages had been made by officials of the Ministry of Health and social security institutions. Officials were influenced by the preferences of stakeholders in the system, such as unions, Congress and state governments, rather than by evidence. In contrast, the recently defined universal healthcare benefits package [8] is divided into clusters of cost-effective interventions. The 10 main service categories are:

- public health education;
- public health outreach;
- ambulatory medical treatments;
- rehabilitation services;
- dental care;
- emergency services;
- acute hospital services;

+ surgical interventions;

+ trauma;

+ expensive treatments for catastrophic illnesses.

The new benefits plan [8] provides essential services in the above areas, but also covers several so-called catastrophic illnesses, including HIV and other medical conditions requiring high-cost technology. Their inclusion was supported by evidence of effectiveness. These diseases are all characterized by a low incidence, a very high cost and random occurrence among the general population, all of which have allowed for actuarial estimates of risk and cost. It was estimated that an average per capita expenditure of US$225 per year would provide for an essential package of 91 medical services [8] as well treatment of the following catastrophic illnesses: leukaemia in children, cervical–uterine cancer, AIDS, respiratory distress syndrome and very low birth weight in newborns. Treatment costs associated with congenital malformations, kidney, corneal and bone marrow transplantation, cancer and major trauma are also covered. In order to increase coverage and expand benefits, additional funding has to be available.

The selection of services and conditions to include within the benefits package was based on: clinical efficacy; incidence and utilization; potential lethality; expert clinical opinion; cost-effectiveness; and social preferences. Clinical protocols for essential services and high-cost illnesses such as HIV were developed, and their associated costs estimated from the number of prevalent and incident cases in the relevant population to compute the resources required for the health plan. The eventual goal is to develop a package of healthcare services aimed at promoting health, preventing disease and providing clinical and surgical treatments for all citizens with no age or gender discrimination.

The HIV epidemic

Epidemiology

The first AIDS case in Mexico was diagnosed in early 1983. By August 1985, there were only 39 reported AIDS cases, but there was a steady increase that was initially believed to have reached its peak in 1993 with approximately 5200 reported AIDS cases, after which the annual number reported stabilized at around 4000. However, after correcting for delay in reporting and undernotification, it is now estimated that the true peak of AIDS cases was likely to have been in 1999 with approximately 6000 cases [9].

Half of all cases in the national AIDS registry are derived from death certificates of individuals who were not diagnosed when they were alive. As a result, there is no epidemiological information on these cases in terms of transmission category or year of diagnosis. In addition, in 1999, the epidemiological surveillance system was decentralized, and notification of AIDS cases fell as a consequence. For instance, in 2002, a programme to recover unreported AIDS cases showed a total of 16,000 unreported cases, while the central files reported only 2000 cases [10].

By June 2003, the reported cumulative AIDS cases reached a total of 69,795, 85% of whom were male (59,228) and 15% female (10,567). The overall male-to-female ratio was 6:1. However, when discounting cases due to blood transfusion, and taking into account only sexually transmitted cases, that ratio rose to 10:1. Therefore, currently the epidemic in Mexico is mainly male, urban and sexually transmitted. However, there are new epidemics as a result of increased secondary heterosexual transmission, for example among injecting drug users (IDUs) in limited areas in the north of the country, clients of sex workers, and men who have sex with both men and women.

The routes of HIV transmission have varied according to gender. Among women, most cases at the beginning of the epidemic were due to blood transfusion; more recently, since blood banks have adopted safety measures, most infections in women have been through sexual transmission. The use of injecting drugs is minimal. HIV transmission among men has mainly involved unprotected homosexual intercourse: 61% of the cumulative AIDS cases in men reported homosexual or bisexual practices. (Fig. 38.1).

The vast majority of AIDS cases (96%) are found in towns and cities with over 2500 inhabitants, and 60% of those living with AIDS reside in six of the country's 32 states, in particular, the Federal District containing Mexico City and contiguous counties from the surrounding State of Mexico; the State of Jalisco, which contains Guadalajara, the second largest city in Mexico; and Veracruz, Puebla and Baja California.

Most AIDS cases (84%) were diagnosed and reported by the social security system, with the remaining cases divided almost equally among the services for the uninsured (SSA) and other sources, including private physicians. Males from larger cities and those who are formally employed are more likely to be insured by the social security institutions. Only 41% of the cumulative reported AIDS cases remain alive. This is not surprising, since almost half of them were identified from death certificates, and others, particularly those diagnosed at the beginning of the epidemic, died before the advent of antiretrovirals [11].

HIV is still primarily an epidemic of urban males who mainly acquire HIV through sex with men or with male or female sex workers, and a minority through injecting drug use. There are, however, emerging trends showing an increase in cases among the general population, especially the unemployed and uninsured, and poorer individuals, also in urban areas, as well as a new epidemic among women infected by their male partners [12].

In January 2004, the estimated number of people living with HIV (PLHIV) in Mexico ranged from 116,000 to 177,000 out of a population of 105 million. Several population surveys have been used to estimate HIV prevalence rates. National representative health surveys showed an

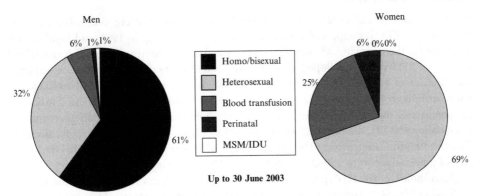

Fig. 38.1 AIDS cases by gender and route of transmission. Source: Registro Nacional de Casos de SIDA.

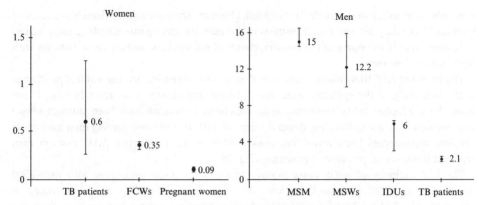

Fig. 38.2 HIV prevalence in selected groups from sentinel studies in Mexico, 1992–1997. Women and men are on different scales. The prevalence in women ranges from 0.09 to 0.06%; the prevalence in men ranges from 2.1 to 15%. The 95% confidence intervals are shown. Source: CENSIDA, Direccíon de Investigacíon, 2004.

estimated prevalence of 0.04% in 1987 and 0.1% in 2000 [13,14]. This had increased to 0.3% by 2003.

Sentinel surveys, while non-representative, have shown higher HIV prevalence rates among men than women. The median estimates from several surveys show the following prevalence rates: 15% among men who have sex with men (MSM); 12.2% among male sex workers (MSWs); 6% among IDUs; and 2% among TB patients. Among women, the most affected groups, as tested in convenience samples, were TB patients (0.6%); female sex workers (FSWs) (0.35%); and pregnant women (0.09%) (see Fig. 38.2).

In summary, the rising HIV epidemic is still highly concentrated in MSM and, to a lesser extent, in FSWs and among IDUs in limited geographical areas. However, risk to female partners of men at risk for HIV infection is increasing.

Treatment and care

Access to antiretroviral drugs came relatively late to Mexico (see Fig. 38.3). For example, zidovudine (AZT) was approved for public funding and use only in 1992, and highly active antiretroviral therapy (HAART) did not become standard care until 1998. The first specialized services for PLHIV were developed within the Mexican Ministry of Health in 1997. A year later, the Minister of Health made the political commitment to provide universal coverage for antiretrovirals in Mexico, but the federal government failed to allocate sufficient funds for the purchase of antiretrovirals, transferring only US$9 million to an *ad hoc* non-governmental organization (NGO), the National AIDS Fund (FONSIDA), which was created specifically to finance access to antiretrovirals. The current federal administration (2000–2006) has declared a goal of universal access to antiretrovirals for all PLHIV by the end of 2006.

The evolution of the HIV epidemic in Mexico and the measures taken in response to it are outlined in Fig. 38.3. Antiretrovirals were first prescribed by private providers for a minority of the richest people in the country, and later by social security providers covering around 50% of the individuals having a clinical prescription for antiretrovirals. The social security

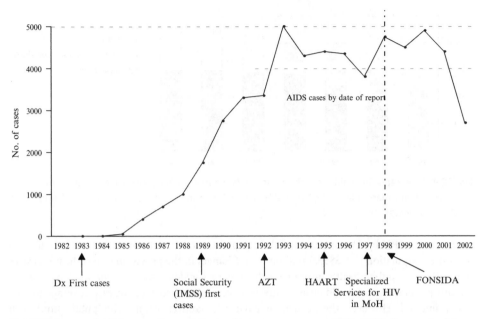

Fig. 38.3 Reported AIDS cases alive and the health system response, 1982–2002. Source: Registro Nacional de Casos de SIDA, June 30, 2002.

institutions were the first to provide public access to HAART. However, the decision to provide antiretrovirals was not based on cost-effectiveness or medical ethics, but rather was due to social mobilization and legal demands for access to antiretrovirals. Beginning in 1991, public services provided by the Ministry of Health (SSA) also purchased and provided antiretrovirals for a limited number of poor patients under research protocols. The coverage for antiretrovirals by mid-2003 was estimated to be between 75 and 90%, and the Ministry of Health's National Centre for AIDS estimated that 99% of PLHIV would have access to antiretrovirals by the end of 2003, including all living AIDS cases and an additional 25,082 people identified as living with HIV but who have not yet developed AIDS (Fig. 38.4).

Specialized care for HIV, including access to antiretrovirals, is provided in 24 states through 89 specialized centres running 119 clinics for testing and counselling for HIV and sexually transmitted infections (STIs). Several factors have contributed to attaining almost universal coverage for antiretrovirals. For instance, there was a decrease in the annual cost of treatment, from US$11,000 per patient [15] to US$4600 per patient in 2002–2003, following negotiations with pharmaceutical companies and their agreement to reduce their prices for government purchases.

The portion of Mexico's population that is without health insurance (about 50%) relies on the Ministry of Health for access to care, but most drugs, including antiretrovirals, are paid for by out-of-pocket expenditures. An increase in public budgets to purchase antiretrovirals for the uninsured population, to substitute out-of-pocket expenditure by public funds, was approved only recently. The 2002 budget for antiretrovirals was approximately US$36.5 million, and this was increased by US$17 million with a view to reaching the goal of universal

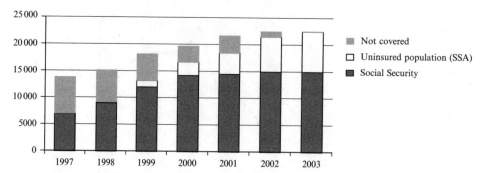

Fig. 38.4 Access to ARVs paid for with public funds. Source: authors' calculations based on unpublished information from the General HIV/AIDS Directorate. Source: Secretaria de Salud (SSA/CENSIDA), Mexico, 2004.

access to HAART by December 2003, bringing the total budget for antiretrovirals for the uninsured population to US$53.5 million [16]. Changes in the provision of healthcare services under the new public health insurance—the *Seguro Popular*—may provide further coverage for this population and could ensure universal access to catastrophic disease coverage for the newly infected. However, the burden of paying for antiretrovirals with public funds will depend on the willingness of the executive branch and Congress to approve special budget appropriations every year, and therefore will depend on social mobilization as well as support from the Ministry of Health.

Better understanding of HIV infection, a more predictable clinical course and the publication of clinical protocols for treatment have made it possible to simplify the treatment and management of HIV patients on an outpatient basis. The streamlining of clinical practices in treating AIDS patients has also helped reduce per-patient costs. Advances in medical therapy and the design of treatment packages that meet international standards have made it possible to define the most cost-effective therapy and make it accessible to a greater number of patients. The purpose of these packages is to achieve access, quality and equity in the supply of antiretroviral ambulatory treatment. Moreover, in regions where the epidemic is stable, costs are more predictable and the budgeting process less complex.

Voluntary counselling and testing

To assure the continuum of care, a programme of HIV testing and counselling was developed to coincide with timely provision of ART and hospital services. The programme has the following components: testing and counselling; ambulatory services (ART, prophylaxis and laboratory monitoring); hospital services for medical complications; and provider development (equipment, infrastructure, education and training).

Prevention

Prevention activities have proved to be a challenge for Mexico's health system. The first successful step in prevention was blood bank safety in 1986–1987. Prevention of mother-to-child transmission (MTCT) of HIV is still poor, depending upon different participating institutions and general access to antiretrovirals. In Mexico, as in many developing countries, the proportion of pregnant women who receive antenatal care at least once is relatively low, mainly due to poor access to health services, the perception that follow-up for healthy pregnancies is unnecessary and utilization of traditional midwives. Thus, the main barrier to preventing MTCT is insufficient access to antenatal care in general, and, therefore, to testing and counselling for women of reproductive age [17].

The administrative separation of preventive, public health and care services has limited prevention and other services for PLHIV. For instance, HIV-infected women do not regularly receive counselling on family planning, and AIDS patients receiving antiretrovirals are not offered advice on preventing transmission. Preventive measures among IDUs are sparse and are seldom provided by the public healthcare system, but rather by NGOs. Unpublished empirical evidence shows that individuals diagnosed as HIV-positive and eligible to receive antiretrovirals may never receive any prevention advice or interventions and are still not being targeted by prevention programmes.

Prevention of sexual transmission of HIV is carried out simultaneously by the healthcare system, civil society and several other actors dealing with sexuality, reproductive health, youth and education, among others. Initially, prevention activities were aimed at the general population, with a focus on women, young women, migrants and the rural population. Only recently has there been a focus on the most vulnerable populations through community-based organizations. The social security system has only developed prevention programmes focused on individuals rather than community-based programmes.

The most recent estimates of expenditure on HIV in Mexico from the National HIV/AIDS Accounts indicate that, of the US$2.07 per capita spent on HIV in 2002, only 20%, or US$0.41 per capita, was spent on prevention. Seventy per cent was spent on provision of care, 10% on administration, and less than 1%—or around US$1 million—on training [18].

The basic package for prevention and promotion includes:

- media campaigns to disseminate health education messages to the general population;
- campaigns targeting groups with high-risk behaviours relative to condom use and safe sex;
- provision of condoms and information to sex workers;
- a blood bank network for HIV screening of blood products;
- expansion of the coverage of STI treatment and quality assurance of these treatments; through the preparation of management protocols and continuing education, and improving drug availability in primary care clinics;
- implementation of needle exchange programmes and equipment disinfection for injecting drug users.

Diagnosis and treatment of STIs

Diagnosis and treatment of STIs is, in the context of HIV, considered to be an important public health and prevention issue [19,20]. Yet, such services are very limited in Mexico and, where they exist at all, are used primarily by young women and housewives, mainly because of the office hours of health establishments. The specialized services to treat STIs disappeared in the mid-1970s, on the expectation that STIs would be treated by family physicians. As a result, STI services are mainly offered during regular office hours, usually mornings, making it difficult for employed men to attend. Health planners have been asked to address this situation so that men and women who are employed and who are hesitant to request leave from their employers for this purpose can have access to STI services. Currently, the only stand-alone STI services are those targeting FSWs. Thus, there is a real need to expand these services to cover other populations vulnerable to HIV, as well as the general population.

The future challenge of financing services

As the HIV epidemic spreads in Mexico, its direct costs challenge the ability of healthcare institutions to provide services for those infected. The social costs are also enormous and affect families and entire communities. Financing varies according to different systems of care; for instance, an uninsured patient might have access to comprehensive care if included in a research project. However, the financial impact on the social security system, which provides resources for approximately 40% of the population in Mexico, and more than 50% of the AIDS cases, could be destabilizing in future. The *Seguro Popular* will provide financial protection to people who are, or have been, uninsured, utilizing federal and state subsidies, and co-payments from individuals according to their socio-economic status. In contrast, other patients attending public clinics may have to face out-of-pocket costs and thus might receive a lower standard of care because of economic barriers. The Mexican system does not generally provide for reimbursement of drug costs, and very frequently there are inadequate supplies of drugs, particularly expensive ones.

On average, the universal provision of a full range of health services has an estimated annual cost of US$12,871 per patient. Both preventive and curative services to mitigate the HIV epidemic are part of the benefits included in this service package. Yet, the annual cost of providing comprehensive services for 10,000 uninsured HIV-infected people has been calculated at US$128.7 million. Due to the high treatment costs associated with HIV, the most equitable way of mitigating the damage caused by this epidemic is to distribute the economic burden across the general population by financing these services, as far as possible, through general tax revenues. However, this may well mean difficult choices about how much to spend on each patient, given the increasing numbers of people likely to be on ART.

Conclusion

Several lessons can be drawn from the Mexican experience regarding both the responses specific to the HIV epidemic and, more generally, healthcare system reform. The government of Mexico concluded that the major challenges facing the health system in Mexico were: providing financial protection in the event of catastrophic illness; improving the quality of care; increasing access to health services; preserving the dignity of the patient; and reducing socio-economic inequalities in healthcare. In response, it created a national System for Social Protection of Health, operated by the *Seguro Popular*. The *Seguro Popular* scheme is considered the most equitable way to pay for costs related to HIV and other catastrophic illnesses because it is largely financed through general tax revenue and, therefore, distributes the economic burden across the whole population. This is an important improvement, given that private insurance does not cover HIV, and the existing social security institutions left half of the population, particularly those living in rural areas, without any health coverage at all.

Nevertheless, several challenges remain. Without major improvements in the area of prevention, and given the cost of antiretrovirals, it is unlikely that the current system can effectively provide adequate and comprehensive care for all those infected with HIV. There is also more work to be done to ensure greater financial protection to families coping with catastrophic illness and to reach the goal of providing ART to everyone who needs it.

The health and human rights agenda has gained enormous importance with the inclusion of HIV in the Ministry of Health's guaranteed package of services, since it is linked to equitable access to health services and therefore to human development. The approval of public funds to pay for such high-cost diseases is linked to the wider process of democratization that Mexico is experiencing. However, effective coverage and the financial sustainability of programmes for HIV will depend on the ability to pool risk and use the purchasing power of the state through a universal system of financing; the performance of Mexico's economy and the country's ability to invest in these treatments; and the ability to maintain democratic progress in the country.

References

1. Human Development Indicators. (2003). www.undp.org.hdi2003, accessed January 27, 2005.

2. Instituto Nacional de Geografía e Informática. Indicadores de Empleo. (2002). URL: http://www.inegi.gob.mx/est/contenidos/espanol/tematicos/coyuntura/coyuntura.asp?t=emp53&c=504.

3. Consejo Nacional de Población. (2002). Indicadores de Salud. URL: http://www.conapo.gob.mx/publicaciones/Cua-salud.htm.

4. Consejo Nacional de Población. (2002). URL: http://www.conapo.gob.mx/00cifras/00indicadores.htm.

5. Secretaría de Salud-México. (2000). Estadísticas e Indicadores. URL: http://pda.salud.gob.mx/msoxps.htm.

6. OECD Reviews of Health Care Systems: Mexico. (2005). Paris: Organization for Economic Co-operation and Development. URL: www.oecd.org.

7. Secretaría de Salud-México. (2000). Programa Nacional de Salud. México. URL: http://www.salud.gob.mx.

8. Avila-Figueroa C, Gómez-Fraga S, Herrera BE, Sousa FA, Lozano AR. (2002). *Estimación de los Costos de Producción de Servicios Clínicos para la Prevención, Diagnóstico y Tratamiento Medico*. Mexico City: Secretaría de Salud.

9. Izazola-Licea JA. (1997). *AIDS: State of the Art: A Review Based on the 11th International Conference on AIDS in Vancouver*. Mexico City: FUNSALUD.

10. Avila FC, McWhinney S, Chequer P *et al*. (1998). *Reconstructing and Predicting the HIV/AIDS Epidemic in Argentina, Brazil, Chile, and Mexico Using Mathematical Modeling*. The End Report. Mexico City: FUNSALUD.

11. Saavedra JA. (2003). State of the AIDS Epidemic in Mexico. National Centre for HIV/AIDS and STIs. Mexico City: Secretaría de Salud. Unpublished.

12. Avila-Figueroa C. (1997). Epidemiology and public health. In: Izazola-Licea JA, ed. *AIDS: State of the Art: A Review Based on the 11th International Conference on AIDS in Vancouver*. Mexico City: FUNSALUD, pp 94–110.

13. Secretaría de Salud, Mexico. (1987). *Encuesta Nacional de Salud (ENSE)*. Mexico City: Secretaría de Salud.

14. Secretaría de Salud, Mexico. (2000). *Encuesta Nacional de Salud (ENSE)*. Mexico City: Secretaría de Salud.

15. Saavedra LJ, Magis RC. (1998). *Costs and Spending on Medical Care of AIDS in Mexico*. CONASIDA: Series Angles of AIDS. Mexico City.

16. Izazola-Licea JA. (2003). *El Financiamiento de las Respuestas Nacionales Contra el SIDA en América Latina y el Caribe y el Flujo de Financiamiento Internacional*. Mexico City: FUNSALUD.

17. Reli K, Bertozzi S, Avila-Figueroa C. (2003). Cost-effectiveness of strategies to reduce mother-to-child transmission in a low HIV-prevalence setting. *Health Policy and Planning* 18(3):290–8.

18. Izazola JA, Avila-Figueroa C, Aran D *et al.* (2002). Country response to HIV/AIDS: National Health Accounts on HIV/AIDS in Brazil, Guatemala, Honduras, Mexico & Uruguay. *AIDS* 16:s66–75.

19. Mills A, Broomberg J, Lavis J, Soderlund N. (1993). *The Costs of HIV/AIDS Prevention Strategies in Developing Countries*. WHO. GPA/DIR/93.2. Geneva: WHO.

20. Ainsworth M, Over M. (1997). *Confronting AIDS: Public Priorities in to Global Epidemic*. World Bank Policy Research Report. New York: Oxford University Press.

Chapter 39

The United States of America

Bruce Fetter[*], Douglas Morgan and Jeffrey Levi[*]

The health system - Bruce Fetter

Political culture

How can the richest country on earth—one that, compared with all other countries in the world, spends the largest proportion of its wealth on healthcare—still leave 16% of its population uninsured[1]? That is one of the major paradoxes concerning this nation of 275 million with a 2001 per capita gross domestic product (GDP) of US$35,200, of which about 15% is spent on health (estimated as 13.9% in [2] and as 14.1% in [3]). Certainly, many patients benefit from the US$1.6 trillion now expended annually, but as long ago as the 1980s, 89% of Americans felt that the US healthcare system needed either fundamental changes or to be completely rebuilt [4]. Since then, politicians and citizens alike have recognized that the system is in crisis, but no solution is in sight.

To understand the US health system, one must touch on the political culture that underlies it, examine the circumstances that have made it different from those of other OECD countries, and trace trends in the way healthcare is funded and how those funds are allocated.

The political culture of US healthcare

Since its establishment and the displacement of its indigenous population, the USA has experienced high levels of immigration. Dominant English speakers imported African slaves, incorporated the inhabitants of former Spanish and Mexican territories in the South-West and regulated the migration of non-English-speaking Europeans, Latinos and, more recently, Asians. Indeed, unlike many Western European nations, the USA has been able to maintain an above replacement-level birth rate, thanks mainly to a very high birth rate among the Latino population [5]. Except for increases in the number of elderly, it should therefore maintain its current age–sex structure.

Unlike the more settled societies of Europe, Americans did not inherit an established healthcare system. Its first modern medical school, Johns Hopkins, did not open until 1893, and scientific standards of medical education were not generally established until the Flexner report of 1910 [6]. In the absence of top-of-the-line physicians, Americans went to the available healers and dosed themselves with patent medicines [7].

US society also lacked traditions of government intervention in healthcare. Indeed, in keeping with practices going back to the eighteenth century founding of the republic, many

* Corresponding authors.
The views expressed in this chapter are those of the authors and are not necessarily those of the organizations they work for, unless specifically stated in the text.

Americans distrusted central government initiatives. The Civil War of 1861–1865 was fought not only over the continuation of slavery but also over disagreements about the proper relationship between the federal government and the states. As late as the 1920s, Massachusetts refused federal money for poor women and children on the grounds that such payments were subversive of the state's authority [8]. Unlike OECD countries such as Britain, France and Germany [2], US aggregate spending on health by all levels of government remained low—16% of National Health Expenditures (NHE) in 1929 and 24% in 1960 [9]. Much of that money came from state and local governments as opposed to the federal government in Washington [10].

At the beginning of the twentieth century, the federal government spent less money on healthcare than did the states, which, in turn, spent less than their municipalities. The leadership of the latter was forced to take action to counter environmental degradation that was every bit as bad as that in European cities at the beginning of the Industrial Revolution. Before the First World War, American municipalities spent relatively large sums on public health, in particular to control infectious disease. States, by contrast, spent most of their health budgets on long-term care for the mentally ill, the developmentally disabled and those suffering from tuberculosis (TB). After the First World War, the federal government increased its expenditures both directly, through the construction of veterans' hospitals, and indirectly, through grants to the states that required matching contributions. Individual states were allowed to tailor programmes to their own needs, provided that they fell within federal guidelines. Municipalities, too, could apply for matching grants, although by the 1970s, they often lacked sufficient revenues to pay their share. By the end of the twentieth century, the relative role of the various levels of government was the reverse of what it had been a hundred years earlier. Federal spending comprised 70% of direct governmental appropriations, which vastly outstripped the 27% of the states and the 3% of the municipalities (3%).

The federal government took a more active role in health financing during the Second World War by exempting from taxation employer and employee payments to private insurers. This indirect subsidy to private insurance, financed through forgone revenues, has persisted to the present [11]. Although limited categories of the indigent and disabled received health benefits through post-war amendments to the Social Security Act of 1935, the real breakthrough to direct federal payments for health services came in 1965 with the enactment of Medicare and Medicaid. Medicare provides universal insurance coverage for all citizens over the age of 65 and for the disabled, but excludes preventive care, outpatient pharmaceuticals and long-term care. Medicaid provides federal matching funds to the states for medical care for the indigent and disabled of all ages and includes the three categories of services excluded from Medicare [12]. Today, if tax exemptions and insurance premiums paid by various levels of government for their employees are added to official estimates of government expenditure for healthcare, government pays for 57% of all US costs [13,14].

Behemoth: US healthcare delivery and its cost

By the 1970s, healthcare in the USA had more or less assumed its current configuration of providers. Hospitals consume the largest share of NHE at 30–40% of the total [9]. Governments own only a minority of them. In 1999, the federal government owned 5% of total units, and state and local governments 23%. The rest are divided between not-for-profit institutions (58%) and investor-owned ones (14%) [15]. At various times—during the 1965–1975 Vietnam War and in 1983—the federal government imposed cost controls that restrained expenditures [16].

After hospitals, physicians and clinical services constitute the next largest expense category, about 22% of NHE. The majority of doctors are in private practice, which explains why NHE hospital accounts include only trainees, recognizing that physicians bill for services separately. Most private practitioners are trained in tertiary care hospitals associated with medical schools, which employ both clinicians and researchers. Paradoxically, the tertiary care hospitals have a clientele that is very different from that seen by the average practitioner. In 1989, the government attempted to control physician costs but succeeded only in reducing the inflation rate for their services from 10 to 5% per annum [16].

To understand this paradox, we must take into account the relationship between the healthcare system and US society as a whole. In any given month, the tertiary centres treat fewer than 0.1% of the American population, while acute primary care hospitals admit approximately 0.8% of the population and 2% are seen as outpatients. About 22% of the population visit a physician's office, and another 7% consult a non-allopathic healer [16]. Most physicians, however, prefer to specialize rather than enter the three categories of primary care: family medicine, general internal medicine and paediatrics. In 1989, only 24% of medical students were training for primary care. Specialists provide primary care for approximately 20% of the population, a practice not discouraged, as in other countries, by legal restrictions that limit access to their services [17]. Still others consult physician's assistants and nurse practitioners.

The third largest expense in the NHE is pharmaceutical products (roughly 9%), including prescription drugs (6%) and over-the-counter items (3%). Although over-the-counter sales remained roughly constant, the cost of prescription drugs rose precipitously between 1995 and 2000, from 6.1% to 9.4% of NHE. This rise was due to direct advertisement to patients and to aggressive promotion by drug representatives to physicians of medications under patent [18].

Health status: the elephant has given birth to a mouse

Given the large sums spent on healthcare, the frequency with which Americans consult physicians and the enormous pharmaceutical industry, one might expect the health of Americans to be the best in the world. By some demographic measures, however, the US performance is mediocre. In 2002, the combined life expectancy at birth was 77.4 years—twentieth out of 30 members in the OECD, 3.5 years behind that of Japan. Infant mortality was 6.7 per 1000, twenty-third in the OECD and nearly double that of Sweden [19]. American performance was better regarding curative procedures. To take one rough indicator, the 5-year survival rate for all diagnosed cancers rose from 46% in 1973 to 60% in 1991 [20]. This compares favourably with a European Union (EU) average of approximately 45% in the period 1990–1994 [21].

The proximate cause of America's mediocre statistical performance is social inequality that leads to uneven access to care. In 1990, African American combined life expectancy at birth was 69.1 years, while that for whites was 76.1, seven years higher. Similarly, the infant mortality rate for African Americans, 18 per 1000, was more than twice as high as that for whites, 7.6 per 1000 [22]. Low socio-economic status has exacerbated these disparities. In the

1980s, for example, the infants of little-educated black mothers were 3.9 times as likely to die during their first year of life as the children of college-educated white mothers [22].

Race and class, however, do not explain all of the inequities of the American system. The poorest Americans have had access to care through Medicaid, as have the elderly and disabled through Medicare. The bulk of working Americans receive medical insurance through their employers, although recent increases in medical costs have reduced the proportion of workers insured and the number of items covered by insurance. The real losers in the US system are the working poor: the young, the self-employed and the non-citizens, who are often Latinos [23]. Medicaid coverage varies widely from state to state, ranging in 1998 from a low 9% of the population without coverage in Nebraska to 25% in Texas [1]. Even uninsured people can obtain care at hospital emergency rooms; the real problem lies in access to clinics, which might provide services to preclude hospitalization [24].

Another barrier to healthcare is cost. In 1996, 23% of the non-elderly population had no coverage for prescription drugs, and in 1998, 27% of the elderly lacked that coverage [16]. Of those with coverage, many cannot afford to make the co-payments not included in their insurers' payments. Although the proportion of healthcare paid out-of-pocket fell from 41% of NHE in 1966 to 15% in 2000, the latter proportion translated to a total of more than US$194 billion [9]. Demands for cash payments had real consequences for the poor. Children whose families lost welfare benefits after the reforms of 1996 were more likely to be hospitalized than those children whose families had retained government insurance protection [22].

The painful necessity of cost control

For half a century, cost control has been a chronic problem in US healthcare. In 1951–1953, expenditure on health amounted to 4.3% of GDP; by 2002, it had risen to 14.9% [2]. The largest relative increases occurred between 1979 and 1982, when the proportion of GDP rose 0.5% *per year*, and between 1985 and 1993, when the proportion of GDP rose 0.4% *per year* [9].

This suggests another factor in the political culture of the USA: politicians are reluctant to use the powers of government to control medical costs. Despite price controls during the Vietnam War and efforts to restrain hospital and physician fees in the 1980s, costs have continued to rise. No single sector has been responsible for this increase; the five largest items in the NHE all reached their maximum percentage of GDP after 1991. Hospital care attained a maximum of 4.8% of GDP in 1992–1993 and then fell back to 4.2% (US$412 billion) in 2000. Physician and clinical services reached a maximum of 3% of GDP in 1992–1995, falling back to 2.9% (US$286 billion) in 2000. The most precipitous increase was in the cost of prescription drugs, which rose from 0.4% of GDP in 1978–1981 to 1.2%, or over US$121 billion, in 2000. Similarly, the administrative and net cost of health insurance rose from 0.1% of GDP before 1958 to 0.8%, or over US$80 billion, in 2000. Finally, dental services rose from 0.3% of GDP in 1948–1953 to 0.6%, or almost US$60 billion in 2000 [9].

A number of cost-cutting measures have been applied to individual sectors, but none has succeeded in controlling health inflation. Medicare and Medicaid have imposed limits on reimbursement to hospitals and physicians, but prices have risen for other clients. Private insurers have organized hospitals and physicians into health maintenance organizations (HMOs) to reduce bills, but their restrictions on service have made them immensely unpopular. Desperate consumers have purchased their prescription drugs abroad, most notably in Canada, where they are sold more cheaply than at home, but the process is cumbersome and pharmaceutical manufacturers resist them at every step.

Nor have political leaders managed to intervene effectively. During his first term in office, President Bill Clinton failed to enact a universal insurance plan that would have come primarily at the expense of the private insurers. President George W Bush and his advisers purvey the nostrum that the system can be made more efficient by removing government entirely from the provision of healthcare and insurance and letting the market determine costs. Legislation enacted late in 2003 that is intended to provide Medicare payments for pharmaceuticals has a number of subversive features. It provides incentives to encourage private insurance companies to compete with Medicare and specifically forbids the government from negotiating with pharmaceutical companies to lower drug costs [25]. One wonders how to end the cozy relationship among the various providers that has already made US healthcare so expensive. Is marching away from the rest of the OECD the answer [8]?

The HIV epidemic - Douglas Morgan and Jeffrey Levi

Epidemiology

In the USA, HIV disproportionately affects racial or ethnic minorities, men who have sex with men (MSM) and injecting drug users (IDUs). While HIV was initially considered to be a predominantly male disease, the proportion of women infected with HIV has been growing rapidly in the last decade (Table 39.1). Almost all those affected by HIV in the USA come from vulnerable minorities; with the acquisition of HIV infection, all face potential and additional stigmatization [26].

Most groups affected by HIV also have legacies of distrust with the public health establishment and the healthcare delivery system. For example, a legacy of distrust between African Americans and public health researchers was created by the infamous Tuskegee experiment, which was conducted in the mid-twentieth century and deliberately permitted African American men to go untreated for syphilis long after effective treatments were available [30]. Until a 2003 Supreme Court decision, homosexual sex was criminalized in a number of states, making the very admission to a state health official of how HIV was transmitted a confession to a crime by confessing to homosexual activity. There is no national legislation and few state laws that protect gay men and lesbians from discrimination, as exists for discrimination based on race, ethnicity, gender and disability, including HIV.

There are also well-documented disparities in access to the healthcare system for racial or ethnic minorities in the USA, as well as MSM and IDUs [31]. This creates particular challenges as the health system asks these stigmatized groups to come forward and be identified for HIV testing and trust its recommendations regarding behaviour changes and healthcare treatment.

Finally, HIV disproportionately affects the poor in the USA, as evidenced by the proportion of people with HIV and AIDS who are eligible for poverty-based healthcare programmes. The federal government estimates that 44% of people living with HIV (PLHIV) are on Medicaid. It is also estimated that at the time of diagnosis, 22% of those with HIV are already on Medicaid. In a country without universal health insurance, and for a disease that

Table 39.1 Demographics

Estimated number of people living with HIV	850,000–950,000
Cumulative AIDS cases, estimated	929,985
Living AIDS cases, estimated	405,926
Annual new HIV infections, estimated	40,000
Proportion of infections among African Americans (proportion of US population)	50% (12%)
Proportion of infections among Latinos (proportion of US population)	15% (14%)
Proportion of infections among whites (proportion of US population)	32% (68%)
Proportion of HIV cases among men who have sex with men	45%
Proportion of HIV cases among injecting drug users	15%
Proportion of HIV cases due to heterosexual contact	34%
Increase in the proportion of AIDS cases among women 1990 to 2003	13–27%

Sources: [27–29].

has very costly, long-term treatment, the additional layer of poverty creates particular challenges for access to appropriate care.

Prevention

HIV prevention efforts to date in the USA have been marked by an emphasis on reaching the affected communities of those at risk and those with HIV with behaviour change messages, and a belief that these messages are most effectively delivered by those who come from these communities. Broad-based national education campaigns, except those to overcome irrational fears of transmission early in the epidemic, have been uncommon.

Most HIV prevention programmes are funded by the US federal government, primarily through the US Centers for Disease Control and Prevention (CDC). CDC is the lead federal public health agency in charge of health promotion activities and disease surveillance. The federal Substance Abuse and Mental Health Services Administration is responsible for substance abuse prevention, a critical component of HIV prevention. This division of labour has created coordination challenges. However, programmes are administered by state and local health departments and community-based organizations, all of which are given flexibility in designing their approaches to preventing further transmission of HIV. The nature of the epidemic varies significantly from state to state—some have high levels of sexual transmission, while others face a larger injecting drug use problem—and the nature of the approach to prevention also varies depending on the targeted population. It is widely held that different approaches are needed for socially diverse populations. For example, prevention programmes will be different for Latinas as opposed to African American MSM.

While flexibility is given to communities in the USA to design their own approaches to HIV prevention, there have been significant restrictions placed on how federal funds may be spent. No federal funds may be spent on syringe exchange programmes (SEPs) for IDUs, despite overwhelming scientific evidence of their effectiveness [32]. Politically, SEPs have been extremely controversial in the USA. While a number of communities have supported such programmes with their own resources, the US Congress has repeatedly forbidden use of federal funds for this purpose. Restrictions are also placed on the content of prevention materials and programmes supported with government funds. Overly explicit references to sexual activity—particularly programmes that address homosexual sex—are generally not permitted.

For over a decade, the US CDC has estimated that there are approximately 40,000 new HIV infections each year. In an effort to reduce this number dramatically, the CDC has recently announced a new direction for US prevention activities [33], placing an emphasis on prevention for those who are HIV-positive, as opposed to those at risk in general, and the integration of HIV prevention into the primary care setting, not unlike efforts for other chronic diseases. This has been met with concern by some in the HIV community, as they fear that other programmes that are community-based and reaching out to those at risk might be cut to make way for this new approach. This concern is premised on the fact that HIV prevention funding in the USA has been relatively flat for a number of years, with prevention often losing out in budget debates to the demand for increased HIV care services. There is a more vocal political constituency in the USA advocating for care and treatment funds; the advocacy for prevention is much weaker. This is reflected in the funding levels for the US CDC's domestic prevention programmes, which have seen marginal declines in the last several years. Funding in fiscal year 2001 was US$795.4 million; in fiscal year 2004, funding was set at US$788.2 million. In contrast, funding for the Health Resources and Services Administration, which funds health services, rose from US$1.7 billion to US$2.045 billion, primarily to support access to new drugs [34].

Treatment and care

Unlike any other chronic disease in the USA, with the exception of end-stage renal disease, HIV care is disproportionately financed by the public sector. A majority of people with HIV use three public programmes to finance their care: Medicaid, which serves certain low-income individuals, including the disabled; Medicare, which serves the elderly and the long-term disabled; and the Ryan White Comprehensive AIDS Resources Emergency (CARE) Act, which serves PLHIV (Table 39.2). About 20,000 people with HIV also get care through the Veterans Health Administration, a US national health service that cares for veterans. A federally funded study found that, of those in regular care in 1996, 44% had their care financed by Medicaid, 6% by Medicare only, though more were dually eligible for Medicaid and Medicare, and 20% were uninsured [J Fleishman, personal communication (2002)]. Only 31% were privately insured; however, an unknown but probably significant number of those with private insurance also accessed publicly funded services if their private insurance coverage was inadequate due, for instance, to insufficient prescription drug coverage.

The centrality of public programmes is also made clear by the levels of spending for HIV. Federal and state spending on Medicaid for HIV-related services was estimated at US$9.3 billion in fiscal 2004; Medicare spending was $2.6 billion and CARE Act spending $2.045 billion in the same time frame, totalling US$13.945 billion [35].

Of these publicly financed programmes, the Ryan White CARE Act is the only one that is dedicated to providing support for care and treatment service for PLHIV. The CARE Act provides support for a continuum of service through a series of grant programmes to local and state governments, HIV primary care providers at either the institutional level or community-based level, and to HIV social service programmes. The CARE Act serves over 500,000 people per year. One component of the CARE Act that has grown in both importance and funding is the AIDS Drug Assistance Program (ADAP). This effort provides funding to 54 eligible states and territories that purchase and distribute HIV-related

Table 39.2 Major US Department of Health and Human Services public programmes financing HIV care in the USA

Programme/spending fiscal year 2004	Funding source	Eligibility	Services
Medicaid/US$5.4 billion in federal spending. On average, states pay another 40% of costs, which would bring total to US$7.56 billion in federal and state spending	Jointly funded and administered by the federal and state governments	Entitlement programme: funding increases to assure access to those who meet eligibility requirement. These vary by state (for the disabled, usually at 74% of the US federal poverty rate of US$9570 for an individual).	Varies by state, most core primary care services, though many states place limits on prescription drugs
Medicare/US$2.6 billion.	Funded and administered by federal government	Entitlement programme: funding increases to assure access to those who meet eligibility requirement. Eligibility criteria are the same nationally: those over 65 and those who are long-term disabled	Full inpatient and outpatient primary care services, with significant co-payments. Most beneficiaries receive no prescription drug coverage
Ryan White CARE Act/US$2.0 billion	Funded by the federal government; administered through grants to states, localities and NGOs.	Discretionary programme: funding is limited to a specific amount determined each year by the US Congress. Eligibility criteria for services determined by localities based on available resources.	Outpatient services of all kinds funded including primary care and social services. Range of services determined by local planning process. Major portion, 33% of funds are set aside for the purchase of HIV-related drugs

Source: [40,41].

Note: other US agencies provide HIV care. The Department of Veterans Affairs and the Department of Defense health systems provide HIV care to their beneficiaries.

pharmaceuticals to eligible clients. The number of US dollars appropriated to this one activity has grown from US$52 million in fiscal 1996 to US$749 million of the fiscal 2004 CARE Act Appropriation. ADAP's proportion of CARE Act funding rose in that same time frame from 7% to 37%, reflecting the growing importance of access to pharmaceuticals in US HIV care. In recent years, almost all increases in the CARE Act's funding have been allocated to the purchase of HIV medications, leaving other services struggling to meet demand. It should be noted that the total spending for AIDS drugs is significantly higher than the ADAP appropriation. Many states—though not evenly throughout the USA—contribute additional funds to their local ADAP programme, increasing available funds by approximately 20% [36]. Even with these new resources, ADAPs throughout the USA have been forced to create waiting lists or adopt other measures that limit access to the programme. As a result, formularies and eligibility criteria vary on a state-by-state basis.

This patchwork of programmes is reflective of the underlying US healthcare system, where responsibility for financing and delivery of services is shared among federal, state and local governments. Thus, for example, the Ryan White CARE Act allocates federal funds for services to high-impact localities (under 'Title I' of the Act) and state health departments (Title II), which either provide services directly or subcontract with non-governmental organizations (NGOs). The CARE Act also provides funding directly from the federal government to NGOs (under Titles III and IV). Together, these programmes attempt to provide a continuum of care-related services for PLHIV. This continuum includes the following:

1. *Primary care medical services.* This includes access to an experienced provider, given research that shows that health outcomes are often better if a member of the care team is more experienced with HIV disease [37,38].

2. *HAART and other drug therapies.* Access to highly active antiretroviral therapy (HAART) is directly associated with the positive changes in mortality and disability rates for people with HIV in the USA. However, with prescription drug coverage often limited or non-existent in private insurance and Medicare, and the high number of uninsured among PLHIV, access to these very expensive prescription drugs is often not assured.

3. *Medical case management services*, including adherence services. Such services are particularly important given the complexity of HIV treatment and the co-morbidities experienced by many people with HIV.

4. *Social case management services.* The social service needs of HIV-positive individuals will vary dramatically, based on co-morbidities and stage of disease, with more intensive HIV-related services needed during end-of-life care, but are often critical to the initiation or maintenance of care treatment.

5. *Behavioural health services.* Many people with HIV need mental health and substance abuse treatment services, both as primary conditions and as they relate to their HIV infection.

6. *Prevention services.* As discussed above, there is growing emphasis in the USA on prevention in the primary care setting. This is considered important both to prevent further transmission of HIV and to address the new concern with superinfection and its potential impact on the efficacy of HAART treatments.

7. *Access to housing services.* A disproportionate number of people with HIV have housing difficulties, including homelessness [39]. These have an impact on the ability of individuals to adhere to treatment regimens and adopt prevention strategies.

8. *Other support or enabling services*, including childcare and transportation.

These services in the USA are provided through the patchwork of public programmes described in Table 39.2. While all are financed in whole or in part with federal funds, tremendous flexibility is given to states and localities in the design of the programmes as they are implemented at the local level. This extends to basic criteria such as income eligibility standards and coverage of basic services. Thus, the breadth of the continuum of services available to an individual with HIV in the USA is very dependent on geography— where you live determines what services you will receive. An individual living in a state with a very generous Medicaid programme and receiving substantial Ryan White CARE Act funds may be eligible for a full set of primary care and social services; if that same individual moved to a state with a less generous Medicaid programme, he or she might be eligible for no public benefits. All systems of healthcare delivery ration access to care and services based on available resources. In the USA, this is compounded by disparities based on geography.

In the mid- to late 1990s, it was generally believed that this array of programmes was able to meet the demand for HIV services, even though access to these services was often a challenge for the individual due to the complexity of the programmes and their eligibility criteria. At the turn of the century, however, there was increasing concern that the system of healthcare delivery was facing particular stresses due to a multiplicity of factors. There is an overall increase in the demand for HIV-related care and related drug treatments due to a steady increase of 40,000 new HIV infections a year; more people with HIV are learning their status earlier as there is more hope about successful treatment; and those already diagnosed are living longer as a result of the success of new treatments. Furthermore, new HIV drugs tend to be additive and very expensive, and co-morbidities, especially hepatitis C virus (HCV), have very costly prescription drug treatments.

Additional pressure results from the peculiarities of eligibility for, and financing of, the programmes. People with HIV are not progressing to disabling conditions as rapidly, if at all. Yet this is the usual pathway to eligibility for the Medicaid and Medicare programmes. As noted above, these are entitlement programmes—funding must increase to meet the demand unless the criteria for eligibility are changed. As states face serious budget crises, they are cutting back on eligibility and benefits under the Medicaid programme, which they co-fund with the federal government. Thus, more and more individuals remain dependent on the services of the Ryan White CARE Act, which do not automatically receive additional money based on demand but require increased appropriations from Congress. Funding for the Ryan White CARE Act has only increased 7% in the last 3 years, with the bulk of that, as noted above, going to the AIDS Drug Assistance Program.

In short, the HIV crisis in the USA has struck particularly vulnerable populations in terms of their ability to access appropriate care and services through the private sector, which is the foundation of US healthcare financing. The result has been the creation of a series of HIV-specific adaptations to the system that are not required in countries with universal access to care guaranteed by the public sector, and the creation of competition between resources devoted to prevention and care that are not issues in other developed countries.

Conclusion

Navigating the complex system of prevention and care in the USA can be challenging for a person with HIV. The USA does not have an integrated healthcare delivery or financing system, even within public sector programmes. Many have noted that the challenges faced by people with HIV are simply a lens through which one can see the larger challenges of the US healthcare system. This is indeed true. However, as challenging as things are for people with HIV, the presence of multiple HIV-specific programmes provides access to more services for poor people with HIV than for those with other chronic conditions. Indeed, while there are probably few lessons to offer other countries regarding HIV care *financing*, given that most other nations rely on a publicly financed system, the US recognition of a need for a broad continuum of services does provide a model for care *delivery* for nations across the world.

References

1. Martin A, Whittle L, Levit K. (2001). Trends in state health care expenditures and funding: 1980–1998. *Health Care Financing Rev* 2(4):111–40.
2. *OECD Health Data 2003*. Paris: OECD.
3. Levit K, Smith C, Cowan C. (2003). Trends in U.S. health care spending (2001). *Health Affairs* 22(1):154–64.
4. Jee M, Or Z. (1999). *Health Outcomes in OECD Countries: A Framework of Health Indicators for Outcome-oriented Policymaking*. OECD Labour Market and Social Policy, Occasional Papers No. 36. Paris.
5. Bachu A and O'Connell A. (2001). *Fertility of American Women: June 2000*. Current Population Reports. Washington, DC: US Census Bureau p 20–543 RV.
6. Ludmerer K. (1985). *Learning to Heal: The Development of American Medical Education*. New York: Basic Books.
7. Young JH. (1961). *The Toadstool Millionaires: A Social History of Patent Medicine in America*. Princeton, NJ: Princeton University Press.
8. Rosenkrantz BG. (1972). *Public Health and the State: Changing Views in Massachusetts*. Cambridge, MA: Harvard University Press.
9. National Health Expenditures. (2002). *Center for Medicare and Medicaid Services*. Office of the Actuary, National Health Statistics Group.
10. Fox DM. (1997). The competence of states and the health of the public. In: Leichter HM. *Health Policy Reform in America: Innovations from the States*. 2nd edn. Armonk, NY: M.E. Sharpe, p29–46.
11. Fox DM. (1993). *Power and Illness: The Failure and Finance of American Health Policy*. Berkeley: University of California Press.
12. Brown L, Sparer M. (2003). Poor program's progress: the unanticipated politics of Medicaid policy. *Health Affairs* 22(1):31–44.
13. Fox DM, Fronstin P. (2000). Public spending on health approaches sixty percent. *Health Affairs* 19(2):271–3.
14. Woolhandler S, Himmelstein DU. (2002). Paying for national health insurance—and not getting it. *Health Affairs* 21(4):88–104.
15. American Hospital Association. (2001). *Hospital Statistics 2001 Edition*. Chicago: Health Forum.
16. Oberlander J. (2003). *The Political Life of Medicare*. Chicago and London: University of Chicago Press.
17. Green LA, Fryer GE, Yawn BP, Lanier D, Dovey SM. (2001). The ecology of medical care revisited. *New England Journal of Medicine* 344(26):2021–25.

18. Ludmerer K. (1999). *Time to Heal: American Medical Education from the Turn of the Century to the Era of Managed Care.* New York: Oxford University Press.

19. Kreling DH, Mott DA, Wiederholt JB. (2001). *Presciption Drug Trends: A Chartbook Update.* Menlo Park, CA: Kaiser Family Foundation.

20. *Historical Statistics of the United States: Millennial Edition.* (1999). Pre-print. Cambridge: Cambridge University Press.

21. Cancer Research UK. (2004). *Cancer in the EU: Survival in the European Union.* URL: http://info.cancerresearchuk.org/canceerstats/cancerineu/survival/.

22. Haines M, Steckel R. (2000). *A Population History of North America.* Cambridge: Cambridge University Press.

23. Hogue CJR, Hargraves MA. (1993). Class, race, and mortality in the United States. *American Journal of Public Health* 83(1):9–12.

24. Starr P. (1987). *The Social Transformation of American Medicine.* New York: Basic Books.

25. Cook JT, Frank DA, Berkowitz C *et al.* (2002). Welfare reform and the health of young children: a sentinel survey in 6 U.S. cities. *Archives of Pediatrics and Adolsecent Medicine* 156(7):678–84.

26. Herek GM, Capitanio JP, Widaman KF. (2002). HIV-related stigma and knowledge in the United States: prevalence and trends, 1991–1999. *American Journal of Public Health* 92(3):371–7.

27. Fleming PL, Byers RH, Sweeney PA, Daniels D, Karon JM, Janssen RS. (2002). HIV prevalence in the United States, 2000, Presented at the 9th Conference on Retroviruses and Opportunistic Infections, Seattle, WA, Abstract 11.

28. US Centers for Disease Control. (2003). *HIV / AIDS in 33 States, 2003.* CDC HIV/AIDS Surveillance Reports, Vol. 15.

29. US Census Bureau. US Census, 2000. Available at: http://www.census.gov/statab/www/.

30. Jones JH. (1981) *Bad Blood: The Tuskegee Syphilis Experiment.* New York: The Free Press.

31. Andersen R, Bozzette S, Shapiro M *et al.* (2000). Access of vulnerable groups to antiretroviral therapy among persons in care for HIV disease in the United States. HCSUS Consortium. HIV Cost and Services Utilization Study. *Health Services Research* 35(2):389–416.

32. Norman J, Vlahow D, Moses L, eds. (1995). *Preventing HIV Transmission: the Role of Sterile Needles and Bleach.* Washington, DC: National Academy Press.

33. CDC. (2004). Advancing HIV Prevention: New Strategies for a Changing Epidemic. Division of HIV/AIDS Prevention, National Center for HIV, STD and TB Prevention, Interim Technical Guidance. URL: http://www.cdc.gov/hiv/partners/ahp.htm. (Accessed March 2005).

34. Kaiser Family Foundation. (2004). Federal Funding for HIV/AIDS: The FY 2005 Budget Request. URL: http://www.kff.org/hivaids/loader.cfm?url=/commonspot/security/getfile.cfm&PageID=31456.

35. Kaiser Family Foundation. (2004). Trends in U.S. Government Funding for HIV/AIDS Fiscal Years 1981 to 2004. URL: http://www.kff.org/hivaids/loader.cfm?url=/commonspot/security/getfile.cfm&PageID=33622.

36. Kaiser Family Foundation. (2004). AIDS Drug Assistance Programs. URL: http://www.kff.org/hivaids/loader.cfm?url=/commonspot/security/getfile.cfm&PageID=36216.

37. Kitahata MM, Koepsell TD, Deyo RA *et al.* (1996). Physicians' experience with the acquired immunodeficiency syndrome as a factor in patients' survival. *New England Journal of Medicine* 334:701–6.

38. Laine C, Markson LE, McKee LJ *et al.* (1998). The relationship of clinic experience with advanced HIV and survival of women with AIDS. *AIDS* 12:417–24.

39. Cunningham WE, Andersen RM, Katz MH *et al.* (1999). The impact of competing subsistence needs and barriers on access to medical care for persons with human immunodeficiency virus receiving care in the United States. *Medical Care* 37:1270–1281.

40. Kaiser Family Foundation. (2005). US Federal Funding for HIV/AIDS: The FY 2006 Budget Request. Menlo Park, CA: Kaiser Family Foundation. Available at: http://www.kff.org/hivaids/loader.cfm?url=/commonspot/security/getfile.cfm&PageID=51641 for spending totals in FY 2004.

41. Centers for Medicare & Medicaid Services. (2005). Baltimore, MD: CMMS. Available at: http://www.cms.hhs.gov/publications/overview-medicare-medicaid/default4.asp for average state match. Accessed May 19, 2005.

Global and National Responses

Chapter 40

The UN response to the HIV pandemic

Eric van Praag[*], Karl L Dehne and Venkatraman Chandra-Mouli

Introduction

It is commonly held that significant conceptual differences within and among international agencies' AIDS policies and strategies hindered an effective response to the epidemic during the 1980s and early 1990s. In fact, one of the reasons for the establishment of the Joint United Nations Programme on HIV/AIDS (UNAIDS) in 1996 was the recognition of the need 'to bring the AIDS activities of six UN agencies into a synergistic effort' [1]. Considerable efforts appear to have been made to harmonize policies and coordinate action since then. Two consecutive unified work plans of UNAIDS and its co-sponsoring agencies have been elaborated [2,3], and various processes of regional strategy development involving UN agencies, bilateral agencies, government representatives and non-governmental organizations (NGOs) embarked upon. A new global AIDS strategic framework [4], which supersedes previous global strategies developed by the World Health Organization (WHO) almost a decade earlier, sets 'guiding principles and leadership commitments that together form the basis for a successful response to the epidemic'. According to the UNAIDS Secretariat's own assessment, 'common ground is increasingly replacing the ideological divides that often hampered previous efforts' [4].

However, little analysis of key features of global AIDS policy and the underlying conceptual differences within and between agencies, and of the extent to which policies have indeed converged, has been carried out. In this chapter, we will examine some historical aspects of the AIDS policy debate within the UN family. In particular, we shall first attempt to show that international AIDS policy has evolved, as had public health policies earlier on, from an emphasis on individual risks and targeted behavioural interventions towards addressing the societal-level determinants of the epidemic. We shall, furthermore, show that international AIDS policies and strategies have changed from an early emphasis on disease control to the promotion of community development, only to swing back later to a biomedical model that embraces new disease control elements such as rapid testing and antiretroviral treatment. Conceptual differences and developments within and between programmes and agencies in intervention approaches will be highlighted to describe further the evolution within the UN community of a balanced HIV response addressing vulnerability and stigma issues while at the same time scaling up access to effective therapies within strengthened health systems.

* Corresponding author.

The views expressed in this chapter are those of the authors and are not necessarily those of the organization they work for, unless specifically stated in the text.

We draw on a large number of WHO, UNAIDS, United Nations Children's Fund (UNICEF) and World Bank policy documents, country strategic plans and our own experiences in policy discussions in both WHO and UNAIDS.

Public health debates before HIV

Disease control versus community empowerment

Most disease control programmes in existence today are ultimately based on principles that guided the successful Smallpox Eradication Programme model, which involves measurable targets of the programme. Secondly, they design a multifaceted strategy to meet these objectives. Lastly, they implement targeted interventions relating to the strategy, or ensure that this is done by appropriate individuals and organizations. Evaluation and monitoring are carried out to determine whether or not the objectives are achieved [5].

If the 1970s saw the eradication of smallpox through the application of a technology-based disease control approach, the decade also heralded the arrival of some revolutionary thinking in public health, which culminated in the Alma-Ata Declaration at the International Conference on Primary Health Care in 1978 [6]. The proponents of this primary healthcare (PHC) approach viewed poor health as due, in large part, to the inequitable distribution of power and wealth. They argued that ill health could not be eradicated by the application of new technologies alone. The solution that they proposed was the vigorous application of a community empowerment approach through full information and participation, to change drastically what they saw as an unacceptable and exploitative situation.

The WHO's historic Alma-Ata Declaration called for international commitment to involve people in the design, choice and delivery of their own healthcare in what was a radical departure from the conventional thinking of that era [6]. The strategic consequences were taken up to the extent possible by many Ministries of Health, the UN agencies, in particular WHO and the United Nations Development Programme (UNDP), and the donor community, in particular the Nordic and Western European countries. As a result, specific units in Ministries of Health were charged with promoting PHC and the establishment of village health committees, supporting training of new multipurpose cadres such as community health workers and strengthening peripheral health units such as dispensaries and PHC centres. At the same time, targeted disease control was promoted as well. A 'selective PHC strategy' was proposed and supported in particular by UNICEF. This strategy viewed Alma-Ata as too idealistic and called for cost-effective interventions to address in the short run the most prevalent and debilitating illnesses with available techniques such as oral rehydration solutions and measles vaccinations [7]. The debate between disciples of the disease control approach and advocates of a more participatory approach to bringing about improvements in health in a broader sense has continued ever since and is well reflected in the structure of WHO and many ministries of health in which divisions responsible for reducing disease burden through targeted technical interventions operate beside divisions devoted to strengthening health systems and primary or community health development.

Not all public health planners and policy-makers have seen the two approaches as fundamentally antithetical, however [8]. Many view multisectoral participation and community involvement as relatively more or less important, depending on the specific health problem, and as a means to an end rather than an end in itself, as the development of the response to HIV within WHO and UNAIDS has shown.

From health education to health promotion

In the area of health education, the mid-1980s saw this shift in perspective from disease control to community development; from an individual and community health education focus towards a societal-level health promotion articulated in an international consensus statement. The Ottawa Declaration defined 'health promotion' as 'the process of enabling people to increase control over and to improve their health' [9,10]. In the same year as the Ottawa declaration, a review of health education approaches in developing countries contrasted the educational, community development approach supported by WHO with the more target-oriented promotional approach supported by UNICEF [11]. The former encompassed a continuum of initiatives that varied from projects that organized community committees as vehicles for collaboration to projects that worked with communities with no prior agenda other than to empower the people. The latter was best seen in social marketing terms, with people considered to be informed consumers of cheap or free and effective immunization and nutrition services rather than individuals to be educated and empowered [11].

The initial response to AIDS

At the same time as the new health promotion concepts were being developed and applied, one of the most serious threats to human health in the twentieth century emerged. However, precisely because HIV infection was new, the initial response had to emphasize the dissemination of information on the nature of the newly detected infection, its modes of transmission and means of avoiding it, as well as anti-discrimination messages to confront 'denial, hysteria and moral panic' [12]. According to the final report of WHO's Global Programme on AIDS (GPA), 'Especially in the earlier stages of the unfolding pandemic,... the development and dissemination of scientifically credible and reliable information on HIV was an invaluable tool in GPA's unrelenting and largely successful effort to advocate a strong and clear public health rationale for protecting the human rights and the dignity of persons living with AIDS' [13].

The initial responses of the GPA and its predecessor, the Special Programme on AIDS (SPA), bore many of the hallmarks of a disease control approach to contain the outbreak of a fatal infectious agent, even though a technological 'fix' was nowhere in sight. According to the earliest Global AIDS Strategy, as outlined in SPA's first progress report, AIDS would be controlled by 'attacking every mode of AIDS virus spread, in every country, using every scientific and educational tool' [14]. HT Mahler, the Director General of WHO at the time, announced: 'In the same spirit that WHO has addressed smallpox eradication, WHO will dedicate its energy, commitment and creativity to the even more urgent, difficult and complex task of global AIDS prevention and control' [14].

Evident from the slogan 'AIDS: a worldwide effort will stop it!', Jonathan Mann, the first Executive Director of GPA, and his team expected considerable results from the control programmes that they helped many countries put in place [15,16]. GPA provided rapid assistance to gather information on the spread of HIV and to develop short- and medium-term National AIDS Control Plans. Funds were easily made available to cover the costs of setting up National AIDS Programme (NAP) infrastructures, surveillance and logistics systems for HIV test kits and condoms, as well as information, education and communication (IEC) programmes. At the same time, the most heavily affected communities in the industrialized countries, for instance gay communities, and healthcare staff and their families in developing countries such as Uganda, had already begun to mobilize themselves, demonstrating what can be considered the earliest community responses to the epidemic [17]

From awareness-raising to behavioural change

Following what GPA's final report calls the emergency stage of the international response to HIV [13] and after, 'well-known and longstanding inadequacies of human resources and infrastructure had hampered a more effective implementation of medium-term plans' [16], the expanding epidemics in Africa, the West and Asia proved that the initial hopes for control had been unrealistic. It was now increasingly recognized that 'technologies' such as value-free information, condoms and drugs to treat sexually transmitted infections (STIs) were valuable, but could not by themselves solve the AIDS problem. AIDS would be around in the foreseeable future. Other important factors fuelling the epidemic needed to be properly understood and effectively dealt with. As the report acknowledges, 'although the early years were spent chasing but never really getting ahead of the virus, there was growth in understanding how to confront it' [13].

A key strategy element that was re-examined during this period was the role of sexual behaviour and how people could be motivated to change it. 'The implementation of effective technologies to prevent HIV-transmission (had) proved to be profoundly complex and difficult; the importance of behavioural factors was underestimated in the early stages of the pandemic' [13]. GPA then systematically assessed behavioural models for their relevance to HIV prevention [18], behavioural scientist posts were created, and in 1991, GPA's Steering Committee on Social and Behavioural Research met for the first time [19]. Growth in the volume of research carried out in this area was subsequently reported upon as one of GPA's achievements [20].

Nevertheless, approaches and strategies implemented in the field continued to vary enormously. In Africa and South Asia, pilot projects using behavioural change approaches among vulnerable populations were successful, although their replication on a large scale was proving difficult [21]. Prevention efforts in low-prevalence regions such as in East Asia, the Pacific, and Central and Eastern Europe mainly took the form of HIV surveillance and the dissemination of infection prevention and control information during the early 1990s [22–24].

The growing emphasis on behavioural change enabled interventions to become more focused. 'Instead of a shotgun approach to selecting targets for change, health educators can now decide in advance on what needs to be considered as a priority area for change and adopt the most appropriate strategies for changing them', one report concluded [18]. 'A shift from a broad thrust to the general public only, to multiple-focused interventions and an increase in involvement of other partners, including NGOs and community groups' was noted in 1990 [23]. Behavioural change interventions began to be directed at sex workers, truckers and other populations at higher risk of HIV exposure on the assumption that for HIV, as for other STIs, the most efficient strategy for reducing the spread was to prevent infections among core transmitters, those with the highest rates of partner change [25].

Vulnerable group behavioural strategies remained controversial, however, both within and outside GPA. These strategies were associated with the risk of overstating the differences between the 'high-risk' and 'mainstream' populations, of focusing exclusively on women as HIV transmitters, of equating unsafe with bad and safe with good behaviours, and of stigmatizing those believed to be in the former behavioural category [26]. Moreover, in some regions, especially in Africa, the opportunity to contain the epidemic by concentrating on inducing behavioural change among high-risk populations had already passed by the early 1990s, as a large proportion of people not belonging to these categories, including many married women, had become infected.

From individual behaviour to societal change

From the early 1990s, it was increasingly recognized that in the absence of a supportive environment, preventing the spread of HIV through the promotion of individual behavioural change was a difficult, if not an impossible, undertaking. As Mann and Tarantola, who guided the development of GPA's original strategy, reflected later on, 'questions inevitably arose about the societal context in which individuals were behaving' and 'as awareness of the economic, political and cultural dimensions of HIV and related behaviours increased, HIV was perceived as resulting from, and therefore defined as, a combination of individual behaviour and societal or contextual forces' [27].

The importance of clear and firm policies protecting marginalized individuals and groups was now frequently stressed. In 1994, Michael Merson, then Director of GPA, pointed out: 'Laws that criminalise homosexuality hinder efforts to reach gay men with information and education. Fear of mandatory testing and detention prevents sex workers and drug users from coming forward for condoms and needles that would protect them' [28].

The revised WHO Global AIDS Strategy of 1993 acknowledged that AIDS was not just a medical or health sector problem, but also a social, cultural and economic one. It emphasized that effective AIDS action could not rely on the technical skills of health cadres alone, and called for the shaping of a multidisciplinary and multisectoral response to the epidemic [29]. Reflecting the greater emphasis on policy development and structural change, the identification of major socio-cultural, economic and political constraints on HIV prevention and the development of strategies to reduce or remove these constraints became distinct elements in GPA's Strategic Plan [30]. It was at this time as well that care was promoted as an essential complement to prevention and, through meeting the medical, social and psychological needs of families affected by HIV, could enhance prevention efforts [31,32].

There was also growing recognition by GPA of the need for national programme planning to achieve greater participation by a broader spectrum of actors. In a move away from the selective disease control programme approach, the integration of national and local HIV programmes into national health systems was discussed [33]. To facilitate this, GPA issued a new set of guidelines on national AIDS planning, including recommendations for national 'consensus-building workshops' involving high-level leaders and decision makers from key sectors, not only health, but also education, social welfare and criminal justice, among others [34]. Almost 60 countries followed these guidelines.

The crucial role that communities have to play in HIV prevention had been strongly endorsed as early as 1992. Building on that, the role that enabling approaches may play in HIV prevention was now discussed in light of the societal-level development approaches espoused by the UNDP, and also with regard to small-scale initiatives for vulnerable individuals, groups and communities [35]. For instance, a GPA newsletter stressed that: 'The community—be it the neighbourhood, the school or college community, a professional group or the smallest support group composed of family or friends—is a uniquely powerful force in societies everywhere, which needs to be harnessed if we are to bring the AIDS pandemic under control' [36]. An exhaustive review of initiatives employing enabling approaches to prevent HIV was carried out. A series of such pilot projects using enabling approaches to prevent HIV among particularly vulnerable groups was initiated, the experiences of which were reviewed, together with similar projects supported by other agencies, by Tawil and colleagues in 1995 [37].

Clearly, without ever reaching the community development end of the policy continuum, GPA's thinking and action had evolved a great deal from its early disease control focus, in light of its own experiences and those of others. Two critical pillars of the Alma-Ata Declaration—multisectoral participation and community involvement—were now central to its agenda. The thrust of the Ottawa Charter, which had called for greater emphasis on 'enabling public policies', on environments and societies rather than merely on individual lifestyle changes, now seemed to be well reflected in its policies, advocacy and research.

Resistance to GPA's policies and strategies: a paradigm shift

Whether rightly or wrongly, many in the international community did not agree with GPA's agenda, especially as 'the ability to translate the new insights into action had lagged behind' [27]. For instance, with regard to poverty as one of the main contextual issues identified, 'public health had difficulty to go beyond pointing to it as a problem' [27]. Moreover, the clear progress made in the analysis of, and reflected in the discourse on, the societal-level determinants and strategies of AIDS as opposed to individual risk behaviours was blurred by persisting inconsistencies between statements that showed a shift in thinking towards an empowerment perspective versus others that revealed a continued commitment to a selective disease control approach. Interventions for a selective approach were easily at hand, while empowerment as a strategy was much more difficult to translate into an effective and sustained intervention.

Various authors noted and reflected upon the shift of paradigms that was occurring during this period. In 1996, an international development journal dedicated an entire issue to AIDS entitled 'Fighting Back: HIV-AIDS and Development', containing long sections on community responses to HIV and AIDS [38]. In the same year, some argued that the AIDS prevention discourse should change in emphasis from individual and group factors that determine behaviours to include systemic, societal and political influences [39], while others found that such a shift had already begun to take place [40]. Summarizing the discussions about 'responses to AIDS by individuals, communities and societies', during the XI International Conference on AIDS in Vancouver that year, Mane et al. confirmed that such a shift in models or paradigms had shaped many of the conference presentations focusing on community empowerment and mobilization [41].

Many health workers coming from a PHC tradition, including the authors of this chapter, saw the opportunity to strengthen further a revival of an updated or redefined Alma-Ata-like approach. The global economic and political climate had changed since the late 1970s and 1980s, but the need for participatory programmes that relate to community health in a comprehensive and holistic way, complementing prevention efforts and care at the individual and community level, had not. Moreover, for those coming from other disciplines and traditions, including development sciences, economics and law, the shift in approaches simply vindicated their view that AIDS was not—and had never been—primarily a disease, but essentially a social, health and development issue that demanded a multisectoral strategy. The newly established UNAIDS programme was expected to spearhead a renewed effort for global advocacy and mobilization. It reduced the emphasis on individual behavioural change and disease control approaches that had been a major part of the former GPA's agenda.

Towards a shared vision

Following on from WHO's GPA, UNAIDS assumed its global leadership and policy-making role in 1996. Created 'to bring the AIDS activities of six UN agencies into a synergistic effort' [1], some of which had hardly been active in AIDS work before, UNAIDS embraced multiple perspectives, striving to build a shared vision of the epidemic and of the required responses to it. However, even though the complementarity of individual behaviour change promotion and strengthened contextual and societal-level responses to the epidemic was no longer controversial, the underlying differences in the views of those of its co-sponsoring agencies, some of which embraced a selective and target-oriented approach to health and others of which favoured a comprehensive development model, had not entirely disappeared.

UNAIDS' co-sponsors

The United Nations Population Fund (UNFPA) had just gone through its own paradigm shift, following the call by the International Conference on Population and Development (ICPD) in Cairo in 1994 to replace family planning programmes that emphasized demographic-specific targets in terms of contraceptive coverage and fertility reduction by the promotion of a comprehensive reproductive health and rights approach, and women's empowerment [42]. Although the translation of its agenda into actionable measures and the provision of comprehensive services has proved difficult [43,44], the ICPD's emphasis on the link between development and gender inequities helped to stimulate the direction of global AIDS policies, as gender became increasingly recognized as an important link in the continuing spread of the epidemic [42].

Drawing on UNDP's experience in development work as well as that from the outcomes of the Cairo conference, Elizabeth Reid, Head of the UNDP HIV Programme in the 1990s, proposed that where an enabling environment existed, change could occur spontaneously; however, outside agencies could also play a valuable catalysing role by helping create the milieu in which change could occur, by ensuring that the required services and supplies were available, and by facilitating dialogue and building consensus [45]. However, if WHO–GPA's prescriptions had been seen by some as narrow and limited, those of UNDP could be seen as unclear with regard to the choice of concrete strategies and activities, and as unlikely to be effective except in the very long term [46]. The UNAIDS Secretariat, aiming to assert itself in its global leadership role, and in anticipation of being asked for demonstrable results of its work by its board and donors, was not willing to place all its eggs in the long-term basket.

Meanwhile, the World Bank, another of UNAIDS' co-sponsors and an important player, embraced an approach that would go beyond individual risk reduction towards addressing the economic and structural causes of the epidemic, but blend it with a decidedly, albeit sophisticated, target-oriented disease control perspective. A comprehensive policy research document was developed that 'draws on three bodies of knowledge: the epidemiology of HIV, public health insights into diseases control, and especially public economics, which focuses on assessing trade-offs in the allocation of scarce resources' [47]. Following discussions with UNAIDS policy-makers and other AIDS experts, several modifications were made to the original draft of the paper, notably the limitations of individual behavioural change strategies were given more prominence than originally planned. Micro-level approaches aiming 'to influence individual choices directly' needed to be complemented by a second, more indirect approach, 'to change the economic and social conditions that make it difficult or impossible for some people to protect themselves from HIV', the document acknowledged. 'Measures pursued by this approach have many other benefits besides reducing the HIV epidemic and they are already on the agenda of most developing governments. The benefits are sometimes more difficult to quantify because of their broad impact. However, these measures (to alter societal norms, raise the status of women and reduce poverty) are highly complementary to policies that directly affect the costs and benefits of risky behaviour' [47].

Arguments also arose over the meaning and importance of 'information'. While most health educators associate 'information' with the old health information dissemination paradigm—with the 'I' in Information, Education and Communication (IEC)—which, on its own, cannot influence or explain behaviours, the economists of the World Bank and many others saw information as an extrinsic determinant of behaviour constituted by 'all types of knowledge, regardless of how it is acquired or shared' [47]. The document therefore took the unprecedented step of explaining in its text what it meant by the provision of 'information', namely the full range of IEC services: information on the facts of transmission and protection; training in skills and motivation; education, such as in schools; and counselling.

The development of HIV policies within UNICEF showed the variety and apparent inconsistencies of its approaches as well. A comprehensive approach had already been adopted in the early 1990s, balancing 'direct' responses—typically in the health sector, such as protection of blood supply, testing and epidemiological monitoring, safe practices in health facilities, promoting access to condoms, and treatment of STIs—with 'indirect multisectoral interventions to address the social and economic conditions that favour the spread of the epidemic' [40]. As one policy document highlights: 'AIDS is fundamentally a development challenge, intermingling issues of poverty, inequality, culture and sexuality in complex ways' [48]. Other passages of the same document, however, reflected not only UNICEF's health promotion, but also its selective PHC emphasis. For instance, social mobilization that had 'brought unprecedented success of the universal child immunization campaign' is alluded to, and efforts to apply approaches 'that relate most directly to achieving measurable gains in the reduction of HIV' [48] are called for. One critical review of UNICEF policies suggested that it might not have sufficiently internalized the HIV threat and proposed, among other strategies, that its support to countries be redirected to poverty reduction and to improving health and basic social services, including condom and essential drug supplies to treat HIV-related conditions. Greater support and direction to regional and country offices with respect to communication for behaviour change as it related to HIV was also proposed [49]. The recently developed UNICEF Medium-Term HIV Strategy 2002–2005 essentially operationalizes these recommendations [50].

In 1994, the WHO saw most of its GPA staff being reallocated to the UNAIDS Secretariat and therefore had to rebuild its capacity to respond to HIV. Building on its comparative strength in the health sector, WHO opted for a policy of mainstreaming, whereby all its departments involved in health promotion and care, health technologies, disease control and health systems integrated specific HIV-related activities into their own programmes. The organization-wide HIV activities were then coordinated by a small unit that provided technical stimulus, monitoring and liaison with UNAIDS and other partners [51]. In this way, community development and health intervention approaches were embraced and supported, although not necessarily blended with HIV-related interventions, while new ones such as HIV treatment could be highlighted and fostered in the WHO's departments.

Vulnerability and an expanded response to the epidemic

Confronted with diverse views among its co-sponsors, the UNAIDS Secretariat thus adopted a broad approach calling for an 'expanded response' to the epidemic that would 'balance strategies focused on risk reduction to slow transmission with those that focus on social and economic policy to reduce vulnerability' [52,53]. In fact, these notions of an 'expanded response' and 'vulnerability reduction' have been the cornerstone of UNAIDS' policy since its inception. As UNAIDS has interpreted them, both imply a shift in emphasis from individual-level analysis and response to enabling policy change and structural interventions, including the required mobilization of leadership to effect these changes. Both concepts also, incidentally, leave room for different interpretations, depending on whether disease control or community development thinking predominates.

The formulation of the 'vulnerability' concept in AIDS policy preceded the establishment of UNAIDS by several years [54,55]. Its explicit introduction into the set of UNAIDS' global objectives, which were otherwise similar to those defined in previous strategic plans, including those developed by WHO's GPA, was mainly meant as a qualitative improvement, to stress the need to go beyond an individual-level perspective. 'In the context of HIV, vulnerability builds on the notion that both personal and collective factors influence the probability of exposure or risk-generating situations and that this influence may vary over time' [52]. However, it may also be interpreted, depending on one's background and ideology, as expanding the risk concept to those at potential or medium risk, such as ordinary young people in a low- or moderately high-prevalence area, rather than those who are at immediate and highest risk, such as sex workers and drug users.

Similarly, the notion of an expanded response to the epidemic can be interpreted in both qualitative and quantitative terms. In addition to scaling up and improving the quality of classic health interventions aimed at providing care and reducing the immediate risk of transmission, and mobilizing the resources for this scale-up, UNAIDS has used the term to propose more initiatives in the health and, especially, social sectors, that may reduce vulnerability in the medium term. These include legislation to prevent discrimination and marginalization, and income-generation programmes and credit schemes particularly for women [52]. 'In the longer term, community development, employment and wealth creation, promotion of equality between men and women, literacy programmes, and the protection of human rights should help address the underlying causes and consequences of the epidemic' [52].

During UNAIDS' initial period, internal debates regarding the terminology contained in official documents beyond these two key concepts—vulnerability reduction and expanded response—had revealed some of the underlying differences in perspective among members of the various schools of thought. For instance, 'intervention,' with its disease control and target connotation, had been replaced by 'action', and 'technical collaboration' temporarily reduced to 'collaboration', only to reappear in its original form in later documents, including the UNAIDS strategic plan [52]. Similar arguments arose over UNAIDS' aim to identify, develop, document and disseminate successful international 'best practice' programmes and projects to stimulate similar action elsewhere. Confronted with the view that there could be no one universally best practice when facing multiple heterogeneous epidemics and context-ually relevant responses, UNAIDS dropped the 'international' and recognized that local processes rather than internationally prescribed methods and expected outcomes were crucial [1,56]. The recently developed UNAIDS strategic planning guidelines, a tool for planners at government, district and community levels, which superseded GPA's national strategic planning guide, are even more cautious, instead mentioning 'best known practices' in other countries and communities from which planners can learn; however, the potential for confusion remains, as most UNAIDS documentation is published in a 'best practice series' [57].

New challenges

Advances in access to highly effective antiretroviral combination therapy are already having a significant impact on global AIDS policies and strategies. Although the impact of therapy on HIV transmission at the individual and community levels is still to be determined, there is increasing evidence that it is not so much the impact of treatments on transmissibility as their perceived or real influence on vulnerability in terms of a reduction of stigma and fatalism that may make a bigger difference. Communities are more active in mobilizing against the epidemic when they are motivated by opportunities for prevention, care, treatment and support [4]. Furthermore, what during the mid-1990s was still rejected as unproven has now been shown to be effective: namely, strategies in which voluntary counselling and testing is the entry to prevention and care [4,58,59]. Botswana, Senegal, Brazil and Thailand were the first countries to adopt formal national AIDS strategies that emphasized universal access to counselling, testing, care and treatment, with the expectation that both those infected and the non-infected might benefit from breaking the silence surrounding HIV [60]. Other countries are in the process of reformulating their national policies and strategies in a similar manner.

Furthermore, the emergence of easily applicable short courses, including single-dose regimens to prevent mother-to-child transmission (MTCT), has revived the debate between those promoting the universal application of a cost-effective technology and those drawing attention to the prior need to address the contextual factors affecting women's—and their children's— risk and vulnerability, including their access to comprehensive reproductive health services [61].

On both these issues, namely, the development of policies and strategies to address the increasingly diverse epidemics and the emergence of affordable HIV combination treatment and simple technologies to prevent MTCT, UNAIDS and its co-sponsors steered a middle course at the end of the 1990s with both targeted interventions and approaches aimed at vulnerability reduction and overall empowerment.

First, a key objective of the unified budget of UNAIDS and its co-sponsors is to reduce the transmission of HIV through the development of programmes 'focused primarily on young people and vulnerable populations' [2,62]. The 2001 Global Strategy Framework reiterated objectives that refer to the education and protection of young people in general, as well as of particularly vulnerable groups [4]. Programmes address individual, institutional and community behaviours or situations that contribute most significantly to HIV transmission and can be modified through targeted programmes, as well as the most significant social and economic factors contributing to individual and community vulnerability to HIV infection [2,62].

Secondly, with regard to treatment and the reduction of MTCT, for instance, UNAIDS and WHO have reorganized their roles again. For example in WHO, a new HIV department was created in 2000 with the key role of making affordable treatment available as soon as possible. Other departments focus on integrated disease management at community level, and others, such as the Reproductive Health Department, aim to strengthen WHO's role in HIV prevention and care for women and newborns. This WHO focus on both integrated and focused health and medical approaches has allowed UNAIDS to emphasize its comparative advantage in coordinating and monitoring its UN agencies and ensuring a multisectoral response. However, UNAIDS and WHO have both cautioned against a too selective treatment approach, stating that while antiretroviral regimens can make a significant contribution, preventive activities at all levels by all sectors remain of paramount importance [2].

Conclusions

The AIDS policies and strategies of international agencies have evolved in light of their own and others' experiences of responding to the epidemic. Their policies and strategies need simultaneously to draw on infectious disease epidemiology, health system strengthening and community development. To date, too many programmes and interventions remain focused on individually defined risk behaviours and treatments, while programmes in which communities are both agents and targets of intervention remain rare [56,63,64]. Policies and strategies are needed that are both population-specific and comprehensive, that blend disease control and community development elements. Through a combination of behavioural and contextual analyses, vulnerable groups and communities can de defined and assessed, including their capacity to self-mobilize and to adopt new norms and technologies. Specific barriers to normative behavioural change that are relevant to specific communities—whether they are primarily defined by location, religion, ethnic affiliation, occupation or shared interests, including sexual preferences—need to be identified. Armed with these insights, tailor-made enabling policies and economic approaches can then be developed successfully. In the same way, communities need to become HIV care- and treatment-prepared because lifelong drug adherence will change daily life. 'It is at the community level that the outcome of the battle against AIDS will be decided' [4]. The challenge for international and UN agencies is to achieve a sufficiently close collaboration to be able to support such a coherent response.

Acknowledgements

We would like to thank Gill Walt for her useful comments, Daniel Taranatola for his extensive review and Harriet Hellar for editorial support.

References

1. UNAIDS. (1997). *Facts About UNAIDS: An Overview.* Geneva: UNAIDS.
2. UNAIDS. (1997). *Unified Budget & Workplan 2000–2001.* Geneva: UNAIDS.
3. UNAIDS. (2001). *Unified Budget & Workplan 2002–2003.* Geneva: UNAIDS.
4. UNAIDS. (2001). *The Global Strategy Framework on HIV/AIDS.* Geneva: UNAIDS.
5. Jamison DJ, Mosley WH, Measham AR, Bobadilla JL, eds. (1993). *Disease Control Priorities in Developing Countries.* New York: Oxford University Press.
6. World Health Organization. (1978). *Alma-Ata: Primary Health Aare.* Health for all Series No. 1, Geneva: WHO.
7. Walsh JA, Warren KS. (1979). Selective primary health care: an interim strategy for disease control in developing countries. *New England Journal of Medicine* 301:18.
8. Rafkin SB, Walt G. (1986) Why health improves: defining the issues concerning 'comprehensive primary health care' and 'selective primary health care'. *Social Science and Medicine* 23:559–66.
9. WHO Regional Office for Europe. (1985). *Health Promotion: Concepts and Principles.* Copenhagen: WHO.
10. WHO/Canadian Public Health Association. (1996). *Ottawa Charter for Health Promotion* 1: 3–5. Ottawa: WHO.
11. World Federation of Public Health Federations. (1986). *Information for Action Issue.* A paper prepared for UNICEF and the Aga Khan foundation. Geneva: WFPHA.
12. Nutbeam D, Blakey V. (1990). The concept of health promotion and AIDS prevention: a comprehensive and integrated basis for action in the 1990s. *Health Promotion International* 5: 233–42.
13. WHO Global Programme on AIDS. (1997). *1987–1995 Final Report with Emphasis on 1994–1995.* Biennium, Geneva: WHO.
14. WHO Special Programme on AIDS. (1987). *Progress Report No. 1, WHO/SPA/GEN 87.1.* Geneva: WHO.
15. Mann J. (1987) In focus: AIDS. *World Health Forum* 8:361–71.
16. Mann JM, Kay K. (1991). Confronting the pandemic: the World Health Organization's Global Programme on AIDS, 1986–1989. *AIDS* 5(Supplement 2):S221–29.
17. Kaleeba N, Kalibala S, Kaseje M *et al.* (1997). Paricipatory evaluation of counselling, medical and social services of the AIDS support organization (TASO) in Uganda. *AIDS Care* 9:13–26.
18. Mehryar AH, Carballo M. (1990). *Models of Behaviour Change: Implications for Research and Intervention Programmes for Prevention and Control of HIV and AIDS.* Geneva: WHO-GPA.
19. World Health Organization. (1992). *Global Programme on AIDS, Report of the Global Commission on AIDS Fifth Meeting, April 1–3, 1992.* (GPA/GCA(5)/92.6). Geneva: WHO.
20. World Health Organization. (1993). *Global Programme on AIDS, Report of the Ninth Meeting of the Management Committee, May 25–27, 1993.* (GPA/GMC(9)/93.12). Geneva: WHO.
21. World Health Organization. (1991). *Global Programme on AIDS, Progress Report* (draft). Geneva: WHO.
22. WHO/ Ministry of Public Health of the People's Republic of China. (1993). *An External Review of the National AIDS Control Programme.* October 18–November 4, 1993. Geneva: WHO.

23. World Health Organization. (1990). *Global Programme on AIDS, Report of the Global Commission on AIDS Third Meeting, March 22–23, 1990.* (GPA/GCA(3)/90.11). Geneva: WHO.

24. Danziger R. (1996). An overview of HIV prevention in central and eastern Europe. *AIDS Care* 8:701–7.

25. Over M, Piot P. (1993). HIV infection and sexually transmitted diseases. In: Jameson DT, Mosley WH, Measham AR, Bobadilla, eds. *Disease Control Priorities in Developing Countries.* New York: Oxford University Press, pp 455–526.

26. O'Shaughnessy T. (1994). *Beyond the Fragments: HIV/AIDS and Poverty, Issues in Global Development, No 1.* Canberra: World Vision Australia, Research and Policy Unit.

27. Mann JM, Tarantola DT. (1998) Responding to HIV/AIDS: a historical perspective. *Health and Human Rights* 2:5–8.

28. Merson MH. (1994). Discrimination Against People Affected by HIV/AIDS. Presented at the 46th Session of the Sub-commission on Prevention of Discrimination and Protection of Minorities of the Commission on Human Rights, Geneva: WHO.

29. World Health Organization. (1992). *The Global AIDS Strategy: WHO AIDS Series 11.* Geneva: WHO.

30. World Health Organization. (1993). *GPA Strategic Plan: 1994–1998.* Geneva: WHO.

31. van Praag E. (1995). The continuum of care: lessons from developing countries. *IAS Newsletter* 3:11–13.

32. Edeid SE, Kahssay HM, van Praag E. (1994). Primary health care approach and the implementation of HIV prevention and AIDS care (editorial). *African Journal of Medical Practice* 1:39–40.

33. Matamora K, Lamboray JL, Laing R. (1991). Integration of AIDS program activities into national health systems. *AIDS* 5(Supplement 1):S193–6.

34. World Health Organization. (1993). *Global Programme on AIDS. National Consensus Workshop on AIDS, Facilitators Guide.* Geneva: WHO.

35. World Health Organization. (1993). Meeting on Enabling Approaches in HIV/AIDS Prevention. *Influencing the Social and Environmental Determinants of Risk, Background Document.* Geneva, WHO.

36. World Health Organization. (1992). *World AIDS Day Newsletter.* Geneva: WHO.

37. Tawil O, Verster A, O'Reilly K. (1995). Enabling approaches for HIV/AIDS prevention: can we modify the environment and minimize the risk? *AIDS* 9:1299–1306.

38. Altman D. (1996). Overview of community responses. *Development* 2:8–16.

39. Gillies P, Tolley K, Wolstenholme J. (1996). Is AIDS a disease of poverty? *AIDS Care* 8:351–63.

40. Parker RG. (1996). Empowerment, community mobilisation and social change in the face of HIV/AIDS. *AIDS* 10(Supplement 3):S27–31.

41. Mane P, Aggelton P, Dowsett G *et al.* (1996). Summary of track D: social science: research, policy and action. *AIDS* 10(Supplement 3):S123–32.

42. United Nations. (1995). *Population and Development, Volume 1: Programme of Action Adopted at the International Conference on Population and Development,* Cairo, September 5–13, 1994. Department for Economic and Social Information and Policy Analysis. New York: UN.

43. Hardee K, Agarwal K, Luke N. (1998). *Post-Cairo Reproductive Health Policies: A Comparative Study of Eight Countries.* Prepared for the Population Association of America meeting, Chicago, April 2–4, 1998. Durham, NC: The Futures Group International, The Policy Project.

44. Dehne KL, Snow R. (1999). *Integrating STI Management into Family Planning Services: What are the Benefits?* Occasional Paper No. 1. Geneva: WHO, Department of Reproductive Health and Research.

45. United Nations Development Programme. (1995). *Development Practice and the HIV Epidemic.* Issues paper 16, New York: UNDP HIV and development programme.

46. Parnell B, Lie G, Hernandez JJ, Robins C. (1996). *Development and the HIV Epidemic. A Forward-looking Evaluation of the Approach of the UNDP HIV and Development Programme.* New York: UNDP.

47. The World Bank/The International Bank for Reconstruction and Development. (1997). *Confronting AIDS, Public Priorities in a Global Epidemic.* New York: Oxford University Press.

48. UNICEF. (1993). *AIDS: The Second Decade. A Focus on Youth and Women.* New York: UNICEF.

49. Dube S. (1999). *The HIV/AIDS Pandemic: An Unprecedented Challenge for UNICEF.* Discussion paper. Geneva: UNAIDS.

50. UNICEF. (2005). *Medium Term HIV/AIDS Strategy: 2002–2005.* New York: UNICEF.

51. World Health Organization. (1999). *WHO's Initiative on HIV/AIDS and Sexually Transmitted Infections (HIS).* WHO/HIS/99.4. Geneva: WHO.

52. UNAIDS. (1995). *Strategic Plan 1996–2000.* Geneva: UNAIDS.

53. UNAIDS. (1997). *Proposed Programme Budget and Workplan for 1998–1999.* Geneva: UNAIDS.

54. Mann JM, Tarantola D, Netter TW, eds. (1992). *AIDS in the World.* Cambridge, MA: Harvard University Press, p325–420.

55. Mann JM, Tarantola D. (1996). *AIDS in the World II: Global Dimensions, Social Roots and Responses.* New York: Oxford University Press, p441–62.

56. UNAIDS. (1998). *Expanding the Global Response to HIV/AIDS Through Focused Action, Reducing Risk and Vulnerability: Definitions, Rationale and Pathways.* UNAIDS Best Practice Collection. Geneva: UNAIDS.

57. UNAIDS. (1998). *Guide to the Strategic Planning Process for a National Response to HIV/AIDS. Introduction.* Geneva: UNAIDS.

58. Voluntary HIV-1 Counselling and Testing Efficacy Study Group. (2000). Efficacy of voluntary counselling in individuals and couples in Kenya, Tanzania, and Trinidad: a randomised trial. *Lancet* 356:103–12.

59. Grant AD, Kaplan JE, De Cock KM. (2001). Preventing opportunistic infections among human immunodeficiency virus-infected adults in African countries. *American Journal of Tropical Medicine and Hygiene* 65:810–21.

60. *The Economist,* 17 August 2001. Botswana Adopts a New Approach to Fighting HIV/AIDS.

61. World Health Organization. (1998). Recommendations on the safe and effective use of short-course ZDV for prevention of mother-to-child transmission of HIV. *WHO Weekly Epidemiological Record* 73:313–20.

62. UNAIDS. (1999). *Overview of Strategy Framework to Assist in the Development of an Integrated Workplan and Budget.* Geneva: UNAIDS.

63. O'Reilly KR, Piot P. (1996). International perspectives on individual and community approaches to the prevention of sexually transmitted disease and human immunodeficiency virus infection. *Journal of Infectious Diseases* 174(Supplement 2):S214–22.

64. van Praag E. (2001). *Planning the Incorporation of Antiretroviral Therapy into Comprehensive Care Programmes, in Improving Access to Care in Developing Countries: Lesson from Practice, Research, Resources and Partnerships.* Paris: Ministère des Affaires Étrangères, WHO and UNAIDS.

Chapter 41

Donor, lender and research agencies' response to the HIV crisis

Chris Simms

Introduction

Although the international donor community (IDC) has long held that governments' failure to confront the HIV pandemic and take clear steps aimed at its prevention and control are key to understanding the severity of today's crisis [1,2], evidence shows that donors themselves did not adequately prioritize and provide effective, timely leadership to tackle the crisis. A significant body of literature, including routine donor evaluations and peer reviews [3,4], raises questions as to the preparedness and capacity of the IDC to respond. Donor aid and the way it was delivered are described as donor-driven, consisting of short-term projects and programmes, lacking community consultation and participation, and evaluated in terms of inputs or disbursements. Furthermore, donor initiatives may have actually reduced access to goods and services aimed at the prevention and treatment of HIV at the individual and community levels. Similarly, review of efforts by the international health research community to deal with such issues as an AIDS vaccine, a 'social vaccine', poor essential health research capacities in developing countries and inequalities in global research spending suggests the response to the pandemic was belated, underfunded and undermined by institutional constraints and the pursuit of Northern agendas over Southern needs.

Level of donor funding targeting HIV

Without a long-term development framework, or even a medium-term instrument such as a Poverty Reduction Strategy (PRS), the IDC had significant influence over priority setting and the development agenda in the 1980s and 1990s. Review of the major health policy movements for the period 1960–2000 shows that strategies of the World Bank ('growth and poverty', poverty alleviation, structural adjustment, 'agenda for reform'), the United Nations (vertical disease control, primary healthcare, 'health systems development') and the European Commission (poverty alleviation, 'rural development', 'integrated development') had 'a heavy influence over policy' that went far beyond financial contributions [5]. Analysis of external aid to the health sector undertaken for the World Bank confirms that overseas development aid (ODA) plays 'a critical role in capital investment, research and strategic planning' in developing countries [6]. In poor countries such as Tanzania, Uganda and Mozambique, where donor contributions constituted 50–70% of public health expenditures, the international donor and lending communities exercised enormous fiscal and policy leverage. For example, as Africa's main development partner and a key member of the international health community, the World Bank reported that it had a special leadership role in fighting HIV. In its seminal document, *Intensifying Action Against HIV*, it acknowledged this role as well as the need that it be held accountable for its stewardship, stating that 'those who look back at this era will judge our institution in large measure by whether we recognized this wildfire that is raging across Africa for the development threat that it is, and did our utmost to put it out. They will be right to do so' [7]. While ultimate responsibility for confronting HIV rests with governments, some analysts conclude that 'donor priorities and financial stringency, at least as much as issues within recipient countries, brought about the past and present low levels of aid funding, which in turn has contributed to the present pandemic' [8].

To the extent that levels of aid funding are an indicator of donors' priorities, expenditure data show that more than a decade had elapsed before donors and lending institutions began to take the fight against HIV seriously. Review of data from the Organization for Economic Cooperation and Development (OECD) Creditor Reporting System (CRS) shows that the worldwide budget of the 22 wealthy donor countries and one donor region [the European Union (EU)] that constitute the Development Assistance Committee (DAC) of the OECD dedicated specifically to controlling AIDS in least-developed and other low-income countries (category 13040) averaged just US$78 million annually between 1990 and 1998 [9]. Only a handful of countries provided funding every year; others, such as Japan, Austria, Luxembourg, Ireland and Portugal, apparently committed no funds toward AIDS. Analysis of Japan's response to HIV, as the world's largest bilateral aid donor, shows that even during the years 2000–2004, 'it fails to give high priority to HIV, including it as one of many targeted infectious and parasitic diseases' [10].

Analysis of the investments made between 1986 and 1996 by the World Bank, the largest contributor to HIV activities, shows that it had 10 stand-alone HIV projects and 51 projects with an HIV component in 27 countries [11]. Bank lending for HIV during these years amounted to a paltry US$552 million. It also appears that it was inequitably distributed across regions—with Brazil, for example, a relatively rich country with a low prevalence rate of less than 1%, receiving US$160 million compared with US$274 million for all of Africa, where some countries, such as Lesotho [12] and Zambia [13], with adult HIV prevalence rates at 26% and 22%, respectively, were virtually ignored until 2000.

Data from the Joint United Nations Programme on HIV (UNAIDS) show that total ODA per HIV-infected person declined by over 50% between 1988 and 1997, to less than US$10 per HIV-infected person. By 1998, the aid effort in sub-Saharan Africa amounted to just over US$3 per HIV-infected person, according to the CRS data. A striking feature of the period was that 'no discernible attempt was made in the 1990s to increase donor flows once it became clear that existing aid flows were insufficient to slow the disease's advance' [14].

In recent years, levels of spending have improved. A new study by the OECD's DAC and UNAIDS demonstrates a clear trend toward rising aid donations to fight HIV [15]. The latest definitive figures, combining the aid efforts of major bilateral and multilateral donors, show an allocation of US$2.2 billion in 2002 to control and combat the pandemic in the developing world. Bilateral aid rose steadily, from US$822 million in 2000 to US$1.1 billion in 2001, and to US$1.35 billion in 2002—a 64% increase over 3 years. Multilateral aid rose from US$314 million in 2000 to US$460 million in 2002, and total contributions to the Global Fund to Fight AIDS, Tuberculosis and Malaria reached US$917 million by the end of 2002, 60% of which will target HIV. Spending on HIV programmes in low- and middle-income countries increased by 20% over 2002 to US$4.7 billion in 2003; government spending alone was about US$1 billion; in 2004, total external and domestic funding reached US$6 billion.

While the inadequacy of donor allocations to HIV before 2000 is self-evident and acknowledged by most donors, some of the most useful data describing this failure are available from the World Bank's Operations Evaluation Department (OED), whose job it is to provide 'independent evaluation' of Bank activities. Of the situations in Zambia and Lesotho noted earlier, for example, OED details the Bank's failure to prioritize and place HIV on the agenda and its consequences. It reports that while the Bank was 'well aware' of the alarming welfare trends caused by HIV in Zambia, health specialists were not successful in persuading 'Bank management to use its influence to bring HIV/AIDS control to the top of the reform agenda through advocacy and inclusion in the macroeconomic dialogue' [13]. OED states that 'earlier advocacy by the Bank, in collaboration with a highly active donor community, might have resulted in a more vigorous and inclusive multisectoral response to HIV/AIDS by GRZ' (Government of the Republic of Zambia) [13]. In the case of Lesotho, OED reports that 'the Bank did not help Lesotho develop the most basic integrated health information system and survey instruments necessary to monitor HIV, leading to underestimation of prevalence and, consequently, of its impact. HIV was not then at the center of the country dialogue and the Bank's 1994 population sector review did not trigger a shift in Bank strategy in the last half of the 1990s towards more actively combating HIV/AIDS' [12]. Given these findings, OED concludes that Lesotho may have been better off without a Bank presence in the health sector [12].

These findings suggest that the donor and lending communities had yet to see the crisis as a development crisis, but rather as a discrete public health challenge. Reviewing levels of donor aid targeting HIV in 1997, the World Bank, in what it called a 'strategic document', *Confronting AIDS: Public Priorities in a Global Epidemic*, states 'these allocations are remarkably large relative to national spending on the same problem and probably in comparison with international spending on any other disease. Perhaps only the international campaign to eradicate smallpox in the 1970s benefited from such a large preponderance of donor funds' [2].

The impact of structural adjustment policies on access to healthcare

The decline of public health delivery systems in many low-income countries in the 1980s and 1990s was associated with economic crisis and the implementation of structural adjustment programmes (SAPs) by the World Bank, the International Monetary Fund (IMF) and some donor agencies. An OED evaluation of 114 adjustment operations in 53 countries for the period 1980–1993 found large reductions in social spending especially in sub-Saharan Africa, where 'during adjustment', spending declined to 76% of 1981 levels, and 'after adjustment' declined to 68% of 1981 levels [16]. These had a prolonged and detrimental impact on governments' ability to respond to the HIV epidemic because effective prevention and control presume a robust health system.

Just as important as the size of the cuts was the way they were implemented. Without proactive steps taken by the international financial institutions (IFIs) to maintain spending that mainly benefited vulnerable groups, large cuts in public health expenditure typically led to the protection of budgets for urban healthcare over rural services, tertiary over primary care, and salaries over operations and maintenance, contributing to the collapse of basic services targeting the poor, such as health education, rural health clinics and outreach services [17].

In retrospect, the World Bank acknowledged that it was a mistake not 'to deal explicitly with the social dimensions of adjustment' and take steps to protect social spending through conditionalities [16]. Similarly, the IMF recognized its failure to take into account the distributional impact of its policies on the lives of ordinary people and to take effective steps to ameliorate these unintended consequences [18]. The World Bank recently reported that 'after a decade and a half of structural adjustment, there seem to be too few positive and sustainable results' [19].

The salient issue identified by the World Health Organization (WHO) is that 'with only a few exceptions, HIV epidemics have hit hardest the countries whose health systems are least able to cope' [20]. Within these countries, the erosion of basic services affected the prevention and control of HIV in various ways: for example, the collapse of health education programmes made it more difficult to inform the citizenry about HIV; also, the decline in essential services undermined the treatment of sexually transmitted infections (STIs)—a high risk factor for the spread of HIV. The interplay between poverty and the epidemic made the poor especially vulnerable to HIV.

> The decline of health, education and other social services implies a loss of opportunities for HIV prevention. People with little or no education (the poor) have poor access to safe sex information. For instance, condom use is associated with higher levels of education. Reduced provision of quality health services also represents a loss of opportunities to control other sexually-transmitted infections, offer reproductive health services, and provide quality care for people infected with HIV-1 [21].

In Mwanza, Tanzania, for example, in the mid-1990s, where there was a reasonable network of dispensaries and health centres compared with more remote sectors, it was found that 'fewer than 10% of symptomatic sexually-transmitted infections occurring in the population were cured by health services. Health staff had been unable to update their skills and knowledge, and health centres were provided with insufficient and inappropriate antibiotics' [22].

Cuts in public health spending in real terms led not only to reduced access to effective HIV healthcare, but also to a deterioration in supervision, monitoring, training and logistics, making some medical practices, such as injections, unsafe and a possible source of HIV transmission. In one study, research into the safety of injections in 19 countries found that in 14 of these, at least 50% of injections were unsafe; of the remaining five countries, rates varied between 21% and 30%; only three countries had no documented problems [23]. Another study that sought to estimate the contribution of unsafe injections to the transmission of HIV suggested that 80,000–160,000 infections may have resulted annually—possibly 2 million infections over 14 years [24]. The World Health Report 2004 reports that 'review of published studies finds that unsafe injections play a minor but significant role in HIV transmissions in sub-Saharan Africa' [20]. Whether or not unsafe injections are a dominant or important mode of HIV-1 transmission remains contentious [25,26].

The impact of health sector reform on prevention and control of HIV

At about the same time that the IDC began making HIV investments, it embarked upon its main policy priority of the next decade, badly needed improvement in the way goods and services were provided and financed through health sector reforms (HSRs) [27,28]. These reforms achieved only modest results due to limited uptake by governments and inadequate planning and implementation by donor and lending agencies. Reforms frequently had the unintended effect of reducing access to effective healthcare, including services aimed at the prevention and control of HIV. For example, with the promotion of cost recovery, it became commonplace to charge users for key HIV services, including the diagnosis and treatment of STIs [29,30], blood transfusion schemes [31] and voluntary HIV counselling and testing (VCT) [32]. Research in Kenya indicates that after the introduction of user-fees at STI referral services, the average monthly attendance of men decreased significantly to 40% of that before fees were levied. Attendance then rose over the next 15-month post-user-charge period, but reached only 64% of the pre-user-charge level [33]. Numerous other studies [34–36] have shown a decrease in utilization of HIV/STI services following the introduction of user-fees, particularly among the poor.

Another strand of reform was healthcare decentralization, which was justifiable as a way of dealing with overly centralized systems that were unresponsive to local health needs. It had mixed results. In 1991, Senegal adopted the district system in the health system, which proved to be an effective framework for the decentralization of HIV activities because it facilitated implementation at the periphery while at the same time including HIV activities in the district's integrated activities package [37]. A recent review of 10 countries in Africa shows that where there was a robust decentralization system in place, these structures facilitated the rapid scaling up of local HIV activities and eliminated the need to create a new framework. This was the case in Ghana and Burkina Faso, while Kenya 'is still struggling to identify a suitable decentralization structure for HIV programmes' [38].

Overall, though, decentralization efforts in the 1990s frequently led to chaotic results. Evaluations show that it was promoted 'without sufficient regard for the administrative or political implications' and that stakeholders 'tended to underestimate the training and technical support needed to help districts undertake their new responsibilities' [39]. The impact of this on Tanzania's HIV services, for instance, was to increase the staff workload beyond their capacity, to the point that they were unable 'to protect themselves and patients from the risk of infection', and were themselves contributing 'to the spread of the infectious disease' [40]. In Ethiopia, decentralization created a federal unit to coordinate health service provision and regional autonomous states in their planning and implementation services. In practice, these bodies do not function, and, due to lack of public service provision, treatment of HIV is done exclusively by non-governmental organizations (NGOs) [37].

Two further reforms that undermined efforts to deal effectively with the epidemic at an early stage were privatization and integration. The private provision of healthcare, an obvious financing alternative in low-income countries, was encouraged by donors without concurrent improvements in regulation and better implementation of existing regulation and training [36]. This had a detrimental effect on the diagnosis and treatment of STIs, where an extensive body of research describes the deficiencies in the quality of private sector care [41–43]. Even if good quality care was available, data show that private practitioners 'have few incentives to provide preventive services' [39] such as treatment of partners, recommending counselling, testing and condom use [44]. Another reform, the horizontal integration of vertical programmes, aimed at improving efficiency, led to efforts to combine HIV/STI programmes with family planning (FP) and maternal and child health (MCH) services. Review of cross-country data from studies undertaken in Ghana, Kenya, Zambia and South Africa [45], consistent with other studies [46–51], shows that integration was misconceived since FP/MCH services are used mainly by married women and children, not by sexually active men and unmarried women. In Zambia, the policy was misguided because the epidemic 'called for an intensive, emergency campaign at a time when disease specific vertical programmes were being dismantled in favor of integrated care' [13]. The opportunity costs and public health implications of these two reforms were enormous.

Constraints on the effectiveness and relevance of donors' responses

Several sources suggest that the quality of donors' responses to the HIV crisis was undermined by systemic, institutional constraints to the point that effective, timely and appropriate measures were probably impossible. Routine donor evaluations and peer reviews on aid effectiveness [3,4], for example, show that during the 1980s and 1990s, the quality of aid and the way it was delivered was neither comprehensive, holistic and long-term nor adequately assessed in terms of outcomes. A recent multi-partner evaluation of donor activities led by the World Bank reported that by the late 1990s, 'concerns were growing about how aid was being used and managed, and about the disappointing impact it was having. The concerns were widespread—at the World Bank and other multilateral agencies, and among bilateral aid agencies, non-governmental organizations (NGOs), and developing country governments' [19]. The reality behind these concerns formed an important part of the context in which the pandemic spread.

Weak targeting and prioritization

A 1998 analysis of the World Bank's HIV activities between 1986 and 1996 looked at 10 stand-alone HIV projects, 51 projects with an HIV component in 27 countries, and a wide range of the Bank's other economic and sector work [11]. It identified three priority areas for government support: information collection, promotion of safer behaviour among those most likely to contract and transmit HIV, and protection for the poorest groups in society from contracting HIV and its consequences. The study found that while all 10 of the HIV projects financed surveillance of HIV and other STIs, 'only a few had indicated a plan to focus these activities on the population groups most at risk in the country' [11]. About 60% of the 51 projects contracted NGOs to provide outreach services to high-risk groups, but 'there is very limited discussion of how these groups had been identified or what additional information was needed to reach them effectively' [11]. Only four of the 10 projects supported condom promotion programmes targeting high-risk groups. While all 10 financed STI treatment, only one planned to focus these services on those at greatest risk. In terms of the poor, only one project provided support for efforts to protect the poorest group in society from contracting HIV or for programmes to mitigate the negative consequences of HIV among those groups. Most of the projects were not based on strong economic analysis.

The 51 projects with an HIV component largely ignored any *ex ante* economic analysis of the proposed AIDS interventions. While the freestanding AIDS projects included some *ex ante* economic analysis, only three prepared adequate cost-benefit analysis. *Ex post* evaluations were only available for four of the eight completed projects, only one of which was classified as 'satisfactory'.

Another key evaluation of the World Bank's Health, Population and Nutrition (HPN) portfolio looked at its investment in 'the best buys in public health and clinical services' for the period 1993–1999, using the criteria of effectiveness, affordability, quality and relevance to the health status of the poor [52]. The 'best buys' for HIV prevention were identified as education on safe behaviour, condom promotion, STI treatment and safe blood supply; for the treatment of STIs, they were case management using syndromic diagnosis and standard treatment algorithms. Of the total 152 HPN projects undertaken, 44 addressed HIV (29%), of which only 10 met the evaluative criteria (23%); for STIs, 51 of the 152 supported STI treatment (34%), of which only seven (14%) met the criteria. Finally, while the World Bank acknowledged that HIV is a multisectoral problem and opportunities existed for interventions in other sectors, there was little evidence that this had occurred.

Lack of multisectoral approach

HIV is a cross-cutting development challenge that warrants a comprehensive and multidimensional response. In the past, the donor community has tended towards supporting short-term, one-dimensional programmes and projects of unknown effectiveness. The OECD DAC finds that Japan is still treating HIV 'as a discrete development challenge of funding related to the health sector, such as research, provision of equipment, counseling, and educational material development. In other words, Japan is yet to see HIV as a cross-cutting challenge that needs to be addressed systematically in many other areas, such as agriculture, rural development, education, public administration, tourism, business development, and so forth' [53]. Most bilateral agencies have moved away from stand-alone HIV projects, having found that an effective prevention and control strategy depends upon a broad multisectoral approach if behaviour and lifestyles were to be affected [54,55]. AusAid, for example, launched a revised HIV Strategy in 2004 that takes a 'more systematic response to HIV across the program, including HIV within country strategies as a cross-cutting issue rather than developing specific HIV projects' [56]. OED data showed that the World Bank, as a rule, 'has not placed sufficient emphasis on addressing determinants of health that lie outside the medical care system, including behavioral change and cross-sectoral interventions' [39]; therefore, it comes as no surprise that Bank 'interventions tended to focus on HIV as a narrow health sector problem rather than multisectoral problem' [52]. OED found that as an institution, the Bank simply had 'neither the incentives nor mechanisms' needed for intersectoral approaches [39].

Lack of consultation between stakeholders and participation by ordinary people and the poor

Another set of constraints that undermined the fight against HIV was the general lack of dialogue, good communication and consultation between stakeholders, including ordinary people and the poor. This may have contributed, in turn, to other weaknesses such as poor donor coordination and failure to develop country-specific responses. The US General

Accounting Office (GAO) assessment of UNAIDS reports that although its success depended upon collegiality, cooperation and consensus, these qualities were not evident in the early years [57]. UNAIDS was more or less imposed on its co-sponsors, 'and there was a certain amount of hostility towards the programme....The cosponsors viewed the Secretariat (of UNAIDS) as competing for funding and were confused by their role within the programme. As a result, until recently, cosponsors were not fully committed either to incorporating HIV into their respective mandates or to participating in UNAIDS. Since cosponsors are accountable to their independent executive board, neither the Secretariat nor the UNAIDS governing board could exercise controlling authority or make the cosponsors effective partners' [57].

As for the bilaterals, it is reported that they were of little assistance when it came time to provide political support and funding to intensify and promote programmes, thus further reducing UNAIDS' effectiveness [57]. The OED reports that the Bank lacks 'strategic and flexible approaches to support the development of intellectual consensus and broad-based coalitions necessary for change' [39]. Most recently, a progress report of the Multi-Country HIV/AIDS Program for Africa (MAP) shows there is 'insufficient partnership or evidence of coordinated collective action among key multilateral, bilateral donors and the UN Theme Group' [58]. It also found 'limited sharing of lessons and experiences among both Bank staff and counterpart teams alike' and concluded that, in view of the fact that ' "learning by doing" underlies the entire approach, a more effective means of sharing MAP experiences is critical' [58].

Because donors seldom take into account beneficiaries' perceptions of health services or how these services relate to their daily lives or even whether they want or use them—what is today called a 'livelihoods approach'—policies and strategies have often lacked what was needed to make them effective and relevant. For example, the negative outcomes of the earlier noted policy of combining HIV/STI and MCH services in settings where men are disinclined to use what are perceived to be female reproductive health services could have been avoided if ordinary people had been consulted [48]. This, as well as failing to consult frontline workers at the village dispensary and clinic, contributed to the failure to reach sexually active men and unmarried women [49]. In its 2002 survey of 43 donors, the Panos Institute found that only 13% had consulted the groups of people actually vulnerable to HIV [59]. It found that notions of consultation and participation in the decision-making process were largely rhetorical; for example, it reported that 'It's very difficult to have participation when you have a deadline of two months or six weeks like in the recent call for applications for the Global Fund. Countries knew in advance that it would be very difficult to develop these proposals so they had teams of consultants come in from the World Bank, UN, everywhere, to develop these proposals without any real participation. They want participation, ownership and so on but then the process is so rapid that it makes this just about impossible' [59]. Regarding Poverty Reduction Strategy Papers (PRSPs) and the International Partnership Against AIDS in Africa (IPAA), it is reported that 'these are very government led. They are all about participation but in name only. They are not very participatory at all, generally they are led by consultants who come in from overseas and direct the process. It's done in a very hurried manner because donors give deadlines that have to be abided by' [59].

The World Bank, too, has failed to consult beneficiaries adequately. A general review of project design documents shows that only 2% estimated consumer response to the proposed intervention [39]. OED reports that, 'although beneficiary surveys and consultations have become more common, only 4 of 224 projects documented the presence of beneficiary decision-making power in project design' [39]. The Bank has been challenged over the last several years to 'reduce constraints and improve institutional support for participation' [60] and embrace the involvement of NGOs, beneficiaries' interest groups and civil society in the formulation and implementation of policy and strategies. [61]. Evaluations of MAP indicate large improvements in consultation at the local level [58].

Monitoring and evaluation

These failures raise questions not only as to why badly conceived reforms would have been recommended in the first place, but why they endured—why immediate measures were not taken to modify or adjust reforms once their negative effects became evident. Part of the answer seems to be that most donors failed to monitor and evaluate outcomes. The Swedish International Development Cooperation Agency (Sida) reports that in India, for example, no mechanism was put in place to evaluate prevention and control activities, and there was no allocation in the NACP budget for monitoring and evaluation (M&E). It concludes that effectiveness was reduced by 'an imperfect and inadequate understanding of what works, which can only come if evaluation procedures are put in place before activities are planned. Unfortunately, other donors have also not insisted on scientific evaluations, though it is now being recognized that there is a need to know whether good money is being thrown after bad' [52]. In a similar vein, the British National Audit Office (NAO) reports that the Department for International Development (DFID) does not know how much it is spending on HIV and has little way of knowing what impact it is having because it is failing to monitor and evaluate impact against objectives set out in its HIV strategy [62]. The US GAO joint evaluation of UNAIDS reports that UNAIDS still 'cannot measure progress towards achieving its objectives or overall results, especially at the country level', despite efforts since 1998 to develop monitoring and evaluation [55]. A separate performance-related instrument, the UNAIDS Unified Budget and Workplan, 'was compiled quickly, did not have high quality indicators' and, 'because it is organized thematically rather than functionally, it is difficult to track or assess UNAIDS' progress in achieving its overall objectives'. It was noted that M&E was constrained by the lack of an evaluative culture within the UN system [55].

As for the World Bank, OED reported that it 'typically focuses on providing inputs rather than clearly defining and monitoring progress towards Health, Population and Nutrition (HPN) development objectives. Because of weak incentives and underdeveloped systems for M&E both within the Bank and borrowing governments, there is little evidence regarding the impact of Bank investments on system performance or health outcomes. The Bank therefore has not used its lending portfolio to systematically collect evidence on what works, what does not, and why' [38]. In the same vein, a recent review of the MAP points out that 'ACTafrica recommends that 5–10% of programme funds be invested in M&E (and) yet the Bank has contributed almost no financial resources to provide M&E technical and implementation support to task teams and clients' [63].

Failure to develop country-specific responses

In the past, HIV initiatives have been inadequately tailored to local needs, reflecting instead standardized institutional solutions. For example, the World Bank was criticized

throughout the 1990s for its formulaic, 'one-size-fits-all' solutions to developmental problems. In 1999, OED reported that 'Bank strategies and policy advice in (the) HPN sector are
too often insufficiently grounded in empirical evidence or institutional analysis of the
country context.... As a result, the Bank has a tendency to promote standard solutions to
health system problems without giving sufficient attention to local institutions or details of
implementation' [33]. Despite the Bank's own analysis showing that projects with poor
economic analysis were at least seven times more likely to perform poorly than were projects
with good economic analysis, the OED concluded that 'few of the HIV Bank projects base
support for interventions explicitly on the principles of public economics or have relied on
sound economic analysis in *ex ante* or *ex post* evaluation' [7]. A recent World Bank interim
review of its HIV Program for Africa reiterates the point that the Bank 'could have analyzed
more systematically the institutional environment and requirements for effective implementation' [63].

A growing trend throughout the 1990s among most bilaterals, with EU nations perhaps being
an exception, was that, rather than focusing on sound country analysis and actual needs,
investments had to be tailored to demonstrate their impact to the public, leading to an
emphasis on achieving quick results through short-term projects. The results-oriented,
'bang-for-the-buck' approaches typified by USAID, which had more to do with achieving
'high visibility' than promoting effective M&E, may not be suitable for dealing with HIV,
which is highly complex and warrants solutions at the local level [59]. The Panos Institute
found that 97% of donors surveyed thought that the bureaucratic need to prove impact, plan
for the short term and strive for administrative efficiency definitely hampered the effectiveness
of their response to HIV [59].

Institutional ideologies

Another factor contributing to the continuation of bad policies that seems to underlie all others
is institutional ideology. The World Bank has often been seen first and foremost as a 'bank' that
measures its success by its disbursements. Remarkably, OED reports that throughout the 1990s,
the Bank's 'core business processes and incentives remained focused on lending money rather
than achieving impact.... Forums for staff to discuss and review progress towards development objectives or recognize and reward evidence of HNP development impact are lacking.
Staff still perceived that rewards were linked primarily to project approval and disbursement'
[39]. This assessment suggests that not only was the Bank constrained by institutional weakness
that led to policies and strategies that may not have been helpful in the fight against HIV, but
was directed by an ethos that lacked the wherewithal to take account of the public health threat
posed by HIV.

Bilaterals, as noted above, are frequently badly hampered by their need to heed the
domestic public's perspective [64]. For example, prevention efforts based on the formula
of ABC—Abstain, Be faithful, use a Condom—are frequently neither relevant nor effective,
regardless of their popularity with the public. Worse yet, of the US government's $15 billion
promised by President George W Bush in the President's Emergency Plan for AIDS Relief
(PEPFAR), only a small portion is being channelled to the Global Fund to Fight AIDS,
Tuberculosis and Malaria (Global Fund) over 5 years. The Global Fund was created in 2002,
having been endorsed by the UN, the leaders of the G8 and African nations, specifically to
meet the needs of those most at risk of AIDS. Duplicating its efforts with an exclusively

American initiative wastes time and resources. This appears to be allowing the US government to pursue its own ideological agenda—for example, by supporting faith-based abstinence efforts rather than programmes for reducing harm through needle exchange and condom distribution campaigns.

Research institutions

Health research is essential for improving health system performance and the health of individuals and populations. It is requisite for achieving many of the United Nation Millennium Development goals, including combating HIV [65], and it is seen as essential for achieving equity in health and development [66]. Some of the important areas that HIV research focuses on are: poor healthcare infrastructure; cost-effectiveness of interventions; 'availability, acceptability and affordability in resource-poor settings'; access barriers; programme implementation; documentation of the shift of HIV to disadvantaged communities; and the social context of interventions [67]. These institutions include international health organizations (WHO, Global Forum for Health Research, Council on Health Research for Development); development banks (World Bank, Asian Development Bank); development agencies (DFID, Sida, USAID); foundations and other research funding agencies (Ford, Rockerfeller, Gates); programme- or disease-based global networks, [International Association of Physicians in AIDS Care (IAPAC)]; thematic initiatives (International AIDS Vaccine Initiative); international research centres (CDC) and university-based institutes; the pharmaceutical industry; and organizations with a regional mandate [African Medical and Research Foundation (AMREF), PAHO].

However, a review of the responses to the HIV crisis by research institutions indicates they lacked a sense of urgency, were severely underfunded or paid little attention to local research priorities. Northern agendas seemed more important than Southern needs—a pattern consistent with the way the international research community has generally responded to the health needs of developing countries over the last several decades. For example, the 1990 landmark Report by the Council on Health Research for Development (COHRED) 'found a major "disequilibrium" between funding investment and the global disease burden—only 5% of total funds ($US30 billion in 1986) was spent on research that addressed the problems of people of low-income countries, who bore 93% of the burden of disease' [68]. It also identified weak research capacity in developing countries, as well as fragmented efforts by international agencies, and recommended 'the use of the "essential national health research" (ENHR), the creation of international facilitating and monitoring support structures, and increased funding on the problems of the poor and disadvantage' [68]. Ten years later, the International Conference on Health Research for Development (ICHRD-2000), whose objective was to assess progress, found that the mobilization of financial resources for ENHR had not materialized and international mechanisms to monitor progress had not followed through [69].

An HIV vaccine

At the Bangkok International AIDS Conference in July 2004, the head of the International AIDS Vaccine Initiative (IAVI), the world's largest single organization devoted to finding a vaccine against HIV, stated that the failure to fund vaccine research adequately was 'a global disgrace'. This failure is all the more problematic given 'a lack of effective, safe, and affordable pharmaceuticals to control infectious diseases that cause high mortality and morbidity among poor people in the developing world' [70]. Analyses of outcomes of pharmaceutical research and development over the past 25 years and review of current public and private initiatives aimed at correcting the imbalance in research and development show that of 1393 new chemical entities marketed between 1975 and 1999, only 16 were for tropical diseases and tuberculosis [70]—the so-called 10/90 gap identified by COHRED [71]. The pharmaceutical industry takes the position that research and development is too costly to invest in likely low-return, neglected diseases. Though it recognizes the urgent need for vaccines against HIV, such investments require sources of financing other than the commercial market if they are to be sustainable [72].

The World Bank AIDS Vaccine Task Force commissioned a study on the perspectives of the biotechnology, vaccine and pharmaceutical industries regarding investment in research and development work on an HIV vaccine with a view to understanding low private investment and exploring potential solutions. In order to raise the levels of private research and development, it recommended a combination of 'push' strategies, which reduce the cost and scientific risk of investment, and 'pull' strategies, which guarantee a market [73]. It found, however, that probably more important than these mechanisms are the actions, leadership and commitment of developing countries—for example, in forging international public–private partnerships for the local testing and development of vaccines.

Social vaccine and knowledge about prevention

Efforts to interrupt the transmission of HIV through prevention programmes have had limited success. UNAIDS (2004) reports that 'prevention programmes reach only one in five of people at risk of contracting HIV', and 'only one in ten pregnant women was offered services for preventing mother-to-child HIV transmission' [74]. Prevention initiatives through 'sustained education, skills training, and support for behavior change', for example, which depend upon appropriate research to inform planners and decision makers with reliable data, have been undermined by the failure to develop ENHR and by fragmented efforts on the part of the IRC. A review of studies of the evidence base in low- and middle-income countries finds that complete cost data were not available in any one country and that the 'costing methods applied and results obtained in this review give rise to questions of reliability, validity and transparency' [75]. Review of nine studies that evaluated the costs and consequences of interventions to reduce mother-to-child transmission in Africa found that information on quantities of resources needed, methods for valuing health outcomes, and unit costs was inadequate. Even basic data on the costs of strengthening the health infrastructure to a reasonable standard to guarantee delivery of interventions were not available [76]. Furthermore, in most developing countries, 'there is not an appropriate scientific infrastructure to support or even validate any HIV prevention programs' [76]. The establishment and maintenance of an adequate scientific infrastructure is of pivotal importance in HIV prevention programmes in developing countries. Laboratories supporting these programmes need to be equipped with essential equipment and trained staff [77].

Strong national health research capacities are the foundation of a global health research endeavour. A notable body of literature shows that, rather than developing local health research capacities, North–South research collaborations were frequently exploitative and characterized as 'scientific colonialism' [71]. Models of international research include the so-called 'Safari model', the 'Courier model' and the 'Mosquito model', all of which entail foreign investigators extracting needed information from a developing country through a variety of means that do not involve significant contributions from local scientists. These methods are now widely recognized as inappropriate and detrimental to the development of local research capacities [78]. Some contend that HIV will provide 'the backdrop for much of the rethinking that is going on with regard to research done by the North in developing countries' [71]. The creation of the African Health Research Forum (AfHRF) in 2003 is seen as one small step taken to address the failure of Northern institutions to provide training or other forms of capacity building while undertaking research in Africa [79].

Research efforts are also influenced by the same constraints that have limited the effectiveness of bilateral and multilateral HIV investments. Issues of coordination, ownership and separate agendas that frequently constrained ODA effectiveness [80] also undermined donor support of research related to HIV. For example, 'in one African country there was a well–designed longitudinal epidemiological study of HIV/AIDS but with relatively little information on behavioral aspects. In the same country another team studied behavioral aspects in detail but in a different site. Apparently, each donor insisted upon having a separate discrete project!' [78]. Few bilateral agencies support research in developing countries—the Canadian International Development Research Centre (IDRC) and the Swedish Agency for Research Cooperation with Developing Countries (SAREC), established in the 1970s, being among the few exceptions. In contrast, the UK's Medical Research Council and the US's National Institute of Health concerned themselves primarily with science, not development, even when they supported research in developing countries [81]. Local and international NGOs, too, have seldom taken research seriously, so that in terms of HIV investment, 'policy makers have no channels of being informed about what is needed, where and how' [54].

In contrast, the World Bank placed 'information collection', including cost-effectiveness of interventions and operational research, at the top of its priority list. Nevertheless, it missed many opportunities to gather information on social and economic aspects of the pandemic and relate them to its own mission. For example, a review of 25 of the World Bank's Country Assistance Strategies (CASs), the main document guiding Bank activities in a borrowing country, shows that it strongly supported measures to improve the status of women and expand levels of girls' education, 'yet not one of them made a link between support for these measures and potentially lowering the transmission of HIV' [11].

These past failures to fund HIV research adequately, to develop local research capacities and to demonstrate that Southern needs are just as important as Northern ones, underscore the need to refocus on the principles of equity, ownership and self-reliance. In the future, experts warn, the international health research community will need to pursue a demand-driven model of research with greater emphasis placed on inclusiveness, and involve all stakeholders, not just research producers—decision makers, users of research and civil society.

Conclusion

In 2000, the international donor and lending communities began a radically new and intensified approach to the fight against HIV based on knowledge management, advocacy, resource development and capacity building, and an emphasis on multisectoral frameworks and working at the community level with local organizations and financing partners. Yet, the challenges remain enormous. Donors will first need to secure an increase in ODA flows from the US$6 billion in 2004 to US$15 billion in 2007. The resurgence of bilateralism and tied aid, which tends to be less effective and only vaguely related to poverty reduction, may threaten prevention and treatment initiatives. The international donor community will be preoccupied with the institutional and administrative constraints on effective spending of aid flows that are widespread in recipient countries—issues related to absorptive capacity, the human resource gap and governance that undermine service delivery. To do this and positively influence governments, particularly the ministries of health and finance, and to take innovative approaches to service delivery, donors will need to pay attention to issues of participation, consultation and coordination as well as monitoring and evaluation.

In terms of identifying the problem, collecting the data and finding a solution, responses to the pandemic in the 1980s and 1990s by the international health research community and the international donor community were obviously inadequate. It can be expected that in this decade, these institutions will be held much more accountable for the quality of their response.

References

1. Ainsworth M, Teokul W. (2000). Breaking the silence: setting realistic priorities for AIDS control in less-developed countries. *Lancet* **356**:55–60.
2. Ainsworth M, Mead Over A. (1997). *Confronting AIDS: Public Priorities in a Global Epidemic.* Oxford: Oxford University Press for the World Bank.
3. World Bank. URL: http://www.worldbank.org/oed/arde (last accessed May 15, 2005).
4. Organisation for Economic Co-operation and Development. URL: www.oecd.org/dac.
5. Perin I, Attaran A. (2003). Trading ideology for dialogue: an opportunity to fix international aid for health. *Lancet* **261**:1216–9.
6. Michaud C, Murray CJ. (1994). External assistance to the health sector in developing countries: a detailed analysis, 1972–90. *Bulletin of the World Health Organization* **72**:639–51. URL: http://www.who.int/bulletin/en/.
7. World Bank. (1999). *Intensifying Action Against HIV in Africa: Responding to a Developmental Crisis, Africa Region.* Washington, DC: World Bank, p7.
8. Attaran A and Sachs J. (2001).Defining and redefining international support for combating the AIDS pandemic. *Lancet* **357**:57–61.
9. OECD, DAC Secretariat. (2000). *Recent Trends in Official Development Assistance to Health.* Paris: OECD.
10. Japan Center for International Exchange. (2004). *Japan's Response to the Spread of HIV.* Tokyo: Japan Center for International Exchange. URL: www.jcie.or.jp/thinknet/policy_studies/hiv.pdf.
11. World Bank. (1998). *HIV Interventions: Ex Ante and Ex Post Evaluation.* World Bank Discussion Paper No. 389. Washington, DC: The World Bank.
12. World Bank and African Development Bank. (2002). *Lesotho: Development in a Challenging Environment, A Joint World Bank and African Development Bank Evaluation* World Bank Operations Evaluation Department and African Development Bank Operations Evaluation Department. Washington, DC and Abidjan.
13. World Bank Operations Evaluation Department. (2002). *Zambia Country Assistance Evaluation, OED Reach,* September 17. Washington, DC: World Bank.
14. Tarantola D, Kieffer MP, Ernberg G, Opuni M, Schwartländer B, Walker N. (1999). *Level and Flow of National and International Resources for the Response for HIV 1996–97.* Geneva: UNAIDS.

15. OECD, Development Assistance Committee (DAC) and the Joint United Nations Programme on HIV (UNAIDS). (2004). Analysis of Aid in Support of HIV Control. Presented at the XV International AIDS Conference, Bangkok, Thailand June 15, 2004.

16. World Bank. (1996). *Social Dimensions of Adjustment: World Bank Experience.* Washington, DC: World Bank, Operations Evaluation Department.

17. World Bank. (1992). Republic of Zambia Public Expenditure Review, Macro, Industry and Finance, Division of Southern Africa Region.

18. Collier P, Gunning JW. (1999). The IMF's role in structural adjustment. *Economic Journal* 109(459): F634–51.

19. World Bank Operations Evaluation Department. (2003). *Toward Country-led Development: A Multi-partner Evaluation of CDF.* Synthesis Report. Washington, DC: World Bank.

20. World Health Organization. (2004). *World Health Report 2004: Changing History.* Geneva: WHO.

21. Buve A, Bishikwabo-Nsarhaza K, Mutangadura G. (2002). The spread and effect of HIV-1 infection in sub-Saharan Africa. *Lancet* 359:2011–7.

22. Buve A, Changalucha J, Mayaud P *et al.* (2001). How many patients with a sexually transmitted infection are cured by health services? A study from Mwanza region, Tanzania. *Tropical Medicine and International Health* 12:971–9.

23. Simonsen L, Kane A, Lloyd J, Zaffran M, Kane M. (1999). Unsafe injection in the developing world and transmission of bloodborne pathogens: a review. *Bulletin of the World Health Organization* 77:789–800.

24. Kane A, Lloyd J, Zaffran M, Simonsen L, Kane M. (1999). Transmission of hepatitis B, hepatitis C, and human immunodeficiency viruses through unsafe injections in the developing world: model-based regional estimates. *Bulletin of the World Health Organization* 77:801–7.

25. Gisselquist D, Minkin SF, Okwuosah A, Salerno L, Minja-Trupin C. (2004). Unsafe injections and transmission of HIV-1 in sub-Saharan Africa. *Lancet* 363:1648.

26. Schmid GP, Buvé A, Mugyenyi P *et al.* (2004). Transmission of HIV-1 infection in sub-Saharan Africa and effect of elimination of unsafe injections. *Lancet* 363:482–88.

27. World Bank. (1987). *Financing Health Services in Developing Countries: An Agenda for Reform.* Washington, DC: World Bank.

28. World Bank. (1993). *World Development Report: Investing in Health.* Washington, DC: World Bank.

29. Forsythe S, Mangkalopakorn C, Chitwarakorn A, Masvichian N. (1998). Cost of providing sexually transmitted disease services in Bangkok. *AIDS* 12(Supplement 2):S73–80.

30. La Ruche G, Lorougnon F, Digbeu N. (1995). Therapeutic algorithms for the management of sexually transmitted diseases at the peripheral level in Cote d'Ivoire: assessment of efficacy and cost. *Bulletin of the World Health Organization* 73:305–13.

31. Hensher M, Jefferys E. (2000). Financing blood transfusion services in sub-Saharan Africa: a role for user fees? *Health Policy and Planning* 15:287–95.

32. Forsythe S, Arthur G, Ngatia G, Mutemi R, Odhiambo J, Gilks C. (2002). Assessing the cost and willingness to pay for voluntary HIV counseling and testing in Kenya. *Health Policy Plan* 17(2):187–95.

33. Moses S, Manji F, Bradley JE, Nagelkerke NJ, Malisa MA, Plummer FA. (1992). Impact of user fees on attendance at a referral center for sexually transmitted diseases in Kenya. *Lancet* 340:463–6.

34. World Health Organization. (1999). *Integrating STI Management into Family Planning Services: What are the Benefits?* Geneva: WHO.

35. World Health Organization. (2002). *Adolescent Friendly Health Services: An Agenda for Change.* Geneva: WHO.

36. Mills A, Brugha R, Hanson K, McPake B. (2002). What can be done about the private health sector in low-income countries? *Bulletin of the World Health Organization* 80:325–30.

37. Mbengue C, Gamble Kelley A. (2001). *Funding and Implementing HIV Activities in the Context of Decentralization: Ethiopia and Senegal.* Bethesda, MD: Abt Associates Inc., Partnership for Health Reform.

38. The World Bank. (2004). *Experience in Scaling-up Support to Local Response in Multi-country AIDS programs (MAP) in Africa.* Environmentally and Socially Sustainable Development (ESSD) Regional Program on HIV/AIDS in collaboration with AIDS Campaign Team for Africa (ACTafrica). World Bank.

39. The World Bank. (1999). *Investing in Health: Development Effectiveness in Health Nutrition and Population Sector.* Washington, DC: World Bank, Operations Evaluation Department.

40. John Snow, Inc. (2001). *Tanzania: Situational Assessment of Logistics Systems for Public Health Commodities at Selected Districts and SDP.* Dar es Salaam, Tanzania: Family Planning and Logistics Management, John Snow Inc.

41. Brugha R, Zwi A. (1999). Sexually transmitted disease control in developing countries: the challenge of involving the private sector. *Sexually Transmitted Infections* 75:283–5.

42. Trostle J. (1996). Inappropriate distribution of medicines by professionals in developing countries. *Social Science and Medicine* 42:1117–20.

43. Adu-Sarkodie YA. (1997). Antimicrobial self-medication in patients attending a sexual transmitted diseases clinic. *International Journal of STDs and AIDS* 8:456–8.

44. World Health Organization. (1999). *Interpreting Reproductive Health.* Geneva: WHO.

45. Lush L, Cleland J, Walt G, Mayhew S. (1999). Integrating reproductive health: myth and ideology. *Bulletin of the World Health Organization* 77:771–7.

46. Walraven GE. (1996). Primary reproductive health care in Tanzania. *European Journal of Obstetrics Gynecology and Reproductive Biology* 69(1):41–5.

47. Dehne KL, Snow R, O'Reilly KR. (2000). Integration of prevention and care of sexually transmitted infections with family planning services: what is the evidence for public health benefits? *Bulletin of the World Health Organization* 78:628–39.

48. Fleischman K, Foreit KH, Agarwal K. (2002). When does it make sense to consider integrating STIs and HIV services with family planning services? *International Family Planning Perspectives* 28(2). URL: http://www.guttmacher.org/pubs/journals/2810502.html.

49. Lush L, Walt G, Cleland J, Mayhew S. (2001). The role of MCH and family planning services in HIV/STD control: is integration the answer? *African Journal of Reproductive Health* 5(3):29–46.

50. Mayhew S. (1996). Integrating MCH/FP and STD/HIV services: current debates and future directions. *Health Policy Plan* 11:339–53.

51. Peterse I, Swartz L. (2002). Primary health care in the era of HIV: some implications for health systems reform. *Social Science and Medicine* 55:1005–13.

52. Claeson M, Mawji T, Walker C. (2000). *Investing in the Best Buys: A Review of the Health, Nutrition and Population Portfolio, FY 1993–99.* Washington, DC: World Bank.

53. OECD Development Assistance Committee. (2004). *Peer Review of Japan.* Paris: OECD, p30.

54. Gupta I, Panda S, Motihar R. (2003). *HIV and Development in India: Background Study for the Swedish Country Strategy for India.* Delhi: Sida.

55. Kilian A. (2002). *HIV control in Kabarole District, Uganda.* Eschborn, Germany: GTZ.

56. OECD Development Assistance Committee. (2004). DAC Peer Review: Main Findings and Recommendations. Australia: OECD.

57. United States General Accounting Office. Report to the Chairman: Subcommittee on African Affairs Committee of Foreign Relations, US Senate. (2001). *Global Health: Joint UN Program on HIV Needs Strengthened Country-level Efforts and Measure Results.* Washington, DC: US General Accounting Office.

58. World Bank, Operations Evaluation Department. (2001). *The US$500 Million Multi-country HIV Program for Africa (MAP).* Progress Review Mission FY01, Washington, DC: World Bank.

59. The Panos Institute. (2002). *Critical Challenges in HIV Communication.* A Panos-London Perspective Paper. London: Panos Institute.

60. World Bank, Operations Evaluation Department. (2000). *Participation in Development Assistance.* Precis No. 209, p4.

61. World Bank, Operations Evaluation Department. (2000). *The Drive to Partnership Aid Co-ordination and the World Bank.* Precis No. 201, p4.

62. National Audit Office. (2004.) *Responding to HIV.* Report of the Comptroller and Auditor General of the Department for International Development. London: the Stationery Office.

63. World Bank. (2004). *Interim Review of the Multi-country HIV Program for Africa.* Washington DC: World Bank.

64. Rogerson A, Hewitt A, Waldenberg D. (2004). *The International Aid System 2005–2010: Forces for and Against Change.* London: Overseas Development Institute (ODI).

65. Sadana R, Pang T. (2003). Health research systems: a framework for the future. *Bulletin of the World Health Organization* 81:222–3.

66. Jacobs M, de Haan S. (2003). Health research systems: an evolving framework. *Bulletin of the World Health Organization* 81:624.

67. Global Forum for Health Research. *Analytical Work: Diseases and Conditions: HIV.* URL: http://www.globalforumhealth.org/pages/index.asp.

68. Neufeld V, Sitthi-Amorn C. (2000). *After the Bangkok Meetings—Opportunities for INCLEN.* Manila: The Inclen Trust.

69. Council on Health Research for Development (COHRED). (2000). *Health Research for Development: The Continuing Challenge.* Discussion paper prepared for the International Conference on Health Research for Development, Bangkok October 2000.

70. Trouiller P, Olliaro P, Torreele E, Orbinski J, Laing R, Ford N. (2002). Drug development for neglected diseases: a deficient market and a public-health policy failure. *Lancet* 359: 2188–94.

71. Tan-Torres Edejer T. (1999). North–South research partnerships: the ethics of carrying out research in developing countries. *British Medical Journal* 319:438–41.

72. Andre FE. (2002). How the research-based industry approaches vaccine development and establishes priorities. *Developmental Biology* 110:25–9.

73. Batson A, Ainsworth M. (2001). Private investment in AIDS vaccine development: obstacles and solutions. *Bulletin of the World Health Organization* 79(8):721–7.

74. UNAIDS. (2004). *Report on the Global AIDS Epidemic (2004), Executive Summary.* Geneva: UNAIDS.

75. Walker D. (2003). Cost and cost-effectiveness of HIV prevention strategies in developing countries: is there an evidence base? *Health Policy and Planning* 18(1):4–17.

76. Scotland GS, van Teijlingen A, Edwin R *et al.* (2003). A review of studies assessing the costs and consequences of interventions to reduce mother-to-child HIV transmission in sub-Saharan Africa. *AIDS* 17(7):1045–52.

77. Gomez-Roman VR. (2003). HIV prevention programs in developing countries are deficient without an appropriate scientific research infrastructure. *AIDS* 17(7):1114–6.

78. Lucas AO. (2001). *International Collaboration in Health Research*. Commission on Macroeconomics and Health (CMH). Working Paper Series Paper No. WG2:2. Geneva: CMH, p6.

79. Ramsay S. (2002). African health researchers unite. *Lancet* 360:1665–6.

80. Walt G, Pavignani E, Gilson L, Buse K. (1999). Health sector development: from aid coordination to resource management. *Health Policy Plan* 14:207–18.

81. Freeman P, Miller M. (2001). *Scientific Capacity Building to Improve Population Health: Knowledge as a Global Public Good*. Commission on Macroeconomics and Health. Working Paper Series Paper No. WG2:3. Geneva: CMH, p9.

Chapter 42

Financing HIV: the roles of international financial institutions

Maureen Lewis[*] and Susan Stout

Introduction

Decades after the first warnings about the coming epidemic, HIV is at last one of the highest priority issues on the global agenda. The direst predictions have come true, with the disease ravaging development prospects across the globe. Prevention through behavioural change or a vaccine remains elusive in many settings.

The loss of a large segment of prime-age adults, particularly women, devastates households in the short to medium term. Long-term losses in human capital formation pose a further risk that influences the inter-generational transfer of knowledge and creates macroeconomic threats, particularly in the most deeply affected countries of sub-Saharan Africa [1]. Halting transmission of this highly adaptable virus continues to prove politically intractable, further endangering countries where it has not yet become a generalized epidemic, particularly the former Soviet Union—notably Russia—and South and East Asia.

Though lower prices are reducing the cost of treatment, the issue of cost is itself dwarfed by the operational challenges of developing and delivering services of sufficient quality and sustainability to avoid unleashing new, drug-resistant strains of the virus. Governments face an enormous list of implementation challenges whose scale and complexity make prioritization politically, as well as managerially, difficult [2].

Rapid increases in the funds now available for HIV, though long awaited, also raise some critical questions. Can low-income countries effectively utilize the massive amount of resources required, or even the amounts already pledged and committed, given their fragile healthcare systems and the gaps in overall institutional capacity? What kind and how much development assistance is needed to win the fight against AIDS?

The role of the international financial institutions (IFIs) is of particular relevance, given their influence on government investment priorities. Despite assumptions to the contrary, the World Bank and the International Monetary Fund (IMF) place no ceilings on government spending. There is a range of possibilities consistent with macroeconomic stability and fiscal responsibility. Both institutions are far more concerned with good government and the effective management of money, especially the efficient disbursement of funds. How much money is expended, how quickly, whether it can be absorbed and spent well, and whether such spending has economic and management implications, are the fundamental drivers of IFI involvement.

* Corresponding author.
The views expressed in this chapter are those of the authors and are not necessarily those of the organizations for which they work, unless stated in the text.

This chapter focuses on the role of IFIs, the effects of increased spending on macroeconomic and fiscal health, the constraints to this additional spending and, finally, the implications for the IFIs and other actors in reaching the twin objectives of sound economic policy and development effectiveness in the effort to halt transmission of HIV and improve the treatment of AIDS.

Financing the fight against HIV

The United Nations Joint Programme on HIV/AIDS (UNAIDS), along with its co-sponsoring members such as the World Bank, is working with major foundations and the private sector to mobilize the resources required to address the HIV pandemic [3]. Several recent estimates of the costs associated with prevention, and especially treatment, suggest that US$10.5 billion would be required in 2005, rising to US$20 billion in 2007. The latter figure alone is more than twice the US$7 billion allocated annually to overall development assistance (ODA) for health. This has led to a focus on rapid and large-scale resource mobilization at the international level. The current value of commitments exceeds US$4.7 billion [4].

Six funding streams currently support the financing of HIV programmes: (i) domestic public spending; (ii) bilateral assistance; (iii) multilateral agencies such as the World Bank; (iv) the Global Fund to Fight AIDS, Tuberculosis and Malaria (Global Fund), which combines public and private giving, including bilateral donors; (v) the private sector, including philanthropic donations such as those of the Gates and Clinton Foundations; and (vi) household out-of-pocket spending. Bilateral assistance is projected to grow faster than the other sources, primarily as a result of the US$15 billion scale-up by the USA for 15 priority countries over 5 years under the President's Emergency Plan for AIDS Relief (PEPFAR). The second most significant source is anticipated to be the Global Fund.

Figure 42.1 summarizes trends in the different resources available for HIV. Both the number of sources and the levels of commitment show rapid increases, which together are closing in on estimated resource needs. Funding is heavily concentrated in a relatively small number of countries. Donors are supporting activities in 140 countries, but about 72% of this funding is allocated to 25 countries, mostly in the highly affected countries in Africa and the Caribbean [5]. Major recipients have seen major increases in HIV support in the last few years.

The rapid scale-up of external resources is placing pressure on countries to absorb this money effectively. The targeted sectors, notably ministries of health (MoHs), are often the least institutionally equipped to expand rapidly and effectively. These institutions generally have neither the authority nor the necessary access to senior finance and planning officials to integrate their requirements effectively into national policy-making and budget allocations. The pressures on MoHs are especially high because they retain responsibility for absorbing and managing the bulk of international AIDS funding.

The challenge of financing the response to HIV is thus two-edged: responding to the level of financial requirements, and ensuring that the very large amounts of resources being made available are quickly and effectively absorbed.

The roles of the IMF and World Bank in relation to HIV

Established after the Second World War, the IMF and World Bank were intended to provide a framework for international economic cooperation and development to foster a stable and prosperous global economy. They have complementary mandates.

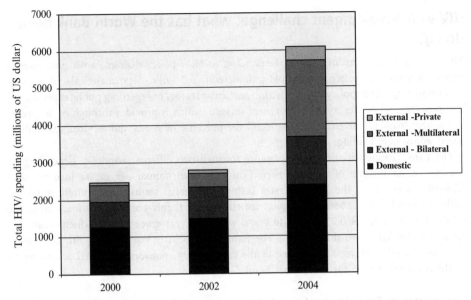

Fig. 42.1 Trends in HIV financing by source: developing world total. The figures for the private sector only reflect international NGOs. Domestic financing includes public and private sources. Sources: OECD, UNAIDS, 2005.

The IMF serves as the lender of last resort for countries, with much of its work comprising preventive measures in monitoring macroeconomic performance. It extends loans of 3–4 years to countries facing severe macroeconomic problems, and 10-year loans at 0.5% interest to the poorest countries. These countries lack the creditworthiness to obtain commercial loans. The short-term nature of the loans reflects the stopgap nature of financing provided to bring a country's economy out of crisis, rather than for long-term stability. Conditions accompany loans to ensure that countries adopt policies and programmes that will return them to financial viability so they can resume growth and repay the IMF. Financing is not provided for particular sectors or projects, but for general support of a country's balance of payments to bolster international reserves, thereby creating the financial space for the government to address the underlying economic problems.

The International Bank for Reconstruction and Development (IBRD), more commonly known as the World Bank, was set up to promote long-term economic development. The World Bank Group, which includes the IBRD, the International Finance Corporation (IFC) and the International Development Association (IDA), is concerned mainly with longer-term development and poverty reduction issues. Its activities include lending to developing countries and countries in transition to finance sectoral projects, often linked to reforms in those same sectors, as well as broader structural reforms, which influence change and affect segments of the economy or government activities. Budget management falls within the mandate of both the World Bank and the IMF, but only the Bank deals directly with individual sectors such as health or education.

HIV as a development challenge: what has the World Bank been doing?

The Bank uses three major tools in responding to HIV: policy dialogue with ministries of finance, line ministries such as the MoH and, increasingly, civil society; analytical and advisory services to help clarify policy options within particular sectors or regarding public expenditures and poverty; and concessional development finance, which it provides through both specific investment loans for investments that entail the purchase of goods and services, and policy-based, adjustment lending.

The Bank channels its financial assistance through two different windows, depending on the per capita income of the borrower. Countries with annual per capita incomes over US$860 borrow from the Bank at rates below commercial terms. The poorest countries, with incomes below US$860 per capita, are eligible for highly concessional loans from the IDA at interest rates of 0.75% over 40 years, with a 10-year grace period, which means the loans are effectively two-thirds grant. The Bank also works in partnership with the United Nations and other players. It was one of the co-founding sponsors of UNAIDS, and serves as the financial trustee for the Global Fund.

Overview of Bank's work on HIV

The Bank first became involved with HIV in the late 1980s, and has since provided more than US$2.2 billion for 91 projects (Figure 42.2) [6]. Its initial efforts were managed within the Bank's overall programme on health, with interventions mostly forming components of larger health loans.

The Bank's earliest large-scale investments in HIV were in Brazil and India. Recent evaluations of both efforts provide several key lessons. The Brazil investments successfully supported

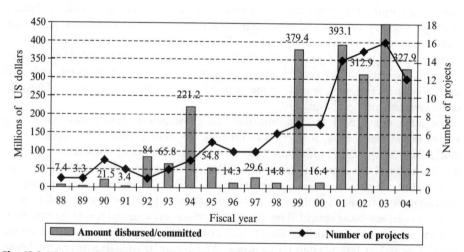

Fig. 42.2 HIV commitments and number of HIV projects, by fiscal year of approval (HIV projects and HIV components greater than US$1 million, including projects in health, education and social protection). Source: World Bank, 2005.

improvements and further expansion of state-of-the-art prevention activities, maintaining a focus on high-risk groups. The project established sexually transmitted infection (STI)/HIV coordination units in 150 municipalities in all 27 states, with enhanced services for diagnosis, treatment and care. Both stages of the project, AIDS I and II, contributed significantly to capacity development at the state and municipal levels. Bank assistance in Brazil also stimulated a competitive grants programme that strengthened the capacity of non-governmental organizations (NGOs) and funded outreach to high-risk groups, considerably expanding programme scope and coverage.

The evaluation of the Bank's work in India concluded that the project had advanced the government's response to HIV by several years and largely put in place the institutional mechanisms at the national and state levels on which a broader response could be launched. In particular, the project greatly improved the safety of the blood supply; established nationwide epidemiological surveillance of HIV; enlisted the mass media and NGOs in increasing awareness of HIV; piloted prevention interventions targeting groups at high risk of spreading HIV, such as sex workers, truck drivers and injecting drug users (IDUs); and trained thousands of health providers in HIV/STI care and prevention [7].

These experiences, along with other ongoing operations, also reflect some common weaknesses. Information gaps, weak disease surveillance systems—a particular failure of the Brazil programme—and limited monitoring and evaluation at the country level make it impossible to assess the epidemiological impact of these interventions accurately. However, there are clearly plausible links to the recorded results, which suggest the effectiveness of prevention efforts, while also highlighting the need to tackle some complex organizational and institutional issues. The Bank recently expanded its efforts through a new multi-country HIV initiative.

What is MAP?

The World Bank's Multi-Country HIV/AIDS Program (MAP) represents a significant departure from traditional Bank lending instruments. It is an ongoing effort designed to permit rapid identification and scale-up of successful experiences. With a focus on learning by doing, it allows for the sharing of experiences within and between countries.

MAP aims to strengthen national HIV strategies through a national institutional framework that would include different sectors. A high-level National HIV/AIDS Coordinating (NAC) body representing all major stakeholders would be responsible for mobilizing resources, monitoring the epidemic and coordinating, but not implementing, programmes and policies through grants to public and private entities. MAP has provided more than US$1.2 billion to 29 countries, including all the IDA eligible countries in Africa.

The impact of MAP has been mixed. On the positive side, the focus on the establishment of mechanisms to mobilize a deep and wide response to the epidemic has facilitated the flow of funds and, to a lesser degree, the availability of technical advice in several countries. The National HIV/AIDS Commission in Ghana, for instance, was able to channel resources to more than 2600 small civil society organizations throughout the country. Ethiopia, Kenya, Uganda and other countries have made similar progress; and over 30,000 subprojects have received assistance across the whole of Africa.

Early on, weak administrative and managerial systems translated into slow disbursement of funds, limited monitoring and virtually no evaluation. Multiministerial decision making within the national councils also had the unintended effect of sidelining MoHs, leading to a vacuum in health leadership. This problem became even more pronounced when other ministries turned to the health ministry for support [8]. More recent achievements have seen disbursements at 95% of forecasts, well above other World Bank project levels, and significant amounts received by MoHs. It is estimated that MoHs will ultimately receive around two-thirds of all MAP funding. Nonetheless, there is an emerging consensus that the Bank needs to focus more attention on providing analysis and advice on the technical content of subgrants, and on the institutional needs of health systems that support HIV programmes.

HIV as a macroeconomic and fiscal challenge: the roles of the IMF and World Bank

HIV has come to transcend all aspects of household and national priorities, especially in the hardest-hit countries. While macroeconomic models suggest limited impacts, the economic effects are becoming obvious, both in terms of national economic losses and in terms of resource allocation and public management.

Planned increases in new funding for HIV represent a significant rise in aid flows for a single cause. However, large financial inflows for any single issue, however critical, can destabilize an economy and pose serious macroeconomic challenges that both the Bank and the IMF have a mandate to address [9]. Heller and Gupta [10] analyse the macroeconomic impacts of tripling official development assistance, a figure close to the amount projected by UNAIDS as required for the disease. The macroeconomic effects depend on the size of the economy and the level of imports, with smaller economies being more vulnerable. Several major risks confront countries expected to receive significant new monies.

Inflation

A large infusion of money financing local goods and services that cannot be adequately absorbed quickly can lead to inflation. Good economic management can contain inflation to a degree, but experience in Ghana in the 1980s suggests the limited effectiveness of even good policies in small countries when the inflows are large [11].

Exchange rate appreciation

A sudden infusion of foreign exchange can lead to an appreciation of the exchange rate, a decline in the competitiveness of domestic production and a loss of exports, thereby harming a major engine of economic growth. If all foreign exchange were spent on importation of antiretroviral drugs, the macroeconomic effects would be minimal because it would not affect local pharmaceutical markets or a government's ability to control monetary policy.

In Uganda, where ODA grants grew by 3.5% of gross domestic product (GDP) between 1995 and 2000, despite prudent fiscal management, the stubborn appreciation of the exchange rate made exports more costly, depressing demand for agricultural exports. A recent analysis of the situation suggests a complex set of effects due to increased flows in small developing countries. An increase in net aid in any sector will lead to a rise in the exchange rate, a drop in exports and a decline in rural incomes in the short run, but a possible reversal in the long run, provided the aid is not devoted to recurrent government expenditures. Unfortunately, this tends to be the case with funds made available for HIV since they finance services, which are almost entirely reliant on recurrent cost [12]. This suggests a trade-off between more donor money and maintaining farmer incomes. If spending on HIV raises productivity, that helps to mitigate the negative effects of large inflows. However large the level of HIV financing, it alone would be unlikely to create an exchange rate crisis. It is HIV spending on top of other inflows that can cause problems.

Sustainability

The inherent uncertainty in continued donor funding raises important questions about sustainability of funding and its predictability. A study of 72 countries found that over time, volatility in aid flows exceeds that in tax revenues and tends to rise and fall along with government budgets, undermining efforts at long-term planning because funding cannot be assured [13]. Fluctuations in resource flows complicate hiring of full-time public sector staff, since they cannot simply be made redundant when funds run low. Likewise, sustained treatment for HIV patients cannot be assured when the resources to keep the programmes operating vary from year to year. Interruptions in treatment can also induce dangerous drug resistance, so the sustainability of funding becomes critical in efforts to extend the lives of HIV patients. It is important to note that fiscal issues would emerge if the flow of subsidized drugs were to be discontinued, leaving the government to finance the ongoing drug therapies.

Inadequate absorptive capacity

Recipient countries often lack the health infrastructure, management and personnel, as well as the flexibility to increase expenditures and the delivery of services efficiently or comply with the financial reporting requirements that accompany aid. This poses a serious obstacle to the efforts of IFIs to address HIV and is discussed more fully below. The magnitude of each of these risks varies with individual country circumstances, but they define the issues that countries and the IFIs must grapple with in balancing economic requirements and the need to tackle HIV.

Constraints on effective spending of increased aid flows

The suddenness of resource availability has found recipient countries unprepared to scale up, given their institutional and administrative weaknesses. This section illustrates the problem of absorptive capacity by comparing anticipated aid flows with current levels of government expenditure, and elaborates on the management and human resource constraints encountered in spending additional resources in the hardest hit countries. A related initiative of the Joint Learning Institute identifies the gap in human resources as the major impediment to adequate spending and service delivery in Africa [14,15]. While no doubt a contributing factor, the effectiveness of human resource use plays an equally important role.

External financing levels and absorptive capacity

Figure 42.3 summarizes the trends in public health spending and external HIV financing for some of the hardest-hit African countries. The volatility in foreign assistance flows was such that averaging these over 3 years was necessary to capture the real trends in HIV monies. Dramatic shifts have occurred in external flows. In Ethiopia, Mozambique and Uganda, foreign assistance and loans for HIV were equivalent to about half of all health spending in 2000–2001 [16]. Between 2000/2 and 2002/4, external funding increased significantly in all of

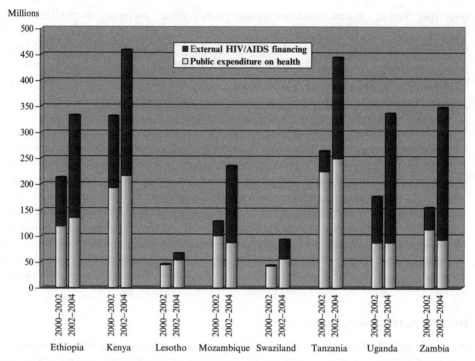

Fig. 42.3 Trends in public health funding and external financing for HIV, 2000–2004. Source: OECD/ DAC; UNAIDS; country public expenditure reviews, various years.

the countries, with Kenya experiencing the smallest increase at 75%. Lesotho and Swaziland have risen dramatically from very modest bases, but it has meant funding increases of well over 1000%, big shifts in resources for small countries.

External funding for the disease is beginning to dwarf overall public health expenditures in several countries. As Fig. 42.3 shows, the level and rate of change in the ratio of public health to external HIV funding between 2000/1 and 2003/4 are impressive.

The divergence is dramatic for all the countries, and particularly so in Uganda, where government spending on health remained constant while external funds for HIV climbed 180%. In Mozambique, public health budgets declined while external funds for HIV jumped 435%, thereby overwhelming health spending. With the exception of Tanzania, in 2002–2004 external HIV support in each of the included countries exceeded domestic spending on health services. The data indicate a clear move from healthcare systems financed by African governments and donors to ones that finance and concentrate on HIV, with declining resources and attention to mainstream healthcare services.

Besides the macroeconomic implications of increased aid, the effort needed to respond effectively to additional external flows is also daunting. It requires reorganizing the delivery and management of health services, integrating HIV more directly in public health services, hiring or contracting additional staff, accommodating dozens of new partners, and expanding infrastructure, and doing so while meeting fiduciary requirements. Indeed, government controls and procedures meant to ensure fair and transparent government—especially with regard to hiring, procurement and contracting services—often get in the way of such rapid change. To place the needed shifts in perspective, it should be remembered that it took the UK a full 2 years to draw up plans to absorb an additional 50% in public health spending. Poor countries are required to increase the scale of their operations even faster, and they lack the infrastructure and capacity to respond quickly. Thus, rapid increases in new monies pose challenges as well as benefits in the national fight against HIV.

Management and human resource capacity

Funding represents a critical but insufficient element in scaling up to fight HIV. Countries need the capacity to manage, spend and monitor additional donor inflows [10,17], but they face significant institutional and governance constraints in doing so [18–20]. Institutions in the poorest developing countries, especially those in the health sector, reveal gaps in basic management and oversight. Inadequate capacity translates into low efficiency and effectiveness of spending, and the lack of accountability means that poor performance goes unaddressed.

The cost of human resources represents over half of the overall costs of healthcare, even in industrialized countries. In lower-income countries, it can reach 90% of health spending. The HIV crisis affects the supply of healthcare providers, as they too are affected by the epidemic. AIDS incidence adds costs through absenteeism of healthcare workers who are too ill to come to work, their use of medical and death-related benefits, and the costs of hiring and training replacement staff for those who die. Evidence from Malawi shows annual absenteeism at 65 days for those with full-blown AIDS, and 15 days for those with HIV [17]. Another key factor that adds to the problem of inadequate human resources is that of sharply increased migration of health workers from countries with high HIV prevalence, reducing their availability at a time when demand is rising in high-prevalence settings.

Poor governance, including corruption and weak financial and personnel management in public health systems, adds to costs and lowers the productivity of existing staff [21]. Household surveys show that in some countries, patients are often required to provide under-the-table payments to health workers for treatment at public clinics [22]. An exercise in tracking public funds from ministries of finance showed that local capture, leakage and bureaucratic impediments prevented resources from reaching the frontline in many African countries. In Ghana, only 20% of non-salary funds ever reached the local clinics [23]. A recent multi-country study recorded absenteeism at primary healthcare clinics in non-AIDS-afflicted countries of 28–42% [24], and in Bangladesh, a survey found that absenteeism among physicians averaged 34%, reaching 74% at the larger clinics [25]. An earlier study in a major public hospital in the Dominican Republic could account for only 12% of physician time over a 2-week period [26]. In a Ugandan study, medical staff were absent over 85% of the time. That, combined with a 76% leakage rate for drugs and common informal payments for 'free' care, compromised quality and access to healthcare despite an adequate complement of staff [27]. The oversupply of physicians in countries such as Egypt and Pakistan has not translated into more effective or accessible healthcare services, suggesting that more than just hiring additional staff will be needed to improve performance in the health sector. These governance challenges bring into question the value of simply increasing staffing in the absence of serious efforts to bolster management and accountability.

A potentially pernicious effect of inadequate staffing is that poorly designed or under-resourced treatment programmes lead to low levels of adherence to complex treatment regimens. If drugs are not administered according to strict protocols, resistant strains of the virus can develop, jeopardizing treatment options for all [28]. Some degree of chaos and a period of adjustment generally accompany major expansions or shifts of service delivery in scaling up. Antiretroviral treatment (ART) services would be no exception, but the ability of the virus to mutate constantly and adapt to changing circumstances and the public-good nature of minimizing resistant strains suggest the need for particular care and attention to protocols and ART management.

Expanding the prevention and treatment of HIV must focus on better management at all levels, improved financial oversight and strengthened accountability for public spending, which can both expand and improve service delivery through addressing issues such as staff absenteeism and productivity, and financial leakages and irregularities.

Framework for reconciling the development and fiscal challenges of HIV

The surge in funding for HIV will inevitably affect government expenditure allocations. Countries and donors have agreed to a process of country prioritization across government needs, and a definition of an affordable package of government programmes. HIV spending is addressed within this framework. On the one hand, new resources for HIV are being made available and often require both government management of the funds and matching public funds. On the other hand, the rise in external resources relieves the public sector of some aspects of HIV costs.

The major development partners have endorsed the Poverty Reduction Strategy Paper (PRSP) and the Medium Term Expenditure Framework (MTEF) as the basic tools for, respectively, prioritizing and allocating both domestic and external financing. The IMF's Poverty Reduction and Growth Facility (PRGF) follows from these broader initiatives and defines the IMF's resource commitments to a country as well as the policy actions needed from its government. PRSPs provide a shared set of priorities for bilateral and multilateral donors. The MTEF offers discipline to the needs and priorities in the PRSP and a context for assessing financial trade-offs when setting priorities. The guidelines provided are general and serve to clarify financial priorities based on country preferences. The MTEF also places public investments in context, taking into account how much a government thinks should be spent on roads or healthcare or agricultural extension services. While still evolving, these tools provide a context and forum for donor exchange and alignment with country priorities, as well as an accountability mechanism for all concerned.

Scaling up to spend and manage increased aid flows is expensive for countries. However, the expected cost and effort are not always anticipated by countries, donors or the IFIs. Part of the challenge for the financial institutions is to find ways to help countries integrate these issues within their overall budget and priority setting processes.

IMF policy and HIV

The IMF plays no direct role in addressing HIV since its mandate requires it to ensure macroeconomic and fiscal stability rather than deal with individual sectors such as health. However, its work with overall spending, conducted with the ministries of finance and economy, does affect budget management and sector policies. The IMF has acknowledged the need for fiscal flexibility to accommodate increased spending for HIV.

A recent IMF policy document notes that 'under the PRSP approach, countries with sound poverty reduction strategies and public expenditure management systems should benefit from higher aid flows', specifically noting transfers from the Global Fund, bilateral donors and philanthropic organizations. It further specifies that these increased aid flows can be accommodated 'where they can be spent productively without undermining macroeconomic stability or fiscal and external debt sustainability', and that 'consideration will need to be given to whether there is sufficient absorptive capacity in the economy, as well as administrative capacity within the government to accommodate these flows' [29].

This policy, while highlighting the importance of a particular health issue, also places responsibility for how much to spend, and on what, entirely on member governments. It does not specify actions but merely defines parameters that promote basic principles. It points to priority funding but does not identify any hard and fast rules on what these priorities should be, or where governments should restrict spending.

The IMF has overarching policies to keep governments solvent, such as exchange rate policies to promote growth and exports, and fiscal discipline to ensure that governments do not spend beyond their means. Government compliance with such conditions can translate into reduced social spending because this is among the largest items in government budgets. Such cuts are often socially or politically unpopular.

It is noteworthy that where the IMF is not actively engaged with governments in lending programmes, HIV donors are scarce. Zimbabwe offers the best example, where much-needed HIV monies have been scaled back because the country is too risky for donors precisely because the IMF and its policy prescriptions have been ignored. The challenge lies in balancing short- and long-term priorities while maintaining financial solvency. HIV adds another important dimension to balancing this equation.

Government actions and IMF policy

The IMF's decision-making procedures and spending restrictions are often criticized as hostile to promoting investment in social sectors such as health and education [30]. However, country circumstances and actions can sometimes be more complicated than they appear. Box 42.1 offers a good example of disorganization in the Zambian government that resulted in a fiscal crisis. Rising resource needs for HIV coincided with a realization that the government was overextended. Scale-up efforts to cope with the rising tide of funds for the disease were directly affected. Severe austerity measures, framed with the assistance of the IMF and World Bank, became necessary to restore fiscal order. The crisis could have been avoided if there had been transparency in government finances and prudent budgetary allocations. Another lesson that emerged was the need for MoHs to act proactively in close coordination with ministries of finance so that the planning of programmes runs alongside work on how they will be financed.

A different story unfolded in Uganda, where significant inflows for HIV created difficulties for the Central Bank due to the timing and nature of the resources and the level of domestic, rather than international, debt. The Global Fund grant arrived outside of the government's budget cycle, and it was not part of the agreed MTEF. On the public debt side, the Bank of Uganda characterized the free money as 'too costly to absorb' [M Obwona, personal communication, 2004]. The government froze the 2002/3 budget for the MoH,

Box 42.1 Zambia: government policy, the IFIs and the fight against HIV

The Zambian HIV epidemic has contributed to government woes as it saps the civil service, raises costs of healthcare with HIV and opportunistic infection (OI) care, and leaves large numbers of orphans in its wake. With 16% of the population and 30% of pregnant women diagnosed as HIV-positive [31], there is no doubt that Zambia faces a crisis. HIV is estimated to have reduced annual economic growth by 1% per year as the epidemic spread unchecked. Efforts to scale up HIV spending have met with a series of setbacks.

Zambia's economic growth has averaged more than 4% in the last 5 years. Although this is not fast enough to reduce poverty in line with the UN's Millennium Development Goals, it represents a sharp improvement over a decade of 1.4% annual growth and declining per capita income [32]. Progress has been made towards macroeconomic stability. However, wage increases in the public sector have been a source of increasing pressure on the fiscal deficit and hence on domestic borrowing and interest rates. Government spending on civil service salaries increased from 5.4% of GDP in 1999 to 8% in 2002.

In 2003, the government granted wage increases and related allowances that would have increased the wage bill to over 10% of the GDP—a wage bill Zambia could ill afford, and well out of line with sound international practice and affordable government (see graph). Generous pension and redundancy payment obligations, which cost roughly 12 years of salary per separated staff [33], led ministries to delay retirements, instead keeping existing staff on the payroll and hiring more. All government bodies hired with impunity, without the knowledge of the Ministry of Finance, ignoring rules about hiring and salaries. No records of the hiring were maintained, and 'ghost workers' proliferated.

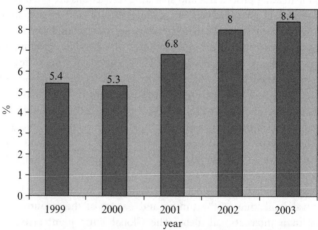

Zambian civil service spending as a percentage of GDP, 1999–2003.

Source: IMF, 2005

The large projected budget overrun threw fiscal policy into disarray, precluding a new 3-year PRGF arrangement after the last PRGF arrangement expired in March 2003. A staff-monitored programme, which was extended to June 2004, served to bring policies back on track for a new PRGF arrangement. These developments delayed progress toward completion of the Heavily Indebted Poor Countries (HIPC) Initiative. It also required the government to renegotiate agreements with public employee unions to bring public spending under control. A Dutch grant for retrenchment costs also allowed the government to shed 7000 civil servants.

With assistance from the World Bank and the IMF, Zambia has sought to frame a solution that could: (i) meet macroeconomic priorities; (ii) address the challenges of governance, public expenditure management and financial accountability; and (iii) ensure that public staffing needs are met, especially in education and health. The newly agreed PRGF specifically addresses staffing issues, supporting limits in the total wage bill that maintain overall public sector staffing costs at 8% of GDP without putting limits on hiring. Recent retirements and redundancies will permit hiring increases, but the rules and priorities regarding how many to hire, and in which sectors, are left to the Zambian government. The World Bank has specifically noted the need to increase efforts and spending on prevention and treatment for HIV [32].

instructing it to 'turn down funding from overseas donors that does not fall within the government's priorities' [34].

In this instance, the constraint was not one of absorptive capacity, but the requirements of sound monetary policy. Without controlling government spending, the government would undermine its ability to control the money supply. The government took a stand to protect its economy without reliance on advice from either the IMF or the World Bank. In both countries, the ultimate decision lay with the national government. In Zambia, both IFIs took a stand on the parameters of national spending, which had a direct effect on the use of HIV funds, but neither institution prescribed what actions government should take.

Implications and actions

The international donor community's largesse comes in response to alarms rung by UNAIDS and others who have seen first hand the devastation caused by the disease. Billions of dollars have been mobilized; the challenge now is to ensure that the monies can be used and absorbed effectively and positive outcomes be assured both in containing HIV and in macroeconomic management.

Large amounts of financing and first-rate advice can achieve little unless countries themselves choose to take charge. The World Bank, IMF and other players can only support what must ultimately be government policy, commitment and action. This remains the fundamental component of effective interventions and satisfactory outcomes for countries, IFIs and other public and private donors. With that as background, this section lays out the implications of the above discussion and suggests areas for further action by the IFIs in particular, but also for other donors and governments who are directly involved as partners in the overall effort.

The IFIs have realized the magnitude of the HIV problem, but, while they acknowledge the imperative to do more on both prevention and treatment, they face challenges in reconciling these needs with prudent macroeconomic policy. In seeking acceptable solutions, at least some of the government spending constraints can be addressed through innovative options.

First, purchasing and donating drugs in kind, as many philanthropic organizations do, would avoid the financial flow problems, since the product would not be bought and sold on the local market but donated and distributed. It therefore would not interfere in principle with fiscal or monetary policy management, nor have any impact on inflation. As a significant component of ART, it could provide a simple alternative to the government importing drugs.

Secondly, since funding flows are concentrated across a relatively short period, the sustainability of funding could be ensured through a transparent Stabilization Fund whereby governments would accept the funds and use the resources flexibly over time. This would avoid the sharp increase in foreign exchange associated with big annual disbursements. Given the chronic nature of HIV infection and the need to maintain ART over the lifetime of patients, extending funding over a longer period and arranging funding in line with capacity would strengthen a country's ability to manage external flows and provide HIV care at the same time.

The experiences of resource-rich countries such as Azerbaijan, Chad and Norway in handling sudden increases in oil revenues, similar to the surge in HIV funds, are instructive. These countries sequestered oil revenues in special stabilization funds to manage their financial resources better and prevent a flood of spending that would undermine good fiscal management. Botswana's experience with putting aside diamond earnings is another example. The IFIs already have experience in assisting governments in undertaking such efforts and could be called upon in this instance to help countries manage their HIV inflows sustainably.

Thirdly, a 'tax' of, say, 10% on all external HIV funds could be levied to pay for the upgrading of the healthcare system. This is a cost donors appear reluctant to underwrite, even though the bulk of the new monies relies on the health system to be effective. Such a tax would spread the cost of scaling up among donors and ensure that governments alone were not paying out of their already scarce funds. The World Bank could manage the necessary transactions, if needed, and support government efforts to expand and restructure their health systems.

Fourthly, both the World Bank and the IMF need to reinforce their standard roles. The IMF can and should continue to work with countries on sound macroeconomic and fiscal management in the face of increased public spending on HIV. It also needs to help governments place the priority of HIV in a broader spending context and assist them in carving out the needed fiscal space for additional health spending in the face of the pandemic. Closer coordination with the World Bank that has more experience with sectoral issues can help to broker a better alignment between ministries of finance and health. Without such collaboration, the opportunity to influence the key levers of government may be lost.

The World Bank is uniquely placed to do more in working with governments at both the economy and sectoral levels to find acceptable solutions to issues confronting the health sector. The World Bank has a comparative advantage, relative to other institutions, to take on the broader agenda of improving budget management, public sector reform and their implications for the management of the health sector. Building on its experience with HIV, the Bank should continue to contribute resources, but also help to focus both borrower and donor attention on easing the administrative and capacity constraints that slow disbursements. For example, the Bank could serve as honest broker in discussions between ministries of finance and health to persuade the former to fund healthcare or accept donor funds, and the latter to give priority to financing and performance issues.

As part of its objective of promoting better governance, the World Bank has a responsibility to better understand the ways to ensure that governments are accountable for the information and services they provide to their citizens. The Bank's effort to enhance the role of local and civil society in providing and managing these services should be reinforced. Sound evaluations to guide programme adjustments and future endeavours must also be supported. The Bank must also encourage innovation (again, with evaluations) to see how best to reconcile demands and constraints in healthcare delivery for, but not restricted to, HIV. Innovations could include providing day beds, assistance with contracting, vouchers, and the use of supervised paraprofessionals.

Finally, IFIs are not well equipped to take on all roles. For example, the IMF has neither the expertise nor the mandate to coordinate donors or play the role of broker between donors and governments. It also has a limited role in sectoral issues such as health. As for the World Bank, it cannot lend to the private sector directly, nor can it solve health system problems in the short term. Its capacity focuses on the longer term, and while defined vertical programmes can produce positive impacts in the short run, overall health system performance and capacity are challenging, long-term projects. By focusing on their respective comparative advantages and encouraging innovative thinking, the two institutions can work together with countries to be a positive force for change in the worldwide fight against the HIV pandemic.

Acknowledgements

Our thanks to Martha Ainsworth, David Andrews, Nancy Birdsall, Peter Heller, Markus Haacker, Keith Hanson, John Hicklin, Mattias Lundberg, Todd Moss, Isabel Rocha-Pimenta, Richard Rowden and Sudhir Shetty for helpful comments, and to Lisa Regis of UNAIDS for assistance with the data. Bilal Siddiqi, Rachel Block, Shweta Jain and Sebastian Sotelo provided able research assistance. The authors alone are responsible for any remaining errors. The views and observations expressed here are those of the authors, and do not necessarily represent the views or policy of the World Bank. The support of the Bill & Melinda Gates Foundation is gratefully acknowledged.

References

1. Bell C, Devarajan S, Gersbach, H. (2004). Thinking about the long-run economic costs of AIDS. In: Haacker M, ed. *The Macroeconomics of HIV/AIDS*. Washington, DC: International Monetary Fund, p96–133.

2. Ainsworth M, Teokul W. (2000). Breaking the silence: setting realistic priorities for AIDS control in less-developed countries. *Lancet* 356:55–60.

3. UNAIDS. (2004). *Financing the Expanded Response to AIDS*. UNAIDS/04.39E. Prepublication Draft. Geneva: UNAIDS.

4. Commission on Macroeconomics and Health (CMH). (2001). *Macroeconomics and Health: Investing in Health for Economic Development*. Geneva: World Health Organization. URL: http://www.cid.harvard.edu/cidcmh/CMHReport.pdf.

5. Organization for Economic Cooperation and Development (OECD). International Development Statistics (IDS) online: databases on aid and other resource flows. URL: http://www.oecd.org/dataoecd/50/17/5037721.htm.

6. Ainsworth M. (2004). Monitoring and Evaluation of National HIV/AIDS Programs: Lessons Learned from Four Developing Countries. Presented at the XV International AIDS Conference, Bangkok, July 11–16, 2004.

7. World Bank Operations Evaluation Department. (2003). India: National AIDS Control Project. Project Performance Assessment Report (Credit 2350). Washington, DC: World Bank. Available at: http://www.worldbank.org/oed/aids/New-India AIDS PPAR-Final.pdf.

8. Putzel J. (2004). The global fight against AIDS: how adequate are the national commissions? *Journal of International Development* **16**:1129–40.

9. Younger S. (1992). Aid and the Dutch disease: macroeconomic management when everybody loves you. *World Development* **20**:1587–97.

10. Heller P, Gupta S. (2002). *Challenges in Expanding Development Assistance*. IMF Policy Discussion Paper No. 02/5.

11. Adenauer I, Vagassky L. (1998). Aid and the real exchange rate: Dutch disease effects in African countries. *Intereconomics* **33**(4):177–85.

12. Adam C, Bevan D. (2003). *Aid, Public Expenditure and Dutch Disease*. The Centre for the Study of African Economies Working Paper Series, Paper 184.

13. Bulir A, Javier Hamann A. (2003). Aid volatility: an empirical assessment. *IMF Staff Papers* 50 No. 1:64–89.

14. Chen L, Evans T, Anand S *et al.* (2004) Human resources for health: overcoming the crisis. *Lancet* **364**:1984–90.

15. Joint Learning Initiative. (2004). *Human Resources for Health*. Boston, MA: Harvard University.

16. Martin G. (2003). *A Comparative Analysis of the Financing of HIV/AIDS Programmes in Botswana, Lesotho, Mozambique, South Africa, Swaziland and Zimbabwe*. Report prepared for the Social Aspects of HIV/AIDS and Health Research Programme. Human Sciences Research Council.

17. Haacker M. (2004). The impact of HIV/AIDS on government finance and the public service. In: Haacker M, ed. *The Macroeconomics of HIV/AIDS*. Washington, DC: International Monetary Fund, p167–81.

18. Kumaranayake L, Watts C. (2001). Resource allocation and priority settings of HIV/AIDS interventions: addressing the generalized epidemic in sub-Saharan Africa. *Journal of International Development* **13**:451–66.

19. Mills A, Hanson K, eds. (2003). Expanding access to health interventions in low and middle income countries: constraints and opportunities for scaling up. Special issue of *Journal of International Development* **15**(1).

20. Over M. (2004). Impact of the HIV/AIDS epidemic on health sectors. In: Haacker M, ed. *The Macroeconomics of HIV/AIDS*. Washington, DC: International Monetary Fund, pp 311–344.

21. Kauffman D, Kraay A, Zoido-Lobatón P. (1999). *Governance Matters*. World Bank Discussion Paper No. 2196.

22. Lewis M. (2006). *Governance and Corruption in Public Health Systems*. Washington, DC: Center for Global Development Working Paper No. 78.

23. World Bank. (2000). *Ghana Governance and Corruption Survey, Evidence from Households, Enterprises and Public Officials*. Africa Region. Washington, DC: World Bank.

24. World Bank. (2003). *World Development Report 2004: Making Services Work for Poor People*. Washington, DC: World Bank and Oxford University Press.

25. Chaudhury N, Hammer J, Kremer M, Muralidharan K, Rogers H. (2006). Missing in Action: Teachers and Health Workers in Developing Countries. *Journal of the European Economic Association* (in press).

26. Lewis M, La Forgia G, Sulvetta M. (1997) Measuring public hospital costs: empirical evidence from the Dominican Republic. *Social Science and Medicine* **43**:221–34.

27. McPake B, Asiimwe D, Mwesigye F *et al.* (1999). Informal economic activities of public health workers in Uganda: implications for quality and accessibility of care. *Social Science and Medicine* **49**:849–65.

28. Over M, Heywood P, Gold J, Gupta I, Hira S, Marseille E. (2004). *HIV/AIDS Treatment and Prevention in India: Modeling the Cost and the Consequences.* Washington, DC: World Bank.

29. International Monetary Fund. (2003). *Aligning the Poverty Reduction and Growth Facility (PRGF) and the Poverty Reduction Strategy Paper (PRSP) Approach: Issues and Options.* IMF Policy Development and Review Department. URL: http://www.imf.org/external/np/prsp/2003/eng/042503.pdf.

30. Burkhalter H. (2004). Misplaced help in the AIDS fight. Editorial. *Washington Post,* May 25.

31. Central Statistical Office (Zambia), Central Board of Health (Zambia), and ORC Macro. (2003). *Zambia Demographic and Health Survey 2001–2002.* Calverton, MD: Central Statistical Office, Central Board of Health, and ORC.

32. World Bank. (2004). *Zambia: Country Economic Memorandum. Policies for Growth and Diversification.* World Bank Report No. 28069-ZA. Washington, DC: World Bank.

33. World Bank. (2004). *Zambia: Public Expenditure Management and Financial Accountability Review. A World Bank Country Study.* Washington, DC: World Bank, p112–23.

34. Wendo C. (2002). Uganda stands firm on health spending freeze. *Lancet* **360**:1847.

Chapter 43

Fiscal and macroeconomic aspects of the HIV pandemic

Markus Haacker

Introduction

Health is a key aspect of development, and it also affects other development objectives, such as education and material living standards. HIV undercuts economic development in many ways [1,2]. Increased mortality associated with HIV is resulting in changes in the composition of the population, with increasing numbers of orphans in many affected countries. In the absence of formal or informal insurance mechanisms, and in light of the stigma associated with the epidemic, the epidemic impoverishes households of people living with HIV (PLHIV). These adverse effects on the microeconomic level can also have important implications for economic development [3].

This chapter is concerned with the implications of HIV on 'public policy', which comprises all areas of government activities, including but beyond the administration of health systems, the delivery of public health services, or the national response to HIV. The first of the chapter's three sections studies the impact of HIV on the ability of governments to provide public services. In countries facing an HIV epidemic, this is compromised because HIV results in a slowdown in government revenues and in higher mortality among public servants, while personnel costs increase. Concurrently, irrespective of the form the national response to HIV takes, the demand for some public services such as health and social services increases.

The second section discusses the fiscal dimension of the national response to HIV. In particular, the financing of health expenditures in low-income countries, both generally and in the context of HIV, is considered. The national response frequently involves a substantial increase in public spending, at least on a sectoral level, and a commitment of future resources. To ensure the sustainability of the programme, and to avoid disruptions owing to funding shortfalls, it is necessary to secure adequate and predictable financing. From the perspective of a ministry of finance, it is also important to understand the financial commitments implied by the national response, and to incorporate it in budget plans. The issue of fiscal sustainability is therefore discussed.

The response to HIV also has important macroeconomic implications, beyond mitigating the macroeconomic costs of the epidemic, owing to reduced incidence of infections and improved availability of treatment, which are addressed in the third section. The response to HIV raises issues of absorptive capacity, especially since much of the HIV-related spending is concentrated in the health sector, facing capacity and human resource constraints. HIV-related aid flows may affect the balance of payments and the composition of aggregate demand. If the exchange rate appreciates as a consequence of the increased availability of

The views expressed in this chapter are those of the author and should not be interpreted as those of the International Monetary Fund.

foreign currency, this can have an adverse effect on exports and the domestic production of tradable goods. However, the form of the macroeconomic adjustment depends on the fiscal stance and the way in which the Central Bank accommodates the increased supply of foreign currency associated with larger aid flows.

The social and economic impact

A discussion of the social and economic impact of HIV is beyond the scope of this chapter, and is provided in this book by Quinlan and Whiteside (Chapter 3). Here, we provide a selective discussion to highlight some of the challenges governments are facing.

The most commonly used measure of the economic impact of HIV is its impact on gross domestic product (GDP) and GDP per capita. While there is a consensus that HIV causes a slowdown of GDP growth due to its adverse effect on productivity and production costs, the effect on GDP per capita is less clear. A more detailed discussion of the various approaches that have been used to analyse the impact of HIV on GDP, GDP per capita or economic growth is provided elsewhere [3]. Here, we discuss the recent growth experience of the countries with the highest HIV prevalence rates. Figure 43.1 shows the evolution of GDP per capita in those countries since 1970.

Based on the experience of these countries, HIV seems not to have resulted in a dramatic drop in GDP per capita. The only country for which a slowdown in the growth of GDP per capita is discernible over the last years is Zimbabwe, and other reasons in addition to HIV are likely to have been operative there. However, compared with other African countries, growth in GDP per capita in the seven countries covered recently has not been impressive. Average growth of GDP per capita for the whole of Africa was more than 2% for the period 1994–2001 compared with the period 1984–1994 [purchasing price parity (PPP)]. For the

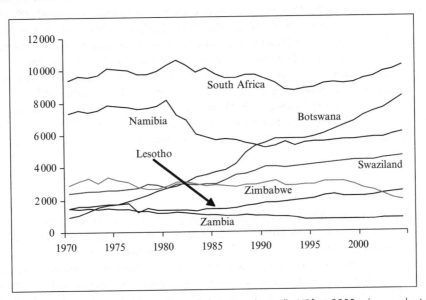

Fig. 43.1 GDP per capita for countries with high HIV prevalence (in US$ at 2000 prices, evaluated at PPP exchange rates). Source: [5].

seven countries, however, growth of GDP per capita increased only by 0.3% over the same period, or 1.3% if Zimbabwe is excluded. Thus, it appears that the experience in the worst-affected countries is consistent with some modest impact of HIV on the GDP per capita growth rate.

It seems, therefore, that the impact of HIV on material living standards as measured by GDP per capita is, on average, relatively small. Nevertheless, a decline in the growth rate of overall GDP, reflecting slower growth or a contraction of the working-age population, has important consequences for government policy. As the domestic tax base is more or less directly related to the level of GDP, domestic revenues grow more slowly. Looking further ahead, a slowdown in GDP also has important consequences for the sustainability of public debt.

Most of the implications of HIV for public policy, however, arise from its impact on the individual or household level. First, the welfare costs of HIV arise primarily from increased morbidity and mortality, and go much beyond any losses in terms of material living standards. Estimates of the costs of increased mortality dwarf any available estimates of the costs on material living standards [4]. Estimates of welfare losses are useful because they put estimates of the costs of HIV in terms of GDP into perspective and provide a framework to integrate the losses associated with increased HIV-related mortality into an economic analysis.

The impact of HIV is very uneven across individuals and households, which has profound policy implications. The magnitude of the social impact of HIV and the challenges governments face as a consequence is proportional to the number of orphans generated as a consequence of their HIV epidemic. Increases in mortality among the working-age population are paralleled by an increasing number of children who become orphans (Table 43.1). In some countries, the number of orphans has already doubled or tripled. Moreover, available projections suggest that by 2010, the number of orphans will increase to around 20% of the youth in Botswana, Lesotho, South Africa, Swaziland, Zambia or Zimbabwe. It is important to note that these are averages for all youth under 17 years of age. As orphan rates among the very young are very low, this implies the existence of much higher orphan rates among teenagers. The challenges to public policy are manifold. Orphans tend to live in poorer households, especially as the number of orphans may exceed the capacities of families and communities to care for them adequately. Government may, therefore, engage in social policy measures to ease the burden on foster families or to support orphan-led households. Access to education is reduced (Table 43.1), especially in countries where enrolment rates are already low.

The impact on public servants

The impact of HIV on public servants may mirror the overall impact on the overall working-age population [8]. However, where HIV prevalence affects socio-economic groups differently, the impact on public servants could be different from the population average.

Most directly, HIV results in increased mortality and morbidity among government employees. As government employees become ill, absenteeism increases or their productivity on the job declines. For example, Grassly and others [9] estimated that absenteeism amounted to an average of 1.3 months annually per HIV-infected employee, with each infected worker experiencing 12–14 episodes of illness before the terminal illness [10].

Table 43.1 HIV and orphans in several African countries

Country	Orphans as share of the young population, 2003[*]		Dependency ratio		Orphans' school attendance rate relative to non-orphans
			Households with children but no orphans	Households with orphans	
	All	**AIDS**			
Botswana	15.1	10.6	1.4	1.7	0.99
Côte d'Ivoire	13.3	6.2	1.4	1.5	0.83
Ethiopia	13.2	3.4	1.5	1.6	0.60
Malawi	17.5	8.7	1.5	2.0	0.93
South Africa	10.3	4.5	1.4	1.7	0.95
Uganda	14.6	7.5	1.7	2.3	0.95
Zimbabwe	17.6	13.5	1.4	2.2	0.85

[*]Young population defined as persons aged 0–17.
Sources: [6,7].

For an HIV prevalence rate of 20%, this would translate into a rate of absenteeism of 2.2%. Another source of absenteeism is funeral attendance. Increased attrition is also associated with an increase in vacancy rates, which has a similar effect on the delivery of public services to that of increased absenteeism.

A second dimension through which increased attrition affects the efficiency of public services is the loss of skills, coupled with the costs of training. As staff members can be expected to remain in service for a shorter time period, the training costs to maintain qualified staff members rise. For example, if staff attrition rises from 5% to 7%, the time government employees can be expected to remain in service decreases from 20 to 14 years, while the costs of training to maintain qualified staff rises by 40%, assuming that each staff member receives some initial training. Increased mortality among staff results in fewer government employees reaching the age and experience they would normally attain to fill the most senior positions. As a consequence, critical positions in government need to be filled by less experienced or qualified staff. Based on estimated mortality rates for the Zambian population, the percentage of staff entering the public service at age 20 that can be expected to survive until age 50 drops from 80% to 40% [11].

Demand for government services

Whether or not the government pursues a proactive policy on HIV, it is likely to face an increase in the demand for public services, most notably in the health sector, but also in areas such as social services and education. This is most clearly formulated in terms of the demand for HIV-related health services. Estimates of the financial resource requirements for expanding the treatment of opportunistic infections and improving access to antiretroviral treatment (ART) are provided in Table 43.2. Coverage rates for the different forms of treatment will presumably differ among these countries, as will the ability of each country's health services to expand medical care. The estimated costs are based on a coverage rate for the care for opportunistic infections of 10% in 2003, rising to 50% by 2010. For ART, it is assumed that the number of patients receiving the treatment through public health services is negligible in 2003 and that coverage rises to 50% by 2010 [11].

Table 43.2 Indicative estimates, in percentage of GDP (unless otherwise stated) of the costs of HIV-related health services, 2010

	Total HIV-related health services, 2010	Of which: costs of ART, 2010	Total health expenditure, 2001	Total health expenditure, 2001 (US$ per capita)	Public health expenditure, 2001	Total government expenditure, 2001	Domestic government revenue, 2001
Botswana	0.8	0.6	6.6	202	4.4	40.8	41.9
Côte d'Ivoire	1.4	1.0	6.2	39	1.0	16.6	17.0
Ethiopia	9.7	7.0	3.6	3	1.5	29.1	18.8
Haiti	0.8	0.6	5.0	23	2.7	10.0	...
Lesotho	3.8	2.8	5.5	21	4.3	43.0	40.8
Malawi	7.8	5.7	7.8	13	2.7	33.1	18.4
Mozambique	6.6	4.8	5.9	12	4.0	34.6	13.3
Namibia	1.4	1.0	7.0	121	4.7	30.1	31.9
South Africa	0.6	0.4	8.6	225	3.6	26.8	24.3
Swaziland	1.3	1.0	3.3	39	2.3	30.7	26.9
Tanzania	2.5	1.8	4.4	12	2.1	16.1	11.4
Uganda	2.2	1.6	5.9	15	3.4	19.8	10.9
Zambia	3.9	2.8	5.7	20	3.0	32.1	19.1
Zimbabwe	3.3	2.4	6.2	44	2.8	37.6	27.1

Sources: [5, 12] and author's estimates.

Overall, the costs of attaining these levels of HIV-related health services are substantial for all the countries covered in Table 43.2, ranging from 0.6 to 9.7% of GDP. These differences in cost stated as a percentage of GDP partly reflect differences in income per capita. Therefore, two of the countries with very high HIV prevalence, Botswana and South Africa, are among those that could conceivably substantially finance expanded access to treatment. However, even for these countries, the financial burden is daunting from a sectoral perspective, corresponding in South Africa to 17% of the health budget and over 2% of total government expenditure. On the other hand, the required expenditure exceeds 5% of GDP for three countries—Ethiopia, Malawi and Mozambique—and exceeds total public health expenditure as a percentage of GDP in 2001 for these and four other countries, namely Côte d'Ivoire, Tanzania, Zambia and Zimbabwe.

The indirect fiscal costs of HIV

While the costs of a national response to HIV can be very substantial, an understanding of the impact of HIV on public finances also requires an assessment of the indirect costs of HIV. In addition to the directly HIV-related expenditures on prevention and treatment, there are indirect costs related to those expenses that are not covered by a specific HIV line item in the government budget. While the dividing line between direct and indirect expenditures is sometimes blurred—for instance, investments in health infrastructure or orphan support—it is a useful distinction to make, because external grants are primarily available for direct HIV-related expenditures, and not for the indirect costs. Thus, while indirect expenditures are lower than the costs of an effective response to HIV, they are disproportionately important in terms of their impact on the fiscal balance and thus public policy.

The most important of such indirect costs are increases in personnel expenditures caused by increased mortality and morbidity, such as pensions to surviving dependants or medical benefits. In case of pensions and other death-related benefits, it is important to look at the net rather than the gross effect. While pensions or one-off benefits for surviving dependants increase, fewer government employees reach retirement age and outlays for old-age pensions therefore decline. However, the net effects on the costs of pensions and death-related benefits are likely to be positive, as death-in-service benefits are typically higher for employees dying early, relative to their previous contributions. One study from Swaziland [13], for example, estimated that the overall costs of the pension scheme would rise by 2–4% of the government's payroll, or 0.3–0.6% of GDP. Other indirect costs include rising medical benefits, although these may be accounted for and financed as part of the national response to HIV; the costs of increased absenteeism, which may take the form of efficiency losses rather than a fiscal cost; and various other forms of social expenditure.

Debt sustainability

Additional pressure on government finances arises from the dynamics of the accumulation of public debt. The most common measure of a country's indebtedness is the *Debt/GDP ratio*. An increase in the government deficit, by increasing Debt (D), would result in a rise in this ratio, whereas an increase in GDP (Y) would reduce it. The evolution of the *Debt/GDP ratio* can be described by:

Percentage change in $\qquad [\frac{D}{Y}] = r + f\frac{Y}{D} - g - n \qquad\qquad$ (1)

where r = the interest rate on public debt; f = the government deficit, including grants, but excluding interest on public debt; g = the rate of growth of GDP per capita; and n = the population growth.

The rate of GDP growth thus is equal to $g + n$. Suppose that the government aims to maintain the *Debt/GDP ratio* at some level $[\frac{D}{Y}]^*$. This requires that the fiscal does not fall below a level given by:

$$f = (g + n - r)\,[\tfrac{D}{Y}]^* \qquad (2)$$

As HIV results in a slowdown in economic growth, i.e. as g, n or both decline, it has some implications for the fiscal balance required to sustain the *Debt/GDP ratio* that is deemed sustainable. For example, if the government aims to keep this ratio at 50% of GDP, and if GDP growth $(g + n)$ declines by one percentage point, this would require a fiscal adjustment of 0.5% of GDP. For some of the worst-affected countries, the US Bureau of Census estimates that population growth (g) has declined by 1.5–2%; even maintaining moderate levels of public debt of 20–30% of GDP would require an adjustment in the fiscal balance of 0.3–0.6% of GDP.

These examples demonstrate how an economic slowdown tightens the scope for public spending while, in the context of HIV, the government also faces considerable additional demands. Taking a longer perspective, the government may therefore respond to the needs associated with a health emergency and temporarily run a higher fiscal deficit. The evolution of public debt is then described by equation (1). To ensure that the national response to HIV is ultimately sustainable, the eventual level of public debt implied by the government's programme would have to be sustainable in order to avoid a disruption of services in the future. The programme thus needs to be embedded in a medium- or longer-term financial plan.

Summary

Our analysis so far has set the stage for a discussion of the fiscal and macroeconomic aspects of the response to HIV. It shows how HIV erodes the government's human and financial resources, while the demand for government services increases. In countries facing severe epidemics, HIV represents a significant challenge for the management of government finances and public services. The design of policies to respond to the epidemic thus needs to be mindful of the fact that this takes place in a context where the government's fiscal position is under pressure, owing to the epidemics' direct and indirect costs, and, in the longer run, as it becomes more difficult to sustain the level of public debt.

Some fiscal aspects of the response to HIV

In many countries, the national response to HIV involves changes in public expenditures that are significant compared with the government's budget overall, or which imply a substantial increase in expenditures in a particular sector, such as health services. Some of the fiscal aspects of HIV have already been discussed in terms of the demand for government services, or the implications for the sustainability of public debt. Here, the fiscal dimension of increased HIV-related expenditures is explored further.

In terms of the financing of the response to HIV, the situation differs across countries. Not only does the extent to which public health services are financed externally differ substantially across countries, but there are also important differences in the mix between public and private financing within countries.

The perception of HIV as a serious global health crisis has translated into a strong response by the international community. As issues regarding the response to HIV transcended the expertise of any UN agency, UNAIDS was established to coordinate the global response, and the Global Fund to Fight AIDS, Tuberculosis and Malaria (Global Fund) was set up as a specialized agency that provides financing for national responses to HIV. The Global Fund is largely financed by grants from public sources. UNAIDS estimates that spending on HIV in 135 low- and middle-income countries reached US$6 billion in 2004, of which US$3.7 billion was financed by external grants, and that on current trends, international disbursement will reach US$7 billion by 2007, contributing to an increase of around US$10 billion. About half of the estimated costs of scaling up HIV activities in low- and middle-income countries would go towards prevention-related activities, one-third towards treatment and care, and 10% towards orphan support. These are averages, and different countries with different epidemics and different HIV prevalence rates will spend resources differently.

While the level of funding available still lags far behind what UNAIDS deems necessary for a comprehensive response to HIV, external finance has enabled some of the countries experiencing severe HIV epidemics to increase spending on HIV substantially. For Ethiopia, Kenya, Malawi, Mozambique, Swaziland, Tanzania, Uganda and Zambia, externally financed HIV spending accounted for all or most of the increases in health spending between 2000/2 and 2002/4. In Uganda and Zambia, externally financed HIV spending now exceeds total domestically financed public health expenditures [14]. Even though not all of these additional expenditures finance additional health services, these numbers suggest that the increase in expenditures on the sectoral level can be very substantial.

In light of the key role of the health sector in countries with severe epidemics, it is important to note that the financing of health services differs significantly across countries. The share of public expenditure in total health expenditure varies across the countries covered, from 16% in Côte d'Ivoire to 79% in Lesotho. Most public health expenditure is financed by either taxation or external resources. One exception is Thailand, where public health insurance plays an important role. For countries with a relatively low income per capita, external assistance is an important source of financing. In Malawi it accounts for 87% of public health expenditure, and 41% of total health expenditure.

A second important difference across countries is the availability of private health insurance ('pre-paid private financing', see Table 43.3). For many of the countries, the share of private out-of-pocket health expenditure is high by international standards, especially as a proportion of total private health expenditure. This reflects the relatively minor role of private health insurance in many low-income countries. Correspondingly, for Botswana, Namibia, South Africa and Zimbabwe—countries with a relatively well-developed insurance sector—private out-of-pocket health expenditure is less important.

These discrepancies across countries are relevant in terms of financing the response to HIV, particularly for prevention, treatment and care. In the absence of some form of health insurance, households are hard pressed or would find it impossible to pay, particularly for the costs of treatment. In many low-income countries, private health insurance is limited to the public sector and parts of the private sector, frequently only covering small—and often the most affluent—population groups. In this situation, the public health sector, or publicly financed private health providers, have a key role in expanding access to treatment to lower-income groups, and thereby ensuring against a reduction in material living standards associated with the epidemic.

Table 43.3 The financing of health services, various countries, 2001

	Total US$ per capita	Total % of GDP	Public % of total	Public: external resources % of public expenditure	Private % of total	Private out-of-pocket % of total	Private out-of-pocket % of private expenditure	Private pre-paid % of private expenditure
Botswana	202	6.6	66.2	0.6	33.8	11.9	35.3	64.7
Brazil	222	7.6	41.6	1.2	58.4	37.4	64.1	35.9
Côte d'Ivoire	39	6.2	16.0	20.0	84.0	75.3	89.7	10.3
Ethiopia	3	3.6	40.5	84.7	59.5	50.4	84.7	15.3
Haiti	23	5.0	53.4	80.3	46.6	21.1	45.3	54.7
Lesotho	21	5.5	78.9	7.6	21.1	21.1	100.0	0.0
Malawi	13	7.8	35.0	75.7	65.0	28.4	43.7	56.3
Mozambique	12	5.9	67.4	54.7[1]	32.6	12.8	39.3	60.7
Namibia	121	7.0	67.8	5.6	32.2	5.8	17.9	82.1
South Africa	225	8.6	41.4	1.0	58.6	13.0	22.1	77.9
Swaziland	39	3.3	68.5	11.5	31.5	31.5	100.0	0.0
Tanzania	12	4.4	46.7	63.2	53.3	44.3	83.1	16.9
Thailand	69	3.7	57.1*	0.2	42.9	36.5	85.0	15.0
Uganda	15	5.9	57.5	43.1	42.5	22.7	53.4	46.6
Zambia	20	5.7	53.1	91.7	46.9	33.7	71.8	28.2
Zimbabwe	44	6.2	45.3	17.2	54.7	28.6	52.2	47.8

*Including 26.8% of total public health expenditure financed by the social security system.
Source: [12].

Detailed data like those presented in Table 43.3 are not available for the financing of HIV-related health expenditure. However, Martin [15] analysed the financing of HIV-related public expenditure in Botswana, Lesotho, Mozambique, South Africa and Swaziland. Her findings showed that the role of external finance for HIV-related expenditure is even more pronounced than that for general health expenditure. With the exception of South Africa, which receives very little external aid, external financing accounted for between 79 and 85% of HIV-related public expenditure in these countries. This is also in line with UNAIDS' global estimates of the financing of HIV-related spending in low- and middle-income countries, according to which over 60% of HIV-related expenditures were financed by international disbursements. As these countries include Brazil and South Africa, which account for a substantial proportion of domestically financed spending, this means that the proportion of external financing is much higher for many low-income countries.

Domestic financing

While external financing plays an important or even dominant role in financing the national response to HIV in many countries, some of the costs need to be financed from domestic revenues or additional borrowing. While in some countries the entire costs of the response to HIV may be financed by external grants, donors would expect a higher share of domestic financing from countries with higher levels of GDP per capita. For example, the World Bank differentiates the terms of its loans according to a country's gross national income (GNI) per capita, and restricts access to its most concessional type of loans to low-income countries (GNI of US$765 per capita or less). The Global Fund uses income categories similar to those established by the World Bank. For example, the Fifth Call for Proposals stipulates that partnerships from countries classified as 'Low Income' by the World Bank are fully eligible to apply for support from the Global Fund, whereas low middle-income countries (GNI between US$765 and US$3035 per capita) and high middle-income countries (GNI between US$3035 and US$9385 per capita) have to provide 10–20% and 20–40%, respectively, of domestic financing. Moreover, in middle-income countries, the Global Fund only underwrites proposals that target poor and vulnerable populations.

More broadly, the issue of domestic financing arises because external financing is generally available only for specific projects or programmes, which would not cover all of the costs of the HIV epidemic to the government. For example, the government would have to finance higher costs of medical and death-related benefits, and other costs related to higher mortality among staff.

In terms of raising additional resources to finance the national response to HIV, it is useful to distinguish between general tax revenues and private financing for specific services. The scope for raising additional tax revenues is generally limited. Even if inefficiencies in the collection of taxes exist or the domestic tax base is relatively narrow, addressing those shortcomings is time-consuming and can be politically difficult. Also, raising taxes can further squeeze the profitability of businesses that are already coping with the adverse impacts of HIV on their employees.

If the scope for raising additional revenues is limited, the government may have to resort to cuts in other areas of expenditure. However, these cuts are problematic if they compromise other expenditure programmes that are desirable from a development perspective, and they may draw resistance from line ministries or other interest groups involved. Nevertheless, while the inherited allocation of expenditures reflects a political consensus about spending priorities, the demand pressures associated with a health emergency may provide an impetus for shifting this consensus and addressing inefficiencies in the delivery of public services or reducing low-priority expenditures. Such items could include a 'revision of existing subsidy programmes, spending cutbacks on defense and internal security, or police, reduced foreign travel or embassy expenses, or rationalization of elements of the civil service that are of low (or zero) productivity (e.g. the frequent problem of overstaffing or even ghost workers)' [16].

Fiscal sustainability

The concept of fiscal sustainability 'relates to the capacity of a government, at least in the future, to finance its desired expenditure programmes, to service any debt obligations, and to ensure its solvency' [16]. From another perspective, fiscal sustainability implies that the allocation of resources is optimal not only within the budget for a given year, but also over time. Below, we will first address issues regarding the sustainability of public spending in the context of HIV in general; then we will discuss some issues specific to externally financed expenditures.

The issue of fiscal sustainability was already introduced in our discussion of the sustainability of public debt. The key lessons from that discussion are that HIV has a negative impact on the fiscal balance, irrespective of the modalities of the national response to HIV, and that in an environment where GDP growth is weakening, the government would eventually have to tighten the fiscal balance in order to sustain a level of public debt that is deemed sustainable. Thus, the HIV epidemic is associated with a tightening of government finances in the longer run.

However, within the planning horizon of a national response to HIV, which, for practical purposes, rarely exceeds 5 years, other considerations are also relevant. First, in many countries, external grant financing substantially contributes to financing the expansion in government expenditures. Secondly, it is common that governments adapt the fiscal stance to accommodate temporary fluctuations in government finances or particular pressing needs. Examples include anti-cyclical fiscal policy, and the management of oil or diamond revenues, part of which may be invested rather than spent, or higher spending in emergency situations such as wars or post-conflict reconstruction.

In light of the pressing needs associated with an HIV epidemic and the risks to welfare and economic development, the government may decide to finance the costs of the national response to HIV, to the extent that it is not financed by grants, but by higher borrowing. However, in the interest of the sustainability of the programmes underwritten by higher borrowing and government spending overall, it is important that the national response to HIV be integrated into a medium-term financial plan. Such a plan needs to specify anticipated government revenues and expenditures, including the national response to HIV, and ensure that expenditure programmes, within an annual budget and over time, reflect the government's priorities.

Fiscal sustainability issues also arise in the context of external financing. External grants typically underwrite particular projects or programmes, with disbursements tied to the stage of implementation. Where grants underwrite broader programmes rather than specific one-off projects, their time horizon seldom exceeds 2 or 3 years. In terms of planning the national response to HIV, this is problematic, as its time horizon substantially exceeds this time frame.

Furthermore, the type of expenditures underwritten by HIV-related grants differs from those supported by other forms of development finance. The latter is typically geared towards capital expenditures or capacity building. In this case, the grant underwrites at least part of the initial investments, whereas the government covers the maintenance or operating costs. This means that after the initial investment phase, supported by external grants, the financial exposure to the government is limited. In the context of the national response to HIV, however, the situation is different, as the grants are geared towards current expenditures, such as salaries or medical purchases. This means that the government carries a higher financial risk in case a grant is not renewed or alternative sources of external financing are not identified to sustain the programme.

To ensure that HIV-related activities 'on the ground' are fully consistent with the objectives of the national response to HIV, it is therefore important that there be a strong national coordinating mechanism—a necessity recognized within the UNAIDS framework of 'The Three Ones'. This includes a National HIV Programme that provides the basis for coordinating the work of all partners, and a National AIDS Coordinating Authority with a broad-based multisectoral mandate. In countries where the size of the response to HIV is significant from a macroeconomic or fiscal perspective, it is important that the agreed HIV Action Framework be adequately integrated into the government's medium-term fiscal planning. It is also important that the HIV Action Framework be consistent with the government's macroeconomic and fiscal policy objectives. This requires that the ministry of finance take an active part in the formulation of the national HIV Action Framework, to help develop the medium-term budgetary implications of the national response to HIV and ensure that adequate financing, from domestic or external sources, is available to underwrite the programme.

In terms of fiscal sustainability, it is also important to differentiate between grants and loans. Grant-financed expenditures raise sustainability issues only if the expenditures underwritten by the grant at some stage need to be financed in some different way, so that what is grant financed today nevertheless implies a potential future financial liability. This is also the case with loan-financed expenditures; however, the loans eventually have to be repaid, which adds to the future financial liabilities associated with the response to HIV.

Another important issue that needs to be taken into account is that the government's resources and the need for public spending in the future depend on the success of the national response to HIV. As increasing prevention efforts result in a decline in the incidence of new infections, this means that the number of people requiring various forms of treatment will eventually decline and the adverse social and economic effects of HIV will be mitigated.

This issue has been explored by Masha [17] in a study motivated by Botswana's national response to HIV. The study compares projections included in a study by the Botswana Institute for Development Policy Analysis (BIDPA) [18] and those implied by the targets of Botswana's National Strategic Framework (NSF) on HIV [19]. The BIDPA study is a very thorough impact analysis, also covering indirect expenses associated with HIV not accounted for in the NSF, such as social expenditure and higher personnel costs, and fiscal savings associated with lower numbers of students. The NSF spells out a comprehensive programme to reduce the incidence of new infections and expand access to treatment; consequently, spending on health and prevention, and in some other areas, exceeds that projected by BIDPA. By 2010, the NSF envisages greatly reduced mortality rates, primarily as a result of

Table 43.4 Indirect fiscal gains (% of GDP) from Botswana's National Strategic Framework on HIV, 2010

	BIDPA (2000)	NSF (2003)	Indirect fiscal gains
Health/prevention	3.5	5.0	–
Social expenditure	1.5	0.7	0.8
Public service	0.8	0.3	0.5
Education	-0.3	-0.1	-0.2
Other	-0.2	3.0	–

Source: [17].

increased access to ART. The fiscal savings associated with the NSF were calculated on the basis of BIDPA's estimates of the indirect expenses, which were scaled down in line with lower mortality rates. Masha (Table 43.4) found that by 2010, the fiscal savings in the areas of social expenditure and public services, partly offset by higher education spending, amounted to 1.1% of GDP, or 14% of the costs of the entire NSF. These estimates, however, certainly understate the savings involved, as they do not include the savings within the areas of health and prevention. In particular, going beyond 2010, successful prevention efforts would eventually result in a substantial decline in treatment costs.

Some macroeconomic aspects of the response to HIV

There are three principal types of issues arising in terms of the macroeconomic consequences of an expanded response to HIV. First, the response to HIV may entail an increase in demand for particular services or aggregate demand that is inconsistent with the productive capacity of the economy. Secondly, increased aid flows may skew the balance of payments and may result in an appreciation of the exchange rate. Thirdly, large aid flows have implications for monetary policy, as the Central Bank has different options to accommodate the increased supply of foreign currency, and these, in turn, have important macroeconomic implications.

Bevan [20] discusses a fourth dimension—the impacts on the institutional and political framework arising if high aid inflows 'induce aid dependency, weakening a government's capacity to generate domestic resources, and undermining the democratic process'. In light of the very specific programmes underwritten by HIV-related grants, these issues are less important in the present context than in other areas of development assistance and are not discussed here.

Before considering the various macroeconomic implications of increased aid flows, one aspect they have in common should be discussed: the scale of the effect depends, of course, on the size of the aid flows, but also on the way in which aid is used. This can involve imports of goods, frequently investment goods; in the context of HIV, aid could also finance medical supplies, including antiretroviral drugs, imports of services such as foreign consultants, purchases of domestic goods, services from domestic suppliers and salaries of domestic staff. To the extent that external aid is used for the importation of goods and services, the macroeconomic effects are mitigated, the inflow of currency is partly offset by the payment for these imports, the direct effects on domestic demand are mitigated, and the size of the net inflow of foreign currency, and therefore the monetary policy challenge, is reduced.

Absorptive capacity

Absorptive capacity needs to be considered in terms of the relationship between aggregate supply, the economy's productive capacity (Y), and aggregate demand. The latter is generally divided into the government's domestic demand (denoted by G), private expenditure ($C + I$, for consumption plus private investment) and the excess of exports (X) over imports (M).

In general, the inflationary impact of aid-financed expenditures depends on how well it is used, in terms of enhancing economic development and thus the productive capacity of the economy. The national response to HIV can have a positive effect on Y. First, most of the positive effects of HIV-related spending serve to mitigate the adverse impact on Y. If anything, Y would therefore decline in our framework. Secondly, many of the economic benefits of a national response to HIV, most notably those of increased prevention efforts, materialize only over time and would not have any immediate effect on Y.

The national response to HIV results in an increase in government expenditure, unless the increased government spending on HIV is financed by a reallocation of expenditures. If it is financed out of additional taxation or domestic borrowing, the increase in G is largely offset by a decline in $C + I$. If it is financed from external resources, the macroeconomic adjustment is more complex. One possibility is that this will have an inflationary effect and will eventually crowd out private expenditure ($C + I$, consumption plus private investment—Fig. 43.2), for example as real interest rates rise ('Case 1' in Fig. 43.2). Another possibility is that the imbalance in the balance of payments results in an appreciation of the exchange rate. The increase in government spending would then be offset by a decline in net exports ($X - M$, exports minus imports—'Case 2' in Fig. 43.2). In the longer run, an assessment of the macroeconomic consequences becomes more complex, as the productive capacity of the economy also depends on investment and the success of the national response to HIV. This is beyond the scope of this chapter [17].

It is first important to note that HIV-related expenditures, while large from a sectoral perspective, still constitute only a small proportion of GDP and usually are not the largest part of external aid. Thus, HIV may exacerbate any issues regarding the domestic absorption of external aid on the macroeconomic level, but would not give rise to such problems by itself. Secondly, this macroeconomic view misses out on many of the complexities of developing the national response to HIV. The reason for this is that HIV-related spending is relatively narrowly focused on particular sectors and—at least in the area of the delivery of health services—requires services with very specific skills whose availability can be limited. Another important constraint is managerial capacity, or, where services are delivered by different providers in a decentralized fashion, the coordination of activities in the context of rapidly expanding HIV programmes; these tasks also require very specific and scarce skills.

Institutions such as the World Health Organization (WHO), in developing strategies to respond to the HIV epidemic, have taken into account the existing capacity constraints in key

$$\text{Case 1:} \quad \underset{\text{(fixed)}}{Y} \quad = \quad \underset{\text{(up)}}{G} \quad + \quad \underset{\text{(down)}}{I+C} \quad + \quad X\text{–}M$$

$$\text{Case 2:} \quad \underset{\text{(fixed)}}{Y} \quad = \quad \underset{\text{(up)}}{G} \quad + \quad I+C \quad + \quad \underset{\text{(down)}}{X\text{–}M}$$

Fig. 43.2 Increased government expenditure and macroeconomic adjustment.

sectors. For example, the Commission on Macroeconomics and Health emphasized the need for decentralized provision of health services [21], thereby reducing the needs for the scarcest, most highly trained category of health personnel. Similarly, the WHO/UNAIDS '3 by 5' initiative, which aimed to expand access to ART rapidly, included a strong training component.

One factor that can either exacerbate or ease the shortages of staff in the health sector is international migration. International migration is in many ways a positive phenomenon, allowing emigrants to attain incomes higher than they would earn in their home countries, while remittances of expatriates can contribute to raising living standards in their home countries. At the same time, the prospect of health services in some of the countries facing severe HIV epidemics being overwhelmed by the additional demands, while trained nurses or doctors leave that country to accept higher-paying positions abroad, raises some awkward questions.

It is important to note that migration also occurs within sub-Saharan Africa and even involves countries from outside the region. For example, about half of the doctors working in the public health sector in Swaziland are expatriates, while, according to anecdotal evidence, many Swazi health professionals work abroad. Thus, while sub-Saharan Africa as a whole experiences a 'brain drain' of health professionals, there is some evidence that countries experiencing catastrophic health situations are able to attract health professionals from other countries, thus mitigating the very tight constraints on the availability of domestic health professionals. One consequence, of course, is a higher rate of brain drain from poorer countries within the region, thus exacerbating the scarcity of health personnel in those countries.

While training staff is a time-consuming proposition and subject to capacity constraints on the level of training institutions, there are two additional ways to increase the availability of trained personnel: increasing retention rates and improving the efficiency of the public service [22]. Of particular relevance to this discussion is that both propositions would probably require increases in salaries of health personnel, and thus have an impact on the fiscal balance. In the public sector, substantial salary increases granted to one group of public servants might result in claims from other branches of the public service. Thus, the fiscal implications of addressing bottlenecks in the health sector can be wider.

Increased aid flows, the balance of payments and the exchange rate

Increased aid flows, to the extent that the respective funds are not directly spent on imports of goods or services, bring about a change in the balance of payments and an inflow of foreign currency. It does not make a big difference if increased aid flows come in the form of grants or concessional loans. However, in terms of the balance of payments, the former are accounted for as a transfer, while the latter are accounted for as a loan.

The supply of foreign currency on the domestic market thus increases, and the price of foreign currency declines. In other words, the domestic currency appreciates.

As a consequence, domestic exports become less competitive, and the export sector may contract. For countries exporting products such as oil, timber or mining products, where royalties or rents from resource extraction account for a significant proportion of government revenues, an appreciation of a country's currency can also have a direct impact on the fiscal balance. This could reduce the value of royalties in domestic currency terms, and, as costs are denominated in domestic currency, the economic rents from resource extraction could decline. At the same time, it becomes cheaper to import, and as domestic buyers switch to imported goods, the demand for domestically produced goods declines.

This adverse impact of aid on exports is referred to as 'Dutch disease'. Historically, the term was coined to describe the economic effects of revenues from oil exploitation on the Dutch economy. Its economic and political significance arises partly from its distributional effects. Profit margins of exporters are squeezed to the extent that some may go out of business, and any changes in the prices of export goods are likely to translate into income losses to farmers or workers in the export sectors. Conversely, there are beneficiaries of aid, such as, for example, the recipients of goods and services and those gaining employment directly or indirectly as a consequence of higher aid flows. As the latter are usually not the same as those who suffer income losses, this can result in political conflict. 'Dutch disease' also has a longer-term dimension. To the extent that exports are an engine of growth and broad-based development, a loss in competitiveness and, consequently, a decline in exports would have a negative impact on a country's development prospects. However, HIV-related aid also finances expenditures that are productivity- and thus growth-enhancing by mitigating the adverse impacts of HIV, and these effects need to be taken into account in an assessment of the impact of increased aid flows on competitiveness.

Monetary policy and inflation

Monetary policy can have some impact on how the macroeconomic adjustment to higher aid flows plays out. This can be illustrated using two basic policy scenarios. In one scenario, the Central Bank does not buy any foreign exchange, and in the second scenario, the Central Bank does buy foreign currency. The actual policy taken by the Central Bank, of course, may be somewhere in between. Also, the Central Bank has more policy instruments at its disposal than described in the second example, and could therefore achieve similar objectives somewhat differently.

In the first case, the Central Bank does not buy any foreign exchange, which is a policy referred to as a 'free float'. This means that the increased supply of foreign currency results in a drop in the price of foreign currency on the domestic market, resulting in an appreciation of the domestic currency, with exports becoming less competitive and imports becoming cheaper. This case is described above in the section on the balance of payments and need not repeated here. We just note for reference that the bulk of the adjustment is borne by the export sector or domestic producers of products competing with imported goods.

Alternatively, the Central Bank may buy some or all incoming foreign currency, thereby accumulating foreign currency reserves, and at the same time increasing the domestic money supply. This would have an expansionary effect, as liquidity in the economy increased, credit became cheaper and aggregate demand increased. Eventually, inflation would start to rise, and consequently, while the exchange rate remained constant, domestic products would become more expensive than foreign products, exports less competitive, and imports cheaper. This would mean an outcome very similar to the scenario described above, although the adjustment in the real exchange rate, or prices in the domestic economy, compared with prices in other countries, might take more time to develop and be accompanied by an inflationary period.

If the Central Bank aimed to keep inflation under control, or if it were concerned about the effect that an appreciation of the country's exchange rate would have on the economy, it could pursue a somewhat different policy and 'mop up' the additional liquidity by issuing treasury bills, or some other measures, such as increasing the commercial banks' reserve requirement. As banks or the general public purchase treasury bills, the liquidity in the economy and the availability of credit decline, and domestic interest rates rise. This has an adverse impact on investment and consumption, and aggregate demand would thus decline. As a consequence, the inflationary impact would be less severe, and the impact on net exports less pronounced. One possible effect of this policy, however, is that the increase in domestic interest rates would put additional pressure on the government budget, as it also implies an increase in interest on the government's domestic debt.

Some concluding remarks

Our discussion set out from an analysis of the impact of HIV on government's capacities, through its economic impact, to loss of human lives and fiscal costs. The main body of the chapter, however, describes the fiscal and economic dimension of the *response* to HIV, especially in countries facing severe epidemics or receiving considerable amounts of external aid. Most importantly, the chapter aims to help develop appropriate and effective health system responses to the HIV pandemic. In this context, our analysis is relevant from several different perspectives.

First, it describes the constraints to governments facing an HIV epidemic among the population, and thus formulates the background against which a national response to HIV is implemented. The epidemic not only erodes the government's human resources, but also has a negative impact on government finance. While various studies do address some aspects of the fiscal impact of HIV, this is not normally done in an integrated fashion, nor is it included in the costing of a national response to HIV.

Secondly, the epidemic—and the modalities of the national response—have significant implications for government finances, and these are not fully understood so far. To ensure that the allocation of resources reflects the government's objectives, both within a given budget and over time, it is important that the costs of HIV be properly estimated and included in the budget and longer-term fiscal planning.

Finally, in light of the large scale of the national response to HIV and the rapid increases in expenditures envisaged, and to ensure that the national response is *sustainable*, it is essential that this be adequately planned. This involves recognizing existing capacity constraints and developing strategies to overcome them—a common theme in efforts to formulate recipes to address the epidemic, and referred to in the discussion of absorptive capacity. In terms of government finances, it involves projecting the impact of HIV and the costs of the national response to HIV, identifying sources of external financing and estimating the domestic financing requirements. Where there is uncertainty about the availability of financing, it is important to specify those risks and develop contingency plans to ensure that key services are maintained.

References

1. Haacker M. (2004a). *The Macroeconomics of HIV/AIDS*. Washington, DC: International Monetary Fund.
2. Haacker M. (2004b). HIV/AIDS: the impact on the social fabric and the economy. In: Haacker M, ed. *The Macroeconomics of HIV/AIDS*. Washington, DC: International Monetary Fund, pp 41–95.

3. Bell C, Devarajan S, Gersbach H. (2004). Thinking about the long-run economic costs of HIV/AIDS. In: Haacker M, ed. *The Macroeconomics of HIV/AIDS* Washington, DC: International Monetary Fund, pp 96–133.

4. Crafts N, Haacker M. (2004). Welfare implications of HIV/AIDS. In: Haacker M, ed. *The Macroeconomics of HIV/AIDS*. Washington, DC: International Monetary Fund, pp 182–197.

5. International Monetary Fund. (2004). *World Economic Outlook Database—September 2004*. Washington, DC: International Monetary Fund. Available online at: http://www.imf.org/external/pubs/ft/weo/2004/04/data/index.htm.

6. Joint United Nations Programme on HIV/AIDS (UNAIDS), United Nations Children's Fund (UNICEF), and US Agency for International Development (USAID). (2004). *Children on the Brink 2004*. Geneva, New York and Washington.

7. United Nations Children's Fund (UNICEF). (2003) *Africa's Orphaned Generation*. New York: UNICEF.

8. Epstein BG. (2004). The demographic impact of HIV/AIDS. In: Haacker M, ed. *The Macroeconomics of HIV/AIDS*. Washington, DC: International Monetary Fund, pp 1–40.

9. Grassly NC, Desai K, Pegurri E *et al.* (2003). The economic impact of HIV/AIDS on the education sector in Zambia. *AIDS* 17(7):1039–44.

10. Government of Malawi and United Nations Development Programme (UNDP). (2002). *The Impact of HIV/AIDS on Human Resource in the Malawi Public Sector*. Lilongwe, Malawi.

11. Haacker M. (2004c). The impact of HIV/AIDS on government finance and public services. In: Haacker M, ed. *The Macroeconomics of HIV/AIDS*. Washington, DC: International Monetary Fund, pp 198–258.

12. World Health Organization. (2004). *World Health Report 2004*. Geneva: WHO.

13. JTK Associates. (2002). *The Impact of HIV/AIDS on the Central Agencies of the Government of Swaziland*. Mbabane, Swaziland.

14. Lewis M. (2005). Addressing the Challenge of HIV/AIDS: Macroeconomic, Fiscal and Institutional Issues. Unpublished draft.

15. Martin HG. (2003). *A Comparative Analysis of the Financing of HIV/AIDS Programmes in Botswana, Lesotho, Mozambique, South Africa, Swaziland, and Zimbabwe*. Pretoria, South Africa: Human Sciences Research Council.

16. Heller PS. (2005). *Understanding Fiscal Space*. IMF Policy Discussion Paper No. 05/4. Washington, DC: International Monetary Fund.

17. Masha I. (2004). An economic assessment of Botswana's National Strategic Framework on HIV/AIDS. In: Haacker M, ed. *The Macroeconomics of HIV/AIDS*. Washington, DC: International Monetary Fund, pp 287–310.

18. Botswana Institute for Development Policy Analysis (BIDPA). (2000). *Macroeconomic Impacts of the HIV/AIDS Epidemic in Botswana*. Gaborone, Botswana.

19. Botswana National AIDS Coordinating Agency. (2003). *Botswana National Strategic Framework for HIV /AIDS 2003–09*. Gaborone, Botswana.

20. Bevan D. (2005). An Analytical View of Aid Absorption: Recognizing and Avoiding Macroeconomic Hazards. Paper presented at the Seminar on Foreign Aid and Macroeconomic Management, Maputo, March 14–15, 2005. Washington DC: International Monetary Fund.

21. Commission on Macroeconomics and Health. (2001). *Macroeconomics and Health: Investing in Health for Economic Development*. Geneva: World Health Organization.

22. Over M. (2004). Impact of the HIV/AIDS epidemic on the health sectors of developing countries. In: Haacker M, ed. *The Macroeconomics of HIV/AIDS*. Washington, DC: International Monetary Fund, pp 311–344.

Chapter 44

Trade, intellectual property and access to affordable HIV medicines

Julian Fleet[*] and Béchir N'Daw

Introduction

The relationship between international trade and intellectual property rules and access to HIV medicines has been the subject of considerable attention and controversy in recent years. Issues concerning the relationship between trade rules and intellectual property rights on the one hand, and public health and access to medicines on the other, are not limited to HIV and AIDS. However, it is fair to say that the threat to human security posed by AIDS, and the social movement surrounding the epidemic, have greatly heightened attention to intellectual property issues not only in the context of HIV and AIDS, but also in relation to other major diseases and public health in general.

The United Nations Security Council, whose primary responsibility under the United Nations Charter is the maintenance of international peace and security, has considered AIDS on its public agenda four times since January 2000. The concern of the Security Council, which had never before focused its agenda on a health or even a social and economic development issue, underscores the exceptional threat created by HIV to human societies in many hard-hit countries. Exceptional threats beg for exceptional responses. This dictum applies not least with regard to trade and intellectual property rights and the response to AIDS.

The purpose of this chapter is fivefold. First, this chapter situates intellectual property issues within the context of efforts to expand on a vast scale access to HIV medicines. Secondly, it summarizes recent developments regarding the affordability of HIV medicines generally. Thirdly, the chapter surveys the major international trade and intellectual property agreements that affect the ability of governments, non-governmental organizations (NGOs) and international organizations to procure HIV medicines at affordable prices. Fourthly, we present a few concrete examples of the ways in which these agreements are or are not being utilized by governments to expand access to HIV treatment. Lastly, we trace some of the more important recent regional, bilateral and national developments in international trade and intellectual property rules.

Background and context

By the end of 2004, UNAIDS and the World Health Organization (WHO) estimated that about 40 million people were living with HIV [1]. More than 20 million people have died of AIDS since the beginning of the epidemic. Most of this HIV-related disease and death, and

* Corresponding author.

the ensuing social and economic crises in high-prevalence countries, can be delayed, and in many cases averted, through antiretroviral treatment (ART). Although this treatment does not eliminate HIV, and thus does not provide a permanent cure for HIV infection, the combining of three or more antiretroviral drugs, which has been routinely done since 1996, has dramatically reduced HIV-related morbidity and mortality and greatly prolonged and improved quality of life for those people living with HIV (PLHIV) who can afford or otherwise gain access to them.

Governments and their country's civil society partners have made important progress in recent years in expanding access to HIV treatment. The international community is succeeding in mobilizing far greater commitment to treatment among donor and developing country governments alike. Among the most important initiatives has been the establishment of new sources of international financing for treatment, such as the World Bank's Multi-Country HIV AIDS Program (MAP) and Treatment Acceleration Project (TAP), The Global Fund to Fight AIDS, Tuberculosis and Malaria (Global Fund), and initiatives such as the WHO/UNAIDS '3 by 5'. The latter had an ambitious target. The campaign was launched on World AIDS Day 2003 by WHO and UNAIDS to promote access to ART to at least 3 million people in developing and transitional countries by the end of 2005.

Despite this progress, many people continue to die unnecessarily. In 2004 alone, 3 million died of AIDS [1], the same as in the two previous years. Of the estimated 6.5 million people in developing and transitional countries urgently needing HIV ART, just under 1 million—only 15% of those in need—had access to it by June 2005 [2]. As early as September 2003, the Director-General of the WHO, the Executive Director of UNAIDS and the Executive Director of the Global Fund declared the lack of HIV treatment in developing countries to be a global public health emergency [3]. Such dire circumstances call for *exceptional* measures to expand access to HIV prevention and care services on a vast scale [4].

Achieving, or coming close to, the WHO/UNAIDS target of 3 million people on ART by the end of 2005, not to mention the ultimate goal of universal access, requires *exceptional* efforts in a number of areas. These include technical public health interventions to promote rational selection and use of HIV medicines; sustained international and domestic financing for treatment; adequate human resources and infrastructure in the health and social services sectors; and, not least, affordable HIV medicines and diagnostics [5].

Affordability of HIV medicines

While the affordability of medicines and diagnostics is only one of several factors affecting access to HIV treatment in developing countries, it is an important one. Medicines of importance to PLHIV include antiretrovirals, antibiotics, antifungal agents and other pharmaceuticals used to treat opportunistic infections. Diagnostics include HIV antibody tests, CD4 tests and HIV viral load tests [6]. For resource-constrained governments in poor countries, the purchase price of these products directly affects the number of patients that can be treated [7]. Countries such as Cameroon and South Africa are using local funds to support HIV treatment services: savings in the use of hospital services and procurement of medicines can be reallocated to support training of desperately needed health workers, strengthening of health system infrastructure or to address other pressing development needs.

The price of HIV medicines is also of concern to multilateral and bilateral donors. The World Bank, the Global Fund and the US President's Emergency Plan for AIDS Relief (PEPFAR) are providing unprecedented amounts of international donor funds for HIV treatment in developing countries. Over half of the monies in the Global Fund's approved AIDS grants are for procurement of medicines and commodities [8]. Thus, for example, it is not surprising that the procurement policy of the Global Fund encourages its beneficiaries to procure at the 'lowest possible price' and to utilize the flexibilities in the multilateral trade and intellectual property rules to obtain lower prices. The Global Fund's procurement policy states that 'The Fund encourages Recipients to comply with national laws and applicable international obligations in the field of intellectual property, including the flexibilities provided in the TRIPS agreement and referred to in the Doha Declaration, in a manner that achieves the lowest possible price for products of assured quality' [9].

Although a few originator 'brand name' drugs are priced lower than their generic counterparts, a recent study by the US Government Accountability Office found that, on the whole, price differences between brand name and generic antiretrovirals 'could translate into hundreds of millions of dollars of additional expense when considered on the scale of . . . (the PEPFAR) . . . goal of treating two million people by the end of 2008' [10]. PEPFAR's procurement of generic antiretrovirals has been limited by its decision to require quality assessment and approval by its own US Food and Drug Administration for medicines purchased with its funds [10].

A number of factors contribute to the price of antiretrovirals and other essential medicines, and several strategies may be employed to promote the affordability of these products. These include:

- differential pricing by pharmaceutical companies through which they may offer lower prices for lower- and middle-income country markets [11];
- generic competition and local production, including from major manufacturers of generic HIV medicines located in developing countries such as Brazil and India;
- voluntary licensing arrangements between originator pharmaceutical companies holding; patent rights to the product and generic manufacturers in countries such as India, Kenya and South Africa;
- reduction and elimination of tariffs and taxes.

These strategies, aided by effective and relentless activism of PLHIV and their allies in civil society, resulted in dramatic decreases in the prices of antiretrovirals in the year 2000, and significant, but more marginal, reductions thereafter. The least expensive WHO-recommended first-line triple antiretroviral combination on offer to low-income countries announced by research-based industry is currently priced at approximately US$460 per person per year. The least expensive price for a generic combination, announced by the Clinton Foundation, is approximately US$140–US$150 per person per year. The Global Fund's *Purchase Price Report*, which made public a significant amount of actual transaction data based primarily on procurement by UNICEF and the International Dispensary Association, has reported transactions as low as US$168 per patient-year for the purchase of antiretrovirals [12].

Of course, even at these dramatically lower prices, antiretrovirals remain unaffordable for the vast majority of individuals living with HIV in developing countries. With price levels approaching the average annual per capita income of many resource-poor countries, international donor support remains crucial. Notwithstanding the increased affordability of antiretroviral medicines, prices for middle-income developing countries, second-line antiretroviral regimens and next-generation products remain a major preoccupation to donors, developing countries, PLHIV and most other stakeholders. Data from the Global Fund's *Purchase Price Report* suggest that prices in low-income countries were broadly consistent with 'access' prices publicized by the pharmaceutical companies. However, in middle-income countries, prices varied considerably and were often very high, higher than what would seem reasonable given the income levels of those countries. Similarly, with regard to molecules in second-line regimens, prices offered by the same company to neighbouring countries were highly variable. For instance, didanosine (ddI) was priced between US$146 and US$1577 per patient-year in Benin, Cambodia, the Central African Republic and Serbia [Ashwin Vasan, personal communication (2005); and 13].

Intellectual property and access to HIV medicines

Much of the public discourse about patents, prices and access to HIV treatment has been filled with obfuscation and even disinformation by both sides of a polarized debate. Those whose economic interests or ideologies are served by strong intellectual property protection often unduly diminish the relationship between patents on HIV medicines and affordable access to HIV treatment, or even conjure up their own unduly narrow definition of generic medicines. Attaran and Gillespie-White, using a methodology of adding the total number of possible product patents that could have been issued in Africa, erroneously concluded that because many antiretrovirals are not patented in many African countries, patents have little to no impact on access, despite the fact that a greater number of patents have been applied for and issued in strategic countries with manufacturing capacity such as South Africa [14]. In a recent paper from the Hudson Institute, Adelman *et al.* erroneously claimed that certain HIV medicines are not 'really generics' because they are 'made in India and Thailand ... (and) are copied and manufactured for developing countries' [15]. Conversely, some anti-globalization campaigners seem to oppose intellectual property protection as a matter of economic ideology. At the same time, many of those working in government, international organizations, academia, civil society and the private sector are simply striving for a more balanced intellectual property system that, while stimulating innovation, serves the overriding concern of the public interest and public health, and especially the needs of the poor to have access to affordable essential medicines.

The term 'intellectual property' broadly refers to the legal rights afforded to inventors, writers and other artists, and other creators to control the use of their scientific, literary, artistic and other creative inventions and works. Fields of intellectual property include patents, copyright and trademarks. The most important field relating to access to pharmaceuticals is patents.

A patent is a document issued following an application by a national patent office or other competent government authority that describes an invention and creates a legal right to exclusive control over the use of the invention for a specified period of time. Patents are national in scope and must be requested separately in each country where the right is sought, except where regional patent bodies have been established, for example, the African Regional Intellectual Property Organization (ARIPO) based in Harare, Zimbabwe, and the Organisation Africaine de la Propriété Intellectuelle based in Yaoundé, Cameroon. Patents are often referred to as creating a 'negative right' because, rather than giving the owner a 'positive right' to make or use the patented product, it allows the patent holder to exclude all others from manufacturing, selling or otherwise using the protected product.

The requirements for patentability include the stipulation that the product or process: (i) be new; (ii) involve an inventive step; and (iii) be capable of industrial application. Member States, however, may exclude inventions from patent protection in order to protect public safety, including the protection of human, animal or plant life or health, and may further exclude diagnostic, therapeutic and surgical methods for the treatment of humans and other forms of life.

Although patents and other forms of intellectual property [16] are only one factor affecting the purchase price of pharmaceuticals, it cannot be denied that patent rights, and the trade laws and intellectual property agreements in which they are enshrined, play an important role in pricing and overall access to HIV-related pharmaceuticals.

The government of Brazil, for example, has released data showing a reduction during the period 1996–2002/3 in the prices of antiretrovirals that the government was producing locally by an average of 87%, compared with a reduction of only 47% during the same time period for antiretrovirals that were patented in Brazil and were being imported [17]. More recently, it was reported that some 70% of the Brazilian government's budget for purchasing antiretrovirals is being spent on four molecules patented in Brazil [18].

Patents feature heavily among the preoccupations of government officials and major multi-lateral procurement agencies. For example, at the annual WHO World Health Assembly meeting in May 2005, the delegate of the Government of the Bahamas, on behalf of all the Caribbean Community and Common Market (CARICOM) countries, described a 'potential crisis' in the Caribbean if countries are 'held hostage to the prices of a single manufacturer' in the procurement of antiretrovirals [19]. UNICEF, which purchases an increasingly large volume of antiretrovirals for developing countries, has identified the lack of readily available and reliable information about patent coverage as a major problem in its procurement work [20].

UNAIDS is not opposed to the granting of patent rights in industrialized countries. In a recent policy speech at the London School of Economics, the Executive Director of UNAIDS, Dr Peter Piot, cast the issue as follows:

> An exceptional response to AIDS demands a new compact between the pharmaceutical industry and the world's poor. A just compact involves two elements. One is to give the pharmaceutical industry patent monopoly and good profits in rich countries—this is essential because new antiretroviral drugs are desperately needed all the time. The second is allowing poorer countries to legally manufacture and sell generics... [4].

Patents in high-income countries provide important incentives for innovative research and development of new HIV medicines and, hopefully, the invention of HIV vaccines. In the absence of a vaccine or a cure, with serious problems of resistance and toxicity, and with the critical need for the development of simpler dosing forms for adults and more palatable and simpler antiretroviral formulations for children, innovation remains a crucial element in the response to AIDS. While patents are not the only conceivable incentive for innovation—and the problem of insufficient research for neglected diseases in developing countries has led to calls for alternative or complementary approaches such as a research treaty among governments [21]—patents today are an important incentive to promote research and development in the private pharmaceutical sector and, increasingly, in academic institutions.

It is essential, however, that intellectual property rights be considered in the context of other social interests, not least access to affordable medicines and the human rights concerning health and scientific progress [22,23]. Access to medicines is now widely regarded as part and parcel of Article 12 of the International Covenant on Economic, Social and Cultural Rights, which recognizes the human right to 'the enjoyment of the highest attainable standard of physical and mental health . . .', and Article 15, recognizing the right of everyone to 'enjoy the benefits of scientific progress and its applications . . .' [24]. The United Nations Commission on Human Rights has issued a number of resolutions on intellectual property and access to HIV medicines [25].

The WTO intellectual property agreements: balancing innovation and access

The three main World Trade Organization (WTO) agreements relating to trade, intellectual property and access to HIV medicines and other essential pharmaceuticals are: (i) the Agreement on Trade-Related Aspects of Intellectual Property Rights (the TRIPS Agreement); (ii) the Declaration on TRIPS and Public Health (the Doha Declaration); and (iii) the August 30, 2003 Decision.

These multilateral trade and intellectual property rules can, and are intended to, promote both innovation and access to pharmaceutical products. Recognizing this and referring expressly to 'generic drugs', 'pharmaceutical policies and practices' and 'intellectual property regimes', United Nations Member States in their 2001 *Declaration of Commitment* of the UN General Assembly Special Session on HIV/AIDS sought to 'promote both innovation and the development of domestic pharmaceutical industries consistent with international law' [26].

The TRIPS Agreement, a 'founding component' of the WTO and contained in an Annex to the overall WTO Agreement, was reached 'against a backdrop of diplomatic efforts to upgrade global intellectual property protection' [27]. TRIPS sets out minimum international norms for patent protection and other categories of intellectual property required of all WTO Member States, which numbered 148 in May 2005. Its standards concerning the availability and scope of patent rights provide that patents shall be available for products and processes in all fields of technology, including pharmaceuticals [28].

Among the key obligations of the TRIPS Agreement is the provision that the term of patent protection shall be at least 20 years from the filing date of the patent application [29]. At the time the TRIPS Agreement was reached, in 1994, the municipal law of many developing countries provided far shorter patent terms, 5 or 10 years, and many developing countries did not offer any patent protection whatsoever for pharmaceuticals or other fields of technology. Brazil, for example, the first developing country to guarantee free access to ART, did not provide for patent protection for medicines until 1996. This was an important factor in the ability of the government of Brazil to manufacture locally, in public and private sector pharmaceutical companies, numerous antiretrovirals for which patent protection may otherwise have been sought by innovator companies.

In addition to extending the coverage of patents and strengthening the scope of patent rights, however, the TRIPS Agreement provides important flexibilities—sometimes referred to as 'public health safeguards'—that allow governments to authorize the use of patented products subject to certain conditions. This 'use of the patented product', commonly known as 'compulsory licensing', includes manufacturing, sale, import and, with some limitation, export. Compulsory licences may be issued for many reasons.

While an application for a compulsory licence normally must be preceded by an attempt to negotiate a voluntary licence on reasonable commercial terms within a reasonable period of time, considerable latitude is available to states in deciding the circumstances under which they may be authorized [27]. Three circumstances are specified in the Agreement for which prior negotiation or notice with the patent-holder is not required: (i) national emergency; (ii) circumstances of extreme urgency; and (iii) non-commercial public use.

Few countries, however, have made use of the compulsory licensing flexibility in the TRIPS Agreement to achieve more affordable antiretroviral medicines. Indonesia, Malaysia, Mozambique, Zambia and Zimbabwe are some exceptions. In October 2004, Indonesia issued a compulsory licence for government use of lamivudine and nevirapine. Malaysia issued a compulsory licence in October 2003 for didanosine, zidovudine and a lamivudine/zidovudine combination, limited to imports for the public hospital sector. Mozambique has issued a compulsory licence for local production of a triple fixed-dose combination product consisting of lamivudine, stavudine and nevirapine. Based on reasons of 'national emergency', Zambia issued a compulsory licence for a triple fixed-dose combination of lamivudine, stavudine and nevirapine. In 2002, the Minister of Justice of Zimbabwe declared a 'national emergency' to enable the government to license the manufacture or use of 'any patented drug, including any antiretroviral drug, used in the treatment of persons suffering from HIV/AIDS . . .' or to import 'any generic drug used in the treatment of persons suffering from HIV/AIDS or HIV/AIDS-related conditions' during the period of emergency [30]. In South Africa, following a finding by the national Competition Commission that the multinational companies GlaxoSmithKline and Boehringer Ingelheim had contravened the national competition laws, a settlement agreement was reached that provided for additional and more extensive voluntary licensing of the products concerned both in South Africa and for export to other sub-Saharan African countries.

In negotiations with multinational pharmaceutical companies whose products are protected by patents in Brazil, the government of Brazil has threatened to issue compulsory licences if the companies refused to offer prices that the government considered affordable. The most recent example came in June 2005, when the President and Minister of Health announced that the antiretroviral lopinavir/ritonavir produced by Abbott Laboratories was 'of public interest' and that the government would produce this medicine in its public pharmaceutical manufacturing facilities if the company did not agree to negotiate a voluntary licence for local production. At the time of writing, however, the government had not issued a compulsory licence for the product concerned, and the terms of any agreement between the government and Abbott Laboratories had not been made public.

Nevertheless, although the WHO has declared that lack of HIV treatment in developing countries constitutes a 'global public health emergency' [31], with potential negative political and economic implications such as negative publicity for a country's tourism industry, many countries have been reluctant to declare a 'national emergency' on account of AIDS or other public health problems, perhaps for reasons concerning stigma as well as for economic interests such as maintaining tourism industries.

The compulsory licensing grounds of public non-commercial use may thus prove more acceptable to governments in future. Under this prong of Article 31 of the TRIPS Agreement, governments in countries whose public health system or medical services provide HIV medicines free of change or with no commercial gain—countries such as Brazil, Ethiopia, Malawi, Senegal, South Africa, India and Thailand—can authorize a licensee to manufacture, sell or import generic versions of the medicine, notwithstanding any valid patents that may have been issued in the country.

Whatever grounds may be used for the granting of a compulsory licence, Article 31 of the TRIPS Agreement requires that a number of conditions be met. These include, *inter alia*, the payment of 'reasonable remuneration' in the form of royalties to the patent-holder, and ensuring the availability of judicial or other independent review.

If there were any doubts concerning the rights of governments to utilize the compulsory licensing provisions of the TRIPS Agreement to protect the public health of their peoples and to promote access to affordable medicines for all, the WTO Declaration on the TRIPS Agreement and Public Health (the 'Doha Declaration') put these doubts to rest [33]. While the TRIPS Agreement itself provides in Article 8 that governments may 'adopt measures necessary to protect public health...' as long as these measures are consistent with TRIPS, the Doha Declaration reinforces the primacy of public health interests in the application of these multilateral trade and intellectual property rules. The Declaration emphasizes in Paragraph 4 that 'the TRIPS Agreement does not and should not prevent Members from taking measures to protect public health' and that 'the Agreement can and should be interpreted and implemented in a manner supportive of WTO Members' rights to protect public health and, in particular, to promote access to medicines for all' [33].

Similarly, while TRIPS Article 31 had always permitted governments to grant compulsory licences and to determine the grounds for their granting, the Doha Declaration, in Paragraph 5, makes explicit that 'public health crises, including those relating to HIV/AIDS, tuberculosis, malaria and other epidemics, can represent a national emergency or other circumstances of extreme urgency' within the meaning of Article 31 of the TRIPS Agreement [33].

The Declaration also contributed to the resolution of a long-running issue concerning the legal principle known as 'exhaustion' underlying another flexibility that is inferred, or at least not prohibited, by the TRIPS Agreement, namely parallel importing. 'Exhaustion' of patent rights is considered to occur when the patent-holder sells the product for the first time. The patent rights end upon the first sale by the patent-holder, allowing the first buyer to resell the product elsewhere. If this first buyer resells the product to someone in another country, this is called 'parallel importing', also known as 'grey market imports'. Parallel imports are thus goods brought into a country that were legitimately placed on the market in a different country. Although TRIPS states that the WTO dispute body cannot be used to resolve disputes about exhaustion, the Doha Declaration, in Paragraph 5, makes more explicit that exhaustion, or parallel importing, is a matter that WTO Members have the discretion to regulate at the national level.

In perhaps the only substantive change from the TRIPS Agreement, the Doha Declaration, in Paragraph 7, provides a blanket extension until the year 2016 of the transition period within which least-developed countries must offer patent protection for pharmaceuticals. Depending upon their income levels and the level of patent protection already available in the country, WTO Member States were given different periods of time to apply the TRIPS Agreement. While high-income countries were required to comply by January 1, 1996, certain developing countries were given until January 1, 2000 or January 1, 2006, and least-developed countries were given until January 1, 2016, with the possibility of exceptions on a case-by-case basis. With the extension of this transition period by the Doha Declaration by 10 years, least-developed countries are under no obligation to provide patent protection for HIV medicines and other pharmaceuticals until 2016. Thus, least-developed country governments have the discretion, at least within the WTO multilateral trade rules, to ensure access to generic HIV medicines within their countries.

One important issue that was not resolved immediately by the Doha Declaration, however, concerned the ability of countries without adequate pharmaceutical manufacturing capacity to source generic medicines from manufacturers who would export to them under a compulsory licence. Article 31(f) of the TRIPS Agreement provides that products made or sold under a compulsory licence should be 'predominantly' for the supply of local domestic markets. This limitation is important because many developing countries do not have manufacturing capacities of their own and must rely on imports from low-priced generics producers in other countries if the compulsory licensing provision is to be meaningful for them. The ministers meeting in November 2002 at the Fourth WTO Ministerial Conference in Doha could not reach agreement on how to address this problem. Instead, in Paragraph 6 of the Declaration, the ministers instructed the WTO Council for TRIPS 'to find an expeditious solution to this problem and to report to the General Council before the end of 2002' [32]

WTO August 30, 2003 Decision

Although the ministers' deadline of December 31, 2002 was not met, in August 2003 a multilateral consensus was finally forged among WTO Member States regarding access to affordable medicines for countries without sufficient manufacturing capacity in the pharmaceutical sector. This consensus, also known as Implementation of Paragraph 6 of the Doha Declaration on the TRIPS Agreement and Public Health, covered public health problems in addition to AIDS, which was particularly important for PLHIV, who are prone to a host of opportunistic infections and other diseases—cancers, fungal infections and other killers—that antiretrovirals do not specifically treat.

International organizations such as WHO and UNAIDS urged that the arrangements under the August 30, 2003 Decision of the Council for TRIPS be implemented in the most flexible manner possible, so that developing countries could utilize the system easily and efficiently in their efforts to ensure greater access to HIV medicines for their peoples [J Fleet, Senior Adviser, UNAIDS Secretariat to the WTO TRIPS Council, June 25, 2002, Geneva. Unpublished; and 33]. In a statement to the TRIPS Council, the representative of the WHO emphasized as the central principle that 'the people of a country which does not have the capacity for domestic production of a needed product should be no less protected by compulsory licensing provisions (or indeed other TRIPS safeguards), nor should they face any greater procedural hurdles, compared to people who happen to live in countries capable of producing the product' [34]. Among the solutions being proposed at the time, WHO recommended that reference to the limited exception to patents under Article 30 be considered the one most consistent with this public health principle [35]. The WHO recommendation, however, was not adopted by the WTO.

According to the WTO in the August 30, 2003 Decision, 'WTO member governments broke their deadlock over intellectual property protection and public health.... They agreed on legal changes that will make it easier for poorer countries to import cheaper generics made under compulsory licensing if they are unable to manufacture the medicines themselves' [35].

The August 30, 2003 Decision establishes a waiver of the obligations under TRIPS Article 31(f) and allows any member country to export pharmaceutical products made under compulsory licences to countries that do not have sufficient pharmaceutical manufacturing capacity. The problem of lack of pharmaceutical manufacturing is a real one for countries like those in Southern Africa that are hard-hit by AIDS. For example, of the 15 countries with adult HIV prevalence above 10% at the time the Decision was being negotiated, only South Africa was considered to have adequate capacity to manufacture antiretroviral medicines. In other words, 14 of these 15 hardest-hit countries would have to find sources of supply for generic medicines in exporting countries if they—the very countries in greatest need—were to benefit from compulsory licensing.

The waiver arrangement is designed to cover pharmaceuticals to address all public health problems identified by the Member States concerned. All WTO member countries are eligible to import under this Decision, but 23 developed countries are listed in the Decision as announcing voluntarily that they will not use the system to import, and others indicated they will use the system only to address emergencies. At the time of writing, however, some 2 years after the Decision was agreed on, and notwithstanding patent law reforms undertaken by Canada and Norway intended to allow their generic companies to utilize this arrangement, the WTO has not been notified of a single instance in which such a waiver would be utilized. Thus, the waiver arrangement under the August 30, 2003 Decision must be monitored and evaluated to ensure that it affords an efficient and effective mechanism to address the problems of concerned states. Lack of use of this temporary WTO waiver system by its intended beneficiaries only heightens the need to adopt a more definitive and lasting amendment to address the problem of Article 31(f) in this context. To date, however, talks within the WTO to amend Article 31(f) have been stalled.

Recent developments in national legislation, and regional and bilateral trade agreements

While the TRIPS Agreement sets out minimum international norms for intellectual property protection, it expressly states that 'members may, but shall not be obliged to, implement in their law more extensive protection than is required by this Agreement', sometimes referred to as 'TRIPS-plus' provisions [36]. In 2004 and 2005, both in national legislation and in regional and bilateral trade agreements between developing countries and the USA, developing countries have opted not to avail themselves of the full flexibilities afforded them under the multilateral WTO intellectual property rules. Indeed, a number of countries have adopted 'more extensive' protection than required under the TRIPS Agreement.

For example, in March 2005, the Indian Parliament passed a new law amending the Patent Act 1970 [37]. The amendments to the Patent Act were intended to address India's obligations by bringing it into compliance with the TRIPS Agreement at the end of its transition period. In order to meet its WTO obligations to comply with TRIPS for patent protection in the pharmaceutical sector by January 1, 2005, the Indian government had passed a temporary ordinance at the end of December 2004.

The passage of the Indian Patent Bill by Parliament in March 2005 ushered in a new patent regime in India under which product patents for pharmaceutical products are now available under Indian law. Up to then, India had provided patent protection only for pharmaceutical processes, allowing its important generic pharmaceutical industry to formulate and manufacture antiretrovirals and other medicines by alternative steps, otherwise known as 'reverse engineering'.

During the legislative process, the Indian Parliament ultimately deleted some provisions in the temporary ordinance that would have resulted in more extensive patent protection than required under the TRIPS Agreement. However, the final law did include an important TRIPS-plus provision: a 3-year waiting period for the issuance of a compulsory licence. This waiting period is not required by the TRIPS Agreement. By failing to retain the full flexibilities permitted by the multilateral rules, the Indian legislative proposals unnecessarily undermine the ability of the Indian generic pharmaceutical industry to supply developing countries with affordable generics. At present, about half of the people on HIV treatment in developing countries are using generic antiretrovirals. The Indian generic industry is the source of most of these medicines in Africa and Asia. Thus, the impact of the Indian patent amendments on access to generic antiretrovirals will be profound.

Similarly, a number of developing countries have entered into regional and bilateral trade agreements with the USA that have intellectual property protection at their core and include provisions for more extensive patent protection than required by TRIPS. These include Guatemala, Honduras, Nicaragua, Costa Rica, El Salvador and the Dominican Republic through the Central American Free Trade Agreement (CAFTA), as well as separate agreements with Chile, Jordan and Morocco. Among the more extensive protection provided in these agreements are the use of national drug regulatory agencies to enforce patents, whereas previously this function was left to the judiciary; longer patent periods; new patents for 'new uses'; limitations on compulsory licensing; and additional restrictions on pharmaceutical test data known as 'data exclusivity' [38]. The Andean states in South America (Columbia, Ecuador, Venezuela, Peru, Bolivia and Argentina), Thailand and even Member States of the Southern African Customs Union (South Africa, Botswana, Lesotho, Swaziland and Namibia), with the highest HIV prevalence rates in the world, are reportedly negotiating similar agreements.

Conclusion

The main messages of this chapter are:

1. Innovation of products for the prevention and treatment of HIV is crucial, and intellectual property rights can provide an important incentive for such innovation.

2. The HIV epidemic requires an exceptional response, including in the area of intellectual property: where intellectual property rights pose a barrier to access to affordable HIV-related medicines, intellectual property rights, which vest in individual persons or corporations, must be subordinate to the human rights concerning health and access to medicines for all [39].

Global trade and intellectual property rules—the WTO TRIPS Agreement, Doha Declaration and August 30, 2003 Decision—offer governments considerable flexibility to expand access to more affordable generic HIV medicines. These flexibilities include compulsory licensing, the absence of any requirement for least-developed countries to issue patents on pharmaceuticals until 2016, and some flexibility for countries with insufficient pharmaceutical manufacturing capacity to source lower-cost generic medicines through exports under a compulsory licence. With few exceptions, however, these flexibilities are not being utilized by developing and transitional countries.

National governments are failing to incorporate the full flexibilities available into their national patent laws. Some, like India, a leading producer of generic HIV medicines, are including in their national laws more extensive patent protection than required by the WTO. Others, such as in Latin America, are entering bilateral or regional trade agreements with the USA that may undermine the flexibilities that are their right under the global rules, impede the ability of those countries to expand access to lower-cost generic medicines and, in turn, diminish the fulfilment of the human rights related to health and scientific progress to which their citizens are entitled.

The lack of access to HIV treatment in developing and transitional countries has been declared a national emergency. In some countries, more than one-third of the adult population is infected with HIV, a treatable but otherwise fatal virus. Faced with such a calamity, no responsible government leader of a high-income country in the Americas, Europe or Asia and the Pacific would tolerate an international property regime that makes it significantly more expensive, and thus more difficult, to get lifesaving medicines to their people. Imposing such a regime on the governments of poorer countries creates unnecessary obstacles to treatment, and only serves to tarnish legitimate intellectual property rights.

References

1. UNAIDS. (2004). *Epidemiological Update*. Geneva: UNAIDS.

2. World Health Organization. (2005). *3 by 5 Progress Report*. Geneva: WHO.

3. World Health Organization. (2004). *3 by 5 Progress Report, December 2003–June 2004*. Geneva: WHO.

4. Piot P. (2005). *Why AIDS is Exceptional*. London: London School of Economics, February 8, 2005.

5. World Health Organization. (2004). *WHO Medicines Strategy, Countries at the Core, 2004–2007*. Geneva: WHO.

6. UNICEF, UNAIDS, WHO, MSF. (2004). *Sources and Prices of Selected Medicines and Diagnostics for People Living with HIV/AIDS*. A Joint UNICEF–UNAIDS–WHO–MSF Project. Geneva.

7. World Bank. (2004). *Technical Guide for HIV/AIDS Medicines and Related Supplies: Contemporary Context and Procurement*. Washington, DC: World Bank, p63.

8. Global Fund to Fight AIDS, Tuberculosis and Malaria. (2004). *Annual Report 2004*. Geneva: Global Fund.

9. Global Fund to Fight AIDS, Tuberculosis and Malaria. (2002). *Report of the Third Global Fund Board Meeting, October 10–11, 2002*. Geneva: Global Fund.

10. United States Government Accountability Office. (2004). *Global Health, U.S. AIDS Coordinator Addressing Some Key Challenges to Expanding Treatment but Others Remain*. Washing DC:GAO 04-784, July 2004.

11. WHO/UNAIDS. (2002). *Accelerating Access Initiative Progress Report*. Geneva: WHO/UNAIDS.

12. Global Fund to Fight AIDS, Tuberculosis and Malaria. (2005). *The Global Fund Purchase Price Report*. Geneva: Global Fund. Available online at www.theglobalfund.org.

13. Médecins Sans Frontières. (2005). *Untangling the Web of Price Reductions*, 8th edn. Campaign for Access to Essential Medicines. Available online at www.accessmed-msf.org.

14. Attaran A, Gillespie-White L. (2001). Do patents for antiretroviral drugs constrain access to AIDS treatment in Africa? *Journal of the American Medical Association* 286:1886–92.

15. Adelman CC, Norris J, Weicher SJ. (2005). *The Full Cost of HIV/AIDS Treatment.* White Paper, 2nd edn. Washington, DC: Hudson Institute, p2.

16. World Intellectual Property Organization. (1998). *Intellectual Property Reading Material.* Geneva: WIPO Publication No. 476(E).

17. National AIDS Programme/Ministry of Health, Brazil. (2003). *Update on the HIV Epidemic.* Brasilia: Ministry of Health.

18. Costa H. (2005). Compulsory licensing of the lopinavir–ritonavir combination. Press conference by the Minister of Health or Brazil held at the UN. Geneva: June 27, 2005.

19. World Health Organization. (2005). Scaling Up Treatment and Care Within a Coordinated and Comprehensive Response to HIV/AIDS. Intervention of the Government of the Bahamas on Behalf of CARICOM Caribbean countries 24 May 2005. 58th World Health Assembly Agenda Item 13.19, Implementation of resolutions (progress reports). Geneva: WHO.

20. United Nations. (2005). Intervention of Ms Hanne Bak Pedersen, UNICEF, Meeting of United Nations and intergovernmental agencies on intellectual property on access to HIV medicines, Geneva, February 11, 2005.

21. Love J. (2005). Sign-on letter to the World Health Organization (WHO) Commission on Intellectual Property, Innovation and Health (CIPIH). Consumer Project on Technology. Geneva: WHO.

22. World Trade Organization. (1999). *Statement of UNAIDS at the Third WTO Ministerial Conference.* Geneva: UNAIDS. Available online at www.unaids.org.

23. World Health Organization. (1999). Globalization and access to drugs, perspectives on the WTO/ TRIPS Agreement. *Health Economics and Drugs.* DAP Series No. 7.

24. United Nations. (1996). *International Covenant on Economic, Social and Cultural Rights.* Adopted and opened for signature, ratification and accession by the General Assembly, Resolution 2200A (XXI), December 16, 1996.

25. UN Commission on Human Rights. (2005). *Access to Medication in the Context of Pandemics Such as HIV/AIDS, Tuberculosis and Malaria.* Resolution of the 61st Commission on Human Rights, E/CN.4/RES/2005/23, 4/15/2005.

26. United Nations (UNGASS). (2001). *Declaration of Commitment.* United Nations General Assembly Special Session on HIV/AIDS, June 2001, paragraph 55.

27. Maskus KE. (2000). *Intellectual Property Rights in the Global Economy.* Washington, DC: Institute for International Economics, 1 and 16.

28. World Trade Organization. (1994). Agreement on Trade-related Aspects of Intellectual Property Rights (TRIPS Agreement), article 27. Geneva: WTO.

29. World Trade Organization. (1994). Agreement on Trade-related Aspects of Intellectual Property Rights (TRIPS Agreement), article 33. Geneva: WTO.

30. Parliament of Zimbabwe. (2002). General Notice 240 of 2002, Patents Act [Chapter 26:03], Declaration of Period of Emergency (HIV/AIDS). Notice 2002, PA Chinamasa, Minister of Justice, Legal and Parliamentary Affairs. Harare: Parliament of Zimbabwe.

31. UN General Assembly on HIV/AIDS. (2003). WHO–UNAIDS Announcement (Briefing/Press Conference) September 22, 2003.

32. World Trade Organization. (2001). *Declaration on the TRIPS Agreement and Public Health.* WTO document WT/MIN(01)/DEC/W2. Geneva: WTO.

33. World Trade Organization. (2004). Statement of UNAIDS at the Fifth WTO Ministerial Conference, Cancun, Mexico September 10–13, 2004. Geneva: WTO.

34. WTO Council for TRIPS. *Statement by the Representative of WHO,* Geneva, September 17, 2002.

35. World Trade Organization. (2003). Decision removes final patent obstacle to cheap drug imports. *WTO News* Press Release: Press/350/Rev.1. August 30, 2003. Geneva: WTO.

36. World Trade Organization. (1994). Agreement on Trade-Related Aspects of Intellectual Property Rights (TRIPS Agreement), article 1. Geneva: WTO.

37. Ministry of Law and Justice, Government of India. (2005). The Patents (Amendment) Act No. 15 of 2005. April 4, 2005. New Delhi: Government of India.

38. Médecins Sans Frontières. (2004). *Access to Medicines at Risk across the Globe—What to Watch Out for in a Free Trade Agreement with the United States.* Fact sheet for the 2004 World Health Assembly, May 14, 2004.

39. United Nations Secretary-General. (2003). *Access to Medication in the Context of Pandemics such as HIV/AIDS.* Report of the Secretary-General. E/CN.4/2003/48, January 16, 2003.

Chapter 45

Country-level public–private partnerships for successful HIV treatment programmes

Jasper Bos[*], Onno Schellekens and Arie de Groot

Introduction

Public–private partnerships (PPPs) for healthcare have recently attracted great interest as a tool to achieve improvements in efficiency, consumer choice and accessibility to healthcare [1–4]. In this chapter, we will cover both practical and theoretical implications of PPPs. First, we start with a theoretical explanation of the reasons why public and private institutions engage in partnerships. Next, we will provide an overview of a number of influential multinational PPPs for HIV. In the remainder of this chapter, we will draw attention to the potential role that local PPPs could play in the creation of a strengthened, sustainable health infrastructure in sub-Saharan Africa.

Rationales for engaging in PPPs

Many definitions for PPPs exist, but all definitions emphasize the shared goal that actors need to possess. For instance, 'PPPs are institutionalized forms of cooperation of public and private actors that work together towards a joint target' [1–4], or, to cite another definition: 'PPPs are a sort of collaboration where the strengths and resources of public and private partners are fully explored in order to pursue shared goals' [5]. These definitions are very broad but give less insight into the reasons participants may have for engaging in such a partnership. PPPs can consist of any combination of non-governmental organizations (NGOs), government bodies, multilateral organizations and the private sector, and all participants will have their own reasons for engaging in partnerships. In this section, we will provide some theoretical arguments about how both public and private institutions can benefit from partnerships.

The case for the private sector

One of the main objectives of the private sector is to maximize profits, which requires a constant balance between investments, price, volume, costs, risk and timelines. The private sector is less willing to carry out projects when there is an imbalance between these parameters. To allow a comparison between future benefits and projected costs, the net present

* Corresponding author.

value framework can be used. We will use this framework to emphasize the effects of public sector participation on the willingness of the private sector to carry out certain projects. The net present value (NPV) of an investment can be calculated as follows [6]:

(1) $NPV = I_0 - \Sigma (E_t - A_t) \times (1/(1-r))^t$

where I_0 = the initial investment at $t = 0$; E_t = all (expected) benefits of the project ($E_t = P \times v$, with P = price and v = sales volume); A_t = all expenses required for carrying out the project; t = the timing of costs and benefits; and r = the risk adjusted discount rate.

If the NPV is positive, the project is expected to be profitable and could be interesting to pursue. As appears from this framework, a number of parameters influence the decision to carry out the project. These are:

- the amount of investment required;
- the expected sales volume of the product, influenced by regulation of demand;
- the maximum allowed price per product;
- the expenses required for product manufacturing or distribution (for instance extra difficulties to offer products or services in a developing country);
- the timing of benefits and costs;
- the risk-adjusted discount rate.

The participation of the public sector in private projects may result in changes in one or more of these parameters. Consequently, this may lead to a positive change in NPV, rendering the project worthwhile to carry out for the private sector. This change in NPV may be caused by a number of mechanisms, which are displayed in Table 45.1.

The most important effects of public sector participation in a project are either related to the investment costs or based on regulatory issues. Since high investments are often necessary in new technologies and the market for healthcare is characterized by complex regulation, it is clear to see that the private sector might benefit from PPPs in health. Aside from these

Table 45.1 Possible influences of PPPs on the parameters of the net present value framework

Parameter	Example of government contribution
Amount of investment required	Lowering of investments by cost sharing between public and private sector
	Using pre-existing capacity (e.g. medical infrastructure)
	Lowering investments by providing tax credits
Expected sales volume	Regulation of demand by government interference or legislation
Maximum price of the product or service	Regulation of price by government (for instance, by the waiving of taxes and import duties of medical equipment)
Expenses of product manufacturing or distribution	Share distribution or manufacturing costs between partners
Timing of benefits and costs	Advance purchase commitments and advance payments
The risk-adjusted discount rate	Shared interest of both public and private sector decreases risks of unexpected government interference

Source: original research.

reasons, sometimes private sector actors may wish to engage in partnerships for ethical reasons or because of pressure from stakeholders, as with, for example, corporate responsibility projects, in which private companies invest in the upgrading of private or public medical services to ensure that not only employees but also the community can receive HIV treatment and care.

Rationales for NGOs to engage in PPPs

NGOs, especially foreign NGOs, usually operate in a complex environment where the regulatory boundaries are set by the local governments and the capacity to operate may be provided or enhanced by both the public and private sector, in terms of both resources and infrastructure. The objective of NGOs, as not-for-profit organizations, is usually related to reaching certain social goals, such as better health for the poor, which might be easily shared with local governments. Participation in PPPs may, given the complex environment and the lack of capacity of both the public and the private sector, increase the chances of NGOs reaching their objectives.

Rationales for the public sector to engage in PPPs

In general, the main objective of the public health sector is the provision of health services that benefit the population. The focus is not necessarily to operate as efficiently as possible against the lowest possible costs, but to maximize the output for a given budget. For the public sector, a partnership will be worth pursuing if the products are believed to be of vital importance to the community as a whole, and if the public sector, on its own, (i) is not able to produce all of the products or services; or (ii) believes that results can be produced more efficiently by, or in cooperation with, the private sector. Especially in developing countries, certain aspects of health and healthcare might benefit from these kinds of partnerships [1–3]. For instance, the development of therapeutics for diseases that are only endemic in developing countries is the major objective of a growing number of PPPs.

An alternative definition of PPPs in health

In industrialized countries, it is common for a share of the medical services to be publicly financed but contracted out to the private sector. These arrangements would not fit the traditional definition of a PPP, since the public and private sectors do not necessarily share the same goals and objectives. However, it is questionable whether the rationales for engaging in PPPs truly involve this 'common shared goal', or if PPPs are not just institutionalized arrangements between the public and private sectors, including NGOs, with shared risks and responsibilities. All these arrangements are symbiotic, i.e. based on mutual benefit. For instance, the public sector is rewarded for the partnering by improvements in cost-efficiency, programme performance and the sharing of risks and responsibilities [1,7], while the private sector benefits from better investment potential and the ability to make a profit. As Scharle noted, the reasons for private sector participation in a PPP are such that 'a good return on investment is definitely an essential consideration from the private sector perspective' [8]. NGOs are rewarded for engaging in PPPs by increases in resources, and they might also become less vulnerable to government intervention by partnering with the public and private sectors.

Given the inherent difference in objectives of both the public and private sectors, it might be more useful to define PPPs not as those partnerships that 'pursue shared goals', but rather as partnerships in which: (i) the respective parties have a mutual benefit from partnering; (ii) the partnership is necessary for the fulfilment of the project; and (iii) responsibilities and risks are shared. For instance, infrastructure and telecom projects that are carried out with private sector participation in developing countries are usually viewed as PPPs [1], but it is unlikely that there is truly a shared goal that drives the participants. The extension of the definition of PPPs to include these contractual relationships allows us to assess the role of private partners in participation and contracting partnerships for HIV as well.

Examples of PPPs for HIV

PPPs can be found on any level in the healthcare system, from large international level partnerships to partnerships that are mostly concerned with the local implementation of projects involving local partners. Also, as seen in Table 45.2, PPPs can be found on any functional level in the healthcare system, ranging from partnerships that are designed for product development to partnerships that are involved in the strengthening of local healthcare systems in developing countries or the exchange of knowledge.

In the following sections, we will provide examples of existing PPPs that focus on HIV. A number of these examples are also featured in the database of PPPs of the Initiative on Public–Private Partnerships in Health (IPPPH) and can be found at http://www.ippph.org.

Partnerships for disease control: product development

A number of partnerships focus on research and development of new antiretrovirals or new preventive interventions. One of the most well known is the International AIDS Vaccine Initiative (IAVI), focusing on the development of a successful HIV vaccine (Box 45.1).

Other examples of partnerships for product development are the Alliance for Microbicide Development (AMD), the International Partnership for Microbicides (IPM) and the Microbicides Development Program, all of which have as their mission to accelerate the development of a successful microbicide that prevents the transmission of HIV.

Both the IPM and the AMD focus on increasing funding for research, raising awareness and leveraging partnerships for the development of microbicides. The Microbicides Development Program is a partnership that operates in order to facilitate clinical trials of microbicides in developing countries. A clinical phase III trial is expected to start soon in multiple locations.

Table 45.2 Categories of current public–private partnerships (PPPs) for health

Category	Level of partnership
Partnerships for disease control: product development	International
Partnerships for disease control: product distribution	National–international
Partnerships for strengthening health services	International
Partnerships for health programme coordination	International, sectoral or regional
Country level partnerships	National, sectoral or regional
Private sector coalitions for health	International–national/regional
Partnerships for product donation	International–national

Source: adapted from [9].

Box 45.1 The International AIDS Vaccine Initiative (IAVI)

IAVI is a consortium consisting of representatives of the pharmaceutical industry, universities and governments. Its objective is to accelerate access to a safe and effective HIV vaccine. IAVI supports this goal through strategic planning and awareness activities, as well as real investments in novel HIV vaccine approaches from both the public and the private sectors. Currently, IAVI owns royalty-free licences on a number of candidate vaccines to ensure the affordability of an effective vaccine.

Sources: www.IAVI.org, www.IPPH.org.

Partnerships for disease control: product distribution

A partnership worth noting is the Accelerating Access Initiative (AAI). The AAI has succeeded in a significant lowering of the prices for antiretroviral therapies (ARTs) for certain developing countries. The partnership provides a framework for countries to gear up and implement ART programmes (Box 45.2).

While the AAI has succeeded in bringing down the costs of branded antiretrovirals, the Clinton HIV/AIDS Initiative has negotiated supplier agreements for low-priced generic antiretrovirals and medical diagnostics (Box 45.3).

Partnerships for strengthening health services

The Namibia HIV/AIDS Alliance is a local partnership for the treatment of HIV patients (Box 45.4).

One of the largest public antiretroviral treatment campaigns in sub-Saharan Africa, the treatment programme of the government of Botswana is the result of the collaboration between the Bill & Melinda Gates Foundation, Merck & Co Inc. and the Government of Botswana. Although scaling up this initiative to include all those in need might be a challenge, given the total demand of over 110,000 people in need of ART in Botswana, this initiative shows the possibilities of PPPs for building capacity for ART in sub-Saharan Africa (Box 45.5). Also, an increasing number of multinational organizations have invested in setting up public or private health treatment programmes for their employees and depend-

---

Box 45.2 The Accelerating Access Initiative (AAI)

The AAI is facilitated by UNAIDS, working with the World Health Organization (WHO), the World Bank, the United Nations Children's Fund (UNICEF), the United Nations Population Fund (UNFPA) and six research-based pharmaceutical companies: Abbott Laboratories, Boehringer Ingelheim, Bristol-Myers Squibb, GlaxoSmithKline, Merck & Co Inc. and F Hoffman-la Roche. Its aim is to increase sustained access to good quality interventions involving committed governments, industry, the UN agencies, development organizations, NGOs and people living with HIV. Currently, over 20 countries have completed national plans and have agreed preferential prices with the individual companies.

Source: UNAIDS, 2004.

Box 45.3 The Clinton HIV/AIDS Initiative

The Clinton Foundation, in collaboration with the Global Fund to Fight AIDS, Tuberculosis and Malaria, the World Bank and UNICEF, aims to extend access to antiretroviral drugs and diagnostics to countries in which these organizations are working. The Clinton Initiative has reached agreements with five large manufacturers of generic therapeutics—Aspec Pharmacare Holdings Ltd, Cipla Ltd, Hetero Drugs Ltd, Ranbaxy Laboratories Ltd and Matrix Laboratories Ltd—and the world market leaders on diagnostics—Bayer Diagnostics, Beckman Coulter, Inc., BD, bioMérieux and Roche Diagnostics—to price their products up to 80% lower than the current market prices. These prices are available for projects that meet the Clinton HIV/AIDS Initiative criteria of the guarantee of payment, the conducting of long-term tenders and the security of drug distribution.

Source: [10].

ants. Well-known examples of companies that have initiated such programmes are, among others, Anglo-American, Celtel, Heineken, Daimler-Chrysler, Diageo, SNV and the Dutch embassies in Africa. The number of companies providing these services is rapidly increasing, especially in South Africa. A large number of South African companies provide some form of HIV services to their employees. These HIV programmes, while only benefiting those employed by the company and their relatives, will help build local capacity and bring valuable knowledge.

Partnerships for global health coordination

The Global Fund to Fight AIDS, Tuberculosis and Malaria is an alliance of UN agencies, developing countries, donor governments, private corporations and NGOs [12] (Box 45.6).

Box 45.4 The Namibia HIV/AIDS Alliance

The Namibia HIV/AIDS Alliance is a partnership for the treatment of HIV and AIDS patients embedded in a primary care health insurance in Namibia. It is a partnership between: a local private sector health maintenance organization (Diamond Health Services), foreign NGOs (Stop AIDS Now!, PharmAccess Foundation and HIVOS), the Namibian Red Cross and an organization of people living with HIV, Elongo Eparu. This programme is financed by the Dutch Postcode Lottery and approved by the Namibian government. Diamond Health Services acts as the implementing partner. PharmAccess has initiated the programme and performs the administrative and medical quality control as well as the local coordination, whereas HIVOS runs the treatment literacy programme. The Red Cross is involved in home-based care of the patients, and Stop AIDS Now! is responsible for the overall international coordination. The programme aims at lower- to middle-income people, staff of the Namibian Red Cross and members of Lironga Eparu. In cooperation with the Namibian Business Coalition against HIV/AIDS (NABCOA), it also aims to remove barriers for companies to buy health insurance for their employees by subsidizing health care.

Source: IPPPH database (www.ippph.org).

Box 45.5 The antiretroviral treatment programme in Botswana

The PPP is formalized as the not-for-profit organization ACHAP (African Comprehensive HIV/AIDS Partnerships). ACHAP assisted with the implementation of the national HIV strategy, including the development of a national monitoring and evaluation system and a needs assessment toolkit that is guiding HIV and AIDS interventions at the district level. ACHAP has also been involved in human capacity building and training of healthcare and other personnel, and has initiated HIV education and awareness programmes. In 2003, approximately 9000 people were enrolled in the treatment programme [11]. This PPP aims to be a model for future PPP responses in sub-Saharan African countries and offers assistance with both antiretroviral treatment and prevention programmes. It is a collaboration between The Merck Foundation/Merck & Co., the government of Botswana and the Bill & Melinda Gates Foundation.

Source: IPPPH database (www.ippph.org).

Other international health partnerships

A number of other international health partnerships exist that at least partly focus on HIV. For instance, the Hope for African Children Initiative (HACI) is an effort to alleviate the challenges faced by millions of African infants who have become orphans due to HIV or are currently living with HIV (Box 45.7).

Private sector coalitions for health

A number of private sector coalitions have emerged that are dedicated to defining the role of the private sector in the fight against HIV. For instance, the Global Business Coalition on HIV is an alliance of international business that focuses on raising awareness of the role that the private sector can play in combating HIV. The Global Business Coalition consists of a large number of private sector companies but also non-profit organizations such as UNAIDS and the World Economic Forum (Box 45.8). Initially, the support for the GBC came from the

---

Box 45.6 The Global Fund to Fight AIDS, Tuberculosis and Malaria

The purpose of the Global Fund to Fight AIDS, Tuberculosis and Malaria is to attract and disburse resources in the fight against these diseases through the use of innovative funding mechanisms. The Global Fund works as a financing mechanism, and proposals to the Fund have to be submitted through country-specific coordinating bodies (country coordinating mechanism, or CCM). Ideally, these CCMs would ensure that both local governments and the private sector actively participate in the development of health improvement programmes, promoting the establishment of PPPs. In reality, the public sector tends to heavily dominate the CCMs. Until now, the Global Fund has attracted US$4.7 billion and has committed US$3 billion towards health programmes that focus on the fight against AIDS, TB and malaria [13]. The Global Fund is financed by governments, the private sector, and private institutional and individual donors.

Box 45.7 The Hope for African Children Initiative (HACI)

The HACI is a partnership of six large humanitarian organizations: CARE, Plan International, Save the Children, the Society for Women and AIDS in Africa, the World Conference on Peace and Religion, and World Vision. This partnership is funded by the Bill & Melinda Gates Foundation. The activities of this partnership are mostly related to raising international and local awareness of the fate of these children.

Source: IPPPH database.

Bill & Melinda Gates Foundation, the Open Society Institute and the United Nations Foundation. Now the major source of funding comes from membership fees. These organizations are PPPs, since they provide a public service, namely the prevention and treatment of HIV, not only to their employees, but also to their dependants and the community.

A number of regional organizations exist that focus on the role of the private sector in

---

Box 45.8 The Global Business Coalition (GBC) on HIV

The activities of the GBC on HIV include public advocacy, education and research on the role of the private sector. The GBC also tries to increase business action, such as the distribution of condoms or the provision of voluntary counselling and testing services, by sharing knowledge on workplace HIV programmes.

Source: IPPPH database.

---

combating HIV. For example, Sida Entreprises in France targets African subsidiaries of French companies and advocates an increased business response against HIV. Numerous smaller business coalitions exist in African countries that are also concerned with HIV, such as the Namibian Business Coalition Against HIV/AIDS (NABCOA) and the South African Business Coalition Against HIV/AIDS (SOBCOA).

Partnerships for product donation

Partnerships also exist in which pharmaceutical companies donate therapeutics to local governments in sub-Saharan Africa. One example is the Diflucan Partnership Programme (Box 45.9).

Box 45.9 The Diflucan Partnership Programme

Pfizer has donated Diflucan®, an antifungal therapeutic that is used for the treatment of opportunistic infections such as cryptococcal meningitis or candidiasis. The distribution of the therapeutic is done in collaboration with local NGOs and local governments. The objectives of the programme are to reach as many patients as possible in sub-Saharan Africa and to train healthcare workers in treating and diagnosing opportunistic infections. The programme has already donated Diflucan to governments and NGOs in a large number of countries and is currently expanding to Asia and Latin America.

Another example of a PPP for product donation is the CARE programme, in which Roche Pharmaceuticals sponsors a treatment programme and donates antiretroviral medication to HIV patients in four countries in sub-Saharan Africa (Box 45.10).

Country-level partnerships

Most partnerships that have been mentioned throughout this section involve local organizations and local governments. However, most of these partnerships have been initiated and are 'owned' by the international community. Partnerships that have been initiated by local government or institutions in sub-Saharan Africa are less well known by the international community. For instance, the IPPPH database on PPPs in health contains information on 92 PPPs, but none of them are country-level partnerships in which the only participants are local stakeholders. Some of the experiments that have been conducted with contracting out of health services—for instance, in Zimbabwe or Tanzania—could be seen as forms of country-level partnerships, but these types of arrangements have not been introduced in most countries in sub-Saharan Africa. Other examples of country-level PPPs are, for instance, the subsidies that African governments give to mission hospitals, which are run by NGOs. These are a form of PPP, since governmental and private (fee-for-service and donations) resources are combined to provide healthcare through private, NGO-owned hospitals. Other examples exist as well; consider the initiatives of local business and healthcare providers to deliver voluntary counselling and testing (VCT) services to the community.

Box 45.10 Cohort programme to evaluate access to antiretroval therapy and education (CARE)

CARE is a pilot programme resulting from a joint effort of PharmAccess Foundation and F Hoffman-LaRoche Ltd, and approved by local governments. It is designed to provide antiretroviral drugs along with comprehensive clinical care in low-resource and low-cost settings in Africa. The programme runs in Abidjan in Côte d'Ivoire, Dakar in Senegal, Nairobi in Kenya and Kampala in Uganda. In total, 200 antiretroviral-naïve patients who are unable to afford antiretrovirals will be provided with highly active antiretroviral treatment (HAART). This programme is designed to assess the feasibility of providing HAART to patients in Africa. The programme also includes education programmes to increase general knowledge of HIV and AIDS, as well as HIV awareness, prevention strategies and treatment adherence.

Source: www.pharmaccess.org.

The potential of local PPPs for HIV prevention and treatment

In the previous section, we indicated that a number of PPPs have increased the affordability and access to HIV care and treatment. However, there is still an enormous gap between the number of people in direct need of HIV treatment and the number of people who actually receive treatment in sub-Saharan Africa. It is estimated by the World Health Organization (WHO) that by the end of 2004, as few as 325,000 people were receiving treatment in sub-Saharan Africa [14]. Now that the procurement procedures are beginning to fall into place, it is time actually to implement programmes 'owned' by local communities on a large scale. The need for local support of programmes is emphasized by recent research by the IPPPH, which examined the role of large PPPs on pharma-based drug access programmes [15]. The IPPPH concluded that drug donation or large price reductions are very useful contributions, but in themselves are not sufficient to initiate and support national disease control programmes. The IPPPH therefore stressed the need for operational support of these programmes on a national level. In this section, we will elaborate on how local PPPs for health could contribute to increasing access to care and strengthening the medical infrastructure.

Local PPPs to increase existing health capacity

The strengthening of health systems in sub-Saharan Africa is considered a prerequisite for increasing access to ART [16]. As a consequence, next to the costs of providing ARTs, large investments would need to be made in health delivery systems to ensure the necessary capacity. The contracting out of a part of the healthcare delivery to the private health sector might be an answer to solve gaps in coverage quickly, or partially. These contracts might not only lead to increases in capacity, but might also improve the efficiency of the programmes [17]. Research in Zimbabwe has shown that the contracting out of hospital services can lead to more cost-efficient care without sacrificing quality [17]. In almost all Western societies, this contracting out of a significant part of healthcare delivery is very common. Also, these types of contracts have played a major role in the healthcare reforms that have been carried out in a large number of developing countries outside sub-Saharan Africa, mainly in Asia and Latin America, and are often seen as a quick and simple solution to solve gaps in coverage [18]. Another benefit of contracting out donor-funded healthcare delivery to the private health sector would be that it might trigger investments in health, improving access to care. The contracting out of services could be formalized by PPPs, in which both the public and private sectors commit themselves to deliver their part of the services needed to execute a health programme. Under these arrangements, the conditions of contracting and the minimal quality requirements of the private health sector could also be leveraged. For instance, NGOs could become part of the PPP and provide quality control services.

The capacity of the healthcare delivery system might also be increased by PPPs between local businesses and the health sector. For instance, existing private company responses to HIV, such as workplace HIV treatment programmes, could be used as a catalyst for expanding treatment programmes beyond employees only. These programmes are often carried out in private health clinics, or in public health clinics that also serve a private or corporate clientele. In these clinics, significant knowledge regarding the treatment of HIV is available, and laboratory facilities are often in place. A PPP could formalize the transfer of knowledge from these clinics to other clinics that focus on the public sector. Also, arrangements could be made for the sharing of clinics and laboratory facilities, thereby reducing a major barrier to the provision of HIV treatment. An example of such collaboration between the public and private sector is seen in Rwanda (Box 45.11).

Other areas could also benefit from a stronger public–private interaction—for instance, the procurement and supply-chain management of antiretrovirals, human resource capacity building, information management and health research services [5]. These are all areas in which the private sector has proven experience, and partnerships may increase the efficiency of services.

Box 45.11 **Public and private sector collaboration in Rwanda**

In Rwanda, a local brewery, a subsidiary of Heineken, started a treatment programme for its employees in 2001. This successful programme has generated both knowledge and infrastructure to expand access to antiretroviral therapy. To increase access to antiretroviral treatment for the general public, the brewery is now outsourcing its antiretroviral treatment facilities in order to facilitate antiretroviral treatment through public and private services on a larger scale. This collaboration is funded by the Dutch government and coordinated by an international NGO.

Source: PharmAccess Foundation.

Innovative PPPs may increase local investment in healthcare

Innovative participation structures, such as donor-funded health insurance in which donors pay the extra premium associated with covering HIV expenses, could also increase the capacity of local health systems. In sub-Saharan Africa, most of the health insurance schemes focus on the part of the population that is formally employed. Consequently, an insurance arrangement in which donors would pay the premium of HIV coverage in an insurance scheme would initially focus on this group. These formal sector employees indeed have a limited form of income, but the impact of HIV on the household is still very high and treatment is often unaffordable to them. This population is largely overlooked by donor agencies but comprises an important part of a country's economy. To prevent such schemes from adding to poverty and inequality, these structures should be combined with schemes that target the poor. For instance, health insurance companies could be compensated for low-income and high-risk patients through an equalization fund [19]. These funds could be co-financed by the donor community and governments. In time, this principle might also be used to support smaller, community-based mutual health organizations (MHOs), thereby increasing access to care in rural, poor areas [20]. The experience with community health insurance schemes funded in part by public funds and run by local clinics in the context of primary healthcare and reproductive services has shown that community health insurance schemes can both be profitable and increase access to care [21–23]. Stimulation of these types of schemes may be a first step towards accessible, more efficient healthcare.

The limited role of local PPPs in sub-Saharan Africa

As we have argued in the previous sections, there is potential for local PPPs to facilitate the implementation of HIV programmes and increase the medical infrastructure. In some countries in sub-Saharan Africa—for instance, Tanzania, Zimbabwe, South Africa and Zambia—governments are already experimenting with some form of public–private arrangements [4]. However, these local partnerships, including contracting arrangements, have not been introduced in the majority of sub-Saharan African countries and are not the primary focus of the donor community. In our view, the lack of local partnerships might be caused by, among other things, the private health sector's limited eligibility for funding, a lack of trust and the lack of strict regulation of the private health sector.

The limited eligibility of the private sector for funding

Healthcare in Africa is predominantly organized through the state, although a large share of private spending is done in the private health sector [4,23]. Therefore, states tend to disburse the available donor funds through the quasi-public sector. As a consequence, private sector programmes are, in general, less likely to be accepted as primary recipients of funding, even if the majority of private health spending is done in the private sector [24]. The focus of institutional donors on the public sector as the primary recipient of funding might thus lead to an exclusion of the private sector, especially since the public sector generally redirects only a very small portion of the donor funding to the private health sector [24]. Increasing funding for the private health sector and stimulating the contracting out of health delivery services to the private sector could increase efficiency and trigger local investments, as well as reduce unfair competition between the public and private health sectors. For instance, employers will hesitate to invest in private or public–private HIV care facilities if the government provides, or claims to provide, this service for free. This reluctance to invest in HIV treatment for employees is seen in Nigeria and Ghana, where some large multinational companies are not paying for HIV treatment for their employees because this is supposedly covered by the government scheme. Unfair competition may also be induced by the controlling powers of local governments. For instance, governments often control drug importation and distribution, and in some countries private sector clinics have to pay more for medication than subsidized public sector clinics do, such as in Rwanda. The issue of unfair competition is one that needs to be acknowledged and addressed by donor organizations. Stimulating local PPPs in which risks and responsibilities of the programme are shared between the public and private sectors could reduce the effects of unfair competition.

The lack of regulation and quality of the existing private healthcare sector

A crucial element for the successful establishment of PPPs will be the level of trust between partners and the quality of services provided by the private health sector. An existing culture gap between the public and private sectors may reduce the chances of launching successful PPPs. For instance, the fear within the public sector that the private sector's only interest is in making a profit may create mistrust [25], especially since some of the mechanisms used to maximize profits may conflict with the goals of better health, such as reducing costs by reducing the size of the workforce [25–27]. Also, there is a lack of strict regulation of the quality of the private healthcare sector on a national level. For instance, in Tanzania and Mozambique, most existing regulations aim at securing entry and minimum quality and are not specifically adapted to discipline the private healthcare sector [4]. This lack of national regulation may contribute to some of the common problems associated with the private health sector, such as overcharging, lack of quality [28,29] and the unfair recruitment of public sector staff. An important task for the international community, including NGOs and governments, would be to pressure sub-Saharan African governments to adopt and enforce strict regulation of the private health sector. In this respect, partnerships between the public and private health sectors could be a first step towards more a uniform healthcare delivery system.

Discussion

In the last few years, a number of high-profile international PPPs have emerged in areas ranging from product development, such as the IAVI, to the implementation of treatment programmes for a wide variety of diseases. These initiatives show that important goals can be—and already have been—achieved if the public and private sectors join forces. In this chapter, we have highlighted the potential of local-level PPPs. Public–private arrangements where the private health sector augments the public system are used in nearly all health systems in developed countries and have been introduced with success in many developing and middle-income countries in Asia and Latin America [1]. Still, these arrangements are seldom used in sub-Saharan African countries and are not currently the focus of the donor community.

In our opinion, PPPs present good opportunities for the scaling-up of treatment and prevention programmes; they may enable the use of all capacity and are likely to trigger private investments in healthcare. Enabling investment in healthcare in sub-Saharan Africa is of utmost importance, since it was recently estimated that around US$72 billion per year, or roughly eight times the amount of all current foreign aid for this region, would be needed to upgrade sub-Saharan public health systems to the level of South Africa's [24]. These figures not only indicate that enormous amounts of funding are required for adequate HIV treatment and care, but also clearly underscore the need for innovative approaches. Given the potential impact of PPPs on the provision of HIV treatment, it should be ensured that PPPs become a necessary ingredient for the expansion of HIV treatment programmes in developing countries.

Acknowledgements

The authors wish to thank Rich Feeley for commenting on draft versions of this chapter.

References

1. Jamali D. (2004). Success and failure mechanisms of public private partnerships (PPPs) in developing countries: insights from the Lebanese context. *International Journal of Public Sector Management* 17:414–30.
2. Reich M. (2000). Public–private partnerships for public health. *Nature Medicine* 6:617–620.
3. The World Bank. (1993). *World Development Report 1993: Investing in Health.* Washington, DC: The World Bank.
4. Kumaranayake L, Lake S, Mujinja P, Hongoro C, Mpembeni R. (2000). How do countries regulate the health sector? Evidence from Tanzania and Zimbabwe. *Health Policy Planning* 15:357–67.
5. Widdus R. (2001). Public–private partnerships for health: their main targets, their diversity and their future directions. *Bulletin of the World Health Organization* 79:213–30.
6. Locher C, Mehlau JI, Wild O. (2004). *Towards Risk Adjusted Controlling of Strategic IS Projects in Banks in Light of the Basel II.* Proceedings of the 37th Hawaii International Conference on System Sciences, p1–6.
7. Pongsiri N. (2002). Regulation and public–private partnerships. *International Journal of Public Sector Management* 15:487–95.
8. Scharle P. (2002). Public–private partnerships as a social game. *Innovation* 15:227–52.
9. Reich M, ed. (2002). *Public–Private Partnerships for Public Health.* Cambridge, MA: Harvard University Press. Available online at http://www.hsph.harvard.edu/hcpds/partnerbook/.
10. *The Clinton HIV/AIDS Initiative.* Press release June 4, 2004. Available at: http://www.clintonpresidentialcenter.org/aids-initiative5.htm.

11. Center for Strategic and International Studies. (2004). *Botswana's Strategy to Combat HIV/AIDS. Lessons for Africa and President Bush's Emergency Plan for AIDS Relief.* Washington, DC: Center for Strategic and International Studies. Available at: http://csis.org/africa/0401_BotswanaHIV.pdf.

12. Brugha R, Walt G. (2001). A global health fund: a leap of faith. *British Medical Journal* 323:152–3.

13. The Global Fund to Fight AIDS, Tuberculosis and Malaria. A Force for Change: The Global Fund at 30 months. http://www.theglobalfund.org/en/about/publications/forceforchange/ (Accessed: February 5, 2005).

14. World Health Organization. (2004). *'3 by 5' Progress Report.* Geneva: WHO and UNAIDS.

15. Caines K, Lush L. (2004). Impact of Public–Private Partnerships Addressing Access to Pharmaceuticals in Selected and Low and Middle Income Countries: A Synthesis Report from Studies in Botswana, Sri Lanka, Uganda and Zambia. http://www.ippph.org/index.cfm?page=/ippph/publications&thechoice=retrieve&docno=101 (Accessed February 3, 2005).

16. Buve A, Kalibala S, McIntyre J. (2003). Stronger health systems for more effective HIV/AIDS prevention and care. *International Journal of Health Planning and Management* 18:S41–51.

17. McPake B, Hongor C. (1995). Contracting out of clinical services in Zimbabwe. *Social Science Medicine* 41:13–24.

18. Palmer N. (2000). The use of private-sector contracts for primary health care: theory, evidence and lessons for low-income and middle-income countries. *Bulletin of the World Health Organization* 78:821–9.

19. Söderland N, Khosa S. (1997). The potential of risk equalisation mechanisms in health insurance: the case of South Africa. *Health Policy and Planning* 12:341–53.

20. Dror DM, Preker AS.(2002). *Social Reinsurance, a New Approach to Sustainable Community Health Financing.* Washington, DC: World Bank and ILO.

21. Walraven GEL. (1995). Health insurance in rural Africa. *Lancet* 345:520.

22. Feeley R. (2000). The Role for Insurance Mechanisms in Improving Access to Private Sector Primary and Reproductive Health Care. Commercial Market Strategies Project. Available at: www.cmsproject.com. (Accessed: September, 10, 2004).

23. Criel B. (1999). The Bwamanda hospital scheme: effective for whom? A study of its impact on hospital utilisation patterns. *Social Science Medicine* 48:897–911.

24. England R. (2004). The private sector is vital. *Lancet* 364:1033–4.

25. Buse K. (2004). Governing public–private infectious disease partnerships. *The Brown Journal of World Affairs* 10:225–41.

26. Buse K, Walt G. (2000). Global public–private partnerships: part 2—what are the health issues for global governance? *Bulletin of the World Health Organization* 78:699–709.

27. Hancock T. (1998). Caveat partner: reflections on partnership with the private sector. *Health Promotion International* 13:193.

28. Brugha R. (2003). Antiretroviral treatment in developing countries: the peril of neglecting private providers. *British Medical Journal* 326:1382–4.

29. Mills A, Brugha R, Hanson K, McPake B. (2002). What can be done about the private health sector in low-income countries? *Bulletin of the World Health Organization* 80:325–30.

Chapter 46

Developing human resources for the HIV pandemic

Norbert Dreesch, Mario R Dal Poz*, Gulin Gedik, Orvill Adams and Timothy Evans

Challenges for health systems and delivery models

At the beginning of the twenty-first century, health systems in both highly industrialized and developing countries are increasingly pluralistic, with diversified public, private, non-governmental organization (NGO), community and home provision of care leading to greater complexity of health service organization. At the same time, political stewardship is often weak and challenged by strong interest groups.

Little progress has been made to reduce inequities in access to care. Financing of health services poses problems due to changes in the burden of disease and population characteristics. In the highly industrialized countries, aging and retirement of the 'baby-boom' generation leave an insufficient number of younger people available to work in the health and social service sectors. In turn, this pressure for services in high-income countries increases the demand for health personnel from the developing world, where in some countries an epidemiological transition is under way, bringing with it increased demand for services and human resources due to chronic diseases and the need for communicable disease control. Diseases such as HIV exert pressure on already overstretched human resources in developing countries.

Reducing poverty and improving equity of access to health services are among the declared Millennium Development Goals (MDGs). However, the increasingly pluralist nature of health systems in developing countries presents real challenges and problems for policy and service delivery coordination. The national health-stewardship capacity is often too weak to steer service delivery properly. Insufficient health budgets add to the complexities.

With the additional demands generated by the HIV epidemic, many governments in resource-poor settings can respond only by allowing increasing numbers of well-intentioned NGOs and other providers to assume essential service provision functions. This further complicates proper national coordination of all stakeholders involved. Strong incentives from various international donors to seek innovative, public or private, for-profit and not-for-profit solutions have emerged to find solutions to these perceived deficiencies and ensure equity of access to care for all members of society, regardless of ability to pay.

Globalization and international finance and credit agency priorities towards containment of public sector expenditures in low-income countries have had an impact on health policy options over the past decade. The adoption of macroeconomic policies under structural

* Corresponding author.

adjustment programmes has usually called for strict fiscal stringency and led to widespread capping of public sector spending.

In countries with high levels of public sector health coverage, and with human resources often consuming over 60% of health budgets, the consequences have been dire. These have included widespread reductions in facility and equipment maintenance, the impossibility of increasing staffing levels in response to population growth and diseases such as HIV, and high levels of dependency on national and international NGOs and bilateral support to provide health services.

Fiscal stringency can also pose problems in the absorption of available human resources. Anecdotally, it is reported that there are 3000 trained nurses in one African country who are not currently employed in the health sector, primarily because expenditure and establishment ceilings mean that the public sector does not, in effect, have a demand for their services, although they are certainly needed based on technical criteria (M Wheeler, personal communication, 2003). Private sector employment possibilities are presumably limited by the stagnation of personal incomes, in line with the overall stagnation of the economy witnessed in many parts of Africa.

Given the slow erosion of organizational and administrative capacity in many developing countries over the past decades, even if funds are made available, effective expenditure limits are defined by the absorptive constraints of the health system. In countries where the greatest challenges for scaling up antiretroviral therapy (ART) are encountered, health systems face two major challenges: the malfunction of the service system and the HIV epidemic. The former is a long-term development problem, while the HIV epidemic undermines system development efforts. Thus, although the problems are closely related, they demand solutions that should be undertaken simultaneously: a gradual strengthening of the service system in conjunction with urgent and effective action to control the epidemic. It should be noted that the heavier the burden of AIDS, the more the health system will be weakened and the fewer the resources that will be available to treat other major diseases, resulting in weakened capacity of health systems to reduce overall morbidity and mortality.

Human resources issues related to the HIV pandemic are intimately related to general trends in population and health workforce development. Some of the known issues and shortcomings can be summed up as follows:

♦ years of neglecting to plan for human resources in light of aging populations and the increased volume of long-term care needs in the industrial world [1];

♦ recruitment of care personnel from the developing world as a rapid and highly cost-effective solution to human resources shortages in industrialized countries, leading to a net outflow of human resources from poor countries with continuing high levels of population growth and associated care and prevention needs, including for HIV;

♦ massive impact of HIV on an already overburdened health workforce;

♦ low morale caused by poor working conditions; lack of incentives to stay in the health workforce;

♦ years of seeing ever-swelling numbers of people living with HIV (PLHIV) filling up more and more hospital beds without any sign of a cure.

New initiatives such as the Global Fund to Fight AIDS, Tuberculosis and Malaria and the US President's Emergency Plan for AIDS Relief (PEPFAR) have mobilized substantial new re-sources. The World health Organization (WHO)/UNAIDS multi-partner initiative to provide

3 million people living with HIV with access to ART by 2005—the '3 by 5' initiative—has recently added additional impetus [2]. Many high-burden countries are now funded to implement ambitious new interventions in HIV prevention and care. Unfortunately, those countries are also the ones whose trained human resources have been most heavily hit by HIV. It is increasingly clear that new programmes can be implemented only with new capacity in both infrastructure and human resources.

Until recently, very little work had been done to consider what staff time and skill levels were needed, now and in the future. Without this information and steps to fill the estimated human resource gaps, the target of putting 3 million people on ART by the end of 2005, for example, would be difficult to achieve. Site visits conducted by WHO and a survey undertaken by the MDG Task Force on HIV of the United Nations Secretary-General in 2003 have shed light on the distribution of tasks between care providers in the ART cycle, members of the community and volunteers from among PLHIV [3].

One possible short-term initiative discussed in some circles is the targeted provision of ART to core groups such as teachers and health workers. This is now an accepted part of the '3 by 5' strategy, and the advantages, disadvantages and ethical dilemmas of this approach have been resolved so that immediate treatment action can start on a highly targeted basis. However, more evidence still needs to be obtained in order to develop feasible planning strategies to halt HIV's inroads into the development process of entire nations. For the health sector, scenario modelling on the basis of the data cited below may help countries to address their educational intake and training needs better than they can at present.

Labour market impact

At the level of both preventive and curative services, women tend to constitute the largest component of the health workforce from primary to tertiary care in many countries. It is therefore important for health and human resource planning to know about the spread of HIV among adult women. UNAIDS figures indicate the spread among adult women shown in Table 46.1 [4].

WHO/UNAIDS figures show that in seven of these 10 regions, heterosexual transmission is one of the main routes for spreading the disease. In terms of labour market needs and supply, infection rates among people in the prime of life are worrying in many countries: '...in 1999,

Table 46.1 Percentage of HIV-positive adult women, end 2001

Sub-Saharan Africa	55%
North Africa and Middle East	40%
South and South-East Asia	35%
East Asia and Pacific	20%
Latin America	30%
Caribbean	50%
Eastern Europe and Central Asia	20%
Western Europe	25%
North America	20%
Australia and New Zealand	10%

Source: UNAIDS 2001 [4].

80 per cent of newly infected people in Rwanda, the United Republic of Tanzania, Uganda and Zambia were aged between 20 and 49 years' [5].

On the simple assumption that these infection rates could be reflected in the health professions, the need for adjustments to workforce planning is evident, as labour in the health sector is likely to be affected disproportionately because of the high number of women in the sector. Productivity losses in this most crucial service sector will be felt widely if patients have to spend more time off work queuing up to receive medication due to lack of staff. In high-burden HIV countries, this could affect productivity and economic development.

In terms of assessing the impact of HIV on the health sector workforce, it is possible to identify the likely effect on the stock of current workers (Tables 46.2 and 46.3). It is apparent that the impact on all sources of inflow and outflow, with the exception of normal retirement, is likely to contribute to an increased outflow and decreased inflow, with a net decline in the

Table 46.2 Likely impact of HIV on inflows to the formal health sector workforce

Type of possible inflow from stock	Likely trend if increasing impact of HIV	Reasons
New entrants from in-country training	DOWN	Choose less stressful alternative jobs/careers
Returnees from other employment/non-employment	DOWN	Stay in less stressful alternative jobs/careers/ situations
International recruits	DOWN	Stay in less stressful alternative jobs/careers/situations

Source: J. Buchan, personal communication.

overall numbers. As data become available from specific countries, it will be possible to quantify the overall effect and the likely impact of each component over time.

The decline in the formal health workforce will lead to more demand for care from the informal sector and family members. The informal sector will also be affected directly and indirectly by HIV and will have to face an increasing burden.

Table 46.3 Likely impact of HIV on outflow from the formal health sector workforce

Type of possible outflow from stock	Likely trend if increasing impact of HIV	Reasons
Normal retirement	DOWN	Fewer workers live to normal retirement age
Move to non-health employment	UP	Indirect impact: more workers leave for 'safer' employment/less stressful employment
Move to non-employment	UP	Indirect impact: more workers leave because of 'fear' of HIV
Long-term illness	UP	Direct impact of HIV
Death	UP	Direct impact of HIV

Source: J. Buchan, personal communication.

Impact of HIV on staff availability and workload in healthcare

The impact of HIV on the delivery of health services has reached alarming levels in many high-prevalence countries, particularly in sub-Saharan Africa. A vicious cycle has been emerging since the early 1990s: it appears that morbidity and mortality among service staff affected by HIV have reduced staff numbers to below critical levels in some countries most affected, although precise data on the size of the problem are lacking.

Insufficient replacement staff and losses in whole age groups of professionals such as nurses, doctors, pharmacists and teachers, combined with increasing demand for care, are likely to have a serious impact on societal development in the countries most affected by HIV. The lack of teaching personnel will reduce the capacity to train replacement staff.

The Food and Agriculture Organization of the United Nations (FAO) estimates that some countries have already lost more than 20% of their agricultural workers [6], and similar losses could be incurred based on infection rates quoted for nurses [7]. Figures quoted by the World Bank when it launched its Education For All initiative painted an alarming picture for HIV infection rates, with South Africa at 12%, Zambia 20%, and parts of Malawi and Uganda at over 30% of the population. Table 46.4 illustrates mortality among teachers in selected countries [8].

However, a recent study in Botswana, Malawi, Namibia, South Africa, Uganda, Zambia and Zimbabwe—some of the countries most affected by HIV—indicates that teacher mortality is well below the population average. In addition, HIV-related mortality may have peaked around the mid- to late 1990s and is apparently in decline in some of the most affected countries, possibly due to behaviour change and the increased availability of antiretroviral drugs [10].

At the same time, some studies indicate that hospital bed occupancy rates have reached 190% since the epidemic started to unfold, for example at Kenyatta Hospital in Nairobi [11–13]. Increased need for testing and follow-up of possibly HIV-infected patients has also been noted as an additional burden on already overstretched staff, thus increasing the overall workload requirements [14].

Increases in HIV-related illnesses such as tuberculosis (TB) add to the staff workload in the countries most affected. About one-third of TB, for example, is estimated to be associated with HIV, adding to the general increase in TB worldwide [15]. In some high-burden countries, an unprecedented increase in reported cases was observed between 1985 and 2002. Table 46.5

Table 46.4 HIV and teacher mortality

Country	Teacher deaths	Comment/other information
Central African Republic	85% attributed to HIV during 1996 and 1998	On average, dying 10 years before retirement age
Zambia	1996: 680	
	1998: 1300	First 10 months of 1998
Kenya	1995: 450	
	1999: 1500	1999: 20–30 teacher deaths from AIDS monthly in one province

Source: World Bank 2002 [9].

Table 46.5 Percentage increase in TB notification between 1985 and 2002

Country	% increase in absolute number, 1985–2002
Botswana	277
Central African Republic	830
Kenya	667
Egypt	755
Indonesia	778
Belize	332
Papua New Guinea	54
Kyrgyzstan	216

Source: WHO 2004 [15].

indicates the order of magnitude of the increased diagnostic and treatment needs in a number of countries that have had substantially increased numbers of notified TB cases.

It is not known whether country workforce plans took these increases in the burden of disease into account when establishing workload staffing norms for facilities. In this context, it is also important to note the prolonged periods of staff sick leave due to HIV infection. Yet labour legislation in many countries prevents replacement of these staff members until they die. Thus, services that already lose staff due to migration to other countries or attrition due to low staff morale are also faced with the inability to replace staff for long periods of time. In addition, the time for training existing staff for HIV prevention and care will increase workload requirements. Furthermore, insufficient planning for human resources for health in the past has meant that countries have insufficient replacements for cohorts of staff reaching retirement age.

Concern in the area of occupational health has also been expressed. Perceived and real increased risks associated with HIV patient care need to be explored as recruitment and retention factors. The Global Burden of Disease analysis shows that 40% of both hepatitis B and hepatitis C in healthcare workers is due to needlestick injuries, with HIV infection estimated at 5% [16]. Some studies have attempted to measure the HIV infection risks for several occupational groups, but no systematic review has been undertaken to assess the impact on workforce losses and the consequent adjustments to planning targets [17].

In some countries, initiatives have been taken to increase student intake by 20% per annum in order to offset anticipated losses due to disease impact and migration (Leana R Uys, personal communication, 2003). Whether or not this will lead to correct replacement numbers is not clear, in view of the small body of knowledge currently available. This indicates great concern over the need to plan for replacements and additional staff. It does, however, happen in the context of a larger crisis in education and training of the health workforce which is characterized by:

- lack of planning and overlapping training activities between programmes, and poor evaluation of outcomes;
- scarcity of educational institutions, faculty and educational materials.

This situation calls for capacity building in many developing countries and strengthening the stewardship function of the state and its health and educational institutions. Furthermore, there is need for improvements in standards, regulation and accreditation. At the same time, educational innovations have to be pursued. This should include modification of teacher skills, knowledge, competencies and attitudes through an educational process. Similarly, the development of team capacities and team work, and not only individual approaches, needs to be fostered.

Impact of HIV on service delivery

The HIV epidemic increased the burden on existing facilities, particularly in the developing world. Wide variations in the quality of inpatient and outpatient service use have been observed in different European countries. These differences ranged from 4.3 days per patient-year for patients in the chronic stage of HIV in Greece to 159.8 days for patients in the late stage of the disease in Spain. A longitudinal study in five hospitals in different African countries showed that the proportion of beds occupied by HIV-positive patients varied between 50% and 70% [12]. In Tanzania, AIDS patients spent, on average, 18 days in hospital against 6 days for all other patients. Two district hospitals were forced to increase bed capacity by constructing new wards to accommodate increasing numbers of AIDS-related admissions. The hospitals were forced to create HIV counselling units that used the available nursing staff, again increasing the workload [13].

Increased admissions, prolonged stay for AIDS patients, increased expenditure on drugs for treatment of opportunistic infections, purchase of HIV reagents, treatment of sick staff and expenses related to the funerals of health workers all increase the burden on already stretched health budgets. A case study of the possible impact of HIV in Kenya estimated an increase of about 46% in costs for the same quality of healthcare due to the increased number of patients and other expenses such as diagnostic and treatment requirements [18]. A study in Uganda showed that HIV has more than doubled the health sector's recurrent expenditures since the epidemic started [19].

Hospital staff in high-burden HIV countries are overwhelmed by increases in workload. As well as the increased demand, staff have had to accommodate further shortages through illness or death of other staff members and absences in order to attend funerals, care for sick relatives and attend training seminars and workshops. The increasing number of tests performed to diagnose HIV or screen blood for transfusion threatens to overwhelm laboratory staff.

At the same time, patients who are infected and have severe symptoms claim to be neglected at hospitals and not given the best services. Health workers, for their part, complain that the lack of protective clothing and equipment is a major hindrance to providing the appropriate services in many cases. Given the effects of HIV they have both experienced and witnessed, they are understandably reluctant to put their families, themselves and their non-HIV-infected patients at risk.

A study conducted by the US Centers for Disease Control (CDC) reported that, of the 23,951 AIDS cases reported up to December 31, 2001, a total of 57 cases (0.2%) were documented as occupationally acquired HIV among people with a history of having worked in healthcare, and a further 138 (0.6%) were classified as possibly acquired occupationally [20]. Despite the objective evidence that occupational risk is low for health workers if they have ready access to protective gear and to training about prevention of infection, these basic means of prevention tend to be absent in the most affected countries.

There is urgent need to make protective clothing and equipment more widely available. More studies are needed on infection risk and personnel behaviour under circumstances in which essential equipment is absent.

Service delivery and HIV continuum of care

To manage the challenge of HIV better, countries need to strengthen various aspects of their health systems. Specific investments in strengthening health systems may improve the capacity of the system to plan and deliver services. Reforms at the sector level may strengthen incentives for efficiency; these include, for example, introduction of contractual relationships, decentralization of decision making, increased autonomy for health providers and integration of services.

Investment in systems can also help the sector absorb additional resources. System-wide changes are required, and managers and health professionals need more autonomy and performance incentives to improve outcomes. The need to reform the health sector is therefore widely accepted, and it has figured on the policy agenda of most countries for a long time.

Decentralization

Decentralization is frequently an essential part of health reform. The process of decentralization can include devolution of decision-making power over parts of the national health budget to regional and district levels of health administration, and transferring authority to local government to make decisions on service organization and staffing patterns of primary and other healthcare facilities. Although decentralization may not lead to short-term improvements in output with the present resource levels, it is often seen as a prerequisite for a future system when more resources are available [21]. Decentralizing services and strengthening local decision-making power are important elements of the system in scaling up ART to attain '3 by 5' targets, since the autonomy given to local decision makers creates space for innovation, community participation and adaptation of public services to local circumstances, all of which are assumed to be conducive to successful implementation [22].

However, evidence of the potential impact of decentralization on the implementation of vertical programmes, as against a whole service delivery system, is mixed. Some studies show that in low-income countries, decentralization is associated with higher rates of immunization coverage [22,23], while in others, the expected benefits of decentralization have not been achieved and the delivery of some vertical programmes worsened after decentralization. In Zambia, for example, a decline in immunization rates, which started before decentralization, did not reverse after increased funds were made available accompanied by decentralization [24]. In two pilot districts in Uganda, districts still lacked the capacity to increase allocation of funds to maternal and child health (MCH) services after decentralization. Moreover, user-fees, though entirely decided upon by districts, reduced the use of MCH services [25].

In delivering ART, similar problems may appear. For example, in South Africa, it has been shown that rigid bureaucracies inherited from the apartheid government may have hampered the implementation of many HIV policies developed at the end of the apartheid era. More recently, however, the decentralized health system allowed some doctors at provincial level to administer antiretroviral drugs at a time when national policy was against it [26]. In late 2003, a policy of broadening access to ART on a national scale was introduced, but its impact on service delivery remains to be seen.

Integration

Integration of components of health programmes at various system levels is another common reform policy that has implications for ART. Integration can be seen as offering ART within a routine primary care context with no specific clinic sessions or facilities designated to serve ART. By not singling out specific service and clinic hours, this kind of integration could reduce stigma and fear. Integration can also be seen in this context as combining hitherto separate clinical sessions, such as for TB and HIV, with the intention of reducing the number of clinical visits.

There has been ongoing discussion on the merits of providing priority interventions vertically or in an integrated way that is potentially relevant to HIV programmes. Some systematic reviews of integration of vertical programmes concluded that there is no strong evidence of outcome differences between vertically provided programmes and integrated ones. However, it would appear that integration has the important advantage of producing a less costly form of service delivery [27]. When it comes to the overall health system, lack of integration has been implicated as the cause of problems such as patients getting lost, delays or failure to provide needed services, and less than optimal outcomes [28,29]. However, it has also been argued that some vertical elements are needed *within* an integrated, universal system [30].

In resource-poor settings, some argue that there is a risk, with a highly integrated system, that resources will be spread so thinly across different services and horizontal functions such as supervision, logistics and training, that activities will fail to reach the minimum quantity and quality to have any impact on health. This risk is greater in a decentralized, integrated system, if it is not drastically reduced in size, than in systems comprising different disease-specific programmes that could allow one programme to fail without a serious effect on others. Below a certain resource level, the service outputs of integrated systems are therefore likely to be lower than systems based on vertical health programmes [21], since vertical programmes prevent resources from 'leaking' into less important areas. Ultimately, the challenge is to strike the right balance between the benefits and shortcomings of either approach for designing patient-oriented—and at the same time, highly cost-effective—ART programmes.

Continuity of care

Programme and human resources planning must take into account the nature of HIV as a chronic disease, giving rise to the need for a wide range of preventive and lifelong care services. It would appear important to organize ART services that are integrated into existing health facilities, thereby allowing the use of facilities at all levels and ensuring continuity of care.

Different stakeholders

Another challenge for the health system will be the integration of different stakeholders, such as the private sector, NGOs and communities, into the system. Contracting out some health services in low- and middle-income countries to private sector providers is sometimes suggested as a mechanism to increase coverage and efficiency. However, the need then arises for development of mechanisms for contracting and for strengthening the regulatory framework, both of which have proved problematic.

The increased attention to ART may also challenge health systems with increased and disproportionate flows of funds. On the one hand, the absorption capacity of the system could be challenged with the rapid increase of funds, but the rest of the services might deteriorate while special attention is paid to ART. On the other hand, the '3 by 5' initiative could be seized upon as an opportunity to develop the whole health system better.

Human resource requirements for HIV ART continuum of care

A disease as devastating as HIV has added a different dimension to planning for human resources in the health sector. As a result of its spread among the healthcare workforce, there is a crisis stemming from years of inadequate investment in health services infrastructure and human resources development. This calls for:

- a multi-skilled workforce equipped with socio-medical intervention knowledge;
- different types of staff to respond to HIV prevention and care tasks;
- a new role for community members, including PLHIV, in chronic care for ART;
- national, regional and district level management of integrated interventions for HIV, TB, malaria, etc.;
- incentive systems to retain the health workforce;
- innovative public/private service delivery models to reach ART coverage goals;
- new models of care leading to the need to adjust distribution of staff across systems levels;
- changes in health labour legislation to accommodate changes in roles and functions.

Different approaches to human resources deployment in ART delivery

Case studies from different countries highlight the workforce implications of specific ways of organizing HIV healthcare delivery. Various approaches have been developed to deliver ART to people with HIV, ranging from national strategies on ART delivery using public sector facilities, to community-based approaches and involvement of the private sector and national or internationally supported NGOs, research sites, mission institutions and innovative company-based employee and family member care schemes.

For example, various national sections of Médecins Sans Frontières (MSF) support well-developed pilot projects providing ART in developing countries. In April 2000, MSF South Africa set up three HIV clinics within township health centres in Khayelitsha, Cape Town. In 2001, they began to offer ART to people with advanced HIV.

The clinics are located within community health centres and provide a package of comprehensive HIV services that include counselling, support, prophylaxis, treatment of opportunistic infections, ART and referrals. The staff initially consisted of one physician, one nurse and one lay counsellor. An additional nurse and lay counsellor have since joined the teams.

This service model puts the nurse workforce at centre stage of ART care and is thought to be appropriate to the realities of the healthcare setting in South Africa. After 2 years of experience, the programme has shown that ART can be provided in primary healthcare settings in resource-limited countries. The success of the clinics suggests that an important component of successful ART programmes includes community participation [31].

Haiti's *Clinique Bon Sauveur*, established in 1998 by Partners in Health and the Haitian organization Zanmi Lasanté, is a model of what NGOs and international cooperation can accomplish. The clinic provides a basic minimum package for HIV that includes highly active antiretroviral treatment (HAART) using directly observed therapy (DOT) through community health workers, monthly support meetings for patients, social support to families, milk substitutes and ART for prevention of mother-to-child transmission

(PMTCT) of HIV, and post-exposure prophylaxis for professional accidents and people who have been raped. The clinic uses basic laboratory analysis and clinical criteria rather than CD4 counts or viral load testing for the initiation of ART. By 2002, more than 4000 HIV-positive people had been monitored at the Clinique Bon Sauveur, and over 400 people living with HIV had started DOT with ART, based on laboratory and clinical criteria [32].

Government initiatives in providing ART are not well documented in the literature, with the exception of Brazil's National AIDS Control Programme. In several sub-Saharan African countries, progress is being made at the government level. In Uganda, 35,000 people were estimated to be receiving ART in September 2004. A system for increasing ART nationwide is being developed and includes a plan of action developed with all partners, using community members, mechanisms for training and guidelines for treatment and care [33].

Kenya is another country that has drawn up legislation related to ART and has imported antiretrovirals, and in September of 2004 was estimated to have 17,000 patients on ART. Thirty start-up centres have been identified, and plans are under way to equip them with appropriate staff. Training materials are in place, and there is a plan to train additional staff.

During the same period, Botswana's national antiretroviral programme had more than 30,000 patients on ART in 23 public sites and private practices. In Benin, an initiative to access antiretrovirals has been in place since early 2002. Since then, 50 patients have started ART.

Existing national programmes highlight the management needs in establishing ART programmes: sufficient numbers of well-trained doctors, nurses and other healthcare workers are urgently needed, and clinical and laboratory facilities are required, along with distribution systems and social support services.

Brazil has provided a success story through its implementation of an effective prevention programme and ensuring universal access to ART. The Ministry of Health invested in infrastructure improvements to have laboratories ready to test throughout the country, with allocations for laboratory staff training, equipment purchase and the provision of reagents. The Ministry of Health also established procedures for the accreditation of public hospitals and expanded the hospital network for the care of HIV-infected patients. With the creation of the Alternative Assistance Programme, professionals were trained in HIV care, and funds were transferred to state and municipal governments to assist patients with different levels of need. Multidisciplinary teams that served the needs of both patients and their families typically provided these services. In the period between 1996 and 2001, the average admissions per patient per year dropped from 1.7 to 0.3, with 358,000 hospitalizations prevented, which resulted in savings of more than US$1 billion. All ART medications registered in Brazil became increasingly accessible. ART medication costs were reduced as a result of Ministry of Health investment in Brazilian-owned drug manufacturers that today supply 50% of all ART medication used in the country [34,35].

An analysis of 41 sites in 10 countries [36] found that ART has been provided in a multitude of settings: government facilities, with or without NGO support, employer-based schemes, university-affiliated research sites, and private practice. Almost all the sites visited were, in one way or another, part of the existing government or medical school infrastructure—for example, for determination of CD4 cell counts, training or other elements of the care process.

ART was found to be delivered in both dedicated and integrated HIV prevention and care clinics. At some sites, the facility manager had decided to combine the TB and HIV/ART clinics to establish a logical care flow. In many countries, NGOs expanded their sites in order to contribute to wider access throughout all provinces or districts. For example, MSF Belgium and France were already expanding their ART programmes at sites in Rwanda and Cambodia after only 1 month of operation (N Dreesch, unpublished report; S Essengue, unpublished report). Most of these programmes were found to be cooperating with government, district or national level facilities and establishing dedicated clinics on hospital premises. In Thailand and Cambodia, expanding access to ART was an extension of ongoing HIV prevention programmes that had been initiated when the dimension of the problem became apparent during the late 1980s and early 1990s.

Workplace initiatives constitute another approach to ART delivery. They may cover employees and their nuclear families for life, even after the employee leaves the company. In the context of scale-up of ART, these initiatives constitute a responsible response by major societal stakeholders—companies that generate wealth and income and have a natural interest in maintaining the best levels of health among their workforce.

Roles and functions facing staff in HIV control and treatment

Scaling up access to ART poses a considerable challenge to existing service delivery systems and human resources deployment. The staff currently engaged in the whole range of services offered in public, NGO and private facilities needs to be trained and reoriented towards delivery of antiretroviral care.

The services needed for the control and treatment of HIV range from prevention and care services, including voluntary counselling and testing (VCT), PMTCT, diagnosis and treatment of opportunistic infections and other HIV-related illnesses, to other support services. These services are intrinsically related to monitoring activities, drug distribution, psychological support, adherence and safe-sex behavioural counselling and nutrition education, even for patients without complications. All these tasks demand service provider time and, with more patients taken on, existing staff will be inadequate if the conventional model of service delivery is used.

In various countries, existing HIV prevention and infectious disease services have been expanded or remodelled to accommodate additional service needs. In Thailand, the existing system of 'anonymous' outpatient department clinics was adjusted to start treating patients. In order to reduce the additional time demands on staff, a system of 'patients' clubs'—groups of PLHIV—was used to bring patients on ART into the care process. Through this volunteer system, PLHIV are part of the clinic treatment staff, providing pre-counselling, peer group advice and monitoring of adherence, home visits with the ability to refer patients back for follow-up, and other psychosocial support. This patient-community support reduces the time pressures on clinical staff, since a large share of the monitoring tasks is transferred to the volunteers (N Dreesch, unpublished report, 2003).

In Rwanda, most ART initiatives include the community, volunteers, associations of PLHIV and their families in the process of treatment and patient follow-up, under the supervision of nurses and social workers. This is similar to the model observed in Thailand, where government policy actively supports the role of PLHIV in the care process, as volunteers working side-by-side with nurses for clerical, pre-counselling and follow-up and in-home visit tasks. At other sites, only a very limited role was foreseen for the group of PLHIV within the facilities themselves (S Essengue, unpublished report, 2003).

Figure 46.1 illustrates the wide range of staff, including PLHIV, involved in drug adherence counselling and, where this was undertaken in Thailand and Cambodia, the range of healthcare settings.

This illustrates the struggle that country health services face in trying to identify the most rational and time-efficient way to provide these essential services. It also shows the multitude of entry points to a single service and further underlines the need to continuously evaluate the service functions assigned to particular members of the care team in order to improve efficiency. For example, at Site 1, adherence counselling could move to a larger pool of adherence counselling providers once a sufficient number of PLHIV became stable on treatment and could join the ranks of service providers as volunteers. This would relieve both the current Site 1 physician and social worker from this task during the emergency scale-up operation. One could argue that this may save healthcare costs while passing them on to PLHIV, who would thus be prevented from pursuing other, possibly income-generating activities. However, the PLHIV participating in the care process could be given a subsidy for their services.

Capacity building for HIV care

Training needs

Increasing access to services implies the transfer of knowledge to existing service providers in all sectors and those currently training to work in healthcare. Figure 46.2 illustrates the various components that address the training needs that must be attended to for scale up strategies to be effective.

The process of identifying staff training needs for scale-up includes:

• addressing ART policy, rules, regulations and professional associations' views and policies;

• review of public or private delivery of services;

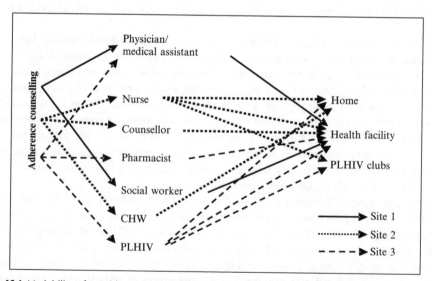

Fig. 46.1 Variability of providers and settings for the delivery of adherence and counselling tasks at three sites. Source: WHO/HRH, 2004.

- review of policy and legal documents governing human resources and training, and regulations governing skills application;
- the model of ART care;
- staff composition (doctors, nurses, laboratory technicians, lay counsellors, pharmacists and others);
- an inventory of total health system personnel and its distribution by category (physicians, nurses and others);
- gender distribution and age composition of the workforce;
- certification rules and licences to practise.

The stocktaking exercise should further include:

- the review of data on unemployed health personnel;
- distribution of staff by sector—public, private or NGO;
- distribution of personnel by programmes [TB, integrated management of childhood illness (IMCI) and others];

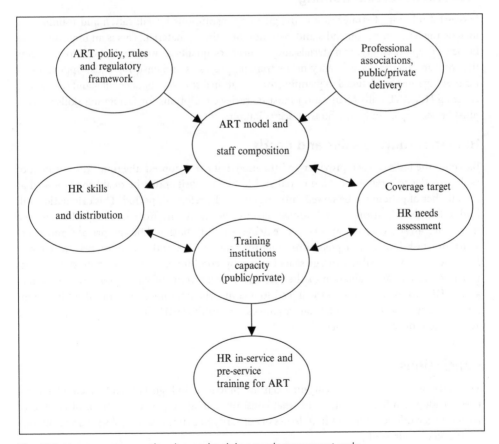

Fig. 46.2 Human resources planning and training needs assessment cycle.

- urban and rural distribution of staff by type of facility;
- volunteer network analysis and scale-up possibilities for ART;
- strategies to re-engage health workers or arrangements with the private for-profit sector for contracting in or out.

Review of education and training capacity and development of training options

Training capacity must be sufficient to respond to potentially large knowledge-transfer needs. Pre- and in-service training capacity must be reviewed, demand and adequacy of current human resource development plans must be forecast, and access to lecturers and tutors and training capacity at national and other system levels will need to be identified. Further important information would be added by evaluating the capacity and quality of teaching institutions, such as through their accreditation, and assessing options for developing modern distance-learning systems, including telemedicine.

Pre- and in-service training

Successful roll-out of strategies for strengthening institutions for education and training will include the harmonization and standardization of training material. This is an important task in view of rapidly emerging materials and the need for quality assurance. Options for reducing the costs and increasing efficiency in the training processes and ensuring equal opportunities for training must be included in planning for educational scale-up. Finally, rules and regulations covering HIV ART skills certification must be reviewed. Options for facilitating skills transfer must be accompanied by methods of accreditation.

Human resources skills and needs

Based on the tasks of each provider and the model of care adopted, the time commitment of each provider to a patient during initial and follow-up visits must be established, as well as the number of patients to be served until the end of the reference period. This calculation will lead to the identification of total human resource needs. It will further be helpful to create a matrix of staff skills across various service delivery points, both public and private, and assess skills and task-integration possibilities across programmes and public or private sectors. Identification of possible synergies achievable by combining tasks and staff skills across programmes and an evaluation of the role and contributions of volunteers, lay counsellors and PLHIV to the ART process will lead to a comprehensive identification of both current staff capacity to scale up and human resources for health (HRH) bottlenecks hampering the achievement of coverage targets.

Conclusions

The health workforce of the twenty-first century practising in high-burden HIV countries will need to adopt a different concept of what constitutes an appropriate allocation of healthcare roles between different types of staff. Issues of authority to define health problems and solutions must also be addressed.

A team approach that is based on the model of one set of knowledge bearers who have the power to define and solely authorize interventions for care must be abandoned in favour of a model that includes patients, family and other members of the community. This will significantly change the way diseases such as HIV can be tackled.

It is clear that the current model will not be able to accommodate the massive increase in access to treatment and care needed for scale-up of HIV programmes. Instead, a reorientation of staff and an enlarged spectrum of providers of care are needed. This will have to include new roles for existing service providers as well as new providers within a continuum of care covering prevention and treatment. It will also require adjusting education and training systems, for example to include community members.

At the international level, stakeholders will need to collaborate to find ways to support these developments. It has become clear that existing programmes for training and education have not yielded the expected results in terms of population health. Whether it be the creation of medical schools throughout the developing world or the abundance of bilateral and multilaterally supported training programmes, the impact has often been minimal or has led to negative developments such as emigration of skilled members of the health workforce.

There is thus a great need to rethink the current models of care, who the caregivers should be and what roles different professional staff and community members should play. Combating HIV calls for innovative, socially responsible and flexible approaches to human resources development and use.

Acknowledgements

The authors wish to thank Sigrid Dräger for editorial assistance during the final preparations of the chapter.

References

1. Alexander JA, Ramsay JA, Thomson SM. (2004). Designing the health workforce for the 21st century. *Medical Journal of Australia* 180:7–9.

2. WHO. (2003). *Perspectives and Practice in Antiretroviral Treatment.* Geneva: World Health Organization.

3. Hirschhorn L, Oguda L, Fullem A, Dreesch N. (2004). *Human Resource Requirements for Providing Antiretroviral Therapy in Resource Poor Settings.* Working paper for the United Nations Millennium HIV/AIDS Task Force, JSI Research and Training. Boston: John Snow, Inc.

4. UNAIDS. (2001). *Fact Sheets. HIV/AIDS in Africa.* Geneva: Joint United Nations Programme on HIV/AIDS.

5. Lisk F. (2002). Labour market and employment implications of HIV/AIDS. In: *ILO, Programme on HIV/ AIDS and the World of Work.* Working Paper, Vol. 1. Geneva: International Labour Organization, p1–15.

6. FAO. (2001). HIV/AIDS devastating rural labour force in many African countries, says FAO. URL: http://www.fao.org/WAICENT/OIS/PRESS_NE/PRESSENG/2001/pren0130.htm (accessed February 8, 2005).

7. Kinoti, SN. (2003). Impact of HIV/AIDS on the Health Workforce. Paper presented at World Bank Seminar Series on Human Resources for Health. Support for Analysis and Research in Africa Project, Academy for Educational Development. Washington, DC. URL: http://info.worldbank.org/etools/bspan/PresentationView.asp?PID=590&EID=289 (accessed February 21, 2005).

8. The World Bank. (2002). *Education and HIV/ AIDS: A Window of Hope.* Washington, DC: The World Bank, p1–79.

9. World Bank. (2002). *HIV/AIDS Blunts Progress in Getting all Children into School by 2015.* Press release no. 2002/298/HD. Washington, DC: World Bank.

10. Bennell, P. (2004). The impact of the AIDS epidemic on teacher mortality in sub-Saharan Africa. URL: http://www.eldis.org/fulltext/teachermortality.pdf (accessed February 8, 2005).

11. Arthur G, Bhatt SM, Muhindi D, Achiya GA, Kariuki SM, Gilks CF. (2000). The changing impact of HIV/AIDS on Kenyatta National Hospital, Nairobi from 1988/89 through 1992 and 1997. *AIDS* 11:1625–31.

12. WHO. (2003). *The WHO and UNAIDS Global Initiative to Provide Antiretroviral Therapy to 3 Million People with HIV/AIDS in Developing Countries by the End of 2005.* Department of HIV/AIDS. Geneva: World Health Organization.

13. Malecela-Lazaro M, Mwisongo A, Makundi E *et al.* (2001). *HIV/AIDS Impact on Health Services in Tanzania.* Dar es Salaam: National Institute for Medical Research Health Systems and Policy Research Department.

14. Wilkinson D, Floyd K, Gilks CF. (1998). Antiretroviral drugs as a public health intervention for pregnant HIV-infected women in rural South Africa: an issue of cost-effectiveness and capacity. *AIDS* 12:1675–82.

15. WHO. (2004). Global Tuberculosis Control—Surveillance, Planning, Financing. WHO report WHO/HTM/TB/2004.331 URL: http://www.who.int/tb/publications/global_report/en/, (accessed February 8, 2005).

16. WHO. (2002). *The World Health Report 2002. Reducing Risks, Promoting Health Life.* Geneva: World Health Organization.

17. Tawfik L, Kinoti S. (2001). *The Impact of HIV/AIDS on the Health Sector in Sub-Saharan Africa: The Issue of Human Resources.* Washington, DC: USAID, Bureau for Africa, Office of Sustainable Development. Support for Analysis and Research in Africa (SARA) Project. URL: http://www.dec.org/pdf_docs/PNACP346.pdf (accessed February 8, 2005).

18. Gilks C, Floyd K, Haran D, Kemp J, Squire B, Wilkinson D. (1998). *Care and Support for People with HIV/ AIDS in Resource-poor Settings.* Health and population occasional paper. London: Department for International Development.

19. Jjemba HM, Madraa E, Lutalo T. (1998). The impact of HIV/AIDS on the health sector in Uganda. International Conference of AIDS 12:944.

20. United States Centers for Disease Control and Prevention. (2002). Surveillance of Healthcare Personnel with HIV/AIDS, as of December 2002 URL: http://www.cdc.gov/ncidod/hip/Blood/hiv-personnel.htm (accessed February 8, 2005).

21. Hanson K, Ranson MK, Oliveira-Cruz V, Mills A. (2003). Expanding access to priority health interventions: a framework for understanding the constraints to scaling up. *Journal of International Development* 15(1):1–14.

22. Khaleghian P. (2003). *Decentralization and Public Services: The Case of Immunization.* World Bank Policy Research Working Paper 2989. Washington, DC: World Bank.

23. Schwartz JB, Guilkey DK, Racelis R. (2002). *Decentralization, Allocative Efficiency and Health Services Outcomes in the Philippines.* MEASURE Evaluation Working Paper WP-02-44. Chapel Hill, NC: University of North Carolina.

24. Jeppson A. (2001). Financial priorities under decentralization in Uganda. *Health Policy and Planning* 16:187–92.

25. Mwesigye F. (1999). *Priority Service Provision Under Decentralization: A Case Study of Maternal and Child Care in Uganda.* Small Applied Research No. 10, Partnerships for Health Reform Project. Bethesda, MD: Abt Associates Inc.

26. Parkhurst J. (2003). National responses to HIV/AIDS: the importance of understanding context. *Journal of Health Service Research and Policy* **8**:131–3.

27. Briggs C, Capdegelle P, Garner P. (2001). Strategies for integrating primary health services in middle- and low-income countries: effects on performance, costs and patient outcomes. *Cochrane Database of Systematic Reviews*(4): CD003318. DOI: 10.1002/ 14651858.CD003318.

28. Berwick D. (1991). Controlling variation in health care: a consultation from Walter Shewhart. *Medical Care* **29**:1212–25.

29. Brodsky J, Habib J, Hirschfeld M. (2003). *Policy Issues in Long-term Care*. Geneva: World Health Organization.

30. Magnussen L, Ehiri J, Jolly P. (2004). Comprehensive versus selective primary health care: lessons for global health policy. *Health Affairs (Milwood)* **23**:167–76.

31. Médecins sans Frontières South Africa, Department of Public Health at the University of Cape Town, and Provincial Administration of the Western Cape, South Africa. (2003). Antiretroviral Therapy in Primary Health Care: Experience of the Khayelitsha Programme in South Africa. Perspectives and Practice in Antiretroviral Treatment. Geneva: World Health Organization URL: http://www.who.int/ hiv/pub/prev_care/en/South_Africa_E.pdf (accessed February 8, 2005).

32. Mukherjee J, Farmer P, Léandre F *et al.* (2003). *Access to Antiretroviral Treatment and Care: The Experience of the HIV Equity Initiative, Cange, Haiti*. Perspectives and Practice in Antiretroviral Treatment. Geneva: World Health Organization, p1–16.

33. Amolo Okero F, Aceng E, Madraa E, Namagala E, Serutoke J. (2003). *Scaling up Antiretroviral Therapy: Experience in Uganda*. Perspectives and Practice in Antiretroviral Treatment. Geneva: World Health Organization.

34. Levi G, Vitoria M. (2002). Fighting against AIDS: the Brazilian experience. *AIDS* **16**:2373–83.

35. Bastos FI, Kerrigan D, Malta M, Carneiro-da-Cunha C, Strathdee SA. (2001). Treatment for HIV/ AIDS in Brazil: strengths, challenges, and opportunities for operational research. *AIDScience*. URL: http://www.aidscience.com/Articles/ aidscience012.asp (accessed February 8, 2005).

36. WHO. (2004). Scaling up HIV/AIDS Care: Service Delivery and Human Resources Perspectives. Department of Human Resources for Health. Geneva: World Health Organization. URL: http:// www.who.int/hrh/documents/en/HRH_ART_paper.pdf (accessed February 14, 2005).

Chapter 47

The contribution of civil society

José M Zuniga

Introduction

Speaking at an international conference on HIV in July 2003, Anthony S Fauci, Director of the US National Institute of Allergy and Infectious Disease (NIAID), included a remarkable slide in his retrospective presentation entitled 'Twenty Years of HIV Science' [1]. The slide featured an undated photograph depicting a protestor holding a sign on which was scrawled an angry exclamation: 'Dr Fauci, you are killing us!' Far from being angry with the demonstrator, the renowned scientist and administrator, who has dedicated most of his career to waging battle against the very disease for which the protester wanted greater scientific and societal commitment, was, in effect, praising him. Indeed, Dr Fauci was making a point about the important role that civil society—in this case activism—has played in shaping HIV science and medicine.

The moment is worth noting for the simple fact that it points to a way in which HIV is without historical precedent. Organizations of citizens, including those living with HIV and those advocating on their behalf, have coalesced to demand services and policy changes from healthcare systems and, when those systems have been lacking, to provide services themselves on a scale that is quite novel. Never before have civil society organizations (CSOs)—defined as any group of individuals that is separate from government and business—done so much to contribute to the fight against a global health crisis, or been so included in the decisions made by policy-makers.

Civil society has certainly been involved in efforts to eradicate or mitigate the effects of diseases in the past. Eusebius, the historian of the early Christian church, was boastful about the tendency of the followers of Christ to care for the sick, even during plagues [2]. The founding of the Red Cross in Geneva in 1863 was an important moment for CSO involvement in the promotion of health and medical treatment [3]. CSOs, including the Rockefeller Foundation, were instrumental in the fight against malaria during the early part of the twentieth century [4]. The March of Dimes, an American organization created to raise money for development of a poliomyelitis vaccine, represented a tremendous outpouring of civic engagement and contributed directly to the successful efforts of researcher Jonas Salk in 1954–1955 [5].

The CSO involvement that one sees in the case of HIV, however, is arguably larger than any of these in both breadth and depth. It is broader in terms of sheer numbers, with one on-line database listing more than 3100 AIDS service and advocacy organizations in 150 countries [6]. It is deeper in terms of the impact that these organizations have made, involving themselves directly in the creation of scientific knowledge, the shaping of public policy and the provision of medical and support services.

The high level of AIDS activism can be partially traced to the demographic profile of affected populations and the manner in which HIV affects the body. Most often infected are young adults, a population that tends to fill the ranks of activist organizations of all types and that is not likely simply to acquiesce in the face of such life challenges. Moreover, even before effective treatment was available in developed countries, an HIV diagnosis usually did not mean immediate death, but two or more years of relatively good health before death. The same can be said of developing countries, at least where diagnostic testing is relatively common and where minimal nutritional levels can be assured. This circumstance provides both a window of opportunity for activism and the incentive to accomplish a great deal in a relatively short amount of time.

Added to these more or less accidental by-products of the average age of people living with HIV (PLHIV), and the years that the untreated disease allows them, is the 'social movement spillover' from other struggles for civil or human rights and social justice. In the USA, and arguably in many other Western countries, the group initially most affected by HIV disease—men who have sex with men (MSM)—drew on the strategies and newfound confidence of the movement for gay rights and the emphasis on self-empowerment that was part of the women's movement of the 1970s [7]. On the global front, the movement for treatment access in the developing world finds common cause and motivation with movements that advocate other social justice measures on behalf of the citizens of economically poor countries, such as cancellation of foreign debt and the promotion of trade rules focused on development and human rights.

However, it would be wrong to locate all the factors that have encouraged AIDS activism as lying outside the stated motivations of activists themselves. The fact is that healthcare systems in developed countries were slow to mount responses, with an average of 2–4 years between first diagnoses and official public awareness campaigns [8]. Also, to this day, financial and social barriers to drug availability, along with insufficient political commitment, keep treatment for HIV and numerous other diseases inaccessible to most people in the developing world.

The direct involvement of CSOs in the treatment and care of PLHIV is partially related to the nature of the pandemic. Less tied to bureaucracy than the more institutionalized actors in domestic healthcare systems and intergovernmental organizations (IGOs), CSOs operate more nimbly and are often better able to respond quickly to needs created by HIV. This can be true in the case of local CSOs, which are more attuned to the community, or international CSOs, which are able to transfer and employ global expertise and monetary resources better than many domestic health systems can do unaided.

Advocacy and activism in developed countries

> We condemn attempts to label us as 'victims,' a term which implies defeat, and we are only occasionally 'patients,' a term which implies passivity, helplessness, and dependence upon the care of others. We are 'People With AIDS [9].

Those two declarative sentences make up the preamble to the Denver Principles, written and unveiled by a PLHIV at a June 1983 forum held in that US city. The Principles demanded protection of human and civil rights and the inclusion of HIV-positive people in the forging of policies that affected them. They asked for support against discrimination, and that PLHIV, and their lifestyles, not be blamed for the HIV epidemic. They called upon PLHIV to 'choose their own agenda', 'plan their own strategies' and 'be involved at every level of decision-making' [10].

The Denver Principles constitute an early and characteristic example of the demand for inclusion and partnership that has been evident in civil society responses to HIV. Activists and advocates have successfully challenged societal reactions, government and corporate policies, and even scientific methods. They have forced re-evaluations and policy changes from the early years of the epidemic through to the present.

Perhaps the most important case in point is the shift in public health doctrine and societal attitudes regarding sexually transmitted infection (STI). The traditional public health approach to handling infectious diseases called for isolation, surveillance, mandatory testing and rigorous contact notification protocols—in short, limitations to an individual's civil and human rights. These limitations were justified on the grounds that protecting the physical health of all members of society was arguably a greater concern than protecting the liberty of an individual. When confronted with an STI epidemic, the public at large, often via official government policy, also employed moralism, according to which the infected person was blamed for his or her illness and for spreading the disease.

However, shortly after the first reports of the disease that would become known as 'acquired immune deficiency syndrome', or 'AIDS', activists rallied to reject draconian policies as well as public shaming. Their speaking out significantly changed the tone of the public discourse around HIV, and, more profoundly, influenced the practice of public health science and policy. Rather than blaming individuals for 'immoral' behaviour, experts began to recognize and address the societal circumstances that rendered individuals vulnerable and promoted the spread of HIV infection—for example, prejudice, lack of information, poverty and limited life choices. In many countries, and in the predominant theorizing of academics and policy experts, protecting the human and civil rights of PLHIV came to be seen as an essential aspect of disease control, marking the first time in the history of public health that reinforcing such protections was taken up as part of a strategy for preventing the spread of an infectious disease. By 1987, the World Health Organization (WHO) had officially adopted this rights-based approach, and it remains the standard for preventive interventions worldwide [11].

HIV-specific CSOs have also influenced official policy in the realm of treatment. Groups such as the AIDS Action Council, a US advocacy organization established in February 1985 to advocate the rights of people with HIV and lobby for increased government funding, were joined in March 1987 by the AIDS Coalition to Unleash Power (ACT UP) in aggressive efforts to influence the course of US public policy on HIV. Started in New York as the brainchild of activist and playwright Larry Kramer, ACT UP, and associated organizations such as the Treatment Action Group (TAG), advanced concerted and dramatic efforts with impressive results. Educating themselves on policy formation and the nuances of clinical trials alike, and combining what they had learned with a passion to save lives, activists challenged orthodoxy on issues of drug pricing, the US government's approval process for new medications and the research agenda.

ACT UP took on Burroughs Wellcome, patent-holder of azidothymidine (AZT), the first antiretroviral drug to demonstrate some antiviral efficacy in suppressing HIV, and, along with pressure from sympathetic members of the US Congress, persuaded the company to reduce its price from US$10,000 to US$8000 per annum in 1987, and further to US$6500 in 1989 [12]. Activists also challenged the US Food and Drug Administration (FDA), in simultaneous street protests and face-to-face debates with government administrators. They spoke up against policies that limited access to drugs that had been proven safe and might be effective. They rejected the requirement that patients not take prophylaxis for opportunistic infections while enrolled in antiretroviral therapy (ART) trials. They argued that placebo-controlled studies did not produce sufficient additional data to warrant condemning to death those patients who did not receive the active drug [13]. Bowing to activist pressure, the FDA changed its policy, and the revision has remained in place. Later, ACT UP demanded and won seats for community members on the committees of the AIDS Clinical Trials Groups (ACTGs), effectively involving itself in the process of setting the research agenda [14,15]. ACT UP also demanded that treatment protocols be amended to include women, a group whose medical needs had been largely ignored in clinical trials and federal policy. Although life-threatening and obviously the result of HIV infection, female-specific opportunistic infections were not considered 'AIDS-defining' by medical and public officials [16]. While there was resistance along the way, many if not most in the scientific and policy establishment, including Dr Fauci, came to value the contributions made by PLHIV and their advocates [17,18]. Given the international influence of US policy decisions and scientific research on HIV, particularly in the first decade [19], the impact was global.

Ten years after its founding, ACT UP's membership had decreased, and the organization that had boasted local chapters in 54 cities and 10 countries in 1991 was down to 12 chapters by 1997. Although the challenge of treatment and prevention in the USA was far from over, and many contentious battles were yet to be fought, much had been gained. More effective treatment was available, and a new government entitlement, the Ryan White Comprehensive AIDS Resources Emergency (CARE) Act, had been authorized by the US Congress and signed into law by a politically conservative US President, George HW Bush, at the urging of activists, to subsidize care and treatment for the majority of Americans living with HIV. Many of the activists who cut their teeth learning about prevention and treatment issues in ACT UP were now 'institutionalized', operating within the system in paid positions. Better healthcare options and a stake in the decision-making process for PLHIV, along with a recognition of the importance of CSO involvement, had largely been attained in the USA, and indeed most of the developed world [20].

Advocacy and activism in developing countries

As CSO involvement in the fight against HIV in developed countries was changing form, activism in developing countries, particularly on the issue of access to treatment, was beginning to accelerate. Civil society activity on HIV in much of the developing world had been muted throughout the 1980s for a variety of reasons. In Africa, the years before 1990 are often referred to as the 'lost decade' in the fight against HIV. Under-reporting of incidence and prevalence, due both to generally less robust healthcare systems and to hesitancy on the part of political leaders to face the economic consequences of reporting real numbers, among other concerns, meant that the population at large was less aware of the crisis in its midst, and therefore less able to mount civil society responses [21]. In many non-democratic countries, organization by civil society, and particularly activism, was officially discouraged, if not outright illegal. In most developing countries, a spontaneous civil society response to HIV was unlikely because the epidemic did not disproportionately affect a marginalized group that already had organizational or political cohesion and a reasonable degree of legal protection, as had been the case with the gay male community in Western Europe, the USA and several other developed countries [22]. Conditions of poverty, of course, also created barriers to civil society engagement.

Nonetheless, CSO involvement in fighting HIV began to pick up speed in many developing countries in the late 1980s and early 1990s. In Southern and Central Africa, this often happened through the infusion of foreign funding, primarily in the areas of HIV awareness and education [23,24]. By the mid 1990s, an extensive collection of CSOs was active in Latin America, particularly in human rights-related work [25]. In Thailand, the national chapter of the Red Cross, the Buddhist monastic community and organizations that had been established to assist sex workers were offering care for PLHIV as well as coordinated prevention interventions [26].

However, profound challenges to governments, IGOs and national healthcare systems—the reshaping of policies through CSO activism and advocacy—came a bit later. Brazil was an exception among many other developing countries in that its CSO response to the AIDS epidemic began early and was robust, especially after the country received a substantial World Bank loan in 1992 that enabled it to provide grants to 600 separate AIDS service organizations [27,28]. Citing the 1988 Brazilian Constitution, which guarantees healthcare to all citizens, this highly mobilized CSO community was able to apply pressure on its government to provide opportunistic infection prophylaxis and AZT monotherapy in 1991 and, in 1996, a range of antiretroviral drugs—including the newly developed protease inhibitors (PIs)—to provide combination antiretroviral regimens. To reduce costs, the government began local production of generic antiretroviral drugs [29].

Results over the next few years were very impressive, with prevention of an estimated 90,000 deaths, 60,000 AIDS cases and 358,000 AIDS-related hospital admissions by 2002. Even when balanced against the relatively high cost of drug production and clinical use, the reduction in out-patient and hospital expenses was estimated to have saved US$200 million [30].

The example that Brazil gave the world of a developing country, albeit a middle-income developing country, willing and able to subsidize ART, provided an impetus for a growing international movement for treatment access. Events unfolding in South Africa in the late 1990s added to the momentum.

A 1997 law requiring the South African government to honour its constitutional mandate to provide healthcare to all its citizens sparked heated debate over the consequent legal ability of interested parties to import or manufacture cheaper generic drugs, including antiretroviral drugs, against typically observed patent protections. A resulting lawsuit, filed in 2001 by the national Pharmaceutical Manufacturers Association (PMA), which challenged the law on the grounds that it was too broad and unfairly targeted pharmaceutical companies, sought to prevent the government from permitting the import and manufacture of these cheaper generics. Only 2 years before, the administration of US President Bill Clinton had first challenged the implications of the law when its US Trade Representative (USTR) placed South Africa on its '301 watch list', essentially a threat of economic sanctions in the face of the government's pending decision on the issue of generic drugs. Both instances, first the US trade threat and subsequently the PMA legal action, served to ignite outrage from, and subsequent advocacy by, South African civil society and international civil society communities. South Africa's Treatment Action Campaign (TAC), founded in 1998, began protesting in earnest at US diplomatic offices shortly after the beginning of the USTR review. A coalition of US organizations, including ACT UP chapters and TAC's US-based partner, Health Gap, simultaneously applied pressure on the Clinton Administration, including direct pressure on US Vice President Al Gore, then in his campaign for the US presidency. The USTR removed the sanctions threat in less than a year, citing the need to protect public health in times of medical emergency over and above intellectual property rights. Similarly, within 2 months of its file date in 2001, the PMA ultimately decided to drop its legal action, facing similar forms of domestic and international civil society pressure. By this point, a large global coalition of organizations was heavily involved in drug access issues [31,32], and the stage was set for a major turning point in international attitudes toward expanded access to ART in the developing world.

That moment came in July 2000 at the XIII International AIDS Conference in Durban, South Africa, the first of these biennial events to be hosted by a developing country—and a country which most profoundly felt the impact of its AIDS epidemic. Several medical and public policy experts cite this conference as the time they began to think of ART in materially poor countries as feasible rather than impossible. Developments came quickly thereafter. In 2001, Médecins Sans Frontières (MSF) received agreement from an Indian pharmaceutical firm to produce generic antiretroviral drugs, reducing their price to a potentially more manageable US$350 per annum. The South African pharmaceutical association dropped its lawsuit against the government, and several international pharmaceutical corporations began to cut their prices in the developing world through an Accelerating Access Initiative (AAI) [33].

In response to a US complaint to the World Trade Organization (WTO) that Brazil's threats of compulsory licences for patented antiretroviral drugs violated the Trade Related Intellectual Property Rights (TRIPS) agreement, global CSOs agitated in support of Brazil, and United Nations agencies began to define access to HIV-treating drugs as a human right. The USA dropped its complaint on June 25, 2001, the same day that a United Nations General Assembly convened a Special Session (UNGASS) on HIV to ratify the Declaration of Commitment on HIV/AIDS, formally establishing the basis for the creation of a Global Fund to Fight AIDS, Tuberculosis, and Malaria (Global Fund). Brazilian President Fernando Henrique Cardoso credited international civil society, saying, 'I have no doubt in my mind that this favourable outcome was decisively influenced by global public opinion' [34]. Other commentators have agreed, going as far as crediting CSOs with influencing the change in opinion of medical experts that ART in the developing world was practicable [35,36].

Two years later, during his January 28, 2003 State of the Union address, US President George W Bush, heavily influenced by religious CSOs, announced the President's Emergency Plan for AIDS Relief (PEPFAR), a massive foreign aid programme to provide US$15 billion over 5 years to combat HIV in 12 African and two Caribbean nations. In November 2003, after continued civil society pressure and planning assistance from several CSOs, including the Clinton Foundation HIV/AIDS Initiative (CHAI) and the Pangaea Global AIDS Foundation, the South African government agreed to begin massive roll-out of ART in public sector hospitals [37].

Outstanding challenges for civil society advocacy

At the time of writing, most national governments remain uncommitted to providing ART, nor do they have a plan in place for making it widely available to their HIV-positive citizens. No developing country's government has issued a demand for compulsory licensing of essential medicines, despite a long sought-after change to WTO rules to allow such procedures, won in August 2003 [38]. Few have taken advantage of voluntary pharmaceutical price reductions, such as the Merck & Co. price reductions for its non-nucleoside reverse transcriptase inhibitor, efavirenz [39]. There is reason to believe that the USA continues to pressure other governments not to adopt the use of generic antiretroviral drugs [40], and the Global Fund launched by the United Nations to facilitate access to

ART across a continuum of HIV care is not receiving the full support required to ensure its sustainability [41].

With regard to government commitment, the South African government's treatment pledge appears to be stalled, with poorly explained delays to the roll-out of ART. The new bureaucracy created for PEPFAR has also been slow in establishing itself, with the first disbursal of funding to CSO service providers taking place over a year after the Bush Administration first announced its contribution to the global fight against HIV in early 2003. The official plan for PEPFAR appears to place even more of an emphasis than was originally intimated on abstinence-only prevention methods and would also seem to preclude the use of generic medicines, again despite claims that the policy would not restrict them [42]. In the face of these developments or lack thereof, while the effectiveness of CSO advocacy has been demonstrated in the past, it will need to be proven once more.

In looking to the way in which the global CSO community will need to respond to these ongoing challenges, it is important to note that, while the impact of past CSO efforts must be judged as key to many important achievements in the development and expansion of HIV treatment, there are also legitimate arguments pointing to negative long-term effects of some policies in which PLHIV and their advocates exercised decisive influence. For example, in the African context of much higher incidence and prevalence rates than were ever seen in Western countries where the concept of voluntary counselling and testing (VCT) was developed, perhaps HIV antibody testing should be made more routine [43]. AIDS chronicler Randy Shilts famously argued that bathhouses in the USA, where HIV was spread to thousands in the gay male community in the 1980s, were allowed to remain open because individuals who did not understand the enormity of the situation or, in some cases, had ulterior motives, misguidedly organized to prevent their being closed [12].

Additionally, questions are sometimes raised about whether CSOs truly speak for the broad HIV-positive community in their various settings, or if activists represent a radical fringe, influential beyond their numbers thanks to organizational ability. Such concerns are inevitable but do not undermine the importance of empowering civil society to be active in giving direction to the fight against HIV. Shifting contexts and new information will always require that policies and procedures be reconsidered. If the ability of interested parties to influence decision making in a democratic society is occasionally a double-edged sword, that does not negate the importance of people being allowed, and even encouraged, to take part. Certainly, more recent global efforts such as the International Treatment Preparedness Programme, a WHO-led initiative delivered through an initial US$1 million grant administered by the US-based Tides Foundation, will provide evidence as to whether many of these past lessons will be heeded in the future, and whether the relative merit of certain criticisms of CSO-based activities warrants greater consideration.

Civil society service provision

As with advocacy and activism, civil society has played a remarkably significant role in the direct provision of HIV services, and for many of the same reasons. Among those most often cited are governments' hesitancy to address politically sensitive issues, and certain strengths common to CSOs, such as connections within communities, lack of bureaucratic ties that slow response times and impede innovation, access to marginalized groups, and cost-effectiveness [44]. Also influential was the historical coincidence of the emergence of HIV and the dominance of certain policy theories that emphasized the need to support civil society on the one hand and retreat from public sector service provision on the other: the 'good government' agenda, the New Public Management, and structural adjustment policies [45].

Civil society responses that are usually pointed to as success stories include that of the gay male community in San Francisco, to which interested parties from all over the world flocked in the 1980s to study the 'San Francisco model' of community-based support services and awareness initiatives [46,47]. In the developing world, Uganda's CSO community, along with a political leadership that was supportive of a frank societal discussion of HIV and its modes of transmission, are partly responsible for that country's famous decline in prevalence rate. The AIDS Support Organisation (TASO), which has employed innovative methods of self-empowerment to train local volunteers, is perhaps the best example of this response [48]. It has also been argued that the somewhat uncoordinated conglomeration of non-state actors that necessarily took on local prevention interventions when the health system was incapable was more effective because its messages were locally tailored and community-specific [49].

However, in the case of medical care, and particularly large-scale ART roll-out, there is a compelling need for national coordination. More than one observer has warned against 'treatment anarchy' in the absence of such governmental orchestration [50,51], and, in the case of Uganda, the same disorder in the health system that was serendipitous for HIV prevention has proved to be a barrier to ART scale-up, as officials have had difficulty synchronizing the contributions of local and international NGOs, for-profit providers and the public sector [52]. Similarly, Botswana's ambitious ART roll-out did not meet its goal for the number of patients on treatment by the first year, partly because of fragmentation in the health system [53].

This situation can lead to conflict between CSOs and government. Ideally, CSOs have an interest in remaining independent and close to the community, as these are some of the factors that contribute to their effectiveness, though there might also be requirements for accountability to international donors or foreign board members. For their part, governments have an interest in promoting nationally driven programmes and may resent CSOs, particularly foreign ones, as a special or outside interest group.

Cognizant of the need to balance governmental coordination and oversight with civil society inclusion, the Global Fund's leadership, for example, delegated the job of crafting grant proposals and overseeing their implementation to country coordinating mechanisms (CCMs) made up of 'representatives from both the public and private sectors, including governments, multilateral or bilateral agencies, non-governmental organizations, academic institutions, private businesses, and people living with the diseases' [54].

The results have not always been perfect. The question of whether CSO and government representatives really share power in the CCMs remains unanswered. The government of South Africa, for instance, quarrelled with the Global Fund in 2002 over a planned disbursement of funding directly to the province of KwaZulu-Natal instead of to the federal government [55]. There have been allegations of government domination of CCMs in Latin American and Caribbean countries [56], and the Ukrainian Ministry of Health simply did not spend its grant, failing to place patients on ART despite the urgency of doing so [57].

Regardless of these difficulties, however, the Global Fund's inclusion of CSOs demonstrates a laudable dedication to multisectoral and participatory processes that have been shown to be effective over the course of the pandemic. Moreover, it reflects the reality that global scale-up of ART will not be possible without the involvement of CSOs. Ideally, ART would always be delivered in fully modern medical facilities, with a low ratio of patients to physicians and other healthcare professionals. That is simply not feasible in many countries in the short term, however, and CSOs have been instrumental in demonstrating that alternative strategies for delivering ART can be effective now.

Indeed, Family Health International (FHI), a group that has coordinated HIV treatment programmes in several developing countries, posits that 'fast and foreign' interventions can provide treatment in the short term, while 'slow and steady' efforts to develop national healthcare infrastructure are undertaken simultaneously [58]. CSOs providing such treatment programmes, even as conventional wisdom held that ART in resource-poor developing countries was not possible, have worked in conjunction with CSO activism to force a reappraisal of accepted thinking. The Brazilian example demonstrated that ART could be delivered in a middle-income, developing country, while CSO programmes, most prominently those coordinated by MSF, demonstrated similar results in countries and regions that were economically worse off.

Deliberately setting out both to provide treatment for its own sake and to 'assess and demonstrate the feasibility of antiretroviral therapy in a range of resource-poor settings', MSF has successfully provided treatment to 5000 patients in Asia, Africa, Eastern Europe and Latin America, learning valuable lessons about the importance of factors such as broad governmental strategy, political will and generic competition to make drug prices affordable [59]. Most importantly, demonstrating the feasibility of ART in these economically burdened settings helped to change the thinking of experts, to transform global access to ART into something that *could* be accomplished and, therefore, *must* be accomplished with all deliberate speed [60]. The result has been a notable shift in emphasis from the feasibility of ART scale-up in the developing world to one focused on strategies to overcome the serious financial obstacles that stand in the way of accomplishing this on the scale required. Local healthcare systems are not all that they should be, but CSOs can help to fill the gaps and save lives that would otherwise be lost.

An initiative advanced by the WHO/UNAIDS as part of its pledge to have 3 million people in the developing world on ART by 2005 (the '3 by 5' initiative), calls for what would probably be the most radical inclusion yet of civil society in the provision of medical services [61]. The plan to use PLHIV and other community health workers to administer ART in directly observed therapy (DOT) interventions draws on the example of a successful programme of the same design in Haiti [62]. It remains to be seen whether this model can be effective on a global scale or if governments and CSOs will adopt this model as a strategy, but that such a model can be considered feasible is testament to the manner in which civil society has earned a place as a partner in anti-AIDS strategies.

Conclusion

Was Dr Fauci right to give credit to activists in his presentation on the history of HIV science? Or, to put it more broadly, has the considerable role played by civil society in the global fight against HIV been of general benefit to the effort? If so, can it continue to be effective? One hesitates to pass judgement or make predictions when the work is so far from over, but it seems safe to answer these questions in the affirmative.

With regard to provision of services, a moral imperative for addressing the HIV pandemic and the destruction it has wrought means that we have no choice but to draw upon the strength of CSOs. We may regret that many governments remain unwilling to engage effectively with politically sensitive issues, such as injecting drug use, sex work and gender discrimination. However, even as we implore national leaders to change their policies, CSOs can address these areas here and now. Moreover, the close ties to communities that CSOs offer mean that they are often the best suited to advance such work.

We might also lament that health systems in so many developing countries are not strong or emboldened enough to provide ART without foreign assistance. However, while we take on the relatively slow task of building or rebuilding national healthcare infrastructures and redressing domestic staffing shortages, we must simultaneously employ the ability to mobilize quickly to provide expertise—a signature trait of CSOs. That 95% of the world's 40 million PLHIV do not currently have access to ART compels us to do so with all possible speed.

With regard to CSO activism and advocacy, the very fact that these statements about the need to expand treatment are widely accepted among the global medical and health policy communities is an example of its positive effects. The empowerment of PLHIV, and their advocates, has meant that scientists, medical professionals and policy-makers have been continually called upon to assure that their work takes into account the perspective of the individual who is living with HIV, and reflects the urgency of a life-and-death matter. That is not to say that the women and men who choose a career in healthcare are insensitive to such concerns. It would also be incorrect to say that they have abandoned data-driven analysis and evidence-based decision making. However, we have seen how CSOs, themselves making arguments based on the facts at hand, have forced re-evaluations of matters that were considered settled. In each case, from established methods of disease control, to protocols for clinical trials, to drug pricing, to the feasibility of ART in the developing world, new consensuses have been reached that reflect both good policy and humanitarian concerns. Continued diligence in this respect, and open and honest discussion about the relative merit of certain criticisms of CSO advocacy strategies and the smaller cadres of advocates who often shape them, will be critical in steering community efforts clear of peril.

We have already seen that respect for civil liberty, openness and democratic processes positively influenced the course of HIV prevention and treatment in various countries, including the USA, Brazil, South Africa and Uganda. In other countries, state secrecy and the repression of civil society influence have exacerbated the incidence and discouraged redress of health system inadequacies. The history of AIDS epidemics in Russia and China, to cite but two examples, reminds us that HIV disease flourishes where those who suffer are prevented from speaking out and acting on their own behalf. While it is disheartening to point to yet another hurdle standing in the way of the world finally controlling the pandemic, failure to democratize the response fully surely stands as such a barrier.

References

1. Fauci AS. (2003). 20 Years of HIV Science. Keynote Lecture, Extraordinary Plenary Session, July 14, 2003. Delivered at 2nd IAS Conference on HIV Pathogenesis and Treatment. July 13–16, 2003. Paris.
2. Eusebius. (324/5). Ecclesiastical History, VII, 21–22. Quoted in McNeil HM. (1976). *Plagues and Peoples*. New York: Doubleday.
3. Buckingham CE. (1964). *For Humanity's Sake: The Story of the Early Development of the League of Red Cross Societies*. Washington, DC: Public Affairs Press.

4. Harrison G. (1978). *Mosquitoes, Malaria, and Man: a History of the Hostilities Since 1880*. New York: EP Dutton.

5. Seavey NG, Smith JS, Wagner P. (1998). *A Paralyzing Fear: The Triumph over Polio in America*. New York: TV Books, L.L.C.

6. National AIDS Manual Organizations search. Accessed March 1, 2004, online at http://www.nam.-co.uk/search/worldmap.asp.

7. Bayer R. (1991). *Private Acts, Social Consequences: AIDS and the Politics of Public Health*. New Brunswick, NJ: Rutgers University Press.

8. Mann, JM. (1992). Foreword to *AIDS in the Industrialized Democracies: Passions, Politics, and Policies*. New Brunswick, NJ: Rutgers University Press.

9. Callan M, Turner D. (1997). A History of the People with AIDS Self-Empowerment Movement. *Body Positive* X(12). Accessed March 4, 2004, online at http://www.thebody.com/bp/dec97/dec97-ix.html.

10. Siplon PD. (2002). *AIDS and the Policy Struggle in the United States*. Washington, DC: Georgetown University Press.

11. Gruskin S, Hendriks A, Tomasevski K. (1996). Human rights and responses to HIV/AIDS. In: Mann J, Tarantola D. eds. *AIDS in the World II*. Oxford: Oxford University Press, pp 326–340.

12. Shilts R. (1987). *And the Band Played On: Politics, People, and the AIDS Epidemic*. New York: St. Martin's Press.

13. Eigo J, Harrington M, McCarthy M. (1988). *FDA Action Handbook*. 1988. New York: ACT UP. Accessed March 10, 2004, online at http://www.actupny.org/documents/FDAhandbook1.html.

14. Bayer R, Oppenheimer GM. (2000). *AIDS Doctors: Voices from the Epidemic*. Oxford: Oxford University Press.

15. Montagnier L. (2000). *Virus*. New York: WW Norton & Company.

16. Corea G. (1992). *The Invisible Epidemic: The Story of Women and AIDS*. New York: Harper Collins.

17. Freiberg P. (1997). After 10 years, ACT UP now fights dwindling membership; Protest Group had remarkable influence on US AIDS policy. *The Washington Blade*. March 14, 1997. Accessed March 3, 2004 online at http://www.aegis.com/news/wb/1997/wb970303.html.

18. Byar DP, Schoenfeld DA, Green SB *et al.* (1990). Design considerations for AIDS trials. *New England Journal of Medicine* 323:1343–8.

19. Merigan TC. (1990). You can teach an old dog new tricks: how AIDS trials are pioneering new strategies. *New England Journal of Medicine* 323:1341–3.

20. Associated Press. (1997). AIDS Activists Mark 10th Year. March 24. 1997. Online at http://www.aegis.com/news/ap/1997/ap970318.html.

21. Mupedziswa R. (1998). AIDS in Africa: past, present, and future. In: AIDS in Africa: The Social Work Response. Harare: *Journal of Social Development in Africa*, School of Social Work, University of Zimbabwe.

22. O'Malley J, Nguyen VK, Lee S. (1996). Nongovernmental organizations. In: Mann J, Tarantola D. eds. *AIDS in the World II*. Oxford: Oxford University Press, pp 341–361.

23. Morna CL. (1990). Southern African NGOs seize the initiative. *WorldAIDS* 12:5–9.

24. Burja J, Baylies C. (2000). Responses to the AIDS epidemic in Tanzania and Zambia. In: Burja J, Baylies C, eds. *AIDS, Sexuality and Gender in Africa: Collective Strategies and Struggles in Tanzania and Zambia*. London: Routledge, pp 25–58.

25. Joint United Nations Programme on HIV/AIDS. (1998). NGO Perspectives on Access to HIV-related Drugs in 13 Latin American and Caribbean countries. 1998. Geneva: UNAIDS. Accessed March 2, 2004, online at http://www.unaids.org /publications/documents/health/access/una98e25.pdf.

26. Beyrer C. (1998). *War in the Blood: Sex, Politics and AIDS in Southeast Asia.* London and New York: Zed Books.

27. Osava M. (2001). NGOs the driving force behind AIDS policy. *Inter Press Service.* December 9, 2001. Accessed March 2, 2004, online at http://www.aegis.com/news /ips/2001/ip011208.html.

28. Connor C. (2000). Contracting non-governmental organizations for HIV/AIDS: Brazil case study. Special Initiative Report No. 30. Partnerships for Health Reform. Accessed March 1, 2004, online at http://www.phrplus.org/Pubs/Sir30.pdf.

29. Galvão J. (2002). Access to antiretroviral drugs in Brazil. *Lancet* **360**:1862–5.

30. Teixera PR, Vitória MA, Barcarolo J. (2003). The Brazilian experience in providing universal access to antiretroviral therapy. In: Moatti JP, Coriat B, Souteyrand Y, Barnett T, Dumoulin J, Flori YA, eds. *Economics of AIDS and Access to HIV/AIDS Care in* Developing Countries. Issues and Challenges. Paris: ANRS, pp 69–88.

31. Zuniga JM. (1998). Challenges of Providing Limited Access to AIDS Drugs in Four Less-Industrialized Nations. Plenary address. November 15, 1998. In: Program and Abstracts of the 2nd International Conference on Healthcare Resource Allocation for HIV/AIDS. November 15–19, 1998. Cancún, Mexico.

32. Oxfam. (1999). *World Trade Rules and Poor People's Access to Essential Drugs.* Policy Briefing Paper. November 1999.

33. World Health Organization. (2002). Accelerating Access Initiative: Widening Access to Care and Support for People Living with HIV/AIDS. Progress Report. June 2002. Geneva: World Health Organization/Joint United Nations Programme on HIV/AIDS. Accessed February 10, 2004, online at http://www.who.int/hiv/pub/prev_care/isbn9241210125.pdf.

34. Cardoso FH. (2003). Keynote address. July 13, 2003. 2nd IAS Conference on HIV Pathogenesis and Treatment. July 13–16, 2003. Paris.

35. Rosenberg T. (2001). Look at Brazil. *New York Times Magazine.* January 28, 2001. Accessed March 3, 2004, online at http://www.accessmed-msf.org/prod /publications.asp?scntid=3082001232234&contenttype=PARA&.

36. Bazell R. (2003). How AIDS treatment for poor countries became possible. Slate. Online at http://slate.msn.com/id/2089907. 3 pages. Accessed March 3, 2004.

37. Schoofs M. (2003). South Africa changes course with aggressive AIDS plan. *Wall Street Journal.* November 19, 2003. Accessed March 10, 2004, online at http://www.aegis.org/news/wsj/2003/WJ031104.html.

38. Duparcq E. (2004). Poor countries fail to take advantage of WTO accord on AIDS drugs. Agence France-Presse, March 7, 2004. Online at http://www.aegis.org./news/afp/2004/AF040330.html. 2 pages. Accessed March 12, 2004.

39. Kaisernetwork. (2004). Merck's discounted antiretroviral drug efavirenz not approved for use in many developing countries. *Kaiser Daily HIV/AIDS Report.* March 3, 2004. Accessed March 5, 2004, online at http://www.kaisernetwork.org/daily_reports/print_report.cfm?DR_ID=22474&dr_cat=1.

40. Kristof ND. (2003). Death by dividend. *New York Times.* November 22, 2003. Accessed March 10, 2004, online at http://www.globalexchange.org/campaigns/ftaa/1313.html.

41. Associated Press. (2004). Lack of money endangers UN plan to treat HIV/AIDS. March 17, 2004. Accessed March 18, 2004, online at http://www.aegis.com/news/ap/2004/ap040329.html.

42. Office of the United States Global AIDS Coordinator. February 23, 2004. The President's Emergency Plan for AIDS Relief: US Five-Year Global HIVAIDS Strategy. Accessed March 2, 2004, online at http://www.state.gov/documents/organization/29831.pdf.

43. Repke HH, Ayensu S. (2001). *HIV/AIDS: Knowledge Protects: New and Specific Approaches to Contain the Spread of HIV in Developing Countries.* Potsdam: Strauss Verlag GmbH.

44. Sehgal PN. (1991). Prevention and control of AIDS: the role of NGOs. *Health Millions* 17(4):31–3.

45. Clayton A, Oakley P, Taylor J. (2000). Civil Society Organizations and Service Provision. 2000. Geneva: United Nations Research Institute for Social Development, Civil Society, and Social Movements. Programme Paper No. 2. Accessed February 14, 2004, online at http://www.unrisd.org/80256B3C005BCCF9/(httpPublications)/19AB2640214382A380256B5E004C94C5?OpenDocument.

46. Arno PS. (1986). The nonprofit sector's response to the AIDS epidemic: community-based services in San Francisco. *American Journal of Public Health* 76:1325–30.

47. Kirp D, Bayer B. (1992). The second decade of AIDS: the end of exceptionalism (Conclusion). In: Kirp DL, Bayer B, eds. *AIDS in the Industrialized Democracies: Passions, Politics, and Policies.* New Brunswick, NJ: Rutgers University Press, pp 361–384.

48. DeJong J. (2001). TASO: An Example of the Evolution of Scaling Up Strategies. In: DeJong J, *A Question of Scale? The Challenge of Non-Governmental Organisations' HIV/AIDS Efforts in Developing Countries.* New York: The Population Council, pp 39–40.

49. Parkhust J, Ssengooba F, Serwadda D. (2003). Uganda: HIV Epidemic and the Healthcare System's Response. In: Program and Abstracts of the 6th International Conference on Healthcare Resource Allocation for HIV/AIDS: Healthcare Systems in Transition. October 13–15, 2003. Washington, DC.

50. Moatti JP, Barnett T, Souteyrand Y, Flori YA, Dumoulin J, Coriat B. (2003). Financing efficient HIV care and antiretroviral treatment to mitigate the impact of the AIDS epidemic on economic and human development. In: Moatti JP, Coriat B, Souteyrand Y, Barnett T, Dumoulin J, Flori YA, eds. *Economics of AIDS and Access to HIV/AIDS Care in Developing Countries: Issues and Challenges.* Paris: ANRS, pp 247–265.

51. Zuniga JM. (2003). Avoiding treatment anarchy. *IAPAC Monthly* 9(8):175. Accessed March 10, 2004, online at http://www.iapac.org/home.asp?pid=76&toolid=2&itemid=302.

52. Birungi H, Mugisha F, Nsabagasani X, Okuonzi S, Jeppsson A. (2001). The policy on public–private mix in the Ugandan health sector: catching up with reality. *Health Policy and Planning* 16(Supplement 2):80–7.

53. Lush L, Darkoh E and Ramotlhwa S. (2006). Botswana. In: Beck EJ, Mays N, Whiteside A, Zuniga JM, eds. *The HIV Pandemic: local and global implications.* Oxford: Oxford University Press, p 181–197.

54. Global Fund to Fight AIDS, Tuberculosis, and Malaria. Country Coordinating Mechanisms. Accessed March 2, 2004, online at http://www.theglobalfund.org/en/apply/mechanisms/.

55. Nolen S. (2002). Global Fund fights AIDS with tied hands. *Globe and Mail (Toronto).* October 5, 2002.

56. Stern R. (2003). The Global Fund and treatment access in Latin America: a critical view. *Global Fund Observer (GFO) Newsletter* 16:3–4. Accessed March 2, 2004, online at http://www.aidspan.org/gfo/archives /newsletter/Issue16.pdf.

57. Brown D. (2004). AIDS fund suspends payments in Ukraine. *Washington Post.* January 31, 2004.

58. van Praag E. (2003). Scaling up care with antiretroviral therapy. In: Program and Abstracts of the 6th International Conference on Healthcare Resource Allocation for HIV/AIDS: Healthcare Systems in Transition. October 13–15, 2003. Washington, DC.

59. Médecins Sans Frontières, World Health Organization, UNAIDS Secretariat. (2003). *Surmounting Challenges: Procurement of Antiretroviral Medicines in Low- and Middle-income Countries.* Geneva: World Health Organization. Accessed February 10, 2004, online at http://www.accessmed-msf.org/documents/procurementreport.pdf.

60. Keeton C. (2003). Drug scheme shows roll-out can work. *Sunday Times* (Johannesburg). December 7, 2003. Accessed February 10, 2004, online at http://www.suntimes.co.za/2003/12/07/news/cape/nct03.asp.

61. Kasper T, Coetzee D, Francoise L, Boulle A, Hildebrand K. (2003). Demystifying antiretroviral therapy in resource-poor settings. *Essential Drugs Monitor* 32:21–2.

62. Farmer P, Leandre F, Mukherjee J, Gupta R, Tarter L, Kim JY. (2001). Community-based treatment of advanced HIV disease: Introducing DOT-HAART (Directly Observed Therapy with Highly Active Anterotrovival Therapy). *Bulletin of the World Health Organization* 79:1145–51.

Chapter 48

The role of community involvement in HIV programmes in South Africa

RA Roberts, A Hickey* and Z Rosner

Introduction

The involvement of civil society organizations (CSOs) and community-based organizations (CBOs) in the global response to the HIV epidemic is unparalleled in public health history. The successful impact of such mobilization is nowhere more evident than in South Africa, where these organizations have had tremendous success in shaping the response to HIV in one of the world's highest burdened countries. Using the Treatment Action Campaign (TAC) and the AIDS Budget Unit (ABU) at the Institute for Democracy in South Africa (IDASA) as case studies, we briefly look at the government's relationship with CSOs, the cooperation amongst these organizations and how these various parties interact to combat the effects of HIV on the country.

CSOs and CBOs serve a variety of functions in South Africa. From parliamentary monitoring and public service accountability to caring for orphans, home-based care (HBC) and financial oversight, CSOs and CBOs are indispensable to the country's HIV response. In particular, HBC services have received much attention from the government. The Department of Health first prioritized home-based care in 2001, subsidized CBOs involved with HBC, and brought these CBOs together in a national conference held in 2002 [1]. At the beginning of 2005, the government recognized the importance of the more than 1700 CBO projects that provide HBC for the nearly half a million South Africans with AIDS, and allotted over US$80 million to create more than 120,000 jobs for HBC workers over the next 5 years [2,3]. This indirect support of CBOs involved with HBC provides long-awaited affirmation of their efforts and addresses the imminent need for a large number of paid HBC workers, since most are currently volunteers [4,5].

While the government has embraced the role of CSOs or CBOs in dealing with the HIV epidemic, it has not always done so in agreement with CSOs or CBOs. Some friction stems from personality clashes, such as the 1999 closure of an umbrella organization of 28 CBOs in Mpumalanga because the provincial Health Minister had a falling out with a staff member associated with the organization [6]. More often, however, the relationship is stretched when CSOs and CBOs call upon government to alter its policy towards HIV significantly, and no organization has called upon the government of South Africa to do that more than the TAC.

Structure and work of the TAC

Since its inception on December 10, 1998, when 20 members held a day-long fast at St. George's Cathedral in Cape Town, the TAC has had a tumultuous relationship with government. This is

* Corresponding author.

not surprising, considering the political climate surrounding HIV in South Africa and the fact that TAC's main objective is to campaign for greater access to treatment for all South Africans by raising public awareness and understanding about issues surrounding the availability, affordability and use of HIV treatments. This approach includes starting programmes that educate, treat and mobilize people living with or affected by HIV, as well as pressuring government and pharmaceutical companies to ensure that medicine is accessible to those who need it. TAC operates on the assumption that prevention, treatment and care must involve the entire community and are inextricably linked to empowering those communities.

The TAC has grown from a small group of activists to a movement of more than 10,000 members with over 200 functioning branches in six of the nine South African provinces. TAC branches can be found in diverse areas, from rural parts of KwaZulu-Natal to cosmopolitan Cape Town. Branch members are people from the community who want to make an impact on the HIV epidemic. They include people of all ages who are living with HIV or AIDS, as well as those who are HIV-negative. Branches hold meetings on a regular basis and elect members who will represent the branch at either district or provincial level. This ensures that lines of communication are established throughout all regions of the country with the aim of capturing the most accurate and robust stream of feedback possible.

TAC's branch activities are broad and involve a number of approaches to fighting HIV. These often complement the TAC's national agenda, but also include programmes separate from its more publicized national campaigns. Local approaches include education about the science of HIV and treatment requirements, treatment literacy, setting up support groups, monitoring the roll-out of antiretroviral drugs, helping local clinics become accredited for the distribution of HIV medicines and pressuring local government to respond better to the needs of those living with HIV.

In addition, TAC branches help foster a community where people can speak openly about their experiences with HIV without fear of stigmatization. Community members are encouraged to ask questions about what it means to be HIV-positive, where they can go for help, and what to expect if they are starting treatment. These communal discussions serve to clear up confusion and create knowledgeable citizens who feel empowered to aid TAC in its struggles. Destigmatization of HIV in South Africa has also been aided by the 'HIV Positive' T-shirts worn by TAC members and allies as well as the organization's insistence that the epidemic receive media and political attention.

Community and civil society involvement in policy development

Drug pricing campaigns to improve treatment access

In October 2000, the TAC launched the Christopher Moraka Defiance Campaign Against Patent Abuse. The campaign was launched with the goal of obtaining more affordable drugs for the people who need them most, and marked the beginning of TAC's interaction with the pharmaceutical industry. Christopher Moraka was a TAC member who lived openly with AIDS. He fell ill with systemic thrush that can be treated with Pfizer's flucanozole (Diflucan®), but he died because he could not afford the medicines he needed.

At the time, Pfizer's drug cost R30 (US$4.71) in the public sector, R80 (US$12.06) in the private sector and R2 (US$0.31) on the generic market. Patent laws were directly impeding the treatment and care of people living with HIV (PLHIV), and TAC saw the need for broader involvement on drug pricing. TAC demanded that Pfizer lower its drug price to R4 (US$0.62)or issue a voluntary licence. When Pfizer offered to donate Diflucan to treat those with the less common cryptococcal meningitis infection but not systemic thrush, TAC continued its public and political pressure on the company to meet its original demands. This included letters to the company's CEO, as well as a highly publicized trip to Thailand by TAC volunteers who smuggled generic versions of fluconazole back to South Africa.

In response, Pfizer initiated legal action against TAC for patent infringement, but withdrew its efforts amidst the public's vociferous support for TAC. The drug company eventually agreed to donate Diflucan to the public sector for treatment of systemic thrush and cryptococcal meningitis, but it did not issue a voluntary licence, nor did it lower its drug price to R4 per capsule. TAC, in conjunction with other organizations, still imports generic fluconazole from Thailand for use in the public sector as stocks of Pfizer's version continue to run out in clinics and hospitals.

Though TAC's demands were not fully met in this campaign, it set a precedent for how TAC would mobilize various sectors of society in future campaigns through partnerships and coalitions. The Christopher Moraka campaign involved community pressure in achieving fairer prices for essential medicines and was strengthened by partnerships with the AIDS Law Project (ALP), Médecins Sans Frontières (MSF) and other organizations such as the Congress of South African Trade Unions (COSATU) and Oxfam. The bolstering of campaigns through partnership is a salient feature of TAC's approach to effecting change. By aligning itself with a variety of movements, broader cross-sections of society are enlisted in TAC's struggle for health rights.

The international impact was also especially important. TAC's partner organizations in the USA, such as the Health Global Access Project (HealthGAP) and ACT UP, campaigned against Pfizer's profiteering. Furthermore, the public outcry in response to Pfizer's legal action against TAC demonstrated that pharmaceutical companies are not invincible, and it is now clear that the right to make a profit will not be accepted complacently while people are dying.

Role of civil society in monitoring HIV funding flows

While TAC received much of the credit for the success of the Christopher Moraka campaign, it relied on financial information from other CSOs to bolster its arguments. Civil society organizations have played a key role in undertaking research and advocacy that address the critical financing issues related to governmental and non-governmental responses to HIV in South Africa. With multiple grants from the Global Fund to Fight AIDS, Tuberculosis and Malaria (Global Fund) in operation in the region, the launch of the President's Emergency Plan for AIDS Relief (PEPFAR) grant programme, and ongoing inflows from bilateral aid and donor agencies, the influx of external funds targeting the fight against HIV in southern Africa has grown considerably. Although the great majority of spending on HIV in the region is donor-funded, financial commitments from the National Treasury are still tremendously important. Government budgets are a fundamental tool in the implementation of public policy, as they set out the allocation of public resources. Often the government budget serves as a more telling indicator of the priority accorded to fighting HIV by the government than official policy or legislation. Furthermore, despite the size of donor inflows, investment from domestic revenues, as reflected in the government budget, is still a critical ingredient for sustainability of any government programme.

In South Africa, non-governmental organizations (NGOs) provide independent research and analysis of these HIV funding flows. Furthermore, there are good examples of civil society organizations using this HIV allocation and expenditure information for *advocacy* purposes. Through budget advocacy, civil society organizations can hold their governments accountable for how domestic and international HIV funds are being utilized within their countries, and press for increased domestic resources to fight HIV.

Using budget research and analysis to track government prioritization of HIV

The ABU at the IDASA is an example of a CSO producing research that tracks government prioritization of HIV in the budget. Since 2001, the ABU has conducted vigorous research, informed and shaped by policy and budget developments, on HIV-specific government allocations and actual expenditure [7–9]. HIV budget monitoring has played a role in illuminating and informing government and civil society alike on the overall resource envelope available for HIV in South Africa, and the priority accorded to the epidemic in the government budget [10].

This research provides evidence of massive increases in national government transfers to provincial departments for HIV. These increases translate into two- or threefold increases in budgets year on year, and thus create tremendous pressure on line managers to spend, often at the expense of clear plans and monitoring and evaluation systems (Fig. 48.1).

What is the potential impact of this research, and how can it contribute to government's response to the epidemic? ABU releases their research in various outputs such as *Budget Briefs*, reports, presentations and newspaper articles. The research has provided HIV advocacy groups, including the TAC, with data for their efforts to increase government resource allocation to fight the epidemic. The allocation data allow for analysis of the sufficiency of the budgeted funds compared with available costing data, as well as their allocative efficiency. In South Africa, despite the existence of a multisectoral integrated plan for fighting the epidemic, the HIV-specific budget is still clearly dominated by the health sector. This calls into question the

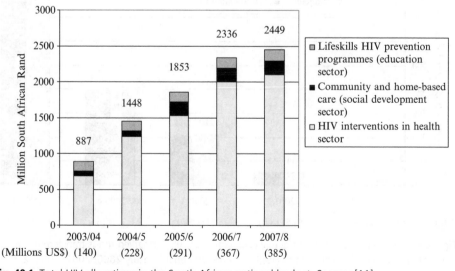

Fig. 48.1 Total HIV allocations in the South African national budget. Source: [11].

appropriateness of the mix of interventions funded and the balance achieved between prevention, treatment and care.

Monitoring expenditures on HIV programmes

While analysis of budget *allocations* sheds light on the prioritization of government's response, monitoring *actual expenditure* against budgeted allocations provides a measure of the efficiency of funding channels used to deliver financial resources to the implementing government body. Actual expenditure analysis also gives invaluable information on where the bottlenecks are.

By regularly producing analyses of provincial spending patterns on HIV grants from national government, ABU makes provincial spending patterns more transparent and simultaneously makes the information easily available to advocacy groups that can take it forward and hold government officials to account for slow spending. After ABU's 2002 research discovered poor spending of HIV conditional grant money, the report was widely publicized, garnering front page space in three newspapers. Government officials were held to account and compelled to provide information and answers on radio shows, in press conferences and at government meetings.

Figure 48.2 shows how spending on HIV conditional grant funds by provinces has improved significantly since the poor spending record reported by ABU in the first year of the programme, 2001. Using this research, evidence-based recommendations are made to National Treasury and Department of Health on effective funding mechanisms for HIV.

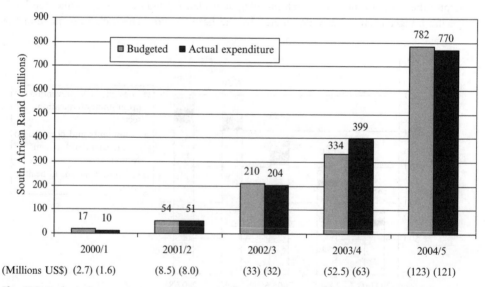

Fig. 48.2 Budgeted amounts versus actual expenditure of HIV earmarked funds transferred from national to provincial Departments of Health. Source: National Treasury 2000, 2001, 2002, 2003, 2004 [12].

Community and NGO involvement in policy implementation

Promoting access to information regarding government's antiretroviral treatment plan

While financial transparency enables CSOs in South Africa to make recommendations on and assess the progress of the government's HIV response, the country's Constitution is one of the most important tools used by CSOs to bring about real change. The progressive nature of South Africa's Constitution has enabled the TAC increasingly to incorporate legal approaches into its fight for affordable medicines for PLHIV and ensure their basic rights. In its legal challenges, TAC has partnered with the AIDS Law Project (ALP), a CSO offering legal assistance on HIV-related issues. One of the more representative examples of this approach is the freedom-of-information case in which TAC successfully forced the Minister of Health to release information about proposed time lines and progress on the implementation of the antiretroviral roll-out.

The TAC found that the Operational Plan on Comprehensive Care and Treatment for HIV and AIDS referred to an item, 'Annexure A', which was not made public by the government and was essential to determine the progress of the antiretroviral roll-out. This delayed the implementation of the plan, made it more difficult for NGOs such as TAC to aid in the roll-out, and resulted in thousands of unnecessary deaths of people with AIDS who were not given antiretrovirals. Ultimately, TAC's legal engagement with the government led to the revelation that the documents referred to existed in draft form only and had never been approved.

The primary significance of this court case, however, is not solely the fact that the Minister was withholding information, but rather that the government was acting as an impediment to working alongside CSOs in rolling out the Operational Plan at the expense of South Africans' lives. As the TAC made clear in its presentation to the court, its goal was to force the Minister of Health to reveal a schedule for the roll-out in order to allow civil society and stakeholders to prepare adequately and aid in the plan's implementation. More importantly, TAC was attempting to give those in need of antiretrovirals a sense of how soon their health might possibly improve.

Countries in which government has supported the roll-out of antiretrovirals, such as Brazil, have had more success with implementation. There are over 90,000 people on treatment in Brazil, and the government has been open to sharing information with other countries looking to confront their HIV epidemics [13]. In South Africa, however, the government appeared to make promises about antiretroviral roll-out while, in reality, it had not finalized an implementation plan.

Role of civil society in tracking roll-out of ARV treatment programmes

As evidenced by the fluconazole campaign and the freedom-of-information case, the community of NGOs in South Africa working in the arena of HIV offers a good example of research organizations and advocacy groups creating strong links to maximize the impact of their efforts. The economical division of labour between research-oriented and advocacy-based NGOs is exemplified in the relationship between the TAC and the ABU. Over the past 2 years, ABU and TAC have developed a cooperative relationship, with ABU providing technical assistance and budget information, and also training TAC staff in provincial and branch offices as well as the National Executive Committee. As part of its effort to provide ready assistance and budget information when needed, ABU has assisted TAC and the ALP with information for court documents and advocacy efforts with respect to provincial expenditure records and drug procurement policy and budgets.

The TAC and other civil society groups have played a critical role in mobilizing support for the roll-out of antiretroviral treatment (ART) in South Africa, and continue to cooperate via various mechanisms to monitor the implementation of the programme and support the roll-out.

The momentum for implementation of ART culminated in 2003, following the formation of a Joint Health and Treasury Task Team tasked with costing and weighing options for the provision of ART by the government. In August 2003, the South African Cabinet instructed the Department of Health (DoH) to develop a 'detailed operational plan' for antiretroviral roll-out; 3 months later, Cabinet approved the Operational Plan [14].

The following year's budget saw R300 million (approximately US$47 million) allocated to provinces for the first year (2004/5) of antiretroviral roll-out [15,16]. Given the urgency of the epidemic, the limited resources available and the significant difference in prevalence rates between provinces, the distribution of these funds among the nine provinces was a critical issue closely watched by the ABU. Of the total antiretroviral allocation, KwaZulu-Natal, Gauteng and Eastern Cape received the largest shares: 21%, 15% and 14%, respectively. How does the HIV disease burden of each province compare with their share of the total funds available for their ART programme?

Figure 48.3 illustrates the provincial share of the total antiretroviral conditional grant funds relative to the provinces' share of the total estimated number of people with AIDS in 2004, according to the Actuarial Society South Africa's (ASSA) 2000 provincial model. KwaZulu-Natal, Gauteng and Mpumalanga received less of the total antiretroviral conditional grant funds than they should have, based on the estimated number of people living with AIDS in those provinces. However, the Western Cape, a wealthier province with strong infrastructure and fewer backlogs, and with around 2% of the total estimated number of people with AIDS in South Africa, received 8% of the antiretroviral conditional grant funds. Notably, the 2005/6 budget allocations retained the same distribution between the provinces.

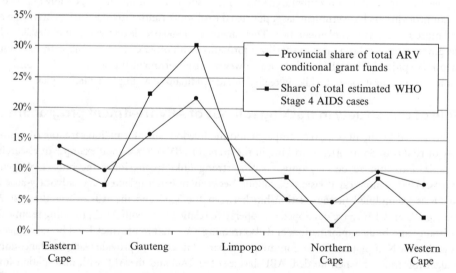

Fig. 48.3 Provincial shares of total antiretroviral (ARV) conditional grant funds compared with provincial HIV burden. Source: [7,17].

The National Treasury and the DoH were responsible for determining the allocation unit costs and provincial shares of total AIDS cases as a starting point for deciding the provincial split, but then adjusted the distribution to take other factors into account. [18]. Those considerations included the varying abilities of provinces to absorb the added funds, the need to cover basic infrastructure costs in low-population provinces, and the need to build the capacity of under-resourced or underspending provinces.

The ABU continued to track which provinces were able to utilize the funds and roll out the programme. Their spending analyses show that aggregate conditional grant spending has improved, but some provinces are still lagging behind. Roll-out has varied considerably across provinces due to readiness, capacity and political will. Tender processes and delays in start-up have created 'lumpy' spending. It also appears that absorption capacity is a more significant constraint to the roll-out than availability of funds. Well-developed, well-resourced provinces are able to utilize resources faster than poorer provinces that still need to improve their service delivery systems. It is becoming clear that the ability of provinces to spend the funds available is a pivotal issue, as well as the willingness of provincial governments to prioritize HIV programmes and ART in their own budget processes.

For these reasons, spending must be closely monitored so that the government is kept on track. This is where civil society can play a critical role in monitoring of public expenditure in order to enhance government commitment and promote more efficient and effective service delivery. The Joint Civil Society Monitoring Forum is a powerful example of this type of effort. The Forum, including TAC, AIDS Legal Network (ALN), Health Systems Trust (HST), the Centre for Health Policy (CHP), MSF and IDASA's ABU, was formed in June 2004 to monitor implementation of the public sector ART programme. ABU's contribution to the joint resolutions of the Forum is the analysis of allocations and expenditure related to the programme, as well as recommendations on how implementing bodies could better access or utilize resources that are already available. This strengthens the impact of the overall results of the Civil Society Monitoring Forum because it enables the integration of financial and non-financial indicators. Too often such a link is not made, and expenditure figures are not tied to impact on services.

The Forum operates on the belief that the successful roll-out of the antiretroviral programme requires government–civil society collaboration and effective monitoring of antiretroviral roll-out by civil society. In a context in which civil society and government relations may be strained, the inclusion of budget analysis in the Forum's activities also facilitates information sharing on the budget between government and the Forum. Using official budget documents as well as provincial interviews, ABU conducts updated analyses of antiretroviral funding and the extent to which antiretroviral resources are being utilized. Such exercises are very important because they empower both government and civil society with information on progress and challenges relating to spending on the antiretroviral programme. Joint resolutions are also put together by Forum members, including budget information, which serve to draw lines of responsibility for dealing with the challenges and improving service delivery.

In summary, applied budget work by CSOs such as the ABU is rooted in our understanding and experience that greater civil society participation in the budget process serves to strengthen the link between public priorities, such as HIV and AIDS, and the allocation of public resources. Our experience in capacity building and training has demonstrated that improved knowledge of the budgeting system increases civil society participation in the budget process. Furthermore, improved civil society participation helps to shape public resource allocation. As a result, better planning when it comes to budgeting and service delivery ultimately increases the effectiveness of those programmes, providing improved prevention, treatment, care and support services to the infected and affected individuals and households.

TAC and local action in treatment, prevention and care

As a research-oriented CSO, the efforts of the ABU are focused on the national and provincial levels, whereas the TAC operates both nationally and at the community level. Locally, TAC has focused on policies and activities that directly affect the lives of members living in the community. This local community involvement can be divided into two categories. The first, direct treatment and counselling for PLHIV, has become a major component of TAC's work through its Treatment Project. The Treatment Literacy programme is the second category, which involves the dissemination of HIV-related information to those in the community most affected by the epidemic.

The Treatment Project

Apart from the support networks that TAC branches provide, one of the deepest impacts that TAC has had on local communities has been through its Treatment Project. The Treatment Project provides antiretroviral medicines to activists and members of the community who are in need of treatment through a network of partner doctors and pharmacists. For each member of TAC who is treated, there is also a non-TAC member of the same community who is sponsored by the Project in order to avoid ethical issues. Community members are selected according to need and potential to meet treatment requirements; money donated to the Treatment Project is allocated to help them obtain a slot at public facilities. Treatment for members of the TAC is administered by the Treatment Project itself. In treating people with AIDS, the Treatment Project commits itself to providing treatment for 5 years and never selects a patient without having 3 years' worth of funds allocated for that patient.

The Treatment Project developed as members of TAC saw too many of their own activists dying because they could not afford antiretrovirals or other medicines to treat opportunistic infections. The loss of experienced and beloved members of the organization meant that the TAC needed to find a way to provide medication if it was to continue fighting for the rights of HIV-positive South Africans. Because of the underlying values of the TAC, the Treatment Project could not provide only private medical access to its members without also finding a way to supplement the public health infrastructure. By helping the public sector to match each TAC member receiving antiretrovirals with an HIV-positive person in the community, the Treatment Project is helping to build the health systems and proving that receiving ART is possible in resource-poor settings.

The impact of the Treatment Project has been significant. The Treatment Project currently has over 100 people on treatment and is working to increase that number to 1000 in the near future. TAC's Treatment Project has particularly appealed to people who want to support HIV campaigns. Most recently, large-scale funds have been raised for the project through the publication of *Telling Tales*, a book edited by Nobel Prize laureate Nadine Gordimer, and through the launch of an annual concert in cooperation with Levi Strauss & Co. The Treatment Project is growing to include more participants while staying true to TAC's goal of providing antiretroviral medications to those who need them in the public sector.

Treatment Literacy

Direct community involvement has also been supplemented through TAC's Treatment Literacy work, which includes publication of materials aimed at educating the public about HIV and AIDS, providing information about counselling and testing sites, and making sure that people understand what taking antiretroviral medicines entails. The Treatment Literacy programme has published a TAC booklet entitled *HIV in our Lives*, which provides guidance to people living with HIV, including advice on how to get tested, what types of feelings you should expect if you are diagnosed with the disease, basic information about the virus, common opportunistic infections, eating healthily and where to find support. Other publications by the Treatment Literacy programme include *A Guide to Treating Opportunistic Infections for People Living with HIV/ AIDS*; *Pregnancy and HIV: A Practical Guide*; a fact sheet on tuberculosis (TB) and HIV co-infection, and a pamphlet on prevention of mother-to-child transmission of HIV. More recently, the Treatment Literacy programme has produced a series of informative posters on various opportunistic infections and their treatments as well as a series on antiretrovirals. These posters are displayed throughout the country at TAC branches, public health clinics, churches, meeting halls and in the offices of partner organizations such as MSF and the Congress of South African Trade Unions (COSATU).

These materials are used in conjunction with treatment literacy workshops where TAC members are trained to be treatment literacy practitioners. These workshops range from half-day crash courses to week-long retreats that cover a range of topics such as the science of HIV, basic biology and human anatomy, health rights, global governance, nutrition, opportunistic infections, antiretrovirals and side effects. Treatment Literacy Practitioners (TLPs) are then able to help educate other TAC members and the general public about HIV. Through branch meetings and support groups, TLPs hold open discussions about the biological workings of HIV, the importance of getting tested, what HIV-positive people can expect when starting treatment, and other related issues. The Treatment Literacy programme addresses these issues head-on and works to counteract the misinformation that often pervades poor communities with low levels of education.

There are two important aspects of the Treatment Literacy programme that supplement TAC's work. The first is the programme's obvious mission—educating the public on what it is like to live with HIV or AIDS and on how to control the disease. The Treatment Literacy programme has been successful in training dedicated educators from within the community who are able to spread these messages very effectively at local level. Through this approach, the Treatment Literacy programme is demonstrating that such knowledge can be used and disseminated in resource-poor settings, thereby counteracting the argument that people living in such settings cannot understand the complexities of HIV treatment. Such views are embodied most prominently by Andrew Natsios, former head of the US Agency for International Development (USAID), who suggested that Africans were incapable of taking antiretrovirals because they could not tell the time [19]. Treatment-literate TAC members are able to understand when they need to take their medications.

The second aspect of the Treatment Literacy programme is tied to the fact that knowledge is directly connected to empowerment. The Treatment Literacy programme has empowered community members so that they feel able to understand treatments and are no longer so dependent upon their doctors. We have found that this knowledge transfer is facilitated by using community members as TLPs because people are much more trusting and willing to listen to someone they can identify with, as opposed to an outsider. Furthermore, TLPs have a perspective more closely aligned with the people they are teaching than doctors or nurses have, and they capitalize on their familiarity with the day-to-day issues of PLHIV in order to make the information relevant.

Increasing the number of informed citizens is central to controlling the HIV epidemic, especially in a country with a poor healthcare system. South Africa's health system is in crisis, with only one doctor for every 5000 people [20]. Nurses and doctors are overworked and often do not have enough time to explain fully to their patients what HIV is. There are now clinics with trained HIV counsellors, but getting to this point has been slow, and there are still far too few.

The Treatment Literacy programme, through educating on a community level, provides support to the public health sector. Patients are able to understand why they are falling ill, and community members who know about HIV can ensure that their local clinics have the necessary medications and trained staff to administer HIV treatment properly. Knowledgeable patients can interact with their healthcare providers with more dignity and can demand treatments by name if need be. Treatment-literate community members also help to ensure that the roll-out of antiretrovirals will be successful.

Community action

The TAC's national agenda largely stems from its local work. For example, Lorna Mlofana, a TAC treatment educator from Khayelitsha, was sexually assaulted and murdered after a group of young men found out that she was HIV-positive. In response, in November 2004, the TAC-Khayelitsha district initiated a month of action to stop the abuse of women and children. The action included a number of activities and culminated in a gathering of 1000 TAC activists from the Khayelitsha area. Among the demands at this meeting was a call for the establishment of a rape centre, which the government had promised the September before. Because over 40% of rapes in the Western Cape occur in Khayelitsha, there was an immediate need for local services. Through this community action, the Director of HIV in the Western Cape promised to make the Simelela clinic an acute rape centre.

Other community actions have also been very important. A number of TAC branches, dissatisfied with their public health facilities, have called on their provincial governments to improve the management and infrastructure of these clinics. Clinics with a chronic under-supply of certain medicines have also been singled out by TAC branches with the aim of improving access to treatment for the general community. More recently, TAC branches have had to counteract misinformation campaigns regarding antiretroviral medication and the TAC itself. Branches provide factual information to concerned community members and have played a role in ensuring local media outlets do not carry advertisements that make false claims about antiretrovirals and TAC.

Problems and challenges

While the TAC has had remarkable success in its short history, it is also prudent to acknowledge the difficulties and failures that the organization has undergone. It is from these lessons that TAC continues to evaluate and redefine itself, and therefore the organization views these 'problems' as indispensable to its improvement. Other organizations may be able to avoid certain pitfalls by taking note of the following challenges that TAC has faced.

South Africa's HIV epidemic disproportionately affects the black population of the country, which, in turn, creates a wedge in the psyche of many non-black South Africans. Members of these groups may not feel as though the epidemic in the country is their concern, since their populations do not suffer to the same extent as the black population. While TAC firmly understands that HIV is not class- or race-specific, many of its programmes and efforts are restricted to the more impoverished and vulnerable communities within South Africa. In turn, TAC is viewed by some sectors of society as primarily a voice for the poor and black communities. This branding of the organization undermines its greater goal of improving the health of the country as a whole and shedding light on the disastrous role HIV plays in South Africa.

It is difficult for TAC to address the most pressing HIV-related needs of South Africans without focusing on the communities in which the HIV is most prevalent. Furthermore, support for TAC within the more well-to-do communities is often tacit at best, which has as much to do with the history of South Africa as it does with the low prevalence of HIV in these areas. To counteract this imbalance, TAC has recently adjusted its campaign efforts to include a wider segment of society. Examples include the placement of white and coloured people in Treatment Literacy posters to visually underscore HIV's colour-blindness. More potently, TAC has taken on a more aggressive approach with the South African media. Every week, stories related to TAC's activities can be found in the South African newspapers with the widest circulation, and TAC makes regular use of press conferences. This regular discourse with the media ensures that members of society who are not direct beneficiaries of TAC's work are nonetheless apprised of the organization's activities.

As in many CSOs and CBOs in the HIV field, women make up the majority of TAC's staff and membership [21]. While this is related to cultural issues, the lack of male responsibility for HIV as evidenced by gender discrepancy in these organizations is a serious hindrance to the long-term containment of HIV in South Africa. In addition, TAC—again like most HIV CBOs— relies on volunteers who are often HIV-positive [22]. Because treatment is still not widely available in South Africa, many members will eventually succumb to the virus. This causes continual emotional hardship within the organization, as well as human resource issues.

Another challenge facing TAC is its relationship with government. While TAC has, at times, overtly supported the national government—for instance, in the Pharmaceutical Manufacturer's Association case against the government—it can also be in direct opposition to the government. On the other hand, TAC often works amicably with provincial governments. For example, the Western Cape province supported TAC's antiretroviral roll-out demands and circumvented the national DoH in order to provide antiretrovirals while the central government's tender awaited finalization. When TAC held its People's Health Summit in May 2005, leading officials from the Western Cape DoH attended and engaged in discussions. This inconsistent response from government highlights one of the largest obstacles to TAC's goals. No matter how successful TAC and other organizations are in the short term, the HIV epidemic in South Africa cannot be controlled without concerted and legitimate support from all levels of government and society.

Conclusion

The impact that CSOs and CBOs have had on South Africa's HIV epidemic is both promising and instructive. Partnership and collaboration among these organizations, as evidenced by the TAC and the ABU at IDASA, for example, have bolstered their individual efforts and strengthened the forces of change that are attempting to influence the course of the HIV epidemic in this country. While the organizations' work may be limited, to an extent, by the national government, government assistance at provincial and district levels indicates that political equivocation is not practised by everyone in government, and provides examples of successful collaboration between CSOs, CBOs and government. Ultimately, these organizations aim to inform and educate the public in order to improve the quality of life for South Africans. When a critical mass is reached, the government will have no choice but to listen to the demands of the people. The CSOs and CBOs involved in HIV work in South Africa will do their best to usher in that time.

References

1. Lebeloe C. (2002). *Report of the First South African National Home/Community Based Care Conference.* Republic of South Africa: National Department of Health. Online at http://www.futuresgroup.com/abstract.cfm/ 3174.

2. Tshabalala-Msimang M. (2005). Monitoring and Evaluation Media Briefing. May 5, 2005. Republic of South Africa: National Department of Health. Online at http:// www.info.gov.za/speeches/2005/05050610451003.htm.

3. *Plusnews.* (2005). South Africa: volunteer caregivers being exploited, says study. January 21, 2005. Health Systems Trust. Online at http://www.hst.org.za/news/20040618.

4. Fox S. (2002). *Integrated Community-based Home Care (ICHC) in South Africa: A Review of the Model Implemented by the Hospice Association of South Africa.* The Centre for AIDS Development, Research and Evaluation (Cadre). Online at http://www.futuresgroup.com/abstract.cfm/3164.

5. Russell M, Schneider H. (2000). *A Rapid Appraisal of Community-based Care and Support Programmes in South Africa.* Johannesburg: Centre for Health Policy, University of Witwatersrand.

6. Cullinan K. (2000). Community Based Care, HST Update #58. Health Systems Trust. Online at http:// www.hst.org.za/uploads/files/upd58.pdf.

7. Dorrington R, Bradshaw D, Budlender D. (2002). *HIV/AIDS Profile in the Provinces of South Africa: Indicators for 2002.* MRC, ASSA, UCT Technical Report. National HIV Prevalence, Behavioural Risks and Mass Media. Household Survey 2002. Cape Town: HSRC Publishers.

8. Guthrie G, Hickey A, eds. (2004). *Funding the Fight: Budgeting for HIV and AIDS in Developing Countries.* Cape Town: AIDS Budget Unit, Idasa Budget Information Service.

9. Hickey A, Ndlovu N, Guthrie T. (2003). *Budgeting for HIV/AIDS in South Africa: Report on Intergovernmental Funding Flows for an Integrated Response in the Social Sector.* Cape Town: AIDS Budget Unit, Idasa Budget Information Service.

10. National Treasury, Republic of South Africa. (2004). *Trends in Intergovernmental Finances: 2000/ 1–2006/7.*

11. National Treasury, Republic of South Africa. (2005). *Estimates of National Expenditure 2005.*

12. National Treasury, Republic of South Africa. Statements of the National and Provincial Governments' Revenue, Expenditure and National Borrowing as at March 31, 2002, at March 31, 2003 and at March 31, 2004. Online at www.treasury.gov.za.

13. Ministry of Health, Brazil. AIDS drugs policy. Online at http://www.aids.gov.br/assistencia/aids_drugs_policy.htm.

14. National Department of Health. (2003). *Operational Plan for Comprehensive HIV and AIDS Care, Management and Treatment for South Africa.* Pretoria: National Department of Health.

15. National Treasury, Republic of South Africa. (2004). *Budget Review 2004.* February 18, 2004.

16. National Treasury, Republic of South Africa. (2004). *Budget Review 2005*. February 23, 2004.

17. National Treasury, Republic of South Africa. (2004). *2004 Division of Revenue Bill.*

18. National Treasury, Republic of South Africa. (2004). *Estimates of National Expenditure 2004.*

19. Attaran A, Freedberg KA, Hirsch M. (2001). Dead wrong on AIDS. *Washington Post.* June 15, 2001.

20. McClelland C. (2002). South African brain drain costing $5 billion—and counting. *Canadian Medical Association Journal* **167**:793.

21. Akintola O. (2004). *A Gendered Analysis of the Burden of Care on Family and Volunteer Caregivers in Uganda and South Africa*. Durban: Health Economics and HIV/AIDS Research Division (HEARD), University of KwaZulu-Natal. Online at http://www.nu.ac.za/heard/research/ResearchReports/2004/Gendered%20Analysis%20of%20Burden%20of%20Care%20-%20Uganda%20%20SA.pdf.

22. Manning R. (2002). *The Impact of HIV/AIDS on Civil Society*. Durban: Health Economics and HIV/AIDS Research Division (HEARD), University of KwaZulu-Natal. Online at http://www.nu.ac.za/heard/research/ResearchReports/2002/ NGO%20Report%20%20Toolkit.pdf.

Strengthening the Response

Chapter 49

Responding effectively to the HIV pandemic

Catherine Hankins[*], Chris Fontaine and Michel Sidibe

The HIV pandemic is an extraordinary kind of a crisis. It is both an emergency and a long-term development issue, and cannot be simply lumped together with the world's many emergencies. HIV is exceptional for many reasons, but primarily because it affects young adults in their most productive years, and because HIV has a long incubation period from infection to manifest disease during which it can be unknowingly transmitted to others. As yet, there is neither a cure nor a vaccine. HIV requires an exceptional response that remains flexible, creative, energetic and vigilant. There is no room for complacency.

Although a cure remains elusive, two decades of tackling HIV have shown that the natural course of the epidemic can be changed with the right combination of leadership and comprehensive action, even in low- and middle-income countries. Forthright national leadership, widespread public awareness and comprehensive prevention efforts at scale have enabled nations such as Uganda and Cambodia to reduce HIV transmission. Decisive action in Thailand averted some 5 million HIV infections during the 1990s. On every continent there are now cities, regions or states where concerted efforts have kept the epidemic at bay.

Starting in 2000, coordinated national and international action slashed the prices of antiretroviral medicines in low- and middle-income countries. In September 2003, at the second UN General Assembly Special Session on HIV/AIDS [1], the World Health Organization (WHO) and the Joint UN Programme on HIV/AIDS (UNAIDS) declared the lack of treatment in low- and middle-income countries a global public health emergency and announced the '3 by 5' Initiative to place 3 million people on antiretroviral treatment (ART) by the end of 2005 [2,3]. This interim target is part of a global movement to mobilize support for vastly expanded—and ultimately universal—treatment access. Universal access to treatment of HIV as a chronic disease will require a significant expansion of healthcare and other social services. Health systems will need strengthening, and concerted efforts will be required to increase respect for human rights. Such a goal may seem lofty, but recent progress shows that it is not impossible. Many countries have incorporated ART into their national HIV plans, setting specific ART coverage targets. Sustained efforts are now under way to make access to these life-prolonging medicines a reality for people living with HIV (PLHIV) who are desperately in need.

* Corresponding author.

The veil of silence and stigma that has crippled efforts to respond to HIV is finally lifting in many countries. Leaders of governments, businesses, and religious and cultural institutions are increasingly coming forward to take action against HIV. The movement of PLHIV has become a global force in the vanguard of social change in responding to the epidemic. The impact of HIV on development prospects in the worst-affected regions is being increasingly recognized, and action is under way to make necessary fundamental shifts in development practice.

This progress cannot be allowed to foster complacency. The international campaign for treatment scale-up has yielded impressive results—access to treatment in low- and middle-income countries increased from 400,000 in June 2004 to 700,000 at the end of 2004 [4,5]. However, the goal of '3 by 5' will not be reached on time, and the road to universal access will be long and hard. More sophisticated monitoring and evaluation of the epidemic's behaviour reveal the scale of the challenge: fewer than one in five people who need prevention services and tools have access to them [6]. Globally, 5–6 million people need antiretroviral medicines now, yet only 12% of them in low- and middle-income countries have access to these drugs.

An unprecedented level of financial resources is now available to tackle HIV, but it is still less than half of what is really needed. Even these funds are not being applied in a fully effective, coordinated manner. In some instances, HIV funding sits idle, blocked in government bank accounts or stalled by rules of international funders. The result: the HIV epidemic is now at a true crossroads. If the world's response to HIV continues in its well-meaning but haphazard and ineffectual fashion, then the global epidemic will continue to outpace the response. This chapter reviews the response to HIV to date at global and country levels, and proposes concrete actions to face the challenges ahead.

Global-level responses

At global level, the response to HIV has increased dramatically in the past decade. The United Nations, its member states, civil society, international foundations, non-governmental organizations (NGOs) and the private sector have all acknowledged the deadly challenge of HIV and taken action.

United Nations

The United Nations system is committed to the effective implementation of the 2001 Declaration of Commitment on HIV which all UN member states signed in 2001 [1]. Twenty-nine individual UN agencies have taken global leadership roles on AIDS in their areas of specialization. UNAIDS now has 10 co-sponsoring agencies working together, with each agency taking the lead in its areas of comparative advantage (Box 49.1).

The UN Secretary-General's four Special Envoys on HIV have increased HIV-related political, donor, civil society and media attention. For example, Nafis Sadik, the Special Envoy for Asia, boosted Nepal's human rights approach to HIV. In several Caribbean countries, Dr George Alleyne, the Special Envoy for the Caribbean, encouraged legal reforms and steps to reduce HIV-related stigma and discrimination. Meanwhile, the UN Special Envoy for Eastern Europe and Central Asia, Dr Lars Kalling, increased awareness of how injecting drug use is a key factor in HIV spread. In Africa, Stephen Lewis, the Special Envoy for that region, joined with James T Morris, Executive Director of the World Food Programme (WFP) and the UN Secretary-General's Special Envoy for Humanitarian Needs in Southern Africa, to raise awareness about Southern Africa's deadly combination of HIV, drought and shrinking human capacity.

> ## Box 49.1 **UNAIDS' Co-sponsoring Agencies**
>
> United Nations Office on Drugs and Crime (UNODC)—injecting drug users
> United Nations Population Fund (UNFPA)—gender and young people
> United Nations Educational, Scientific and Cultural Organization (UNESCO)—education
> United Nations Children's Fund (UNICEF)—orphans, children and mother-to-child transmission
> International Labour Organization (ILO)—HIV and the workplace
> United Nations Development Programme (UNDP)—HIV, governance and development
> World Health Organization (WHO)—treatment and care
> World Bank—Multi-Country HIV/AIDS Program (MAP)
> World Food Programme (WFP)—food security
> United Nations High Commission for Refugees—displaced persons

In 2003, responding to the increasing feminization of the HIV epidemic, UNAIDS launched the Global Coalition on Women and AIDS. It brings together PLHIV, civil society leaders, celebrity activists, NGO representatives and UN figures to facilitate collaboration and to support innovative scaling up of efforts that have an impact on women's and girls' lives. Each of the following seven focal areas of action is convened by a UN agency and a civil society partner:

♦ preventing HIV infection among girls and young women;

♦ reducing violence against women;

♦ protecting girls' and women's property and inheritance rights;

♦ ensuring girls' and women's equal access to treatment and care;

♦ supporting community-based care with a special focus on girls and women;

♦ promoting women's access to new prevention technologies and supporting ongoing efforts towards girls' universal education.

Bilateral contributions

Forty years ago, the Organisation for Economic Co-operation and Development (OECD) called for high-income countries to contribute at least 0.7% of their gross national product to official development assistance, and this goal was adopted by UN Member States. However, so far, only five countries have met this target: Denmark, Luxembourg, The Netherlands, Norway and Sweden. There has been renewed global commitment to work in partnership to achieve the Millennium Development Goals and to overcome conditions fuelling the HIV epidemic, such as poverty, hunger and inequality.

Ensuring there are adequate funds to mount an effective global response to the HIV epidemic has proven difficult. However, in recent years there has been an unprecedented increase in global financial resources. In 1996, when UNAIDS was launched, available HIV funding in low- and middle-income countries totalled US$300 million. This amount represented contributions by bilateral donors, international NGOs and the UN system, notably the World Bank. By 2004, an estimated US$6.1 billion was available for the HIV response that year. Yet this amount is only half of what was required by 2005, and an even smaller proportion of what will be required by 2007 to mount a comprehensive response to HIV in low- and middle-income countries.

Nonetheless, there are some positive signs. The Secretary-General's call in Abuja in 2001 for a 'war chest' to fight HIV, tuberculosis (TB) and malaria led, in January 2002, to the setting up of the Global Fund to Fight AIDS, Tuberculosis and Malaria (Global Fund) as a partnership between governments, civil society and the private sector. Its mandate is to provide new money and create new ways to disburse funds to fight these three diseases that between them kill more than 6 million people every year. As of April 2005, cumulative disbursements had reached US$1.1 billion out of a total commitment in signed grant agreements of US$2.3 billion. This equals 54% of the US$2 billion targeted to be disbursed by the end of 2005 [7]. With approximately US$5.9 billion pledged through 2008, the Global Fund has been a major contributor to the overall increase in resources to fight AIDS, TB and malaria. In terms of funds disbursed to programmes fighting the three diseases, the Global Fund now contributes 20% of the total international investment disbursed to programmes fighting AIDS, 50% of the total disbursed to fight TB and 45% of the total disbursed for malaria.

About 60% of these funds are earmarked for HIV programmes, 23% to malaria and 17% to TB. To date, sub-Saharan Africa, the region with the greatest disease burden and the scarcest resources, has received 60% of the grant money.

By May 2005, US$6.1 billion had been pledged up to 2008 and beyond, and US$3.6 billion had actually been paid into the Global Fund's bank account. However, more donor assistance is urgently needed to close the financing gap in health in the poorest countries of the world [8,9]. To help ease the uncertainty under which the Fund operates, 100 NGOs around the world started the 'Fund the Fight' coalition, a campaign for regular and committed Global Fund supporters.

Also helping to close the gap are the many low- and middle-income countries now making far greater domestic investments on HIV. The World Bank's Multi-Country HIV/AIDS Program for Africa (MAP and TAP), the US President's Emergency Plan for AIDS Relief (PEPFAR), along with real evidence that other donor governments are finally becoming serious about addressing the resource constraints, are all encouraging. The UK International Finance Facility proposal and the French fuel tax initiative are promising developments to ensure more sustainable and predictable donor funding.

However laudable and important all this is, the African countries worst affected by HIV would gain far more in financial resources from the cancellation of debts, from the ending of rich-world agricultural subsidies and trade barriers, and from truly affordable prices for pharmaceuticals. For too many years, billions of dollars annually have gone to servicing debt that African countries could have put to use investing in the AIDS response, education and other critical development fronts.

Public expenditure ceilings, such as those set in Medium Term Expenditure Frameworks, restrict the levels of investment across all sectors needed to mount an exceptional HIV response. The goal of financing an exceptional response needs to be balanced with fiscal and economic discipline and good sense, with solutions found as they have been for post-conflict or post-disaster situations. After the Second World War, the Marshall Plan for Europe required setting aside public expenditure ceilings. A dialogue with the International Monetary Fund and donors was begun in 2004 to emphasize the urgency of finding solutions, creating fiscal space [10] and minimizing macroeconomic effects of large funding flows. There is growing recognition that increased spending on HIV is a capital investment, not just an expenditure item, because such investments focus on restocking and protecting human capital.

The 2002 Monterrey Conference on Financing for Development marked a new step toward international burden sharing to meet key global development challenges. Participating countries made pledges that would translate into an increased official development assistance resource flow from US$58 billion in 2002 to US$75 billion in 2006, or from 0.23 to 0.29% of gross national income. This would provide significant additional funds, but it still falls abysmally short of the 0.7% commitment.

All stakeholders need to continue exploring innovative ways of raising domestic and international resources to deal with shared concerns about the developmental, economic, social and political impact of HIV. In the most-affected countries, HIV has taken its toll on essential development resources and capacities. However, investing in HIV prevention, HIV treatment and impact mitigation has proven to be good development practice and, in some countries, an imperative for national survival. The benefit of investing early to avoid higher costs later is particularly obvious in the case of HIV. Most industrialized countries will need to propose bold increases in their direct assistance to poorer countries for HIV programming. For maximum impact, these must be additional resources and not funds diverted from other priority development programmes aimed at reaching other Millennium Development Goals.

Effectively using increased official development assistance resources calls for all involved to recognize fully the developmental dimensions of HIV, as well as the HIV dimension of development. Countries need to strengthen their national capacity to move towards HIV-sensitive budgeting and to use funds efficiently and effectively. Donor efforts to harmonize practices to reduce transaction costs are a priority for effective use of funds. There must be clear recognition that regular development work forms the basis for virtually all HIV interventions, in addition to ameliorating the conditions that create underlying vulnerability to HIV: addressing poverty and inequity, strengthening physical infrastructure, and building capacity.

Civil society

At global level, civil society has been pivotal in the response to HIV. NGOs such as the International Coalition of AIDS Service Organisations (ICASO), the Global Network of People Living with HIV (GNP+), the International Community of Women living with HIV (ICW) and others have been actively representing their constituencies on the boards of the Global Fund and UNAIDS, as well as on the organizing committees of various international HIV conferences. The International AIDS Alliance conducts studies to synthesize civil society perspectives and undertakes capacity-building initiatives to support local NGO responses. The World AIDS Campaign is a coalition of civil society organizations that supports World AIDS Day activities on December 1 each year along with mobilization around HIV issues throughout the year.

Private sector

Recognizing that the HIV epidemic is profoundly affecting global businesses through its impact on workers, customers and markets, the Global Business Coalition on HIV/AIDS works to increase business involvement in the global HIV response. It helps companies to implement workplace, employee and community prevention, care and support programmes; to use business innovation and flexibility to make HIV programmes more effective; and to carry out business advocacy and leadership promoting greater HIV action and partnerships with governments and communities.

In recent years, public–private partnerships have emerged as a way of redressing the HIV-related resource imbalance between low- and middle-income and industrialized countries. The Global Fund is a prime example. The Accelerating Access Initiative, which helped bring down antiretroviral prices; the International AIDS Vaccine Initiative, which conducts advocacy and research for an HIV vaccine; the International HIV Treatment Access Coalition, which worked to create enabling conditions for treatment scale-up; the Global HIV Vaccine Enterprise, which is fostering concerted action by partners to fast-track development of an HIV vaccine; and the Stop TB Partnership, which addresses TB and TB/HIV issues, are examples of such international partnerships in the HIV field.

Monitoring the global response

As part of follow-up activities to the 2001 UN Declaration of Commitment on HIV/AIDS, the UNAIDS Secretariat and co-sponsors collaboratively developed a series of global, regional and national indicators to measure the world's progress in reaching the Declaration's targets.

In 2003, 103 Member States of the UN provided UNAIDS with national reports on their progress, which formed the basis of a comprehensive assessment of global, regional and national responses to AIDS. It was called the *Progress Report on the Global Response to the HIV/AIDS Epidemic, 2003* [11].

In 2004, key elements of this material were updated further by a study called *Coverage of Selected Services for HIV/AIDS Prevention and Care in Low- and Middle-income Countries in 2003* [6]. These two reports present progress on key global and national indicators in areas such as national response scale-up, resources, eliminating stigma and discrimination, and prevention and treatment programmes.

Examples of key findings include the following: global funding available to respond to HIV almost tripled since 2002, but remains seriously inadequate, and, due to various blockages, is not reaching those who need it most; 38% of countries still have not adopted HIV-related anti-discrimination legislation; only one in five people have access to prevention services, and nearly one-third of countries lack policies that ensure women's equal access to critical prevention and care services. The goal of the UNAIDS report was to spur all stakeholders to generate even greater commitment towards achieving the 2001 UN Declaration of Commitment targets. Information from the UNAIDS Country Response Information System (CRIS), which supports the management of national information, was used to prepare the 2005 report on global progress towards the targets for the UN General Assembly Special Session on AIDS in June 2005 [12].

Country responses

For two decades, the HIV epidemic has been tightening its grip on development. Lack of resources in low- and middle-income countries has hindered their ability to develop effective national responses to their HIV epidemics. Now that funds are beginning to become available, many countries with generalized epidemics face the challenge of ensuring that new resources are efficiently absorbed into a growing and sustainable national HIV response. A major roadblock is the lack of national capacity. A paucity of well-trained individuals, crumbling infrastructure and an absence of modern technology prevents rapid scale-up of HIV initiatives to critical coverage levels. In the hardest-hit countries, HIV-related migration, illness and death are draining precious governmental capacities. This, in turn, contributes to the epidemic's spread, causes other development efforts to fail and creates a vicious cycle.

Even in settings that are more resource-rich, HIV prevention and HIV treatment and care are complex problems that require a complex, multipronged response. Strong national leadership and ownership, good governance, multisectoral planning and coordination, resource mobilization, reinforced capacity to absorb resources and implement programmes, close monitoring and evaluation, and the significant participation of communities, civil society and the private sector are all needed. As more external stakeholders offer assistance, it is increasingly important to create donor harmonization and coherence around national structures, strategic plans, and monitoring and evaluation systems.

The Three Ones

The need for donor harmonization has been of increasing concern as funding flows have increased. Lack of harmonization among donors at country level creates inefficiencies, with the result that precious resources are wasted and people who need help do not receive it. Duplicate efforts by donors are major obstacles to the response against HIV. For example, in several countries in Africa and Asia, there were 50 or more donor HIV planning missions in 2004 alone. With each visit, understaffed agencies push aside pressing work to take donors on site visits. Countries must often satisfy donor conditions that are not a part of their national HIV strategy, and scarce staff time is absorbed filling out paperwork rather than saving lives. Although this problem has long been true of development work in every sector, the exceptional crisis is accelerating donor harmonization and alignment around national priorities.

In April 2004, at a meeting in Washington, DC co-chaired by UNAIDS, the UK and the USA, an historic agreement was reached by donors and low- and middle-income countries to work more effectively together in scaling up national HIV responses. They adopted three core principles for concerted country-level action—the Three Ones (see Box 49.2). The concepts of national ownership, multisectorality, mainstreaming, harmonization and coherence have been combined into these principles, which aim to increase the pace of the HIV response and promote more effective use of resources by clarifying relevant roles and relationships. This demand-driven approach is not surprising, as national HIV programmes of African countries led the development of the Three Ones at the 2003 International Conference on AIDS and STIs in Africa. The principles were later endorsed in January 2005 by 45 heads of state at the African Union Summit in Abuja.

Unfortunately, global agreement on the Three Ones has not translated into global adherence to them. Competing donor priorities, territorialism among multilateral agencies, and host–country infighting has slowed progress. In March 2005, commitment to the Three Ones was renewed at a meeting in London convened by the UK, the USA, France and UNAIDS. A Global Task Team was formed to develop recommendations for new methods and mechanisms to

---

Box 49.2 The three core principles for concerted country-level action: the Three Ones

One agreed AIDS Action Framework that provides the basis for coordinating the work of all partners;
One National AIDS Coordinating Authority with a broad-based multisectoral mandate;
One agreed country-level Monitoring and Evaluation system.

make the Three Ones a reality. It is too early to tell whether this initiative will lead to a significant acceleration in country-level coordination and alignment, but the continued support of the Three Ones is reason for optimism.

Political commitment

Unfortunately, the Three Ones cannot work without a strong national political will to tackle the HIV epidemic. However, in many countries, national leaders refuse even to talk about HIV. The hardest-hit countries in Africa have learned the harsh lesson of inaction. Political commitment has recently increased as the voices of those affected by the epidemic overwhelm those in denial. Still, in many countries where HIV is quickly spreading, such as those in Asia and Eastern Europe, a lack of leadership raises fears that these countries will not adequately address the epidemic until it is too late.

In sub-Saharan Africa, the epidemic's scale is convincing leaders in countries such as Kenya, Botswana, Malawi and Lesotho to take personal responsibility for implementing the national AIDS response [13]. The world's two most populous countries, China and India, have made leadership breakthroughs. Regional entities such as the Association of South-East Asian Nations (ASEAN), the United Nations Economic and Social Commission for Asia and the Pacific, the Pan Caribbean Partnership against HIV/AIDS and the Commonwealth of Independent States (CIS) are active in highlighting HIV as a development issue requiring a multisectoral response. In February 2004, high-level government representatives from 53 countries attended the European Union's Breaking the Barriers Conference in Dublin and pledged to achieve concrete HIV-related targets within Europe and Central Asia.

Traditional and religious leaders can also make an impact. Examples are as diverse as the Great Council of Chiefs in Fiji; the Malian League of Imams and Islamic Scholars; the South Asia Inter-Faith Consultation on Children, Young People and AIDS; the South African Anglican Church; the South African NGO Positive Muslims; the Ramakrishna Centre in Durban; the Hindu Council of Africa; and the Samaritan Ministry in the Bahamas.

Governance

Democratic and efficient development activities depend on good governance, full constituent participation, the rule of law, transparency, community responsiveness, consensus building, equity, effectiveness and accountability. These are complex and interrelated issues, but they have concrete applications. For example, countries with high levels of constituent participation generally have more dynamic national HIV responses. South Africa's recent treatment and care policy changes were spurred on by steady pressure from the country's HIV-positive community, prominent legal and health professionals and many national and international NGOs. An open, participatory governance system allowed for civil society to provoke positive change.

Similarly, the rule of law is based on legislation and regulations, and on citizens being fully aware of their rights and how to protect them within existing legal frameworks and policies [14]. Applying rule of law and good governance concepts to AIDS activities inspires democratic planning and implementation. In 2002, the UN Secretary-General established a Commission on HIV/AIDS and Governance in Africa to combine applied research, policy dialogue and advocacy. The Commission is based at the Economic Commission for Africa in Addis Ababa, Ethiopia. It matches current knowledge gained from HIV responses with knowledge gaps, and works to make good governance relevant to Africa's policy-makers and implementers. In a similar vein, UNDP's South-East Asia HIV and Development Programme has strongly promoted good governance in HIV responses in countries such as China, the Lao People's Democratic Republic and Vietnam [15]. In Eastern Europe, UNDP promotes creating open and inclusive environments. This includes comprehensive, multisectoral policies and innovative partnerships that build trust and reduce stigma to turn back the epidemic.

Civil society

Community groups and civil society organizations that emerge in the HIV response reflect the diversity of those affected by the epidemic. All have a key role to play. Civil society organizations often have innovative approaches to the epidemic and can channel funds to communities, augment state service delivery and monitor national government policies. PLHIV particularly need to be involved in all aspects of the response, from planning and decision making to implementation and review. They should play a major role in ART programmes, particularly in helping people gain access to care and in assisting patients with treatment adherence. Also, when they are supported to play an active role in HIV prevention programmes, they can be particularly effective in making HIV real to peers.

Civil society organizations are most valuable and effective if they work with, rather than in parallel to, governments. Both sides need to be open to partnerships, and it is up to governments to provide a positive environment. Factors that enable these groups to contribute include legal recognition, tax incentives, streamlined contracting regulations and agreed-upon ground rules to involve them in decision making and information sharing. In addition, both sides need to adopt measures to ensure accountability and transparency. At the community level, governments' administrative procedures must be flexible enough to include local NGOs. Legal obstacles need to be overcome. For example, many government agencies in countries of Eastern Europe and the CIS cannot transfer funds to the accounts of NGOs or subcontract programme activities to them [16]. Many NGOs often have their own problems, including inadequate skills and capacity, high staff turnover and a mistrust of authorities that is not always justified. Actions to resolve these issues include improved staff training, dialogue between state and non-state participants and legal frameworks for the activities of NGOs.

Working in partnerships to respond to HIV

National HIV authorities are increasingly turning to formal partnership forums to stimulate non-governmental participation, broaden national ownership of the response and increase transparency. This approach was first developed in Africa under the International Partnership against AIDS in Africa. The concept is now more widespread, but its best examples are still in sub-Saharan Africa. For example, the Uganda AIDS Partnership is a national coordinating mechanism of nine 'constituencies' working on HIV that represent all stakeholders at all levels. They share information and jointly plan and coordinate activities. In neighbouring Kenya, an annual Joint AIDS Programme Review by all stakeholders supports the country's multisectoral response, linking its strategic plan and other important policy-making processes.

Both the World Bank MAP and the Global Fund aim to involve civil society in direct ways. The MAP works through its financing channels to NGOs, while the Global Fund explicitly requires NGOs to participate in its Country Coordinating Mechanisms that prepare proposals for AIDS-related projects.

Working with civil society is a constant process of learning and adapting for everyone involved. Many NGOs do not have enough resources or technical and managerial skills, and need to receive technical and financial support to improve their networking and participating capacity. Governmental partners need to adopt more positive attitudes about working with NGOs [17] and understand the potential fruits of partnerships with them.

Businesses can contribute to the HIV response at different levels, depending on their size, type and location. Their three main contributions are in the form of workplace programmes, leadership and advocacy for HIV work, and partnerships with the community and government for a strengthened response to the epidemic. A business can influence its sourcing partners and distributors as well as companies in other sectors, consumer groups, communities and governments. For example, the Thailand Business Coalition on HIV/AIDS, American International Assurance (Thailand) and the Population Council have directly encouraged 125 Thai businesses to implement HIV prevention programmes by providing life insurance premium bonuses of 5–10% to companies with workplace prevention activities.

The Global Reporting Initiative, which links the world of work to wider questions of governance, has chosen South Africa for the first phase of its efforts to develop international standards for HIV reporting by businesses and other organizations. Project partners include some of the country's major companies and representatives from other interested parties such as labour, government and the Treatment Action Campaign [18,19].

At national and regional levels, the most visible public–private HIV partnerships have involved major pharmaceutical companies. In Botswana, the Ministry of Health, the Bill & Melinda Gates Foundation and the Merck Company Foundation formed an ART programme known as *Masa*, a Setswana word meaning 'new dawn'. By September 2004, more than 32,000 patients were receiving antiretrovirals through the programme [5]. In Romania, a public–private partnership involving the government and six major pharmaceutical companies—Abbott Laboratories, Boehringer Ingelheim, Bristol-Myers Squibb, GlaxoSmithKline, Hoffman-La Roche, and Merck & Co.—has worked on the country's national plan for access to HIV treatment and care. Under the plan, the Romanian government supports HIV patient treatment and care costs from national budgets. The companies have agreed to reduce certain drug prices by between 25 and 87%, or to donate drugs and equipment to measure viral load and CD4 counts.

Businesses are also forming HIV response partnerships with civil society organizations. For instance, in Namibia, Namdeb Diamond Corporation provides support to the *Lironga Eparu* ('learn to survive') organization of PLHIV.

Adhering to the principle of multisectorality through involving public, private and civil society sectors maximizes resources—financial and otherwise—for countries' response to HIV. It allows countries to move away from depending on external support for AIDS activities, and toward national autonomy. The 2001 UN Declaration of Commitment on HIV/AIDS urges diverse stakeholders to be actively involved in national responses [1]. By 2003, countries were expected to establish and strengthen national response mechanisms by involving the private sector, civil society partners, PLHIV and key vulnerable populations. Broad involvement requires coordination if it is to be effective. The Three Ones principles mentioned above isolate the key elements of country level coordination.

UNAIDS surveys have found that many low- and middle-income countries have national frameworks and national coordinating authorities, and they are at least starting to develop national monitoring and evaluation systems. However, the existence of these structures is not sufficient for an effective multisectoral and participatory response.

HIV plans cannot drive coordination if they are not specific. Yet many national frameworks have not been translated into specific work plans with budgets. They are also rarely developed in participation with key stakeholders, especially women's groups, faith-based organizations, district and local authorities and the private sector. An even larger shortcoming is that few of the existing national HIV authorities have the technical capacity they need to fulfil their mandates. A UNAIDS survey of low- and middle-income countries found that only 11% had sufficient technical capacity to coordinate among partners; only 4% had sufficient technical capacity to mobilize and track resources; only 4% had sufficient technical capacity for monitoring and evaluation; and only 8% had sufficient technical capacity strategic information management [20].

The barriers to coordination are both internal and external. In many countries, poorly defined roles between ministries of health and national AIDS councils have caused confusion and conflict, which has slowed national strategy implementation. Government ministries often have little incentive to follow the guidance of national coordinating mechanisms. Many perceive cooperation as a threat because they may lose influence and budgetary control. This has sometimes led to outright jurisdictional battles between national AIDS councils and health ministries. Furthermore, in far too many countries, civil society representatives still do not participate in high-level decision making.

Donors often mix political interests with social interests, which can override national priorities and marginalize groups particularly vulnerable to HIV infection. There is also extreme pressure from donor country legislatures to show results, which can limit harmonization of efforts. However, when bilateral and multilateral donors support and communicate with HIV coordinating bodies and promote the inclusion of civil society, they reinforce the bodies' position as leaders of multisectoral responses. Firm donor support also increases HIV authorities' capacities to create a national monitoring and evaluation system, and to produce strategic information. The Global Fund and the World Bank have embedded these principles in their HIV work, but bilateral support is more uneven [21]. The alignment of bilateral donors is critical to the functioning of truly effective national coordinating bodies. This is a particularly important principle, since ministries of health will play a central role in the global scale-up of ART, but health ministries cannot handle this massive task alone. To expand antiretroviral access rapidly, national HIV authorities need to play a strong coordinating role and involve local governments and civil society.

Mainstreaming HIV into all institutional activities

Institutions ideally address HIV-related issues through 'mainstreaming', ensuring that every relevant development they carry out has an HIV component. Mainstreaming addresses sectoral links to the HIV response, as well as the root causes of the epidemic's spread. For example, as education ministries increase access to education and improve its quality, the provision of HIV education should be mainstreamed into the curriculum. They also need to ensure that young girls have equal access to a broader education to empower them in society and thereby decrease their vulnerability to HIV infection.

Mainstreaming is a key strategy in converting global commitments into national development agendas. The 2001 UN Declaration of Commitment on HIV/AIDS called for a coordinated multisectoral response to HIV within each country and integration of HIV strategies into overall development strategies [1]. The most common development instruments in low- and middle-income countries are the Poverty Reduction Strategy Papers (PRSPs) qualifying them for zero- or low-interest loans or debt relief from the World Bank and International Monetary Fund. A PRSP lays out a country's economic, structural and social objectives and identifies needs for external financing to achieve those objectives. To boost mainstreaming implementation, the International Monetary Fund and the World Bank declared in 2001 that mainstreaming HIV into major development frameworks was a priority. However, at the end of 2004, 29% of the national development plans and PRSPs reviewed by UNAIDS had no HIV-related indicators. In other words, responding to HIV was not a focus of these countries' development efforts [20].

Even in countries that reported mainstreaming of HIV into development work, it is often little more than words on paper. Of the more than 70 countries surveyed, 40% reported that mainstreaming had yet to lead to concrete outputs [20]. Countries that have made progress in mainstreaming HIV into all government sectors include Zambia and Ghana. The Zambian Ministry of Agriculture and Cooperatives staff work with the UN Food and Agriculture Organization to emphasize the epidemic's role in eroding food security, ways that agricultural officials can mitigate that impact with labour-saving technologies and practices, and methods to preserve knowledge, enhance gender equality, improve nutrition for agricultural workers living with HIV, and promote economic and food safety nets [22]. In Ghana, different sectoral HIV funds are placed in the hands of the Ghana AIDS Commission. Each ministry is required to devote 5% of its AIDS budget to mainstreaming. The Ghana AIDS Commission releases the remaining 95% of the budget only after sector managers have agreed to this. This arrangement ensures there is 'buy-in' from the ministries to the mainstreaming process [23].

However, multisectoral responses do not necessarily provide a one-size-fits-all formula. The epidemic's highly varied nature rules out resolving it through detailed global guidelines. In high-prevalence countries, the epidemic touches all of society. National AIDS commissions and other coordinating bodies need to act like 'councils of war' and directly involve the head of state. Countries with lower prevalence also require strong multisectoral prevention and care responses, and they need to use the comparative advantages of individual ministries in addressing the epidemic. Often, health ministers still consider HIV their 'turf', but they do not have the will or strength to catalyse, leverage or lead the necessary comprehensive response.

Decentralization—empowering regions, communities and districts

Decentralization is one of the chief strategies used to improve good governance and development programme implementation. In this process, central governments devolve powers and responsibilities to lower administrative institutions. Decentralization aims to make decision making more democratic, equitable and locally responsive. As a result, the process inspires 'national ownership' along with civil society and private sector involvement in policy-planning.

However, HIV response decentralization has often faltered [24]. UNAIDS found that 10% of surveyed countries had not started a formal decentralization process, and another 51% had started a process but had yet to achieve any concrete results [20]. Governments are used to working within strict hierarchical structures, and the benefits of involving communities are not always clear. At the same time, communities often do not have the necessary representative structures or administrative capacity to participate effectively. A great deal of training and facilitation may be necessary on both sides if they are to work effectively with each other.

Despite the problems, HIV-related decentralization is a reality in countries such as Papua New Guinea, Uganda, the United Republic of Tanzania and Morocco, where local strategic plans have been developed for coordinating activities and monitoring implementation. In Burkina Faso, Ethiopia, Kenya, Ghana and Uganda, the World Bank MAP has helped prevention and care programmes to reach communities and households. In Cambodia, UNDP's Community Enhancement Programme works with the Ministry of Rural Affairs to encourage communes (local districts) to prepare development plans, building local capacity to collect and analyse AIDS data used to support planning and monitoring.

Various country experiences show that strong financial and political investment is needed to create effective district and local coordination bodies. At the local level, capacity gaps pose challenges, much as they do at the national level. There is now an urgent need to develop innovative ways of addressing capacity issues at all levels of health systems, particularly at lower staff levels [25–27]. This situation is becoming even more urgent as access to ART expands.

Strengthening capacity

The HIV epidemic works in a vicious cycle, striking hardest in those countries with the weakest capacity to respond to it. In many countries, HIV is currently depleting technical and administrative capacity faster than it can be replenished. This is creating an unparalleled crisis in human resources, and is reversing many of the development gains made in previous decades.

Even before HIV emerged, public service systems in low- and middle-income countries were struggling to meet their citizens' needs. In the healthcare sector, problems included poor delivery infrastructure; inadequate human resources; poorly defined services, functions, skills and protocols; and inadequate management and administration. In much of sub-Saharan Africa, AIDS has turned these weaknesses into crises.

Capacity building requires funding and political commitment, but it also calls for a broader vision that combines short-term emergency measures with long-term, sustained strengthening of the fundamental institutions of modern statehood. The most immediate requirement is to preserve existing capacity by keeping people alive and healthy. In the worst-affected African countries, no other measure will so quickly and directly arrest the decline in national capacity as providing treatment and care [28]. At the same time, efforts will need to focus on using existing capacity to its fullest as HIV treatment initiatives get up to speed. A wide range of untapped community resources, particularly PLHIV, will need to compensate for formal skills gaps.

Furthermore, additional efforts are required to minimize the 'brain drain'—the migration of trained professional staff to higher-income countries. This phenomenon is most obvious in the health sectors of Southern Africa, where doctors and nurses are emigrating to Australia, Europe, the Gulf countries, Japan and the USA. These countries offer these workers an attractive alternative to the poor conditions and low pay that characterize their own healthcare systems.

South Africa is particularly hard hit by an exodus of doctors and nurses leaving for higher-paid jobs overseas [29,30]. The South African Medical Association estimates as many as 5000 doctors have left the country in recent years. The Democratic Nursing Organization of South Africa says 300 trained nurses leave each month. Zambia is another hard-hit country; it has only 400 practising doctors, whereas it once had 1600 [31].

Some countries, such as the UK, have established codes of conduct to prevent 'poaching'. Improving working conditions and wages in affected countries can also keep health professionals from moving abroad. An International Organization for Migration programme, called

'Migration for Development in Africa', helps African countries to encourage their qualified expatriates to return, and to retain professionals who might otherwise be tempted to leave. The programme operates in Benin, Cape Verde, Ghana, Kenya, Rwanda and Uganda [32].

Rebuilding and increasing capacity

Inadequate training of new health professionals is another major issue. In some cases, the pre-service training of system in hard-hit countries has completely broken down. UNDP's Southern Africa Capacity Initiative is exploring ways to build sustainable capacity across sectors, including local training of professionals in key sectors, use of information technology, non-traditional approaches such as contracting out public service delivery to civil society organizations or international NGOs and contracting the private sector to provide public services.

Botswana has hired foreign professionals to provide much-needed treatment and care and to build local capacity through a training programme carried out in partnership with the Botswana–Harvard AIDS Institute Partnership. Botswana's Ministry of Health also has a training programme called *Kitso* ('knowledge' in Setswana), and private practitioners and health personnel at hospitals run by large mining companies have also been trained. In addition, a 'preceptorship' programme brings HIV experts from top international institutions to mentor national staff [33].

WHO works with the German Agency for Technical Cooperation to help African and European institutions become 'knowledge hubs' in HIV treatment and HIV prevention for regional skills transfer and training. In Uganda, a knowledge hub has been established with the Joint Clinical Research Centre and other leading training providers. Similar knowledge hubs have been established in Eastern Europe and West Africa.

Strategic information for evidence-informed policy and programming

Strategic information is any information that can usefully guide policy and programming decisions. All decision makers facing the tough choices and dilemmas presented by AIDS need evidence-informed policy guidance. For example, decisions about introducing appropriate harm-reduction strategies or combinations of prevention interventions for sexual transmission need to be informed by clear evidence about what works. Needle exchange has been shown to reduce HIV transmission and bring injecting drug users (IDUs) into contact with health and social services, but it is too soon to gauge the effectiveness of supervised injection centres, which hold the promise of reducing HIV transmission among those IDUs most at risk of exposure to HIV. Decisions about how to balance promoting abstinence, delaying sexual debut, reducing the number of sexual partners and encouraging condom use need to be informed by scientific evidence about the effectiveness of each strategy in different contexts, and by young people's and adults' perspectives on what might work best.

If policies and programmes are to reflect the epidemic's realities, countries need the capacity to track the epidemic and analyse trends, understand behavioural patterns, map vulnerable populations, measure social and economic impact, monitor programme indicators, evaluate progress and conduct operations research to refine programmes. Both the short-term and long-term effectiveness of national responses depends on knowing which data are needed, and how to collect, compile, analyse and translate them into strategic information to move policy agendas forward and ensure the most effective programming. In many parts of the world, this 'data-informing decisions' capacity needs strengthening.

UNAIDS works with partners such as WHO, the US Centers for Disease Control and Prevention, Family Health International, the East–West Center and the Futures Group International to build and enhance capacity at country level for modelling and estimation of the epidemic. In 2003, over 300 representatives from national AIDS programmes and the research institutions of 130 countries were trained in skills for capturing, validating and interpreting HIV-related data and in the use of updated modelling methodologies to improve HIV and AIDS estimates. In 2005, 11 workshops around the world refined skills and produced country-level epidemic updates, and UNAIDS established regional Technical Support Facilities to improve country partners' access to timely and quality-assured technical assistance and capacity-building support.

Whereas classic surveillance collects information such as HIV prevalence, AIDS cases and mortality, second-generation surveillance adds risk-behaviour information. Together they help countries to assess the course of their epidemics and decide on strategic responses. Examples of behavioural data collection activities include India's massive 2001–2002 national behavioural survey [34] and the UNAIDS Second-Generation Surveillance Project, funded by the European Community and carried out in partnership with WHO and eight countries in Africa, Asia, the Caribbean and Latin America. Including NGOs in surveillance activities helps provide access to hard-to-reach populations. In Vietnam and Mexico, NGOs facilitated access to IDUs for behavioural research. In the Dominican Republic, the sex workers' association MODEMU, and the gay men's organization *Amigos Siempre Amigos* ('friends always') provided peer interviewers [13].

Indonesia conducted behavioural surveillance in 2003–2004, covering nearly half its provinces and all key populations at higher risk—men who buy sex, sex workers (women, men and transgender), IDUs, men who have sex with men, and youth at higher risk. Robust provincial estimates were developed on the number of people at risk of infection and already infected with HIV. This permitted policy-makers, community groups, NGOs and local AIDS Control Commissions to adapt existing programming to actual conditions. For example, harm-reduction programmes now focus on sexual and injecting risk, since it was found that many male injectors—up to 70% in one major city—have unprotected sex with sex workers. Furthermore, condom promotion programmes have a renewed emphasis on reaching potential clients of sex workers.

Operations research collects and analyses information as programmes are implemented and scaled up. This research uses a systematic approach to 'learning by doing' and captures information in a way that helps programme managers and designers to make the best use of it to improve programmes.

Key questions for treatment scale-up include: how best to avoid drug stock-outs; which are the most useful components of community treatment literacy programmes; how to maintain adherence; which tasks can care providers undertake, and the training needed; how best to keep costs down; which laboratory monitoring is essential; and how to measure the clinical effects of treatment and return to normal function. Operations research can influence policy and programming. For example, Senegal monitored antiretroviral adherence in relation to the costs borne directly by patients and found that the more patients paid on a sliding scale by income, the less adherent they were. These findings influenced Senegal's decision to introduce a universal access, free-of-charge antiretroviral programme [35].

Operations research in prevention can focus on many different aspects of programming, such as comparing results of various methods of offering HIV testing and assessing the effects on stigma of prevention programming. Prevention–treatment integration can influence the effectiveness of both prevention and treatment. For example, ART programmes in Khayelitsha, South Africa; Masaka, Uganda; and Cange, Haiti have helped support prevention activities, documenting increased interest and willingness of community members to come forward for HIV testing [13].

UNAIDS' major priorities include reporting on the impact of the global response and building country capacity to carry out credible monitoring and evaluation. To drive this agenda forward, UNAIDS provides innovative links between monitoring, evaluation research and financial tracking.

Monitoring and evaluation are essential to determining whether programmes are reaching target populations and accomplishing their objectives. Spurred on by UNAIDS since 2001, various stakeholders have come to a consensus on global indicators for various comprehensive response interventions. However, this is just a beginning. It is critical to improve country capacity to measure these indicators, and to use this information to improve programmes so they work effectively.

To build capacity, the comprehensive approach includes training, technical assistance, access to improved guidelines and tools, and helping countries to recruit national expert staff for monitoring and evaluation activities. UNAIDS and other partners, such as the US Government, have conducted regional training sessions. These sessions use a standardized curriculum to teach monitoring expertise, computer database use and ways to present complex data to different audiences. The Global AIDS Monitoring and Evaluation Team, housed at the World Bank, concentrates on helping countries to find and hire local monitoring and evaluation staff and to develop functioning monitoring and evaluation offices. To mentor and assist these efforts, UNAIDS and the US Centers for Disease Control have sent experts to key countries to build on existing efforts and address key monitoring and evaluation information gaps.

Monitoring country responses: commitment and action

Ultimately, leadership must translate into concrete action. UNAIDS monitors the progress of the global AIDS response in various ways, and its AIDS Programme Effort Index is one tool for measuring country-level commitment. The Index was developed by the US Agency for International Development, the UNAIDS Secretariat, the WHO and the US-based Policy Project. It tracks a country's effort in 10 different programme categories, but does not measure actual output such as coverage of a specific service.

The results between the year 2000, based on 40 countries, and 2003, based on 54 countries, show there is a general pattern of improvement [36]. Significant gains in national commitment were recorded in the categories of treatment and care, political support, policy and planning, and programme resources. Improvements in providing resources, and in treatment and care, were particularly notable since these were the lowest-rated components in 2000. The creation of the Global Fund and rising bilateral donor funding levels explain much of the resource component's increase. The increase in care-related efforts probably reflects international donors' new emphasis on treatment access.

In 2003, additional data were collected from 103 countries to track national commitment and action, and policy development and implementation [10]. Although the data showed an increase in the number of countries with comprehensive, multisectoral national HIV strategies and government-led national AIDS coordinating bodies, one striking finding was that resources were often not invested in programme areas with the greatest impact. For example, in several Latin American countries, programmes for IDUs and men who have sex with men were scarce, even though these populations suffered from high HIV infection rates. Similarly, in an Asian country with low general population prevalence (0.3%), high prevalence among IDUs (80%) and sex workers (30%) and evidence that injecting drug use and sex work together accounted for 90% of new infections, interventions to protect IDUs and sex workers were just one of the country's nine strategic priorities. In an African country where general population HIV prevalence was a stable 1.8%, sex worker HIV prevalence was 78% and 82% in the two largest cities, 75% of new infections in men in the capital city were clients of sex workers, and only 0.8% of HIV investments focused on sex work [37].

In some countries, policy and strategic planning has moved ahead, but legislation has not kept up, and regressive or contradictory laws remain on the books. In the context of injecting drug use, some countries with restrictive laws have nonetheless carried out pilot projects involving needle and syringe exchanges, methadone maintenance therapy and condom promotion at entertainment establishments. In the Russian Federation, a recent criminal code amendment allowed for harm-reduction projects to operate legally. Unfortunately, some legal barriers remain—most notably, the ban on substitution therapy [38].

Conclusion

The impacts of HIV on the development capacity of poor countries is significantly undermining their ability to make substantive progress towards the Millennium Development Goals, particularly with regard to poverty reduction, education and health targets, and the care of orphans. Therefore, strengthening the response to HIV must be a central part of development programming and practice. It cannot be overemphasized that HIV is both a global emergency and a long-term development crisis that requires an exceptional and sustained response far beyond the scale of anything the world has seen to date. However, an effective global response will only be achieved if countries own and drive their national responses within their own borders. International financial and technical assistance from UN agencies, donors, bilateral funders, foundations and others is important, but it must be embedded within national responses to be effective.

The cornerstones of nationally led responses to HIV are best summed up by the concept of the 'Three Ones'. The key to success is strengthened and sustained national leadership that includes, engages and empowers all levels of civil society, particularly women. New strategies are needed to deal with the disproportionate impact of the epidemic on women, girls and orphans, including microcredit, school support and food assistance programmes. Empowerment and capacity need to be devolved from national to regional, district and community levels so that people are empowered to be effectively involved in decision making that affects them, and their energy and commitment on the frontlines of the response can be harnessed.

Harmonizing multisectoral responses, donor activities, and monitoring and evaluation will support countries in their national responses. Bottlenecks within both international and domestic systems, which cause delays in the transfer of funding and other resources to the key stakeholders who can best use them, must be overcome. Development instruments and policies need to be reviewed and revised; internationally agreed-upon instruments such as debt relief, tariff removal and PRSPs have the potential to improve health policies, governance and institutions in relation to HIV.

It is critical to develop strategies for radical and innovative approaches to restoring human capacity in the worst-affected countries. These include massive ART programmes; a complete rethinking of how skills will be built, retained and sustained; salary support; and stopping the drain of health and administrative workers to other sectors and to industrialized countries.

Finally, the epidemic is not going to be resolved in the short term; strategists should be looking 10, 20 or even 30 years ahead. Scientific and strategic information to guide the response, accountability mechanisms to track resources and demonstrate that they are being used to their fullest potential, situation assessment and early warning systems with a 'people focus', and dissemination of best practices are all needed to get on top of the epidemic. The response must be on a scale and with a scope to match the epidemic—the world is far from that now.

Acknowledgements

The authors wish to acknowledge Valerie Manda for her assistance with references in the final manuscript.

References

1. United Nations General Assembly. (2001).Twenty-sixth special session, Agenda item 8, 01 43484, Resolution adopted by the General Assembly [without reference to a Main Committee (A/S-26/L.2)] S-26/2. Declaration of Commitment on HIV/AIDS; August 2001. Available at: http://www.un.org/ ga/ aids/docs/aress262.pdf. Last accessed May 25, 2005.

2. WHO/UNAIDS/Global Fund. (2003). Media Pack for the Global Launch of the '3 by 5' Initiative and World AIDS Day, 2003: Global Video and Audio News Release: Transcription of the Statements. Available at: http:// www.who.int/3by5/mediacentre/en/ Broll_3by5launch2003.pdf. Last accessed May 23, 2005.

3. World Health Organization. (2003). *World Health Organization and UNAIDS Unveil Plan to Get 3 Million AIDS Patients on Treatment by 2005.* Press release, 1 December 2003. Available at: http:// www.who.int/ mediacentre/news/releases/2003/pr89/en/.Last accessed May 25, 2004.

4. UNAIDS/WHO. (2004). '3×5' *Progress Report: December 2003 through June 2004.* Geneva: UNAIDS/ WHO. Available at: http://www.who.int/3by5/en/Progressreport.pdf. Last accessed May 23, 2005.

5. UNAIDS/WHO. (2004). '3×5' *Progress Report.* Geneva: UNAIDS/WHO. Available at: http:// www.who.int/3by5/progressreport05/en/. Last accessed May 23, 2005.

6. Futures Group/POLICY Project in cooperation with USAID, UNAIDS, WHO and UNICEF. (2004). *Coverage of Selected Services for HIV/AIDS Prevention, Care and Support in Low and Middle Income Countries in 2003.* Washington, DC: Futures Group/POLICY Project in cooperation with USAID, UNAIDS, WHO and UNICEF June 2004. Available at: www.FuturesGroup.com.

7. Feachem R. (2005). Opening Speech, The Global Fund 10th Board Meeting, Geneva April 21–22, 2005. Available at: http://www.theglobalfund.org/en/about/board/tenth/openingspeechfeachem/. Last accessed May 23, 2005.

8. The Global Fund to Fight AIDS, Tuberculosis and Malaria. (2005). *Investing in The Future: The Global Fund at Three Years.* Geneva: The Global Fund. Available at: http://www.theglobalfund.org/en/ files/ about/replenishment/progress_report_en.pdf. Last accessed May 23, 2005.

9. The Global Fund to Fight AIDS, Tuberculosis and Malaria Pledges. Available at: http:// www.theglobalfund.org/en/files/pledges&contributions.xls. Last accessed May 25, 2005.

10. Heller PS. (2005). International Monetary Fund: Understanding Fiscal Space. Presented at the Joint United Nations Programme on HIV/AIDS, Geneva Switzerland, February 2005.

11. Joint United Nations Programme on HIV/AIDS (UNAIDS). (2003). *Progress Report on the Global Response to the HIV/AIDS Epidemic.* Follow-up to the 2001 United Nations General Assembly Special Session on HIV/AIDS, Geneva: UNAIDS.

12. United Nations General Assembly. (2005). Fifty-ninth session Agenda item 43, Follow-up to the outcome of the twenty-sixth special session: implementation of the Declaration of Commitment on HIV/AIDS. Progress made in the implementation of the Declaration of Commitment on HIV/AIDS, Report of the Secretary-General. April 2005. Available at: http://www.unaids.org/html/pub/publications/external-documents/ga59_sgprogressreport_04apr05_en_pdf.pdf. Last accessed May 25, 2005.

13. Joint United Nations Programme on HIV/AIDS (UNAIDS). (2004). *Report on the Global AIDS Epidemic: 4th Global Report.* Geneva: UNAIDS. Available at: http://www.unaids.org/bangkok2004/report.html. Last accessed May 23, 2005.

14. Hsu L. (2004). *Building Dynamic Democratic Governance and HIV-resilient Societies.* United Nations Development Programme (UNDP)/Joint United Nations Programme on HIV/AIDS (UNAIDS), Bangkok, Thailand, February 2004. Available at: http://www.hiv-development.org/text/publications/OsloPaper.pdf. Last accessed May 23, 2005.

15. UNDP. (2002). *Introducing Governance into HIV/AIDS Programmes: People's Republic of China, Lao PDR and Viet Nam.* UNDP South East Asia HIV and Development Programme, Bangkok, Thailand, June 2002. Available at: http://www.hiv-development.org/text/publications/Good%20Governance.pdf. Last accessed May 23, 2005.

16. UNDP. (2004). *HIV/AIDS in Eastern Europe and the Commonwealth of Independent States: Reversing the Epidemic, Facts and Policy Options.* Bratislava, Slovak Republic: UNDP. Available at: http://rbec.undp.org/hiv/?english. Last accessed May 23, 2005.

17. International HIV/AIDS Alliance. (2004). *Civil Society and the 'Three Ones': A Discussion Paper.* Available at: http://synkronweb.aidsalliance.org/graphics/secretariat/publications/Civil_Society_and_Three_Ones_Eng.pdf. Last accessed May 23, 2005.

18. *The Cape Argus.* (2003). Eskom pledges R5m to provide HIV training to medics. May 8, 2003. Available at: http://www.hst.org.za/news/20030507. Last accessed May 23, 2005.

19. Global Reporting Initiative. (2003). *Reporting Guidance on HIV/AIDS: A GRI Resource Document.* Amsterdam: Global Reporting Initiative. Available at: http://www.globalreporting.org/guidelines/HIV/HIVAIDSpilot.pdf. Last accessed May 23, 2005.

20. Joint United Nations Programme on HIV/AIDS (UNAIDS). (2005). *2004 Key Results Annual Country Reports: An Internal Analysis of 76 Countries.* Geneva: UNAIDS.

21. Joint United Nations Programme on HIV/AIDS (UNAIDS). (2004). *2003 Key Results Annual Country Reports: An Internal Analysis of 71 Countries.* Geneva: UNAIDS.

22. Food and Agriculture Organization of the United Nations/Ministry of Agriculture and Cooperatives of the Republic of Zambia. (2004). *Strengthening Institutional Capacity in Mitigating HIV/AIDS Impact on the Agricultural Sector Potential Mitigation Interventions.* Available at: ftp://ftp.fao.org/docrep/fao/007/y5656e/y5656e00.pdf. Last accessed May 23, 2005.

23. Elsey H, Kutengule P. (2003). *AIDS Mainstreaming: A Definition, Some Experiences and Strategies.* Durban: University of Natal, Health Economics and AIDS Research Division (HEARD) Available at: http://www.sarpn.org.za/documents/d0000271/P263_HIV_Report.pdf. Last accessed May 23, 2005.

24. Lubben M, Mayhew SH, Collins C, Green A. (2002). Reproductive health and health sector reform in developing countries: establishing a framework for dialogue. *Bulletin of the World Health Organization* 80:667–74.

25. Chen L, Hanvoravongchai P. (2005). HIV/AIDS and human resources. *Bulletin of the World Health Organization* 83:243–44.

26. Joint Learning Initiative. (2004). *Human Resources for Health: Overcoming the Crisis.* Cambridge MA: Harvard University Press.

27. Chen L, Evans T, Anand S *et al.* (2004). Human resources for health: overcoming the crisis. *Lancet* 364:1984–90.

28. Piot P. (2005). Why AIDS is Exceptional. Speech given at the London School of Economics. London, UK, February 2005. Available at: http://www.unaids.org/en/ about+unaids/speeches.asp. Last accessed May 23, 2005.

29. Thomson A. (2003). Medical exodus saps South Africa's war on AIDS. *Reuters AlertNet*, May, 2003. Available at: http://www.hivandhepatitis.com/recent/developing/020503t.html. Last accessed May 23, 2005.

30. International Organisation for Migration. (2003). *Mobility and HIV/AIDS in Southern Africa: A Field Study in South Africa, Zimbabwe and Mozambique.* Pretoria: International Organisation for Migration. Available at: http://www.iom.int/en/PDF_Files/HIVAIDS/Southern_africa_hiv.pdf. Last accessed May 23, 2005.

31. Lauring H. (2002). Action needed on brain drain. *Globaleyes*, March, 2002. Available at: http://manila.djh.dk/global/stories/ storyReader$98. Last accessed May 23, 2005.

32. International Organisation for Migration. *Migration for Development in Africa (MIDA).* Available at: http://www.iom.int/MIDA/#specific. Last accessed May 23, 2005.

33. Joint United Nations Programme on HIV/AIDS (UNAIDS). (2003). *Stepping Back from the Edge: The Pursuit of Antiretroviral Therapy in Botswana, South Africa and Uganda.* Geneva: UNAIDS. Available at: http://www.dec.org/ pdf_docs/PNACU828.pdf. Last accessed May 25, 2005.

34. National AIDS Control Organization/Ministry of Health and Family Welfare, Government of India. (2001). *National Baseline High Risk and Bridge Population Behavioural Surveillance Survey.* New Delhi: ORG Center for Social Research.

35. Lanièce I, Mounirou C, Desclaux A *et al.* (2003). Adherence to HAART and its principal determinants in a cohort of Senegalese adults. *AIDS* 17(Supplement 3): S103–8.

36. USAID, UNAIDS, WHO, Policy Project, Futures Group. (2003). *The Level of Effort in the National Response to AIDS: The AIDS Program Effort Index (API)—the 2003 Round.* Washington DC: Futures Group International. Available at: http://www.policyproject.com/pubs/ monographs/API2003.pdf. Last accessed May 23, 2005.

37. ACTafrica and UNAIDS. (2002). Joint MAP Implementation Support Mission Report: Cameroon, Benin, and Central African Republic. Available at:http:// www.worldbank.org/oed/aids/evaluation_-design/ references.html. Last accessed May 25, 2005.

38. WHO/UNODC/UNAIDS. (2005). *Substitution Maintenance Therapy in the Management of Opioid Dependence and HIV/AIDS Prevention.* Geneva: WHO/UNODC/UNAIDS. http://www.who.int/ substance_abuse/ publications/en/PositionPaper_English.pdf. Last accessed: May 23, 2005.

Chapter 50

Some lessons learned

Eduard J Beck* and Nicholas Mays

Between October 1980 and April 1981, five young men in three different Californian hospitals were treated for *Pneumocystic carinii* pneumonia (PCP), two of whom died. These were the first people diagnosed with what the US Centers for Disease Control (CDC) subsequently called AIDS, and they published an early report on their experiences in June 1981 [1]. Twenty-five years later, the number of people infected with and dying from HIV is still increasing and now involves millions of people from all countries and continents around the world. Increasingly, the poor, the young, women and other vulnerable populations tend to be most affected.

This book has brought together the experiences of many authors who have been, and continue to be, directly involved with containing the HIV pandemic, at either country or international levels. Country authors have described the HIV epidemic in their specific country and how their country and its health system responded to the epidemic, while also recognizing how the country's health system had to change in order to deal with the HIV epidemic. As well as providing relevant historical descriptions, authors were asked to identify lessons learned within countries that might guide future strategies, act as a baseline to review developments and inform other countries. The aim was to use the case studies to help answer the four questions posed in the Introduction:

1. Which health systems appear to have done particularly well in responding to their country's HIV epidemic, and which aspects of their health system and of their response appear to have been most influential in this response?

2. Are there examples of countries that appear to be doing better or worse than their overall situation would predict, in terms of their per capita gross domestic product (GDP), prevalence of HIV, quality of health system or other factors? If so, how are these countries managing to do this, and what lessons do such responses have for other countries?

3. Is there anything that can be generalized from the 'effective' responses, either to similar countries in terms of level of development, nature of health system, system of government, history, culture and other relevant factors, or more widely—are there any general factors that are positively or negatively associated with control of the HIV pandemic?

4. Are the 'lessons' that have been drawn from the most celebrated country responses correct, and, if so, are they helpful to a wider range of countries?

This concluding chapter attempts to shed light on these questions—drawing mainly on the material in the country case studies—by discussing the principal elements associated with effective country responses.

* Corresponding author.

The health systems of affected countries are inevitably at the forefront of national responses, and for this purpose both the formal and informal systems, and the private as well as public sectors, have important roles to play. However, as most authors have described, the response to the HIV pandemic requires a wider, multisectoral response, since the pandemic is deeply rooted in the social and economic conditions within and between nations. To address such epidemics successfully, these national and international determinants—which affect behaviours, increase HIV transmission and prevent the implementation of therapeutic services—need to be addressed. The extent and nature of the response required will vary from country to country and continent to continent and will depend on the proportion of the population infected, the type of HIV epidemic and its drivers, the resources available, the ability to deploy those resources effectively through the country's institutions, and the prevailing cultural norms. As a result, it would be misguided to offer a single, simple 'recipe' for an effective response, given the importance of each country's context.

Instead, the focus in what follows is on the main elements commonly found in different countries that have made progress in terms of both treatment and prevention. This is not to say that a successful response is always the product of all the elements described, but rather that each needs to be carefully considered when developing a strategy appropriate to a particular setting, including high-, middle- and lower-income countries. Though there is no attempt to prioritize the different elements, an increasingly salient aspect of a country's response relates to the provision of appropriate health services.

Provision of health services

A recent development has been the international recognition that all countries need to combine preventive interventions with appropriate treatment and care. While high-income countries have been able to provide both preventive and therapeutic HIV services since the 1980s, only in the last 5 years have national policy-makers and those involved with global institutions recognized that middle- and lower-income countries also require effective, efficient, equitable and acceptable preventive and therapeutic HIV services, ideally integrated in a seamless way with related conditions such as tuberculosis (TB) and the health system in general.

There are many reasons for this paradigm shift, in particular more effective advocacy by a variety of pressure groups, reduction in the price of antiretroviral and other drugs, as well as fears that high-burden countries may cause local, regional or international social instability, threatening national and international security. Whether such fears are realistic remains to be determined.

Indeed, there has been considerable progress since the 2000 Durban International AIDS Conference on developing therapeutic services in middle- and lower-income countries. The number of people treated with antiretroviral therapy (ART) in the developing world had increased to an estimated 1 million by June 2005 [2]. Not only have the number of antiretroviral drugs increased over time, their prices have decreased dramatically over the last 5 years, especially in middle- and lower-income countries. ART has both a preventive and therapeutic function: it prevents infection from mother to child, and may play a similar role in adults, depending on the outcome of pending pre-exposure prophylaxis studies; ART also reduces morbidity and mortality in HIV-infected people. In industrialized countries, ART is tailored more closely to individual patient requirements in terms of dosing, pill burden and range of available drugs, while in middle- and lower-income countries, a more public health or population approach is being promoted, determined by economic factors. This is based on deliberate decisions by countries and international organizations such as the World Health Organization (WHO) [3] to restrict the types and number of antiretroviral drugs available through the public sector or non-governmental organizations (NGOs) in these countries in order to keep costs of ART and related support services as low as are consistent with an acceptable quality of life and increased length of survival with HIV.

HIV-related therapeutic services include ART and other drugs for the treatment of opportunistic infections. The drugs themselves are only part of a much broader service infrastructure that is required to scale up HIV therapeutic services. This includes educating those who prescribe ART and those with HIV to ensure optimal prescribing, monitoring and adherence to these drugs, as well as providing appropriate palliative care. The provision of services needs to extend beyond health facilities and, where appropriate, might include home- or community-based care. While healthcare providers in Cuba, Senegal and other middle- and lower-income countries manage the majority of HIV-infected people in a primary care setting, in the USA and Europe this is mostly done in specialist clinics or hospital centres.

Many have welcomed the recent momentum to provide HIV-infected people in middle- and lower-income countries with appropriate treatment and care, including ART. However, if HIV incidence levels are not reduced, the increasing number of new people infected with HIV, combined with fewer people dying from HIV due to ART, will result in more HIV-infected people alive and requiring medical and social services. Apart from humanitarian considerations, increased requirement for HIV services can lead to significant cost increases, as has recently been seen in the USA [4] and the UK [5]. As the complementary nature of HIV therapeutic and preventive services was recognized some time ago [6], the irony of improving HIV treatment and care services is that it strongly reinforces the need to increase prevention efforts, particularly in poorer countries and among both HIV-negative and HIV-positive populations, to prevent the number of people living with HIV (PLHIV) from increasing further. Otherwise, it will be impossible to ensure universal access to ART except in rich countries.

Prevention programmes may be more effective if people are more willing to come forward for testing, knowing that there is treatment available should they test positive. Being on treatment may also be more conducive to safer sex and safer injecting behaviour as well as reducing an individual's infectivity should he or she have unprotected sex. Effective and wide-ranging prevention programmes are required to improve awareness of HIV and how to prevent its spread in the general public and in vulnerable groups. Such programmes will need to be sustained and will require a mix of general population and targeted preventive programmes and public information to stop HIV transmission. Prevention efforts are undermined in situations where the popular perception of who is at risk and how transmission occurs is at odds with reality. The increased availability of treatment may be another means of reducing the stigma attached to HIV and the fear people feel toward the disease, which may contribute to its normalization as a major chronic condition rather than a stigmatized killer disease.

The experiences of haemophiliac populations on various continents and of blood donors in Henan, China and other regions of the world have dramatically and tragically demonstrated the need for uninfected blood and blood products to avoid the spread of HIV. In addition to uninfected blood and blood products, people also need to have access to condoms and uninfected injecting equipment to make their sexual and injecting behaviour safer at an individual and community level. Many countries still lack access to cheap but good quality condoms. Where the epidemic involves injecting drug users (IDUs)—for example, in Russia, Ukraine, Italy and Spain—they require access to sterile needles and syringes. Researchers are also conducting investigations with opiate replacement or substitution programmes. Initiatives in some of these areas are controversial in many countries, including Italy, the USA, Indonesia, China and Thailand, despite evidence that these measures help control the spread of HIV.

Furthermore, as many authors state in this book, there is an urgent need to develop a cost-effective, acceptable HIV vaccine that can be distributed to relevant populations. Given the many technical challenges that exist in this field, there is a very strong case for a much greater international effort involving both public and private sectors. Even a partially effective vaccine would appreciably improve preventive options, yet there are currently few incentives for many businesses to invest in this area, compared with the pharmaceutical industry. For this reason, progress with vaccines is likely to depend on a strong publicly financed effort, in collaboration with those private interests that can be encouraged to think it worthwhile to invest some of their own resources in this field.

Health service infrastructure and human resources

Apart from involving and increasing the number of existing health facilities, new developments should include the establishment of safe injecting sites, voluntary counselling and testing (VCT) sites, as well as antenatal, sexually transmitted infection (STI), and malaria and TB care and support services. Such sites will need to have access to the necessary equipment, laboratory and pharmaceutical support to provide these services, and monitor responses. This will require a functioning referral system, integrating tertiary specialist centres in larger cities with district hospitals and rural health facilities or general practices. This also requires reliable procurement systems and distribution networks for pharmaceutical and laboratory goods.

Apart from providing the relevant physical structure, healthcare staff are also required to provide the actual services in a way that maintains quality and confidentiality. The scale-up of services in many countries, especially in middle- and lower-income countries, is currently constrained by the lack of trained staff and therefore requires training new staff. Many countries have started to train additional professional staff, but retaining existing and new staff will be an equally important task. Most of the staff are trained within the public sector, but many move from rural to urban centres or from the public to the more lucrative private sector or overseas. Retaining healthcare staff is likely to require improved salaries and working conditions, which may also affect other professional groups, and may, therefore, have a general effect on wages, economic competitiveness and the 'fiscal space' that governments enjoy.

High-income countries have had their own health service staffing problems, and countries such as the USA, Canada, the UK and other European countries have been recruiting healthcare staff from a number of middle- and lower-income countries. However, the flow of trained staff is not only from the South to the North; middle- or lower-income countries also compete among themselves to attract the necessary staff. For example, Botswana has been recruiting staff from neighbouring Zambia, Zimbabwe and South Africa, thereby exacerbating staff shortages in these countries.

Efforts to build organizational and staff capacity and capability in the health system and in the wider civil society need to go hand-in-hand. The physical and managerial infrastructure needs to be developed to support the new human resources. For example, the pay-off from better staff training is maximized if the staff are working in a system with appropriate, well-functioning equipment as well as timely, transparent decision making with clear lines of accountability for the use of resources and the quality of services delivered. Similarly, there may be little or no value in increasing the financial resources available without the infrastructure and staff to use them effectively.

Public and private healthcare sectors

As described in this book, in countries such as those of the former Soviet Union, Cuba, the UK and France, the public sector is primarily responsible for HIV-related care. In most countries, however, both public and private sectors are involved. Many HIV-infected people on ART in Uganda are managed by private practitioners, subcontracted by the Ugandan government. Similarly, most HIV-related services in India are provided outside the public sector.

Authors from a number of countries reported that despite incurring greater expense, many people preferred to see private practitioners rather than those working in the public sector when given the choice. This raises issues regarding the relationship between private and public provision, particularly as it relates to ensuring that the private sector supports the goal of equity of access to HIV services in relation to need. While in some countries the private sector is only accessible to those with the private means, in others the government has deliberately involved the private sector and NGOs in order to extend publicly funded provision of ART to an increasing number of patients.

Decentralization of the response

In most countries, there is considerable regional diversity in the prevalence and incidence of HIV infection, in the drivers of the epidemic and, therefore, in the required response. Larger countries often have more diverse epidemics purely because they tend to encompass more diverse economic and social areas. As a result, it makes sense to organize a decentralized response in which local government agencies and other organizations are given considerable freedom in responding to their local epidemics as long as they can show relevance to local circumstances and produce regular and credible information on the impact of their policies and programmes on the epidemic. Under such circumstances, and to enhance effectiveness, local agents will require access to resources to implement the plans, as well as decision-making authority on how to use resources. The expansion of ART to reach more people will require the distribution of health services in divergent settings, from densely populated urban areas to remote, sparsely populated areas in Canada, Russia, Amazonia in Brazil, rural China or Africa. This raises many logistical issues, from geographical isolation and limited access to services, to limitations placed on access for cultural or economic reasons. It also raises the question of whether there are facilities in place where HIV services can be provided, which is often a product of the robustness of the pre-existing health system.

Vertical versus horizontal programmes

Many HIV-infected people in middle- or lower-income countries live in rural areas and rely on local health facilities to provide services. Many of these people also need treatment for TB and STIs. This raises the issue of whether HIV preventive and therapeutic programmes should be separate, 'vertical' programmes not directly linked to other relevant programmes or the general healthcare system. While HIV programmes may start off as vertical programmes, long-term sustainability will require that they become integrated with other relevant services. While in urban centres in middle- and lower-income countries, HIV-infected people can be treated in specialist clinics, rural health facilities treat not only people with HIV infection, but also those with concomitant TB, malaria, other STIs, malnutrition or those who require antenatal or other services [7]. This necessitates integration with existing health services or, at the very least, the development of HIV services closely coordinated with the rest of the local health system. Thus, although specialized, 'vertical' structures are put in place to provide new HIV services in response to short-term targets and related resources, the goal should be to integrate them into the overall 'horizontal' structure as soon as possible, while strengthening the latter in the process.

Wider health system stability and capability facilitates the development of a sustainable response, as shown by Costa Rica's ability to use its well-developed public health system as the basis for its universal antiretroviral programme. This indicates that it is important not to undermine general primary care programmes by attracting key staff into specialist HIV centres. A strong general health system is vital for sensitizing providers and the population to the ways in which the country's epidemic can be controlled, and to their respective contributions to this goal. This is particularly challenging for poorer countries. While industrialized countries have the infrastructure to build HIV-related services into their existing health services, this frame-work is either non-existent or inadequate in many of the African, Asian, Caribbean and Eastern European countries. These countries then face major challenges, particularly in the presence of internationally led, ambitious scale-up programmes with very short-term objectives such as the WHO/UNAIDS '3 by 5' or the US President's Emergency Plan for AIDS Relief (PEPFAR). Such programmes can easily become yet another vertical programme that these countries have to manage alongside other services. This may appear inevitable in settings where 'mainstream' health services are weak. In order to achieve rapid increases in treatment rates, it is tempting for donors and recipient governments to continue setting up stand-alone antiretroviral pro-grammes rather than attempting the more complex task of coordinating the delivery of ART and other HIV services with the existing health services, which may well be of poor quality and need parallel investment. To produce a sustainable response to HIV that can reach those in need, programmes will need to be progressively integrated with the rest of the health system, as demonstrated in Cuba and Thailand.

Community involvement, community-based and civil society organizations

The importance of involving community groups and PLHIV has been demonstrated in a number of countries. South Africa provides a clear example where community groups combined with civil society organizations forced the South African government to provide ART to its citizens. Over the last 25 years, Africa, South and North America, Europe, Asia, the Caribbean and other areas of the world have also demonstrated the importance of involving community and civil society organizations to ensure the establishment and provision of preventive and therapeutic services. Those countries that have directly involved individuals and groups most affected by the epidemic have been more successful in developing effective, efficient, equitable and acceptable preventive and therapeutic HIV services. This suggests that HIV-infected populations or those vulnerable to HIV infection should not be marginalized, but rather brought directly into the process of containing the epidemic in their respective countries. When this happens, governments are less able to ignore the nature and scale of their national epidemics.

For example, countries that deny the existence and severity of their epidemics, or refuse to discuss conditions by which the disease is spread, greatly hamper their ability to slow transmission and respond to the needs of PLHIV. This includes denying the existence of commercial sex work or men who have sex with men (MSM), *a priori* ruling out particular interventions on principle without considering evidence of their effectiveness in risk reduction, such as needle exchange schemes or promoting the use of condoms [8], or stigmatizing or criminalizing vulnerable groups. Such attitudes and behaviours tend to be seen in countries with weaker civil society involvement.

Negative social attitudes toward MSM, for instance, slowed down the response in Barbados. Similarly, the initial lack of openness in China about the extent and nature of the epidemic, stigmatization of risk groups and PLHIV, and discrimination against PLHIV were all associated with a failure to slow down the increase of newly infected people. In Ukraine, IDUs are criminalized to such an extent that those with HIV are reluctant to come forward for treatment for fear of being imprisoned, which then increases their likelihood of infecting others and reduces the accuracy of surveillance. The lack of openness and good data also serves to perpetuate the perception that HIV is a disease exclusively of IDUs, despite its current spread within the general population via heterosexual contact. A similar situation exists in Russia, which also demonstrates a punitive, hostile culture towards IDUs, MSM and PLHIV. As another example, in Argentina, a great deal of preventive effort was initially misdirected at female sex workers rather than MSM, in part because of poor information but also because of the stigma faced by MSM in that country. Denying access to already limited treatment contributes to the general spread of infection and exposes vulnerable groups to higher risks. The experience of Senegal stands in marked contrast: religious and civil society organizations there were mobilized to counter stigma and discrimination. This produced preventive efforts based on risk reduction that drew on a long tradition of involvement in both the health and education sectors. Religious leaders were at the head of campaigns to resist discrimination against PLHIV and groups at high risk.

A pragmatic, realistic approach to combating and responding to the epidemic is characterized by a willingness to explore a variety of prevention strategies, in conjunction with a willingness to recognize publicly the implications of behaviours that may be illegal or socially unacceptable, but which are commonplace and help to spread the epidemic. Such strategies may prevent high-risk behaviour from being driven underground by further criminalization. For example, in addition to mobilizing civil society organizations, Senegal also legalized prostitution, enabling sex workers to receive regular health checks and facilitating the effective promotion of condom use by prostitutes, since they are in regular contact with public health clinics and are willing to come forward for check-ups, HIV tests and support now that their work is not illegal. Such an approach to risk reduction includes efforts to destigmatize HIV and aims to ensure that people with HIV, especially women, enjoy full legal and human rights, free from discrimination. However, such approaches are not universally accepted. There is conflict in Italy, for example, between those who favour a risk-reduction approach to HIV prevention and those who favour promoting sexual abstinence and increasing control of behaviours, such as prostitution and injection drug use, associated with the spread of HIV.

Intersectoral collaboration

Effective governments work not just through their own agencies, but also through regional and local public, private and civil society organizations in the health field and beyond to implement their national strategies. They do this without attempting to prescribe in detail how such organizations should operate, as long as they can show they are contributing positively to achieving national goals and targets in HIV prevention and control. For example, a notable feature of the Ugandan response was the government's willingness to involve, work with and through a large number of local NGOs that it did not directly control but that were trusted by local people. Similarly, in Haiti, civil society organizations and the churches have played a large part in prevention and treatment. In contrast, the lack of a tradition of NGO and civil society involvement in the health systems of former Soviet countries such as Russia and Ukraine is a major handicap today, given that the state health infrastructure has deteriorated badly and that little is available to fill the gaps in provision. NGOs may be better situated than government agencies to lead local prevention initiatives, perhaps because they understand local communities better or because local people may trust them more than government agencies.

Sometimes the intersectoral approach can be a formal partnership or another type of coordinating mechanism that recognizes and encourages the contributions of affected communities and individuals with HIV; civil society, such as community and religious leaders; bodies representing people with HIV, as in Senegal; and business, as well as the government and international agencies. This approach can also focus on wider, 'upstream' issues such as gender power inequities and poverty, as well as more immediate issues such as improving access to ART.

A final element in a collaborative, intersectoral response within countries involves arrangements for 'mainstreaming' the response to HIV. This means putting into place incentives to ensure that all relevant government agencies, such as the ministries of education, transportation, planning, economic development and others, play their part in the response rather than leaving it exclusively to the ministry of health and health sector agencies. There are many ways to encourage this to happen, but they are all predicated upon adequate funding and an ability to provide evidence of practical plans to assist in the response to HIV, as well as some mechanisms to ascertain that these plans have been implemented. For example, the ministry of education might have to prepare viable plans for including key HIV messages within the national school curriculum before funds are released for other educational projects or new programmes closer to the heart of ministers and other officials.

Apart from developments within countries, alliances and increased collaboration are developing across countries, ranging from those among health professionals to complex alliances involving multilateral, bilateral and commercial organizations working with politicians, healthcare professionals, community groups and larger civil society organizations. While in some countries alliances and collaborations have been slow to form, there is evidence that collaboration is increasing along with greater recognition that the successful containment of the pandemic is contingent on a broad, integrated national and international response.

Within this context, the provision of HIV preventive and therapeutic services is not just an 'extra' that governments provide for their populations *if* or *when* it suits them, but are basic human rights [9]. It is striking the number of middle- and lower-income countries that, although having previously experienced a period of military rule or dictatorship, are now committed to developing national anti-HIV strategies. Those societies most successful at containing their HIV epidemics tend to be democratic and have a relatively open and interactive civil society.

Funding HIV therapeutic and preventive services

Many of the low- and middle-income countries studied in this book indicated that it had become more feasible for them to provide their citizens with ART since prices had come down. This occurred partly because of the adoption of differential pricing policies by some pharmaceutical companies, but also through the production of generic antiretroviral drugs, especially in countries such as India, China, Thailand and Brazil. Others, such as Nigeria, are currently planning production of these generic drugs or are actively negotiating with pharmaceutical companies to reduce the price of branded antiretroviral drugs or obtain permission to manufacture selected generics as alternatives to branded drugs.

Some of the NGOs have been able to negotiate special prices with pharmaceutical companies. To date, the Clinton HIV/AIDS Initiative has been the most successful, negotiating US$140 per person per annum for a triple antiretroviral drug combination. However, even that price remains prohibitive, especially for lower-income countries. The cost of drugs is only one part of the costs of providing treatment and care, which include staff costs, laboratory costs and the general cost of running health facilities [10].

Even high-income countries such as Canada and the UK are concerned about the increasing cost of antiretroviral drugs, particularly in light of next-generation drugs such as fusion inhibiters, which are used for salvage therapy and are priced far higher than some of the other drug classes. Furthermore, while the contemporary drug combinations have dramatically reduced morbidity and mortality of HIV-infected people, these drugs do not eliminate HIV and therefore need to be taken for the rest of the person's life, increasing cumulative lifetime costs of providing treatment and care. The current drugs all have unwanted toxic and metabolic effects and, with improper use, can contribute to the onset of antiretroviral drug resistance. Some of these resistant strains are transmissible. This not only affects the health of people on ART, including those who may acquire multidrug-resistant HIV, but it also has economic consequences. Even for middle- or lower income countries, marked variation exists in the cost of the same drugs because of variations in the price of key chemical intermediaries and active pharmaceutical ingredients (APIs) for antiretrovirals that can be obtained from different commercial companies around the world [11]. Furthermore, the amount of APIs available worldwide is currently limited [E Dos Santos Pinheiro, personal communication (2005)]. Even if 3 million people could have been identified and prepared for ART by the end of 2005, the limited amount of APIs available would not have enabled that many people to be treated.

As part of the 'human rights' approach to HIV, WHO and UNAIDS advocate that in middle- and lower-income countries, HIV-infected people should have access to HIV preventive and therapeutic services free-at-the-point-of-delivery. This concerns government officials in many different countries that rely on patient co-payments to raise additional revenues. However, a number of middle- and lower-income countries—such as Brazil, Senegal and Cambodia—are already providing ART free-at-the-point-of-delivery. The July 2005 G-8 meeting in Scotland also endorsed the principle of providing 'universal free HIV services by 2010' [12], which has also been promoted through the 'Free by Five' campaign [13]. How 'universal' will be defined, in terms of the percentage covered of those requiring ART, remains to be agreed on at the time of writing. While this statement is extremely encouraging, the resources required to achieve this will need to follow and be maintained. In addition, it must be remembered that there have been many free-at-the-point-of-delivery TB programmes for some time, and yet they have not necessarily succeeded in reducing the number of people infected with TB because of barriers to accessing services other than user-charges, such as distance, travel costs and loss of income as a result of attending for treatment. Programmes will need to take these factors into account as well as providing free treatment and drugs.

A recent UNAIDS report estimated that to achieve a 75% coverage rate by 2008, US$12.3 billion is required for treatment and care [14]. Add relevant investment in prevention services, services for orphans, programme costs and human resources, and that estimate climbs to US$55.1 billion. For the period 2005–2007, the same report estimated 'the funding gap between resources available and those needed of at least US$18 billion', which 'is likely to be a significant underestimate' [14].

The reported differences in expenditure on preventive compared with therapeutic services in a number of high-income countries covered in this book are disconcerting. Some other countries may have switched expenditures that previously were for preventive services to therapeutic services, as in the case of Mexico. Every country will need to address how HIV preventive and therapeutic services are funded, and what will be appropriate expenditures for these services. Countries will have to look closely at the best financial arrangements for them to ensure that HIV service provision free-at-the-point-of-delivery is sustainable in the longer term. This will require making good use of available resources. Some of these 'risk-sharing schemes' can be based on internal, country sources—for example, personal or corporate taxation, or compulsory social insurance, which could be paid for from increased export earnings—as well as tapping into external sources from bilateral or multilateral donors.

Most high-income countries already have well-developed risk-pooling systems based on a tax-financed national health service or national health insurance, as described in the chapters from the UK, Spain, France and Italy. The USA has a mosaic of coverage that, despite being more expensive, provides significantly lower levels of coverage in terms of access, use and quality of services to some population subgroups than is the case, for example, in European systems. Access to ART, for instance, is not currently assured for all HIV-positive people in the USA: where people live has a big influence on whether or not they will receive ART. However, even the USA provides a high and rapidly growing level of public funding for HIV treatment, care and prevention services compared with other chronic conditions that also disproportionately affect poor and marginalized groups in the population.

Many middle- and lower-income countries are heavily reliant on donors for providing funds for preventive and therapeutic HIV services. Given their current economic status, this may be, for many, a long-term dependency. Because of the financial incentives associated with donor programmes, it is important that countries should be able to maintain a degree of independence from donor organizations and sponsoring countries. These countries should not be reduced simply to serving the needs of donor organizations or their sponsoring countries. Examples have been seen where donor countries have tried to set strict limitations on the services they want '*their* aid' to fund [15], though not all concur with such an approach [16].

Some countries, although they have accepted donor involvement, have made it a point that they—and not the donor community—decide the agenda and pace of their own development through collaboration with the donor community. At the same time, many countries, including affluent countries such as Botswana, are concerned that the international community will develop 'donor fatigue'.

There may be problems with the disbursement of funds from donors to countries, and, once these funds arrive in the respective countries, there may be additional concerns over the allocation of resources to the appropriate areas of the health sector. Furthermore, not many countries or funding bodies have mechanisms in place to track whether resources that are brought into the country reach the areas of the health service where they are most needed. In addition, donor activities need to be harmonized within countries—not only with local professionals and institutions, but also between the different donor organizations.

Government, business and civil society all need to recognize that a large part of spending on HIV, including on local and regional coordination, should be seen as an investment in social and economic development and needs to be connected to a broader response. There is a tendency in finance ministries to view health expenditure as largely consumption spending, unlike spending on things such as transport infrastructure, which is more likely to be seen as a direct contribution to future economic growth. Yet, well-targeted spending on HIV prevention and treatment has a positive effect on human capital, thereby contributing to people's health and their ability to participate productively in the economy. In turn, the economies of many middle- and lower-income countries need to be strengthened so that this labour can be better used, but this is unlikely to occur without the international community giving serious attention to the indebtedness of many poor countries, international trade agreements that are biased against primary producing countries in the South, and wider global social and economic conditions, all of which hold back economies in poor countries and the effective response to HIV globally [12].

Political will and accountability

A sustained high political priority to combating HIV and the conditions in which the epidemic thrives—such as poverty, instability and gender inequity—involves effective and focused leadership at the highest level and is crucial to a successful response to the epidemic. Country governments have to be brave enough to take responsibility for tackling the epidemic in their countries rather than blaming wealthier countries for inaction, and leaders have to stake their personal reputations on their ability to organize an effective response, as has occurred in Uganda and Botswana. The case studies in this book show that there are significant disparities in prevention and treatment, even between democratic countries with similar GDP per capita and similar prevalence of HIV. For instance, the South African ANC government resisted giving HIV a high political priority for some time despite its very high prevalence. This undoubtedly slowed the response. Other sub-Saharan African countries, on the other hand, have given HIV control high priority as part of overall social and economic development efforts. It was apparent in other countries, such as Argentina and Haiti, that with sufficient political will and planning, a reasonably effective response to HIV in the short and medium term could be mounted, even if the society and health system were in disarray.

A number of the country studies also show how improvement in the response, particularly better access to treatment and care, occurred after military governments or civil wars had been brought to an end and more accountable governments had come to power. In Brazil, universal access to ART has become a centrepiece of the public health system set up by a democratic government after a period of military rule [9]. In such circumstances, a commitment to improving population health can be one way for a new democratic regime to establish its credentials with the people. Other countries embarked on the scale-up of HIV prevention and therapeutic services because of an overriding awareness of the increasing incidence in the general population and its likely consequences, or because they became concerned with infection rates in strategically important subpopulations, such as military recruits or school teachers.

Linked to the issue of political will and commitment, it appears that the more a government depends on the support of the people for its survival in office, the more people are able to put pressure on the government and the more amenable the policy process is to the views of interest groups representing those affected by the epidemic. This, then, is more likely to produce a sustained response. The ability of NGOs representing PLHIV to take part in public debate about how the government should respond to the HIV epidemic eventually compelled the South African government to begin the roll-out of ART, despite its earlier resistance to acknowledging the link between HIV and AIDS, and its scepticism about the effectiveness of ART. At a much earlier stage in the pandemic, civil society organizations played a large part in getting the US Government to prioritize HIV programmes, as the chapter on civil society organizations demonstrated.

A single strategic response

The principle of 'The Three Ones' encapsulates the importance of developing a coherent strategic response. The principle includes:

- One national agreed-upon HIV strategy or action plan;
- One national agency or authority with appropriate technical capacity responsible for coordinating the efforts of health and other organizations;
- One national multisectoral monitoring and evaluation system to track the response.

The agreed-upon national strategy for the control of HIV and the treatment and care of PLHIV needs to go beyond aspirations and broad goals to include detailed plans of action and targets to be achieved by particular dates, together with budgets and real resources to underpin the work of all partners involved in the HIV response. A number of countries have elegant aspirational strategies but lack realistic plans with budgets linked to infrastructure and staff to implement the goals in their strategies. For instance, Nigeria's current health system is too weak to implement its HIV strategy to any appreciable extent. Likewise in Indonesia, a weak public health system operating in a context of political and economic crisis undermined their strategic plans.

The single agency generally needs to have a broad mandate that extends beyond that of the health ministry and has a clear agreement with that ministry—and, if necessary, other ministries—on their relative roles. The country case studies have shown how many countries—as disparate as Ethiopia, Nigeria, Russia or Ukraine—lack sufficient accurate, contemporary strategic information to enable policy-makers, healthcare professionals and other relevant groups to devise appropriate programmes and evaluate their outcome and impact. It is a high priority for countries to develop a single, nationwide system capable of monitoring trends and transmission risk factors in the epidemic for a range of population subgroups and geographical areas. They will also need to be able to monitor and evaluate different responses and different combinations of prevention, treatment and care. In particular, sentinel surveillance is essential for an accurate picture of the changing nature of the epidemic and to inform changes in the direction and nature of the response. This could include reinvigorating behavioural interventions with subpopulations that had been targeted previously, as in the UK, or shifting attention to new or emerging risk groups. For example, the response in countries such as Russia and the Ukraine were hampered in a major way not only by the deterioration of the public health infrastructure, but also by the reliance on case reporting and the results of screening unrepresentative populations for an understanding of the nature and dynamics of the epidemic rather than sentinel reporting at a range of locations. Achieving a single system for monitoring and evaluation will require negotiations with donors to encourage them to harmonize their activities and requirements, and link them closely to national HIV strategies.

Methods to monitor and evaluate programmes

It is very important to record, monitor and evaluate the different HIV programmes as well as ascertain to what extent they can be integrated into national health systems. 'The Three Ones' include the development of a single national monitoring and evaluation system in each country. This, in conjunction with information obtained through surveillance, provides the strategic information that policy-makers need at local, subnational, national and global levels to decide which services or programmes to implement, and to monitor and evaluate their success once they have been implemented.

However, over the last few decades, there has been considerable debate as to what constitutes evidence of effectiveness and which methods provide such evidence. This has been a debate between proponents of the use of randomized controlled trials (RCTs) and those who see a place for a range of non-experimental or observational methods, as well as experimental methods or RCTs, as the most appropriate means to evaluate services and programmes. The use, cost and outcome of HIV service provision are increasingly being monitored and evaluated through the use of observational databases, especially in Europe and North America [17], while their utility to monitor and evaluate scale-up of HIV service provision in middle- and lower-income countries is increasingly being recognized [7]. Some of the impetus for their increasing use in industrialized countries [18] has been a perceived imperative for cost containment linked to a growing awareness of unexplained differences in the use of health services by age, gender and geography that persist after controlling for population needs and case severity [19,20]. The remaining variation is generally attributed to unjustifiable differences in clinical practice. As a result, proponents of such observational 'outcomes-based' research on normal clinical practice argue that the results can be used to produce practice guidelines '... which in turn will reduce the pressure for growth and produce a leaner, trimmer health care economy' [21].

Information on the *structure, process, outcome* [22] and *impact* of healthcare provision can now be collected at many levels due to the enormous developments in information technology. This includes activity data on the use of services, drugs prescribed and procedures performed, as well as the outcomes of these interventions. *Outcomes* are changes in health status of individuals attributable to treatments or other interventions, and include biomedical measures—clinical or other markers [20]—as well as more subjective measures of patient wellbeing [23], while *impact* in this context is the *outcome* at the population level.

The use of such databases allows researchers to assess the impact of interventions under real-life conditions. However, since databases reflect the patterns of routine clinical practice, differences between the outcomes of different programmes may be due to unknown differences in patient characteristics rather than true differences between programmes. While *known* sources of confounding can to be controlled for in non-experimental studies, concerns remain about the existence of *unknown* confounders. The ability of observational studies to demonstrate 'real' causal associations between interventions and outcomes remains controversial, with some claiming that their results can [24,25], and others that they cannot [26–28], be as valid as those obtained from well-executed RCTs.

Well-designed RCTs measure the *efficacy* or outcome of an intervention under experimental conditions and only for those populations that are part of the trial (internal validity). Translating the RCT findings to real-life situations (external validity) can be more problematic. This can be because the characteristics of the populations using the intervention in real life are different, or because of the effect of other factors that were not part of the original experimental framework but are nonetheless present in real life [29,30].

This apparent dilemma as to whether to rely on RCTs or observational data is less problematic when it is recognized that a range of complementary randomized and non-randomized approaches are required for monitoring and evaluating programmes. When it is recognized that the scientific process is a cyclical interplay between hypothesis generating and testing, using both verification and falsification or inductive and deductive methods [31,32], then it becomes clear that observational, analytical and experimental studies [33] as well as operational research all have a legitimate role within the process, depending on the purpose of the research and the point reached in the cycle. Imre Lakatos described the research process as a spiral [34]. If the spiral is cylindrical, this, in Lakatos' terms, would be a 'progressive research programme' that produces constructive information; if the spiral is conical, the research programme would, in Lakatos' terms, be degenerating and no longer produce constructive information [34]. This dynamic view of the research process is contrary to the more static view, where the research process is described in terms of a research pyramid [35], in which the information obtained through RCTs is considered to be the 'gold standard' at the apex [36] (Fig. 50.1).

Adopting a dynamic perspective on the research process allows the different methods to be used sequentially as part of a larger research programme. Qualitative and quantitative observational studies (cross-sectional or serial cross-sectional) constitute the main hypothesis-generating studies, while the hypothesis-testing studies comprise analytical studies

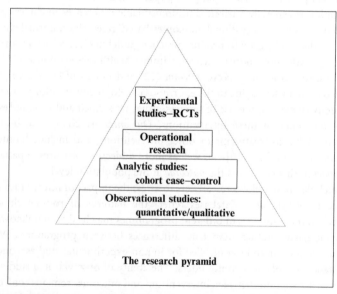

Fig. 50.1 The research pyramid: a static interpretation of the research process based on a hierarchical view of the research methods with the 'gold standard' at its apex.

(case–control and cohort), experimental studies (especially RCTs) and operational research. Operational research, sometimes described as health services research, in this context refers to those studies that are primarily focused on monitoring and evaluating the implementation of specific interventions or programmes in routine healthcare over extended periods of time. Operational research is a 'method of mathematically based analysis for providing a quantitative basis for management decisions' [37]. From this perspective, there is no single hierarchy of research methods, and knowledge is gained by sequential use of complementary research methods (Fig. 50.2).

The analysis of the changing mortality patterns of HIV-infected individuals at the end of the 1980s and beginning of the 1990s provides an example of this dynamic, cyclical process [29]. After the recognition of AIDS in 1981 [1], analytical studies demonstrated the relationship between HIV infection and AIDS as well as the transmission characteristics of HIV. On the basis of these analytical studies, intervention policies were formulated and implemented, including the use of media campaigns to make the public aware of this new health problem. These campaigns encouraged the adoption of 'safer sex' or 'safer shooting' behaviours. The campaigns also encouraged people at risk of infection to be tested for HIV infection, especially after the introduction of the more rapidly performed enzyme-linked immunosorbent assay (ELISA) antibody tests in 1986 [29].

Based on the association between HIV infection and AIDS, pharmaceutical companies started to develop antiretroviral drugs, of which zidovudine (AZT) was their first successful candidate. The efficacy of AZT was demonstrated through phase III RCTs, and the drug was introduced into routine clinical practice in early 1987. Observational studies performed beyond 1987 demonstrated improved survival patterns, with median survival from time of diagnosis of AIDS increasing from 9 to 20 months, which was initially attributed directly to the introduction of AZT [29]. When it became apparent that AZT monotherapy had only limited effectiveness, the discourse changed to ' . . . there is a suspicion that much of the increase in survival after a

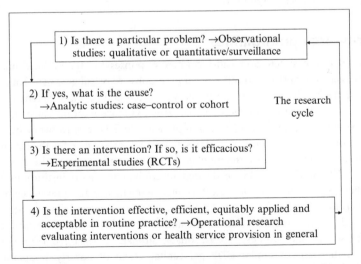

Fig. 50.2 The research cycle: a dynamic interpretation of the research process with the various research methods answering different but complementary questions.

diagnosis of AIDS that has been noted in the developed world results more from the use of prophylaxis against *Pneumocystis carinii* pneumonia than the early treatment of HIV-1 with zidovudine' [38].

After the introduction of AZT into routine clinical practice, observational studies also demonstrated that improved survival was not only related to the use of AZT, but was also due to patients presenting earlier in the course of HIV infection, many of whom had less severe PCP and could be treated earlier with specific anti-PCP therapy [29,39]. Early and regular out-patient attendances before and after the first episode of PCP were independently associated with reducing the likelihood of death, as was being treated with primary or secondary PCP prophylaxis [29,39].

The knowledge gained through this process depended on the complementary and sequential use of a variety of research methods [29]. Observational studies formed the initial baseline from which hypotheses were generated. Analytical studies tested these hypotheses, experimental studies tested the efficacy of a proposed intervention derived from the analytical studies, while operational research monitored and evaluated its implementation and changes over time, including the extent to which the original baseline parameters had changed. Changes to initial baseline parameters led to further analytical studies, and so on, as knowledge was gained.

Since the late 1940s, certainty of medical knowledge in the context of scientific modernity has relied on the pre-eminence of a single approach to knowledge creation [40], in this case the RCT. However, the validity of relying on a single 'gold standard' method of knowledge legitimization has been increasingly questioned, as has the view that scientific theories can be freed from their specific historical and social contexts. Each research method has its own methodological limitations and appropriate applications. When used in conjunction with each other, they can help build a more complete account of a phenomenon, such as an HIV epidemic, than is possible when they are used in isolation. Such an approach provides a more secure methodological basis for monitoring, evaluation and policy formulation than reliance on a single approach such as the RCT.

Future research programmes

The aspects of health system and wider country responses to HIV outlined above are the product of largely descriptive accounts written in response to broad guidance from the editors. They are not the results of systematic primary research comparing different countries' responses. However, they do form the potential basis for more rigorous research designed to answer the overarching question of which approaches to HIV control work best for which population groups in which country contexts. Given the importance for the functioning of a country's health system to reduce the number of new cases and improve the quality of life of people with HIV, studies should be devised in conjunction with institutions within the countries that look at the effect of indicators such as incidence and prevalence of HIV on a range of governmental, health system and civil society features in countries experiencing similar economic and social conditions and with similar levels of resources available for HIV programmes, so that their contexts are reasonably similar. For example, countries might be compared on the basis of similar GDP per capita, extent of poverty, population density, disparities between the status of men and women, extent of recent social disruption and other relevant factors. In order to ensure comparability, the prevalence and incidence of other major lethal and disabling diseases, such as TB and malaria, also need to be taken into account, since they compete for resources and attention with HIV, particularly in re-source-poor settings.

One starting point for defining the explanatory variables could be the features of country responses discussed in this chapter, such as the relationships between HIV programmes and 'mainstream' health services, the availability of accurate, timely strategic information, sustained political attention to HIV and efforts to reduce the stigma associated with HIV. A systematic review of other studies that look at responses to the HIV epidemic focused at the health system level would provide part of the basis for identifying other potentially important explanatory factors.

Empirical data should then be consistently collected within countries for each of the factors identified. This should include data collected routinely through monitoring and evaluation systems, and information initially collected for patient management, some of which can also be used for monitoring and evaluating programmes and routine healthcare provision at health facility, subnational and national levels. When combined with other relevant information, the cost and cost-effectiveness of services provided at these three levels can be estimated and used to provide important contemporary information for policy formulation, implementation and evaluation.

Additional information would also be needed, derived from detailed original research. This is especially likely in relation to some of the more conceptual variables identified as potentially important in this book, such as the relationship and degree of coordination between HIV-specific programmes and the generality of the health system in a country, the degree to which the response is managed in a decentralized way, the extent to which sexual and related matters can be discussed openly, or the nature of the political commitment to HIV control. Some of this research would be demanding, such as understanding cultural 'no-go' areas; some would be more straightforward though still requiring original research, such as collecting data on the extent of civil society organizations' involvement in service delivery and their participation in strategic policy development, or people's entitlements and access to services according to the various public and private insurance arrangements within countries. Comparing performance in similar countries would shed light on the question posed at the beginning of this chapter on which aspects of more and less successful systems' responses appear to have been most influential.

If it proved feasible to compare the effectiveness or cost-effectiveness of the response in a relatively small number of socio-economically similar countries, it would be logical to try the more difficult task of extending this analysis across countries at different socio-economic levels, especially comparing middle- and lower-income settings, in order to see if there are countries that perform better than one might expect given their circumstances, why this may be the case, the contribution of actions within and outside the health system and whether anything can be learned for wider application from the experiences of such countries. Such analyses would have some similarities with the thinking behind the *World Health Report 2000* [41], which attempted to compare the overall performance of the health systems of every country in the world, taking into account the extent to which each system operated in a socio-economic environment conducive or inimical to improving population health. For example, simple adjustments were made to health measures to take account of the average number of years of schooling achieved in each country, on the assumption that the better educated a population, the better its health status should be and the easier the task of the health system. These adjustments were contentious since they altered the performance ranking of some countries very appreciably. The same may occur in relation to HIV control, shedding light on the question posed at the start of the chapter as to whether the lessons drawn from the most celebrated country responses are indeed the correct ones, and whether there are less well-known responses that are more worthy of attention once socio-economic conditions are taken into account.

Though comparative health systems and policy research across countries is difficult to do, it is an essential complement to the ongoing effort of biomedical research to develop and improve HIV drug treatment or to develop potential vaccines. It is also an essential complement to the more targeted evaluative research, which compares the effectiveness of the different, specific HIV programmes that comprise country responses, such as different ways of promoting condom use or different forms of provision for safe injecting by IDUs. All the separate aspects of the response—the staff, laboratories, support services, training schools, drugs, vaccines, counselling, social supports and prevention programmes—have to function together within a system that is adapted to the specific economic, social and cultural context of the country. Without research, analysis and lesson learning at the various levels of the system, the relative contribution and interdependency of each aspect of the response will not be understood, and countries will continue to struggle to contain their HIV epidemics. We hope this book helps to promote this effort.

References

1. US Centers for Disease Control. (1981). Pneumocystis pneumonia—Los Angeles. *Morbidity and Mortality Weekly Reports* **30**:250–2.

2. World Health Organization. (2005). *Progress on Global Access to HIV Antiretroviral Therapy: An Update on '3 by 5'*. Geneva: WHO. http://www.who.int/3by5/fullreportJune2005.pdf (accessed July 11, 2005).

3. World Health Organization. (2004). *Scaling up Antiretroviral Therapy in Resource-limited Settings: Treatment for a Public Health Approach, 2003 Revision*. Geneva: WHO. http://www.who.int/hiv/pub/prev_care/en/arvrevision2003en.pdf (accessed July 20, 2004).

4. Swann C. (2005). Number of Americans with HIV soars past 1m. *Financial Times* June, 14 2005.

5. Beck EJ, Mandalia S. (2003). The cost of HIV treatment and care in England since HAART: part 1. *British Journal of Sexual Medicine* **27**(1):19–23.

6. Beck EJ. (1991). HIV-infection and intervention: the first decade. *AIDS Care* **3**:295–302.

7. Beck EJ, Bailey C, Boucher P, Travers P. (2004). WHO—Electronic Medical Record Meeting, Stanley Hotel, Nairobi Kenya, August 30–31, 2004. Geneva: WHO. Available at www.who.int/KMS/initiatives/EMR-Meeting-Report-2004.pdf.

8. New York Times Editorial. (2005). Despite being largest AIDS funder, US policy on needle exchange makes it 'scoundrel' in HIV/AIDS fight. *New York Times*, June 27, 2005.

9. Galvao J. (2005). Brazil and access to HIV/AIDS drugs: a question of human rights and public health. *American Journal of Public Health* **95**:1–7.

10. Badri M, Maartens G, Mandalia S *et al.* (2006). Cost-effectiveness of Highly Active Antiretroviral Therapy in South Africa. PlosMedicine **3**:e4.

11. World Health Organization. (2004). Sources and Prices of Active Pharmaceutical Ingredients. Geneva: WHO. http://www.who.int/3by5/amds/api.pdf (accessed July 29, 2005).

12. Anonymous. (2005). The Gleneagles Communiqué. http://www.fco.gov.uk/Files/kfile/PostG8_Gleneagles_Communique.pdf (accessed July 8, 2005).

13. Whiteside A, Lee S. (2005). The 'free by 5' campaign for universal, free antiretroviral therapy. *PLoS Med* **2**(8):e227. http://medicine.plosjournals.org/archive/1549–1676/2/8/pdf/10.1371_journal.pmed. 0020227-p-L.pdf (accessed August 7, 2005).

14. UNAIDS. (2005). Resource Needs for an Expanded Response to AIDS in Low and Middle Income Countries. Presented at the Programme Coordinating Board, Geneva 27–29 June 2005. Geneva: UNAIDS. http://www.unaids.org/Unaids/EN/About+UNAIDS/What+is+UNAIDS/UNAIDS+at+country+level/The+Three+Ones/Follow+up+to+Making+the+Money+Work+meeting.asp (accessed July 11, 2005).

15. Sternberg S. (2005). White House changes tune on AIDS groups working overseas. *USA Today*, 9 June 2005. http://www.usatoday.com/news/washington/2005–06–06-us-aids_x.htm (accessed July 7, 2005).

16. Boseley S. (2005). Britain rebuffs call to block anti-AIDS needle exchanges. *The Guardian*, June 28, 2005.

17. Beck EJ, Mandalia S. (2003). The cost of HIV treatment and care in England since HAART: part 2. *British Journal of Sexual Medicine* 27(2):21–23.

18. Elwood P. (1988). Shattuck lecture—outcomes management. *New England Journal of Medicine* 318:1549–56.

19. Black N. (1997). Developing high quality clinical databases. *British Medical Journal* 315:381–2.

20. Epstein AM. (1990). The outcomes movement—will it get us where we want to go? *New England Journal of Medicine* 323:266–70.

21. Wennberg JE. (1990). Outcomes research, cost containment and the fear of health rationing. *New England Journal of Medicine* 323:1202–4.

22. Donabedian A. (1969). *Explorations in Quality Assessment and Monitoring. Volume III. The Methods and Findings of Quality Assessment and Monitoring.* Ann Arbor, MI: Health Administration Press.

23. Lohr KN. (1989). Advances in health status assessment. *Medical Care* 27(Supplement 3): S1–11.

24. Benson K, Hartz AJ. (2000). A comparison of observational studies and randomized, controlled trials. *New England Journal of Medicine* 342:1878–86.

25. Concato J, Shah N and Horwitz RI. (2000). Randomized, controlled trials, observational studies, and the hierarchy of research designs. *New England Journal of Medicine* 342:1887–92.

26. Byar DP. (1991). Problems with using observational databases to compare treatments. *Statistics in Medicine* 10:663–6.

27. Doll R. (1993). Summation of the conference. In: Warren KS, Mosteller F, eds. Doing more harm than good: the evaluation of health care interventions. *Annals of the New York Academy of Sciences* 703:310–3.

28. Bristol HSR. (1994). Collaboration. MRC Health Services Research Initiative: outline of the bid. University of Bristol, p15.

29. Beck EJ. (1998). The Use and Costs of Services and Changing Mortality for AIDS patients Treated at St.Mary's Hospital, London 1982–1991. PhD Thesis. London: Department of Epidemiology and Public Health, Imperial College of Science, Technology and Medicine, University of London.

30. Smith GSS, Pell JP. (2003). Parachute use to prevent death and major trauma related to gravitational challenge: systematic review of randomised controlled trials. *British Medical Journal* 327: 1459–61.

31. Susser M. (1986). The logic of Karl Popper and the practice of epidemiology. *American Journal of Epidemiology* 124:711–8.

32. Ng SKC. (1991). Does epidemiology need a new philosophy? *American Journal of Epidemiology* 133:1073–7.

33. Barker DJP, Rose G. (1984). *Epidemiology in Medical Practice*, 3rd edn. Edinburgh: Churchill Livingstone, p67–108.

34. Lakatos I. (1986). Falsification and the methodology of scientific research programmes. In: Worrall J, Currie G, eds. *The Methodology of Scientific Research Programmes*. Cambridge: Cambridge University Press, p8–101.

35. Olkin I. (1995). Statistical and theoretical considerations in meta-analyses. *Journal of Clinical Epidemiology* **48**:133–46.

36. Cochrane A. (1972). *Effectiveness and Efficiency. Random Reflections on Health Services.* Oxford: The Nuffield Provincial Hospital Trust.

37. Oxford English Dictionary. (Draft Revision June 2004). *Operational Research.* http://dictionary.oed.com/cgi/entry/
00332509?single=1&query_type=word&queryword=operational&first=1&max_to_show=10.

38. Rutherford GW. (1994). Long-term survival in HIV-1 infection. *British Medical Journal* **309**:283–4.

39. Beck EJ, Mandalia S, Miller DL, Harris JRW. (1998). Hospital service intervention and improving survival of AIDS patients, St. Mary's Hospital, London 1982–91. *International Journal of STD and AIDS* **9**:280–90.

40. Habermas J. (1981). Modernity versus postmodernity. *New German Critique* **22**:3–14.

41. World Health Organization. (2000). *World Health Report 2000.* Geneva: WHO.

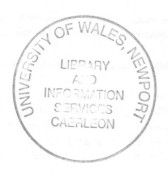

Index